Cancer of
the Breast

THE EDWIN SMITH SURGICAL PAPYRUS
3000–2500 BC (Case 45)

If thou examinest a man having bulging tumors of his breast (and) thou findest that (swellings) have spread over his breast; if thou puttest thy hand upon his breast upon these tumors, (and) thou findest them very cool, there being no fever at all therein when thy hand touches him: they have no granulation, they form no fluid, they do not generate secretions of fluid, and they are bulging to thy hand.

There is no (treatment).

This excerpt from an Egyptian papyrus, translated by J. H. Breasted, is considered the earliest reference to cancer of the breast, for which there was no treatment (Breasted, J. H.: The Edwin Smith Surgical Papyrus. Chicago, University of Chicago Press, 1930).

Fifty centuries later, more than one-third of women treated for breast cancer are cured (Adair et al., 1974).

Cancer of
the Breast

William L. Donegan, M.D., F.A.C.S.
Professor of Surgery
Medical College of Wisconsin
Chairman, Department of Surgery
Sinai Samaritan Medical Center
Milwaukee, Wisconsin

John S. Spratt, M.S.P.H., M.D., F.A.C.S.
Professor of Surgery (Surgical Oncology)
Professor of Community Health
Head, Division of Health Systems
The James Graham Brown Cancer Center
  of the University of Louisville School of Medicine
Louisville, Kentucky
Clinical Professor of Surgery
Uniformed Services University of the Health Sciences
Bethesda, Maryland

W.B. Saunders Company
A Division of Harcourt Brace & Company
Philadelphia   London   Toronto   Montreal   Sydney   Tokyo

W.B. SAUNDERS COMPANY
A Division of
Harcourt Brace & Company

The Curtis Center
Independence Square West
Philadelphia, Pennsylvania 19106

Library of Congress Cataloging-in-Publication Data
Cancer of the breast / [edited by] William L. Donegan, John S. Spratt—4th ed.
p. cm.
Includes bibliographical references and index.
ISBN 0–7216–4694–8
1. Breast—Cancer.   I. Donegan, William L.   II. Spratt, John S. (John Stricklin)   [DNLM: 1. Breast Neoplasms.   WP 870 C2155 1995]
RC280.B8C316 1995
616.99′449—dc20
DNLM/DLC   94–12235

Cancer of the Breast, 4th edition   ISBN 0–7216–4694–8

Last digit is the print number: 9   8   7   6   5   4   3   2   1

Contributors

Douglas M. Ackermann, M.D.
Associate Clinical Professor, Department of Pathology, University of Louisville School of Medicine; Staff Member, Alliant Health Care System (Norton/Kosair Children's Hospitals), Louisville, Kentucky
Microscopic Anatomy of the Breast

Randal N. Arnold, J.D.
Attorney-at-Law, Kluwin, Dunphy, Hinshaw, and Culbertson, Milwaukee, Wisconsin
Medical Malpractice Liability for Errors in Breast Cancer Diagnosis and Treatment

Barbara W. Ashley, R.N., M.S.N.
Faculty Associate, The Johns Hopkins University School of Nursing, and The University of Maryland School of Nursing; Oncology Clinical Specialist, The Johns Hopkins Oncology Center; Clinical Coordinator, The East Baltimore Health Program, The Johns Hopkins Hospital, Baltimore, Maryland
Nursing Care

Ricky J. Ballou, M.S., Ph.D., M.D.
Associate Professor of Anatomy, and Medical Oncology Fellow, University of Louisville School of Medicine, Louisville, Kentucky
Chemosensitivity of Cultured Human Breast Cancer

Sharleen Johnson Birkimer, Ph.D., R.D.
Professor, Department of Health, Physical Education, and Recreation, University of Louisville, Louisville, Kentucky
Nutrition and Breast Disease

Jennifer Dunn Bucholtz, R.N., M.S., O.C.N.
Clinical Specialist, The Johns Hopkins Oncology Center at The Johns Hopkins Hospital, Baltimore, Maryland
Nursing Care

James D. Cox, M.D., F.A.C.R.
Professor of Radiotherapy, and Coordinator, Interdisciplinary Program Development, M. D. Anderson Cancer Center, Houston, Texas
Definitive, Adjuvant, and Palliative Radiation Therapy for Mammary Cancer

William L. Donegan, M.D., F.A.C.S.
Professor of Surgery, Medical College of Wisconsin; Chairman, Department of Surgery, Sinai Samaritan Medical Center, Milwaukee, Wisconsin
Introduction to the History of Breast Cancer; Common Benign Conditions of the Breast; Epidemiology and Etiology; Diagnosis; Staging and Primary Treatment; Surgical Management; Screening and Follow-Up; Multiple Primary Cancers in Mammary and Extramammary Sites, and Cancers Metastatic to the Breast; Local and Regional Recurrence; Breast Carcinoma and Pregnancy; Sarcomas of the Breast; Cancer of the Male Breast

William B. Farrar, M.D.
Associate Professor, and Chief, Division of Surgical Oncology, Department of Surgery, The Ohio State University College of Medicine; Attending Staff Member, The Ohio State University Hospitals, and The Arthur G. James Cancer Hospital and Research Insititute; Courtesy Staff Member, Children's Hospital, and Park Medical Center, Columbus, Ohio
Physiology of the Breast

Joy L. Fincannon, R.N., M.S., O.C.N., C.S.
Instructor, University of Maryland, Baltimore, Graduate School of Nursing; Psychiatric Consultation-Liaison Nurse, The Johns Hopkins Oncology Center, The Johns Hopkins Hospital, Baltimore, Maryland
Nursing Care

John W. Gamel, M.D.
Professor, Department of Ophthalmology and Visual Sciences, University of Louisville School of Medicine; Staff Physician, Department of Ophthalmology, Veterans Administration Medical Center–Louisville, Louisville, Kentucky
Metastasis to the Eye and Ocular Adnexa

Paul K. Gardner, M.D.
Instructor, Department of Neurological Surgery, University of Louisville School of Medicine; and Staff Member, Alliant Health Care System (Norton/Kosair Children's Hospitals), University of Louisville Hospital, and Veterans Adminstration Medical Center–Louisville, Louisville, Kentucky
Neurologic Aspects of Breast Cancers

Janusz J. Godyn, M.D.
Assistant Professor of Laboratory Medicine and Pathology, University of Medicine and Dentistry of New Jersey–New Jersey Medical School; Director, Division of Hematopathology, University of Medicine and Dentistry of New Jersey–University Hospital, Newark, New Jersey
The Genetic Basis for the Emergence and Progression of Breast Cancer

George B. Haasler, M.D.
Associate Professor, Cardiothoracic Surgery, Medical College of Wisconsin; Director, Thoracic Surgery and Lung Transplant Programs, John L. Doyne Hospital; Co-Director, Lung Transplant Program, Children's Hospital of Wisconsin; Attending Staff, Veterans Administration Medical Center; Associate Attending Staff, Froedtert Memorial Lutheran Hospital; Associate Staff, Columbia Hospital, Milwaukee, Wisconsin
Thoracic Surgical Problems in Breast Cancer Therapy

Becky J. Hollingsworth, M.S.S.W.
Director of Support Services, The James Graham Brown Cancer Center of the University of Louisville School of Medicine, Louisville, Kentucky
Community Resources for the Breast Cancer Patient

Leslie E. Hughes, M.B., D.S., F.R.C.S., F.R.A.C.S.
Emeritus Professor of Surgery, University of Wales College of Medicine, Honorary Consulting Surgeon, University Hospital of Wales, Heath Park, Cardiff, United Kingdom
A Unifying Concept for Benign Disorders of the Breast: ANDI

Maurice J. Jurkiewicz, M.D., D.D.S., F.A.C.S.
Professor of Surgery, Emory University School of Medicine; Staff Member, Emory University Hospital, Crawford Long Hospital of Emory University, Scottish Rite Children's Medical Center, Egleston Children's Hospital, Atlanta, Georgia
Breast Reconstruction

Carl G. Kardinal, M.D., F.A.C.P.
Associate Professor of Clinical Medicine, Tulane University School of Medicine, and Louisiana State University School of Medicine; Associate Head, Division of Hematology and Medical Oncology, Ochsner Clinic; Associate Director, Ochsner Cancer Institute, New Orleans, Louisiana
Endocrine Therapy of Breast Cancer

Arthur H. Keeney, M.D., D.Sc.
Distinguished Professor of Ophthalmology, Department of Ophthalmology, University of Louisville School of Medicine; Attending Staff Member, Veterans Administration Medical Center–Louisville, Louisville, Kentucky
Metastasis to the Eye and Ocular Adnexa

Russell A. Klingaman, J.D.
Attorney-at-Law, Kluwin, Dunphy, Hinshaw, and Culbertson, Milwaukee, Wisconsin
Medical Malpractice Liability for Errors in Breast Cancer Diagnosis and Treatment

Sharon L. Krumm, Ph.D., R.N.
Associate Professor, The Johns Hopkins University School of Nursing; Research Associate, The Johns Hopkins University School of Medicine; Director, Oncology Nursing at The Johns Hopkins Hospital, Baltimore, Maryland
Nursing Care

James G. Kuhns, M.D.
Associate Clinical Professor of Pathology, University of Louisville School of Medicine; Staff Member, Alliant Health Care System (Norton/Kosair Children's Hospitals), Louisville, Kentucky
Microscopic Anatomy of the Breast

Richard R. Love, M.D., M.S.
Professor of Human Oncology, and American Cancer Society Professor of Clinical Oncology, University of Wisconsin, Madison, Wisconsin
Prevention of Breast Cancer

Catherine E. Mahaffy, B.S.N., R.N., O.C.N.
Senior Clinical Nurse, The Johns Hopkins Oncology Center, The Johns Hopkins Hospital, Baltimore, Maryland
Nursing Care

John Mahan, M.D.
Resident, Department of Orthopedic Surgery, University of Louisville Hospital, Louisville, Kentucky
Orthopedic Management of Skeletal Metastases

John S. Meyer, M.D.
Visiting Professor of Pathology, Washington University School of Medicine, St. Louis, Missouri; Chief Pathologist, St. Luke's Hospital, Chesterfield, Missouri
Cell Kinetics of Breast and Breast Tumors

John Peter Minton, M.D., M.MSc., Ph.D., F.A.C.S.
Professor of Surgery, and American Cancer Society Professor of Clinical Oncology, Ohio State University; Staff Member, The Ohio State University Hospitals, Columbus, Ohio
Physiology of the Breast

Myron Moskowitz, M.D., F.A.C.R.
Emeritus Professor of Radiology, University of Cincinnati; Attending Radiologist, University of Cincinnati Medical Center, Cincinnati, Ohio
Breast Imaging

Polly A. Newcomb, Ph.D.
Assistant Professor, Department of Human Oncology, University of Wisconsin Medical School, Madison, Wisconsin
Prevention of Breast Cancer

Christian Paletta, M.D., F.A.C.S.
Associate Professor of Surgery, Division of Plastic and Reconstructive Surgery, St. Louis University School of Medicine, St. Louis, Missouri; Staff Member, St. Louis University Hospital, Cardinal Glennon Children's Hospital, John Cochran Veterans Administration Medical Center, St. Mary's Health Center, St. Louis, Missouri
Breast Reconstruction

Carlos M. Perez-Mesa, M.D.
Associate Chief, Department of Pathology, Roswell Park Cancer Institute, Buffalo, New York
Gross and Microscopic Pathology

George H. Raque, Jr., M.D.
Assistant Professor of Neurosurgery, Division of Neurological Surgery, University of Louisville School of Medicine, Louisville, Kentucky
Neurologic Aspects of Breast Cancers

Janell Seeger, M.D., F.A.C.P.
Associate Professor of Medicine, Department of Medical Oncology, University of Louisville School of Medicine, Louisville, Kentucky
Chemotherapy of Breast Cancer

David Seligson, M.D., F.A.A.O.S., F.A.C.S.
Professor and Vice-Chairman, Department of Orthopedics, University of Louisville; Attending Physician, Department of Orthopedics, University of Louisville Hospital, Alliant Health Care Systems (Norton/Kosair Children's Hospitals), Louisville Baptist Hospital, Louisville, Kentucky
Orthopedic Management of Skeletal Metastases

Christopher B. Shields, M.D.
Professor, Department of Neurosurgery, University of Louisville School of Medicine; Staff Member, Alliant Health Care System (Norton/Kosair Children's Hospitals), University of Louisville Hospital, Louisville, Kentucky
Neurologic Aspects of Breast Cancers

Curtis P. Sigdestad, Ph.D.
Professor, Department of Radiation Oncology, The James Graham Brown Cancer Center of the University of Louisville School of Medicine, Louisville, Kentucky
Epidemiology and Etiology

Pippa M. Simpson, Ph.D.
Assistant Professor, and Biostatician, Department of Pediatrics, Wayne State University, Detroit, Michigan
Statistical Methods in Cancer Research

Muthukumaran Sivanandham, Ph.D.
Assistant Professor, Department of Surgery, New York Medical College, Valhalla, New York; Research Manager, Department of Surgery, St. Vincent's Hospital and Medical Center of New York, New York, New York
Immunology, Serum Markers, and Immunotherapy of Mammary Tumors

John A. Spratt, M.D.
Assistant Professor, Department of Surgery, Medical College of Virginia, Virginia Commonwealth University; Staff Surgeon, Medical College of Virginia Hospitals, McGuire Veterans Administration Hospital, Richmond Memorial Hospital, Henrico Doctor's Hospital, Richmond, Virginia
Growth Rates; Statistical Methods in Cancer Research

John S. Spratt, M.S.P.H., M.D., F.A.C.S.
Professor of Surgery (Surgical Oncology), Professor of Community Health, and Head, Division of Health Systems, The James Graham Brown Cancer Center of the University of Louisville School of Medicine, Louisville, Kentucky; Clinical Professor of Surgery, Uniformed Services University of the Health Sciences, Bethesda, Maryland; Active Staff Member, University of Louisville Hospital, Alliant Health Care System (Norton/Kosair Children's Hospitals), St. Anthony Medical Center; Consulting Staff Member, Veterans Administration Medical Center–Louisville, Baptist Hospital East, Jewish Hospital, Humana Hospital–Audubon, Humana Hospital–Suburban, Louisville, Kentucky
Gross Anatomy of the Breast; Epidemiology and Etiology; Growth Rates; Surgical Management; Screening and Follow-Up; Multiple Primary Cancers in Mammary and Extramammary Sites, and Cancers Metastatic to the Breast; Statistical Methods in Cancer Research

George P. Studzinski, M.D., Ph.D.
Professor of Laboratory Medicine and Pathology, University of Medicine and Dentistry of New Jersey–New Jersey Medical School; Attending Pathologist, University of Medicine and Dentistry of New Jersey–University Hospital, Newark, New Jersey
The Genetic Basis for the Emergence and Progression of Breast Cancer

Gordon R. Tobin, M.D., F.A.C.S.
Professor of Surgery, Division of Plastic and Reconstructive Surgery, University of Louisville School of Medicine; Staff Member, University of Louisville Hospital, Veterans Administration Medical Center–Louisville, Alliant Health Care System (Norton/Kosair Children's Hospitals), Jewish Hospital, Louisville, Kentucky
Gross Anatomy of the Breast

Michael T. Tseng, Ph.D.
Professor of Anatomy, and Director, Tumor Evaluation Laboratory, University of Louisville School of Medicine, Louisville, Kentucky
Chemosensitivity of Cultured Human Breast Cancer

Danielle M. Turns, M.D.
Professor (Retired), Department of Psychiatry, University of Louisville School of Medicine, Louisville, Kentucky
Psychosocial Factors

Jean M. Wainstock, M.S., R.N., O.C.N.
Clinical Nurse Specialist, Department of Surgical Oncology, Johns Hopkins Breast Center, Baltimore, Maryland
Nursing Care

Michael J. Walker, M.D.
Associate Professor of Surgery, Division of Surgical Oncology, Department of Surgery, Ohio State University; Attending Surgeon, Arthur G. James Cancer Hospital, and Ohio State University Hospitals, Columbus, Ohio
Physiology of the Breast

Marc K. Wallack, M.D.
Professor, Department of Surgery, New York Medical College, Valhalla, New York; Chairman, Department of General Surgery, St. Vincent's Hospital and Medical Center of New York, New York, New York
Immunology, Serum Markers, and Immunotherapy of Mammary Tumors

David E. Weissman, M.D.
Associate Professor of Medicine, Medical College of Wisconsin, Milwaukee, Wisconsin
Management of Pain

Patti M. Wilcox, R.N., C.S., A.N.P.
Adult Nurse Practitioner, The Johns Hopkins Oncology Center; Faculty Associate, The Johns Hopkins University School of Nursing; Affiliate Staff Member, The Johns Hopkins Hospital, Baltimore, Maryland
Nursing Care

J. Frank Wilson, M.D.
Professor and Chairman, Department of Radiation Oncology, Medical College of Wisconsin; Active Staff Member, John L. Doyne Hospital, Froedtert Memorial Lutheran Hospital, Milwaukee, Wisconsin; West Allis Memorial Hospital, West Allis, Wisconsin; Community Memorial Hospital, Menomonee Falls, Wisconsin; Consulting Staff Member, Zablocki Veterans Administration Medical Center, Children's Hospital of Wisconsin, Lakeview Hospital, and Sinai Samaritan Medical Center, Milwaukee, Wisconsin
Definitive, Adjuvant, and Palliative Radiation Therapy for Mammary Cancer

James L. Wittliff, Ph.D., F.A.C.B.
Professor of Biochemistry, University of Louisville School of Medicine; Director, Hormone Receptor Laboratory, The James Graham Brown Cancer Center of the University of Louisville School of Medicine, Louisville, Kentucky
Hormone and Growth Factor Receptors

Thomas M. Woodcock, M.D.
Professor, Department of Medicine, The James Graham Brown Cancer Center of the University of Louisville School of Medicine, Louisville, Kentucky
Chemotherapy for Breast Cancer

James W. Yates, Ph.D.
Professor, Exercise Physiology Laboratory, University of Louisville School of Medicine, Louisville, Kentucky
The Role of Exercise and Weight Control in Cancer Prevention and Rehabilitation

Constance R. Ziegfeld, M.S., R.N.
Adjunct Faculty Member, University of Maryland, University of Delaware, and Johns Hopkins University; Assistant Director of Nursing, The Johns Hopkins Oncology Center, The Johns Hopkins Hospital, Baltimore, Maryland
Nursing Care

Preface

This book is a project that has spanned three decades of our professional lives and has grown along with our knowledge and experience. It began when we were surgeons at the Ellis Fischel State Cancer Hospital (EFSCH) in Columbia, Missouri, and continued after one of us (WLD) relocated to the Medical College of Wisconsin in Milwaukee, Wisconsin, in 1974 and the other (JSS) to the University of Louisville in Louisville, Kentucky, in 1976. It includes the inspiration of our mentors and the contributions of those who have been our colleagues along the way.

The first edition of *Cancer of the Breast,* published in 1967, was in response to an invitation from J. Englebert Dunphy, M.D., to contribute to a series of monographs entitled *Major Problems in Clinical Surgery.* One of us (JSS) was studying growth rates of cancers, including pulmonary metastases from breast cancer, and the other (WLD) was in the process of reviewing the treatment of breast cancer at EFSCH. This work had been made known to Dr. Dunphy by our friend and mentor, Carl A. Moyer, M.D., who was then Chairman of the Department of Surgery at Barnes Hospital–Washington University Medical Center in St. Louis, Missouri, and in whose program both of us received our surgical training. The first edition was followed by a second edition in 1979 and by a third in 1988. A sustained interest in breast cancer has shaped our professional careers and accounts for this fourth edition.

Our predecessors at EFSCH established the excellent clinical records system and follow-up program that made many of our early studies possible. Physicians, nurses, and administrative and clerical personnel kept the program running, always with more work than resources, to serve the medically indigent cancer victims of Missouri. A biomathematics section was established at EFSCH through a Clinical Center Grant from the National Cancer Institute and was headed by Francis R. Watson, Ph.D., whose logic and Socratic methods gave order and discipline to our early efforts.

After we left EFSCH, our sources of data have included clinical records and clinics at Medical College of Wisconsin–affiliated hospitals and the Breast Cancer Detection Demonstration Project in Louisville, as well as our own clinical practices. Participation in the clinical trials program of the National Surgical Adjuvant Breast and Bowel Project (NSABP) has been a rewarding activity and accounts for emphasis on studies by this group in several chapters of this book. The science and leadership of Dr. Bernard Fisher of the University of Pittsburgh, who chaired this organization continuously for almost four decades and whose life's work changed the "paradigm" of breast cancer, provide a model for us and all who study this disease.

The breast is the single most frequent site of cancer among women in the United States, and efforts to control it are a national priority. Research is intense, and rapid changes are occurring in clinical management. Earlier detection is possible through the use of mammography, and treatment is often feasible through the application of breast-conserving methods. Systemic therapy is integral to modern management. The relationship between cancer and benign breast disease is becoming clearer. These dynamic changes are addressed in the present edition of this text. It is current and more comprehensive than ever before, but it still maintains clinical management as its focus. New and important chapters have been added and address benign breast disorders, microscopic anatomy, oncogenes, cancer prevention, cardiothoracic problems, orthopedic problems, legal issues, pain control, and community resources for the patient with breast cancer. We are pleased to retain the talents of previous contributors, and we welcome a number of new ones whose works enhance this volume. We appreciate the outstanding work of all who have joined this project.

Some regrettable losses deserve mention. Tragic is the untimely death of John Peter Minton, M.D., who brought his enthusiastic, friendly capabilities to both the bedside and the laboratory. John agreed to update his chapter on physiology for this edition but died in an automobile accident on November 27, 1990. We are indebted to his colleagues at Ohio State University for accepting the task of revising his chapter. Also missed will be the friendship and wise counsel of Lauren V. Ackerman, M.D., who died July 28, 1993. Dr. Ackerman, the first pathologist at the EFSCH, set up the clinical and pathologic record system from which we obtained abundant data. We knew him after he came to Barnes Hospital in St. Louis, where he was our teacher and friend.

The editors at W.B. Saunders Company again have done an admirable job of bringing text and illustrations together in a readable and pleasing format. Our secretaries deserve our appreciation for suffering through the preparation of yet another edition. This is particularly true for Susan Albertin, who served as coordinator and whose patient attention to many details was called upon in two previous editions and again in this one. In Louisville, Peggy Dawson, Betsy Hafgan, and Rhonda Hawley provided invaluable assistance.

Finally, we express our gratitude and respect for the many women, and a few men, whom we have been privileged to attend through the years. We hope this book provides information of value to physicians and other health professionals who confront problems of the breast as well as to the people who suffer from them.

WILLIAM L. DONEGAN
JOHN S. SPRATT

Contents

1
Introduction to the History of Breast Cancer

William L. Donegan

Breast cancer is an ancient disease. Breast tumors were described by the Egyptians 3000 years before the birth of Christ. Subsequently, Greek and Roman physicians wrote about breast cancer, and the record of the disease continued through the Middle Ages and into modern times. The excellent histories of Cooper (1941), Lewison (1953), Ackerknecht (1965), Power (1934–1935), Mansfield (1976), and DeMoulin (1983) are valuable resources for this account.

Surgery is the oldest means of treating breast cancer. It has been used in every age of history, yet enthusiasm for it has waxed and waned. Operations have been devised, discarded, rediscovered, changed, and abandoned again in seemingly endless fashion as physicians have sought to employ the science and technology of their times. It is in the growth of knowledge about this disease that the story of surgery for breast cancer takes on meaning and continuity.

The course of events in the history of breast cancer management permits four periods to be identified. The earliest period can be characterized as empirical, and in it treatment was discouraged. Experience had taught that some tumors of the breast were aggravated by operations. Such tumors were best recognized and left undisturbed. In the next period, cancers were considered a systemic disease. Surgical removal might give temporary relief, but it could not be expected to cure a patient. The third period was one of growing optimism, based on the thesis that breast cancer began as a local disease and, if detected early, was curable with local treatment. Finally, in the modern era, the problem has been recognized as more complex than previously appreciated, and new principles of treatment are evolving.

THE EARLY PERIOD

Surgery was not performed for breast cancer in ancient Egypt. The Edwin Smith surgical papyrus, which dates from the Egyptian pyramid age (around 3000–2500 BC) describes eight cases of tumors or ulcers of the breast. Tumors that were hard, were cool to the touch, and contained no fluid were distinguished from inflammations and abscesses; for the former, the writer admitted that "there is no treatment." Reference is made to one patient who was treated by cauterization with a fire stick. The later Ebers papyrus (1600–1500 BC) makes no reference to cancer of the breast.

Indian writings dating to 2000 BC mention the treatment of tumorous growths with surgical extirpation, cautery, and arsenic compounds. Cuneiform tablets of Assyria, with writings that date to this same period, only mention the occurrence of breast cancer.

In an isolated account, Herodotus (484–425 BC) gives Democedes, a Persian physician who lived in Greece at the time, credit for curing the wife of King Darius of a "tumor" of the breast that had ulcerated and spread.

Hippocrates (460–375 BC), the most famous of Greek physicians, mentioned breast cancer only twice and both times darkly. He stated, "A woman in Abdera had a carcinoma of the breast and bloody fluid ran from the nipple. When the discharge stopped, she died." Later, he described what must have been a typical course in a patient: ". . . and hard tumors appear in the breast, some large and some smaller, these do not suppurate, but continually grow harder and harder. From these grow hidden cancers . . . and everything (the patients) eat tastes bitter, and if you give them more to eat, they refuse it, and shut their mouths. They become delirious, their eyes are hard, and they do not see clearly, and pains dart from the breast to the neck and beneath the shoulder blades, thirst seizes upon them, the nipples are dry, and the whole body becomes emaciated . . . When they have gone as far as this, they do not recover, but die of this disease." From his experience he counseled, "It is better not to apply any treatment in cases of occult cancer; for if treated, the patients die quickly, but if not treated they hold out for a long time."

The early Romans performed extensive surgery for cancer of the breast, including removal of the pectoral muscles. The Roman scholar Aulus Cornelius Celsus (42 BC to 37 AD) advised against this practice as well as against the use of caustic medicines, cautery, and excision. He described the evolution of cancer from a benign tumor, which the Greeks called a "cacoëthes," to a carcinoma without ulceration, to an ulcer and, finally, to a "thymium," and counseled that "none of these can be removed but the cacoëthes; the rest are irritated by every method of cure." To distinguish a cacoëthes from a carcinoma, he advised first treating with caustics and, if the symptoms grew milder, proceeding to incision and cautery. If the disease was irritated, however, the transition to carcinoma had already occurred, and only the use of mild medicines was appropriate.

CANCER AS A SYSTEMIC DISEASE

In the second century, Galen (129–200 AD) dominated the field of medicine. The prestige of this famous Greek phy-

1

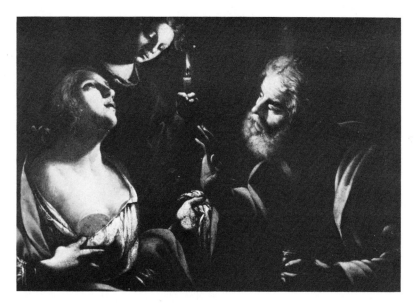

Figure 1-1. The martyrdom of St. Agatha, the patron saint of breast diseases, is preserved in paintings throughout Europe. Christians were severely persecuted during the reign of the Roman emperor Decius (201–251 A.D.), and Quintianus, his governor in Sicily, used this pretext to wreak revenge on this beautiful woman of Catania who true to her Christian beliefs spurned his lustful advances. The tortures she suffered at his hands included amputation of her breasts and ultimately proved fatal. She is often shown with her breasts being cut off or sadly carrying her breasts on a platter. Here, she is visited in her dungeon cell by St. Peter and by the Christ child, who heal her wounds. The complete story is told by Lewison (1950).

sician who worked among the Romans was such that his teachings were perpetuated for 1000 years. Hippocrates earlier had taught that disease was caused "by the particular humor that prevails in the body," blood, phlegm, yellow bile, or black bile." Galen expanded and refined this humoral theory of disease. He attributed cancer to an excess of black bile in the body, calling it "melancholia," a local manifestation of the constitutional disturbance. "Cancerous tumors develop with greatest frequency in the breasts of women," he said, and he noted the particular susceptibility of postmenopausal women. "Such unnatural tumors have their source in the black bile," he continued, "a superfluous residue of the body." The balance of humors in a person's body also accounted for his or her disposition. Excessive black bile made a person sad and morose, not an unlikely combination with cancer. This systemic concept must have corresponded well with what appeared to be the prospects for cure at that time. It was Galen who likened the appearance of cancers to that of a crab, with the large veins extending from all sides giving the appearance of legs.

Nevertheless, Galen excised those tumors that were removable and, apparently appreciating the value of wide removal, recommended excision through the healthy surrounding tissues. "Make accurate incisions surrounding the whole tumor so as not to leave a single root," he counseled. "Let the blood flow and do not check it at once but make pressure on the surrounding veins so as to squeeze out the thick blood." Galen insisted that ligatures invited recurrence in the surrounding tissues and avoided their use.

Leonidus of the Alexandrian school (180 AD) had also learned to place his incisions through normal tissues wide of the tumor but was more concerned than Galen about controlling hemorrhage. Aetius quoted Leonidus, ". . . placing the patient in a recumbent position, I make an incision into the sound part of the breast, above the cancer, and immediately apply the cautery until an eschar is produced to stop the bleeding." He then proceeded to alternately cut and cauterize until the breast was removed, with a final cauterization intended to eradicate any residual tu-

mor. The use of knife and cautery, as described by Leonidus, persisted for more than 11 centuries as did the avoidance of ligatures.

Little surgical progress was made during the Dark Ages. Most medical historians attribute this to the humoral theory of disease taught by Hippocrates and by Galen, the slavish adherence to Galen as the ultimate authority on things medical, and the strong pervasive influence of the church. The Council of Tours in 1162 discouraged surgery as treatment for cancer of the breast. The cruel persecution of St. Agatha, canonized by the early church as the patron saint of women with breast disease, included amputation of the breasts, and this was often depicted in art with the surgical instruments of the day (Fig. 1–1). In consequence, cautery and caustics became the predominant methods of treatment even though it continued to be widely accepted that breast cancer was an incurable disease. Perhaps the blurred distinction between malignant and benign tumors permitted sufficient successes to keep hope alive. Albucasis (936–1013 AD), an Arabian surgeon who produced the first illustrated treatise on cautery, doubted the value of surgery and knew of no case of breast cancer that had been cured. Other notables perpetuated earlier techniques. Lanfrank (1296 AD) in France used the 1100-year-old cut-and-cauterize technique of Leonidus. Ambroise Paré (1510–1590) excised small breast tumors but substituted the application of sulfuric acid for the hot cautery. Large tumors were treated with milk, ointment, and vinegar. Henri de Mondeville (1260–1320) and Guy de Chauliac (1300–1368) both operated on breast cancers that could be widely excised, but the former preferred arsenic and zinc chloride caustic pastes for large tumors. Unorthodox treatments temporarily employed during this time included bisection of the affected breast in an attempt to dissolve the tumor by means of a ligature, which was practiced by Francisco Araceo (1439–1571) in Spain. Compression of the breast with lead plates was used by Lenard Fuchs (1501–1566).

The end of the Middle Ages was marked by extremes. In the 16th century, William Clowes (1560–1634), the physician of Queen Elizabeth I of England, advocated the laying on of hands, and for a time royalty were solicited to touch the afflicted in hopes of healing them. Peter Lower (1597) applied goat's dung, and later James Cook (1614–1688) practiced bleeding from the basilic vein. Some applied frogs, bisected chickens, or fresh parts of other animals to the affected breast with results that remain obscure.

At the same time, innovators began to loosen the bonds of tradition. In Brussels, Andreas Vesalius (1514–1564), the father of modern anatomy, published *De humani corporis fabrica libri septem* in 1543, which corrected the errors of Galen's anatomy and substituted the use of ligatures for hot cautery when excising breast cancers. Jacques Guillemeau (1550–1601) reinstituted removal of the pectoralis major muscle along with the breast. At the school in Salerno, Italy, Marcus Aurelius Severinus (1580–1656) began to remove axillary lymph nodes along with the breast. He, as well as Ambroise Paré earlier, was among the first to appreciate that they were a part of the tumorous process.

The 16th century initiated a resurgence of surgery, and the next two centuries were noteworthy for techniques of mastectomy that were both thorough and efficient in their execution. In a time without anesthesia, the motivation was a mercifully swift amputation of the breast. Johann Scultetus (1595–1645), who published in Ulm a popular compendium of surgical techniques, accomplished this by passing two large needles attached to heavy cords through the base of the breast in opposite directions, and while pulling up on the cords, swiftly amputated the breast with a knife, following which hemostasis was achieved with a cauterizing iron. Wilhelm Fabry (1560–1634), a German barber–surgeon who was a pupil of Vesalius, accomplished the same end with large metal tongs, which, when closed, encompassed the base of the breast with an iron ring. Traction on the instrument then stretched the breast away from the chest wall, permitting it to be amputated swiftly and accurately with a knife. In 1708, Godefrides Bidloo illustrated his own special instruments for swift amputation, which consisted of a knife, a one-pronged fork, and a two-pronged fork. One or both forks were thrust through the base of the breast to transfix it and provide traction before the knife was used (Fig. 1–2). The evolution of this method culminated in 1721 with the technique of Gerard Tabor. Tabor employed a hinged instrument composed of two semicircles with handles which could be clamped around the base of the breast. A curved knife blade hinged at the same fulcrum could be swept through the ring in one stroke, completing the operation in perhaps no more than 1 or 2 seconds. The breast was removed more completely by these procedures than with any earlier technique and many later ones; however, because the resulting wound was large and required many months to heal, these techniques were abandoned in favor of less complete procedures that permitted closure of the skin.

In 1662, Reverend John Ward described an operation that he observed in which, after the skin was cut, the tumor was bluntly separated from surrounding tissues with the hands. On each of the succeeding 2 days, the wound was opened and additional portions of the tumor cut out. The patient died several months later with cancer still present in the breast. It was to discourage such piecemeal operations that Jean Louis Petit (1674–1750), the foremost French

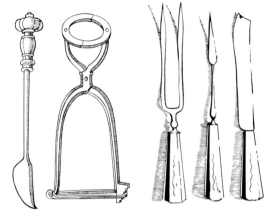

Figure 1–2. Mastectomy instruments used by Fabricus Hildanus *(left)* and by Godefridus Bidloo *(right)* in the 17th century. In each case, the breast was transfixed either with a metal ring on tongs or with forks and then quickly cut away with a knife. (Redrawn from Cooper, W. A.: The history of radical mastectomy. Ann. Med. Hist., 3:36, 1941.)

surgeon of the period, wrote in his *Traite des Operations* concerning carcinoma of the breast that all tissues should be removed in one piece. Although his excision of the breast was less complete than that of Scultetus before him, he urged the removal of all enlarged axillary lymph nodes and of the pectoralis fascia and pectoralis muscle if they appeared to be involved.

During this period, cancer remained conceptually a constitutional disease caused by aberrations of body fluids, variously black bile, components of the blood, excess acid, or too much alkali. It was common for physicians to note that the patient appeared of a "melancholy" disposition, obviously prone to the disease. Local stagnation or coagulation of these fluids, or some other precipitating event, explained the appearance of a "scirrhous," the contemporary term for cancer. The breast was particularly susceptible. DeMoulin (1983) points out that Professor Boerhaave of Leyden (1668–1738) thought trauma ("contusio") that was harmless to the skin was nevertheless sufficient to cause a cancer in the breast. Tight clothes, blows to the breasts, or rough handling of the breasts was suspect. Some blamed local irritation from retention of curdled milk. Many believed that air had a stimulating effect on cancers; Claude-Nicolas Lecat (1700–1768) in Rouen attributed the rapid spread of ulcerating breast cancers to the fact they reached the air and were responding to its putrifying effects. As late as 1912, the following statement on hematoma of the breast appeared in a respected surgical text: "In view of the fact that trauma is a possible cause of malignant disease, a short prophylactic course of x-rays may be advisable" (Handley, 1912). We still hear these echoes from the past from patients who trace the origin of the cancer in their breast to an injury or who express reservations about an operation for fear that it will let air get to the cancer and cause it to spread.

After discovery of the lymphatic system, which resulted from Ascelli's description of lacteals in 1622 and from the description of the thoracic duct by Pecquet, Bartholinus, and Rudbeck in 1651, René Descartes (1596–1650) substituted a lymph theory of the origin of breast cancer for

Galen's black bile theory, and this was perpetuated by John Hunter (1728–1793) in the 18th century. Hunter taught that a defect existed in the lymph, and, where it coagulated, breast cancer made its appearance. This represented little improvement over the black bile theory, but it may have had the effect of promoting the removal of enlarged axillary lymph nodes.

BREAST CANCER AS A LOCAL DISEASE

In the 18th century, a concept that provided hope for surgical cure was introduced. In 1757 in France, Henri François LeDran advanced the theory that cancer began in its earliest stages as a local disease (Fig. 1–3). It spread first via the lymphatics to regional nodes and subsequently entered the general circulation (LeDran, 1757). LeDran's theory offered the possibility that if surgery were performed sufficiently early, it could encompass and cure the disease. Bernard Peyrilhe (1773), as well as other notables of the day, embraced this pivotal concept, and during the next century it gradually replaced the humoral theory of cancer.

The constitutional theory did not die easily. More than a century later, Henry Arnott of St. Thomas Hospital in London still felt obliged to argue for the local origin of cancer

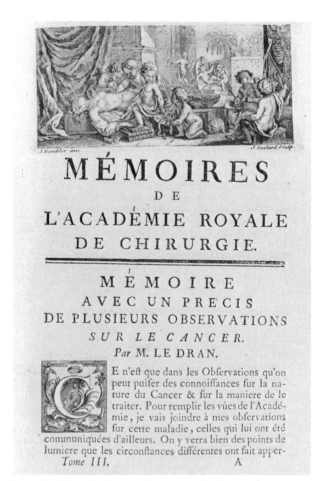

Figure 1–3. The illuminated title page of LeDran's signal paper in 1757 supporting the local origin of breast cancer.

and the value of early surgery (Arnott, 1871). He likened cancer to a thistle in a cornfield. "If this weed be allowed to remain until the flower-head has passed to its stage of ripe, feathery seeds, these are wafted hither and thither, and, taking root, become so intimately and largely mingled with the corn that the complete removal of the nuisance is impossible without greatly endangering the whole crop. But if the original plant be removed at once all this danger is avoided." "Our problem," he said, prescient of future mass screening, "is to discover these tumors before the afflicted one can do so."

With the acceptance of the local theory, the principles of curative surgery sanctioned wide en bloc operations and surgical resection at the earliest possible moment. These principles guided efforts for the next 100 years and kindled unparalleled optimism for surgical cure. In the words of LeDran, "Every cancer begins by the obstruction of one or more glands," and "we may hope for a perfect cure." As early as 1773, Peyrilhe advised an operation that removed the cancerous breast along with the axillary contents and the pectoralis major muscle, the same operation introduced by Halsted more than 100 years later. Jean Louis Petit warned against cutting through the mammary gland and urged removal of the axillary nodes as well as the pectoral fascia and pectoralis muscle if necessitated by the extent of involvement. His contemporary, Lorensius Heister (1683–1758), removed not only the pectoralis major muscle but ribs as well, if necessary, to remove all the tumor.

Advances in science and medicine in the 19th century included the introduction of general anesthesia in 1846, of antisepsis in 1867, and of microscopic pathology. These accrued to the benefit of all surgery. Specific to the treatment of breast cancer, the period was noted for the development of radical surgery and for the discovery that breast cancer was hormone-dependent. In the closing decade of the 19th century, x-rays and radium were discovered, and radiotherapy made its debut.

During most of the 19th century, operations for cancer of the breast were still dangerous, and surgeons continued to be pessimistic about the results. Overwhelming infection was the major cause of operative mortality, being as high as 20% in some series. The selection of obvious cancers for surgery and poor postoperative care contributed to the dismal results. Alexander Monroe (1773–1859) reviewed 60 cases of surgically treated breast cancer at this time and found only four patients free of disease at the end of 2 years. Sir James Paget in 1853 confessed to having never seen a cure and advised that "in deciding for or against the removal of a cancerous breast, in any single case, we may, I think, dismiss all hope that the operation will be a final remedy for the disease." Equally pessimistic, Hayes Agnew (1818–1892) wrote, "I do not despair of carcinoma being cured somewhat in the future, but this blessed achievement will never be wrought of the knife of the surgeon." Robert Liston's opinion in 1840 was that "recourse may be had to the knife in some cases, but the circumstances must be very favorable indeed to induce a surgeon to recommend or warrant him in undertaking any operation for removal of malignant disease of the breast."

In these years, no consistent practice can be found with respect to the amount of skin and breast removed or the

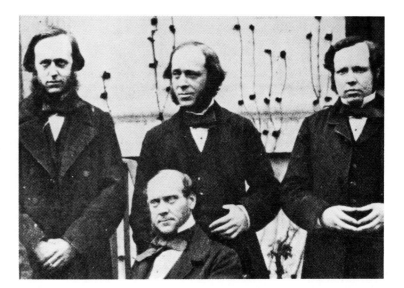

Figure 1–4. Charles Moore *(top center)* supported the local origin of breast cancer theory and authored a classic paper in 1867 advocating routine total en bloc removal of the breast. He is pictured with associates outside of the Middlesex Hospital in London, England. (From the Archives of Middlesex Hospital, London, England.)

removal of enlarged axillary lymph nodes. The ominous nature of the latter was fully appreciated. In Scotland, James Sime observed in 1842, ''it appears that the result of operations for carcinoma when the glands are affected is almost always unsatisfactory, however perfectly they may seem to have been taken away. The reason for this probably is that the glands do not participate in the disease unless the system is strongly disposed to it and consequently their removal, however freely and effectually executed, cannot prevent the patient's relapse.''

A touching account of mastectomy in the early 19th century is recorded by the Scottish surgeon John Brown, who participated as a student (Robbins, 1984). In a fragment of the account, Allie, the patient, enters the operating theater with her husband and their dog, Rab. ''The operating theater is crowded, much talk and fun, and all the cordiality and stir of youth. The surgeon with his staff of assistants is there. In comes Allie; one look at her quiets and abates the eager students. That beautiful old woman is too much for them; they sit down, and are dumb, and gaze at her. These rough boys feel the power of her presence. She walks in quietly, but without haste; dressed in her mulch, her neckerchief, her white dimity shortgown, her black bombazeen petticoat, showing her white worsted stockings and her white carpet-shoes. Behind her was James, with Rab. James sat down in the distance, and took that huge and noble head between his knees. Rab looked perplexed and dangerous; forever cocking his ear and dropping it as fast. Allie stepped up on a seat, and laid herself on the table, as her friend the surgeon told her; arranged herself, gave a rapid look at James, shut her eyes, rested herself on me, and took my hand. The operation was at once begun; it was necessarily slow; and chloroform—one of God's best gifts to his suffering children—was then unknown. The surgeon did his work. The pale face showed its pain, but was still and silent. Rab's soul was working within him; he saw that something strange was going on—blood flowing from his mistress, and she suffering; his ragged ear was up, and importunate; he growled and gave now and then a sharp impatient yelp; he would have liked to have done something to that man. But James had him

firm, and gave him a glower from time to time, an intimation of a possible kick, all the better for James, it kept his eye and his mind off Allie. It is over; she is dressed, steps gently and decently down from the table, looks for James, then, turning to the surgeon and the students, she curtsies, and in a low, clear voice, begs their pardon if she has behaved ill. The students—all of us—wept like children, the surgeon wrapped her up carefully—and, resting on James and me, Allie went to her room, Rab following . . .''

Two forces pushed the concept of radical surgery forward: the theory of local origin and the practical effort to eliminate local recurrence. Ultimately, these two forces reinforced each other. The former culminated in the permeation theory of W. Sampson Handley, and the latter in operations to routinely remove the entire breast, the axillary contents, and finally, the pectoral muscles—in sum, the radical mastectomy of William Halsted.

In 1867 the case for local origin was given renewed impetus by Charles H. Moore at the Middlesex Hospital in London (Fig. 1–4) (Moore, 1867). In a publication entitled ''On the Influence of Inadequate Operations on the Theory of Cancer,'' Moore observed that recurrences after limited operations for breast cancer were generally near the scar and that their pattern suggested centrifugal spread from the original site (Fig. 1–5). He concluded that surgical failure was due not to a systemic diathesis but to failure of the surgeon to remove all local extensions of the disease. His principles of surgical cure are classic:

1. ''It is not sufficient to remove the cancer or any portion only of the breast in which it is situated; mammary cancer requires the careful extirpation of the entire organ. The attempt to save skin which is in any degree unsound is of all errors perhaps the most pernicious, and whenever its condition is doubtful, that texture should be freely removed.''

2. ''In the performance of the operation, it is desirable to avoid, not only cutting into the tumor, but also seeing it. No actually morbid texture should be exposed, lest the active microscopic elements in it be set free and lodge in the wound.''

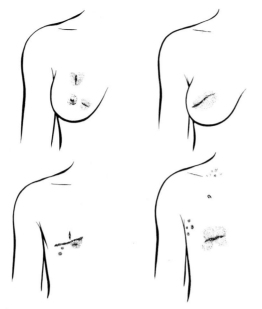

Figure 1–5. Four examples of cases illustrated by C. H. Moore in 1867 show local recurrence of breast cancer after "inadequate operations." The local origin of breast cancer was supported by this evidence, and it provided the foundation for wide en bloc removal of the entire breast as appropriate initial treatment. *Dark lines* indicate excisional scars, and *gray areas* show recurrent carcinoma. (Redrawn from Moore, C. H.: On the influence of inadequate operation on the theory of cancer. Med. Clin. Trans. (Lond.), *32:245, 1867.)

3. "Diseased axillary glands should be taken away by the same dissection as the breast itself, without dividing the intervening lymphatics."

The importance of Moore's paper lies in its evidence for the local origin of breast cancer and for supporting wide removal en bloc of all diseased and suspected tissues as a principle of cure. Moore's operation was widely adopted. Joseph Lister (1827–1912) supported his concept and was perhaps the first to expose the axilla by division of the pectoral muscles. Samuel D. Gross, professor of surgery at Jefferson Medical College in Philadelphia and in Louisville, enlarged it to include removal of the pectoral fascia.

Routine removal of the entire breast is clearly traceable to Moore, and routine removal of the axillary nodes is possibly so. Although originally he referred only to removal of "diseased axillary glands," Moore subsequently stated that they can never be assumed to be healthy (Power, 1934–1935). Surgeons became increasingly aware of the difficulty of determining by palpation whether axillary lymph nodes were involved and, impressed with the frequency of axillary recurrence when they were not included, began to remove them routinely. In Britain, William M. Banks of Liverpool pioneered this practice. In a paper read before the British Medical Association at Worcester in 1882, entitled "Free Removal of Mammary Cancer with Extirpation of the Axillary Glands as a Necessary Accompaniment," he reported 46 cases and said, "In the present paper the principal object is to advocate the removal of the axillary glands as well as the breast in all cases . . . I have been quietly practicing this for 3–4 years" (Banks, 1902). As early as 1871, Küster of Berlin included axillary dissection as an essential part of mastectomy, whether or not lymph nodes could be felt in the axilla during the operation, and Halsted later gave Küster credit for being the first to advocate systematic cleaning out of the axilla (Küster, 1883). Routine axillary dissection dramatically reduced recurrences at that site. Schmid (1887) reported that among 95 cases of recurrence in Küster's series, only one occurred in the axilla.

The pectoralis fascia and its underlying muscle were the next tissues to become suspect, largely through the microscopic research of von Volkman and Heidenhain in Germany. The microscope became a powerful tool in the 19th century (Schlumberger, 1944). In the early decades, many had observed the small "globules" and "corpuscles" that could be found in plant and animal specimens. By 1831, even the nucleus had been described, but it was found inconsistently and was assigned little importance. Not until Schleiden (1838) and Schwann (1847) stressed the importance of the nucleus as integral to these structural elements in plants and in animal tissues, respectively, did the "cell theory" take form. True cells could then be distinguished from various other microscopic features. It was Schwann's professor at the University of Berlin, Johannes Müller, who first described the cellular structure of cancers, the subject of his 1838 landmark publication, "On the fine structure and form of morbid tumors." Interestingly, Müller, the founder of cancer histology, vastly underestimated the importance of his work when in deference to the need for a simple and easy means of diagnosis he penned, "Microscopic and chemical analysis will therefore never become a means of medical diagnosis; it would be ridiculous to wish this or even consider it possible." Widespread efforts to identify a specific cancer cell that would unify the diagnosis of cancer, however, did fail. Concurrent with these events was the belief that cells developed from an amorphus "blastema," a vague concept which persisted despite lack of scientific support and perhaps for want of a satisfactory alternative. It is said to be Robert Remak, professor of anatomy in Berlin, who in 1852 first pointed out that tissues increased by the division of existing cells, but others, who were principally studying embryogenesis, (e.g., von Baer, Kölliker, and Goodsir) had also observed cell division. Rudolph Virchow finally disposed of the blastema theory in his *Die Cellularpathologie,* a collection of twenty lectures delivered in Berlin in 1858 and considered one of the most important medical books of all time. He concluded that all cells were the product of previous cells, and coined the historic aphorism, "omnis cellula e cellula."

Joseph Claude Recamier introduced the concept of metastasis in 1829, and this concept was further refined by the German school. Wilder credits the microscopic research of Thiersch (1822–1895) and of Waldeyer (1836–1921) with the concept that metastases originate from migrating cancer cells rather than by the spread of tumor "juices" and, furthermore, that the cells were liberated from the primary tumor into the lymph and blood by both continuous growth and embolization (Wilder, 1956). To explain the distribution of metastases, researchers became divided between those who considered it an impartial process determined by mechanical entrapment of cells and those who, with Steven

Paget (1889), believed in the theory of "seed and soil" (i.e., cancer cells lodge and grow selectively only at favorable locations).

Germany led in this era of discovery. Von Volkman was one of the first to supplement removal of the breast and axillary contents with routine removal of the fascia of the pectoralis major muscle. In 1875, he explained, "I was led to adopt this procedure because on microscopical examination I repeatedly found when I had not expected it that the fascia was already carcinomatous whereas the muscle was certainly not involved" (Halsted, 1894–1895). Heidenhain's observations went further (Heidenhain, 1889). He reported that he had examined 18 of Küster's mastectomy specimens in which the pectoralis muscle was removed and found unsuspected microscopic invasion of the muscle in three cases. Heidenhain believed that in such cases contraction of the muscle could spread cancer cells throughout the lymphatics of its entire substance. Thus, Heidenhain concluded, "Removal of a piece of the muscle with the tumor is not enough." He recommended that in cases when the cancer had grown into the pectoralis major muscle or was adherent to its fascia, the muscle is to be removed in its entirety.

This thought was extended by William Stewart Halsted, Professor of Surgery at the Johns Hopkins Hospital. Halsted had studied 2 years in Germany and was particularly aware of developments in that country. His contribution to the progress of surgery lay in advocating routine removal of the pectoralis major muscle and in reinforcing the principle of en bloc resection. Said Halsted in 1894, "The pectoralis major muscle, entire or all except its clavicular portion, should be excised in every case of cancer of the breast, because the operator is enabled thereby to remove in one piece all of the suspected tissues. The suspected tissue should be removed in one piece, (1) lest the wound become infected by the division of tissues invaded by the disease, or of lymphatic vessels containing cancer cells, and (2) because shreds or pieces of cancerous tissue might readily be overlooked in a piecemeal extirpation" (Halsted, 1894–1895) (Fig. 1–6).

Halsted's operation removed the entire breast with its overlying skin, the pectoralis major muscle, and the axillary contents; it was initially known as the "complete operation," and ultimately as "radical mastectomy." It was used by Halsted in 1883 in "almost every case" and was mentioned in a publication by him in 1891 entitled "The treatment of wounds with a special reference to the value of the blood clot in the management of dead spaces" (Halsted, 1891). In 1894, he published the results of 50 patients treated since 1889 in this manner in the Johns Hopkins Hospital Reports. Halsted emphasized the dramatic reduction in local recurrences (only 6% in his series) compared with the 56% to 81% reported by surgeons in Europe. By present definitions, 18% of the 50 cases had recurrence in and around the wound at that time. Nevertheless, after 37 years, Lewis and Rienhoff (1932) at Johns Hopkins reported that recurrence locally had risen in the original cases to only 31.5%, still a distinct improvement over previous results.

The radical mastectomy was an idea whose time had arrived. In the same year as Halsted's 1894 report, Willie Meyer, Professor of Surgery at the New York Postgraduate

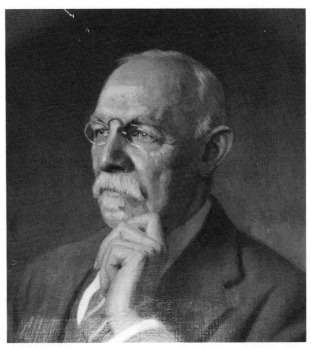

Figure 1-6. William S. Halsted (1852–1922), Professor of Surgery at the Johns Hopkins Hospital in Baltimore, Maryland, achieved markedly improved local control of breast cancer with "radical" mastectomy and standardized surgical treatment in the United States for 75 years with this operation. (Photograph of a painting by Thomas C. Corner. Courtesy of the Alan Mason Chesney Medical Archives of the Johns Hopkins Medical Institutions, Baltimore, MD.)

Medical School, reported a similar operation independently conceived but motivated by the same rationale that Halsted had expressed (Meyer, 1894). As Meyer performed his first operation on September 19, 1894, Halsted preceded him by several years. Only details of the operation varied. Meyer used a diagonal incision, which ultimately became more popular than Halsted's tear drop incision; excised the pectoralis minor muscle rather than dividing it, as Halsted had done (a modification later adopted by Halsted); and dissected the axilla before dividing the breast and muscles from the chest wall, rather than afterwards as in the Halsted procedure. Both surgeons emphasized the necessity of removing a large amount of skin sufficient to require split-thickness skin grafting, a procedure that had recently been developed by Thiersch in 1886.

Was Meyer's method preceded by another? *The Lancet* of February 4, 1893, relates that William Arbuthnot Lane in Britain discussed an operation in which he "took away the whole of the pectoral muscles with the subjacent breast, and then carefully dissected from the vessels and nerves of the axilla every bit of areolar tissue together with the lymphatic vessels and glands" (Clinical Society of London, 1893). He then "urged the advisability of removing the pectoral muscles and fascia forming the anterior wall of the axilla with the lymphatic vessels in relation to it. By these means not only were the primary growth and the cancerous glands removed, but, also, all the lymphatic channels along which infection had extended."

The radical mastectomy soon received conceptual support in the permeation theory of W. Sampson Handley of London, which, at the close of the 19th century, epitomized the biology of breast cancer (Handley and Thackray, 1969). Handley (1906) believed that the "embolic theory" described earlier by Stephen Paget was inadequate to explain the spread of breast cancer. The embolic theory held that metastases resulted from spread of cancer cells through the blood vessels, but it could not explain why some organs were more favorable sites than others or why the pattern varied. It was appreciated that breast cancer often spread to bones, but why it spread to some bones and not to others was uncertain (e.g., metastases were frequent in the axial skeleton but rare distal to the elbow or the knee). Nor did it explain why the pleura and lungs were involved in some cases leaving the bones exempt. To support these doubts, investigations at this time began to suggest that the bloodstream was hostile to cancer cells, rendering them ineffectual and destroying them through thrombosis (Schmidt, 1903). Convinced by his own dissections that lymphatics were the conduits to satellite nodules around breast cancer and to lymph nodes, Handley concluded, "Hence it is no doubt that although carcinoma often obtains access to the blood almost as early as to the lymph, its dissemination takes place almost entirely by the lymphatics and not by the blood vessels." Handley's theory, based on autopsy studies, was that cancers originated at one focus and spread exclusively through lymphatics. The lymphatic spread was by growth in continuity (permeation) rather than embolic and occurred equally in all directions. Regional lymph nodes, which were perfect filters of cancer cells, halted the progress of permeation until the tumor was able to grow through them, and only then were the cells capable of reaching the bloodstream for embolic spread. Hematogenous dissemination happened only very late in the preterminal phase of the disease. Lymphatic permeation occurred principally in deep fascial planes, and seemingly discontinuous metastases were an illusion created by a process of obliterative lymphangitis, which erased the continuity.

Handley's permeation theory was embraced by Halsted, and the two surgeons together gave an enormous impetus to radical extirpative surgery. Theoretically, it was possible even in advanced stages of the disease for a surgeon who was sufficiently aggressive to encompass the cancer and all of its extensions. Said Halsted, "We believe, with Handley, that cancer of the breast in spreading centrifugally preserves in the main continuity with the original growth," and again, "Though the area of disease extends from cranium to knee, breast cancer in the broad sense is a local affection, and there comes to the surgeon an encouragement to greater endeavor with the cognition that the metastases to bone, to pleura, to liver are probably parts of the whole, and that the involvements are almost invariably by process of lymphatic permeation, and not embolic by way of the blood" (Halsted, 1907).

Another of Halsted's practices that became firmly entrenched was biopsy followed by immediate mastectomy. Increasingly aware of the need for accurate diagnosis, he made incisions for biopsy with increasing frequency. Being also aware of the implantability of cancer, he said, "The excision of a specimen for macroscopic or microscopic examination is never resorted to except just before operation" (Halsted, 1907).

The wide scope of Halsted's operation greatly reduced the frequency of recurrence in the surgical area, but it is difficult to establish that it improved the chances of cure. Some of Halsted's cases were not cancers; others were obviously advanced. Bloodgood described one of Halsted's early cases as follows: "The tumor now occupies the entire breast and is adherent to the pectoral muscle. The nipple is retracted. There is a large abscess in the axilla" (Halsted, 1894–1895). In an actuarial analysis performed by the present author, only 8% of his first 50 cases were alive and free of disease at the end of 4 years. Greenough at the Massachusetts General Hospital reported better results with incomplete operations (Greenough et al., 1907). Henderson and Canellos (1980) compared Halsted's cases with earlier untreated cases from the Middlesex Hospital and estimated no more than 12% improvement in survival. Aware of the complexity of the lymphatic system, Rudolph Matas of New Orleans criticized the "complete" operation as not being truly complete. Nevertheless, Halsted's prestige and his influence as a teacher resulted in wide acceptance of his operation in the United States and abroad (Rutkow, 1978). After a period of indiscriminate use, the contraindications to radical mastectomy were defined through the scholarly work of Cushman Haagensen in New York, and improved results understandably proceeded pari passu with more careful case selection and earlier diagnosis (Haagensen, 1971).

In the 20th century, radical surgery reached its zenith. It soon became evident to Halsted that his operation was incomplete, and he extended it by dividing the clavicle and removing the supraclavicular nodes. Occasionally, enlarged internal mammary nodes were removed as well. Halsted abandoned these modifications because removing the supraclavicular nodes seldom cured a patient if metastases were present (10% of cases at 3 years), and the internal mammary nodes could not readily be removed en bloc. With this demonstration that little could be gained by enlarging the operation, radical mastectomy in its original form was widely accepted as the ultimate surgery for cancer of the breast.

In 1922, the year that Halsted died, W. Sampson Handley refocused attention on internal mammary metastases with parasternal biopsies and advocated their treatment with interstitial radium (Handley, 1922). This work was extended by his son, Richard S. Handley, who routinely began to biopsy internal mammary nodes during radical mastectomy in 1946, and in a series of 50 patients found metastases in 38% of the cases (Handley and Thackray, 1949) (Fig. 1–7). The implications were clear: spread of tumor to these nodes doomed fully one-third of all radical mastectomies to failure. In response to this information, the radical mastectomy was extended by a number of surgeons to include the removal of these nodes, an operation which became known as "extended radical mastectomy." Margottini in Italy was the first to do this routinely in 1948 (Margottini, 1952). Soon Urban, Sugarbaker, and others in the United States advocated the removal of the internal mammary nodes en bloc with the remainder of the specimen (Sugarbaker, 1953; Urban, 1964). Because of its logic, feasibility, and safety,

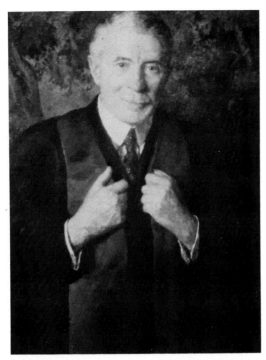 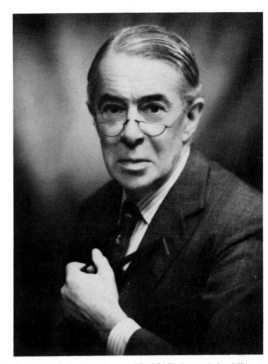

Figure 1-7. The Handleys of London. William Sampson Handley *(left)* (April 10, 1872–March 18, 1962) formulated the permeation theory of breast cancer spread, which supported radical mastectomy. Richard S. Handley, O.B.E. *(right)* (May 2, 1909–June 16, 1984), the son of W. S. Handley, demonstrated the frequency of metastases to internal mammary lymph nodes in operable cases of breast cancer and popularized the modified radical mastectomy. The photographs were kindly supplied by Mrs. R. S. Handley.

this operation was adopted at many centers. Dahl-Iversen and associates in Denmark went further, removing the supraclavicular as well as the internal mammary nodes at the time of mastectomy, but not as an en bloc dissection (Dahl-Iversen and Tobiassen, 1969). Prudente amputated the upper extremity en bloc with mastectomy in an attempt to cure relatively advanced cases, and Wangensteen culminated this progression with "super radical" mastectomy, in which Halsted's procedure was extended to include supraclavicular, internal mammary, and mediastinal lymph nodes, first in two stages and later in one (Prudente, 1949; Wangensteen et al., 1956). Although Wangensteen and colleagues found that 37 (57.8%) of 64 patients with clinically operable breast cancer had nodal metastases beyond the limits of the standard radical mastectomy, they abandoned the procedure because of high operative mortality (12.5%) and the lack of a significant improvement in results.

Radiation therapists in the 20th century inherited and applied the concept of radical en bloc ablation. The discovery of x-rays in 1895 by Wilhelm Conrad Roentgen added an important new tool for the local treatment of breast cancer. While professor of physics at the University of Würzburg, Roentgen noted that an invisible emission from a cathode ray tube caused nearby barium platinocyanide to fluoresce. It also affected photographic plates and penetrated objects impervious to light, including the human body. Because of the rays' uncertain nature, he called them "X-rays." They were later named Roentgen rays after their discoverer, who, for his work, received the Nobel prize in physics in 1901. Intense investigation soon unveiled addi-

tional sources of ionizing radiation. In 1903, the Nobel prize in physics was shared by Pierre and Marie Curie and Henri Becquerel of France. The latter discovered the radioactivity of uranium in 1896, and the Curies isolated radium from uranium ores (pitchblende) 2 years later. Radium and its encapsulated gaseous emission, radon, proved potent sources of gamma radiation that could be placed against or implanted into tumors.

The clinical and biologic effects of the new rays were quickly investigated. Within a year of Roentgen's discovery, Emil Grubbe in Chicago (Grubbe, 1933) and Hermann Gocht in Hamburg (DeMoulin, 1983) used x-rays to treat cases of inoperable breast cancer. These beginnings were unregulated, often inept, and, before the lethal effect of cumulative exposure was appreciated, sometimes tragic; however, the benefits of irradiation became clear. By 1912, radiotherapy was well established; in this year, W. Sampson Handley wrote in a major surgical text, "The principal use of X-rays in breast cancer is as a prophylactic against postoperative recurrence. But even in advanced cases they are often an effective means of relieving pain. I have known pain in the back and thorax to completely disappear for a time after one application of the rays . . . Apart from their analgesic properties," he continued, "X-rays promote the fibrosis and superficial healing of deposits in the skin and subcutaneous tissues. Upon visceral and other deep deposits they have no influence, nor do they appear to delay the course of dissemination" (Handley, 1912). Important landmarks in the progress of radiotherapy included reliable methods for measuring dosage (attributed to Holzknecht of

Vienna in 1902), the introduction of dose fractionation through work at the Curie Foundation in Paris, and development of high-energy "supervoltage" sources.

The story of radiotherapy is one of progressively improving technology, precision, and interest in two questions: Could irradiation improve the results of radical surgery, and Could radical irradiation be substituted for radical surgery? Ionizing irradiation was initially focused on inoperable cases but soon was used to supplement radical operations. Irradiation of the internal mammary and supraclavicular lymph nodes proved more acceptable to surgeons than did extended mastectomies, and the practice of supplementing surgery with irradiation when metastases were found in axillary lymph nodes or when the primary tumor lay medially in the breast became widespread.

The few advocates of simple mastectomy found a champion at midcentury in Robert McWhirter of Edinburgh, who challenged the status quo by reporting that 757 patients with operable breast cancer who were treated with simple mastectomy and irradiation of the supraclavicular, internal mammary, and axillary lymph nodes had a 5-year survival rate (62%) comparable with that being achieved with radical surgery (McWhirter, 1948). McWhirter's work implied that irradiation was effective treatment not only for the internal mammary and supraclavicular lymph nodes but also for axillary nodes. The question then remained whether cancer could be controlled in the breast itself, a question of great cosmetic interest. Early work with radiation implants by Keynes in England and with external beam sources by Baclesse in France indicated that this might be so (Keynes, 1937; Baclesse, 1965). Preliminary efforts in this direction produced 5-year survival rates in operable cases comparable with those for patients treated surgically, but local morbidity was prohibitive (Hochman and Robinson, 1960). High-energy sources introduced in the mid-1950s reduced cutaneous morbidity, and the attractive prospect of breast preservation led inevitably to studies in several centers in which radical irradiation constituted the primary mode of treatment (Prosnitz et al., 1977). Surgery was relegated to local removal of the primary tumor for diagnosis and biochemical analysis and to removal of axillary nodes for staging. The issues of irradiation carcinogenesis, long-term tumor control, and long-term morbidity remained to be answered, but results indicated that irradiation was an alternative to mastectomy for the treatment of many women with breast cancer (Harris et al., 1983).

Lasting clinical observations date from the 1800s. Sir James Paget's description in 1874 of erosion of the nipple as a sign of underlying carcinoma, subsequently designated "Paget's disease," is a model of English brevity. "I believe it has not yet been published," began Paget, "that certain chronic affections of the skin of the nipple and areola are very often succeeded by the formation of scirrhous cancer in the mammary gland. I have seen about fifteen cases in which this has happened, and the events were in all of them so similar that one description may suffice." The article occupies only three pages. The ominous nature of inflammatory changes accompanying breast cancer was documented as early as 1814 by Bell. In 1869, Koltz in Halle described this presentation as a clinical entity, "mastitis carcinomatosa," and it became known as inflammatory breast cancer in the present century. Rigoni-Stern linked breast cancer with nulliparity in 1842 in a study of women in Verona; in his study, he found nuns to be at more than three times the risk of other women (Rigoni-Stern, 1842). The frequency of this "pest" among nuns had been noted earlier in 1713 by Ramazzini in Padua (Haagensen, 1986). Less clinical, but still relevant to the course of surgery, Rotter in 1899 described lymph nodes, later known as "Rotter's nodes," lying along the course of the superior thoracic artery between the two pectoral muscles. The occasional presence of metastases in these nodes provided additional support for surgical removal of both pectoral muscles.

A final heritage from the 19th century was the discovery that breast cancer was hormone-dependent. Sir Astley Cooper had noted in 1836 that the growth of breast cancers sometimes fluctuated with the menstrual cycle. It became known that a temporary regression could occur at menopause. At a surgical congress in Berlin in 1889, Schinzinger stated that the disease grew more slowly in postmenopausal women and even suggested castration as a means for hastening the benefit of menopause. But it was not by this line of reasoning nor was it in England or Germany that the value of castration was demonstrated; instead, it was through G. Thomas Beatson's studies of lactation in Scotland. Beatson learned that lactation in cattle could be prolonged indefinitely by removing the ovaries, and noting the similarity between the proliferation of tissues in the breast with lactation and with cancer, he reasoned that castration might also cause cancer cells to degenerate into milk. In 1896, Beatson reported that surgical castration of two patients with advanced breast cancer produced tumor regression, and for the first time a systemic treatment was available for patients with this disease (Beatson, 1896). Although the operation did not prove curative, one-third of menstruating patients received temporary benefit. Discovery that one organ could influence the function of another through humoral means was also a milestone in physiology and led Starling and Bayliss in London to introduce the concept of "hormones" in 1905. Early in the development of radiation therapy, it was found that ovarian ablation could be accomplished with radiation. Although this avoided surgical risk, the hormonal changes and the accompanying clinical rewards were achieved more slowly. Almost 50 years later, Farrow and Adair (1942) demonstrated the palliative value of castration in men. In rapid succession, Huggins and Bergenstal (1951) demonstrated benefit from adrenalectomy, and Luft and Olivecrona (1953) from hypophysectomy. Not all responded, but in the patients who did, estrogen deletion was generally conceded to be the salient mechanism. Patient selection remained an inexact process until the discovery of estrogen receptors in the 1960s. Estrogen-dependent tumors contained a specific protein in the cellular cytoplasm that selectively bound estradiol (Jensen et al., 1967; McGuire et al., 1975), and its absence in significant quantities identified patients who seldom responded to endocrine ablation. They could be spared the morbidity of useless treatment.

RECENT CONCEPTS

The acceptance of radical mastectomy was virtually complete in the first half of the 20th century. Surgeons generally were convinced that it could not be improved; Halsted had tried to do so and failed. Standard management for breast tumors became hospital admission with biopsy under general anesthesia, frozen section for diagnosis, and immediate radical mastectomy. Deformity of the chest, lymphedema of the arm in many cases, and occasional irradiation-induced sarcomas were small prices to pay for an optimum chance of cure. The feature that most marked developments of the later 20th century was a turbulent re-evaluation of these concepts.

The stimulus had a dual origin. First, it became increasingly apparent that the limits of radical surgery had been reached without achieving cure in at least one-third of patients. Despite the fact that radical mastectomy (or its extensions) was taught in every medical school and was widely practiced, deaths from breast cancer remained undiminished. Second, accumulating knowledge about the biology of breast cancer changed the understanding of this disease, and the new insights explained the therapeutic stalemate. It became evident, for example, that the tumor frequently arose in multiple sites throughout the breast and often spread so early in its course that the period of local confinement had come to an end long before its presence was discovered. Early diagnosis, advocated by physicians through the centuries, became a greater challenge than previously imagined.

The permeation theory of tumor spread was an early casualty. In 1931, Gray massaged contrast material into mastectomy specimens and demonstrated that the lymphatics around the primary tumor, even when axillary nodes contained metastases, were neither obliterated nor filled with cancer cells (Gray, 1938–1939). Thus, in early cases, embolism rather than permeation was the principal method of lymphatic spread. Gray's discovery weakened the en bloc principle of radical surgery and contributed to the rationale for the "modified" radical mastectomy (i.e., removal of the breast and axillary contents while preserving the pectoralis major muscle). The modified mastectomy, essentially the same operation used by Küster and by Banks 70 years earlier, was reintroduced in England in the 1930s by Patey, championed by R. S. Handley, and subsequently pioneered in the United States by Auchincloss and by Madden (Patey and Dyson, 1948; Madden, 1965; Patey, 1967; Handley and Thackray, 1969; Auchincloss, 1970). Because of its cosmetic superiority and equivalent results, it had replaced Halsted's radical mastectomy in the United States by 1975 as the operation most often performed for operable breast cancer (Lazaro et al., 1978; NIH Consensus Development Conference Summary, 1979).

Another blow to the permeation theory was delivered in 1955 by Engell, who demonstrated venous dissemination of cancer cells from early operable tumors—further evidence that early spread was not solely through lymphatics and that venous embolization frequently, if not always, preceded attempts to surgically encompass the diseased tissues. Cure evidently depended on events other than the removal of every tumor cell.

Only a few years later, the Fisher brothers (1967) clearly showed that lymph nodes were not effective barriers to the spread of cancer cells. They demonstrated in rabbits that living tumor cells easily passed through lymph nodes into efferent lymphatics and also probably into veins through lymphaticovenous connections. Not only were lymph nodes poor filters, but in addition cancer cells seemed to pass easily back and forth between the blood vessel and lymphatic systems (Fisher and Fisher, 1966).

Tumor kinetics received increasing scrutiny. Observed gross rates of growth of breast cancers studied by Gershon-Cohen and others permitted theoretic calculations suggesting that breast cancers existed for several years before they reached clinically detectable size (Gershon-Cohen et al., 1963; Bond, 1968). The ample opportunity to metastasize widely during this protracted period of occult growth obviously placed a limit on the absolute curability of breast cancer and supported the case of "predeterminists" of the 1950s (Park and Lees, 1951). In the minds of some investigators, the question of whether invasive breast cancer was ever cured remained open (Mueller and Jeffries, 1975).

The concept of immunologic resistance against tumors also grew and was credited with limited success. As early as 1922, W. Sampson Handley wrote, "There is a considerable body of evidence that lymphatic glands are able to deal with cancer cells in limited doses; Williams especially has drawn attention to the fact that, in days when the axillary glands were not removed with the breast, axillary recurrence was not so frequent as with our present microscopical knowledge of axillary gland invasion we should expect to find it." This observation was confirmed 55 years later by Fisher in a controlled clinical trial (Fisher, 1977). At midcentury, the immunology of cancer was placed on a firmer basis with the demonstration of tumor-related antigens and a measurable host response (Foley, 1953). The intense subsequent research in cancer immunology generated the concept of a dynamic tumor-host interaction that could be influenced by biologic events in favor of one or the other. Circumstantial support for strong host resistance could be found in occasional spontaneous regressions of cancer, long delayed recurrences, and surgical cure in circumstances when this seemed highly unlikely, possibly through the body's ability to destroy small numbers of residual tumor cells. Rapid tumor growth and early death implied poor host resistance. Conceptually, surgery for neoplasia became less akin to the excision of a foreign body than to a means of conducting biologic warfare.

As the initial immune response was vested in regional lymph nodes, the routine removal or irradiation of clinically normal nodes came into question. George Crile, Jr., was prominent among those who opposed radical surgery (Crile, 1971). Impressed with both the morbidity of axillary node dissection and his favorable experience with limited operations at the Cleveland Clinic, Crile maintained that there was no advantage to prophylactic dissection of clinically normal nodes even if they contained occult cancer. Said he, "It is just as effective to defer treatment until the nodes become palpably involved." Bond suggested that prophylactic node dissections might even be detrimental (Bond, 1968). Fisher speculated that if host resistance were reflected in destruction of metastases within nodes, normal nodes might well represent strong host resistance rather than the absence of metastatic spread (Fisher, 1976).

The uncertain biology of the small breast cancers being detected raised questions about the need for routine mastectomy. The rationale for total mastectomy was based not only on the effort to remove all local extensions of cancer but also on the observation that even in early cases, breast cancer arose as a multifocal change throughout the mammary parenchyma (Gallager and Martin, 1969; Schwartz et al., 1980). Nevertheless, the frequency with which these microscopic tumors became clinical cancers during the patient's remaining lifetime was uncertain.

The questions about radical surgery fortunately coincided with the emergence of new scientific tools: the prospective randomized clinical trial and modern statistical analysis. These exercises in clinical discipline, which served to reduce the biases of patient selection that plagued earlier studies, were used initially in England in the 1950s to evaluate the outcome of adjuvant irradiation. In a climate of rising controversy about local treatment, they were widely adopted by concerned physicians.

Early trials focused on treatment of regional nodes. Within a relatively short period, they compared radical mastectomy combined with postoperative irradiation with simple mastectomy combined with postoperative irradiation (Brinkley and Haybittle, 1966; Bergdahl, 1978), radical mastectomy with radical mastectomy combined with postoperative irradiation (Patterson and Russell, 1959), simple mastectomy combined with postoperative irradiation with radical mastectomy (Bruce, 1971), simple mastectomy combined with postoperative irradiation with mastectomy extended to the supraclavicular and internal mammary lymph nodes (Kaae and Johansen, 1969), simple mastectomy with simple mastectomy combined with postoperative irradiation (Murray et al., 1977), radical mastectomy with radical mastectomy plus internal mammary node dissection (Lacour et al., 1976; Veronesi and Valagussa, 1981), and simple mastectomy with radical mastectomy (Fisher et al., 1977). The results were as follows:

1. The stage of disease had a decided influence on survival; variations of local treatment did not.

2. The presence or absence of metastases in regional nodes was of primary prognostic importance, as was the absolute number of nodes involved.

3. Postoperative irradiation reduced local and regional recurrence within treated fields, but without improving survival.

4. Routine removal of axillary lymph nodes or of internal mammary lymph nodes reduced tumor recurrence at these sites without improving survival.

5. Irradiation controlled metastases in regional lymph nodes as did surgical removal.

6. Removal of axillary lymph nodes often resulted in lymphedema of the arm, which was increased further by irradiation of the axilla.

These studies confirmed what surgeons observed almost 100 years earlier—that is, that radical local treatment resulted in improved local and regional control of tumor but unfortunately without influencing survival.

Other clinical trials focused on management of the breast itself. At Guy's Hospital, London, patients were randomized for treatment between local tumor excision or radical mastectomy, each followed by postoperative irradiation. Low doses of irradiation resulted in a high frequency of recurrence in the breast and nodes after the more limited surgical procedure (Hayward, 1977). Studies in Italy and the United States subsequently determined that high doses of irradiation could greatly reduce recurrence in the breast after local tumor removal (Veronesi, 1977; Fisher, 1977).

It is apparent that the two forces responsible for advancing radical surgery reached their limits. The effort to prevent local-regional failures by enlarging the field of operation reached anatomic limits without eliminating mortality. The concept of local origin provides a basis for cure only if diagnosis can be made before dissemination occurs—which means while the disease is still occult—and this remains an imperfect attainment. Recognition that failures were likely the result of early occult dissemination initiated the present era of systemic adjuvant therapy.

The development of mammography is a passage in this history that is too important to omit. It represented a giant leap in early diagnosis. For the first time, breast cancers could be discovered when they were too small to be found on physical examination. Like so many facets of science, its development was at the hands of many. Following Roentgen's discovery of x-rays at the University of Würzburg in 1895, diagnostic radiology developed rapidly. That is, except for examination of the breast. The first radiologic studies of the breast were reported by Salomon from the University of Berlin in 1913, but only on surgical specimens, and although the radiologic signs of carcinoma were accurately described, this information was considered of only academic interest. According to Hoeffken and Lanyi (1977), not until 1927 did Kleinschmidt in Leipzig produce the first roentgenogram of a living breast. In the next decade, clinical investigations were carried out in South America by Dominguez (1930), by Warren in the United States (1930), and by Vogel (1932) in Germany. Some investigators injected air and contrast materials into breasts in an effort to enhance the examination, but images were poor and the results were disappointing. Leborgne, a student of Dominguez, made useful comparisons between mammograms and pathology and described calcifications in the breast in detail (1953); however, at midcentury, only a few enthusiasts such as Goshen Cohen in Philadelphia and Gros in Strasbourg sustained interest in mammography. Not until Robert Egan introduced new techniques to improve soft tissue contrast and detail in 1960 at the M.D. Anderson Hospital in Houston was serious consideration given to widespread use of mammography as a diagnostic device (Egan, 1972). Standardization of technique and widespread training of radiologists followed. At first, emphasis was placed on evaluation of clinically evident breast masses. An important conceptual change occurred in the 1960s, when it was discovered that mammograms also revealed preclinical signs of breast cancer. By this time, the achievements of radical surgery had reached their limits, and early discovery of malignant lesions was clearly needed. This provided an impetus that culminated in the use of mammography for screening large asymptomatic populations. The controlled studies that followed pioneered by Strax and associates in

New York clearly indicated that, when used in conjunction with physical examination, routine periodic mammography reduced mortality from breast cancer (Strax, 1989).

CONCLUSION

After 5000 years, the cause of breast cancer remains unknown, and a practical means of prevention is not at hand. Its incidence continues to rise, and death rates remain undiminished. The clinical descriptions of the ancients are familiar even today. Illustrations in rare and faded volumes show the repetitious story, and in the texts of a century ago, before the dictates of privacy deleted faces, the victims look up from the pages with haunting eyes. Such advanced cases are not as frequent anymore now that earlier diagnosis is possible, but the epidemic continues. New insights are needed.

Bernard Fisher at the University of Pittsburgh has been most instrumental in defining a new model of the disease, a new "paradigm" to replace the outmoded conceptions of Handley and Halsted. The essentials of Fisher's 1981 thesis are that breast cancer is a systemic disease, not in the ancient sense of a diathesis but in that tumor cells regularly disseminate from the primary tumor long before the disease is discovered. Furthermore, the dissemination of malignant cells is not orderly, but rather a disorderly process of embolization that occurs through blood vessels and lymphatics and with free interchange between the two. Finally, a complex (and poorly understood) biologic relationship exists between the patient and her cancer that is often reflected in the lymph node. Regional lymph nodes are not a barrier to tumor cells; metastases in lymph nodes simply confirm that resistance is flagging and that metastases are being permitted throughout the body. "The primary aim of oncologic surgery (with or without aid of radiation therapy) at present," state Fisher and Gebhardt (1978), "seems to be directed toward reducing the tumor burden to a number of viable cells that are entirely destroyable by: (1) host immunologic (and possibly other) factors alone, (2) systemically administered anti-cancer agents, or (3) a combination of both." Unfortunately, the critical reduction and the extent of surgery required to reach it remain obscure. Hayward was more specific. He identified four current obligations of the surgeon: (1) to provide local tumor control, (2) to determine the pathologic status of axillary lymph nodes, (3) to provide tumor tissue for diagnosis and biologic markers, and (4) to provide local treatment that is compatible with systemic adjuvant therapy (Hayward, 1981).

The long evolution to radical surgery was based principally on the clear demonstration that it controlled the local tumor more effectively than limited operations. This benefit cannot be discarded without an equally effective substitute. If the conceptual base was faulty, it must be appreciated that the biology of breast cancer is still imperfectly understood. Much depends on developments in radiation therapy and systemic therapy. Surgery and radiation are both effective local treatments, and a choice between the two may simply be a matter of relative morbidities. In the unlikely event that breast cancers can be routinely discovered in their earliest phases, this choice may be the only decision that is necessary. If systemic therapy proves capable of curing only when the tumor burden is reduced to a minimum, then surgery or irradiation, or some combination of the two, may prove the best means of accomplishing this end. If a totally effective systemic therapy is eventually found, local treatment may become unnecessary altogether.

References

Ackerknecht, E. H.: History and Geography of the Most Important Diseases. New York, Hafner Publishing Company, 1965, pp. 162–173.
Arnott, H.: On the therapeutical importance of recent view of the nature and structure of cancer. St. Thomas Hospital Report, 2:103–122, 1871.
Auchincloss, H.: Modified radical mastectomy: Why not? Am. J. Surg., 119:506, 1970.
Baclesse, F.: Five-year results in 431 breast cancers treated solely by roentgen rays. Ann. Surg., 161:103–104, 1965.
Banks, W. M.: A brief history of the operations practiced for cancer of the breast. Br. Med. J., 1:5–10, 1902.
Beatson, G. T.: On the treatment of inoperable cases of carcinoma of the mamma: Suggestions for a new treatment with illustrative cases. Lancet, ii:104, 1896.
Bergdahl, L.: Simple and radical mastectomy with postoperative irradiation: A controlled trial. Am. Surg. 44:369–373, 1978.
Bond, W. H.: The influence of various treatments on survival rates in cancer of the breast. In Jarrett, A. S. (Ed.): The Treatment of Carcinoma of the Breast. Excerpta Medica Foundation for Syntex Pharmaceuticals (Maidenhead, Berkshire, England), 1968, pp. 24–39.
Brinkley, D., and Haybittle, J. L.: Treatment of stage II carcinoma of the female breast. Lancet, ii:291, 1966.
Bruce, J.: Operable cancer of the breast: A controlled clinical trial. Cancer, 28:1443–1452, 1971.
Clinical Society of London: Effectual method of operating for cancer of the breast. Lancet, i:248, 1893.
Cooper, W. A.: The history of the radical mastectomy. Ann. Med. History, 3:36–53, 1941.
Crile, G. Jr.: Treatment of cancer of the breast: Past, present, and future. Cleve. Clin. Q., 38:47–54, 1971.
Dahl-Iversen, E., and Tobiassen, T.: Radical mastectomy with parasternal and supraclavicular dissection for mammary carcinoma. Ann. Surg., 170:889–891, 1969.
DeMoulin, D.: A Short History of Breast Cancer. Boston, Martinus Nijhoff Publishers, 1983.
Dominguez, C. M.: Estudio radiologico de los descalcificadores. Bol. Soc. Anat. Path., 1:175–180, 1930.
Egan, R. L.: Mammography. 2nd ed. Springfield, IL, Charles C Thomas, 1972, pp. 3–13.
Engell, H. C.: Cancer cells in the circulating blood. Acta Chir. Scand. (Suppl. 201), pp. 1–70, 1955.
Farrow, J. H., and Adair, F. E.: Effect of orchiectomy on skeletal metastases from cancer of the male breast. Science, 95:654, 1942.
Fisher, B.: Some thoughts concerning the primary therapy of breast cancer. Recent Results Cancer Res., 57:150–163, 1976.
Fisher, B.: United States trials of conservative surgery. World J. Surg., 1:327–330, 1977.
Fisher, B.: A commentary on the role of the surgeon in primary breast cancer. Breast Cancer Res. Treat., 1:17–26, 1981.
Fisher, B., and Fisher, E. R.: The interrelationship of hematogenous and lymphatic tumor cell dissemination. Surg. Gynecol. Obstet., 122:791, 1966.
Fisher, B., and Fisher, E. R.: Barrier function of lymph node to tumor cells and erythrocytes: I. Normal nodes. Cancer, 20:1907–1913, 1967.
Fisher, B., and Gebhardt, M. C.: The evolution of breast cancer surgery: Past, present, and future. Semin. Oncol. 5:385–394, 1978.
Fisher, B., Montague, E., Redmond, C., et al.: Comparison of radical mastectomy with alternative treatments for primary breast cancer. Cancer, 39:2827–2839, 1977.
Foley, E. J.: Antigenic properties of methyl-cholanthrene–induced tumors in mice of the strain of origin. Cancer Res., 13:835, 1953.

Gallagher, H. S., and Martin, J. E.: Early phases in the development of breast cancer. Cancer, *24:*1170–1178, 1969.

Gershon-Cohen, J., Berger, S. M., and Klickstein, H. S.: Roentgenography of breast cancer moderating concept of "biologic predeterminism." Cancer, *16:*961, 1963.

Gray, J. H.: The relation of lymphatic vessels to the spread of cancer. Br. J. Surg., *26:*462–472, 1938–1939.

Greenough, R. B., Simmons, C. C., and Barney, J. D.: The results of operations for cancer of the breast at the Massachusetts General Hospital from 1894 to 1904. Trans. Am. Surg. Assoc., *25:*80–102, 1907.

Grubbe, E. H.: Priority in the therapeutic use of x-rays. Radiology, *21:*156–162, 1933.

Haagensen, C. D.: Diseases of the Breast. 2nd ed. Philadelphia, W. B. Saunders, 1971, pp. 622–630.

Haagensen, C. D.: Diseases of the Breast. 3rd ed. Philadelphia, W. B. Saunders, 1986, p. 42.

Halsted, W. S.: The treatment of wounds with a special reference to the value of the blood clot in the management of dead spaces. The Johns Hopkins Hospital Reports, *2:*255–314, 1891.

Halsted, W. S.: The results of operations for the cure of cancer of the breast performed at the Johns Hopkins Hospital from June 1889 to January 1894. The Johns Hopkins Hospital Reports, *4:*297–350, 1894–1895.

Halsted, W. S.: The results of radical operations for the cure of cancer of the breast. Trans. Am. Surg. Assoc., *25:*61–79, 1907.

Handley, R. S., and Thackray, A. C.: The internal mammary lymph chain in carcinoma of the breast: Study of 50 cases. Lancet, *ii:*276, 1949.

Handley, R. S., and Thackray, A. C.: Conservative radical mastectomy (Patey's operation). Ann. Surg., *170:*880, 1969.

Handley, W. S.: Cancer of the Breast and Its Operative Treatment. London, John Murray Publishers, 1906, pp. 1–15.

Handley, W. S.: The breast. *In* Choyce, C.C. (Ed.): A System of Surgery. Vol. 2. New York, Funk & Wagnalls Company, 1912, p. 94.

Handley, W. S.: Cancer of the Breast and Its Treatment. 2nd ed. London, John Murray, 1922, p. 256.

Harris, J. R., Hellman, S., and Silen, W.: Conservative Management of Breast Cancer: New Surgical and Radiotherapeutic Techniques. Philadelphia, J. B. Lippincott, 1983.

Hayward, J. L.: The surgeon's role in primary breast cancer. Breast Cancer Res. Treat., *1:*27–32, 1981.

Hayward, J. L.: The Guy's trial of treatments of "early" breast cancer. World J. Surg., *1:*314–316, 1977.

Heidenhain, L.: Über die Ursachen der localen Krebsrecidive nach Amputation mammae. Verhandlungen der Deutschen Gesellschaft für Chirurgie, Achtzehnter Congress, Berlin, 1889.

Henderson, I. C., and Canellos, G. P.: Cancer of the breast: The past decade. N. Engl. J. Med., *302:*17–30 (Part I), and *302:*787–790 (Part II), 1980.

Hochman, A., and Robinson, E.: Eighty-two cases of mammary cancer treated exclusively with roentgen therapy. Cancer, *15:*670–673, 1960.

Hoeffken, W., and Lanyi, M.: Mammography. Philadelphia, W. B. Saunders, 1977, pp. 1–3.

Huggins, C., and Bergenstal, D. M.: Influence of bilateral adrenalectomy, adrenocorticotrophin, and cortisone acetate on certain human tumors. Science, *144:*482, 1951.

Jensen, E. V., DeSombre, E. R., and Junglblut, P. W.: Estrogen receptors in hormone responsive tissues and tumors. *In* Wissler, R. W., Dao, T. L., Wood, S. (Eds.): Endogenous Factors Influencing Host-Tumor Balance. Chicago, University of Chicago Press, 1967, pp. 15–30.

Kaae, S., and Johansen, H.: Simple mastectomy plus postoperative irradiation by the method of McWhirter for mammary carcinoma. Ann. Surg., *170:*895–899, 1969.

Keynes, G.: Conservative treatment of cancer of the breast. Br. Med. J., *2:*643–647, 1937.

Koltz, H. H.: Über Mastitis Carcinomatosa Gravidarum et Lactantium. Halle, 1869.

Küster, E.: Zur Behandlung des Brustkrebses. Arch. F. Clin. Chirg., *29:*723–753, 1883.

Lacour, J., Bucalossi, P., Cacers, E., et al.: Radical mastectomy versus radical mastectomy plus internal mammary dissection. Cancer, *37:*206–214, 1976.

Lazaro, E. J., Rush, B. F., Jr., and Swaminathan, A. P.: Changing attitudes in the management of cancer of the breast. Surgery, *84:*441–447, 1978.

LeDran H. F.: Memoire avec un precis de plusieurs observations sur le cancer. Memoires de L'academie royale de chirurgie, *3:*1–54, 1757.

Lewis, D., and Rienhoff, W. F. Jr.: A study of the results of operations for the cure of cancer of the breast performed at the Johns Hopkins Hospital from 1889 to 1931. Ann. Surg., *95:*336–400, 1932.

Lewison, E. F.: Saint Agatha, the patron saint of diseases of the breast in legend and art. Bull. Hist. Med. *24:*409–420, 1950.

Lewison, E. F.: The surgical treatment of breast cancer: An historical and collective review. Surgery, *34:*904–953, 1953.

Luft, R., and Olivecrona, H.: Experiences with hypophysectomy in man. J. Neurosurg. *10:*301, 1953.

Madden, J. L.: Modified radical matectomy. Surg. Gynecol. Obstet., *121:*1221, 1965.

Mansfield, C.: Early breast cancer: Its history and results of treatment. *In* Wolsky, A. (Ed.): Experimental Biology and Medicine. Monographs on Interdisciplinary Topics. Vol. 5. New York, Karger, 1976, pp. 2–22.

Margottini, M.: Recent developments in the surgical treatment of breast cancer. Acta Unio Int Contra Cancrum, *8:*176–178, 1952.

McGuire, W. L., Carbone, P. P., and Vollmer, E. P.: Estrogen Receptors in Human Breast Cancer. New York, Raven Press, 1975.

McWhirter, R.: The value of simple mastectomy and radiotherapy in the treatment of cancer of the breast. Br. J. Radiol., *21:*599–610, 1948.

Meyer, W.: An improved method of the radical operation for carcinoma of the breast. Med. Rec., *46:*746–749, 1894.

Moore, C. H.: On the influence of inadequate operations on the theory of cancer: Royal Medical and Chirurgical Society, London. Medica Chirurgical Transactions, *32:*245–280, 1867.

Mueller, C. B., and Jeffries, W.: Cancer of the breast: Its outcome as measured by the rate of dying and causes of death. Ann. Surg., *182:*334–343, 1975.

Müller J.: Über den feinern Bau und die Formen der krankhaften Geschwulste. Berlin, G. Rehner, 1838.

Murray, J. G., MacIntyre, J., Simpson, J. S., and McDonald, A. M.: Cancer research campaign study of the management of "early" breast cancer. World J. Surg., *1:*317–319, 1977.

NIH Consensus Development Conference Summary. The treatment of primary breast cancer: Management of local disease. Vol. 2. No. 5., 1979.

Paget, J.: On the disease of the mammary areola preceding cancer of the mammary gland. St. Bartholomew's Hospital Report, *10:*87, 1874.

Paget, S.: The distribution of the secondary growths in cancer of the breast. Lancet, *ii:* March 23, 1889.

Park, W. W., and Lees, J. C.: The absolute curability of cancer of the breast. Surg. Gynecol. Obstet., *93:*129–152, 1951.

Patey, D. H.: A review of 146 cases of carcinoma of the breast operated on between 1930 and 1943. Br. J. Cancer, *21:*260–269, 1967.

Patey, D. H., and Dyson, W. H.: The prognosis of carcinoma of the breast in relation to the type of operation performed. Br. J. Cancer, *2:*7–13, 1948.

Patterson, R., and Russell, M. H.: Clinical trials in malignant disease. Part III—Breast cancer: Evaluation of postoperative radiotherapy. J. Fac. Radiol, *10:*175–180, 1959.

Power, D.: The history of the amputation of the breast to 1904. Liverpool Medico-Chirurgical Journal, *42/43:*29–56, 1934–1935.

Prosnitz, L. R., Goldenberg, I. S., Packard, R. A., et al.: Radiation therapy as initial treatment for early stage cancer of the breast without mastectomy. Cancer, *39:*917–923, 1977.

Prudente, A.: L'amputation inter-scapulo-mammothoracique (technique et resultats). J. Chir. *65:*729, 1949.

Rigoni-Stern, D.: Fatti statistici relativi alle malattie cancerose che servirono de base alle poche cose dette dal dott. Gior. servire progr. Pat. e Terap., *2:*507, 1842.

Robbins, G. F.: Silvergirl's Surgery—The Breast. Austin, TX, Silvergirl, 1984, pp. 24–29.

Rutkow, I. M.: William Stewart Halsted and the germanic influence on education and training programs in surgery. Surg. Gynecol. Obstet., *146:*602–606, 1978.

Schlumberger, H. G.: Origins of the cell concept in pathology. Arch. Pathol., *37:*396–407, 1944.

Schmid, H.: Zur Statistick der Mammacarcinome und deren Heilung. Deutsche Zeitschrift für Chirurgie, *26:*139–192, 1887.

Schmidt, M. B.: Die Verbreitungswege der Karzinome. Jena, 1903.

Schwartz, G. F., Patchefsky, A. S., Feig, S. A., et al.: Multicentricity of non-palpable breast cancer. Cancer, *45:*2913–2916, 1980.

Strax, P.: Control of breast cancer through mass screening from research to action. Cancer, *63:*1881–1887, 1989.

Sugarbaker, E. D.: Radical mastectomy combined with in-continuity resection of the homolateral internal mammary node chain. Cancer, *6:*969–979, 1953.

Urban, J. A.: Surgical excision of internal mammary nodes for breast cancer. Br. J. Surg., *51:*209–212, 1964.

Veronesi, U.: Conservative treatment of breast cancer: A trial in progress at the cancer institute of Milan. World J. Surg., *1:*324–326, 1977.

Veronesi, U., and Valagussa, P.: Inefficacy of internal mammary node dissection in breast cancer surgery. Cancer, *47:*170–175, 1981.

Vogel, W.: Die Roentgendarstellung der Mammatumoren. Arch. Klin. Chir., *171:*618, 1932.

Wangensteen, O. H., Lewis, F. J., and Arhelger, S. W.: The extended or super-radical mastectomy for carcinoma of the breast. Surg. Clin. North. Am., *36:*1051–1063, 1956.

Warren, S. L.: A roentgenologic study of the breast. Am. J. Roentgen., *24:*113–124, 1930.

Wilder, R. J.: The historical development of the concept of metastasis. J. Mt. Sinai. Hosp., *23:*728–734, 1956.

2 Microscopic Anatomy of the Breast

James G. Kuhns
Douglas M. Ackermann

The mammary glands are modified eccrine glands of the skin located on the anterior chest wall whose ductal and lobular units extend far into the adjacent subcutaneous fat. The gland itself is segmentally divided into 15 to 20 distinct glandular units, or lobes, each of which has a ductal orifice at the apex of the nipple. Prior to puberty, a mammary gland consists of little more than a complex system of ductal structures (Amenta, 1986), a configuration that persists in the male breast throughout life. At puberty, the glands in the female progressively enlarge. The amount of fibrofatty elements increases, the ducts elongate, and small areolar buds form, but full maturation is not attained until pregnancy.

NIPPLE, AREOLA, AND BREAST PARENCHYMA

The areolar region of skin, including the nipple, consists of a keratinizing stratified squamous epithelium with a dense basal melanin deposition, which accounts for the region's dark pigmentation. The adjacent dermis, in contrast to typical skin, contains a radially arranged prominent smooth muscle component that extends longitudinally along the lactiferous ducts. The areola also contains hair follicles, sebaceous and sweat glands, and large modified areolar glands, known as Montgomery's glands, which account for the small elevations on the surface of the areola (Fig. 2–1A and B). With stimulation, the muscle fibers of the areola contract, hardening and elevating the nipple. The nipple is traversed by multiple lactiferous ducts that range from 2 to 4 mm in diameter. These have convoluted walls (to permit high flow) and a squamous lining near the surface exit (see Fig. 2–1C). They commonly create a pocket or vestibule, known as the lactiferous sinus, that lies at the base of the nipple. The ducts and sinuses are lined by a single or double layer of simple columnar epithelial cells. As the ducts ramify deeper into the breast parenchyma, they form smaller ductal units (see Fig. 2–1D). These smaller ducts and ductules are lined by a two-cell layer composed of inner epithelial cells and outer, spindle-shaped mesenchymal myoepithelial cells.

The basic hormonally sensitive and lactational unit of the breast is the terminal ductal-lobular unit. In the resting phase, this unit is lined by cuboidal epithelium that is surrounded by an inactive layer of myoepithelial cells (Figs. 2–2 to 2–6). This unit is embedded in a myxoid loose connective tissue that has a rich capillary supply and that may contain a few lymphocytes, histiocytes, plasma cells, and mast cells. This connective tissue is generally sharply demarcated from the denser, less cellular, and more peripheral supportive collagenous tissue and fat. The cuboidal and myoepithelial cells in different lobular units may appear quite varied, depending on the amount of cytoplasm associated with these cells and their nuclear characteristics. The myoepithelial cells surround the lobule between the inner aspect of the basement membrane and the more superficial cuboidal cells and are arranged in a banding pattern. The sarcoplasma within the myoepithelial cells contains contractile filaments that insert on the hemidesmosomes of the adjacent basement membrane. These intracytoplasmic myofilaments contract when exposed to oxytocin and prolactin, facilitating the excretion of the secretory contents within the lobules.

The lobular units vary from 0.3 to 0.6 mm in diameter and are interconnected by a labyrinth of extralobular terminal ductules. These are hormonally sensitive and may be the site of intraductal hyperplasia. These ductules fuse in a cascading series to form the final 15 to 20 largest ducts of the breast that come together immediately beneath the areola (Snell, 1984; Leeson et al., 1988; Ross et al., 1988; Arey, 1974; Amenta, 1986; Hughes et al., 1988; Karcioglu and Someren, 1985; and Fechner and Mills, 1990).

HORMONAL CHANGES

During the hormonal changes of the menstrual cycle, the lobular unit and its associated terminal duct undergo histologic alterations. During the estrogen (proliferative) phase, especially during the first week of the phase, a proliferation of the cuboidal cells is present, and an occasional mitotic figure is observed. Later, during the progesterone (secretory) phase, active apocrine secretions from the cuboidal cell lining may be observed. The adjacent lobular stroma becomes edematous, and the lumen of the ductules begins to open with secretions. These changes vary from one lobular unit to another (Vogel et al., 1981).

Text continued on page 21

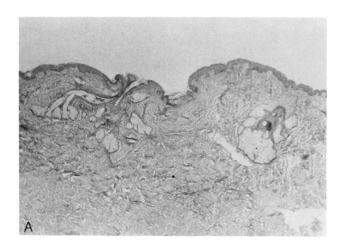

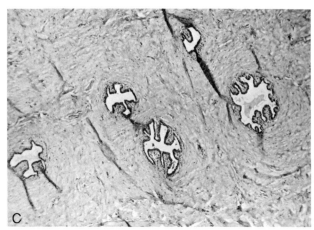

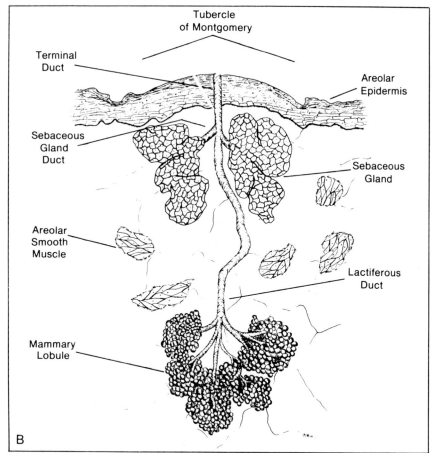

Tubercle
of Montgomery

Terminal
Duct

Areolar
Epidermis

Sebaceous
Gland
Duct

Sebaceous
Gland

Areolar
Smooth
Muscle

Lactiferous
Duct

Mammary
Lobule

B

Figure 2–1. Histologic section *(A)* and reconstruction *(B)* of Montgomery's tubercle of the areola. (Reconstruction reproduced with permission. Smith et al, 1982.) *C,* Ducts of the nipple. A transverse section shows that the ducts are corrugated to permit dilation. The smooth muscle that surrounds them provides continence of secretions and enables the nipple to become erect.

Illustration continued on following page

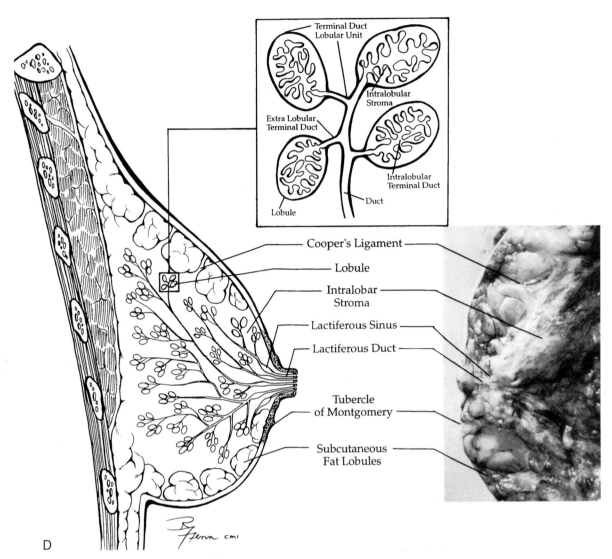

Figure 2–1 *Continued D,* Diagrams and corresponding gross photograph illustrate the location of the terminal lobule, ductules, and fusion of the lactiferous ducts.

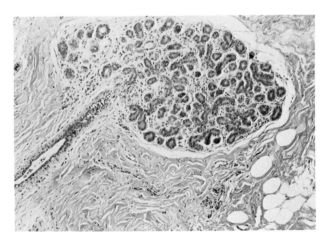

Figure 2–2. This view of a terminal ductal-lobular unit demonstrates the extralobular terminal duct and the lobular unit in a resting phase. (× 65.)

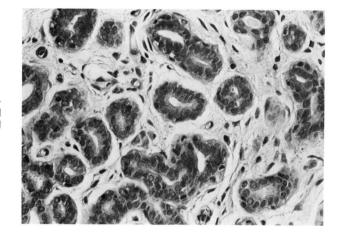

Figure 2–3. A higher magnification view of lobular unit demonstrates the lining cuboidal cells and adjacent myoepithelial cells embedded in a loose myxomatous, richly vascularized intralobular connective tissue matrix. (× 260.)

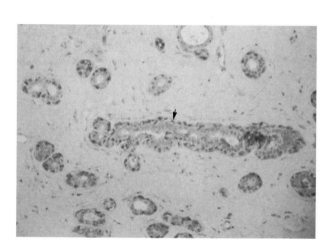

Figure 2–4. In this section, the contractile myoepithelial cells of the ducts *(arrow)* are darkened by a stain for S-100 antigen. Their contraction ejects milk from the ductal system. (Courtesy of Reuben Eisenstein, M.D.)

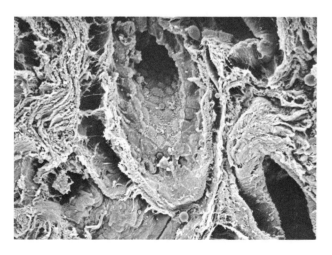

Figure 2–5. Scanning electron microscopy of a portion of a lobule at a high power demonstrates the cuboidal cells of the lobule. (× 1000.)

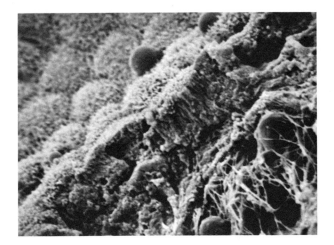

Figure 2-6. Scanning electron microscopy of surface and cut section of cuboidal cells lining lobules. (× 4000.)

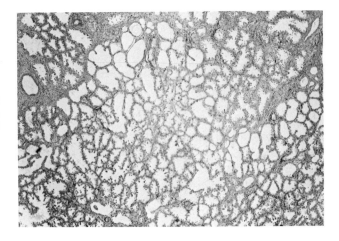

Figure 2-7. This low-power (× 65) view of lactational changes in the breast shows enlargement of the lobular units and the shedding of cytoplasmic vacuoles of protein-lipid complexes into the lumen.

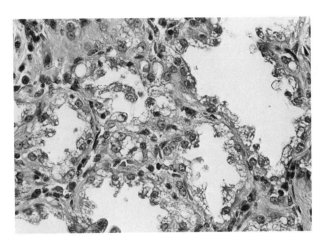

Figure 2-8. Same view as in Figure 2-7, but magnified × 260.

GESTATIONAL AND LACTATIONAL CHANGES

During pregnancy (Figs. 2–7 and 2–8), the lobular units undergo marked proliferation and enlargement. In the third trimester of pregnancy, the perilobular stroma has diminished and is diffusely displaced by hypertrophied lobules that closely approximate each other. Intracytoplasmic fat droplets accumulate within the lobular epithelial cells, and secretions exude into the adjacent lumina (Fechner and Mills, 1990).

As pregnancy continues, a colostrum composed of desquamated epithelial cells and fluid accumulates (Harris et al., 1987); the colostrum is released in the immediate postpartum period. During lactation, the large epithelial cells show vacuoles and small cytoplasmic blebs on the luminal borders. The secretion of the contents within the vacuoles is of an apocrine type, leaving residual cells with scant cytoplasm and prominent nuclei, which produces a hobnail pattern. These stages are variably present within the breast for a period up to 3 months after lactation has ceased. In addition, apoptosis, in which cells are shed into the lumen, is seen during lactation.

POSTMENOPAUSAL CHANGES

The loss of hormonal stimulation produces a decrease in the absolute number of lobular units as well as a diffuse atrophy of the residual lobular units. The loose paralobular and intralobular connective tissue become progressively collagenized and less cellular. These changes of atrophy are variable and incomplete. Some women maintain a premenopausal lobular appearance well into their 70s (Wellings et al., 1976).

References

Amenta, P. S.: Elias-Pauly's Histology and Human Microanatomy. New York, Wiley, 1986.

Arey, L. B.: Human Histology: A Textbook in Outline Form. Philadelphia, W.B. Saunders, 1974.

Fechner, R. E., and Mills, S. E.: Breast Pathology. Chicago, ASCP Press, 1990.

Harris, J. R., Hellman, S., Henderson, I. C., Kinne, D. W. (Eds.): Breast Diseases. Philadelphia, J.B. Lippincott, 1987.

Hughes, L. E., Mansel, R. E., and Webster, D. J.: Benign Disorders and Diseases of the Breast: Concepts and Clinical Management. Philadelphia, Bailliere-Tindall, 1988.

Karcioglu, Z. A., and Someren, A.: Practical Surgical Pathology. Lexington, MA, D. C. Heath & Co, 1985, pp. 553–635.

Leeson, T. S., Leeson, C. R., and Paparo, A. A.: Text/Atlas of Histology. Philadelphia, W.B. Saunders, 1988.

Ross, M. H., Reith, E. J., and Romrell, L. J.: Histology: A Text and Atlas. Baltimore, Williams & Wilkins, 1988.

Smith, D. M., Peters, T. G., and Donegan, W. L.: Montgomery's areolar tubercle. Arch. Pathol. Lab. Med., *106*:60–63, 1982.

Snell, R. S.: Clinical and Functional Histology for Medical Students. Boston, Little, Brown & Co, 1984.

Vogel, P. N., Ageogiadee, N. G., and Fetter, B. F.: The correlation of histologic changes in the human breast with menstrual cycle. Am. J. Pathol., *104*:23, 1981.

Wellings, S. R., Jensen, H. M., and DeVault, M. R.: Persistence of atypical lobules in the human breast may be precancerous. Experientia, *32*:1463, 1976.

3 Gross Anatomy of the Breast

John S. Spratt
Gordon R. Tobin

Ablative cure of mammary carcinoma by surgical or radiation therapy is based on the possibility that viable cancer is limited to the breast or to the breast and the regional lymph nodes. Confinement of cancer to the lymph nodes requires that the cancer cells have arrived in the nodes via afferent lymphatics, that the nodal sinuses have retained the cancer cells, and that some of these cells have survived and are engaged in growth and replication.

If the metastatic foci in the lymph nodes are not removed or destroyed, sustained growth will result in increasing morbidity from uninhibited local progression. Resection of the lymph nodes, therefore, is pertinent to the surgical management of mammary cancer and local control of cancer on the chest wall. Knowledge of the presence or absence of metastases in the lymph nodes is essential in prognostication. The extent of metastatic cancer in lymph nodes is a measure of the propensity of a specific cancer to metastasize.

The design of surgical and radiation therapy has been based largely on an empirical knowledge of the anatomy of the breast and regional lymph nodes. Of equal importance is the functional lymphatic anatomy as studied by injection, by the distribution of lymph node metastases, and by the dissemination of cancer beyond its locoregional confines.

This chapter reviews the pertinent parts of the developmental, topographic, fascial, muscular, neural, lymphatic, and vascular anatomy of the breast and mammary region. Emphasis is placed on the functional anatomy of lymphatics.

DEVELOPMENTAL ANATOMY

Embryologically, the human breast develops in the pectoral portion of an ectodermal thickening extending from the axilla to the vulva bilaterally. This ''milk streak'' is present by the sixth week of fetal life. By the ninth week, most of the line has atrophied except in the pectoral region. Here, the nipple bud appears as a proliferating mass of basal cells.

By the end of the third month of gestation, squamous cells from the surface begin to invade the nipple bud. The mammary ducts develop as downgrowths from this, terminating in lobular buds that proliferate into acini with sexual maturity.

The entire gland develops as a large dermal and subcutaneous organ from a single focus on the skin. This point is pertinent to the lymphatic drainage of the breast. As is true of all embryonal organogenesis, anomalous development can occur at any phase (Geschickter, 1943).

TOPOGRAPHIC ANATOMY

The adult mammary gland is situated principally between the superficial and deep layers of the superficial pectoral fascia of the anterior chest wall, extending roughly from the second to the sixth or seventh anterior intercostal space. This cephalocaudal dimension is 10 to 12 cm on the average, and the gland generally has a maximum thickness of 3 to 5 cm. The fatty layer overlying the parenchyma of the breast makes a variable contribution to the mass of the breast and fluctuates with total body fat.

The nonlactating breast weighs 150 to 200 g; the lactating gland may weigh as much as 400 to 500 g.

The volume of the breast varies widely from individual to individual and from side to side of the chest. Using biostereometric volume measurements of the breast, Loughry and associates (1989) determined that the volume ranged from 21.1 mL^3 to 1932.1 mL^3, with an average of 405.1 mL.^{3} The volumes of the left and right breasts varied by up to 50%; occasionally, the difference was in excess of 200 mL^3, but this degree of variance was restricted to only 3% (18 of 598) of the study population. Over 50% of women have volume differences that exceed 10% of breast volume, and over 25% have volume differences that exceed 20% of volume. These asymmetries are not well perceived by patients, as only one-third of patients who perceive that they have breasts of equal size do, in fact, have breasts with equal measurements.

Breast volume also fluctuates widely with the menstrual cycle. The breast tissue and parenchymal water content has been measured using magnetic resonance imaging in healthy women during different phases of the menstrual cycle (Fowler et al., 1991). The total breast volume, the parenchymal volume, and the water content were lowest between the 6th and 15th days of the cycle. Between the 16th and 28th days, the parenchymal volume increased by 38.9%, and the water content rose by 24.5% and peaked on about the 25th day. Within 5 days of the onset of menses, the parenchymal volume fell by 30.3%, and the water content decreased by 17.5%. In the second half of the cycle, a clear increase in both water and tissue content is observed. The volume changes were smaller in women who were taking oral contraceptives. Parous women had smaller fluctuations than did nulliparous women. These changes paralleled changes observed in the breasts of women undergoing mammoplasties during different phases of the menstrual cycle (Vogel, 1981; and Anderson et al., 1982).

The gland is divided into 15 to 20 lobes, each with an excretory duct passing centrally to the nipple. The nipple, located at about the fourth interspace in youth, contains 15 to 20 orifices of the excretory ducts (Fig. 3–1A).

The breast's most biologically active component is the ductal-lobular unit. Each terminal duct drains a number of lobules, each of which is 1 to 2 mm in diameter (Fig. 3–1B). Each breast is estimated to contain 10^4 to 10^5 lobules. The epithelial lining of the lobule consists of superficial (luminal) A cells. These are involved in milk synthesis. Basal or B cells, also called "chief cells," have stem cell activity. Myoepithelial cells constitute the third type (Parks, 1959). Ductography rarely visualizes lobules (Fig. 3–1C) (Sartorius, 1987; and Diner, 1981).

Passing from the deep layer of superficial fascia on the deep surface of the breast up between the lobes to the corium of the mammary skin are the suspensory ligaments

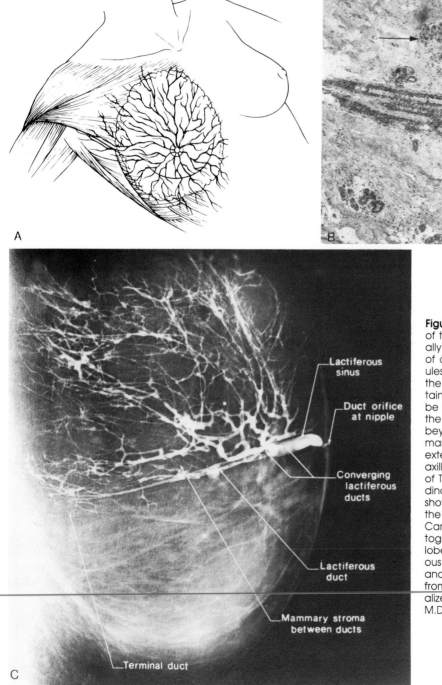

Lactiferous sinus

Duct orifice at nipple

Converging lactiferous ducts

Lactiferous duct

Mammary stroma between ducts

Terminal duct

Figure 3–1. *A,* A schematic representation of the lobes of the breast arranged radially around the nipple. Each lobe consists of a collecting system of ducts and lobules that drains through a single orifice at the nipple. The number of lobes is uncertain and may vary, but it is estimated to be from 15 to 20. This illustration conveys the fact that ducts and lobules can reach beyond the apparent limits of the mammary parenchyma. Often, breast tissue extends for a variable distance into the axilla as the "tail of Spence." (Courtesy of Thomas G. Peters, M.D.) *B,* This longitudinal histologic section of part of a lobe shows lobules *(arrows)* arranged along the duct that drains them. (Courtesy of Carlos M. Perez-Mesa, M.D.) *C,* This ductogram demonstrates the distribution of a lobe within the breast. The large lactiferous sinus is distended by contrast medium and drains a network of collecting ducts from myriad lobules. Lobules are not visualized. (Courtesy of Thomas G. Peters, M.D.)

of the breast (Cooper's ligaments) (Fig. 3–2). The deep layer of the superficial fascia on the undersurface of the breast is separated from the deep fascia by a fascial cleft. The presence of this cleft contributes to the considerable mobility of the breast (Fig. 3–3).

FASCIAL ANATOMY

The mammary gland is contained within the superficial pectoral fascia. This layer of fatty areolar tissue is continuous below with Camper's superficial abdominal fascia and above with superficial cervical fascia.

Superiorly, the lower fibers of the platysma muscle separate the superficial fascia from the deep pectoral fascia. The deep pectoral fascia covers the pectoralis major muscle.

It is attached to the sternum and superolaterally to the clavicle and axillary fascia. Inferiorly, it is continuous with the deep fascia of the abdominal wall.

As the ducts and lobules of the breast arborize through the layers of superficial fascia, they maintain an intimate relation to the skin, particularly near the nipple, and the peripheral extent of the arborization is frequently indistinct. The intimate relation of breast parenchyma to dermis has been used as the basis for justifying the elevation of thin skin flaps and the performance of a wide dissection, as discussed later in chapters covering total mastectomy (Hicken, 1940).

The anatomy of breast parenchyma is relevant to the desire of some to do a "prophylactic" or "preventive" mastectomy in the hope that breast cancer may be pre-

vented. Goldman and Goldwyn (1973) explored this proposition and confirmed that breast tissue remains after subcutaneous mastectomies. They performed subcutaneous mastectomies according to the prescribed technique in cadavers with no known breast pathology. Then, they sampled the subareolar and peripheral tissue that remained. They found that all cadavers had breast tissue beneath the areola and that five of six cadavers had breast tissue at other sites; only one of the six cadavers had no residual breast tissue according to their sampling technique. They cautioned that subcutaneous mastectomy cannot be considered completely prophylactic, as it does not remove all breast tissue. Although they recommended multiple biopsies before the insertion of implants, such a small sample of the total area of resection could be expected to present a considerable sampling error.

The reduction of breast tissue volume cannot be assumed to bring about a proportional reduction in cancer risk. The failure of Klamer and colleagues (1983) to reduce breast cancer in a rat model dosed with a potent breast carcinogen by resecting one entire mammary fold is evidence of this. This observation is also supported by Jackson and associates (1984). In fact, development of breast cancer has been reported after subcutaneous mastectomies that were performed for benign disease (Goodnight et al., 1984; Bowers and Radlauer, 1969). Goodnight and coworkers pointed out that when valid reasons for doing a preventive mastectomy can be identified, a total mastectomy is the minimal operation. They contend that subcutaneous mastectomy as a cancer-preventing procedure must be regarded as an experi-

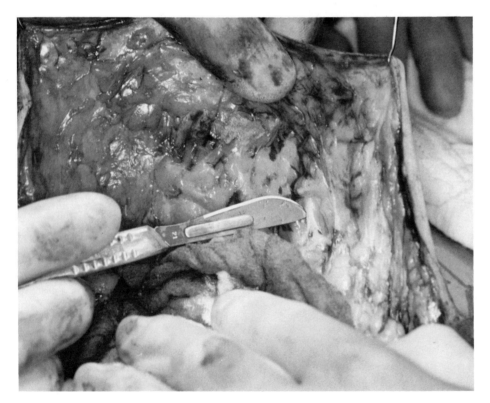

Figure 3–2. The surgeon appreciates Cooper's ligaments as strong bands of dense fascia encountered at mastectomy during elevation of the skin flaps. In this photograph, one of this complex system's attachments can be seen at the tip of the scalpel just before it is transected. (Courtesy of William L. Donegan, M.D.)

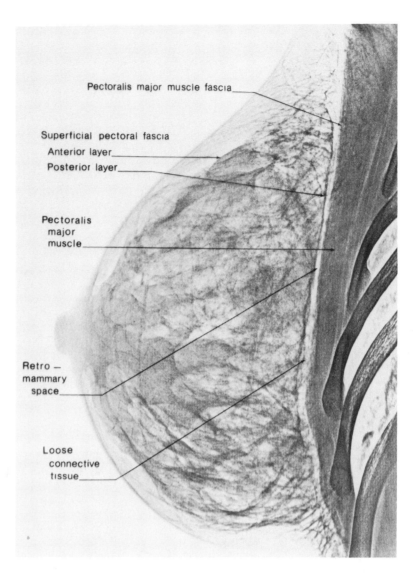

Figure 3–3. This xerogram shows the distribution of mammary tissue lying within the superficial fascia of the anterior chest. The breast is separated from the deep pectoral fascia overlying the muscles by a cleft (retromammary space) that is clearly visible. The periphery of the gland is at a greater distance from the skin than is the central part closer to the nipple, a fact of some surgical significance. (Courtesy of Thomas G. Peters, M.D.)

imental treatment. Prophylactic mastectomy remains a valid concern because it is based on unproved assumptions.

Fascia Deep to the Pectoralis Major Muscle

Deep to the pectoralis major muscle the clavipectoral fascia envelops the pectoralis minor muscle. Superior to the pectoralis minor muscle, it forms a thickened layer of fascia attached to the clavicle. This thickened clavipectoral fascia superior to the pectoralis minor is pierced by the anterior thoracic vessels and nerve and by the cephalic vein. Lateral to the muscle, it attaches to the axillary fascia.

The deep pectoral fascia thickens to form the roof of the axillary space, the axillary fascia. Through the axillary fascia, an opening allows passage of vessels and lymphatics from the breast and the arm. Below and lateral to the pectoralis minor muscle, it fuses with the deep fascia of the anterior surface of the pectoralis major muscle. This fascia continues as a thin cover for the serratus anterior muscle, and it also envelops the axillary vessels, forming the vascular sheath.

The fatty areolar tissue lying between the clavipectoral fascial layers anteriorly, the axillary vascular sheath superiorly, and the thin fascia on the chest wall and deep muscles (intercostal muscles, serratus anterior muscle, coracobrachialis muscle, and subclavius muscle) envelops the large valvular axillary lymphatics from the upper extremity. The axillary lymph nodes lie in proximity to the branches of the great veins in the axilla and are surrounded by fatty areolar tissue (Fig. 3–4*A* and *B*) (Singer, 1935).

MUSCULAR AND NEURAL ANATOMY

The principal muscles encountered in operations on the breast include (1) the pectoralis major, (2) the pectoralis minor, (3) the serratus anterior, (4) the latissimus dorsi, (5) the subscapularis, and (6) the aponeurosis of the external oblique and rectus abdominis. Details regarding the innervation and actions of these muscles are in Table 3–1. The lower fibers of the platysma muscle crossing the clavicle in the superficial fascia, the subclavius, and the coracobrachialis are viewed in the periphery of the surgical field.

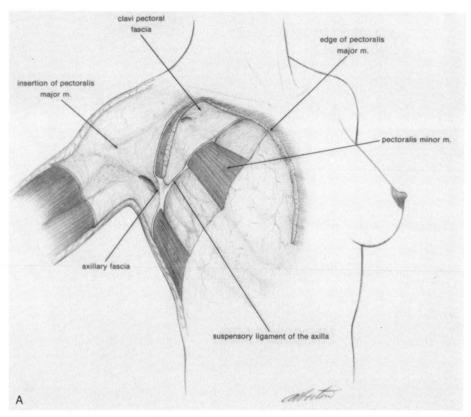

clavi pectoral
fascia

edge of pectoralis
major m.

insertion of pectoralis
major m.

pectoralis minor m.

axillary fascia

suspensory ligament of the axilla

A

Figure 3-4. *A,* Relationship of the fascial compartments and muscles of the pectoral region, breast, and axilla (see text) (Courtesy of William L. Donegan, M.D.). *B,* A sagittal section of the axilla shows the relationship of muscles, blood vessels, and nerves to fascial planes. (Courtesy of Thomas G. Peters, M.D.)

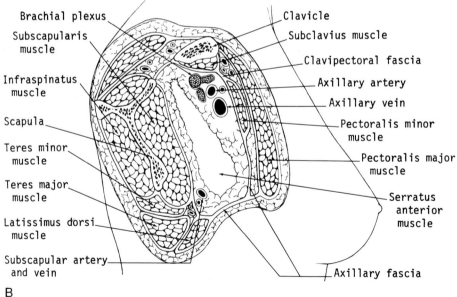

Brachial plexus

Subscapularis
muscle

Infraspinatus
muscle

Scapula

Teres minor
muscle

Teres major
muscle

Latissimus dorsi
muscle

Subscapular artery
and vein

Clavicle

Subclavius muscle

Clavipectoral fascia

Axillary artery

Axillary vein

Pectoralis minor
muscle

Pectoralis major
muscle

Serratus
anterior
muscle

Axillary fascia

B

Table 3–1. MUSCLES RELATING TO OPERATIONS ON THE BREAST

Muscle	Origin	Insertion	Innervation	Action	Significance in Regional Breast Anatomy	Significance in Breast Surgery
Pectoralis major	Medial half of clavicle, sternum, costal cartilages 1 to 6, aponeurosis of the external abdominis oblique muscle	Greater tubercle of the humerus	Medial and lateral pectoral (anterior thoracic) nerves	Flexes, adducts, and medially rotates the arm	1. Major muscle mass posterior to breast 2. Breast parenchyma may grow through retromammary space into the muscle 3. Lymphatics from breast pierce and circumvent the pectoralis major muscle	1. Excised in radical mastectomy 2. Anterior fascia removed in modified mastectomy
Pectoralis minor	External surface of ribs 2, 3, 4, and 5 anteriorly	Coracoid process of the scapula	Medial pectoral (anterior thoracic) nerve	Depresses the shoulder inferiorly	1. Superior portion crosses anterior to axillary sheath, dividing axilla into low, mid, and high portions 2. Interpectoral nodes lie immediately anterior to the pectoralis minor muscle 3. Part of the anterior wall of axilla	1. Division of axilla into low, mid, and high regions allows for accurate location of nodal involvement by neoplasia 2. Excised in radical mastectomy 3. Excised in Patey's modified mastectomy
Subclavius	First rib at costochondral junction	Clavicle, inferior surface	Subclavian nerve	Depresses the clavicle	1. Superficial and deep fasciae are contiguous with the clavipectoral fascia	1. Not seen during mastectomy
Rectus abdominis	Pubic crest	Cartilages of ribs 5, 6, and 7	Same as external abdominis oblique muscle	Flexes the vertebral column; tenses the anterior abdominal wall	1. The inferomedian portion of the breast overlies the fascia of the upper rectus abdominis muscle	1. Fascia of the upper portion exposed during mastectomy
External abdominis oblique	Ribs 5 to 12 interdigitate with serratus anterior muscle	Linea alba, pubis, inguinal ligament, and iliac crest	1. Intercostal nerves 7 to 12 2. Iliohypogastric nerve 3. Ilioinguinal nerve	Muscle of respiration; increases abdominal pressure in micturition, defecation; flexes the vertebral column	1. The inferior portion of the breast parenchyma overlies the external abdominis oblique muscle 2. Part of the pectoralis major muscle arises from the external abdominis oblique muscle	1. Exposed during mastectomy
Serratus anterior	External surface of ribs 1 to 8 anterolaterally	Broadly on anteromedial border of the scapula	Long thoracic nerve	Abducts and laterally rotates the scapula; "fixes" the scapula to chest wall	1. Forms medial wall of axilla 2. Major muscle mass deep to the lateral one-third of the breast	Long thoracic nerve injury causes: 1. Winged scapula deformity 2. Limited arm abduction beyond 90 degrees
Latissimus dorsi	Spinous processes T-6 to T-12, L-1 to L-5, sacrum and iliac crest by the lumbar aponeurosis; ribs 10 to 12	Intertubercular groove of the humerus	Thoracodorsal nerve	Extends, adducts, and medially rotates the arm	1. The superficial and deep fascia of this muscle are contiguous with the axillary fascia 2. Forms part of the posterior wall of the axilla	1. The anterior border of the latissimus dorsi muscle is the most posterior limit of dissection in mastectomy 2. Injury to the thoracodorsal nerve results in paralysis 3. Used as a muscular or myocutaneous flap in reconstruction of the breast
Teres major	Dorsal scapula	Intertubercular groove of the humerus	Subscapular nerve	Adducts, medially rotates, and extends the arm	1. Forms part of the posterior wall of the axilla	
Subscapularis	Scapula (subscapular fossa)	Lesser tubercle of the humerus	Subscapular nerve	Medially rotates and adducts the arm	1. Forms part of the posterior wall of the axilla	1. Nerve injury causes subscapularis palsy
Coracobrachialis	Coracoid process of the scapula	Humerus, medially	Musculocutaneous nerve	Flexes and adducts the arm	1. Forms part of lateral wall of the axilla	1. May be exposed during axillary dissection

(Courtesy of Thomas G. Peters, M.D.)

The pectoralis major muscle, deep to the fascial cleft behind the breast and invested by the deep fascia, has its origin from the medial half of the clavicle, the lateral sternum, the cartilage of the sixth and seventh ribs, and the aponeurosis of the external oblique muscle. From this broad origin, it converges to an insertion on the greater tubercle of the humerus (Fig. 3–5).

The muscle is composed of many segments, which are a phylogenetically preserved expression of internal metamerism in the pectoral girdle. The segments can be separated surgically, as they have independent neurovascular supplies (Tobin, 1985). This has clinical significance for reconstructive surgery (Tobin et al., 1982) and for the technique of modified mastectomy.

The authors have studied the natural cleavage between the clavicular and sternocostal portions of the muscle by fresh cadaver dissections and its use during mastectomies to preserve the pectoralis major muscle innervation. These dissections are illustrated in Figures 3–6 to 3–12. The dissections confirm that the cleavage is visible when the deep pectoral fascia has been reflected laterally. At this point, the cleavage may be opened throughout its length to expose the axillary fascia and axillary fat pad under the deep surface of the pectoralis major muscle. The pectoralis minor muscle is seen beneath this deep fascia. This exposure permits easy, direct visualization of the pectoralis major innervation and permits the surgeon to palpate the axillary fat pad directly for enlarged lymph nodes. The surgeon may perform a dissection of the axillary fat pad with excellent exposure while preserving the innervation and vascularization of the pectoralis major muscle. The surgeon needs a clear understanding of the innervation to do this (Figs. 3–6 to 3–12). The pectoralis major muscle is innervated by the medial and lateral pectoral nerves, also known as the medial and lateral anterior thoracic nerves. Their designation as medial and lateral refers to their origin from the medial and lateral cords of the brachial plexus, not to their position on the chest wall (Gray's Anatomy, 1993). In fact, the medial portion of the pectoralis major muscle is innervated by the lateral pectoral nerve, and the lateral portion of the muscle by the medial pectoral nerve. In some surgical publications, the nerves are named medial and lateral, according to their position on the chest wall; this reverses their designation and leads to some confusion. The traditional names are used in this text. Ordinarily, the lateral pectoral nerve courses medial to the pectoralis minor muscle to reach its destination, and the medial pectoral nerve courses through or lateral to the pectoralis minor muscle. Serra and colleagues (1984) have quantified variations in innervation. They stress the importance of preserving the nerves to the pectoralis major that innervate the lower third of the muscle (the costoabdominal insertions or the lateral segments of the muscle). A schematic drawing of the innervation is provided in Figures 3–13 and 3–14. In Figure 3–15, the distribution of nerves in the dissections of Serra and colleagues is compared with those of Moosman (1980). Without preservation of these nerves, the denervated portions of the pectoralis major muscle become flaccid and atrophic.

The relation of the branches of the medial pectoral nerve to the pectoralis minor muscle is intimate, as is shown in Figure 3–16. The various divisions of the nerve may decussate on either side of the muscle and through its body. The

Text continued on page 34

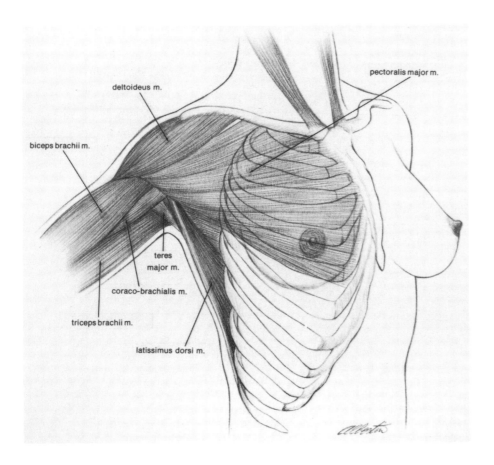

Figure 3–5. Relationship of the pectoralis major muscle to the underlying breast. Note that the breast overlaps the lower border of the pectoralis major muscle. (Courtesy of William L. Donegan, M.D.)

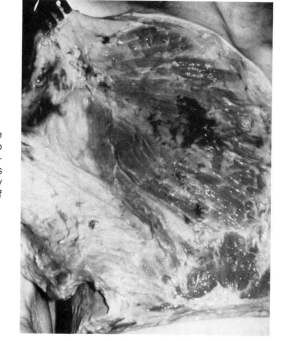

Figure 3–6. The deep pectoral fascia has been resected laterally to the edge of the pectoralis major muscle. The breast is superficial to the deep pectoral fascia and has been reflected laterally. This fascia may be partially reflected from the deep surface of the pectoralis major muscle. This dissection is the same as that performed in modified radical mastectomy to the point at which a retractor can be placed under the free edge of the muscle to pull it anteromedially and expose the axilla.

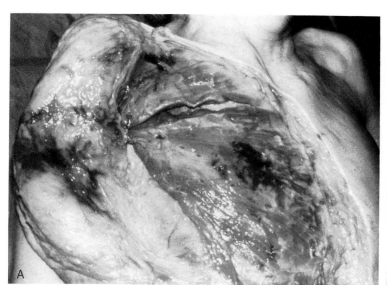
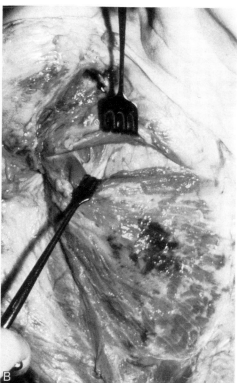

Figure 3–7. The natural cleavage between the clavicular and sternocostal origins of the pectoralis major muscle has been opened *(A)* and is separated by retractors *(B)*. The pectoralis minor muscle shows through the axillary fascia laterally, and the lymph node–bearing axillary fat pad can be seen in *B* medial to the pectoralis minor muscle. At this point, the contents of the axillary fat pad may be palpated with considerable accuracy for firm lymph nodes.

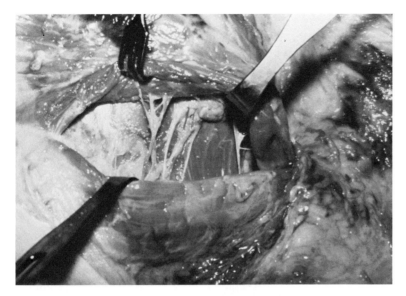

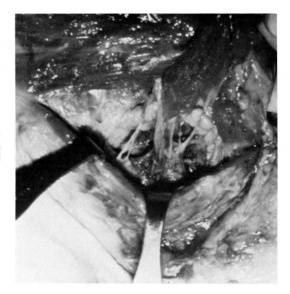

Figure 3–8. By retracting the sternal portion of the pectoralis major muscle inferiorly, the variable number and distribution of nerve branches and their relation to the pectoralis minor muscle can be seen. When a branch transgresses the body of the pectoralis minor, this muscle may have to be dissected away in pieces to preserve it.

Figure 3–9. The pectoralis minor muscle has been transected at its insertion and is being dissected away from the nerves to the pectoralis major muscle. The pectoralis minor is enveloped by the clavipectoral fascia, which may be followed to its origin on the clavicle.

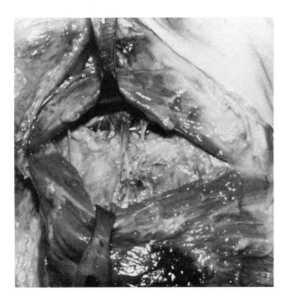

Figure 3–10. The pectoralis minor muscle has now been removed, and the intact branches of the nerves to the pectoralis major muscle are exposed. From this point, the axillary vein may be demonstrated, and the axillary fat.

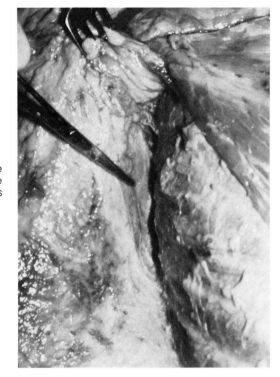

Figure 3–11. The clamp points to the nerve of the serratus anterior muscle just under the fascia adjacent to the chest wall. For this nerve to be preserved, it must be dissected out of the fascia and mobilized from its site of appearance below the axillary vein to its muscular insertion.

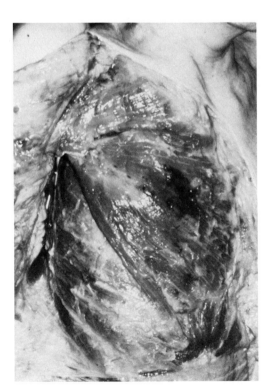

Figure 3–12. The entire breast, axillary fat pad, pectoralis minor muscle with intrapectoral lymph nodes, and the axillary fat pads have been removed, leaving an intact, innervated, and vascularized pectoralis major muscle. The intact nerves to the serratus anterior and latissimus dorsi muscles are seen.

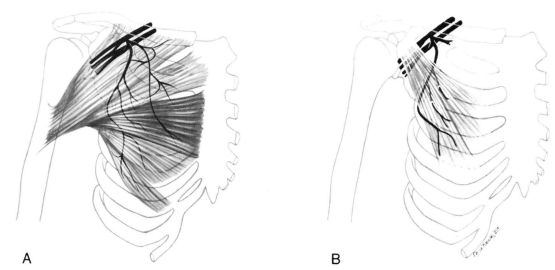

Figure 3–13. *A,* The lateral pectoral nerve innervates the clavicular and sternal origins of the pectoral major muscle. *B,* The medial pectoral nerve descends along the edge of the pectoralis minor muscle, crosses it, innervates it, and courses between the two pectoral muscles to innervate the lower third and the costoabdominal insertions of the pectoralis major muscle. (From Serra, G. E., Maccarone, G. B., Ibarra, P. E., et al.: Lateral pectoralis nerve: The need to preserve it in the modified radical mastectomy. J. Surg. Oncol., *26:*278, 1984. Reprinted with permission.)

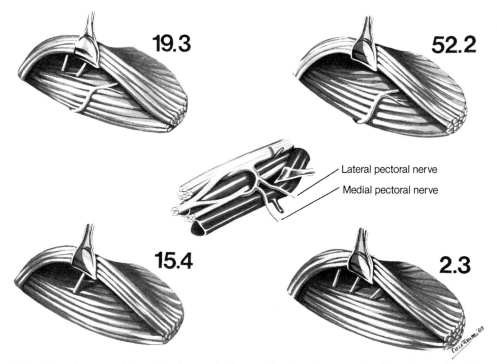

Figure 3–14. Relationships of the medial pectoral nerve to the pectoralis minor muscle. (From Serra, G. E. Maccarone, G. B., Ibarra, P. E., et al.: Lateral pectoralis nerve: The need to preserve it in the modified radical mastectomy. J. Surg. Oncol., *26:*278, 1984. Reprinted with permission.)

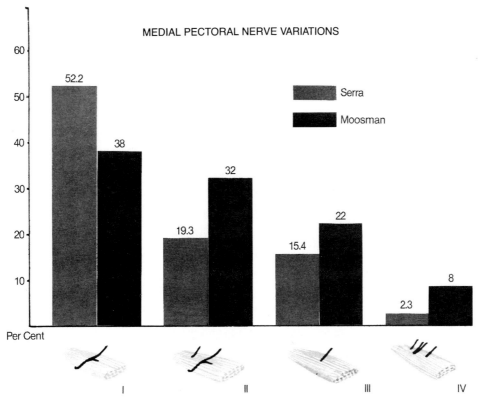

Figure 3–15. Comparison of the dissections of Serra and Moosman quantifying the relationship of the medial pectoral nerve to the pectoralis minor muscle. Numbers indicate percentages. (From Serra, G. E., Maccarone, G. B., Ibarra, P. E., et al.: Lateral pectoralis nerve: The need to preserve it in the modified radical mastectomy. J. Surg. Oncol., *26*:278, 1984. Reprinted with permission.)

Figure 3–16. *A,* The surgical anatomy of the relationship of various nerves to the pectoralis minor muscle after incision of fascia.

Illustration continued on following page

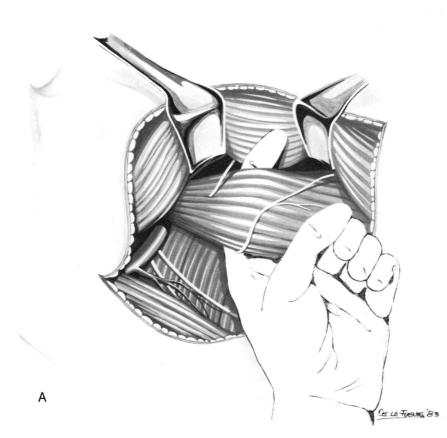

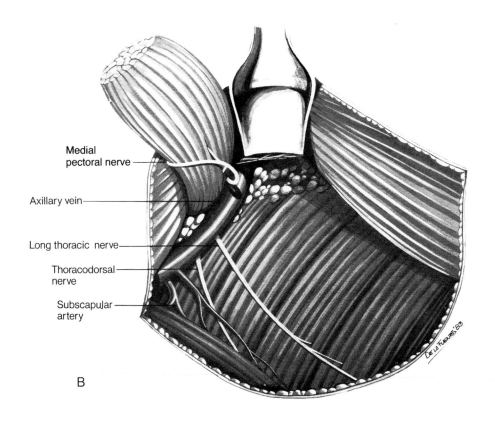

Medial
pectoral nerve

Axillary vein

Long thoracic nerve

Thoracodorsal
nerve

Subscapular
artery

B

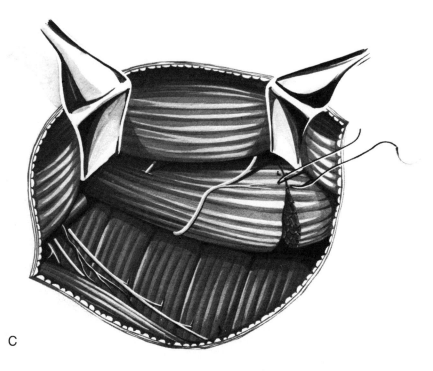

C

Figure 3-16 *Continued B,* The exposure of the axilla is obtained by dividing the origin of the pectoralis minor muscle on the chest wall. *C,* The transected but still innervated pectoralis minor muscle may be sutured to its origin on the thorax at the completion of the axillary dissection. (From Serra, G. E., Maccarone, G. B., Ibarra, P. E., et al.: Modified radical mastectomy technique of E. Scanlon. Int. J. Breast Mammary Pathol., 26:278, 1984. Reprinted with permission.)

body of the muscle may be dissected away from the nerve when the nerve passes through the body of the pectoralis minor muscle. It should be noted that the number of nerve branches is highly variable. Preservation of only one or two branches does not avoid the risk of pectoralis major denervation.

The pectoralis major muscle is mainly innervated by the

lateral pectoral (anterior thoracic) nerve arising from the lateral cord of the brachial plexus. The nerve passes over the first part of the axillary vein medial to the pectoralis minor muscle, and its branches pierce the clavipectoral fascia to enter the deep surface of the muscle.

The pectoralis minor muscle arises from the anterior and medial surfaces of the third, fourth, and fifth ribs (and

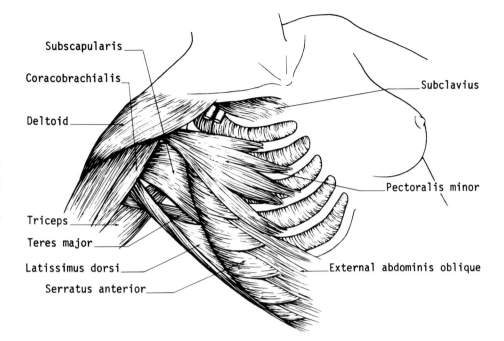

Figure 3–17. In this drawing, the pectoralis major muscle has been removed to illustrate the underlying muscles, most of which are visualized during surgical removal of the breast and axillary lymph nodes. (Courtesy of Thomas G. Peters, M.D.)

Subscapularis

Coracobrachialis

Deltoid

Triceps

Teres major

Latissimus dorsi

Serratus anterior

Subclavius

Pectoralis minor

External abdominis oblique

sometimes the second rib) and inserts as a tendon into the coracoid process of the scapula (Fig. 3–17). Innervation is into the deep surface via the medial anterior thoracic nerve. Except for the loss of soft tissue on the anterior thoracic wall, no measurable disability attends the loss of function of the pectoralis minor muscle. The functional loss following removal of the pectoralis major muscle is small and is well tolerated.

The serratus anterior muscle is important in stabilization of the scapula on the thorax. Its denervation results in a winged scapula, and this palsy can be a source of significant morbidity. For this reason, the nerve to the serratus anterior muscle is preserved in mammary surgery. The muscle arises from the upper nine ribs as a thin sheet with segments corresponding to each rib of origin and with fibers passing superiorly and posteriorly to an insertion into the ventromedial angle and along the ventrovertebral border of the scapula. The lower four points of origin interdigitate with the external oblique muscle.

The nerve to the serratus anterior muscle (the long thoracic nerve or the external respiratory nerve of Bell) arises from the fifth, sixth, and seventh cervical nerves and passes deep to the axillary artery and vein, staying close to each segment of the thoracic wall. As it passes caudally, it gives branches to each segment of the serratus anterior muscle (Tobin, 1993).

The long thoracic nerve is superficial to the deep fascia investing the serratus anterior muscle. When the fascia is stripped away from the serratus anterior during the deep portion of an axillary dissection, the nerve can easily be seen. The fascia adjacent to the nerve must be divided so that the nerve can be isolated from the axillary contents throughout its length.

The latissimus dorsi muscle is of importance in breast surgery because the deep fascia investing the muscle is continuous anteriorly with the axillary fascia and because the nerve to the muscle traverses the axillary contents. The muscle has a broad origin from the lumbar fascia on the back and sweeps forward and superiorly to insert into the intertubercular groove of the humerus.

The anterior edge of the latissimus dorsi muscle is almost vertical in the midaxillary line. This edge marks the dorsal extent of a total mastectomy. Detachment of the investing fascia of the muscle at this edge is equivalent to the detachment of the axillary fascia from its dorsal attachment.

The nerve to the latissimus dorsi muscle (thoracodorsal nerve) arises from the posterior cord of the brachial plexus, appears beneath or dorsal to the axillary vein along the posterior axillary wall, and passes through the lymph node–bearing areolar tissue of the axilla to the upper portion of the muscle. If the latissimus dorsi neurovascular supply is removed, the functional loss is weakened extension, internal rotation, and adduction of the humerus. This is tolerated well by most individuals (Tobin et al., 1980). When possible, the latissimus dorsi neurovascular supply should be preserved by careful dissection, as this both lessens functional loss and preserves the muscle for reconstructive purposes.

The subscapularis muscle, which passes between the subscapular fossa and the lesser tubercle of the humerus, forms the posterior wall of the axilla just inferior or caudal to the axillary vein. In dissecting the fascia from the muscle, it is pertinent to look for and preserve the nerve to the subscapularis muscle, lying on the muscle's upper anterior surface. This muscle produces medial rotation of the arm and assists in flexion, extension, abduction, and adduction of the arm. It helps to stabilize the humerus in the glenoid fossa. A subscapularis palsy can produce significant morbidity.

The external oblique muscle is of consequence because its upper slips of origin interdigitate with the origins of the pectoralis minor and serratus anterior muscles. Medially, its aponeurosis forms the anterior rectus sheath and marks the lower extent of a radical mastectomy. Also, the latissimus dorsi and the rectus abdominis muscles provide skin and muscle flaps that are of value in chest wall reconstruction if local recurrence of tumor requires anterior chest wall resection (Tobin, 1986).

Infrequent muscular anatomy may be encountered. The axillopectoral muscle (Langer's axillary arch) is seen in about 7% of cases (Sisley, 1987). This muscle arises as a slip from the latissimus dorsi muscle and courses anterior to the axillary vein. It must be divided to completely expose the vein (Fig. 3–18A). Less frequently encountered is the sternalis muscle, which courses parallel to the sternum and displaces the origin of the pectoralis major muscle laterally (see Fig. 3–18B).

Cutaneous sensation to the breast is provided by anterior and lateral perforating branches of the segmental nerves. Worthy of mention is that sensation to the nipple is usually supplied by branches of the fourth thoracic nerve (Fig. 3–19).

VASCULAR ANATOMY

The arterial supply to the breast is from multiple sources (Fig. 3–20). The inner quadrants are supplied medially by perforating branches (rami perforantes) of the internal mammary (internal thoracic) arteries that penetrate each intercostal space and the overlying pectoralis major muscle origin along the lateral sternal border, with the second, third, and fourth perforating arteries providing the predominant supply. All quadrants are supplied by multiple skin muscle–perforating branches of the thoracoacromial artery; these penetrate the pectoralis major muscle to enter the deep

surface of the breast. The outer quadrants are supplied by the lateral thoracic (external mammary) artery, which both perforates the lateral segment of the pectoralis major muscle and comes around its lateral border. The outer quadrants are also supplied segmentally by lateral cutaneous branches of the posterior intercostal arteries, with the third, fourth, and fifth arteries providing the predominant supply. All of these arteries connect with each other by collateral branches in the breast and overlying skin. During lactation, arterial diameters and flow increase substantially.

The venous drainage of the breast does not precisely follow the arterial supply in the periareolar region centrally (Fig. 3–21). Here, the veins form an anastomotic circle superficially in the subcutaneous tissue beneath and around the areola. This plexus drains centrifugally toward the periphery via large diameter subcutaneous veins that connect to the veins that accompany the arteries supplying the breast. This superficial venous pattern can often be seen in women with more transparent skin and during lactation, when venous flow increases.

Lymphatic Anatomy

Certain general principles regarding lymphatic anatomy of any site are applicable to the breast. The subepithelial plexus of lymphatics is valveless and is confluent with the subepithelial plexus over the entire body surface. Lymph can flow in any direction in this plexus but does so sluggishly. This subepithelial plexus (sometimes called the "papillary plexus" because of its tuftlike extensions into the connective tissue of the dermal papillae) is connected by vertical lymphatics to a valvular labyrinth of subdermal

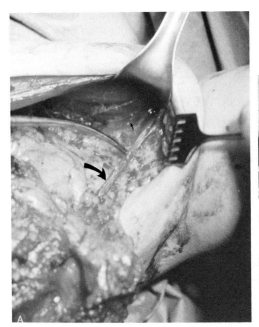
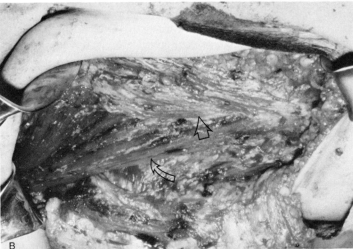

Figure 3–18. *A,* A long, narrow axillary arch muscle encountered during mastectomy is indicated by the clamp and *large arrow.* This muscle arises from the latissimus dorsi muscle and courses anterior to the axillary vein. The lateral edge of the pectoralis major muscle is indicated by the *small arrow.* (Courtesy of William L. Donegan, M.D., 1992.) *B,* A sternalis muscle discovered during mastectomy *(large arrow).* The pectoralis major muscle *(curved arrow)* is shorter than usual and has its origin lateral to the sternalis muscle. The patient's head is to the left. (Courtesy of William L. Donegan, M.D., 1992.)

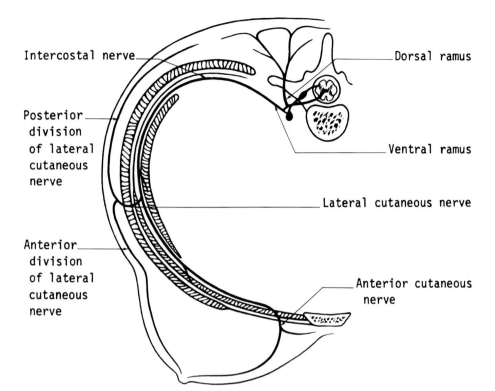

Figure 3–19. Distribution of a segmental nerve and its relationship to the breast. Cutaneous branches of the fourth thoracic nerve generally supply sensation to the nipple. (Courtesy of Thomas G. Peters, M.D.)

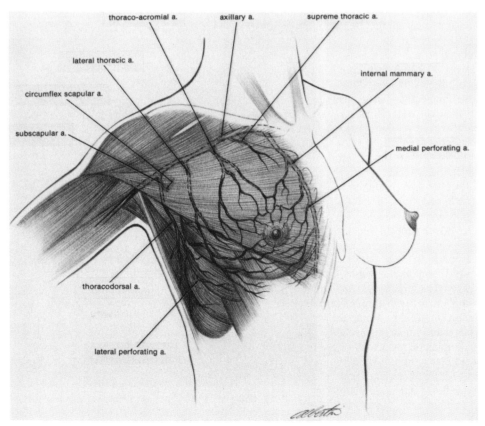

Figure 3–20. Arterial supply of the breast. Branches of the axillary and internal mammary arteries provide arterial blood flow to the breast. The internal mammary artery and the lateral thoracic artery (external mammary artery) approach the breast from the medial side and the lateral side, respectively, whereas the thoracoacromial artery reaches it by penetrating the pectoralis major muscle from behind. (Courtesy of William L. Donegan, M.D.)

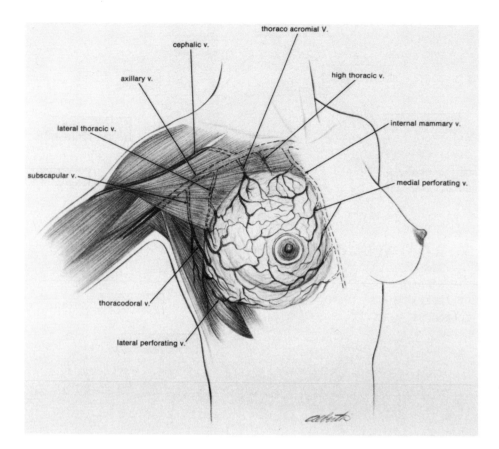

Figure 3–21. Veins of the breast form a prominent subcutaneous network, ultimately carrying blood into the axillary and internal mammary veins. (Courtesy of William L. Donegan, M.D.)

lymphatics. This was well demonstrated by Gray (1939) when he injected mammary skin with Thorotrast.

Centrally, the subepithelial and subdermal plexuses are confluent with the subareolar plexus, which in turn communicates with fine lymphatics of the lactiferous ducts. These lymphatics lie in the loose connective tissue just outside the myoepithelial layer of the duct wall (Bonser et al., 1961). The subareolar plexus also receives lymphatics from the areola and nipple.

The lymphatics paralleling the lactiferous ducts are equivalent to the vertical lymphatics that connect the subepithelial and subdermal lymphatics elsewhere in the body with the deep subcutaneous plexus (Spratt et al., 1965).

The breast is a specialized dermal organ that undergoes most of its growth during puberty. Growth probably occurs within the ducts and lobules by lengthening of existing lymphatics rather than by development of new ones. If lactiferous duct lymphatics are equivalent to the vertical connecting lymphatics, their valve structure would be equivalent, and a unidirectional lymph flow from superficial to deep would exist. Thus, the lymph should flow from the subareolar plexus via the lactiferous duct lymphatics to the perilobular and deep subcutaneous lymphatic plexus. Injection studies refute the older concept that lymph flows centripetally to the subareolar plexus (Turner-Warwick, 1959; Halsell et al., 1965). Rather, lymph flows unidirectionally in valvular lymphatics from superficial to deep and toward the regional lymph nodes.

A technique for appreciating the pattern of lymphatic

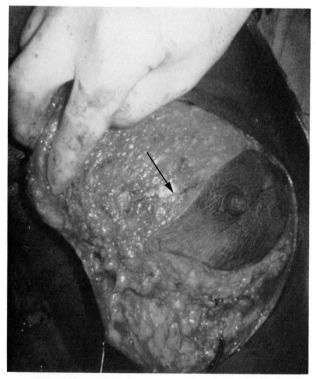

Figure 3–22. Methylene blue dye was injected into the subareolar area and is seen coursing through a lymphatic toward the periphery of the breast *(arrow)*. (Courtesy of William L. Donegan, M.D., 1992.)

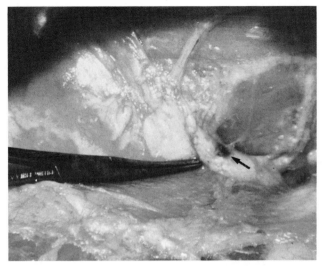

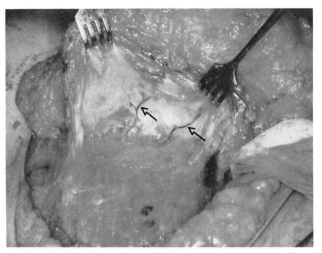

Figure 3–23. Methylene blue dye injected into the breast before mastectomy has stained an interpectoral (Rotter) node, confirming the importance of Rotter's nodes to the lymphatic drainage of the breast. (Courtesy William L. Donegan, M.D., 1992.)

Figure 3–24. Methylene blue dye injected into the breast preoperatively is seen filling two lymphatics (indicated by the *arrows*) that perforate the deep pectoral fascia to disappear into the pectoralis major muscle. (Courtesy of William L. Donegan, M.D., 1992.)

arborization is to inject the breast preoperatively with methylene blue dye. This dye promptly enters the lymphatics and visibly stains them. Examples of this are seen in Figures 3–22 to 3–24. In these dissections, methylene blue dye was injected into the subareolar area. The dye is seen coursing through the para-areolar lymphatics toward the periphery of the breast (see Fig. 3–22). In Figure 3–23, staining of Rotter's interpectoral lymph nodes is seen, confirming the importance of these nodes in the lymphatic drainage of the breast. In Figure 3–24, lymphatics from the breast are seen perforating the deep pectoral fascia to disappear into the pectoralis major muscle.

The functional anatomy of the lymphatics is the most important determinant of the direction of lymph flow. The valvular lymphatics undergo wavelike contractures that "milk" the lymph toward the regional lymph nodes. As a result, intralymphatic cancer cell emboli are rarely seen in unobstructed valvular lymphatics. Reverse flow in valvular lymphatics is possible only in the presence of the dilation that accompanies obstruction to flow. The valvular lymphatics frequently will rupture before permitting reverse flow.

These valvular lymphatics must be regarded as a continuum interconnected as a coarse labyrinth of anastomotic channels (Fig. 3–25). The lymphatics roughly follow the major veins, and the volume of lymph flow is roughly proportional to the volume of blood flow to a particular organ. Normally, lymph can bypass obstructed lymph nodes through the anastomotic channels. Thus, lower nodes can be missed, and the first metastasis may appear at a higher node.

Two other anatomic situations can make lymph nodes ineffective filters. Lymphatics have been observed to empty directly into veins without passing through nodes (Wallace, 1965), and lymph can pass directly into the efferent veins

Figure 3–25. A cleared mastectomy specimen injected preoperatively with iron–Prussian blue. The coarse labyrinth of blood vessels and the less distinct lymphatics accompanying them toward the regional nodes can be seen. (From Turner-Warwick, R. T.: The lymphatics of the breast. Br. J. Surg., *46*:574, 1959. Reprinted with permission.)

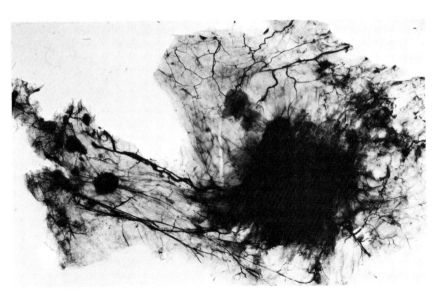

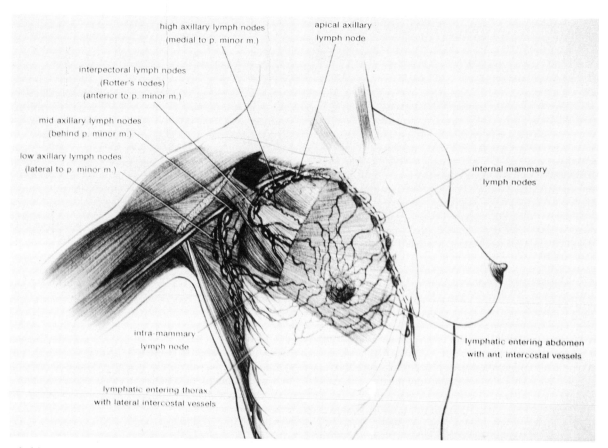

Figure 3–26. Principal lymph node groups, the axillary and internal mammary, tend to parallel the major veins. A coarse labyrinth of valvular lymphatics lying on the deep layer of the superficial fascia constitutes the major afferent lymphatics to these lymph nodes. The deep fascia and muscles have few lymphatics and little relation to the plexus in the superficial fascia that drains the breast. The lymphatics from the plexus in the superficial fascia probably penetrate the muscles only in the few loci penetrated by veins; for example, the acromiothoracic artery and vein perforate the pectoralis major muscle. (Courtesy of William L. Donegan, M.D.)

of lymph nodes instead of into efferent lymphatics (Pressman and Simon, 1961). Neither phenomenon has been demonstrated for the fine lymphatics of the breast.

The lymphatics lying within the deep fascia about muscular compartments (i.e., within the fascia of the pectoralis major muscle) are fine in size and communicate little with the subcutaneous plexus. Studies have shown these lymphatics to be of little or no significance in the spread of mammary cancer (Turner-Warwick, 1959; Auchincloss, 1963).

Other potential routes of spread from the lower and medial portion of the breast might be via the lymphatic plexus on the rectus sheath to the subperitoneal areolar plexus. When metastatic cancer is so obstructive as to produce extensive reflux into the valveless subepithelial plexus, the cancer cells may go to the skin in any direction through this plexus.

Valvular lymphatics of the subcutaneous and intramammary plexi assure unidirectional flow toward lymph nodes in the axilla, to the internal mammary chain, and to intercostal lymph nodes lying posteriorly in a paravertebral position (Fig. 3–26). The supraclavicular and prescalene nodes receive lymph from the breast after it has passed through the axillary and internal mammary groups. The lymph nodes tend to lie in the fat around the bifurcation of major veins.

The proportion of lymph flowing to the paravertebral glands and their significance as a site for primary metastasis from mammary cancer have not been investigated. However, they could be a source of the posterior mediastinal and pleural metastases and the associated pleural effusion that is often seen late in the course of mammary cancer. Lymphatics that follow the lateral perforating intercostal vessels provide access to the paravertebral nodes and perhaps are the cause of the ipsilateral predilection of malignant pleural effusions. Vital dye injected into the mammary parenchyma has been demonstrated in these lymphatics on occasion during mastectomy (Fig. 3–27).

On the basis of the proportion of radioactivity in lymph nodes after intramammary injection with gold (^{198}Au), Hultborn and associates (1955) estimated that only 1% to 3% of the lymph flow from the breast entered the internal mammary lymph nodes. However, colloidal gold went to the internal mammary lymph nodes in small amounts *regardless* of the portion of the mammary gland injected. Supraclavicular nodes were also examined, and radioactivity was found. Some radioactivity was present in the liver as well.

In the study by Hultborn and colleagues (1955), about 97% to 99% of the radioactivity in the lymph nodes was found in the axillary nodes. This lymph node concentration represented only about 10.5% of the ^{198}Au injected because

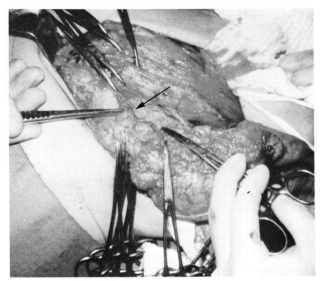

Figure 3–27. Methylene blue dye injected into the breast before the beginning of the mastectomy is shown coursing through a lymphatic *(arrow)* from the laterally reflected breast to enter the chest wall directly, just lateral to the pectoralis major muscle. The patient's head is to the left. (Courtesy of William L. Donegan, M.D., 1992.)

most radioactivity remained at the site of the injection. No assessment of the radioactivity in the posterior intercostal lymph nodes was made. Also, the proportion of flow can vary widely when principal pathways are obstructed, as may be the case in metastatic mammary cancer.

The major, and generally the primary, group of lymph nodes acquiring lymphatic metastases remains the axillary group. The axillary lymph nodes averaged 24 ± 9 (SD) in 195 complete axillary dissections (Level III), with a range of 4 to 51 nodes (personal communication, W. L. Donegan). Fisher and Slack (1970) reported on the total number of axillary nodes removed in radical mastectomy specimens from 2768 patients at 43 institutions. The mean number was 17 when nodes were normal or contained only 1 to 3 metastases. The mean number increased to 21 when 4 or more nodes contained metastases. Eighty-one nodes were found in 1 patient. They have been divided into several subgroups by anatomists. Pickren and coworkers (1965), in clearing axillary lymph nodes for studying the pathologic anatomy of metastases, subdivided the nodes as follows: (1) the highest nodes, including the subclavicular or higher axillary vein group from the apex of the axilla (from beneath the clavicle to the lower border of the pectoralis minor muscle); (2) interpectoral nodes, lying between the pectoralis major and pectoralis minor muscles; (3) the lower axillary vein group, from the lower border of the pectoralis minor muscle to the lateral limits of dissection; and (4) the central group, including the external mammary, paramammary, and scapular nodes (Auchincloss, 1963).

The lymphatics from the posterior breast that accompany the thoracoacromial vessels pass through the interpectoral group en route to the upper axillary chain. Most lymphatics arise in the lobules and pass through the substance of the breast and through the axillary fascia to the external mammary lymph nodes. These lymphatics lie approximately parallel to the lateral thoracic vessels (see Fig. 3–26).

The internal mammary lymph nodes accompany the internal mammary artery and vein. The lymph nodes are found in the intercostal spaces and posterior to the costal cartilages close to the sternum. Variable numbers of lymph nodes exist, but they average 3.8 in number in extended mastectomy specimens. As many as 14 are sometimes found (Donegan, 1972). Most of the nodes are in the upper parasternal area near bifurcations of the intercostal and internal mammary veins.

Afferent lymph vessels are received from the upper abdominal wall and the anterior thoracic wall, and efferent vessels from the anterior diaphragmatic nodes are also received into the internal mammary lymph drainage channels. Efferent lymphatics connect the nodes and terminate above in the various lymphatics that enter the jugular veins. Cross-anastomosis of lymphatics in the retrosternal area between these chains is the rule (Turner-Warwick, 1959; Rouviere, 1938).

The studies by Fisher and Fisher (1966, 1969, and 1972) on the pathophysiology of metastases greatly broadened insight into the complex interrelationships between lymphatic and hematogenous spread and the receptivity of tissues to metastatic growths. The unifying concept derived from their studies is shown in Figure 3–28. The studies support the concept that tumor cells that are primarily lymph-borne may reach the blood vascular system, through which they become further dispersed. These same cells freely circulating in the blood may re-enter the lymphatics and appear in the thoracic duct lymph. In this situation, the two vascular systems are unified.

Cancer cells may be entrapped in regional lymph nodes. They may also enter the blood vascular system within lymph nodes, or they may completely bypass nodes via collateral lymphatics, disseminating by means of the thoracic duct directly into the bloodstream. The ability of tissues to entrap and to allow growth of cancer cells arriving in the capillary beds of the tissues is determined by many variables, both humoral and local.

The conclusion to be drawn from many studies is that local ablative therapy with or without the inclusion of regional lymph nodes is not enough to adequately treat many

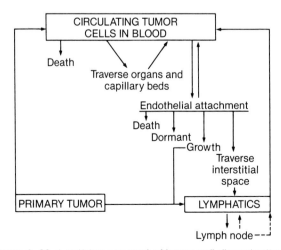

Figure 3–28. A unifying concept of tumor cell dissemination.

cancers. The ease with which cancer cells can spread through lymph and blood vascular conduits as a consequence of the anastomoses between these systems makes many former concepts about the progression of cancer obsolete. Localization at the site of origin and spread to no more than first-order regional lymph nodes are functions of the biologic characteristics of specific cancers, not limitations imposed by the anatomy of the lymph vascular system.

References

Anderson, T. J., Ferguson, D. J. P., and Raab, G. M.: Cell turnover in the "resting" human breast: Influence of parity, contraceptive pill, age, and laterality. Br. J. Cancer, 46:376–382, 1982.

Auchincloss, H.: Significance of location and number of axillary metastases in carcinoma of the breast: A justification for a conservative operation. Ann. Surg., 158:37, 1963.

Bonser, G. M., Dossett, J. A., and Jull, J. W.: Human and Experimental Breast Cancer. Springfield, IL, Charles C Thomas, 1961.

Bowers, D. G. Jr., and Radlauer, C. B.: Breast cancer of prophylactic subcutaneous mastectomies and reconstruction with Silastic protheses. Plast. Reconstr. Surg., 44:541, 1969.

Butcher, H. R., and Hoover, A. L.: Abnormalities of human superficial cutaneous lymphatics associated with stasis ulcers, lymphedema, scars and cutaneous autografts. Ann. Surg., 142:633–653, 1955.

Diner, W. C.: Galactography: Mammary duct contrast examination. Am. J. Radiol., 137:853, 1981.

Donegan, W. L.: Mastectomy in the primary management of invasive mammary carcinoma. In Hardy, J. D. (Ed.): Advances in Surgery, Vol 6. Chicago, Year Book Medical Publishers, Inc., 1972, pp. 1–101.

Fisher, B., and Fisher, E. R.: The interrelationship of hematogenous and lymphatic tumor cell dissemination. Surg. Gynecol. Obstet., 122:791, 1966.

Fisher, B.: Prospects for the control of metastases. Cancer, 24:1263, 1969.

Fisher, E. R., and Fisher, B.: Experimental studies of factors influencing development of hepatic metastases: XVII. Role of thyroid. Cancer Res., 26:2248, 1966.

Fisher, E. R., and Fisher, B.: Effects of x-irradiation of parameters of tumor growth, histology, and ultrastructure. Cancer, 24:39, 1969.

Fisher, E. R., and Fisher, B.: Local lymphoid response as an index of tumor immunity. Arch. Pathol., 94:137, 1972.

Fisher, B., and Slack, N. H.: Number of lymph nodes examined and the prognosis of breast carcinoma. Surg. Gynecol. Obstet., 131:79–88, 1970.

Fowler, P. A., Casey, C. E., Cameron, G. G., et al.: Cyclic changes in composition and volume of the breast during the menstrual cycle, measured by magnetic resonance imaging. Br. J. Obstet. Gynaecol., 97:595–602, 1991.

Geschickter, C. F.: Diseases of the Breast. Philadelphia, J. B. Lippincott, 1943.

Goldman, L. D., and Goldwyn, R. M.: Some anatomical considerations of subcutantous mastectomy. Plast. Reconstr. Surg., 51:501, 1973.

Goodnight, J. E. Jr., Quagliana, J. M. and Morton, D. L.: Failure of subcutaneous mastectomy to prevent the development of cancer. J. Surg. Oncol., 26:198, 1984.

Gray, J. H.: The relation of lymphatic vessels to the spread of cancer. Br. J. Surg., 26:462, 1939.

Halsell, J. T., Smith, J. R., Bentlage, C. R., et al.: Lymphatic drainage of the breast demonstrated by vital dye staining and radiography. Ann. Surg., 162:221, 1965.

Hicken, N. F.: Mastectomy: Clinical pathologic study demonstrating why most mastectomies result in incomplete removal of the mammary gland. Arch. Surg., 40:6, 1940.

Hultborn, K. A., Larsen, K. G., and Raghnult, I.: The lymph drainage from the breast to the axillary and parasternal lymph nodes studied with the aid of colloidal [198]Au. Acta Radiol. (Stockh.), 43:52, 1955.

Jackson, C. F., Palmquist, M., Swanson, J., et al.: The effectiveness of prophylactic subcutaneous mastectomy in Sprague-Dawley rats induced with 7,12-dimethylbenzanthracene. Plast. Reconstr. Surg., 73:249–260, 1984.

Klamer, T. W., Donegan, W. L., and Max, M. H.: Breast tumor incidence in rats after partial mastectomy resection. Arch. Surg., 118:933, 1983.

Loughry, C. W., Sheffer, D. B., Price, T. E., et al.: Breast volume measurement of 598 women using biostereometric analysis. Ann. Plast. Surg., 22:380–385, 1989.

Moosman, D. A.: Anatomy of the pectoral nerves and their preservation in modified mastectomy. Am. J. Surg., 139:883, 1980.

Parks, A. G.: The micro-anatomy of the breast. Ann. R. Coll. Surg. 24:235, 1959.

Pickren, J. W., Rube, J., and Auchincloss, H.: Modification of conventional radical mastectomy: A detailed study of lymph node involvement and follow-up information to show its practicality. Cancer, 18:942, 1965.

Pressman, J. J., and Simon, M. B.: Experimental evidence of direct communications between lymph nodes and veins. Surg. Gynecol. Obstet., 113:537, 1961.

Reichert, F. L.: The regeneration of lymphatics. Arch. Surg., 13:871–881, 1926.

Rouviere, J.: Anatomie des Lymphatiques de l'Homme (Translation by M. J. Tobias). Ann Arbor, MI, Edwards Bros., 1938.

Sartorius, O. W., Morris, P. L., Benedict, D. L., and Smith, H. S.: Contrast ductography for recognition and localization of benign and malignant breast lesions: An improved technique. In Logan, W. W. (Ed.): Breast Carcinoma. Philadelphia, J. B. Lippincott, 1987, p. 281.

Serra, G. E., Maccarone, G. B., Ibarra, P. E., et al.: Lateral pectoralis nerve: The need to preserve it in the modified radical mastectomy. J. Surg. Oncol. 26:278, 1984.

Singer, E.: Fasciae of the Human Body and Their Relations to the Organs They Envelop. Baltimore, Williams & Wilkins, 1935.

Sisley, J. F.: The axillopectoral muscle. Surg. Gynecol. Obstet., 165:73, 1987.

Spratt, J. S., Shiever, W., and Dillard, B.: Anatomy and Surgical Technique of Groin Dissection. St. Louis, C. V. Mosby, 1965.

Tobin, A.-E., Barber, J. H., Slater, A. D., et al.: The anatomic basis for serratus anterior aortic counterpulsation in humans. Plast. Surg. Forum, 44:657–660, 1993.

Tobin, G. R.: Myocutaneous and muscle flaps: Refinements and new applications. Curr. Probl. Surg., 23:315–393, 1986.

Tobin, G. R.: Pectoralis major segmental anatomy and segmentally split pectoralis major flaps. Plast. Reconstr. Surg., 75:814, 1985.

Tobin, G. R., Gordon, J. A., Smith, B., et al.: Preserving motor function by splitting muscle and myocutaneous pedicles. Plast. Surg. Forum, 31:559, 1980.

Tobin, G. R., Spratt, J. S., Bland, K. I., and Weiner, L. J.: One-stage pharyngoesophageal and oral myocutaneous reconstruction with two segments of one musculocutaneous flap. Am. J. Surg., 144:489, 1982.

Turner-Warwick, R. T.: The lymphatics of the breast. Br. J. Surg., 46:574, 1959.

Vogel, P. M., Georgiade, N. G., Fetter, B. F., et al.: The correlation of histologic changes in the human breast with menstrual cycle. Am. J. Pathol., 104:23–24, 1981.

Wallace, S.: Direct communication between a lymph channel in neck and external jugular vein visualized by lymphography and x-ray obtained. In Spratt, J. S., Shieber, W., and Dillard, B. (Eds.): Anatomy and Surgical Technique of Groin Dissection. St. Louis, C.V. Mosby, 1965.

Williams, P. L., Warwick, R., Dyson, M., and Bannister, L. H. (Eds.): Gray's Anatomy. 37th ed. New York, Churchill Livingstone, 1993, p. 1131.

4 Physiology of the Breast

William B. Farrar
Michael J. Walker
John Peter Minton

The structure, size, form, and function of breast tissue result from an intricate combination of hormone signals and ratios that permit epithelial cells to produce and secrete milk for the nourishment and sustenance of infants.

Breasts develop from an ectodermally derived plaque of cells inconspicuously located in the abdominal region. It regresses soon after its appearance at 6 weeks postfertilization except in the anterior thoracic portion of the embryo. The analage of the lactiferous ducts invades the mesodermal connective tissue by 16 to 24 weeks. By 8 months of gestation, the nipple and areola are developed. Breasts of the newborn may secrete a fluid (so-called "witches' milk"), an indication of the responsiveness of these tissues to hormone stimulation.

The breast is a tubuloalveolar gland. By puberty, 15 to 20 ducts are formed; the arborization develops into 10 to 15 lobes, which are separate glands embedded within the breast's fatty stroma.

The secretory units of the breast are the alveoli or saccular invaginations of the lactiferous ducts. It is these secretory units that are so responsive to hormone modulations that promote growth or regression of the breast tissue. Myoepithelial cells form a web around the alveolar structure and along the outside of the interlobular channels. Contraction of the myoepithelial cells is responsible for the emptying ("let-down") or ejection of milk from the lobules into the lactiferous ducts.

Growth of the breast in females at puberty is stimulated by estrogens from the ovaries, but its development is dependent on several hormones. Estrogen alone has no effect; however, in the presence of prolactin, hydrocortisone, growth hormone, and insulin, it causes arborization of the ductal system. Progesterone induces development of terminal ducts and of the lobuloalveolar structure capable of milk secretion. The response to progesterone also requires the presence of growth hormone and insulin. Testosterone inhibits growth of the breasts.

The postpubertal breast may be mature, but it is inactive. A proliferative phase occurs during pregnancy. This is followed by a lactating stage for milk production after parturition, after which regression takes place. An involutional or atrophic phase occurs after lactation ceases and when menopause occurs. Minor physical changes also occur in some women's breasts during the menstrual cycle (Halban, 1905). The premenstrual enlargement is not well understood but is believed to be due to hyperemia and edema.

In the inactive or resting stage, the breast lobules consist of tubules or ducts separated by connective and adipose tissue. The proliferative phase that occurs in pregnancy is associated with major changes. Breast growth early in pregnancy is a hyperplasia of the ductal and secretory elements. Later in pregnancy, hypertrophy of alveolar cells and secretory elements is coupled with decreases in fat and fibrous connective tissue.

During lactation, the cells lining the alveolar sacculations become columnar and look like exocrine cells. These cells deposit their lipids, fluids, carbohydrates, and proteinaceous products into the alveolar lumen. Protein products leave the cells by exocytosis from the cells' apices without loss of cytoplasm. Lipids are transported out of the cells with a significant decrease in cell cytoplasm. Contractions of the myoepithelial cells force the fluid from the alveolar sacculus into alveolar ducts and into the lactiferous ducts and sinuses. The hormonal and neurologic trigger for these myoepithelial contractions is the stimulation from the suckling infant.

Regression, involution, and atrophy follow when the infant's suckling no longer stimulates the breast. Residual alveolar milk products are reabsorbed, and the breast parenchyma involutes and is replaced with increased fat and connective tissue. Macrophages and histocytes are active during this involutional process in the ducts and alveoli.

The process of lactation is controlled by a series of complex hormonal and biochemical events. The levels of progesterone, estrone, estradiol, estriol, prolactin, and placental lactogen all increase during the 40 weeks of gestation (Rigg et al., 1977; Del Pozo and Brownell, 1979; Carr et al., 1981; and Tulchinsky et al., 1972). However, estrogen by itself may not be as important in breast growth as it was initially assumed to be. Progesterone appears to stimulate the growth of lobuloalveolar segments of the breasts while inhibiting secretory activity by blocking the terminal differentiation, which is later induced by prolactin (Davis et al., 1972). Cortisol potentiates the action of prolactin on breast differentiation. Lactation may occasionally be induced in nulliparous women as well as in men by a regular sucking stimulus (Brown, 1978; and Rosner, 1979). Lactogenesis is triggered by a fall in the plasma progesterone levels when the plasma prolactin and breast development are adequate to promote milk secretion (Kuhn, 1969, 1977). At parturition, the levels of placental lactogen disappear rapidly (within hours). Progesterone levels fall more slowly (within several days); estrogen levels decrease over the first week postpartum. Prolactin level falls slowly (>14 days) in the non-nursing mother. In nursing mothers, the prolactin level falls much more slowly, with the decrease usually dependent on the time that the infant nurses (Delvoye et al., 1977; and Hiba et al., 1977). Although placental hormones are suspected of being significant inhibitors of lactation and retained placental fragments delay lactation, prolactin appears to be the hormone most necessary for lactation, and use of the inhibitor bromocriptine can suppress lactation (Brun del Re et al., 1973; and Kuhn, 1977). Occasionally, lactation occurs in women with low prolactin levels. The real trigger for lactation is now believed to be the postpartum decline in progesterone levels along with the long hormonal preparation for lactation that is completed at childbirth (Franks et al., 1977). Nipple neurosensory reflexes to the brain must be triggered to stimulate the secretion of the hormones, oxytocin, and prolactin. Oxytocin stimulates contraction of the myoepithelial cells, producing milk ejection or ''let-down.'' Prolactin drives the synthesis and secretion of milk into the alveolar spaces. Milk production is regulated by infant demand, and prolactin is important in the production of volume (Brun de Re et al., 1973; Aono et al., 1977; Gross and Eastman, 1979; and Kauppila et al., 1981).

Once the stimulus of breast feeding stops, involution begins almost immediately. Milk composition changes rapidly following weaning, with increases in protein, sodium, and chloride concentrations and with a decrease in potassium, lactose, and citrate (Hartmann and Kulski, 1978). Both immunoglobulin A (IgA) and lactoferrin levels increase, and this is related to a deterioration of the blood-milk barriers, which permits plasma to enter alveolar lumina. Blood flow to the breast decreases with involution, and a decline occurs in the release of enzymes necessary for milk production. Alveolar distention is a major factor inducing the cessation of lactation.

Near the menopause, involution results in the disappearance of alveoli and intralobular ducts and in the hyalinization of these structures.

THE HORMONES

The interrelationship of a variety of hormones is very important to breast function. A review of these hormones and their interactions follows.

Oxytocin

Oxytocin is synthesized in pure form in the magnocellular neurons in the supraoptic and paraventricular nucleus of the hypothalamus (du Vigneaud et al., 1954; Morris et al., 1977; and Zimmerman and Defendini, 1977). The fibers of the paraventricular nucleus pass to the supraoptic nucleus, where they join fibers from that nucleus. Together, these fibers travel to the medial eminence of the posterior pituitary gland. Oxytocin, a 10-k protein, is released via the exocytosis of secretory granules (Robinson et al., 1977; Theodosin and Dreifus, 1977; and Amico et al., 1981). Its action is mediated through an electrical potential-producing nerve depolarization prior to milk ejection, as has been shown in experimental animals (Poulain et al., 1977). Oxytocin release may be a conditioned reflex in response to an infant's cry, and release may not occur under conditions of pain or emotional stress (Barowicz, 1978; Clarke and Merrick, 1978; and Moos and Richard, 1979). Oxytocin release can be stimulated by catecholamines when epinephrine and dopamine are injected into the intracerebral ventricle. In contrast, alpha-adrenergic blocking agents and antiagonists block milk ejection. These activities appear to be mediated by the central nervous system. Morphine blocks milk ejection by preventing the release of oxytocin from the nerve terminals in the posterior pituitary gland. Beta-endorphins of pituitary origin modulate oxytocin release within the pituitary gland.

Oxytocin interacts with the myoepithelial cells located in the basement membrane of the alveolus and along the intralobular ducts. Oxytocin binding sites have been localized, and oxytocin receptors are believed to increase in number in the breast and uterus at parturition. Oxytocin apparently acts by phosphorylation of myosin, resulting in the contraction of the myoepithelial cells (Bremel and Shaw, 1978). This contraction is best accomplished by intermittent releases of oxytocin rather than by a continuous secretion, emphasizing the relationship with intermittent suckling of the nipple as a stimulus for milk ejection.

Lactogenic Hormones

Lactogenic hormones are single-chain polypeptides with molecular weights of 21 to 23 kd and include prolactin and growth hormone, both pituitary hormones, and placental lactogen or chorionic somatomammotropin. Prolactin is probably the most important hormone secreted in response to suckling. When it combines with receptors on the milk-secreting cells, it stimulates milk production. Prolactin also stimulates mammary growth and differentiation.

The role of placental lactogens and growth hormone is less clear. The genes for the production of placental lactogen and growth hormone are located on chromosome 17 (Owerbach et al., 1980). The similarity of the primary and intervening sequences of these genes suggests gene reduplication as the origin of these hormones.

Prolactin

Prolactin is synthesized in the mammotropes of the pars distalis of the pituitary on membrane-bound ribosomes, processed in the Golgi membranes, stored in secretory granules, and secreted by exocytosis. Prolactin inhibitory factor (PIF), which is secreted into the pituitary portal blood system by the tubuloinfundibular neurons of the hypothalamus, is controlled by dopamine, estrogens, thyrotropin-releasing hormone, and endorphins (De Hertogh et al., 1975; and Del Pozo and Brownell, 1979). PIF *is* dopamine and thus suppresses the production and release of prolactin by interacting with the dopamine receptor sites on prolactin-producing cells. L-Dopa, which is converted to dopamine, and bromocriptine, a dopamine agonist, interfere with prolactin release. Prolactin messenger ribonucleic acid (mRNA) transcription is inhibited by dopaminergic compounds (Minton and Dickey, 1973; Morris et al., 1977; and Moos and Richard, 1979). Long-term administration of estrogen increases both pituitary and plasma prolactin levels. This results from an increase in the number and activity of pituitary prolactin cells (Lloyd et al., 1975). Chronic elevated estrogen response appears to block the effect of dopamine on prolactin production and produces hypertrophy of pituitary cells, an accumulation of intracellular prolactin-containing granules, and an increase in the content of prolactin transcription-specific mRNA. Estrogen treatment appears to decrease the inhibitory effects of dopamine on prolactin release (Raymond et al., 1978; and Antakly et al., 1980). Estrogen has also been shown to augment prolactin release at the hypothalamus (De Hertogh et al., 1975; and Labrie et al., 1980). Thyrotropin-releasing hormone is not important in prolactin release, although a thyrotropin-releasing hormone infusion can be used to determine prolactin reserve. Both calcium and thyrotropin-releasing hormone are important for inducing electrical activity in prolactin cells and for releasing protein (Sand et al., 1980; and Vincent et al., 1980). Thyrotropin-releasing hormone does augment prolactin mRNA transcription (Raymond et al., 1978; and Potter et al., 1981).

Prolactin release is enhanced by stress, possibly by hypothalamic opiates. The morphine antagonist naloxone decreases prolactin secretion and oxytocin release (Nicoll and Bern, 1972). The dopamine agonist bromocriptine blocks prolactin release, whereas phenothiazine stimulates milk secretion by blocking dopamine synthesis (De Hertogh et al., 1975; Del Pozo et al., 1977; Fluckiger, 1978; and Del Pozo and Brownell, 1979).

Prolactin increases the production of the milk protein casein and increases synthesis of protein mRNA (Guyette et al., 1979; and Teyssot and Houdebine, 1980). Prolactin increases the rate of fatty acid production in breast tissues and also favors the synthesis of medium-chain fatty acids, which are characteristic of lactating breast tissue (Strong et al., 1972; and Wang et al., 1972). Lipoprotein production has yet to be clearly defined.

Prolactin binds to prolactin membrane receptors on the mammary cell surface. Changes in the number of prolactin receptors on mammary cells correlate with the level of serum prolactin and the period of early lactation (Bohnet et al., 1977; and McNeilly and Friesen 1977). Ergot alkaloids block this increase in the number of receptors, and an increase in their number can be produced by injecting prolactin into the system (Djiane and Durand, 1977). Because progesterone blocks the increase in receptor number, the ratio of serum prolactin levels to progesterone levels seems important in modulating increases in the number of receptors. Prolactin receptor levels appear to be dependent on a variety of hormonal concentrations and ratios. Increases or decreases in receptor concentrations change the sensitivity of a cell for milk production. The variations in receptor concentrations imply internalization and processing of hormone receptor complexes.

Prolactin appears to be internalized in the cell to promote a signal for cellular milk production (Nolin and Witorsch, 1976; Nolin, 1978; and Shiu, 1980). Studies support the concept that prolactin is involved in transduction via microtubules to activate casein mRNA and to promote casein synthesis (Houdebine et al., 1979; Houdebine and Djiane, 1980).

Minton began physiologic studies of breast tissue in 1972 in an attempt to clinically decrease circulating prolactin levels in women with breast cancer. Twenty per cent of women with painful bony metastases from breast cancer who were given L-dopa (250 mg every 4 hours) experienced dramatic relief of pain and a subsequent long-term clinical benefit from endocrine ablative surgery (Dickey and Minton, 1972a and b; Minton and Dickey, 1973; and Ferrar et al., 1981). These studies indicated that in some women with metastatic breast cancer, bone pain could be controlled by suppression of serum prolactin levels (Minton, 1974 and 1976). It was suspected that the decrease in bone pain was due to lowering of the cellular metabolism of hormone-sensitive breast cancer cells, with reduced production of pain-producing prostaglandin E_2 (Kibbey et al., 1979). Studies in experimental animals subjected to hormonal manipulation and prolactin suppression demonstrated significant changes in intratumor prostaglandin levels, which correlated with tumor regression (Foecking et al., 1982 and 1983).

Human Placental Lactogen

Human placental lactogen levels rise continually throughout pregnancy. Hypoglycemia and the mass of the placenta are the only factors that change levels of placental lactogen (Bigazzi et al., 1979). Bromocriptine does not change them. Human placental lactogen seems to have a role similar to that of prolactin in lactation, but the major role of this hormone must be related to breast growth and differentiation during pregnancy, as the decrease in its concentration is rapid after the placenta is delivered at parturition.

Estrogens, Progesterone, and Adrenocortical Hormones

Estrogens, progesterone, and adrenocortical hormones play a role in the modulation of the lactogenous hormones. Estrogens stimulate mammary growth but inhibit milk secretion, yet they promote prolactin secretion by the anterior pituitary gland (McManus and Welsch, 1980).

Estrogens

Estrogens are responsible for the proliferation of mammary epithelium, especially in the ductal portions of the gland. Nearly all studies show a relationship between estrogen and intact pituitary function for satisfactory mammary growth (Edwards et al., 1979; and Leclerg and Heuson, 1979). A correlation between the concentrations of these hormones has been made with plasma estradiol-17β and prolactin levels at puberty, pregnancy, and menarche, and in association with oral contraceptive use (Robyn et al., 1977; Hertz et al., 1978).

Estrogens bind with the estrogen receptors in breast tissue. Strong evidence supports that combining estrogens with prolactin can produce and promote a galactorrhea syndrome (Antunes et al., 1977). Interestingly, estrogen is produced in normal breast tissues as well as in breast cancer tissue (Edwards et al., 1979). Excessive estrogen production does stop lactation and is associated with a decrease of prolactin level in the mammary epithelial cells, suggesting interference with prolactin binding to the cell by the internalization or modulation of prolactin receptor sites (Lemarchand-Beraud et al., 1977).

Progesterone

Progesterone appears to synergize with estrogen and prolactin to produce full lobuloalveolar development of the gland, but it inhibits milk secretion during pregnancy. Progesterone prevents an accumulation of enzymes necessary for the terminal differentiation of breast cells for lactation but actively promotes breast growth. Progesterone in combination with estrogen is responsible for lobuloalveolar development during pregnancy and prevents an increase of lactose in breast tissue in pregnancy (Folley and Malpress, 1948; Kuhn, 1977; Cowie, 1978; and Topper and Freeman, 1980). In addition, progesterone inhibits the prolactin-induced rise of alpha-lactalbumin in breast tissue during pregnancy (Turkington and Hill, 1969; and Speake et al., 1976). Progesterone also decreases prolactin-induced rises in casein and inhibits glucose oxidation and conversion to lipids (De Hertogh et al., 1975; Greenbaum et al., 1978; Rosen et al., 1978; and Teyssot and Houdebine, 1980). It is speculated that progesterone inhibits the process of breast epithelial differentiation by inhibiting the binding of cortisol and preventing glucocorticoid potentiation of prolactin (Ganguly et al., 1982). In addition, progesterone may modify ribosomal RNA and casein mRNA synthesis (Teyssot and Houdebine, 1980). Progesterone binding sites appear to decrease significantly during lactation, accounting for the absence of progesterone effect on the breasts during lactation.

Glucocorticoids

Lactation cannot be initiated or sustained in the absence of glucocorticoids. Current speculation is that withdrawal of progesterone at parturition allows cortisol to exert a stimulus for lactation. Glucocorticoid receptors bound with glucocorticoids translocate to the nucleus after binding, but progesterone can bind this receptor, preventing translocation and blocking the action of glucocorticoids (Shyamala, 1975; and Shyamala and Dickson, 1976). Glucocorticoids increase the accumulation of casein and casein mRNA when breast tissue is exposed to prolactin (Mills and Topper, 1970; Devinoy and Houdebine, 1977; and Bolander and Topper, 1979). When prolactin is absent, little activity is present (Devinoy and Houdebine, 1977).

Insulin, Thyroid Hormones, and Growth Factors

Insulin is an important requirement for the growth of mammary epithelial cells in tissue culture, but it does not seem to play an important role in development of breast tissue. Insulin is important in lipid synthesis, regulating the transport of glucose into the acinar cells (Robinson et al., 1978). Not only is the availability of glucose affected by insulin, but also glucose metabolites such as lactate and pyruvate influence the fatty acid production of lactating epithelial cells (Bartley and Abraham, 1976).

Thyroid hormone is involved in mammary growth and lactation, but its role is more permissive than regulatory (Lyons, 1958). For example, in the presence of low concentrations of prolactin, thyroxine promotes lobuloalveolar development (Singh and Bern, 1969). High doses of thyroxine shut the system down (Vonderhaar, 1979). Prostaglandins act as one of the factors by which preparturition inhibits secretion.

Several growth factors are involved in normal growth and development of the breast. Transforming growth factor-alpha and epidermal growth factor are both able to promote local lobuloalveolar development in vitro when implanted as slow release pellets into the mammary gland of mice (Vanderhaar, 1987). Transforming growth factor-beta inhibits development of mammary ducts around an implant but has no effect on distant tissues (Silberstein, 1987). The interaction of several other growth factors, namely insulin-like growth factor, platelet-derived growth factor, and fibroblast growth factors, and how they influence development of the glandular and stromal elements of the breast are currently being investigated.

LACTATION

The mechanisms of milk production involve five different pathways. The first four are transcellular pathways: (1) protein, citrate, calcium, phosphate, and lactose all leave the cell through exocytosis in Golgi-derived secretory vesicles; (2) milk fat is secreted in the form of milk fat globules; (3) water, sodium, potassium, and chloride are secreted across the cell membranes; and (4) immunoglobulins such as IgA and other plasma proteins exit by pinocytosis or exocytosis. In the fifth pathway, leukocytes, sodium, and plasma protein may enter the milk by a paracellular route or between the membranes of the lactating cells. Each alveolar unit creates about 1 or 2 mL of milk per gram of tissue per day. Milk is stored adjacent to the cells that produce it, and when myoepithelial cells contract, the milk passes rapidly through the ductal system and out of the breast. Little of the milk is reabsorbed in transit. Exocytosis is the process by which most milk components leave the cells. The amino acid sequences of milk proteins are coded in nuclear deoxyribonucleic acid which is transcribed into mRNA. The latter passes to the cytoplasm, where it translates to ribosomes bound to the rough endoplasmic reticulum. As proteins are synthesized, amino acids are inserted into the sequence across the endoplasmic reticular membrane. Carbohydrate groups are added according to the appropriate sequence. The product is then transferred to a Golgi system for sorting and storage. Calcium, phosphates, and citrate enter the Golgi vesicles from the cytoplasm. Inside the Golgi vesicles, calcium and phosphates combine with caseins and phosphoproteins and form aggregates or micelles. Lactose is formed in the Golgi system from an interaction of the membrane-bound galactosyl transferase and alpha-lactalbumin. Lactose osmotically attracts water into the Golgi vesicles. The vesicles, containing lactose, water, milk protein, calcium, phosphates, and citrates, pass to the apical membrane of the cell, fuse, and are released into the lumina.

Triglycerides are synthesized in the cytoplasm and smooth endoplasmic reticulum of alveolar cells and coalesce into large droplets. These droplets become enveloped in apical plasma membranes and separate as fat globules. Sodium, potassium, and water move into the secretory vesicle in response to osmotic gradients. Chloride and bicarbonates may have active transport systems at the apical membranes to account for the electrolyte disequilibrium (Peaker, 1977 and 1978; and White et al., 1981).

The composition of milk changes dramatically in the first 5 days of lactation. Initially, the breasts secrete precolostrum, which has high concentrations of sodium chloride, lactoferrin, and immunoglobulins. Colostrum, which is high in immunoglobulins, is secreted for the first 5 days after delivery. Finally, milk containing high lactose levels is secreted. Milk proteins are alpha-lactalbumin (30%), lactoferrin (10–20%) casein (40%), and IgA (10%). Other proteins include IgG, IgM, isozyme, and serum albumin. Less concentrated proteins found in milk include a variety of binding proteins, hormones, and epidermal growth factor, vitamin B_{12}–binding protein, folate-binding protein, prolactin, and milk fat globule membrane protein. In addition, over 30 enzymes have been identified in human milk. Most of these enzymes are secretions of the Golgi apparatus (Jenness, 1974; Mather and Keenan, 1975; Waxman and Schreiber, 1975; Payne et al., 1976; Bezkorovainy, 1977; Carpenter, 1980; Mather et al., 1980; Samson et al., 1980; and Sandberg et al., 1981).

Casein accounts for 40% of the protein secreted by the human breast (Jenness, 1979). Alpha- and beta-caseins contain proline residues and a negatively charged carboxyl and phosphate end group that commonly interacts with calcium. The opposite end is hydrophobic. Alpha-lactalbumin, derived from lysosomes, is a cofactor in lactose synthesis and a major source of lactose. Lactoferrin is an iron-binding protein that resembles transferrin. It is concentrated in colostrum and is bacteriostatic and bacteriocidal by binding iron necessary for bacterial replication (Weinberg, 1978). IgA is present early in lactation, but IgG and IgM are less concentrated in human milk. Serum albumin is present at a concentration of 2 mg/mL in colostrum, but this ratio changes to 0.5 mg/mL in later stages (Phillippy and McCarthy, 1979). Milk fat globule membranes are enveloped by apical plasma membranes. Xanthine oxidase and butyrophilin are proteins associated with milk fat globule membrane. These proteins have been found only in the apical surface of mammary epithelium (Franke et al., 1981).

Methylxanthine and Benign Breast Disease

The measurement of cyclic adenosine monophosphate (cAMP) levels in normal breast tissue, fibrocystic breast tissue, and breast cancer tissue by Minton and associates

suggested a significant increase in cancer tissue (Minton et al., 1979; and Ferrar et al., 1981). The cAMP increase in these tissues was not due to an increase in phosphodiesterase, which allegedly inhibits the breakdown of cAMP production (Foecking et al.; 1980; Elliot et al., 1981; and Minton et al., 1981a). The elevated adenylate cyclase level pointed to the possibility of an endogenous hormonal influence on the activation of the cAMP system, but an analysis of serum estrogen levels did not show a significant difference. Because painful, swollen, and lumpy breasts ("fibrocystic disease") were associated with elevated cAMP levels and protein kinase activities, a program aimed at abstention from cAMP-activating agents was undertaken (Minton et al., 1979).

Women with "fibrocystic breast disease" were asked not to consume methylxanthine-containing products, such as coffee, tea, colas, and chocolate. After a few months (less in younger women), both pain and lumps began to resolve, and improvement persisted as long as the patients abstained from methylxanthine (Minton et al., 1981a). In some women, even after total abstention from caffeine products, symptoms began to recur. In other women, no clear improvement was seen (Minton and Abou-Issa, 1986). A careful diet diary showed that women whose disease had resolved made subtle changes in their eating patterns. Women whose symptoms were reactivated had begun to consume foods containing an increased proportion of tyramines. For some patients, these were foods that they had neither liked nor eaten frequently prior to abstaining from methylxanthines. Most women could not explain their new preference. Some noted they experienced a "high" or "kick" from tyramine-containing foods. Tyramine-containing foods include cheese, wine, beer, spices, nuts, mushrooms, bananas, and other less commonly consumed products, such as pickled herring. In general, these are the food products people with high blood pressure are asked to avoid because of their adverse effects on hypertension.

Other factors, such as nicotine use and emotional and physical stresses, were also found to reactivate symptoms (Fig. 4–1). The changes in breasts after consumption of tyramines led Minton to measure serum catecholamine levels. He found that methylxanthines, nicotine, and tyramines can elevate serum catecholamines and increase catecholamine release in humans. Methylxanthine and catecholamine levels were measured in women with no breast disease, those with fibrocystic changes, and those with breast cancer. The results showed that women with benign and malig-

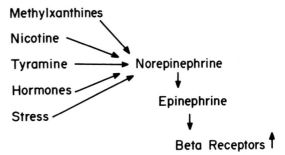

Figure 4–1. Graphic presentation of the factors that may promote fibrocystic changes.

Table 4–1. SERUM METHYLXANTHINES (NG/ML) AND CATECHOLAMINES (PG/ML) IN CONTROLS COMPARED WITH WOMEN WITH MASTALGIA AND BREAST CANCER

	Control	Cyclic Mastalgia	Noncyclic Mastalgia	Breast Cancer
Age	30.4 ± 2.0	33 ± 1.6	42.6 ± 2.8	60.8 ± 3.3
Number	17	30	6	7
Caffeine	2567.8 ± 490	2256.7 ± 327.9 NS	3341 ± 934.5 NS	4949 ± 1016.8 S (193%)
Theobromine	413.6 ± 36.4	588.8 ± 89.8 NS	850.2 ± 246.5 5 S (205%)	819.3 ± 132.2 SSS (198%)
Total methylxanthines	3294.9 ± 517.2	3184.4 ± 412.2 NS	4728.8 ± 907.9 NS	6321.6 ± 1189.4 SS (192%)
Epinephrine	275.6 ± 54.6	1121.2 ± 222.1 SSS (406%)	1623.6 ± 291.1 SSS (589%)	991.5 ± 695.2 NS
Norepinephrine	403.7 ± 61.2	511.9 ± 49.4 S (127%)	907.5 ± 313.2 S (224%)	514.2 ± 55.5 NS
Dopamine	1250.6 ± 265.1	588.8 ± 64.2 SSS (47%)	577 ± 77.1 S (46%)	342.6 ± 60 SSS (27%)
Dopa	267.5 ± 66.4	2673 ± 31.8 NS	340.5 ± 38 NS	540.0 ± 84 S

Abbreviations : NS (not significant): $P > 0.05$; S: $P < 0.05$; SS: $P < 0.01$; SSS: $P < 0.005$.

nant breast disease had a higher level of circulating catecholamines than women without breast disease when circulating levels of methylxanthines were the same (Table 4–1). This observation suggests a different sensitivity to caffeine or catecholamine release in women with breast disease. The level of dopamine, the prolactin-inhibiting factor, was lower in patients with high catecholamine levels; this provides a rationale for the higher prolactin levels in the breast cancer patients observed by Malarkey and colleagues (1977, 1983). Methylxanthine-stimulated release of catecholamines and increased levels of circulating catecholamines would have no clinical importance unless receptor activity in the breast tissue for these hormones could be demonstrated. An analysis of the beta-adrenergic receptor sites in normal and benign breast conditions was done to determine whether the receptor concentrations were the same in women with fibrocystic changes and normal breast tissue. A significant increase was demonstrated in fibrocystic breast tissue compared with normal breast tissue. In addition, there appeared to be a supersensitivity to the interaction of catecholamines with beta-adrenergic receptors that induced an avalanche of adenylate cyclase activity. This increased cAMP ultimately produced the excess of fluid and fibrosis in breasts deemed to be affected by fibrocystic changes (Fig. 4–2). The possibility that a predisposition for increased beta-receptor concentrations is genetic rather than induced needs further clarification, as does the possibility

that sensitivity may vary, depending on other hormone concentrations (e.g., estrogens) during the menstrual cycle.

Animal studies pointed out a cancer-promoting relationship between fat consumption at 40% to 45% of total calorie intake per day and breast cancer when animals consuming caffeine were exposed to a carcinogen (Minton et al., 1981a). A series of animal studies evaluated beta-glucuronidase as well as other cancer promoting agents as a carrier of potential carcinogens. It was observed in rats that lowering endogenous serum beta-glucuronidase with D-glucaric acid reduced the anticipated effects of known carcinogens (Walaszek et al., 1986). Women with fibrocystic changes have concentrations of beta-glucuronidase in cyst fluid that vary tenfold in different cysts. In addition, current studies show that women with breast disease fall into two major categories, those with high and those with low serum beta-glucuronidase levels (Fig. 4–3).

Women with breast disease fit the stress profile (Bammer and Newberry, 1981). If these women have a genetic mechanism that promotes secretory activity in breast tissue as a result of endogenous catecholamine stimulation (Fig. 4–1), and if a subset of these women have high circulating beta-glucuronidase levels and can concentrate carcinogens consumed in an American diet high in fats, nitrates, and transformed hydrocarbons, it is then possible that carcinogenic agents are transported to the ducts of the breast where cancer is produced. Caffeines consumed by sensitive indi-

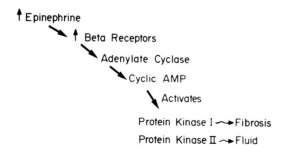

Figure 4–2. Graphic presentation of the response of fibrocystic breast tissue to beta-receptor activation.

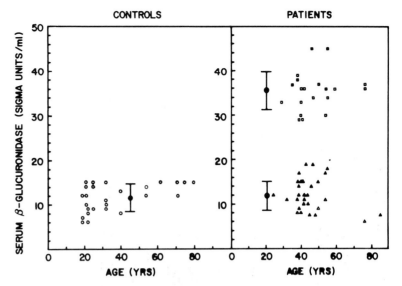

Figure 4–3. Distribution of serum β-glucuronidase levels in Sigma units/ml in patients with fibrocystic breast changes and controls.

viduals who release excessive catecholamines may cause a double effect, decreasing immune surveillance by natural killer cells involved in cancer surveillance (Tonneson et al., 1985; and Blazar et al., 1986). Then, cancer cells may propagate unchallenged by the individual's immune defense mechanisms. The end result is a situation in which the growth of malignant cells is promoted in susceptible individuals.

References

Amico, J. A., Seif, S. M., and Robinson, A. G.: Oxytocin in human plasma: Correlation with neurophysin and stimulation with estrogen. J. Clin. Endocrinol. Metab., *52:*988, 1981.

Anderson, N. G., Powers, M. T., and Tollaksen, S. L.: Proteins of human milk. I. Identification of major components. Clin. Chem. N.Y., *28:*1045, 1982.

Antakly, T., Pelletier, G., Zeytinoglu, F., and Labrie, F.: Changes of cell morphology and prolactin secretion induced by 2-Br-x-ergocyptine, estradiol, and thyrotropin-releasing hormone in rat anterior pituitary cells in culture. J. Cell. Biol., *86:*377, 1980.

Antunes, J. L., Housepian, E. M., Frantz, A. B., et al.: Prolactin-secreting pituitary tumors. Ann. Neurol., *2:*148, 1977.

Aono, T., Shioji, T., Shoda, T., et al.: The initiation of human lactation and prolactin response to suckling. J. Clin. Endocrinol. Metab., *44:*1101, 1977.

Bammer, K., and Newberry B. H. (Eds.): Stress and Cancer. Toronto, C. J. Hogrefe, 1981.

Barowicz, T.: Inhibitory effect of adrenaline on oxytocin release in the ewe during the milk-ejection reflex. J. Dairy Res., *46:*41, 1978.

Bartley, J. C., and Abraham, S.: The absolute rate of fatty acid synthesis by mammary gland slices from lactating rats. J. Lipid Res., *17:*467, 1976.

Bezkorovainy, A.: Human milk and colostrum proteins: A review. J. Dairy Sci., *60:*1023, 1977.

Bigazzi, M., Ronga, R., Lancranjan, I., et al.: Pregnancy in an acromegalic woman during bromocriptine treatment: Effects on growth hormone and prolactin in the maternal, fetal and amniotic compartments. J. Clin. Endocrinol. Metab., *48:*9, 1979.

Blazar, B. A., Rodrick, M. L., O'Mahony, J. B., et al.: Suppression of natural killer-cell function in humans following thermal and traumatic injury. J. Clin. Immunol., *6:*26, 1986.

Bohnet, H. G., Gomez, F., and Friesen, H. G.: PRL and estrogen binding sites in the mammary gland of the lactating and non-lactating rat. Endocrinology, *101:*1111, 1977.

Bolander, F. F., Jr., and Topper, Y. J.: Relationships between spermidine, glucocorticoid and milk proteins in different mammalian species. Biochem. Biophys. Res. Commun., *90:*1131, 1979.

Bremel, R. D., and Shaw, M. E.: Actomyosin from mammary myoepithelial cells and phosphorylation by myosin light chain kinase. J. Dairy Sci., *61:*1561, 1978.

Brown, R. E.: Relactation with reference to application in developing countries. Clin. Pediatr., *17:*333, 1978.

Brun del Re, R., del Pozo, E., de Grandi, P., et al.: Prolactin inhibition and suppression of puerperal lactation by Br-ergo cryptine (CB154). A comparison with estrogen. Obstet. Gynecol., *41:*884, 1973.

Carpenter, G.: Epidermal growth factor is a major growth promoting agent in human milk. Science, *210:*198, 1980.

Carr, B. R., Parker, C. R., Jr., Madden, J. D., et al.: Maternal plasma adrenocorticotropin and cortisol relationships throughout human pregnancy. Am. J. Obstet. Gynecol., *139:*416, 1981.

Clarke, G., and Merrick, L. P.: A tentative identification of the synaptic transmitters involved in the neural regulation of oxytocin release. J. Physiol., *277:*19, 1978.

Cowie, A. T.: Backward glances. *In* Yokoyama, A., Mizuno, H., and Nagasawa, H. (Eds.): Physiology of Mammary Glands. Baltimore, University Park Press, 1978, p. 43.

Davis, J. W., Wilkman-Coffelt, J., and Eddington, C. L.: The effect of progesterone on biosynthetic pathways in mammary tissue. Endocrinology, *91:*1011, 1972.

De Hertogh, R., Thomas, K., Bietlot, Y., et al.: Plasma levels of unconjugated estrone, estradiol and estriol and of HCS throughout pregnancy in normal women. J. Clin. Endocrinol. Metab., *40:*93, 1975.

Del Pozo, E., Hiba, J., Lancranjan, I., et al.: Prolactin measurements throughout the life cycle. *In* Crosignani, P. G., and Robyn, C. (Eds.): Prolactin and Human Reproduction. London, Academic Press, 1977, p. 61.

Del Pozo, E., and Brownell, J.: Prolactin: I. Mechanisms of control, peripheral actions and modification by drugs. Horm. Res., *10:*143, 1979.

Delvoye, P. , Demaegd, M., Delogne-Desnoeck, Jr., et al.: The influence of the frequency of nursing and of previous lactation experience on serum prolactin in lactating mothers. J. Biosoc. Sci., *9:*447, 1977.

Devinoy, E., and Houdebine, L.-M.: Effects of glucocorticoids on casein gene expression in the rabbit. Eur. J. Biochem., *75:*411, 1977.

Dickey, R. P., and Minton, J. P.: Levodopa relief of bone pain from breast cancer. N. Engl. J. Med., *286:*843, 1972a.

Dickey, R. P., and Minton, J. P.: L-Dopa effect on prolactin, follicle-stimulating hormone, and luteinizing hormone in women with advanced breast cancer: A preliminary report. Am. J. Obstet. Gynecol., *114:*266, 1972b.

Djiane, J., and Durand, P.: Prolactin-progesterone antagonism in self-regulation of prolactin receptors in the mammary gland. Nature, *266:*641, 1977.

du Vigneaud, V., Ressler, C., Swan, J. M., et al.: The synthesis of oxytocin. J. Am. Chem. Soc., *76:*3115, 1954.

Edwards, D. P., Chamness, G. C., and McGuire, W. L.: Estrogen and progesterone receptor proteins in breast cancer. Biochim. Biophys. Acta, *560:*457, 1979.

Elliot, J., Abou-Issa, H., Foecking, M. K., et al.: Cyclic nucleotides as predictors of benign to malignant progression of breast disease. Breast, *7:*6, 1981.

Ferrar, J. J., Reiches, N. A., and Minton, J. P.: Endocrine ablation in breast cancer patients who have failed cytotoxic therapy. J. Surg. Oncol., *18:*231, 1981.

Fluckiger, E. W.: Lactation inhibition by ergot drugs. *In* Yokoyama, A., Mizuno, H., and Nagasawa, H. (Eds.): Physiology of Mammary Gland. Baltimore, University Park Press, 1978, p. 71.

Foecking, M. K., Minton, J. P., and Matthews, R. H.: Progressive patterns in breast diseases. Med. Hypotheses, *6:*659, 1980.

Foecking, M. K., Kibbey, W. E., Abou-Issa, H., et al.: Hormone dependence of dimethylbenz(a)anthracene-induced mammary tumor growth; correlation with prostaglandin E2 content. J. Natl. Cancer Inst., *69:*433, 1982.

Foecking, M. K., Abou-Issa, H., Webb, T., et al.: Concurrent changes in growth-related biochemical parameters during regression of hormone dependent rat mammary tumors. J. Natl. Cancer Inst. *71:*773, 1983.

Folley, S. J., and Malpress, F. H.: Hormonal control of lactation. *In* Pincus, G. (Ed.): The Hormones. Vol. 1. New York, Academic Press, 1948, p. 745.

Franke, W. W., Heid, H. W., Grund, C., et al.: Antibodies in the major insoluble milk fat globule membrane-associated protein: Specific location in apical regions of lactating epithelial cells. J. Cell. Biol., *89:*485, 1981.

Franks, S., Kiwi, R., and Nabarro, J. D. N.: Pregnancy and lactation after pituitary surgery. Br. Med. J., *1:*882, 1977.

Ganguly, R., Majumder, P. K., Ganguly, N., et al.: The mechanism of progesterone-glucocorticoid interaction in regulation of casein gene expression. J. Biol. Chem., *257:*2182, 1982.

Greenbaum, A. L., Sochor, M., and McLean, P.: Regulation of mammary gland metabolism, pathways of glucose utilization, metabolic profile and hormone response of a modified mammary gland cell preparation. Eur. J. Biochem., *878:*505, 1978.

Gross, B. A., and Eastman, C. J.: Prolactin secretion during prolonged lactational amenorrhoea. Aust. N.Z.J. Obstet. Gynaecol., *19:*95, 1979.

Guyette, W. A., Matusik, R. J., and Rosen, J. M.: Prolactin-mediated transcriptional and post-transcriptional control of casein gene expression. Cell, *17:*1013, 1979.

Halban, J.: Die innere Secretion von Ovarium und Placenta und ihre Bedeutung fur die Function der Milchdruse. Arch. Gynaek., *75:*353, 1905.

Hartmann, P. E., and Kulski, J. K.: Changes in the composition of the mammary secretion of women after abrupt termination of breast feeding. J. Physiol., *275:*1, 1978.

Hertz, J., Anderson, A. N., and Larsen, J. F.: Correlation between prolactin and progesterone, oestradiol 17B and oestriol during early human pregnancy. Clin. Endocrinol., *9:*97, 1978.

Hiba, J., Del Pozo, E., Genazzani, A., et al.: Hormonal mechanism of milk secretion in the newborn. J. Clin. Endocrinol. Metab., *44:*973, 1977.

Houdebine, L.-M., Djiane, J., and Clauser, H.: Endocrinologie—rôle des lysosomes, des micro-tubules, et des microfilaments dans le mécanisme de l'action lactogène de la prolactine sur la glande mammaire de lapine. C. R. Acad. Sci. Ser. D., *289:*679, 1979.

Houdebine, L.-M., and Djiane, J.: Effects of lysomotropic agents, and of microfilament- and microtubule-disrupting drugs on the activation of casein-gene expression by prolactin in the mammary gland. Mol. Cell. Endocrinol., *17:*1, 1980.

Jenness, R.: The composition of milk. In Larson, B. L., and Smith, V. R. (Eds.): Lactation: A Comprehensive Treatise. Vol. III. New York, Academic Press, 1974, p. 3.

Jenness, R.: The composition of human milk. Semin. Perinatol., *3:*225, 1979.

Kauppila, A., Kivinen, S., and Ylikorkala, O.: Metoclopramide increases prolactin release and milk secretion in puerperium without stimulating the secretion of thyrotropin and thyroid hormones. J. Clin. Endocrinol. Metab., *52:*436, 1981.

Kibbey, W. E., Bronn, D. G., and Minton, J. P.: Prostaglandin synthetase and prostaglandin E2 levels in human breast carcinoma. Prostaglandins and Medicine, *2:*133, 1979.

Kuhn, N. J.: Progesterone withdrawal as the lactogenic trigger in the rat. J. Endocrinol., *44:*39, 1969.

Kuhn, N. J.: Lactogenesis: The search for trigger mechanisms in different species. Symp. Zool. Soc. (Lond.), *41:*165, 1977.

Labrie, F., Ferland, L., Di Paolo, T., et al.: Modulation of prolactin secretion by sex steroids and thyroid hormones. *In* MacLeod, R., and Scapagnini, U. (Eds.): Central and Peripheral Regulation of Prolactin Function. New York, Raven Press, 1980, p. 97.

Leclerg, G., and Heuson, J. C.: Physiological and pharmacological effects of estrogens in breast cancer. Biochim. Biophys. Acta, *560:*427, 1979.

Lemarchand-Beraud, T., Reymond, M., Berthier, C., et al.: Effects of oestrogens on prolactin and TSHA secretion in women. *In* Crosignant, P. G., and Robyn, C. (Eds.): Prolactin and Human Reproduction. London, Academic Press, 1977, p. 135.

Lloyd, H. M., Meares, J. D., and Jacobi, J.: Effects of oestrogen and bromocryptine on in vivo secretion and mitosis in prolactin cells. Nature, *255:*497, 1975.

Lyons, W. R.: Hormonal synergism in mammary growth. Proc. R. Soc. Lond. Ser. B, *149:*303, 1958.

Malarkey, W. B., Schroeder, L. L., Stevens, V. C., et al.: Disordered nocturnal prolactin regulation in women with breast cancer. Cancer Res., *37:*4650, 1977.

Malarkey, W. B., Kennedy, M., Allred, L. E., et al.: Physiologic concentrations of prolactin can promote growth of human breast tumor cells in culture, J. Clin Endocrinol. Metabol., *56:*673, 1983.

Mather, I. H., and Keenan, T. W.: Studies on the structure of milk fat globule membrane. J. Membr. Biol., *21:*65, 1975.

Mather, I. H., Tamplin, C. B., and Irving, M. G.: Separation of the proteins of bovine milk-fat-globule membrane by electrofocusing with retention of enzymatic and immunological activity. Eur. J. Biochem., *110:*327, 1980.

McManus, M. J., and Welsch, C. W.: DNA synthesis of benign human breast tumors in the untreated athymic "nude" mouse. Cancer, *45:*2160, 1980.

McNeilly, A. S., and Friesen, H. G.: Binding of prolactin to the rabbit mammary gland during pregnancy. J. Endocrinol., *74:*507, 1977.

Mills, E. S., and Topper, Y. J.: Some ultrastructural effects of insulin, hydrocortisone, and prolactin on mammary gland explants. J. Cell Biol., *44:*310, 1970.

Minton, J. P.: Prolactin and human breast cancer. Am. J. Surg., *128:*628, 1974.

Minton, J. P.: Precise selection of breast cancer patients with bone metastasis for endocrine ablation. Surgery, *80:*513, 1976.

Minton, J. P., and Abou-Issa, H.: Fibrocystic breast disease—its management and explanation. *In* Najarian, J. S., and Delaney, J. P. (Eds.): Advances in Breast and Endocrine Surgery. Chicago, Year Book Medical Publishers, 1986, p. 15.

Minton, J. P., and Dickey, R. R.: Levodopa test to predict response of carcinoma of the breast to surgical ablation of endocrine glands. Surg. Gynecol. Obstet., *136:*971, 1973.

Minton, J. P., Abou-Issa, H., Elliot, J. B., et al.: Biochemical subgrouping of benign breast disease to define premalignant potential. Surgery, *90:*652, 1981a.

Minton, J. P., Foecking, M. K., Webster, D. J. T., et al.: Response of fibrocystic disease to caffeine withdrawal and correlation of cyclic nucleotides with breast disease. Am. J. Obstet. Gynecol., *135:*157, 1979.

Minton, J. P., Walaszek, Z., Schooley, W., et al.: β-Glucuronidase levels in patients with fibrocystic breast disease. Br. Cancer Res. Treat., *8:*217–222, 1986.

Moos, F., and Richard, P.: The inhibitory role of β-adrenergic receptors in oxytocin release during suckling. Brain Res., *169:*595, 1979.

Morris, J. F., Sokol, H. W., and Valtin, H.: One neuron-one hormone. Recent evidence from Brattleboro rats. *In* Moses, A. M., and Share, L. (Eds.): International Conference on the Neurohypophysis. New York, Karger, 1977, p. 58.

Nicoll, C. S., and Bern, H. A.: On the actions of prolactin among the vertebrates: Is there a common denominator? *In* Wolstenholme, G. E. N. and Knight, J. (Eds.): Lactogenic Hormones, Ciba Foundation Symposium. Edinburgh, Churchill Livingstone, 1972, p. 299.

Nolin, J. M.: Target cell prolactin. *In* McKerns, K. W. (Ed.): Structure and Function of the Gonadotropins. New York, Plenum Press, 1978, p. 151.

Nolin, J. M., and Witorsch, R. J.: Detection of endogenous immunoreactive prolactin in rat mammary epithelial cells during lactation. Endocrinology, *99:*949, 1976.

Owerbach, D., Rutter, W. J., Martial, J. A., et al.: Genes for growth hormone, chorionic somatomammotropin and growth hormone-like gene are on chromosome 17 in humans. Science *209:*289, 1980.

Payne, D. W., Peng, L.-H., Pearlman, W. H., et al.: Corticosteroid-binding proteins in human colostrum and milk and rat milk. J. Biol. Chem., *251:*5272, 1976.

Peaker, M.: The aqueous phase of milk; Ion and water transport. *In* Peaker, M. (Ed.): Comparative Aspects of Lactation. New York, Academic Press, 1977, p. 113.

Peaker, M.: Ion and water transport in the mammary gland. *In* Peaker, M. (Ed.): Lactation: A Comprehensive Treatise. New York, Academic Press, 1978, p. 437.

Phillippy, B. O., and McCarthy, R. D.: Multi-origins of milk serum albumin in the lactating goat. Biochim. Biophys. Acta, *584:*298, 1979.

Potter, E., Nicolaisen, A. K., Ong, E. S., et al.: Thyro-tropin-releasing hormone exerts rapid nuclear effects to increase production of the primary prolactin mRNA transcript. Proc. Natl. Acad. Sci. USA, *78:*6662, 1981.

Poulain, D. A., Wakerly, J. B., and Dyball, R. E. J.: Electrophysiological differentiation of oxytocin and vasopressin-secreting neurons. Proc. R. Soc. Lond., Ser. B, *196:*367, 1977.

Raymond, V., Beaulieu, M., Labrie, F., et al.: Potent antidopaminergic activity of estradiol at the pituitary level on prolactin release. Science, *200:*1173, 1978.

Rigg, L. A., Lein, A., and Yen, S. S. C.: Pattern of increase in circulating prolactin levels during human gestation. Am. J. Obstet. Gynecol., *129:*454, 1977.

Robinson, A. G., Seif, S. M., Huellmantel, A. B., et al.: Physiologic and pathologic secretion of neurphysins in the rat. *In* Moses, A. M., and Share, L. (Eds.): International Conference on the Neurohypophysis. New York, S. Karger, 1977, p. 136.

Robinson, A. M., Girard, J. R., and Williamson, D. H.: Evidence for a role of insulin in the regulation of lipogenesis in lactating rat mammary gland. Biochem. J., *176:*343, 1978.

Robyn, C., Delvoye, P., Van Exter, C., et al.: Physiological and pharmacological factors influencing prolactin secretion and their relation to human reproduction. *In* Crosignani, P. G., and Robyn, C. (Eds.): Prolactin and Human Reproduction. London, Academic Press, 1977, p. 17.

Rosner, M. D.: Galactorrhea in men. J.A.M.A., *1:*1327, 1979.

Rosen, J. M., O'Neal, D. L., McHugh, J. E., et al.: Progesterone-mediated inhibition of casein mRNA and polysomal casein synthesis in the rat mammary gland during pregnancy. Biochemistry, *17:*290, 1978.

Samson, R., Mirtle, C., and McClelland, D. B. L.: The effect of digestive enzymes on the binding and bacterio-static properties of lactoferrin and vitamin B_{12} binder in human milk. Acta Paediatr. Scand., *59:*517, 1980.

Sand, O., Haug, E., and Gautvik, K. M.: Effects of thyroliberin and H-aminopyridine in action potentials and prolactin release and synthesis in rat pituitary cells in culture. Acta Physiol. Scand., *108:*247, 1980.

Sandberg, D. P., Begley, J. A., and Hall, C. A.: The content, binding, and forms of vitamin B_{12} in milk. Am. J. Clin. Nutr., *34:*1717, 1981.

Sapag-Hagar, M., and Greenbaum, A. L.: Adenosine $3':5'$-monophosphate and hormone interrelationships in the mammary gland of the rat during pregnancy and lactation. Eur. J. Biochem., *47:*303, 1974.

Shiu, R. P. C.: Processing of prolactin by human breast cancer cells in long term tissue culture. J. Biol. Chem., *255:*4278, 1980.

Shyamala, G.: Glucocorticoid receptors in mouse mammary tumors: Specific binding to nuclear components. Biochemistry, *14:*437, 1975.

Shyamala, G., and Dickson, C.: Relationship between receptor and mammary tumor virus production after stimulation by glucocorticoid. Nature, *262:*107, 1976.

Silberstein, G. B., and Daniel, G. W.: Reversible inhibition of mammary gland growth by transforming growth factor β. Science, *237:*291–295, 1987.

Singh, D. V., and Bern, H. A.: Interaction between prolactin and thyroxine

in mouse mammary gland lobulo-alveolar development in vitro. J. Endocrinol., *45:*579, 1969.

Speake, B. K., Dils, R., and Mayer, R. J.: Regulation of enzyme turnover during tissue differentiation. Interactions of insulin, prolactin and cortisol in controlling the turnover of fatty acid synthetase in rabbit mammary gland in organ culture. Biochem. J., *154:*359, 1976.

Strong, C. R., Forsyth, I., and Dils, R.: The effects of hormones on milk-fat synthesis in mammary explants from pseudo-pregnant rabbits. Biochem. J., *128:*509, 1972.

Teyssot, B., and Houdebine, L.-M.: Role of PRL in the transcription of B-casein and 28S ribosomal genes in the rabbit mammary gland. Eur. J. Biochem., *110:*236, 1980.

Teyssot, B., and Houdebine, L.-M.: Role of progesterone and glucocorticoids in the transcription of the B-casein and 28-S ribosomal genes in the rabbit mammary gland. Eur. J. Biochem., *114:*597, 1981.

Theodosin, D. T., and Dreifus, J. J.: Ultrastructural evidence for exo-endocytosis in the neurohypophysis. *In* Moses, A. M., and Share, L. (Eds.): International Conference on the Neurohypophysis. New York, S. Karger, 1977, p. 88.

Tonnesen, E., Brinklov, M. D., Schou, O. A., et al.: Natural killer cell activity in a patient undergoing open-heart surgery complicated by an acute myocardial infarction. Acta Pathol. Microbiol. Immunol. Scand. [C], *93:*229, 1985.

Topper, Y. J., and Freeman, C. S.: Multiple hormone interactions in the developmental biology of the mammary gland. Physiol. Rev. *60:*1049, 1980.

Tulchinsky, D., Hobel, C. J., Yeager, E., et al.: Plasma estrone, estradiol, progesterone, and 17-hydroxyprogesterone in human pregnancy. Am. J. Obstet. Gynecol., *112:*1095, 1972.

Turkington, R. W., and Hill, R. L.: Lactose synthetase: Progesterone inhibition of the induction of x-lactalbumin. Science, *163:*1458, 1969.

Vincent, J. D., Dufy, B., Gourdji, D., et al.: Electrical correlates of prolactin secretion in cloned pituitary cells. *In* MacLeod, R., and Scapagnini, U. (Eds.): Central and Peripheral Regulation of Prolactin Function. New York, Raven Press, 1980, p. 141.

Vonderhaar, B. K.: Local effects of EGF-, TGF-, and EGF-like growth factors on lobuloalveolar development of the mouse mammary gland in vivo. J. Cell. Physiol., *132:*581–584, 1987.

Vonderhaar, B. K.: Lactose synthetase activity in mouse mammary glands is controlled by thyroid hormones. J. Cell Biol., *82:*675, 1979.

Walaszek, Z., Hanausek-Walaszek, M., Minton, J. P., et al.: Dietary glucarate as anti-promoter of 7,12-dimethylbenz(a)anthracene-induced mammary tumorigenesis. Carcinogenesis, 7:1464, 1986.

Wang, D. Y., Hallowes, R. C., Bealing, J., et al.: The effect of prolactin and growth hormone on fatty acid synthesis by pregnant mouse mammary gland in organ culture. J. Endocrinol., *53:*311, 1972.

Waxman, S., and Schreiber, C.: The purification and characterization of the low molecular weight human folate binding protein using affinity chromatography. Biochemistry, *14:*5422, 1975.

Weinberg, E. D.: Iron and infection. Microbiol. Rev., *42:*45, 1978.

White, M. D., Ward, S., and Kuhn, N. J.: Composition, stability and electrolyte permeability of Golgi membranes from lactating rat mammary gland. Biochem. J., *200:*663, 1981.

Yang, J., Guzman, R., Richards, J., et al.: Growth factor- and cyclic nucleotide-induced proliferation of normal and malignant mammary epithelial cells in primary culture. Endocrinology, *107:*35, 1980.

Zimmerman, E. A., and Defendini, R.: Hypothalamic pathways containing oxytocin, vasopressin and associated neurophysins. *In* Moses, A. M., and Share, L. (Eds.): International Conference on the Neurohypophysis. New York, S. Karger, 1977, p. 22.

5

Nutrition and Breast Disease

Sharleen Johnson Birkimer

The notion that what a person eats may be involved in the development of cancer is not a new one; it was discussed in the Middle Ages. In the past decade the public and the scientific community have become very interested in the relationship between dietary components and cancer. An understanding of the role of nutrients in the initiation and promotion of oncogenic cells is important in preventing and managing cancer in humans.

In investigating possible dietary causes of cancer, research has taken two basic forms: epidemiologic investigations and animal studies of whether nutrients are capable of influencing tumor development when consumed in amounts that are within the typical human intake (National Research Council, 1982, 1989a; Rivlin, 1982).

For women in most Western countries breast cancer is the most prevalent cancer. Epidemiologic and experimental evidence indicate that diet is a major etiologic factor, especially after menopause. Most of the research has focused on dietary fat and the possible role of obesity; however, the possible role of protein, various vitamins and minerals, and methylxanthines has also been investigated. Epidemiologic researchers try to associate individual dietary risk factors with the occurrence of disease in a defined population. These studies have been called the most challenging and controversial in cancer epidemiology (Lyon et al., 1983).

Epidemiologic studies can be used to circumvent two limitations of laboratory research in which animal models are used. First, the results can be applied directly to humans; the findings need not be extrapolated from one species to another. Second, because the levels and patterns of exposure to the dietary components occurred in humans, there is no need to interpolate from the artificially high levels frequently used in laboratory animal models.

Epidemiologic studies, however, introduce ethical issues. One cannot add known carcinogens to the diet or remove well-established protective factors. Major changes in diet cannot be allowed during study periods. Bias can enter into the selection of study participants. The women being studied may not be representative of the female population. A major difficulty is the long latency period between the first exposure to the dietary component and the development of breast disease.

METHODS OF COLLECTING DIETARY INFORMATION

Epidemiologists and nutritionists have several methods for collecting dietary information. Some, based on government food production and disappearance statistics, collect group data only indirectly and involve no personal contact with subjects. Other methods assess the nutrient intake of individuals or groups by interview or questionnaire. Each method has strengths and weaknesses. The choice depends on many factors. The primary method of indirectly collecting group data involves calculating the national per capita food consumption by using food balance sheets or food disappearance data. The researcher compares the rates of various types of cancer with the national per capita disappearance of a particular nutrient, such as fat. The researcher must assume an equal distribution of food among the population—and that the amount of food that disappeared was consumed (Armstrong and Doll, 1975; Miller, 1977; National Research Council, 1982; Graham, 1986; Bingham, 1991).

The household food inventory is a more direct method At the beginning of the period, someone records the types and amounts of all food in the house. A record is kept of food purchased and of food consumed away from the home. At the end of the study period, another inventory is performed. Individual dietary data—diet recall, food records or diaries, diet history—better represent what food is actually consumed. The strengths and weaknesses of each form of diet record have been discussed in a number of reviews (Becker et al., 1960; Houser and Bebb, 1981; Sorenson, 1982; Lyon et al., 1983) and book chapters (Willett, 1990a; Witschi, 1990). No method is universally regarded as the most valid and reliable one, and data obtained by one method should be compared advisedly to data obtained by another. Conflicting conclusions in studies may be due to methods that are poorly designed and controlled.

OBESITY

Studies of relationships between obesity and breast cancer are difficult because the association between dietary fat, total calorie intake, and obesity is complex. A gram of fat contains more than twice the kilocalories of a gram of protein or carbohydrate. A diet rich in fat is also commonly high in total kilocalories and may lead to obesity. There also is no universally adopted definition of obesity. In animal studies restricted calorie intake frequently reduced mammary tumors, but the effect could be due to the reduction in consumption of some macronutrient. Reducing the quantity of the usual feeding mixture could reduce the amounts of vitamins and minerals consumed. Obesity may also influence premenopausal women differently than it does postmenopausal women (de Waard, 1964; Reddy,

1986; Albanes, 1987*a;* Osler, 1987; Tornberg et al., 1988; Pathak and Whittemore, 1992).

Animal experiments have taken on importance in the last few years, owing to the lack of definitive human studies (Freedman et al., 1990). Since early in this century calorie restriction has been known to suppress tumor formation. Tannenbaum and coworkers in the 1940s and 1950s reported a consistent reduction in mammary tumors in underfed animals, increased survival time for animals fed a low-calorie ration, and an increase in number of tumors in mice fed a high-fat diet (Tannenbaum, 1947). This work was corroborated by numerous laboratories. Albanes (1987*a*), who reviewed 45 animal experiments on tumor incidence in calorie-restricted rodents, calculated an average decrease in lifetime cumulative tumor incidence of 61%.

Welsch and associates (1990) were able to find no significant differences in the mean number of mammary carcinomas per rat in rats fed diets that contained 5% fat versus 20% fat when caloric intake was restricted to 12% less than ad libitum. Freedman and Clifford (1991), however, believed Welsch's group (1990) overstated the effect of calorie consumption and suggested that the fat effect may be greater with ad libitum feeding than with restricted feeding. Freedman and colleagues (1990) reviewed 100 animal experiments and concluded that higher calorie and fat intake each, independently, increased the incidence of mammary tumor formation but that the effect of calorie intake was more significant.

Early studies of human obesity addressed overweight, as opposed to true obesity (i.e., excess body fat). Overweight was related to deviation from ideal body weight as determined by height (de Waard et al., 1964). Investigators now use Quetelet's index or body mass index (BMI) because obesity can be measured independently of height (Berkowitz et al., 1985; Shun-Zhang, et al., 1990; Simard et al., 1990). This index may be expressed as weight (in kilograms) divided by height (in centimeters or meters) squared (de Waard et al., 1977). The criteria for obesity vary because there is no universally accepted BMI level. A BMI range of 20 to 24.9 is considered normal (Burton and Foster, 1985; Pi-Sunyer, 1988).

A 1985 National Institutes of Health consensus conference (Burton and Foster, 1985) recommended using simple height-weight charts for initial assessment of obesity. They distinguished between tables of *average* heights and weights and weight-for-height tables designed to reflect the lowest mortality rate. The latter are usually labeled *desirable* or *ideal* weights. They suggested the 1959 Metropolitan Life Insurance tables of desirable weight for individuals with a family history or current presence of a disease or with risk factors complicated by obesity. The more liberal 1983 Metropolitan Life Insurance tables could be used for those without these factors. The BMI is a valuable measure in studies of desirable weight. Other studies have evaluated breast cancer risk with skin fold measurements and elbow width (Schapira et al., 1991*a*).

Researchers have recently become interested in *where* body fat is carried. Sellers' group (1992) showed an association between increased central body fat and breast cancer. This observation could provide an explanation for con-

flicting results of previous research. Sellers' group (1992) found that fat pattern predicted the development of postmenopausal breast cancer principally for women with a family history of the disease. A distinctive pattern of body fat may be related to low levels of sex hormone–binding globulin levels in premenopausal breast cancer patients and increased testosterone levels in postmenopausal cases (Schapira et al., 1991*b*).

Benign Breast Disorders

Being thin may increase the risk of developing benign breast disorders (BBDs). Berkowitz and coworkers (1985) found an association between a low Quetelet index and chronic cystic mastopathy in premenopausal and postmenopausal women, but the association was stronger in premenopausal women. Hislop and Elwood (1981) found the association only in women older than 30 years. Although Brinton and associates (1981) did not analyze the data by menopausal status, they too reported an association between a low Quetelet index and BBD. In the Canadian National Breast Screen Study the Quetelet index for women with fibrocystic changes was significantly lower than that of women with breast cancer, but not lower than that of the control subjects (Simard et al., 1990).

Parazzini and colleagues (1984) were not able to demonstrate a linear relationship between BMI and BBD. The lack of consistency in selection of controls, somewhat different criteria for BBDs, and the fact that breast lumps are difficult to detect in women who have more adipose tissue may account for this discrepancy.

Breast Cancer

Epidemiologic research has shown a relationship between the total kilocalories available in a country and mortality from breast cancer (Armstrong and Doll, 1975; Gray et al., 1979). Since a large number of kilocalories can lead to obesity a correlation between excess body fat and breast cancer in postmenopausal females is not surprising. In 1964 de Waard and his coworkers proposed that premenopausal and postmenopausal breast cancer might be two different diseases. They suggested that increased risk in premenopausal women was the result of abnormal ovarian function and that cancer in postmenopausal women was the product of increased estrogen production in excess body fat. In the 1970s, de Waard published several studies showing that postmenopausal women with breast cancer weigh more than their cohorts without cancer. Later, de Waard and colleagues (1977) attributed half of the differences in breast cancer incidence between regions in Holland where the incidence was high and one in Japan where it was low to differences in body height and weight. Much of the correlation is removed if an adjustment is made for the correlation of height and weight. de Waard concluded that overweight, as defined by the Quetelet index, is not so much a risk factor as being both heavy and tall. Having a large body surface area increases the relative risk of breast cancer in postmenopausal women.

The majority of studies report opposite effects of weight on breast cancer risk in premenopausal and postmenopausal women. Eight of fourteen studies found obesity to be protective in premenopausal women and a risk factor for postmenopausal subjects.

Staszewski (1977) studied 900 breast cancer cases and 581 control subjects. The risk was 48% greater for women over 50 years of age who weighed more than 80 kg as compared with those who weighed less than 60 kg. Premenopausal women who weighed 70 to 79 kg had a slightly lower relative risk than women who weighed less than 60 kg. The Quetelet index data showed similar results. Le Marchand and associates (1988) found that a lower Quetelet index at adolescence (but not absolute body weight) was related to premenopausal cancer. A heavy adult weight and weight gain during the adult years were associated with postmenopausal cancer. Interpretation of the findings of Pathak and Whittemore (1992) and Yuan and colleagues (1988) is less straightforward. Pathak and Whittemore (1992) compared the incidence of breast cancer in two countries where the incidence of breast cancer is high, three where it is moderate, and two where it is low. They reported an increasing risk of breast cancer as the Quetelet index increased in postmenopausal women in all the countries. The relationship in premenopausal women, however, varied by country. A Quetelet index over 24 was protective in the United States and Wales. The authors speculated that the differences might reflect differences in the location of the fat in women in various countries.

Willett and researchers at the Channing Laboratory in Boston, Massachusetts, reported one of the few prospective investigations of weight and risk of breast cancer in premenopausal women (Willett et al., 1985). They sent follow-up questionnaires in 1978 and 1980 to the 121,964 married female registered nurses in 11 large U.S. states who had returned a 1976 questionnaire in which they reported their current weight, height, history of cancer diagnoses, and known risk factors for breast malignancy. The risk of breast cancer was 34% lower among women who were in the highest quintile of the Quetelet index. The authors attributed this excess incidence among lean premenopausal women to the relatively greater likelihood of early diagnosis in lean women.

Premenopausal women who weigh in the upper weight categories or are in the upper Quetelet index divisions commonly have a risk ratio of 0.5 when compared with premenopausal women who weigh less or are in lower Quetelet index divisions (Le Marchand et al., 1988). A low adult Quetelet index was associated with an increased risk of premenopausal breast cancer in a study done principally with women who belonged to the Mormon church, but a high index at age 12 years was associated with an increased risk of cancer. The odds ratio, adjusted by multiple regression analysis for other factors that may influence the risk of breast cancer, was over 2.4 for women who had a high Quetelet index level at age 12 years, providing some evidence for an effect of early obesity on premenopausal cancer. Many workers have found a risk ratio of 2.0 or more to be associated with increased weight or higher Quetelet index in postmenopausal women (Staszewski, 1977; Helmrich et al., 1983). Other reports found the risk ratio was

below 2.0, but increased weight or a higher Quetelet index was still associated with increased cancer risk (Kelsey and associates, 1981). The research team led by Saxon Graham (1991) reported increasing adjusted odds ratios with each increment in the Quetelet index, but the levels reached only 1.8.

Being overweight did not emerge as a risk factor in a case-control study done by Lubin and colleagues in Israel (1985a). The premenopausal women and early postmenopausal women did not have a significant difference in BMI, but the postmenopausal women aged 60 years and older did have a significantly higher BMI. These women had at least twice the risk of developing breast cancer when compared to postmenopausal women who had a lower BMI. The premenopausal women with breast cancer that were 40 years old had a significantly lower BMI than the surgical controls. These results support the hypothesis that being underweight for height may be a risk factor for premenopausal women. The Lubin study used weight *prior to* the illness as the "recent weight." This is a better research tool than weight at the time the cancer was diagnosed, which was used by Brisson and coworkers (1984). A potential problem with the Lubin study, however, is that height and weight data were reported by the participants. Other researchers have not been able to find a difference in breast cancer incidence based on the height or weight of the subjects (Burch et al., 1981). Zumoff and Dasgupta (1983) were able to relate obesity to breast cancer only in populations previously known to have a high incidence of obesity. No relationship was found between obesity and breast cancer in populations with a low incidence of obesity. The investigations were done in a variety of countries, which may account for varying results.

Whittemore and associates (1985) found an association between breast cancer risk and increased weight for height during college years, but not 20 to 30 years later. They suggested that weight does not directly influence the risk of developing breast cancer, though it may directly reflect early diet or exercise patterns. The follow-up study of women examined in the National Health and Nutrition Examination Survey I (NHANES I) research project also suggested a potential role for early eating habits (Swanson et al., 1988). Adult height, a possible reflection of nutrient intake early in life, was the only anthropometric value associated with an increased risk of breast cancer. Choi and colleagues found a strong association between postmenopausal cancer and an increase in weight between the time of menopause and diagnosis (Choi et al., 1978). A large case-control study in the San Francisco, California, area found that the relationship began earlier. In this study, an increase in the Quetelet index from age 20 years to the age at interview was one of the strongest predictors of postmenopausal cancer (Paffenbarger et al., 1980). Other investigators confirmed the reports and documented that an increase in weight throughout adult life is associated with an increased risk of postmenopausal cancer (Hislop et al., 1986; Le Marchand et al., 1988). A loss in weight throughout adult life may actually decrease the risk (Lubin et al., 1985a). An effect of early obesity on premenopausal cancer is more difficult to document. One report found the commonly reported inverse relationship between premenopausal cancer and a woman's Quetelet index at age 18 years and as an adult (Pryor et al., 1989). However, the Quetelet index levels at age 12 years were positively related to premenopausal breast cancer. A Canadian study (Hislop et al., 1986) found that women who had been heavy as a child, as a teenager, or as an adult had less premenopausal cancer.

Some investigators have shown that being tall was a risk factor, but adjusting the height for weight generally decreased the risk (Tornberg et al., 1988; Albanes and Taylor, 1990). Some found the risk only in premenopausal or postmenopausal women. A follow-up of the NHANES I study (Swanson et al., 1988) found that the risk of breast cancer was associated only with increased stature and elbow width.

Obesity and Prognosis

Factors that initiate breast cancer may also influence prognosis. Several studies have shown a relationship between body weight and breast cancer mortality. Women in the lowest weight categories, in most of the studies, had the longest survival time or the best prognosis as measured by tumor size or extent of lymph node involvement (Donegan et al., 1978; Boyd et al., 1981; Tartter et al., 1981; Newman et al., 1986; William et al., 1988; Coates et al., 1990; Schapira et al., 1991*a*). Other researchers have found no relationship (Heasman et al., 1985; Hebert and Toporoff, 1989). A 32-year follow-up on subjects participating in the Framingham Heart Study reported that *fluctuations* in body weight had a greater effect on morbidity from all types of cancer than stable weight (Lissner et al., 1991). Breast cancer was not singled out. Tartter's group (1981) found that women who weighed less than 150 lb prior to a mastectomy had a 5-year, disease-free survival rate of 67%, compared with a 49% survival rate for women who weighed more than 150 lb. When body weight and presurgery serum cholesterol levels were both considered, women who weighed more than 150 lb and had a high serum cholesterol value had a significantly shorter survival time than women who weighed less and had a low serum cholesterol level. In 1981, Boyd showed that a body weight of 64 kg (140.8 lb) was a significant dividing line for differences in survival. Women who weighed less than 64 kg survived longest. For Donegan and coworkers (1978) the cutoff point for nonrecurrence of cancer was 58 kg (130 lb) or less, especially if the women did not have axillary lymph node metastases. The authors were able to follow some patients for 24 years after mastectomy. Eberlein and colleagues (1985) reported significantly longer disease-free and survival times for 316 women with breast cancer who weighed less than 64 kg when they first came to the National Cancer Institute. The effect of weight was reduced to statistically insignificant levels when the number of involved nodes and age were included in the analysis.

Several studies analyzed the relationship between the Quetelet index and survival rates (Donegan et al., 1978; Eberlein et al., 1985; Gregorio et al., 1985). All indicated that longer survival time was associated with a low Quetelet index. In one study (Schapira et al., 1991*a*) women who carried excess fat in the upper body, as opposed to the abdominal and thigh regions, appeared to have a more favorable prognosis as measured by less lymph node involvement, smaller tumors, and higher levels of estrogen receptors. Sohrabi and colleagues (1980) and others came to the conclusion that obesity was related to tumor size and node status, but not independently to poor prognosis.

Women frequently gain weight during chemotherapy (Heasman et al., 1985; Huntington, 1985). In a Canadian study designed primarily to observe changes in body weight during adjuvant chemotherapy for breast cancer, Heasman and coworkers (1985) reported no association between a mean weight gain of 4.3 kg and disease recurrence. This was also true for Quetelet index and body surface area, and with and without adjustment for other prognostic factors. Body weight, Quetelet index, and body surface area had no linear relationship to survival. Levine and associates (1991) explored the psychological and biologic factors that led to weight gain in 32 women undergoing chemotherapy. The mean weight gain was 1.8 kg in 2 months of treatment. A follow-up 2 years later showed a mean gain of 6.03 kg in the 27 women who had gained weight. The 12 women who experienced a recurrence gained an average of 1.20 kg, as compared with a gain of 6.53 kg for women who had no recurrence. Thus, weight gain was a predictor of possible remission at 2 years. Decreases in distress, anxiety, and obsessive-compulsive behaviors were associated with increases in weight. The investigators hypothesized that when women had completed chemotherapy they felt less anxious and began to eat more. A group of nurses studied weight gain in 73 women after they underwent definitive surgery (DeGeorge et al., 1990). The women who tended to respond to external eating cues gained the most. They concluded that the gain is controllable through kilocalorie reduction and exercise. Weight gain by 545 women receiving adjuvant therapy following mastectomy for node-positive breast cancer was also reported by Camoriano's group (1990). The median weight change for postmenopausal women following 60 weeks' therapy was 3.6 kg; for premenopausal women the gain was 5.9 kg, as compared to only 1.8 kg for women in both menopausal categories who did not receive treatment. After 6½ years' follow-up, the premenopausal women who had gained more than the median amount of weight at 60 weeks had a relapse rate 1.5 times greater, and a risk of death 1.6 times greater, than the women who were below the median. Relapse and death rates in postmenopausal women were not related to weight gain.

The race of the woman and her nutritional status may interact to govern her survival (Coates et al., 1990). A cohort of 1491 white and 469 Black women in Georgia who had breast cancer were followed for at least 5 years following diagnosis. The Black women tended to have more advanced disease at diagnosis, more lymph node involvement, and shorter survival times than the white women. They also had higher Quetelet index values and lower levels of serum albumin and hemoglobin than did the white women within each stage of disease. The excess mortality among the Black women with Stage III disease was reduced to only 1.14, however, when adjustments were made for the differences in Quetelet index, serum albumin, and hemoglobin. The authors concluded that only a part of the difference in survival between the races could be accounted for by nutritional status; the residual differences in extent of disease at each stage also probably contribute.

LIPIDS

Of all the dietary components that have been associated with breast cancer, lipids have received the most attention. The relationship between a diet high in simple lipids (commonly called dietary fat), especially the polyunsaturated fatty acids, and mammary carcinogenesis has been known since the 1940s. A relationship between polyunsaturated fatty acids and breast cancer is not as clearly demonstrated in human studies as it is in animal work (Hems, 1978). Saturated fatty acids have been more commonly associated with breast cancer in recent human studies (Toniolo et al., 1989*b;* Zaridze et al., 1991). Most human studies have not found an association between the derived lipid, cholesterol, and breast disease (Katsouyanni et al., 1986, 1988; Hirohata et al., 1987). Enthusiasm for a lipid–breast cancer association has waned in recent years. Numerous review articles have been written that reassess the animal and human data. Almost universal agreement exists on a relationship between dietary fat and breast cancer in animal, international correlation, and migrant studies, but case-control and cohort studies provide less compelling evidence.

Animal Experiments

Evidence collected over the last 50 years makes it clear that animals fed high-fat diets develop mammary tumors more readily than those fed low-fat diets (Freedman et al., 1990; Ip, 1990; and Welsch, 1992). The other major finding is the role of polyunsaturated fatty acids in enhancing mammary tumor development (Abraham et al., 1984; Gabor et al., 1985; Sundram et al., 1989; Fischer et al., 1992). All major investigations done after the early 1970s show an awareness of the possible influence of the type of dietary fat on breast cancer development. Saturated fatty acids and the omega-3 series of fatty acids have inhibitory effects, whereas linoleic acid may increase tumorigenesis. Researchers have difficulty separating the effects of total fat from those of various types of fat: A low-total-fat, high–linoleic acid diet does not have the detrimental effects of a diet high in both total fat and linoleic acid.

Epidemiologic Evidence

Several international studies show an association between per capita fat disappearance and breast cancer incidence or mortality (Carroll, 1975; Gray et al., 1979; Rose et al., 1986). Though they are called *food consumption data,* they actually represent food disappearance data. These studies are of interest for generating hypotheses, but data must be interpreted cautiously because they assume equal distribution of food within the population, their quality varies from country to country, and it is not possible to control for confounding variables.

In the 1960s, Lea (1966) conceived that the international differences in breast cancer incidence might be influenced by differences in environmental temperature. Since environmental temperature influences what foods are grown and consumed he examined the consumption of various dietary components in 23 countries. He found a high correlation between dietary fat disappearance and age-adjusted death rate. Armstrong and Doll (1975) determined consumption in some 32 countries, and found that breast cancer incidence ($r = 0.79$) and mortality ($r = 0.89$) were positively correlated with total fat consumption. Gray and coworkers (1979) also showed a positive correlation between the incidence of breast cancer and total fat of 0.78 and a correlation of 0.93 for mortality rates. Armstrong (1976) was not able to relate the increase in breast cancer incidence and mortality in the United States, England, and Wales to fat consumption. Kolonel and associates (1983) suggested that dietary fat was probably only a weak risk factor for breast disease in Hawaii. Rose and colleagues (1986) showed that a positive correlation between total fat intake and breast cancer mortality in 30 countries was stronger for postmenopausal than for premenopausal women. The correlation could be attributed to animal fat intake; no correlation was seen between vegetable fat sources. Israel was an exception, where animal fat intake is low but the mortality rate high. The authors attributed this to the wide variation of breast cancer among the various ethnic groups there. A joint Italian–United States epidemiologic study also reported a relationship between high dietary fat, especially saturated fatty acids, and an increased incidence of breast cancer (Taioli et al., 1991). The consumption of pasta was three times greater in southern Italy than in the United States, and the southern Italians got most of their fat from the oleic acid in olive oil, a monounsaturated fatty acid, whereas in the United States more linoleic acid, a polyunsaturated fatty acid, is used.

The risk for women who emigrate from a country with a low incidence of breast cancer to one with a higher incidence gradually approaches that in the new country. Several studies have suggested that the change is related to dietary habits (Wynder, 1980; Kolonel et al., 1983; Mettlin, 1984). Unfortunately, many migrant studies collect mortality data rather than incidence data, and most do not collect dietary information (Prentice et al., 1989). Another problem is time lag between the diet changes and the manifestation of cancer. Dietary changes may need to occur in childhood to alter the cancer rate of postmenopausal women (London and Willett, 1989). Prentice and Sheppard (1989), however, were able to explain 90% of the variation in breast cancer rates based on per capita fat consumption during periods only 5 years earlier. Breast cancer mortality in the southern region of Italy is 30% to 50% lower than in the northern regions. Toniolo and colleagues (1989*b*) evaluated the effect on breast cancer incidence of internal migration from southern to northern Italy. The sample size was small, but when adjusted for nondietary confounding variables, they determined that place of birth was not as important a factor as diet in breast cancer incidence.

Japan has one of the lowest rates of breast cancer mortality, and the United States one of the highest; the second and third generations of Japanese women who emigrated to the United States display a higher breast cancer mortality rate than the original generation who emigrated (Tominaga, 1985). The increasing age-adjusted death rates for breast cancer in Japan may be related to the increased per capita intake of fat, as the Japanese diet becomes more westernized (Kato et al., 1987). Prentice and associates (1989) calculated a risk of 3.0 for Japanese women in the United States, as compared to women who had remained in Japan. Not all studies have been able to attribute the difference to dietary components. Hirohata and colleagues, in Fukuoka, Japan, were not able to report any difference in total fat, saturated fat, oleic acid, linoleic acid, animal protein, or dietary protein in a case-control study of hospitalized breast cancer patients matched with one hospital and one neighborhood control (Hirohata et al., 1985, 1987). Women who emigrated from Asia and Africa to Israel showed a similar rise in the incidence of breast cancer as they moved from a low-risk to a high-risk area. In this group even the original generation who emigrated showed a rise as they adopted the lifestyle patterns, including the eating habits, of their new country (Modan et al., 1975; Kakar and Henderson, 1985). The breast cancer mortality rate of Polish immigrants appears to approach those of the United States (Staszewski and Haenszel, 1965), United Kingdom (Adelstein et al., 1979), and Australia (Staszewski et al., 1971) within one generation. Similar trends in Italian immigrants to the United States (Haenszel, 1961) and to Australia (Margetts et al., 1981) has been reported.

Other authors have studied breast cancer mortality trends within a small geographic area. The British wartime experience provided a time of reverse Westernization of the diet. During World War II, the fat, sugar, and meat content of the diet in England and Wales decreased. These changes correlated with a reduction in breast cancer mortality rates two decades later. Within the United States, age-adjusted breast cancer mortality rates have been associated positively with consumption of dairy products and negatively with eggs (Gaskill, et al., 1979). One must assume stable eating habits to relate dietary components from the mid-1960s to early 1970s to cancer death rates in 1969 to 1971. Mettlin and colleagues (1990) found that breast cancer patients drank more milk, especially whole milk, than controls.

Case-Control Studies

Of 25 case-control studies published since 1985 that examine diet and risk of breast cancer 10 found a statistically significant relationship between a high level of total dietary fat and the risk of breast cancer. Studies by van't Veer and associates (1989a, 1991) reported a decreased risk with a diet low in total fat and high in fiber and fermented milk. Others (Toniolo et al., 1989b; Zaridze et al., 1991) found an increased intake of fatty acid, but not total dietary fat, associated with increased risk of breast cancer.

In general, food groups rich in fat show a better association with risk than the level of total dietary fat or the type of fatty acids (Hulka, 1989). Animal protein foods (Toniolo et al., 1989a), eggs (Iscovich et al., 1989), meat (Hislop et al., 1986; La Vecchia et al., 1989; Ingram et al., 1991), poultry and fish (Simard et al., 1990), and food groups rich in animal fat (Richardson et al., 1991) all contain significant amounts of fat and were shown to increase the risk of breast cancer. Grains (Pryor et al., 1989), low-fat dairy products and "noncitrus" fruit (Iscovich et al., 1989), and vegetables (La Vecchia et al., 1989; Simard et al., 1990) are all

associated with a decreased risk. Exceptions are found. Iscovich and colleagues (1989) and Pryor and associates (1989) found a decreased risk of breast cancer associated with whole milk or dairy fat. Another report (van't Veer et al., 1990a) found a decreased incidence associated with fermented milk, but not regular milk, when the data were adjusted for fat content of the diet. Many researchers did, however, find an increased risk of breast cancer associated with an increase in total dietary fat (Shun-Zhang et al., 1990; van't Veer et al., 1990a; Richardson et al., 1991), saturated fat (Toniola et al., 1989a,b; Richardson et al., 1991; Zaridze et al., 1991), and monounsaturated fat (Shun-Zhang et al., 1990; Richardson et al., 1991). In general, the relationship was not as significant as that with food groups. Total fat or the type of fatty acids was not associated with risk in several other studies (Rohan et al., 1988; Graham et al., 1991).

Inconsistent results may be due to wide variations in the number of foods on questionnaires. Inaccurate recall also causes variations in results (London and Willett, 1989; Schatzkin et al., 1989a). Nondietary factors are not always determined and their influence on risk is unknown (Rohan and Bain, 1987; Berrino and Muti, 1989). Considering the heterogeneity of the research designs, it is remarkable that so many of these investigations found a relationship between dietary fat and risk of breast cancer.

Two early studies indicating that total fat may be a significant risk factor were done with Canadian women. Miller and associates (1978) interviewed 488 breast cancer patients and 488 well-matched controls using diet history, a food frequency questionnaire, and 24-hour recall. The subjects consumed more total kilocalories, total fat, saturated calories, oleic acid, linoleic acid, and cholesterol than did controls. The second Canadian study (Lubin et al., 1981) showed higher risk ratio factors than the first one. Researchers in Israel (Lubin et al., 1986), United States (Mettlin et al., 1990), Italy (LaVecchia et al., 1987), China (Shun-Zhang et al., 1990), Canada (Simard et al., 1990), Netherlands (van't Veer et al., 1990a), Australia (Ingram et al., 1991), and France (Richardson et al., 1991) all have found total fat, or foods rich in fat, to be associated with increased risk. In addition researchers in the United States (Brisson et al., 1989), Italy (Toniolo et al., 1989b), and Russia (Zaridze et al., 1991) found a positive relationship between a high intake of saturated fatty acids (but not total dietary fat) and breast cancer. Greek workers (Katsouyanni et al., 1986, 1988) found a modest increase in risk associated with monounsaturated fatty acids, but not total dietary fat. Howe and coworkers (1990) combined the original data from 12 case-control studies and concluded that saturated fat (and possibly monounsaturated fat) was associated with an increased risk of breast cancer in postmenopausal women.

Total fat, the type of fatty acids, and food groups high in fat were not associated with a significant breast cancer risk in studies done in Japan (Hirohata et al., 1985), Hawaii (Hirohata et al., 1987), Australia (Rohan et al., 1988), Argentina (Iscovich et al., 1989), and the United States (Graham et al., 1991). In addition, researchers in Greece (Katsouyanni et al., 1988), United States (Brisson et al., 1989), Italy (Toniolo et al., 1989b), and Russia (Zaridze et al., 1991) found a positive relationship between a type of fatty acid, but not total dietary fat, and an increase in breast cancer. Additional studies reported prior to 1985 (Graham et al., 1982; Phillips and Snowdon, 1983) also concluded that dietary fat could not be considered a risk factor. These studies were done in a wide variety of geographic areas with women of widely varying eating habits. Thus, one cannot immediately attribute the opposing conclusions to cultural differences. The studies reported by Hirohata's group in Japan (1985) and Hawaii (1987) are frequently quoted in support of the hypothesis that dietary fat is not related to breast cancer.

All except one of these research teams reported on the adult diet. The focus of the study by Pryor and associates (1989) was on adolescence. After adjusting for traditional risk factors, decreased premenopausal breast cancer risk was actually associated with an "adolescent diet" high in fat.

The ability to replicate findings at a later date in the same population adds reliability to results. Graham and colleagues demonstrated this capability in two large-scale case-control studies using subjects in western New York. The 1982 study failed to show an increased risk of breast cancer associated with animal fat, vegetable fat, or total fat consumption. Almost a decade later Graham and associates (1991) also failed to find any relationship between fat intake and breast cancer.

Assuming that spouses ate similar diets, Nomura and colleagues (1978) studied the diets of 86 Japanese men married to women who had breast cancer and compared their diets to those of 6774 Japanese men married to women without breast cancer. Based on personal records of the frequency with which various foods were eaten, the spouses of women with breast cancer consumed more meat, butter, margarine, and cheese, corn, and wieners than did the control spouses.

Mammary Tissue

Conflicting evidence for a role for fat in causing breast cancer risk comes from case-control studies using mammary tissue samples. Fatty acid profiles of subcutaneous fat from 53 women undergoing surgery at Guy's Hospital in London, England (Caleffi et al., 1987), did not reveal differences between the control women and breast cancer cases. These results were similar to those from the Israeli study (Eid and Berry, 1988) of adipose tissue obtained from 85 sequential patients undergoing breast biopsy. The fat did not differ in women with carcinoma, fibroadenoma, or other types of breast disease. The lack of difference in fatty acid composition may be due to the absence of wide variation in the fatty acid composition of the diet of the cases and the controls. Hill and Wynder (1987) reported a significantly greater amount of linoleic and stearic acid and a significantly lower amount of palmitic and oleic acid in tissue from American postmenopausal patients as compared with Japanese cases. No difference was found in the fatty acid composition of breast tissue in premenopausal Japanese and American women.

Prospective Studies

Prospective studies involve following a group of women over a period of time. Time and cost are two reasons few prospective studies are conducted. Only two since 1985 (Vatten et al., 1990; Howe et al., 1991a) reported a relationship between diet and risk. The women in the NHANES I Epidemiological Follow-up Study cohort actually provided evidence for a protective effect of high fat intake in premenopausal women. The Nurses' Health Study (Willett et al., 1992) showed a similar trend among both premenopausal and postmenopausal women. The largest of these prospective studies, by Willett and associates (1992), involved 89,494 nurses who were followed for 8 years. A 61-item food-frequency questionnaire was used to determine the nutrient content of the nurses' diets. During the follow-up, 1439 cases of breast cancer were diagnosed among the 89,494 subjects. After adjusting for known determinants of breast cancer, the relative risk of developing breast cancer did not differ for women in the highest quintile of calorie-adjusted total fat intake and those in the lowest quintile. The risk was actually lower in the higher quintiles than at the lowest quintile. Women who got less than 29% of their total kilocalories from fat had the highest relative risk of breast cancer. Similar results were found for saturated fatty acids, linoleic acid, and cholesterol. The menopausal status of the women did not make a difference in their relative risk. This well-done prospective study discourages the hypothesis that the amount of fat in a woman's diet is the most significant factor in the development of breast cancer. A study of 34,388 postmenopausal women from Iowa (Kushi et al., 1992) produced conflicting results. After adjustment for known risk factors, a "modest" positive association was found between total dietary fat and polyunsaturated fatty acid intake and breast cancer. However, three other statistical procedures involving energy adjustment failed to support a positive association. A study in the Netherlands (van den Brandt et al., 1993) also involved only postmenopausal women, but the observations reported by the authors are similar to those of the NHANES I study and the observations on the women from Iowa.

Type of Fat

Food-frequency questionnaires are seldom specific enough to obtain an accurate estimate of saturated, monounsaturated, and polyunsaturated fatty acids, so it is not surprising that most studies fail to find an influence on risk for a type of fatty acid. Howe (1991a) found that monounsaturated fatty acids increased risk. Eight of their twelve case-control studies that estimated fatty acid by degree of saturation found some relationship with breast cancer. The consumption of monounsaturated fatty acids (Katsouyanni et al., 1986, 1988; Shun-Zhang et al., 1990) and saturated fatty acids (Brisson et al., 1989; Toniolo et al., 1989a,b; Richardson et al., 1991; Zaridze et al., 1991) were marginally associated with an increased risk of breast cancer. A large intake of polyunsaturated fatty acids tended to decrease the risk in one study (Zaridze et al., 1991).

Nutritionists currently recommend that less than 30% of

an individual's total kilocalories come from fat. No prospective studies adequately address the incidence of breast cancer in diets this low in fat. Future prospective studies may need to be carried on longer because it is not clear where in the life cycle the influence of dietary factors is greatest.

Fat and Prognosis

The fat in the diet of women with breast cancer may be related to survival. Morrison and colleagues (1976) suggested the low level of dietary fat normally found in the Japanese diet may be an explanation for the longer survival time for Japanese women with breast cancer as compared with American women. Kyogoku and associates (1992) provided support for this hypothesis when they were not able to report a relationship between the 1-, 5-, and 10-year survival rates from breast cancer and dietary fat in 212 Japanese breast cancer patients who underwent surgical procedures between 1975 and 1978. The greater amount of linoleic acid found in breast tissue of American postmenopausal breast cancer patients when compared with postmenopausal Japanese women with breast cancer (Hill and Wynder, 1987) may be a factor in the shorter relapse-free survival time for American women. Linoleic acid is a precursor of arachidonic acid and prostaglandins that may be associated with increased risk of breast tumors. In contrast, Verreault and colleagues (1988) provided evidence that polyunsaturated fatty acids reduce—and saturated fat increases—the percentage of postmenopausal patients who have involved nodes.

Serum Lipids and Breast Disease

Although hypercholesteremia is a well-recognized risk factor for atherosclerosis, any relationship to cancer is less clearly established. Studies have reported lower (Vatten and Foss, 1990; Potischman et al., 1991), higher (Bani et al., 1986; Cowan et al., 1990), and no different (Keys et al., 1985; Howson et al., 1986) serum cholesterol levels in breast cancer cases than in controls. The positive relationship reported by Dyer and coworkers (1981) in a large, Chicago-based study needs to be interpreted cautiously (Rose and Shipley, 1980). A 20-year Swedish cohort study of 46,570 women younger than 75 years does not show a clear trend in the relationship between breast cancer risk and serum cholesterol (Tornberg et al., 1988). Women under 50 years of age showed a negative correlation. A few studies (Howson et al., 1986; Potischman, et al., 1991) investigated a relationship between cholesterol and the stage of breast cancer. Tartter (1981) found high body weight combined with high serum cholesterol to be associated with advanced stages, but neither factor alone showed an association. Howson (1986) could not identify a relationship between breast cancer stage and serum cholesterol. Potischman and colleagues (1991) found a high level of serum triglycerides in breast cancer patients, especially in association with a low serum beta-carotene level. Boyd and others (Boyd et al., 1982; Brisson et al., 1982; Wolfe et al.,

1987) found mammographic evidence of dysplasia to be associated with higher levels of high-density lipoprotein type C and with a family history of breast cancer. Women with dysplasia had lower serum triglyceride levels, but this association was removed when a history of breast cancer was taken into consideration. Boyd and McGuire (1990) concluded that some of the differences in the high-density lipoprotein type C levels of populations is due to the association of a greater total intake of dietary fat and of polyunsaturated fatty acids with higher high-density lipoprotein type C levels.

Mechanisms

Increased risk of breast cancer related to early menarche, nulliparity, late first full-term pregnancy, and late menopause (Moore et al., 1983) suggest hormonal involvement in mammary carcinogenesis, and fatty acids are the metabolic precursors of reproductive hormones. Several articles have addressed mechanisms by which dietary fat, hormones, and breast cancer may interact (Welsch, 1987; Williams and Dickerson, 1987; Hagerty et al., 1988; Carroll and Parenteau, 1991). The most common theory is that dietary fats modify endogenous hormone status, and the alterations can enhance or retard tumor development. Estrogens and prolactin are the major hormones. Plasma prolactin levels generally decrease with increasing parity (Kwa et al., 1981). Meyer and coworkers (1986) found elevated serum prolactin in 41 premenopausal women with breast cancer, and Ingram and colleagues (1990) reported a twofold increase in prolactin levels. Postprandial levels of prolactin are higher in the women with Stage II disease than in those with Stage I disease (Goettler et al., 1990). Other research includes the possible role of lipid in alteration of cell-mediated cytotoxicity (Thomas and Erickson, 1985), inhibition of mammary intercellular communication by fatty acids (Aylsworth et al., 1984), use of antioxidants to inhibit lipid-induced mammary carcinogenesis, and the transfer of growth factors from adipose tissue of the mammary gland to the glandular tissue (Carroll and Parenteau, 1991).

Data on the ability of high levels of fat in the diet to affect hormone levels are conflicting (Welsch, 1987; Carroll and Parenteau, 1991). Experimental evidence does show the ability of fat to influence serum and urine hormone levels. Reducing dietary fat from 35% to 21% of total kilocalories significantly reduced serum total estrogens, estrone, and estradiol in premenopausal women with cystic breast disease and cyclic mastalgia (Rose et al., 1987); a low fat diet reduced total and weakly bound plasma estradiol in 73 postmenopausal women without breast disease who were not using exogenous hormones (Prentice et al., 1990). Shultz and associates (1987), however, could find no difference in plasma and urine hormone levels between vegetarians (who consumed 28% of their energy as fat) and nonvegetarians (36%). However, within the nonvegetarian group, serum prolactin levels increased with an increase in total fat. Ingram and coworkers (1989) could not change estradiol by lowering the fat content from 40% to 20% of total kilocalories. Vegetarians do have significantly lower plasma levels of estradiol-17β than nonvegetarians (Barbosa et al., 1990).

PROTEIN AND CARBOHYDRATE

Only the macronutrients—protein, lipid, and carbohydrate—contribute kilocalories to the diet, and the percentage of kilocalories in the diet from one macronutrient influences the percentages of the other two. If the kilocalories intake from protein and fat is higher than average, carbohydrate will represent a smaller proportion. Because nutrients are so interrelated in food, it is frequently difficult to separate the respective influences of dietary protein, carbohydrate, and lipids on breast disease. Foods rich in animal protein are commonly also rich in fat.

It is not surprising, then, that large portions of foods rich in both dietary protein and lipids are frequently positively correlated with breast cancer (Toniolo et al., 1989*a*; Shun-Zhang et al., 1990). Refined sugar is positively related to the breast cancer mortality rate because the women in industrialized nations whose diet is rich in fat and protein usually also consume a lot of refined sugar (Lubin et al., 1981). Prentice and colleagues (1988), however, did not find a relationship between per capita consumption of either protein or carbohydrate and breast cancer incidence in 21 countries. The dietary intake of protein and carbohydrate did not influence the mammographic patterns in Canadian women with breast cancer as compared to control women in the Canadian National Breast Screening Study (Brisson et al., 1989).

Protein

Few studies report actual protein consumed in grams for breast cancer patients and control subjects. Shun-Zhang and associates (1990) reported that patients consumed significantly more protein per day (mean = 67 g) than controls (mean = 61 g). When the higher total kilocalories and fat consumed by patients were taken into consideration, however, the difference disappeared.

Diet researchers commonly use animal products, milk, or meat as categories. Some (Vatten and Foss, 1990; Ingram et al., 1991; Richardson et al., 1991) report a positive relationship between one or more of the categories and breast cancer; others (Hirohata et al., 1987; Mills et al., 1988; Iscovich et al., 1989; Mills et al., 1989) do not. Some of the differing results may be attributable to the amount of meat and cheese consumed. The fat in an ounce of meat or cheese can vary from 1 to 8 g (Pennington and Church, 1985). Some differences could be in the wide range of individual fat consumption per day. In an Italian study (La Vecchia et al., 1987), the risk of developing breast cancer was significant only when the women consumed more than 7 portions of meat a week.

Van't Veer (1991), however, found a negative association with breast cancer and fermented milk products, even after adjusting for the amount of fat in the diet. Perhaps, the microorganisms in fermented milk products have a protective role that is more powerful than the amount of total

fat. Le and associates (1986) reported a negative relationship between yogurt consumption and breast cancer but a positive association between high-fat cheese consumption and the fat consumed in milk. These results support the theory that fermented milk products may produce fewer gut bacteria that synthesize carcinogens than do unfermented products.

Carbohydrate

Fiber is the carbohydrate that has received most attention in relation to breast disease. Most studies report an association between increased dietary fiber and decreased risk of breast cancer (Hebert et al., 1989; Pryor et al., 1989; van't Veer et al., 1990*b*). One of the difficulties in interpreting these data is that diets rich in fat are usually low in fiber; thus it is hard to separate the influence of fat from that of fiber. The high fat and fiber content of the Finnish diet, however, supports an important role for high fiber, because the breast cancer mortality rate is lower there than in countries where the typical diet is low in fiber and high in fat (Adlercreutz et al., 1986). Graham and colleagues (1982) and the Nurses' Health Study (Willett et al., 1992) could report no effect for dietary fiber on breast cancer risk. No studies report a negative influence of fiber.

Several studies postulate a role for fiber in estrogen metabolism. The literature generally supports an inverse relationship between dietary fiber and breast cancer. Goldin (1982, 1986) and Barbosa (1990) and their groups reported higher fecal excretion of estrogens and lower plasma concentrations of estrogens associated with high fiber intake. Rose (1990) hypothesizes, "Dietary fat promotes intestinal reabsorption of estrogens by enhancement of deconjugating enzyme activity, whereas intraluminal fiber retards this process." One study (Rohan et al., 1990) suggested a decrease in benign proliferative epithelial disorders of the breast associated with intake of much fiber. A diet high in fiber may contribute to the more favorable prognosis for women who have had surgery for breast cancer (Holm et al., 1989).

Animal Data

Very little animal work has focused on protein or carbohydrate intake. Carroll (1975) did an extensive review and concluded that dietary protein had little, if any, effect on the formation of mammary tumors. The conflict between epidemiologic data and Carroll's review is probably due to the ability of animal researchers to "fine-tune" rations for energy content. Cohen's group (1991) indicated that dietary fiber could protect against N-nitrosomethylurea (U)–induced rat mammary tumors when rats were fed a high-fat diet. The fiber did not influence serum estradiol-17β levels, a finding in opposition to the human data (Barbosa et al., 1990; Rohan et al., 1990). Serraino and Thompson (1992) reported inconsistent effects on rat mammary tumorigenesis when they supplemented a high-fat corn oil diet with 5% flaxseed flour. The flaxseed-supplemented diet reduced the size of tumors only when it was fed in the promotional stage or throughout the experiment, not when fed during initiation. The authors speculated that the results may be due to the antiestrogenic effect of the high fiber (lignan) content of the flaxseed.

VITAMINS AND MINERALS

Most of the epidemiologic and animal research relating dietary components to breast disease has focused on the role of lipids and excess body fat; the role of the micronutrients, vitamins, and minerals has received little attention.

Vitamin A

Vitamin A is the name for a diverse collection of chemical compounds. The naturally occurring retinoid forms found predominantly in animal foods are retinol (the alcohol), retinaldehyde (the aldehyde), and retinoic acid (the acid form). The precursor forms, the carotenes, are found in plant foods, especially green or yellow ones. Carrots, broccoli, and acorn squash are all rich in carotenes. Only about 50 of the approximately 500 carotenoids that exist are actually precursors of retinol. Beta-carotene is the most active of these carotenes. Most of the carotene is converted to retinol in the intestinal mucosal cells (National Research Council, 1989b). Approximately 6 μg of beta-carotene is required to produce 1 μg of retinol, but the actual amount apparently depends on dietary intake: under conditions of low dietary intake of carotenes the rate of conversion to retinol is much higher. Excess carotene is stored mostly in body fat. Retinol is mobilized from the liver and transported to the target tissues in a complex of retinol, retinol-binding protein, and transthyretin (formerly called prealbumin). There appear to be cell-surface receptors on the target cells that recognize retinol-binding protein and permit the entry of retinol (Hunt and Groff, 1990).

The Recommended Dietary Allowance (RDA) of vitamin A for nonpregnant, nonlactating females older than 11 years is 800 μg of retinol equivalents (RE) per day. One RE is defined as 1 μg of all-*trans*-retinol, 6 μg of all-*trans*-beta-carotene, or 1.2 μg of other pro–vitamin A carotenoids (National Research Council, 1989b; Hunt and Groff, 1990). Before 1974, the RDA for vitamin A was measured in International Units (IU), and 800 RE is approximately 4000 IU. The advantage of using RE as the unit of measurement is that it takes into account the variations in absorption and metabolism of the various forms of vitamin A. Some food charts and food labels still list vitamin A in terms of IU and assume that animal foods contain retinol and plant foods provide the vitamin in the beta-carotene form. Research articles in breast disease usually still state dietary vitamin A in IU because many nutrient databases, especially those in Europe, still use this unit of measurement.

Because vitamin A is stored in the liver, it is not essential that the RDA be consumed every day. When consumed in excess, vitamin A is known to be toxic. The daily intake of vitamin A needed and how long this much must be consumed before toxic levels are reached varies among persons, but toxic symptoms have been associated with a daily intake of as little as 15,000 μg of retinol from a combination of food and supplements. Dietary carotene generally is not thought to be toxic, but an alarming yellowing of the skin may occur if large amounts of foods rich in beta-carotene are consumed (Bendich and Langseth, 1989).

Experimental work with animals shows that retinoids inhibit the carcinogenic process in mammary cells. McCormick and coworkers (1980, 1983) and Holtzman (1988) demonstrated an inhibition of mammary cancer when retinyl acetate was fed to rats. Grubbs and associates (1977) inhibited the incidence of 7,12-dimethylbenz(a)anthracene–induced benign and cancerous mammary tumors with the synthetic retinoid, retinyl methyl ether. Takahashi and Biempica (1985) suggested the possibility of using vitamin A to prevent mammary metastasis by inhibiting the production of collagenases. Lacroix and colleagues (1990) were able to slow the progression of mammary tumors in ovariectomized rats. Nagasawa (1984) found a different effect. He reported an increase in the incidence of both pregnancy-dependent and autonomous mammary tumors in mice that were fed vitamin A. All of the experimental mice developed mammary tumors by 13 months of age, as contrasted with 57.9% of control mice. The animal data generally support the ability of beta-carotene to inhibit mammary tumors (Rettura et al., 1983; Seifter et al., 1984).

Reports on human breast disease and vitamin A are difficult to compare. Some investigators reported on dietary carotene or retinol (Iscovich et al., 1989; van't Veer, 1990b, 1991); others studied the plasma carotene or plasma retinol levels of breast cancer patients and of controls (Marubini et al., 1988; Potischman et al., 1991). Vegetables as a food group, and not the actual retinol or carotene intake, were the focus of studies in Greece (Katsouyanni et al., 1986), Italy (La Vecchia et al., 1987), and Canada (Simard et al., 1990).

The results are as diverse as the methods. An increase in dietary beta-carotene significantly decreased the risk of breast cancer (La Vecchia et al., 1987; Rohan et al., 1988), decreased estrogen receptor–negative breast cancers, but not estrogen receptor–positive ones (Cooper et al., 1989), and reduced high-risk images on mammograms (Brisson et al., 1989). Beta-carotene was weakly protective against breast cancer in another report in which total calorie intake was taken into consideration (Iscovich et al., 1989). For Greek women (Katsouyanni et al., 1988) high consumption of vitamin A, retinol, or carotene was protective against breast cancer. Several investigators found no relationship between either vitamin A or beta-carotene intake and breast cancer in case-control comparisons (Potischman et al., 1990; van't Veer et al., 1991). The risk of breast cancer varied very little with vitamin A intake in an Australian study reported by Rohan and colleagues (1988) and in an Italian study by Marubini and coworkers (1988).

Little work has been reported on benign breast disorders. Vitamin A supplements were protective against the development of proliferative breast disease but not against severe atypias and borderline carcinoma in the Canadian National Breast Screening Study (Hislop et al., 1990). No relationship was found between retinol or beta-carotene and proliferative epithelial disorders (Rohan et al., 1990; Potischman et al., 1990). Vitamin A may be a useful treatment for the pain of benign breast disorders in women who are not responsive to methylxanthine withdrawal or analgesics (Band et al., 1984). When 12 premenopausal women with measurable pain from benign breast disease were treated with 30,000 RE (150,000 IU) vitamin A per day for 3 months, nine patients reported a marked improvement in breast pain, and five had a complete or partial decrease in measurable breast masses. Unfortunately, mammographic parenchymal patterns remained unchanged and half the subjects developed toxicity.

Most studies indicate no relationship between breast cancer and plasma retinol (Russell et al., 1988; Potischman et al., 1990) or beta-carotene (Schrijver et al., 1987; Marubini et al., 1988). Wald and colleagues (1984) found a tendency for serum beta-carotene levels to be lower in patients with breast cancer than in controls; Marubini and associates showed increased cancer risk as blood retinol levels increased.

Interactions between serum retinol and carotenes may have varying results. Potischman and associates reported no relationship between serum retinol and breast disease except in women with low beta-carotene levels. In this group risk for breast cancer increased as serum retinol increased within the lowest quartile of beta-carotene levels. The lower serum beta-carotene levels found in breast cancer patients may be the result, not the precursor, of the disease. Potischman's group (1990) reported decreasing beta-carotene levels in the serum at later stages of the disease, possibly owing to lower dietary intake of vitamin A. Some researchers report a relationship between dietary intake and serum retinol level (Marubini et al., 1988) or serum carotene level (Marubini et al., 1988; Potischman, 1990). Schrijver and colleagues (1987) found the amount of carotenoids in the diet was reflected in plasma carotenoids, but total vitamin A intake was not related to plasma retinol. A British study could not find a relationship between the stage of cancer and serum beta-carotene levels (Wald et al., 1984).

Vitamin D

Preliminary evidence exists that vitamin D might reduce the incidence of breast cancer. Garland and his colleagues found a negative association between vitamin D from exposure to sunlight and the development of breast cancer (Garland et al., 1990). The annual age-adjusted mortality rate for breast cancer varied from 17 to 19 per 100,000 in the South and Southwestern United States to 33 per 100,000 in the Northeastern states. Similar results were reported by Gorham's group (1989). Women with vitamin D receptors in breast tissue may have a better survival rate than those who lack them (Colston et al., 1989). Animal studies suggest that vitamin D inhibits the growth of breast cancer cell cultures (DeLuca and Ostrem, 1980; Eisman et al., 1980; Abe et al., 1991), but the diets of Canadian women with breast cancer contained more vitamin D than those of controls (Simard et al., 1991).

Vitamin E

Vitamin E is really a mixture of at least eight compounds, including tocopherols and tocotrienols. By international agreement, natural alpha-tocopherol is designated RRR-alpha-tocopherol, and the synthetic compound is all-rac-alpha-tocopherol. Since 1980, the vitamin activity in the RDA has been expressed in milligrams of alpha-tocopherol equivalents (TE). TE take into consideration the potency of the various forms of vitamin E. The RDA for a nonpregnant, nonlactating female 11 years of age or older is 8 mg alpha-TE. The amount of vitamin needed in the diet increases with the intake of polyunsaturated fatty acids. It has not been possible to devise a formula to relate vitamin need to intake of polyunsaturated fatty acids. As a result, the RDA is based on the amount needed to support blood levels of vitamin E that are considered adequate. Again, IU still are sometimes used in current literature. Conversion of IU to milligrams depends on the form of tocopherol, but 1 mg of the acetate form of the synthetic compound is equal to 1 IU of alpha-tocopherol. Most food composition tables list only the alpha-tocopherol content of foods, so it is difficult to relate intake to TE (Guthrie, 1986).

The best-researched role of vitamin E is as an antioxidant in plant and animal tissue, especially those containing polyunsaturated fatty acids. In the absence of adequate antioxidants, excessive free radicals may form from the oxidation of unsaturated fatty acids and damage the tissue (Guthrie, 1986). Selenium is also an endogenous antioxidant because it is an essential component of glutathione peroxidase, one of the major enzymes involved in protecting cells against oxidative tissue damage (Chow, 1979). The higher the level of polyunsaturated fatty acids in the diet, the greater is the need for an antioxidant to prevent tissue damage (Witting, 1969). At least one species of animal (hens) appears to require no antioxidant at all if its diet is low enough in fat (Bieri et al., 1960).

The roles of selenium and vitamins A, C, and E in the antioxidant process, and in prevention of cancer, have been reviewed by several authors (Kakar and Henderson, 1985; McCay, 1985; Kline and Sanders, 1991; Vitamin E Research Service, 1991).

Harman (1969) and Lee and Chen (1979) showed some reduction in tumors in animals fed vitamin E, but other researchers (Beth et al., 1987) were not able to do so. Only one large-scale human study (Wald et al., 1984) has investigated the role of vitamin E in the prevention of breast cancer. The investigations by Schrijver and colleagues (1987) and Gerber and associates (1989) compared dietary vitamin E for patients and control subjects. No difference was found by either group. The unexpectedly high serum vitamin E level of women with breast cancer observed by Gerber's group (1988, 1989) was attributed to their intake of linoleic acid and vitamin E in sunflower oil. Several reports concern the use of vitamin E for benign breast disorders. Abrams (1965) found vitamin E useful in relieving some of the symptoms of menopause. Two other investigators (London et al., 1978; Sundaram et al., 1981) reported a positive response to vitamin E in women with mammary dysplasia. Others have found no effect for vitamin E in the treatment of benign breast disease (Ernster et al., 1985; Meyer et al., 1990). Ernster and colleagues conducted a 2-month, double-blind, randomized clinical trial in which 37 women took 600 mg alpha-tocopherol and 36 women took a placebo. Meyer and associates (1990) also used 600 mg of alpha-tocopherol in a 3-month trial in 105 women whose benign breast disease had been confirmed by mammography. Both concluded vitamin E had no effect.

Selenium

Most of the literature on selenium in carcinogenesis was published in the last 15 years (Newberne and Saphakarn, 1983). Combs and Clark (1985) concluded, "Almost all of these investigations have found high-level [selenium] treatments to cause at least moderate (15% to 35%) reductions in tumor incidence." Selenium treatments were ineffective in reducing tumors in only eight studies. Several authors observed a decrease in spontaneous (Schrauzer et al., 1978) or chemically induced (Ip et al., 1985, 1992; Maruyama et al., 1991) mammary tumors when animals were fed selenium or when it was added to a selenium-deficient diet (Harr et al., 1972). The addition of selenium is especially beneficial if the animal's diet is rich in polyunsaturated fat (Ip and Sinha, 1981). Other authors (Takada et al., 1992) report that a combination of vitamin E and selenium inhibits 7,12-dimethylbenz[a]anthracene (DMBA)–induced mammary tumors. After adding selenium to the high-fat diet of rats before and after the administration of DMBA, Ip (1981) concluded that the element had a prophylactic effect on both the initiation and the promotion phases of carcinogenesis, but continuous consumption is necessary. Selenium was able to inhibit the reappearance of mammary tumors that had regressed after ovariectomy. His data suggest that selenium may function not only as a chemopreventive agent but as an adjuvant chemotherapeutic. Horvath and Ip (1983) found that vitamin E supplementation alone was ineffective in reducing the incidence of DMBA tumors. The addition of selenium, however, significantly reduced tumor incidence. Selenium supplementation alone did not. Horvath and Ip (1983) and Medina and coworkers (1983) all found that the anticarcinogenic action of selenium could not be attributed to the role of selenium in glutathione peroxidase activity. This may be because the enzyme itself is the limiting factor. It is already operating near its maximal capacity, and additional selenium cannot further increase activity. Food scientists may be able to increase the selenium content of vegetables and potentiate the anticarcinogenic properties of selenium. Ip and colleagues (1992) were able to enhance the anticarcinogenic capability of selenium-rich garlic by incorporating more selenium into garlic cultivated in a greenhouse. Stoewsand and colleagues (1989), however, were not successful in further reducing the incidence of mammary cancer in animals fed brussels sprouts by adding more selenium to them.

Epidemiologic studies show conflicting evidence for a relationship between selenium and breast cancer. Using food disappearance data, Schrauzer and colleagues (1976, 1977a,b) have correlated per capita intake of selenium with cancer mortality rates in more than 20 countries. They found an inverse relationship between selenium intake and several cancers, including breast cancer. Using pooled blood from healthy donors in 22 countries, they found a inverse relationship between serum selenium level and breast cancer. In case-control studies McConnell and colleagues (1980) and Schrijver and associates (1987) found that patients had significantly lower serum selenium levels than control subjects. Basu and coworkers (1989) also found lower serum selenium levels in breast cancer patients when they compared the levels in 30 breast cancer patients, 29 women with benign breast disease, and 30 control subjects. Shamberger and coworkers (1973), Meyer and Verreault (1987), and Knekt and his colleagues (1991), however, could not report a relationship between selenium levels in the blood of breast cancer patients and of control subjects. Researchers in the prospective Nurses' Health Study (Hunter et al., 1990) found no differences in the selenium content of toenail clippings from women who developed breast cancer during the 53 months of the study and those who did not.

The evidence for a relationship between vitamin E and breast disease is not as compelling as for selenium. It is difficult to make a recommendation with certainty, but presently women should be encouraged to include in their diets foods rich in vitamin E and in selenium.

No RDA has been established for selenium, but the National Academy of Sciences considers 58 to 288 μg to be in the adequate and safe range. The selenium content of plant foods depends on the soil in which they were grown. Animals develop selenium poisoning if they graze predominantly on plants growing in selenium-rich soil (Guthrie, 1986). Since humans consume food grown in a wide range of soils, they are not likely to develop selenium toxicity unless they supplement their diets with large amounts. As little as 2.5 to 3.8 mg of selenium may produce harmful effects (Underwood, 1973; Young and Richardson, 1979).

Other Vitamins and Minerals

Very little research has been done on other vitamins and minerals. The most comprehensive study by Schrijver and colleagues (1987) found that levels of 25-OH-vitamin D and copper were lower in untreated breast cancer patients than in control subjects. The breast cancer patients and controls had similar serum folic acid, vitamin B_{12}, and zinc levels, but serum levels of ferritin and copper were higher in the postmenopausal patients. The latter finding is different from the reports of Dabek and coworkers (1992), who found that the premenopausal women with breast cancer had higher serum copper levels than the premenopausal controls, but there was no significant difference between the two groups of postmenopausal women.

An interesting subject for future research is the possible protective role of table salt. Pawlega, in Cracow, Poland (1989), asked women to complete a 44-item food-frequency questionnaire as part of a case-control study and found a negative association between salt intake and breast cancer risk. Pawlega speculated that it might be the selenium or iodine in the salt that exerted the protective effect. Considerable attention has been focused on ascorbic acid (vitamin C) in preventing cancer (Cameron et al., 1979; Newberne and Saphakarn, 1983), but little has been reported concerning its possible role in breast cancer. Graham and coworkers (1982) found no relationship between ascorbic acid intake and breast cancer. Since portion sizes of food were not estimated, one can only say the breast cancer patients did not differ in their frequency of consuming foods rich in ascorbic acid. The biologic mechanism(s) by which ascorbic acid might assist in the prevention or treatment of breast cancer are a matter of speculation. Ascorbic acid prevents scurvy, but research has also shown that ascorbic acid may be important in many biochemical systems. Ascorbic acid is used in the synthesis of collagen and of some hormones and neurotransmitters, including norepinephrine, epinephrine, and serotonin; as a detoxifier of some carcinogens; and as a possible protector of vitamins E and A from oxidation (Block and Menkes, 1989; Henson et al., 1991).

ETHANOL

Beginning the early 1980s, large-scale epidemiologic studies attempted to relate alcohol consumption to breast cancer. Large case-control studies with 1000 or more cases and a like number of control subjects (Le et al., 1984; Harvey et al., 1987; La Vecchia et al., 1989; Kato et al., 1989) have shown increases of up to three times in the relative risk of breast cancer for women who drank alcohol. Two prospective studies reported in 1987 (Schatzkin et al., 1987; Willet et al., 1987*b*) and one in 1988 (Hiatt et al., 1988) also found statistically significant relationships between alcohol consumption and the development of breast cancer. These results were obtained when the traditional risk factors, such as hormone status, obesity, and number of children, were taken into consideration. Other large-scale case-control studies, however, have found none (Harris and Wynder, 1988; Chu et al., 1989). Two prospective studies (Hiatt and Bawol, 1984; Schatzkin et al., 1989*b*) also did not. Some conflict may be attributed to sampling differences. For example, about 5% of the women in the California study (Hiatt and Bawol, 1984) consumed more than three drinks per day. In a study by Byers and Funch (1982), the largest amount of alcohol consumed was less than one drink per day. Le and coworkers (1984) included women with cholelithiasis in their control subjects, but La Vecchia and colleagues (1985*a*) considered women with cholelithiasis to be ineligible because of the association with obesity and multiparity, two factors known to influence breast cancer. A review of these studies indicates that the studies reporting a positive relationship are more likely to have used hospital controls. Women who consume alcohol may be more likely than women who do not to be admitted to the hospital for other diseases. The type of alcohol may be a factor. Wine and stronger alcoholic drinks may increase the risk more than beer, even when the amount of pure alcohol is equivalent (Richardson et al., 1989). Conversely, Willett and colleagues in the Nurses' Health Study (1987) and Harvey and associates (1987) found that beer and hard liquor elevated the risk of breast cancer but wine did not influence the risk. Most studies reported an increasing risk with increased alcohol consumption, but Hiatt and Bawol (1984), van't Veer and associates (1989*b*), and Toniolo and colleagues (1989*c*) found alcohol consumption only increased the risk of breast cancer if the consumption was above levels of intake commonly considered moderate. Other

studies (Harvey et al., 1987; O'Connell et al., 1987; Hiatt et al., 1988) did not control for other dietary variables, such as fat. Schatzkin and colleagues (1989*c*) reported any positive association between alcohol and the risk of breast cancer disappeared when dietary fat intake was taken into consideration. Menopausal status and age at menopause are not stated in most of the studies. The Russian study reported by Zaridze and colleagues (1991) and the cohort study in Northern California (Hiatt et al., 1988) reported that alcohol significantly increased risk for postmenopausal women, but not premenopausal ones. O'Connell and coworkers (1987) found a protective effect of low alcohol consumption as compared to abstinence in premenopausal women. Drinking more than three drinks a day, however, increased the risk in premenopausal women. Comprehensive surveys of the literature were compiled in the late 1980s and early 1990s (Howe et al., 1991*b*). Three (Graham, 1987; Longnecker et al., 1988; Stampfer et al., 1988) concluded that the consumption of alcohol is associated with risk of breast cancer. The fourth review (Howe et al., 1991*b*) confirmed a relationship between alcohol consumption and breast cancer but concluded that the relationship had public health consequences only if the women drank 40 g or more of pure alcohol per day. This quantity is less than four drinks of hard liquor, three or four beers, or three or four glasses of wine a day.

No clear-cut body of evidence relates alcohol consumption to breast cancer, but as numerous studies from different countries show a positive association between the two even when traditional risk factors are taken into consideration, it might be concluded that alcohol consumption, especially at a high level, probably does influence the risk of breast cancer.

CAFFEINE

Methylxanthines include caffeine, theophylline, and theobromine. All are purine-based compounds commonly found in plant foods. Coffee, tea, soft drinks, chocolate, and some over-the-counter drugs contain methylxanthines, whether as a natural constituent or as an additive. Caffeine is found in coffee, tea, chocolate, and the kola beans used in soft drinks. Tea also contains theobromine and theophylline; and cocoa contains theobromine in addition to caffeine (Graham, 1978).

Minton generated interest in methylxanthines, especially caffeine, as a risk factor for benign or malignant breast disorders and mastodynia in 1979 (Minton et al., 1979*a,b*). Research studies, however, yielded inconsistent results. Three reviews of the literature concluded that there is little scientific basis for associating caffeine intake with chronic cystic mastopathy and other forms of benign breast disorders (Curatolo and Robertson, 1983; Pozniak, 1985; Levinson and Dunn, 1986). An additional review summarizing the results reported by 10 research teams (Bullough et al., 1990) found that only 4 reported a positive relationship between methylxanthine consumption and fibrocystic changes. Pozniak (1985) and Lubin and Ron (1990) reviewed the literature on caffeine or methylxanthine-containing beverages and breast cancer. Both concluded there was no relationship.

An animal experiment that involved DMBA-induced breast cancer in rats (Minton et al., 1983) showed that caffeine and unsaturated fatty acids in the diet enhanced the development of mammary tumors by decreasing latency time and increasing the incidence of multiple tumors. A series of studies by Minton and colleagues at Ohio State University showed that when caffeine and other beverages containing methylxanthine were eliminated from the diet of women who had clinical evidence of fibrocystic changes, a majority experienced disappearance of the symptoms (Minton et al., 1979a, 1981). Women with and without breast disease did not differ significantly on past methylxanthine exposure, with the exception of chocolate consumption; the percentage of women with chronic cystic mastopathy who had consumed chocolate was slightly more than the proportion of control women. A 1-year clinical trial of caffeine restriction (Russell, 1989) indicated that restriction of caffeine was an effective means of reducing breast pain associated with fibrocystic changes. However, only 113 (81.9%) of the 147 women actually reduced their caffeine consumption, and only 69 (61%) experienced relief or reduction in breast pain. Thus, they could document reduction in, or relief from, pain in only 47% of the original subjects.

As the result of a questionnaire given to these women seeking information about their family history of breast disease, the researchers believed that women with chronic cystic mastopathy may have a genetic predisposition to breast disease. Using graphic stress telethermometry to precisely measure the course of the breast disease, Brooks's group (1981) confirmed Minton's reports of improvement in chronic cystic mastopathy when methylxanthines were restricted. An Italian study (La Vecchia et al., 1985b) also showed a positive association between methylxanthine consumption and dysplastic disease of the breasts, but not fibroadenomas. The association gained strength with the duration of methylxanthine consumption. Coffee drinkers had an increased risk of carcinoma but not of fibroadenomas (Mansel et al., 1982).

Several case-control studies have shown a relationship between caffeine consumption and various forms of benign breast disorders (Lawson et al., 1981; Ernester et al., 1982; Boyle et al., 1984; Odenheimer et al., 1984). In two of these studies (Lawson et al., 1981; and Ernester et al., 1982) the association was so modest that their data added little support to the claim. Boyle and coworkers (1984) found an association only with chronic cystic mastopathy and not with fibroadenomas or other benign breast problems. Using discordant twins in a case-control study of risk for benign disorders allowed Odenheimer and colleagues (1984) to control for genetic and early environmental factors. They found a positive association with coffee consumption. The association, stronger in monozygotic than in dizygotic twins, lends further support to a genetic factor in benign disorders.

Two prospective studies (Snowdon and Phillips, 1984; Jacobsen et al., 1988) and numerous case-control studies (Lawson et al., 1981; Lubin et al., 1981; Le, 1985; Lubin et al., 1985b; Rosenberg et al., 1985; Katsouyanni et al., 1986; La Vecchia et al., 1986; Schairer et al., 1987; Rohan

and McMichael, 1988; Iscovich et al., 1989; La Vecchia et al., 1992) have not shown a relationship between caffeine consumption and breast cancer. Two of these studies (Le, 1985; Schairer et al., 1987) reported an *inverse* relationship between caffeine consumption and breast cancer. All except one (La Vecchia et al., 1992) assumed coffee to be the main source of caffeine in the diet. La Vecchia and associates reported on only *tea* and cancer risk. Most of the studies controlled for other known breast cancer risk factors. Only Rohan and McMichael (1988) specifically included an estimate of methylxanthines in medicine in the analysis. Rohan and McMichael (1988) and Schairer and colleagues (1987) analyzed results by menopausal status. Neither group observed a significant relationship between methylxanthine intake and breast cancer in postmenopausal women, but Rohan and Michael (1988) found one in the premenopausal subjects. Other reports have not supported a relationship (Le, 1985; Rosenberg et al., 1985; Parazzini et al., 1986; Schairer et al., 1987; Simard et al., 1990). Simard and associates (1990) did find that women with fibrocystic changes consumed more tea and coffee than women with breast cancer, but not more than the controls.

Correlation studies present contrasting findings. Stocks (1970) reported a strong positive correlation between *tea,* but not coffee, consumption and breast cancer in 6 of the 10 countries with the highest breast cancer rates. Armstrong and Doll (1975) found a nonsignificant positive correlation between caffeine and breast cancer incidence and mortality rates in 32 countries. Phelps and Phelps (1988) reported a significant positive correlation between caffeine consumption and breast cancer mortality in 44 countries; though, when they controlled for fat intake, the correlation became negative.

Reviewers have expressed reservations about some of the methods used in these studies. Some apparently did not ask about the use of pills containing caffeine (Ernster, 1981; Simard et al., 1990) or about sources of caffeine other than coffee (Katsouyanni et al., 1986) or tea (La Vecchia et al., 1992). Ernster and coworkers (1982) stated that observer bias could have been a factor in their study. Sample sizes vary. Only 20 women with benign breast disorders completely abstained from methylxanthines in one of the studies reported by Minton and associates (Minton et al., 1979a). The number of subjects in the case-control studies varied from 120 cases and 120 controls (Katsouyanni et al., 1986) to 1510 cases and 1882 controls (Schairer et al., 1987). The studies with the most subjects are not necessarily better designed. Some of the variation in results could have resulted from subject selection and the assumption that "a cup" was 5 or 6 ounces (Lubin et al., 1985b). This may not be accurate. Boyle (1984), Rosenberg (1985), and Iscovich (1989) and their groups were among the few to say they had asked women to distinguish between caffeinated and decaffeinated coffee and tea consumed. Some interviewers (Le, 1985; Iscovich et al., 1989) assessed only recent caffeine consumption, which might not be an accurate measure of earlier habits. The brand and method of preparation influence the caffeine content of coffee and tea. Instant freeze-dried coffee has less than half the caffeine content of automatic dripolator coffee; the caffeine content of tea varies by more than 100%, depending on brand and brewing time (Bunker and McWilliams, 1979). An analysis of the caffeine content of 86 home-prepared beverage samples showed much variation in caffeine content per cup (Gilbert et al., 1976).

It is, finally, not possible to draw any definite conclusions about the nature of the relationship between methylxanthine consumption and breast disease. The present evidence, however, leads one to conclude that methylxanthine ingestion does not increase the risk of breast cancer. More discriminating data are needed on the possible influence of methylxanthines on fibrocystic changes. Therefore, it seems prudent to advise women with breast pain or tenderness or with known fibrocystic changes to try to eliminate all methylxanthines from their diet for at least 6 months to determine their impact on symptoms.

GUIDE TO FOOD CHOICES

There is no basis for suggesting major modification in the diets of women as a means of preventing breast diseases. There does seem to be sufficient evidence, however, to make the following suggestions:

1. Women should maintain, or attain, their "ideal" weight. Unfortunately, scientists will probably never agree on the correct weight for each individual woman. The Metropolitan height and weight tables (Metropolitan Life Foundation, 1983) and the Quetelet index (Khosla and Lowe, 1967) are guidelines commonly used in publications. The Metropolitan weights are those associated with the lowest mortality rates for men and women from age 25 to 50 according to height and body frame. Longevity may not, however, be the best criterion for "ideal" body weight. Women who live near a university or sports medicine research center may be able to have their percentage of body fat estimated using the hydrostatic weighing procedure (Katch et al., 1967). This procedure allows one to estimate the amount of body fat and lean body mass and determine a suggested weight for the woman based on the percentage of her body that is fat. Unfortunately, the ideal percentage of fat is not known.

2. The percentage of kilocalories in most American women's diets that come from fat should be reduced. Thirty per cent of kilocalories from fat is a commonly suggested goal (National Research Council, 1982). Thirty per cent may not be low enough, however, because research has not shown a decrease in breast cancer when women followed a diet that supplied no more than 30% of kilocalories from fat. Epidemiologic evidence leads one to believe that perhaps 20% would be a better goal. A carefully selected low-fat diet also reduces the incidence of other diseases, such as coronary heart disease (Report of National Cholesterol Education Program Expert Panel, 1988). Scientific data do not provide a strong basis for suggesting a change in the type of fat from saturated fatty acids to polyunsaturated fatty acids, as is commonly suggested, but animal research suggests that a diet high in polyunsaturated fatty acids is correlated with breast cancer. The human epidemiologic data, however, are less conclusive (Hems, 1978). Some data suggest benefit from a reduction in dietary cholesterol.

3. Women should consume a diet that meets the RDA for protein, vitamins, and minerals (National Research Council, 1989b).

4. Moderate consumption of alcohol or abstinence is advised. Caffeine-containing beverages need to be restricted only for women who respond to high caffeine intake with sore or tender breasts.

These guidelines are similar to the Dietary Guidelines for Americans suggested by the United States Department of Agriculture (1985). They also suggest that a sensible diet should contain adequate starch and fiber and not too much sugar and sodium. The data do not suggest that these changes can modify breast disease, but nothing suggests that they are harmful.

A dietary counselor can help a woman evaluate her current diet and suggest changes in her eating patterns. Counseling is available from registered dietitians and nutritionists at most hospitals and at many medical clinics. National and local cancer societies also have resources.

References

Abe, J., Nakano, T., Nishii, Y., et al.: A novel vitamin D_3 analog, 22-oxa-1,25-dihydroxyvitamin D_3, inhibits the growth of human breast cancer *in vitro* and *in vivo* without causing hypercalcemia. Endocrinology, *129:*832, 1991.

Abraham, S., Faulkin, L. J., Hillyard, L. A., et al.: Effect of dietary fat on tumorigenesis in the mouse mammary gland. J. Natl. Cancer Inst., *72:*1421, 1984.

Abrams, A. A.: Use of vitamin E in chronic cystic mastitis. N. Engl. J. Med., *272:*1080, 1965.

Adami, H. O., Rimsten, A., Stenkvist, B., et al.: Influence of height, weight and obesity on risk of breast cancer in an unselected Swedish population. Br. J. Cancer, *35:*787, 1977.

Adelstein, A. M., Staszewski, J., and Muir, C. S.: Cancer mortality in 1970–1972 among Polish born migrants in England and Wales. Br. J. Cancer, *40:*464, 1979.

Adlercreutz, H., Fotsis, T., Bannwart, C., et al.: Determination of urinary lignans and phytoestrogen metabolites, potential antiestrogens and anticarcinogens in urine of women on various habitual diets. J. Steroid. Biochem., *25:*791, 1986.

Albanes, D.: Caloric intake, body weight, and cancer: A review. Nutr. Cancer, *9:*199, 1987a.

Albanes, D.: Total calories, body weight, and tumor incidence in mice. Cancer Res., *47:*1987, 1987b.

Albanes, D., and Taylor, P. R.: International differences in body height and weight and their relationship to cancer incidence. Nutr. Cancer, *14:*69, 1990.

Armstrong, B.: Recent trends in breast-cancer incidence and mortality in relation to changes in possible risk factors. Int. J. Cancer, *17:*204, 1976.

Armstrong, B., and Doll, R.: Environmental factors and cancer incidence and mortality in different countries, with special reference to dietary practices. Int. J. Cancer, *15:*617, 1975.

Aylsworth, C. F., Jones, C., Trosko, J. E., et al.: Promotion of 7,12-dimethylbenz(a)anthracene-induced mammary tumorigenesis by high dietary fat in the rat: Possible role of intercellular communication. J. Natl. Cancer Inst., *72:*637, 1984.

Band, P. R., Deschamps, M., Falardeau, M., et al.: Treatment of benign breast disease with vitamin A. Prev. Med., *13:*549, 1984.

Bani, I. A., Williams, C. M., Boulter, P. S., et al.: Plasma lipids and prolactin in patients with breast cancer. Br. J. Cancer, *54:*439, 1986.

Barbosa, J. C., Shultz, T. D, Filley, S. J., et al.: The relationship among adiposity, diet, and hormone concentrations in vegetarian and nonvegetarian postmenopausal women. Am. J. Clin. Nutr., *51:*798, 1990.

Basu, T. K., Hill, G. B., Ng, D., et al.: Serum vitamin A and E, beta-carotene, and selenium in patients with breast cancer. J. Am. Coll. Nutr., *8:*524, 1989.

Becker, B. G., Indik, B. P., and Beeuwkes, A. M.: Dietary intake methodologies—a review. Tech. Rep., University of Michigan, School of Public Health Ann Arbor, Office of Research Administration, 1960.

Bendich, A., and Langseth, L.: Safety of vitamin A. Am. J. Clin. Nutr., *49:*358, 1989.

Berkowitz, G. S., Kelsey, J. L., LiVolsi, V. A., et al.: Risk factors for fibrocystic breast disease and its histopathologic components. J. Natl. Cancer Inst., *75:*43, 1985.

Berrino, F., and Muti, P.: Mediterranean diet and cancer. Eur. J. Clin. Nutr., *43* (Suppl. 2): 49, 1989.

Beth, M., Berger, M. R., Aksoy, M., et al.: Effects of vitamin A and E supplementation to diets containing two different fat levels on methyl-nitrosourea-induced mammary carcinogenesis in female SD-rats. Br. J. Cancer, *56:*445, 1987.

Bieri, J. G., Briggs, G. M., Pollard, C. J., et al.: Normal growth and development of female chickens without dietary vitamin E or other antioxidants. J. Nutr., *70:*47, 1960.

Bingham, S. A.: Limitations of the various methods for collecting dietary intake data. Ann. Nutr. Metab., *35:*117, 1991.

Birt, D. F.: Dietary fat and experimental carcinogenesis: A summary of recent in vivo studies. *In* Poirer, L. A., Newberne, P. M., and Pariza, M. S. (Eds.): Advances in Experimental Medicine and Biology: Essential Nutrients in Carcinogenesis. Vol. 206. New York, Plenum Press, 1986, pp. 69–84.

Block, G., and Menkes, M.: Ascorbic acid in cancer prevention. *In* Moon, T. E., and Micozzi, M. S. (Eds.): Nutrition and Cancer Prevention: Investigating the Role of Micronutrients. New York, Marcel Dekker, 1989, pp. 341–388.

Boyd, N. F., and McGuire, V.: Evidence of association between plasma high-density lipoprotein cholesterol and risk factors for breast cancer. J. Natl. Cancer Inst., *82:*460, 1990.

Boyd, N. F., Campbell, N. F., Germanson, T., et al.: Body weight and prognosis in breast cancer. J. Natl. Cancer Inst., *67:*785, 1981.

Boyd, N. F., O'Sullivan, B., Campbell, J. E., et al.: Mammographic signs as risk factors for breast cancer. Br. J. Cancer, *45:*185, 1982.

Boyle, C. A., Berkowitz, G. S., LiVolsi, V. A., et al.: Caffeine consumption and fibrocystic breast disease: A case-control epidemiologic study. J. Natl. Cancer Inst., *72:*1015, 1984.

Brinton, L. A., Vessey, M. P., Flavel, R., et al.: Risk factors for benign breast disease. Am. J. Epidemiol., *113:*203, 1981.

Brisson, J., Merletti, F., Sadowski, N. L., et al.: Mammographic parenchymal patterns of the breast and breast cancer risk. Am. J. Epidemiol., *115:*428, 1982.

Brisson, J., Morrison, A. S., Kopans, D. B., et al.: Height and weight, mammographic features of breast tissue, and breast cancer risk. Am. J. Epidemiol., *119:*371, 1984.

Brisson, J., Verreault, R., Morrison, A. S., et al.: Diet, mammographic features of breast tissue, and breast cancer risk. Am. J. Epidemiol., *130:*14, 1989.

Brooks, P. G., Gart, S., Heldfond, A. J., et al.: Measuring the effect of caffeine restriction on fibrocystic breast disease. The role of graphic stress telethermometry as an objective monitor of disease. J. Reprod. Med., *25:*279, 1981.

Bullough, B., Hindi-Alexander, M., and Fetouh, S.: Methylxanthines and fibrocystic breast disease: A study in correlations. Nurse Pract., *15:*36, 1990.

Bunker, M. L., and McWilliams, M.: Caffeine content of common beverages. J. Am. Diet. Assoc., *74:*28, 1979.

Burch, J. D., Howe, G. R., and Miller, A. B.: Breast cancer in relation to weight in women age 65 years and over. Can. Med. Assoc. J., *124:*1326, 1981.

Burton, B., and Foster, W. R.: Health implications of obesity: An NIH consensus development conference. J. Am. Diet. Assoc., *85:*1117, 1985.

Byers, T., and Funch, D. P.: Alcohol and breast cancer. Lancet, *1:*799, 1982.

Caleffi, M., Ashraf, J., Rowe, P. H., et al.: Comparison of fatty acid profiles of subcutaneous fat from women with breast cancer, benign breast disease and normal controls. Anticancer Res., *7:*1305, 1987.

Cameron, E., Pauling, L., and Leibovitz, B.: Ascorbic acid and cancer: A review. Cancer Res., *39:*663, 1979.

Camoriano, J. K., Loprinzi, C. L., Ingle, J. N., et al.: Weight change in women treated with adjuvant therapy or observed following mastectomy for node-positive breast cancer. J. Clin. Oncol., *8:*1327, 1990.

Carroll, K. K.: Experimental evidence of dietary factors and hormone-dependent cancers. Cancer Res., *35:*3374, 1975.

Carroll, K. K., and Parenteau, H. I.: A proposed mechanism for effects of diet on mammary cancer. Nutr. Cancer, *16:*79, 1991.

Choi, N. W., Howe, G. R., Miller, A. B., et al.: An epidemiologic study of breast cancer. Am. J. Epidemiol., *107:*510, 1978.

Chow, C. K.: Nutritional influence on cellular antioxidant defense systems. Am. J. Clin. Nutr., *32:*1066, 1979.

Chu, S. Y., Lee, N. C., Wingo, P. A., et al.: Alcohol consumption and the risk of breast cancer. Am. J. Epidemiol., *130:*867, 1989.

Coates, R. J., Clark, W. S., Eley, J. W., et al.: Race, nutritional status, and survival from breast cancer. J. Natl. Cancer Inst., *82:*1684, 1990.

Cohen, L. A., Kendall, M. E., Zang, E., et al.: Modulation of N-nitroso-methylurea-induced mammary tumor promotion by dietary fiber and fat. J. Natl. Cancer Inst., *83:*497, 1991.

Colston, K. W., Berger, U., and Coombes, R. C.: Possible role for vitamin D in controlling breast cancer cell proliferation. Lancet, *1:*188, 1989.

Combs, G. F., and Clark, L. C.: Can dietary selenium modify cancer risk? Nutr. Rev., *43:*325, 1985.

Combs, G. F. Jr., and Combs, S. B.: The nutritional biochemistry of selenium. *In* Darby, W. J., Broquist, H. P., and Olson, R. E. (Eds.): Annual Review of Nutrition. Palo Alto, Calif., Annual Reviews, 1984, p. 257.

Cooper, J. A., Rohan, T. E., Cant, E. L. et al.: Risk factors for breast cancer by oestrogen receptor status: A population-based case-control study. Br. J. Cancer, *59:*119, 1989.

Cowan, L. D., O'Connell, D. L., Criqui, M. H., et al.: Cancer mortality and lipid and lipoprotein levels. The Lipid Research Clinics Program Mortality Follow-Up Study. Am. J. Epidemiol., *131:*468, 1990.

Curatolo, P. W., and Robertson, D.: The health consequences of caffeine. Ann. Intern. Med., *98:*641, 1983.

Dabek, J. T., Hyvönen-Dabek, M., Härkönen, M., and Adlercreutz, H.: Evidence for increased non-ceruloplasmin copper in early stage breast cancer serum. Nutr. Cancer, *17:*195, 1992.

DeGeorge, D., Gray, J. J., Fetting J. H. et al.: Weight gain in patients with breast cancer receiving adjuvant treatment as a function of restraint, disinhibition, and hunger. Oncol. Nurs. Forum, *17*(3 Suppl):23, 1990.

DeLuca, H. F., and Ostrem, V.: The relationship between the vitamin D system and cancer. Adv. Exp. Med. Biol., *206:*413, 1980.

de Waard, F.: Breast cancer incidence and nutritional status with particular reference to body weight and height. Cancer Res., *35:*3351, 1975.

de Waard, F., and Baanders-van Halewijn, E. A.: A prospective study in general practice on breast-cancer risk in postmenopausal women. Int. J. Cancer, *14:*153, 1974.

de Waard, F., Baanders-van Halewijn, E. A., and Huizinga, J.: The bimodal age distribution of patients with mammary carcinoma. Cancer, *17:*141, 1964.

de Waard, F., Cornelis, J. P., Aoki, K., et al.: Breast cancer incidence according to weight and height in two cities of the Netherlands and in Aichi Prefecture, Japan. Cancer, *40:*1269, 1977.

Donegan, W. L., Hartz, A. J., and Rimm, A. A.: The association of body weight with recurrent cancer of the breast. Cancer, *41:*1590, 1978.

Dyer, A. R., Stamler, J., Paul, O., et al.: Serum cholesterol and risk of death from cancer and other cause in three Chicago epidemiological studies. J. Chronic Dis., *34:*249, 1981.

Eberlein, T., Simon, R., Fisher, S., et al.: Height, weight, and risk of breast cancer relapse. Breast Cancer Res. Treat., *5:*81, 1985.

Eid, A., and Berry, E. M.: The relationship between dietary fat, adipose tissue composition, and neoplasms of the breast. Nutr. Cancer, *11:*173, 1988.

Eisman, J. A., McIntyre, I., Martin, T. J., et al.: Normal and malignant breast tissue is a target organ for 1,25-$(OH)_2$ vitamin D_3. Clin. Endocrinol., *13:*267, 1980.

Ernester, V. L.: The epidemiology of benign breast disease. Epidemiol. Rev., *3:*184, 1981.

Ernster, V., Goodson, W. H. III, Hunt, T. K., et al.: Vitamin E and benign breast "disease": A double-blind randomized clinical trial. Surgery, *97:*490, 1985.

Fischer, S. M., Leyton, J., Lee, M. L., et al.: Differential effects of dietary linoleic acid on mouse skin-tumor promotion and mammary carcinogenesis. Cancer Res., *52*(Suppl):2049s, 1992.

Freedman, L. S., and Clifford, C. K.: Enhancement of mammary carcinogenesis by high levels of dietary fat and its association with ad libitum feeding (Correspondence). J. Natl. Cancer Inst., *83:*299, 1991.

Freedman, L. S., Clifford, C., and Messina, M.: Analysis of dietary fat, calories, body weight, and the development of mammary tumors in rats and mice: A review. Cancer Res., *50:*5710, 1990.

Gabor, H., Hillyard, L. A., and Abraham, S.: Effect of dietary fat on growth kinetics of transplantable mammary adenocarcinoma in BALB/c mice. J. Natl. Cancer Inst., *74:*1299, 1985.

Garland, F. C., Garland, C. F., Gorham, E. D., et al.: Geographic variation in breast cancer mortality in the United States: A hypothesis involving exposure to solar radiation. Prev. Med., *19:*614, 1990.

Gaskill, S. P., McGuire, W. L., Osborne, C. K., et al.: Breast cancer mortality and diet in the United States. Cancer Res., *39:*3628, 1979.

Gerber, M., Cavallo, F., Marubini, E., et al.: Liposoluble vitamins and lipid parameters in breast cancer. A joint study in northern Italy and southern France. Int. J. Cancer, *42:*489, 1988.

Gerber, M., Richardson, S., Crastes-de-Paulet, P., et al.: Relationship between vitamin E and polyunsaturated fatty acids in breast cancer. Nutritional and metabolic aspects. Cancer, *64:*2347, 1989.

Gilbert, R. M., Marshman, J. A., Schwieder, M., et al.: Caffeine content of beverages as consumed. Can. Med. Assoc. J., *114:*205, 1976.

Goettler, D. M., Levin, L., and Chey, W. Y.: Postprandial levels of prolactin and gut hormones in breast cancer patients: Association with stage of disease, but not dietary fat. J. Natl. Cancer Inst., *82:*22, 1990.

Goldin, B. R., Adlercreutz, H., Gorbach, S. L., et al.: Estrogen excretion patterns and plasma levels in vegetarian and omnivorous women. N. Engl. J. Med., *307:*1542, 1982.

Goldin, B. R., Adlercreutz, H., Gorbach, S. L., et al.: The relationship between estrogen levels and diets of Caucasian American and Oriental immigrant women. Am J. Clin. Nutr., *44:*945, 1986.

Gorham, E., Garland, C. F., and Garland, F. C.: Acid haze air pollution and breast and colon cancer mortality in 20 Canadian cities. Can. J. Public Health, *80:*96, 1989.

Graham, D. M.: Caffeine—its identity, dietary sources, intake and biological effects. Nutr. Rev., *36:*97, 1978.

Graham, S.: Hypotheses regarding caloric intake in cancer development. Cancer, *58:*1814, 1986.

Graham, S.: Alcohol and breast cancer. N. Engl. J. Med., *316:*1211, 1987.

Graham, S., Hellmann, R., Marshall, J., et al.: Nutritional epidemiology of postmenopausal breast cancer in Western New York. Am. J. Epidemiol., *134:*552, 1991.

Graham, S., Marshall, J., Mettlin, C., et al.: Diet in the epidemiology of breast cancer. Am. J. Epidemiol., *116:*68, 1982.

Gray, G. E., Pike, M. C., and Henderson, B. E.: Breast cancer incidence and mortality rates in different countries in relation to known risk factors and dietary practices. Br. J. Cancer, *39:*1, 1979.

Gregorio, D. I., Emrich, L. J., Graham, S., et al.: Dietary fat consumption and survival among women with breast cancer. J. Natl. Cancer Inst., *75:*37, 1985.

Grubbs, C. J., Moon, R. C., Sporn, M. B., et al.: Inhibition of mammary cancer by retinyl methyl ether. Cancer Res., *37:*599, 1977.

Guthrie, H.: Evaluation of Nutritional Status. *In* Guthrie, H. (Ed.): Introductory Nutrition. 6th ed. St. Louis, C. V. Mosby, 1986, p. 478.

Haenszel, W.: Cancer mortality among foreign born in the United States. J. Natl. Cancer Inst., *26:*37, 1961.

Hagerty, M. A., Howie, B. J., Tan, S., et al.: Effect of low- and high-fat intakes on the hormonal milieu of premenopausal women. Am. J. Clin. Nutr., *47:*653, 1988.

Harman, D.: Dimethylbenzanthracene induced cancer: Inhibiting effect of dietary vitamin E. Clin. Res., *17:*125, 1969.

Harr, J. R., Exon, J. H., Whanger, P. D., et al.: Effect of dietary selenium on *N*-2-fluorenyl-acetamide (FAA)–induced cancer in vitamin E supplemented, selenium depleted rats. Clin. Toxicol., *5:*187, 1972.

Harris, J. R., Lippman, M. E., Veronesi, U., et al.: Breast cancer. N. Engl. J. Med., *327:*319, 1992.

Harris, R. E., and Wynder, E. L.: Breast cancer and alcohol consumption. A study in weak associations. J. A. M. A., *259:*2867, 1988.

Harvey, E. B., Schairer, C., Brinton, L. A., et al.: Alcohol consumption and breast cancer. J. Natl. Cancer Inst., *78:*657, 1987.

Heasman, K. Z., Sutherland, H. J., Campbell, J. A., et al.: Weight gain during adjuvant chemotherapy for breast cancer. Breast Cancer Res. Treat., *5:*195, 1985.

Hebert, J. R., and Toporoff, E.: Dietary exposure and other factors of possible prognostic significance in relation to tumour size and nodal involvement in early-stage breast cancer. Int. J. Epidemiol., *18:*518, 1989.

Helmrich, S. P., Shapiro, S., Rosenberg, L., et al.: Risk factors for breast cancer. Am. J. Epidemiol., *117:*35, 1983.

Hems, G.: The contributions of diet and childbearing to breast-cancer rates. Br. J. Cancer. *37:*974, 1978.

Henson, D. E., Block, G., and Levine, M.: Ascorbic acid: Biological functions and relation to cancer. J Natl. Cancer Inst., *83:*547, 1991.

Hiatt, R. A., and Bawol, R.: Alcohol beverage consumption and breast cancer incidence. Am. J. Epidemiol., *120:*676, 1984.

Hiatt, R. A., Klatsky, A. L., and Armstrong, M. A.: Alcohol consumption and the risk of breast cancer in a prepaid health plan. Cancer Res., *48:*2284, 1988.

Hill, P., and Wynder, E. L.: Comparison of mammary adipose fatty acid composition in Japanese and American breast cancer patients. Eur. J. Cancer Clin. Oncol., *23:*407, 1987.

Hirohata, T., Nomura, A. M., Hankin, J. H., et al.: An epidemiological study of the association between diet and breast cancer. J. Natl. Cancer Inst., *78:*595, 1987.

Hirohata, T., Shigematsu, T., Nomura, A. M., et al.: Occurrence of breast cancer in relation to diet and reproductive history: A case-control study in Fukuoka, Japan. J. Natl. Cancer Inst. Monogr., *69:*187, 1985.

Hislop, T. G., and Elwood, J. M.: Risk factors for benign breast disease: A 30-year cohort study. Can. Med. Assoc. J., *124:*283, 1981.

Hislop, T. G., Band, P. R., Deschamps, M., et al.: Diet and histologic types of benign breast disease defined by subsequent risk of breast cancer. Am. J. Epidemiol., *131:*263, 1990.

Hislop, T. G., Coldman, A. J., Elwood, J. M. et al.: Childhood and recent eating patterns and risk of breast cancer. Cancer Detect. Prev., *9:*47, 1986.

Holm, L. E., Callmer, E., Hjalmar, M. L., et al.: Dietary habits and prognostic factors in breast cancer. J. Natl. Cancer Inst., *81:*1218, 1989.

Holtzman, S.: Retinyl acetate inhibits estrogen-induced mammary carcinogenesis in female ACI rats. Carcinogenesis, *9:*305, 1988.

Horvath, P. M., and Ip, C.: Synergistic effect of vitamin E and selenium in the chemoprevention of mammary carcinogenesis in rats. Cancer Res., *43:*5335, 1983.

Houser, H. B., and Bebb, H. T.: Individual variation in intake of nutrients by day, month, and season and relation to meal patterns: Implications for dietary survey methodology. *In* National Research Council, Committee on Food Consumption Patterns: Assessing Changing Food Consumption Patterns. Washington, DC: National Academy Press, 1981, p. 155.

Howe, G. R., Friedenreich, C. M., Jain, M., et al.: A cohort study of fat intake and risk of breast cancer. J. Natl. Cancer Inst., *83:*336, 1991*a*.

Howe, G. R., Hirohata, T., Hislop, T. G., et al.: Dietary factors and risk of breast cancer: Combined analysis of 12 case-control studies. J. Natl. Cancer Inst., *82:*561, 1990.

Howe, G., Rohan, T., Decarli, A., et al.: The association between alcohol and breast cancer risk: Evidence from the combined analysis of six dietary case-control studies. Int. J. Cancer, *47:*707, 1991*b*.

Howson, C. P., Kinne, D., and Wynder, E. L.: Body weight, serum cholesterol, and stage of primary breast cancer. Cancer, *58:*2372, 1986.

Hulka, B. S.: Dietary fat and breast cancer: case-control and cohort studies. Prev. Med., *18:*180, 1989.

Hunt, S. M., and Groff, J. L.: The Vitamins. *In:* Advanced Nutrition and Human Metabolism. St. Paul, MN, West Publishing Co., 1990, pp. 226–231.

Hunter, D. J., Morris, J. S., Stampfer, M. J., et al.: A prospective study of selenium status and breast cancer risk. J.A.M.A., *264:*1128, 1990.

Huntington, M. O.: Weight gain in patients receiving adjuvant chemotherapy for carcinoma of the breast. Cancer, *56:*472, 1985.

Ingram, D., Bennett, F., and Wood, A.: Estradiol binding to plasma proteins after changing to a low-fat diet. Nutr. Cancer, *12:*327, 1989.

Ingram, D. M., Nottage, E. M., and Roberts, A. N.: Prolactin and breast cancer risk. Med. J. Aust., *153:*469, 1990.

Ingram, D. M., Nottage, E., and Roberts, T.: The role of diet in the development of breast cancer: A case-control study of patients with breast cancer, benign epithelial hyperplasia and fibrocystic disease of the breast. Br. J. Cancer, *64:*187, 1991.

Ip, C.: Prophylaxis of mammary neoplasia by selenium supplementation in the initiation and promotion phases of chemical carcinogenesis. Cancer Res., *41:*4386, 1981.

Ip, C.: Quantitative assessment of fat and calorie as risk factors in mammary carcinogenesis in an experimental model. Prog. Clin. Biol. Res., *346:*107, 1990.

Ip, C., and Sinha, D. K.: Enhancement of mammary tumorigenesis by selenium deficiency in rats with a high polyunsaturated fat intake. Cancer Res., *41:*31, 1981.

Ip, C., Carter, C. A., and Ip, M. M.: Requirement of essential fatty acid for mammary tumorigenesis in the rat. Cancer Res., *45:*1997, 1985.

Ip, C., Lisk, D. J., and Stoewsand, G. S.: Mammary cancer prevention by regular garlic and selenium-enriched garlic. Nutr. Cancer, *17:*279, 1992.

Iscovich, J. M., Iscovich, R. B., Howe, G., et al.: A case-control study of diet and breast cancer in Argentina. Int. J. Cancer, *44:*770, 1989.

Jacobson, E. A., James, K. A., Frei, J. V., et al.: Effects of dietary fat on long-term growth and mammary tumorigenesis in female Sprague-Dawley rats given a low dose of DMBA. Nutr. Cancer, *11:*221, 1988.

Kakar, F., and Henderson, M.: Diet and breast cancer. Clin. Nutr., *4:*119, 1985.

Katch, F., Michael, E., and Horvath, S.: Estimation of body volume by underwater weighing: Description of simple inexpensive method. J. Appl. Physiol., *23:*811, 1967.

Kato, I., Tominaga, S., and Kuroishi, T.: Relationship between westernization of dietary habits and mortality from breast and ovarian cancers in Japan. Jpn. J. Cancer Res., *78:*349, 1987.

Kato, I., Tominaga, S., and Terao, C.: Alcohol consumption and cancers of hormone-related organs in females. Jpn. J. Clin. Oncol., *19:*202, 1989.

Katsouyanni, D., Trichopoulos, D., Boyle, P., et al.: Diet and breast cancer: A case-control study in Greece. Int. J. Cancer, *38:*815, 1986.

Katsouyanni, K., Willet, W., Trichopoulos, D., et al.: Risk of breast cancer among Greek women in relation to nutrient intake. Cancer, *61:*181, 1988.

Kelsey, J. L., Fisher, D. B., Holdferd, T. R., et al.: Exogenous estrogens and other factors in the epidemiology of breast cancer. J. Natl. Cancer Inst., *67:*327, 1981.

Key, T. J., Darby, S. C., and Pike, M. C.: Trends in breast cancer mortality and diet in England and Wales from 1911 to 1980. Nutr. Cancer, *10*(1–2):1, 1987.

Keys, A., Aravanis, C., Blackburn, H., et al.: Serum cholesterol and cancer mortality in the Seven Countries Study. Am. J. Epidemiol., *121:*870, 1985.

Khosla, T., and Lowe, C. R.: Indices of obesity derived from body weight and height. Br. J. Prev. Soc. Med., *21:*122, 1967.

Kline, K., and Sanders, B. G.: Anti-tumor proliferation properties of vitamin E. *In* Jacobs, M. M. (Ed.): Vitamins and Minerals in the Treatment of Cancer. Boston, CRC Press, 1991.

Knekt, P., Aromaa, A., Maatela, J., et al.: Serum selenium and subsequent risk of cancer among Finnish men and women. J. Natl. Cancer Inst., *82:*864, 1991.

Kolonel, L. N., Nomura, A. M., Hinds, M. W., et al.: Role of diet in cancer incidence in Hawaii. Cancer Res., *43*(Suppl.):2397, 1983.

Kushi, L. H., Sellers, T. A., Potter, J. D., et al.: Dietary fat and postmenopausal breast cancer. J. Natl. Cancer Inst., *84:*1092, 1992.

Kwa, H. G., Cleton, F., Bulbrook, R. D., et al.: Plasma prolactin levels and breast cancer: Relation to parity, weight and height, and age at first birth. Int. J. Cancer, *28:*31, 1981.

Kyogoku, S., Hirohata, T., Nomura, Y., et al.: Diet and prognosis of breast cancer. Nutr. Cancer, *17:*271, 1992.

Lacroix, A., Doskas, C., and Bhat, P. V.: Inhibition of growth of established *N*-methyl-*N*-nitrosurea–induced mammary cancer in rats by retinoic acid and ovariectomy. Cancer Res., *50:*5731, 1990.

La Vecchia, C.: Nutritional factors and cancers of the breast, endometrium and ovary. Eur. J. Cancer Clin. Oncol., *25:*1945, 1989.

La Vecchia, C., Decarli, A., Franceschi, S., et al.: Alcohol consumption and the risk of breast cancer in women. J. Natl. Cancer Inst., *75:*61, 1985*a.*

La Vecchia, C., Decarli, A., Franceschi, S., et al.: Dietary factors and the risk of breast cancer. Nutr. Cancer, *10:*205, 1987.

La Vecchia, C., Franceschi, S., Parazzini, F., et al.: Benign breast disease and consumption of beverages containing methylxanthines. J. Natl. Cancer Inst., *74:*995, 1985*b.*

La Vecchia, C., Negri, E., Parazzini, F., et al.: Alcohol and breast cancer: Update from an Italian case-control study. Eur. J. Cancer Clin. Oncol., *25:*1711, 1989.

La Vecchia, C., Negri, E., Franceschi, S., et al.: Tea consumption and cancer risk. Nutr. Cancer, *17:*27, 1992.

La Vecchia, C., Talamini, R., Decarli, A., et al.: Coffee consumption and the risk of breast cancer. Surgery, *100:*477, 1986.

Lawson, O. H., Jick, H., and Rothman, K. J.: Coffee and tea consumption and breast disease. Surgery, *90:*801, 1981.

Le, M. G.: Coffee consumption, benign breast disease, and breast cancer (Letter to the editor). Am. J. Epidemiol., *122:*721, 1985.

Le, M. G., Hill, C., Kramar, A., et al.: Alcoholic beverage consumption and breast cancer in a French case-control study. Am. J. Epidemiol., *120:*350, 1984.

Le, M., Moulton, L., Hill, C., et al.: Consumption of dairy produce and alcohol in a case-control study of breast cancer. J. Natl. Cancer Inst., *77:*633, 1986.

Lea, A. J.: Dietary factors associated with death-rates from certain neoplasms in man. Lancet, *2:*332, 1966.

Lee, C., and Chen, C.: Enhancement of mammary tumorigenesis in rats by vitamin E deficiency. Proc. Am. Assoc. Cancer Res. Am. Soc. Clin. Oncol., *20:*132, 1979.

Le Marchand, L., Kolonel, L. N., Earle, M. E., et al.: Body size at different periods of life and breast cancer risk. Am. J. Epidemiol., *128:*137, 1988.

Levine, E. G., Raczynski, J. M., and Carpenter, J. T.: Weight gain with breast cancer adjuvant treatment. Cancer, *67:*1954, 1991.

Levinson, W., and Dunn, P. M.: Nonassociation of caffeine and fibrocystic breast disease. Arch. Intern. Med., *146:*1773, 1986.

Lissner, L., Odell, P. M., D'Agostino, R. B., et al.: Variability of body weight and health outcomes in the Framingham population. N. Engl. J. Med., *324:*1839, 1991.

London, S., and Willett, W.: Diet and the risk of breast cancer. Hematol. Oncol. Clin. North Am., *3:*559, 1989.

London, R. S., Solomon, D. M., London, E. D., et al.: Mammary dysplasia: Clinical response and urinary excretion of 11-deoxy-17-ketosteroids and pregnanediol following alpha-tocopherol therapy. Breast, *4:*19, 1978.

Longnecker, M. P., Berlin, J. A., Orza, S. M., et al.: A meta-analysis of alcohol consumption in relation to risk of breast cancer. J.A.M.A., *260:*652, 1988.

Lubin, F., and Ron, E.: Consumption of methylxanthine-containing beverages and the risk of breast cancer. Cancer Lett., *53:*81, 1990.

Lubin, F., Ron, E., Was, Y., et al.: Coffee and methylxanthines and breast cancer: A case-control study. J. Natl. Cancer Inst., *74:*569, 1985*b.*

Lubin, F., Ron, E., Wax, Y., et al.: A case-control study of caffeine and methylxanthines in benign breast disease. J. A. M. A., *253:*2388, 1985*c.*

Lubin, F., Ruder, A. M., Wax, Y., et al.: Overweight and changes in weight throughout adult life and breast cancer etiology. Am. J. Epidemiol., *122:*579, 1985*a.*

Lubin, F., Wax, Y., and Modan, B.: Role of fat, animal protein, and dietary fiber in breast cancer etiology: A case-control study. J. Natl. Cancer Inst., *77:*605, 1986.

Lubin, J. H., Burns, P. E., Blot, W. J., et al.: Dietary factors and breast cancer risk. Int. J. Cancer, *28:*685, 1981.

Lyon, J. L., Gardner, J. W., West, D. W., et al.: Methodological issues in epidemiological studies of diet and cancer. Cancer Res., *43* (Suppl.):2392, 1983.

Mansel, R. E., Webster, D. J. T., Burr, M., et al.: Is there a relationship between coffee consumption and breast disease? Br. J. Surg., *69:*295, 1982.

Margetts, B. M., Hopkins, S. M., Binns, C. W., et al.: Nutrient intakes in Italian migrants and Australians in Perth. Food Nutr., *38:*7, 1981.

Marubini, E., Decarli, A., Costa, A., et al.: The relationship of dietary intake and serum levels of retinol and beta-carotene with breast cancer. Results of a case-control study. Cancer, *61:*173, 1988.

Maruyama, H., Watanabe, K., and Yamamoto, I.: Effect of dietary kelp on lipid peroxidation and glutathione peroxidase activity in livers of rats given breast carcinogen DMBA. Nutr. Cancer, *15:*221, 1991.

McCay, P. B.: Vitamin E: Interactions with free radicals and ascorbate. *In* Olson, R. E., Beutler, E., and Broquist, H. P. (Eds.): Annual Review of Nutrition. Palo Alto, Calif., Annual Reviews, 1985, p. 323.

McConnell, K. P., Jager, R. M., Bland, K. I., et al.: The relationship of dietary selenium and breast cancer. J. Surg. Oncol., *15:*67, 1980.

McCormick, D. L., Burns, F. J., and Albert, R. E.: Inhibition of rat mammary carcinogenesis by short dietary exposure to retinyl acetate. Cancer Res., *40:*1140, 1980.

McCormick, D. L., Sowell, Z. L., Thompson, C. A., et al.: Inhibition by retinoid and ovariectomy of additional primary malignancies in rats following surgical removal of the first mammary cancer. Cancer, *31:*594, 1983.

Medina, D., Lane, H. W., and Tracey, C. M.: Selenium and mouse mammary tumorigenesis: An investigation of possible mechanisms. Cancer Res., *43* (Suppl.): 2460, 1983.

Metropolitan Life Foundation: Height and weight tables. Stat. Bull., *64:*2, 1983.

Mettlin, C.: Diet and the epidemiology of human breast cancer. Cancer, *53:*605, 1984.

Mettlin, C. J., Schoenfeld, E. R., and Natarajan, N.: Patterns of milk consumption and risk of cancer. Nutr. Cancer, *13:*89, 1990.

Meyer, F., and Verreault, R.: Erythrocyte selenium and breast cancer risk. Am. J. Epidemiol., *125:*917, 1987.

Meyer, F., Brown, J. B., Morrison, A. S., et al.: Endogenous sex hormones, prolactin, and breast cancer in premenopausal women. J. Natl. Cancer Inst., *77:*613, 1986.

Meyer, E. C., Sommers, D. K., Reitz, C. J., et al.: Vitamin E and benign breast disease. Surgery, *107:*549, 1990.

Miller, A. B.: Role of nutrition in the etiology of breast cancer. Cancer, *39:*2704, 1977.

Miller, A. B., Kelly, A., Choi, N. W., et al.: A study of diet and breast cancer. Am. J. Epidemiol., *107:*499, 1978.

Mills, P. K., Annegers, J. F., and Phillips, R. L.: Animal product consumption and subsequent fatal breast cancer risk among Seventh-day Adventists. Am. J. Epidemiol., *127:*440, 1988.

Mills, P. K., Beeson, W. L., Phillips, R. L., et al.: Dietary habits and breast cancer incidence among Seventh-day Adventists. Cancer, *64:*582, 1989.

Minton, J. P., Abou-Issa, H., Reiches, N., et al.: Clinical and biochemical studies on methylxanthine-related fibrocystic breast disease. Surgery, *90:*299, 1981.

Minton, J. P., Abou-Issa, H., Foecking, M. K., et al.: Caffeine and unsaturated fat diet significantly promotes DMBA-induced breast cancer in rats. Cancer, *51:*1249, 1983.

Minton, J. P., Foecking, M. K., Webster, D. J., et al.: Response of fibrocystic disease to caffeine withdrawal and correlation of cyclic nucleotides with breast disease. Am. J. Obstet. Gynecol., *135:*157, 1979*a*.

Minton, J. P., Foecking, M. K., Webster, D. J., et al.: Caffeine, cyclic nucleotides, and breast disease. Surgery, *86:*106, 1979*b*.

Modan, B., Barell, V., Lubin, F., et al.: Dietary factors and cancer in Israel. Cancer Res., *35:*3503, 1975.

Moore, D. H., Moore, D. H. II, and Moore, C. T.: Breast carcinoma etiological factors. Adv. Cancer Res., *40:*189, 1983.

Morrison, A. S., Lowe, C. R., MacMahon, B., et al.: Some international differences in treatment and survival in breast cancer. Int. J. Cancer, *18:*269, 1976.

Nagasawa, H.: Stimulation of neonatal treatment with vitamin A of spontaneous mammary tumor development in GRS/A mice. Breast Cancer. Res. Treat., *4:*205, 1984.

National Research Council, Committee on Diet, Nutrition and Cancer: Diet, Nutrition and Cancer. Washington, D.C., National Academy Press, 1982.

National Research Council, Committee on Diet and Health: Diet and Health: implications for reducing chronic disease risk. Washington, DC, National Academy Press, 1989*a*.

National Research Council, Food and Nutrition Board: Recommended Dietary Allowances. 10th ed. Washington, DC, National Academy Press, 1989*b*.

Newberne, P. M., and Saphakarn, V.: Nutrition and cancer: A review, with emphasis on the role of vitamins C and E and selenium. Nutr. Cancer, *5:*107, 1983.

Newman, S. C., Miller, A. H., and Howe, G. R.: A study of the effect of weight and dietary fat on breast cancer survival time. Am. J. Epidemiol., *123:*767, 1986.

Nomura, A., Henderson, B. E., and Lee, J.: Breast cancer and diet among the Japanese in Hawaii. Am. J. Clin. Nutr., *31:*2020, 1978.

O'Connell, D. L., Hulka, B. S., Chambless, L. E., et al.: Cigarette smoking, alcohol consumption, and breast cancer risk. J. Natl. Cancer Inst., *78:*229, 1987.

Odenheimer, D. J., Zuzunegui, M. V., King, M. C., et al.: Risk factors for benign breast disease: A case-control study of discordant twins. Am. J. Epidemiol., *120:*565, 1984.

Osler, M.: Obesity and cancer. A review of epidemiological studies on the relationship of obesity to cancer of the colon, rectum, prostate, breast, ovaries, and endometrium. Dan. Med. Bull., *34:*267, 1987.

Paffenbarger, R. S., Kampert, J. B, and Chang, H. G.: Characteristics that predict risk of breast cancer before and after the menopause. Am. J. Epidemiol., *112:*258, 1980.

Parazzini, F., La Vecchia, C., Riundi, R., et al.: Methylxanthine, alcohol-free diet and fibrocystic breast diseases: A factorial clinical trial. Surgery, *99:*576, 1986.

Parazzini, F., La Vecchia, C., Franceschi, S., et al.: Risk factors for pathologically confirmed benign breast disease. Am. J. Epidemiol., *120:*115, 1984.

Pathak, D. R., and Whittemore, A. S.: Combined effects of body size, parity, and menstrual events on breast cancer incidence in seven countries. Am. J. Epidemiol., *135:*153, 1992.

Pawlega, J.: Does salt protect against breast cancer (Letter to the editor)? Nutr. Cancer, *12:*197, 1989.

Pennington, J. A. T., and Church, H. N.: Bowes and Church's Food Values of Portions Commonly Used. 14th ed. Philadelphia, J. B. Lippincott, 1989.

Phelps, H. M., and Phelps, C. E.: Caffeine ingestion and breast cancer. A negative correlation. Cancer, *61:*1051, 1988.

Phillips, R. L., and Snowdon, D. A.: Association of meat and coffee use with cancers of large bowel, breast, and prostate among Seventh-day Adventists: Preliminary results. Cancer Res., *43* (Suppl.):2403, 1983.

Pi-Sunyer, F. X.: Obesity. *In* Shils, M. E., and Young, V. R. (Eds.): Modern Nutrition in Health and Disease. 7th ed. Philadelphia, Lea & Febiger, 1988, p. 796.

Potischman, N., McCulloch, C. E., Byers, T., et al.: Breast cancer and dietary and plasma concentrations of carotenoids and vitamin A. Am. J. Clin. Nutr., *52:*909, 1990.

Potischman, N., McCulloch, C. E., Byers, R., et al.: Associations between breast cancer, plasma triglycerides, and cholesterol. Nutr. Cancer, *15:*205, 1991.

Pozniak, P. C.: The carcinogenicity of caffeine and coffee: A review. J. Am. Diet Assoc., *85:*1127, 1985.

Prentice, R. L., and Sheppard, L.: Validity of international, time trend, and migrant studies of dietary factors and disease risk. Prev. Med., *18:*167, 1989.

Prentice, R. L., Kakar, F., Hursting, S., et al.: Aspects of the rationale for the Women's Health Trial. J. Natl. Cancer Inst., *80:*802, 1988.

Prentice, R. L., Pepe, M., and Self, S. G.: Dietary fat and breast cancer: A quantitative assessment of the epidemiological literature and a discussion of methodological issues. Cancer Res., *49:*3147, 1989.

Prentice, R., Thompson, D., Clifford, C., et al.: Dietary fat reduction and plasma estradiol concentration in healthy postmenopausal women. J. Natl. Cancer Inst., *82:*129, 1990.

Pryor, M., Slattery, M. L., Robison, L. M., et al.: Adolescent diet and breast cancer in Utah. Cancer Res., *49:*2161, 1989.

Reddy, B. S.: Dietary fat and cancer: Specific action or caloric effect. J. Nutr., *116:*1132, 1986.

Report of the National Cholesterol Education Program Expert Panel on Detection, Evaluation and Treatment of High Blood Cholesterol in Adults. Arch. Intern. Med., *148:*36, 1988.

Rettura, G., Duttaqupta, C., Listowsky, P., et al.: Dimethylbenz(a) anthracene (DMBA) induced tumors; prevention by supplemental β-carotene (BC) (Abstract). Federation Proceedings, *42:*786, 1983.

Richardson, S., de Vincenzi, I., Pujol, H., et al.: Alcohol consumption in a case-control study of breast cancer in southern France. Int. J. Cancer, *44:*84, 1989.

Richardson, S., Gerber, M., and Cenee, S.: The role of fat, animal protein and some vitamin consumption in breast cancer: A case-control study in southern France. Int. J. Cancer, *48:*1, 1991.

Rivlin, R. S.: Nutrition and cancer: State of the art relationship of several nutrients to the development of cancer. J. Am. Coll. Nutr., *1:*75, 1982.

Rohan, T. E., and Bain, C. J.: Diet in the etiology of breast cancer. Epidemiol. Rev., *9:*120, 1987.

Rohan, T. E., and McMichael, A. J.: Methylxanthines and breast cancer. Int. J. Cancer, *41:*390, 1988.

Rohan, T. E., Cook, M. G., Potter, J. D., et al.: A case-control study of diet and benign proliferative epithelial disorders of the breast. Cancer Res., *50:*3176, 1990.

Rohan, T. E., McMichael, A. J., and Baghurst, P. A.: A population-based case-control study of diet and breast cancer in Australia. Am. J. Epidemiol., *128:*478, 1988.

Rose, D. P.: Dietary fiber and breast cancer. Nutr. Cancer, *13:*1, 1990.

Rose, G., and Shipley, M. J.: Plasma lipids and mortality: A source of error. Lancet, *1:*523, 1980.

Rose, D. P., Boyar, A. P., Cohen, C. et al.: Effect of a low-fat diet on hormone levels in women with cystic breast disease. I. Serum steroids and gonadotropins. J. Natl. Cancer Inst., *78:*623, 1987.

Rose, D. P., Boyar, A. P., and Wynder, E. L.: International comparisons of mortality rates for cancer of the breast, ovary, prostate, and colon, and per capita food consumption. Cancer, *58:*2363, 1986.

Rosenberg, L., Miller, D. R., Helmrich, S. P., et al.: Breast cancer and the consumption of coffee. Am. J. Epidemiol., *122:*391, 1985.

Russell, J. J., Thomas, B. S., and Bulbrook, R. D.: A prospective study of the relationship between serum vitamins A and E and risk of breast cancer. Br. J. Cancer, *57:*213, 1988.

Russell, L. C.: Caffeine restriction as initial treatment for breast pain. Nurse Pract., *14:*36, 1989.

Schairer, C., Brinton, L. A., and Hoover, R. N.: Methylxanthines and breast cancer. Int. J. Cancer, *40:*469, 1987.

Schapira, D. V., Kumar, N. B., Lyman, G. H., et al.: Abdominal obesity and breast cancer risk. Ann. Intern. Med., *112:*182, 1990.

Schapira, D. V., Kumar, N. G., Lyman, G. H., et al.: Obesity and body fat distribution and breast cancer prognosis. Cancer, *67:*523, 1991*a*.

Schapira, D. V., Kumar, N. G., and Lyman, G. H.: Obesity, body fat distribution, and sex hormones in breast cancer patients. Cancer, *67:*2215, 1991*b*.

Schatzkin, A., Carter, C. L., Green, S. B., et al.: Is alcohol consumption related to breast cancer? Results from the Framingham Heart Study. J. Natl. Cancer Inst., *81:*31, 1989*b*.

Schatzkin, A., Greenwald, P., Byar, D. P., et al.: The dietary fat–breast cancer hypothesis is alive. J.A.M.A., *261:*3284, 1989*a*.

Schatzkin, A., Jones, D. Y., Hoover, R. N., et al.: Alcohol consumption and breast cancer in the epidemiologic follow-up study of the First National Health and Nutrition Examination Survey. N. Engl. J. Med., *316:*1169, 1987.

Schatzkin, A., Piantadosi, S., Miccozzi, M., et al.: Alcohol consumption and breast cancer: A cross-national correlation study. Am. J. Epidemiol., *18:*28, 1989*c*.

Schrauzer, G. N.: Selenium and cancer; a review. Bioinorg. Chem., *5:*275, 1976.

Schrauzer, G. N., White, D. A., and Schneider, C. J.: Cancer mortality correlation studies. III. Statistical associations with dietary selenium intakes. Bioinorg. Chem., *7:*23, 1977*a*.

Schrauzer, G. N., White, D. A., and Schneider, C. J.: Cancer mortality correlation studies. IV. Associations with dietary intakes and blood levels of certain trace elements, notably Se-antagonists. Bioinorg. Chem., *7:*35, 1977*b*.

Schrauzer, G. N., White, D. A., and Schneider, C. J.: Selenium and cancer: Effects of selenium and of the diet on the genesis of spontaneous mammary tumors in virgin inbred female C3II/St mice. Bioinorg. Chem., *8:*387, 1978.

Schrijver, J., Alexieva-Figusch, J., van Breederode, N., et al.: Investigations on the nutritional status of advanced breast cancer patients. The influence of long-term treatment with Megestrol Acetate or Tamoxifen. Nutr. Cancer, *10:*231, 1987.

Seifter, E., Rettura G., and Levenson, S. M.: Supplemental B-carotene (BC); prophylactic action against 7,12-dimethylbenz(a)anthracene (DMBA) carcinogenesis (Abstract). Fed. Proc., *43:*662, 1984.

Sellers, T. A., Kushi, L. H., Potter, J. D., et al.: Effect of family history, body-fat distribution, and reproductive factors on the risk of postmenopausal breast cancer. N. Engl. J. Med., *326:*1323, 1992.

Serraino, M., and Thompson, L. U.: The effect of flaxseed supplementation on the initiation and promotional stages of mammary tumorigenesis. Nutr. Cancer, *17:*153, 1992.

Shamberger, R. J., Rukovena, E., Longfield, A. K., et al.: Antioxidants and cancer. I. Selenium in the blood of normals and cancer patients. J. Natl. Cancer Inst., *50:*863, 1973.

Shultz, T. D., Wilcox, R. B., Spuhler, J. M., et al.: Dietary and hormonal interrelationships in premenopausal women: Evidence for a relationship between dietary nutrients and plasma prolactin levels. Am. J. Clin. Nutr., *46:*905, 1987.

Shun-Zhang, Y., Rui-Fang, L., Da-Dao, Xu, et al.: A case-control study of dietary and nondietary risk factors for breast cancer in Shanghai. Cancer Res., *50:*5017, 1990.

Simard, A., Vobecky, J., and Vobecky, J. S.: Nutrition and lifestyle factors in fibrocystic disease and cancer of the breast. Cancer Detect. Prev., *14:*567, 1990.

Simard, A., Vobecky, J., and Vobecky, J. S.: Vitamin D deficiency and cancer of the breast: An unprovocative ecological hypothesis. Can. J. Pub. Health, *82:*300, 1991.

Snowdon, D. A., and Phillips, R. L.: Coffee consumption and risk of fatal cancers. Am. J. Public Health, *74:*820, 1984.

Sohrabi, A., Sandoz, J., Spratt, J. S., et al.: Recurrence of breast cancer. Obesity, tumor size, and axillary lymph node metastases. J.A.M.A., *244:*264, 1980.

Sorenson, A. W.: Assessment of nutrition in epidemiologic studies. *In* Schottenfeld, D., and Fraumeni, J. F. Jr. (Eds.): Cancer Epidemiology and Prevention. Philadelphia, W. B. Saunders, 1982, p. 434.

Stampfer, M. J., Colditz, G. A., and Willett, W. C.: Alcohol intake and risk of breast cancer. Compr. Ther., *14:*8, 1988.

Staszewski, J.: Breast cancer and body build. Prev. Med., *6:*410, 1977.

Staszewski, J., and Haenszel, W.: Cancer mortality among Polish born in the United States. J. Natl. Cancer Inst., *35:*292, 1965.

Staszewski, J., McCall, M. G., and Stenhouse, N. S.: Cancer mortality in 1962–1966 among Polish migrants to Australia. Br. J. Cancer, *25:*599, 1971.

Stocks, P.: Cancer mortality in relation to national consumption of cigarettes, solid fuel, tea and coffee. Br. J. Cancer, *24:*215, 1970.

Stoewsand, G. S., Anderson, J. L., Munson, L., et al.: Effect of dietary brussels sprouts with increased selenium content on mammary carcinogenesis in the rat. Cancer Lett., *45:*43, 1989.

Sundaram, G. S., London, R., Manimekalai, S., et al.: Alpha-tocopherol and serum lipoproteins. Lipids, *16:*223, 1981.

Sundram, K., Khor, H. T., Ong, A. S. H., et al.: Effect of doter palm oils on mammary carcinogenesis in female rats induced by 7,12-dimethylbenz(a)anthracene. Cancer Res., *49:*1447, 1989.

Swanson, C. A., Jones, D. Y., Schatzkin, A., et al.: Breast cancer risk assessed by anthropometry in the NHANES I epidemiological follow-up study. Cancer Res., *48:*5363, 1988.

Taioli, E., Nicolosi, A., and Wynder, E. L.: Dietary habits and breast cancer: A comparative study of United States and Italian data. Nutr. Cancer, *16:*259, 1991.

Takada, H., Hirooka, T., Hatano, T., et al.: Inhibition of 7,12-dimethylbenz(a)anthracene-induced lipid peroxidation and mammary tumor development in rats by vitamin E in conjunction with selenium. Nutr. Cancer, *17:*115, 1992.

Takahashi, S., and Biempica, L.: Effects of vitamin A and dexamethasone on collagen degradation in mouse mammary adenocarcinoma. Cancer Res., *45:*3311, 1985.

Tannenbaum, A.: Effects of varying caloric intake upon tumor incidence and tumor growth. Ann. NY Acad. Sci., *49:*5, 1947.

Tartter, P. I., Papatestas, A. E., Ioannovich, J. et al., Cholesterol and obesity as prognostic factors in breast cancer. Cancer, *47:*2222, 1981.

Thomas, I. K., and Erickson, K. L.: Lipid modulation of mammary tumor cell cytolysis: Direct influence of dietary fats on the effector component of cell-mediated cytotoxicity. J. Natl. Cancer Inst., *74:*675, 1985.

Tominaga, S.: Cancer incidence in Japanese in Japan, Hawaii and Western United States. J. Natl. Cancer Inst. Monogr., *69:*81, 1985.

Toniolo, P., Protta, F., and Cappa, A. P. M.: Risk of breast cancer, diet and internal migrations in northern Italy. Tumori, *75:*406, 1989*b*.

Toniolo, P., Riboli, E., Protta, F., et al.: Calorie-providing nutrients and risk of breast cancer. J. Natl. Cancer Inst., *81:*278, 1989*a*.

Toniolo, P., Riboli, E., Protta, E., Charrell, M., et al.: Breast cancer and alcohol consumption: A case-control study in Northern Italy. Cancer Research, *49:*5203, 1989*c*.

Tornberg, S. A., Holm, L. E., and Carstensen, J. M.: Breast cancer risk in relation to serum cholesterol, serum beta-lipoprotein, height, weight, and blood pressure. Acta Oncol., *27:*31, 1988.

Underwood, E. J.: Trace elements. *In* Toxicants Occurring Naturally in Foods. 2nd ed. Washington, DC, Food and Nutrition Board, National Academy of Sciences, 1973, p. 43.

United States Department of Agriculture: Dietary Guidelines for Americans. 2nd ed. Home and Garden Bulletin 232. Washington, DC, U.S. Government Printing Office, 1985.

van den Brandt, P. A., van't Veer, P., Goldbohm, R. A., et al.: A prospective cohort study on dietary fat and risk of postmenopausal breast cancer. Cancer Res., *53:*75, 1993.

van't Veer, P., Dekker, J. M., Lamers, J. W. J., et al.: Consumption of fermented milk products and breast cancer: A case-control study in the Netherlands. Cancer Res., *49:*4020, 1989*a*.

van't Veer, P., Kok, F. J., Hermus, R. J., et al.: Alcohol dose, frequency and age at first exposure in relation to the risk of breast cancer. Int. J. Epidemiol., *18:*511, 1989*b*.

van't Veer, P., Kok, F. J., Brants, H. A., et al.: Dietary fat and the risk of breast cancer. Int. J. Epidemiol., *19:*12, 1990*a*.

van't Veer, P., Kolb, C. M., Verhoef, P., et al.: Dietary fiber, beta-carotene and breast cancer: results from a case-control study. Int. J. Cancer, *45:*825, 1990*b*.

van't Veer, P., Van Leer, E. M., Rietdijk, A., et al.: Combination of dietary factors in relation to breast-cancer occurrence. Int. J. Cancer, *47:*649, 1991.

Vatten, L. J., and Foss, O. P.: Total serum cholesterol and triglycerides and risk of breast cancer: A prospective study of 24,329 Norwegian women. Cancer Res., *50:*2341, 1990.

Verreault, R., Brisson, J., Deschenes, L., et al.: Dietary fat in relation to prognostic indicators in breast cancer. J. Natl. Cancer Inst., *80:*819, 1988.

Vitamin E Research and Information Service: Role of the antioxidants in cancer prevention and treatment. Vitamin E Research Summary, LaGrange, IL, September, 1991.

Wald, N. J., Boreham, J., Hayward J. L., et al.: Plasma retinol, beta-carotene and vitamin E levels in relation to the future risk of breast cancer. Br. J. Cancer, *49:*321, 1984.

Welsch, C. W.: Enhancement of mammary tumorigenesis by dietary fat: Review of potential mechanisms. Am. J. Clin. Nutr., *45:*192, 1987.

Welsch, C. W.: Relationship between dietary fat and experimental mammary tumorigenesis: A review and critique. Cancer Res., *52*(Suppl):2040s, 1992.

Welsch, C. W., House, J. L., Herr, B. L., et al.: Enhancement of mammary carcinogenesis by high levels of dietary fat: A phenomenon dependent on ad libitum feeding. J. Natl. Cancer Inst., *82:*1615, 1990.

Whittemore, A. S., Paffenbarger, R. S., Anderson, K., et al.: Early precursors of site-specific cancers in college men and women. J. Natl. Cancer Inst., *74:*43, 1985.

Willett, W.: The search for the causes of breast and colon cancer. Nature, *338:*389, 1989.

Willett, W. C.: Overview of nutritional epidemiology. *In* Willett, W. (Ed.): Nutritional Epidemiology. New York, Oxford University Press, 1990*b*.

Willett, W. C.: Food frequency methods. *In* Willett, W. (Ed.): Nutritional Epidemiology. New York, Oxford University Press, 1990*a*.

Willett, W. C., and MacMahon, B.: Diet and cancer—an overview. N. Engl. J. Med., *310:*697, 1984.

Willett, W. C., Browne, M. L., Bain, C., et al.: Relative weight and risk of breast cancer among premenopausal women. Am. J. Epidemiol., *122:*731, 1985.

Willett, W. C., Hunter, D. J., Stampfer, M. J., et al.: Dietary fat and fiber in relation to risk of breast cancer. J.A.M.A., *268:*2037, 1992.

Willett, W. C., Stampfer, M. J., Colditz, G. A., et al.: Dietary fat and the risk of breast cancer. N. Engl. J. Med., *316:*22, 1987*a*.

Willett, W. C., Stampfer, M. J., Colditz, G. A., et al.: Moderate alcohol consumption and the risk of breast cancer. N. Engl. J. Med., *316:*1174, 1987*b*.

William, G., Howell, A., and James, M.: The relationship of body weight to response to endocrine therapy: Steroid hormone receptors and sur-vival of patients with advanced cancer of the breast. Br. J. Cancer, *58:*631, 1988.

Williams, C. M., and Dickerson, J. W.: Dietary fat, hormones and breast cancer: the cell membrane as a possible site of interaction of these two risk factors. Eur. J. Surg. Oncol., *13:*89, 1987.

Witschi, J. C.: Short-term dietary recall and recording methods. *In* Willett, W. (Ed.): Nutritional Epidemiology. New York, Oxford University Press, 1990.

Witting, L. A.: The oxidation of alpha-tocopherol during the autoxidation of ethyl oleate, linolenate, and arachidonate. Arch. Biochem. Biophys., *129:*142, 1969.

Wolfe, J. N., Saftlas, A. F., and Salane, M.: Mammographic parenchymal patterns and quantitative evaluation of mammographic densities: a case control study. Am. J. Roentgenol., *148:*1087, 1987.

Wynder, E. L.: Dietary factors related to breast cancer. Cancer, *46*(Suppl.):899, 1980.

Wynder, E. L.: Amount and type of fat/fiber in nutritional carcinogenesis. Prev. Med., *16:*451, 1987.

Wynder, E. L.: Strategies toward the primary prevention of cancer. Lucy Wortham James clinical research award lecture. Arch. Surg., *125:*163, 1990.

Young, V. R., and Richardson, D. P.: Nutrients, vitamins and minerals in cancer prevention—facts and fallacies. Cancer, *43*(Suppl. 5):2125, 1979.

Yuan, J., Yu, M. C., Ross, R. K., et al.: Risk factors for breast cancer in Chinese women in Shanghai. Cancer Res., *48:*1949, 1988.

Zaridze, D., Lifanova, Y., Maximovitch, D., et al.: Diet, alcohol consumption and reproductive factors in a case-control study of breast cancer in Moscow. Int. J. Cancer, *48:*493, 1991.

Zumoff, B., and Dasgupta, I.: Relationship between body weight and the incidence of positive axillary nodes at mastectomy for breast cancer. J. Surg. Oncol., *22:*217, 1983.

Zumoff, B., O'Connor, J., Levin, J., et al.: Nonobesity at the time of mastectomy is highly predictive of 10-year disease-free survival in women with breast cancer. Anticancer Res., *2:*59, 1982.

Appendix I

1983 Metropolitan Height and Weight Tables for Men and Women (According to Frame, Ages 25–59)

Height (In Shoes)†		Weight in Pounds in Indoor Clothing*			Height (In Shoes)†		Weight in Pounds in Indoor Clothing*		
Feet	Inches	Small Frame	Medium Frame	Large Frame	Feet	Inches	Small Frame	Medium Frame	Large Frame
Men					Women				
5	2	128–134	131–141	138–150	4	10	102–111	109–121	118–131
5	3	130–136	133–143	140–153	4	11	103–113	111–123	120–134
5	4	132–138	135–145	142–156	5	0	104–115	113–126	122–137
5	5	134–140	137–148	144–160	5	1	106–118	115–129	125–140
5	6	136–142	139–151	146–164	5	2	108–121	118–132	128–143
5	7	138–145	142–154	149–168	5	3	111–124	121–135	131–147
5	8	140–148	145–157	152–172	5	4	114–127	124–138	134–151
5	9	142–151	148–160	155–176	5	5	117–130	127–141	137–155
5	10	144–154	151–163	158–180	5	6	120–133	130–144	140–159
5	11	146–157	154–166	161–184	5	7	123–136	133–147	143–163
6	0	149–160	157–170	164–188	5	8	126–139	136–150	146–167
6	1	152–164	160–174	168–192	5	9	129–142	139–153	149–170
6	2	155–168	164–178	172–197	5	10	132–145	142–156	152–173
6	3	158–172	167–182	176–202	5	11	135–148	145–159	155–176
6	4	162–176	171–187	181–207	6	0	138–151	148–162	158–179

(Source of basic data: Build Study, 1979, Society of Actuaries and Association of Life Insurance Medical Directors of America, 1980. Copyright 1983, Metropolitan Life Insurance Company. Reprinted with permission.)
*Indoor clothing weighing 5 lb for men and 3 lb for women.
†Shoes with 1-inch heels.

1983 Metropolitan Height and Weight Tables for Men and Women on Metric Basis (According to Frame, Ages 25–59)

Height (In Shoes)† Centimeters	MEN Weight in Kilograms (In Indoor Clothing)*			Height (In Shoes)† Centimeters	WOMEN Weight in Kilograms (In Indoor Clothing)*		
	Small Frame	Medium Frame	Large Frame		Small Frame	Medium Frame	Large Frame
158	58.3–61.0	59.6–64.2	62.8–68.3	148	46.4–50.6	49.6–55.1	53.7–59.8
159	58.6–61.3	59.9–64.5	63.1–68.8	149	46.6–51.0	50.0–55.5	54.1–60.3
160	59.0–61.7	60.3–64.9	63.5–69.4	150	46.7–51.3	50.3–55.9	54.4–60.9
161	59.3–62.0	60.6–65.2	63.8–69.9	151	46.9–51.7	50.7–56.4	54.8–61.4
162	59.7–62.4	61.0–65.6	64.2–70.5	152	47.1–52.1	51.1–57.0	55.2–61.9
163	60.0–62.7	61.3–66.0	64.5–71.1	153	47.4–52.5	51.5–57.5	55.6–62.4
164	60.4–63.1	61.7–66.5	64.9–71.8	154	47.8–53.0	51.9–58.0	56.2–63.0
165	60.8–63.5	62.1–67.0	65.3–72.5	155	48.1–53.6	52.2–58.6	56.8–63.6
166	61.1–63.8	62.4–67.6	65.6–73.2	156	48.5–54.1	52.7–59.1	57.3–64.1
167	61.5–64.2	62.8–68.2	66.0–74.0	157	48.8–54.6	53.2–59.6	57.8–64.6
168	61.8–64.6	63.2–68.7	66.4–74.7	158	49.3–55.2	53.8–60.2	58.4–65.3
169	62.2–65.2	63.8–69.3	67.0–75.4	159	49.8–55.7	54.3–60.7	58.9–66.0
170	62.5–65.7	64.3–69.8	67.5–76.1	160	50.3–56.2	54.9–61.2	59.4–66.7
171	62.9–66.2	64.8–70.3	68.0–76.8	161	50.8–56.7	55.4–61.7	59.9–67.4
172	63.2–66.7	65.4–70.8	68.5–77.5	162	51.4–57.3	55.9–62.3	60.5–68.1
173	63.6–67.3	65.9–71.4	69.1–78.2	163	51.9–57.8	56.4–62.8	61.0–68.8
174	63.9–67.8	66.4–71.9	69.6–78.9	164	52.5–58.4	57.0–63.4	61.5–69.5
175	64.3–68.3	66.9–72.4	70.1–79.6	165	53.0–58.9	57.5–63.9	62.0–70.2
176	64.7–68.9	67.5–73.0	70.7–80.3	166	53.6–59.5	58.1–64.5	62.6–70.9
177	65.0–69.5	68.1–73.5	71.3–81.0	167	54.1–60.0	58.7–65.0	63.2–71.7
178	65.4–70.0	68.6–74.0	71.8–81.8	168	54.6–60.5	59.2–65.5	63.7–72.4
179	65.7–70.5	69.2–74.6	72.3–82.5	169	55.2–61.1	59.7–66.1	64.3–73.1
180	66.1–71.0	69.7–75.1	72.8–83.3	170	55.7–61.6	60.2–66.6	64.8–73.8
181	66.6–71.6	70.2–75.8	73.4–84.0	171	56.2–62.1	60.7–67.1	65.3–74.5
182	67.1–72.1	70.7–76.5	73.9–84.7	172	56.8–62.6	61.3–67.6	65.8–75.2
183	67.7–72.7	71.3–77.2	74.5–85.4	173	57.3–63.2	61.8–68.2	66.4–75.9
184	68.2–73.4	71.8–77.9	75.2–86.1	174	57.8–63.7	62.3–68.7	66.9–76.4
185	68.7–74.1	72.4–78.6	75.9–86.8	175	58.3–64.2	62.8–69.2	67.4–76.9
186	69.2–74.8	73.0–79.3	76.6–87.6	176	58.9–64.8	63.4–69.8	68.0–77.5
187	69.8–75.5	73.7–80.0	77.3–88.5	177	59.5–65.4	64.0–70.4	68.5–78.1
188	70.3–76.2	74.4–80.7	78.0–89.4	178	60.0–65.9	64.5–70.9	69.0–78.6
189	70.9–76.9	74.9–81.5	78.7–90.3	179	60.5–66.4	65.1–71.4	69.6–79.1
190	71.4–77.6	75.4–82.2	79.4–91.2	180	61.0–66.9	65.6–71.9	70.1–79.6
191	72.1–78.4	76.1–83.0	80.3–92.1	181	61.6–67.5	66.1–72.5	70.7–80.2
192	72.8–79.1	76.8–83.9	81.2–93.0	182	62.1–68.0	66.6–73.0	71.2–80.7
193	73.5–79.8	77.6–84.8	82.1–93.9	183	62.6–68.5	67.1–73.5	71.7–81.2

(Source of basic data: Build Study, 1979, Society of Actuaries and Association of Life Insurance Medical Directors of America, 1980. Copyright 1983, Metropolitan Life Insurance Company. Reprinted with permission.)
*Indoor clothing weighing 2.3 kg for men and 1.4 kg for women.
†Shoes with 2.5-cm heels.

How to Determine Your Body Frame By Elbow Breadth

To make a simple approximation of your frame size:

Extend your arm and bend the forearm upwards at a 90° angle. Keep the fingers straight and turn the inside of your wrist toward the body. Place the thumb and index finger of your other hand on the two prominent bones on either side of your elbow. Measure the space between your fingers against a ruler or a tape measure. (For the most accurate measurement, have your physician measure your elbow breadth with calipers.) Compare this measure with the measurements shown below.

These tables list the elbow measurements for men and women of medium frame at various heights. Measurements lower than those listed indicate that you have a small frame while higher measurements indicate a large frame.

Men				Women			
Height (In 1-inch Heels)	Elbow Breadth (Inches)	Height (In 2.5-cm Heels)	Elbow Breadth (cm)	Height (In 1-inch Heels)	Elbow Breadth (Inches)	Height (In 2.5-cm Heels)	Elbow Breadth (cm)
5'2"–5'3"	2½"–2⅞"	158–161	6.4–7.2	4'10"–4'11"	2¼"–2½"	148–151	5.6–6.4
5'4"–5'7"	2⅝"–2⅞"	162–171	6.7–7.4	5'0"–5'3"	2¼"–2½"	152–161	5.8–6.5
5'8"–5'11"	2¾"–3"	172–181	6.9–7.8	5'4"–5'7"	2⅜"–2⅝"	162–171	5.9–6.6
6'0"–6'3"	2¾"–3⅛"	182–191	7.1–7.8	5'8"–5'11"	2⅜"–2⅝"	172–181	6.1–6.8
6'4"	2⅞"–3¼"	192–193	7.4–8.1	6'0"	2½"–2¾"	182–183	6.2–6.9

(Source of basic data: Data tape, HANES I—Anthropometry, goniometry, skeletal age, bone density, and cortical thickness, ages 1–74. National Health and Nutrition Examination Survey, 1971–75, National Center for Health Statistics.

6 A Unifying Concept for Benign Disorders of the Breast: ANDI

Leslie E. Hughes

ANDI (Aberrations of Normal Development and Involution) is presented as a terminology and as a framework for understanding benign breast disorders (BBDs) (Hughes et al., 1987). It is based on two main principles. First, most BBDs arise as a result of the dynamic changes occurring in the breast through the three main periods of reproductive life: breast development (the early reproductive period), the mature reproductive period, and involution. Second, most of these disorders can be seen as a spectrum that extends from the normal process to overt disease; between these extremes lie conditions so common in frequency and so modest in severity that use of the term "aberration" to describe them seems more appropriate than use of the term "disease."

The ANDI concept is gaining increasing acceptance as a framework to describe clinical features and pathology using terms that are consistent with current understanding of pathogenesis. It has wide implications in relation to the accuracy of terminology and the understanding of BBDs; these implications extend to management of the disorders. The ANDI concept has been adopted by a multinational, multidisciplinary working party (Hughes et al., 1992). This chapter presents the thinking and principles underlying the concept, which are described in greater detail elsewhere (Hughes et al., 1989).

It is difficult to justify the neglect accorded to BBDs by clinicians; however, this neglect is not altogether surprising in view of the great amount of attention that breast cancer has received as a result of the anguish and stress associated with its diagnosis and treatment. BBDs deserve an equal standing because they underlie 90% of clinical consultations involving the breast. Unless they are managed effectively—that is, on the basis of sound understanding—these disorders are associated with much patient stress and impairment of a patient's familial relationships. Appreciation of pathophysiology is always the basis of sound management, and it is here that the difference between breast cancer and BBDs is apparent.

Breast cancer is universally understood on the basis of a unified concept that has both longitudinal and horizontal elements. The longitudinal element extends from premalignant conditions to microinvasion, to local extension, and to nodal and distant spread. The horizontal elements cover a variety of histologic types, including lobular, ductal, and anaplastic and their variants, as well as biologic factors such as hormone receptor status and growth factors. In terms of pathogenesis, the basic etiology of breast cancer remains obscure; however, it is known to result from a number of influences—genetic, hormonal, and chemical—that act on the deoxyribonucleic acid (DNA) of a cell. Thus, when a female patient presents with breast cancer, she can be categorized within this overall framework. This allows initiation of a therapeutic strategy that is appropriate to her individual circumstances. Furthermore, an analysis of the factors that may have led to her cancer can be made.

The situation is very different in patients with benign conditions for which no such framework exists. Each condition tends to be seen as an individual entity and is assessed in isolation and is managed empirically. Because there is no encompassing framework against which these disorders can be set, the important borderline between "normal" and "disease" statuses has remained blurred. This sometimes results in inappropriately radical management for a condition that may now be recognized as lying toward the normal end of the spectrum. I would suggest that a woman who presents with a benign condition can be categorized within a framework as easily as can the woman who presents with breast cancer.

The main advantages of the ANDI concept are as follow:

1. It provides a clear terminology that addresses clinical and histologic aspects individually, facilitating communication between surgeon, radiologist, pathologist, and patient.

2. It relates clinical findings to pathogenesis. This is important in assessing clinical significance and in enhancing understanding of the individual components of BBDs.

3. By stressing the borderline between normal and abnormal conditions, it facilitates the placing of an individual case within the overall framework; this leads to appropriate management.

4. It emphasizes the normality or near-normality of most BBDs, justifying the use of the term "disorder" rather than "disease"; the latter term is retained for a small, well-defined subgroup of BBDs.

First, the development of this concept is best considered against the background of the problems associated with present attitudes and with the advances in understanding that underlie the ANDI concept. Next, it is appropriate to consider the concept's implications for managing BBDs.

THE PROBLEMS ASSOCIATED WITH TRADITIONAL CONCEPTS OF BENIGN BREAST DISORDERS

Poor Understanding of Pathogenesis

Pathogenesis is often poorly understood. Examples of this are seen in the conventional attitudes with regard to fibroadenomas, breast macrocysts, and fibrocystic disease. Fibroadenomas are by convention regarded as benign tumors and are treated as such—that is, by mandatory surgical excision. The failure to see macrocysts in the context of the normal variant—the cystic involution of lobules—leaves them to be regarded as a potential form of malignancy (although rare) and, hence, to be excised if they recur. The view that fibrocystic disease is a pathologic condition, defined as a histologic entity rather than as a physiologic disturbance, has resulted in many frustrating studies that have attempted to determine whether this clinical condition has premalignant potential. A further example is the confusion of duct ectasia with macrocysts; this lack of understanding arises from a failure to recognize cysts as lobular in origin and duct ectasia as ductal in origin (Azzopardi, 1979).

Loose Terminology

For 200 years, individual workers in this field have tended to produce their own nomenclatures, usually with little regard for the terms used by previous clinicians. Each has devised terms that stress particular aspects of the condition. Earlier clinicians often used clinical terms, such as "chronic mastitis." Terms used by later specialists tended to reflect the biopsy appearance of symptomatic lesions (e.g., "fibrocystic disease," "hyperplastic cystic disease"), but did not fully describe the range of histologic appearances in asymptomatic breast tissue. Over 40 names have been used to describe the variety of conditions covered by the old term "chronic fibrocystic disease," and other BBDs have been treated in similar fashion (Table 6–1). It is hardly surprising that much confusion among clinicians has occurred when communicating with one another and even more so when clinicians have attempted to communicate concepts to clinicians in other specialties, to radiologists, and to pathologists.

Inappropriate Correlation of Clinical Features with Histologic Changes

In the past, a patient with a clinical abnormality was subjected to local biopsy and to analysis of the histologic changes that correlated with that clinical episode, assuming that a causal relationship existed. Hence, processes such as fibrosis, cyst formation, adenosis, mild epithelial hyperplasia, and lymphocyte infiltration have come to be regarded as indicators of disease and symptom-related. A number of detailed histologic studies of normal breasts have shown that this view is unfounded (Sandison, 1962). It must now

Table 6–1. CONFUSION OF TERMINOLOGY—SOME OF THE NAMES USED FOR COMMON BENIGN BREAST DISORDERS

Cyclic Nodularity
Fibrocystic disease
Fibroadenosis
Cystic hyperplasia
Chronic cystic mastitis
Chronic mastitis
Chronic mastopathy
Schimmelbusch's disease
Duct Ectasia/Periductal Mastitis
Variant of cystic disease
Plasma cell mastitis
Varicocele tumor
Secretory disease
Mastitis obliterans
Comedomastitis
Giant Fibroadenomatous Tumors
Giant fibroadenoma
Cystosarcoma phyllodes
Phyllodes tumor
Serocystic disease of Brodie
Juvenile fibroadenoma

be accepted that the changes classically regarded as fibrocystic disease can be found in normal asymptomatic breasts or in a symptomatic breast distant to the site of symptoms and thus lie within the spectrum of normality. The pathologist's practice of reporting these histologic changes to justify the clinician's decision for performing biopsy may be responsible in large degree for the continuing attribution of the condition to disease.

The "Nondisease" Concept

The recognition that the histologic changes of fibrocystic disease are normal has led to a reaction in the opposite direction—that is, that fibrocystic disease does not exist (i.e., it is a nondisease [Love et al., 1982]). Although such an attitude is useful in denying the putative association between fibrocystic disease and cancer, it can be a disservice to women who suffer from BBDs and who may have symptoms of distressing severity. Many clinicians regard BBD as synonymous with fibrocystic disease and use the nondisease concept to label patients as neurotic. A more comprehensive understanding of BBDs as expressed through the ANDI concept recognizes that painful nodularity has a physiologic basis that can validate the reality of the condition as a cause of morbidity (Kumar et al., 1984). Furthermore, the range of BBDs is far too wide to be encompassed by an all-embracing term such as "fibrocystic disease."

All of these problems can be related to a poor appreciation of the pathogenesis of BBDs and to a poor appreciation of the spectrum of normal and abnormal within the breast during a woman's reproductive life. Such an appreciation is critical to an understanding of BBDs and to the ANDI concept; therefore, it is dealt with in some detail in this chapter.

THE PHYSIOLOGIC STRUCTURAL CHANGES WITHIN THE NORMAL BREAST

Although the broad concepts of the hormonal changes within the breast that are associated with development, menstruation and pregnancy, and the menopause have been well appreciated, the details of the physiologic control and structural changes are less widely understood. However, some important studies have added greatly to our knowledge of these subjects. Two surgeons played a crucial role in elucidating the clinical significance of lobular development and involution (Hayward and Parks, 1958; and Parks, 1959), whereas another surgical group demonstrated the physiologic basis of painful nodularity (Kumar et al., 1984; and Kumar et al., 1985). Davies has elucidated periductal inflammatory change and its significance (Davies, 1975). Histologic studies of large normal population groups defined the range and incidence of ''pathologic'' changes in the normal breast (Sandison, 1962; and Sloss et al., 1957), while others defined in detail the spectrum of hyperplastic changes and its association with cancer (Dupont and Page, 1985; and Wellings et al., 1975). These and similar studies have clarified the spectrum of normality, providing a background for defining histologic abnormality.

This background knowledge of the spectrum of normal processes within the breast is of the greatest importance and can be summarized as follows (it is dealt with in detail in a later section):

The Premenarchal Breast

During the period preceding menarche, the breast consists of only a few small ducts behind the nipple. The breast is not subject to disorder or disease during this period unless it is abnormally stimulated by hormonal influences—maternal influences in the neonatal period, or inappropriate hormonal production at a later point.

The Perimenarchal Period (Early Reproductive Life)

Although the perimenarchal period is dominated by the process of ductal extension and lobular development, the extent of lobular variability was not appreciated until the publication of Parks's study (Parks, 1959). Parks described a spectrum ranging from normal lobules to giant lobules and subclinical fibroadenomas that demonstrated no histologic difference between large lobules and small fibroadenomas. Furthermore, small fibroadenomas were shown to be more common than was clinically recognized, demonstrating the existence of a continuum from normal lobule to clinical fibroadenoma. Thus, clinically detectable fibroadenoma is seen as the ''tip-of-the-iceberg'' end of a spectrum of normal lobular development—not as a specific entity of a benign tumor—and fibroadenoma can be seen to conform to the terminology of aberrations in normal development.

The Reproductive Period of Cyclic Changes

The monthly cyclic changes in the breast, and the more radical changes superimposed by pregnancy, have long been appreciated; however, the detail of the histologic changes associated with menstruation (Vorherr, 1974) have received less study than may be realized. Pregnancy-associated changes in the breast illustrate the factors predisposing a woman to a BBD. Although the stimulus of pregnancy and lactation and the withdrawal of the stimulus at weaning are intense, the changes of involution after pregnancy are surprisingly patchy and variable—in fact, the changes of pregnancy may persist for years. This observation illustrates the fundamental focal variation in the hormonal responsiveness of many endocrine target organs. Such variation within the breast, compounded by repeated cyclic change, provides a ready explanation for the histologic changes in stroma and glandular tissue found in the normal breast that have previously been labeled as fibroadenosis. The more complex changes of sclerosing adenosis may also arise in this way.

Despite this acceptance of structural changes in the breast resulting from cyclic stimulation and regression during reproductive life, no histologic explanation of the premenstrual pain and nodularity that form such a large part of the clinical spectrum of BBD yet exists. Although edema would seem to be an obvious cause, breast pain is not associated with changes in total body water (Preece et al., 1975), and methodologic difficulties exist in quantifying local edema. Of greater importance to our understanding of BBDs is the fact that a physiologic abnormality can be demonstrated in patients with severe premenstrual pain (Kumar et al., 1984). These patients can be shown to have exaggerated prolactin release on hypothalamic stimulation. This indicates the need to consider functional or physiologic aspects equally as important or even more important than structural changes in assessing BBDs.

Involution

Since the changes of perimenopausal involution are protracted (taking place possibly from 35 to 55 years of age) and are complex (involving all elements of the breast), it is not surprising that minor disorders of involution are frequently seen. Periductal inflammatory changes may lead to contrasting sclerosis or weakening of the duct wall. The former may be a normal mechanism for duct involution, whereas the second results in ductal ectasia. Lobular involution normally consists of an orderly loss of both lobular epithelium and stroma; this leads to the simple disappearance of the whole lobule or to its replacement by a ghost of hyaline fibrotic tissue. In contrast, lobular involution may take the variant pattern of cystic lobular involution, as described by Parks (1959). In this process, the acini within a lobule distend to become microcysts, which in turn may provide the basis for the development of macrocysts. Although the process is not completely understood, the interrelationship of the epithelium and specialized lobular stroma is vital. As long as some lobular stroma persists, the

Table 6–2. CLASSIFICATION OF THE MORE IMPORTANT BENIGN CONDITIONS

Period	Main Clinical Presentation
Menarche 　Lobular development	Fibroadenoma
Reproductive life 　Cyclic changes of 　menstruation and 　pregnancy	Pain and nodularity
Menopause 　Period of involution	Macrocysts Duct ectasia Periductal mastitis Nipple retraction Epithelial hyperplasias

microcystic involution may revert to normal involution (Azzopardi, 1979). Presumably, it is the premature disappearance of this stroma, or perhaps blockage of the efferent ductule, that converts microcystic involution (normal) into gross cyst formation (aberration).

Furthermore, Parks found epithelial hyperplasia to be commonly observed during the perimenopausal period; this was the case in other studies as well (Sloss et al., 1957; and Wellings et al., 1975). Hyperplastic changes are sufficiently common to be regarded as normal and may regress after the menopause. Thus, the major areas of BBD—duct ectasia and periductal inflammation, macrocyst formation, and epithelial hyperplasia—may all be seen as arising on the basis of normal involutional processes.

THE DEFINITION OF CLINICAL SYNDROMES OF BENIGN BREAST DISORDERS

In parallel with the fostering of understanding of normal and abnormal processes in the breast, greater appreciation of clinical aspects of BBDs has resulted from clinics dedicated to the study of these disorders (Hughes et al., 1989). These have led to more accurate definition of clinical syndromes, such as a detailed classification of breast pain, to clarification of periductal mastitis, and to an appreciation of the benign significance of macrocysts and the nipple discharge of duct ectasia. This clarification of clinical syndromes has highlighted the tendency of most common BBDs to be associated with one of the three main phases of reproductive life (Table 6–2). This sets the scene for a broad framework to encompass the spectrum of BBDs.

THE UNDERLYING PRINCIPLES OF THE ANDI CONCEPT AND TERMINOLOGY

The four main principles underlying the concept of ANDI are presented in Table 6–3. Most BBDs are related to the normal processes during the three main periods of reproductive life (see Table 6–2).

Table 6–3. THE PRINCIPLES UNDERLYING THE ANDI CONCEPT

1. Most benign disorders are related to normal processes of reproductive life.
2. There is a spectrum that ranges from normal to aberration and, sometimes, to disease.
3. The definition of normal and abnormal is pragmatic.
4. The ANDI concept embraces all aspects—symptoms, signs, histology, and physiology.

Early Reproductive Period (Fibroadenoma)

Simple fibroadenoma is a common condition of early reproductive life, with its peak incidence during lobular development in women aged 15 to 25 years. It is conventionally considered a benign tumor of the breast; the alternative concept—that it is a minor aberration of the normal process of lobular development—is so central to the ANDI concept that it is useful to consider the evidence in detail (Table 6–4).

Parks (1959) showed that the concept of "normal lobule" or "clinical fibroadenoma" was invalid. A continuum exists that relates normal lobules and lobules of increasing size to subclinical and, finally, clinical fibroadenoma. Each of these is much more common than is seen clinically, and most normal breasts show giant lobules or microfibroadenomas. Fibroadenomas do not grow progressively as do benign tumors. Most reach a size of between 1 and 2 cm and either remain static or regress. They show marked hormonal sensitivity—a sensitivity that is of a greater degree than is usually seen with benign neoplasms. Thus, a fibroadenoma that is present during pregnancy will lactate in the puerperium. Should a fibroadenoma escape the surgeon's knife, it will involute at the menopause, ending as a mass of hyaline fibrous tissue, perhaps with calcification.

All of these factors are more characteristic of and consistent with an aberration of the normal lobular growth process than with a benign tumor.

Mature Reproductive Period

The dominant clinical presentation in this period is cyclic pain and nodularity. Although many studies have shown that no histopathologic basis exists for this condition, a physiologic aberration can be demonstrated: an increase in stimulated prolactin release (Kumar et al., 1984). Again, there is a clinical spectrum of severity of symptoms ranging from the absence of symptoms to mild premenstrual discomfort to occasional pain of great severity.

Table 6–4. EVIDENCE THAT SIMPLE FIBROADENOMA IS AN EXAMPLE OF ANDI, NOT OF A BENIGN TUMOR

1. A continuum exists between normal lobule, large lobule, subclinical fibroadenoma, and clinical fibroadenoma.
2. All of the entities in 1 are histologically similar.
3. Fibroadenoma is hormone-responsive.
4. Fibroadenomas are self-limiting.

Involution

In this period, the main clinical presentations are macrocysts and the histologic presentation of epithelial hyperplasia. A less common problem is nipple discharge associated with duct ectasia.

In view of the complexity of the processes associated with involution of lobules and ducts, it is hardly surprising that aberrations should be common. Hayward and Parks (1958) described the process of microcystic lobular involution—a minor variation of normal lobular involution—that can be seen in most normal breasts if it is sought. It provides an explanation for the development of macrocysts. Thus, the spectrum from normal lobular involution through microcystic involution to macrocyst formation shows similarity to the development of fibroadenoma and to lobular development.

Ductal dilatation can be explained as damage from the periductal infiltrate that is so often seen around ducts, whereas the common benign nipple retraction of the menopausal period can be attributed to excessive damage with fibrosis and subsequent scar contraction.

The Spectrum from Normal to Aberration and, Sometimes, to Disease

The spectrum from normal to aberration to disease has been illustrated in relation to the manifestation of fibroadenoma, cyclic pain and nodularity, and macrocysts. It is an important part of the ANDI concept, replacing the old idea that one dealt either with normality or disease. Although it is clear that the spectrum from normality to aberration is a continuum, at present there is no similar clear-cut evidence that the aberration-to-disease end of the spectrum, when it is reached, is also a continuum. For example, there is no evidence that giant fibroadenoma develops from a normal fibroadenoma; the two entities may be separate conditions ab initio. Likewise, no definite evidence exists to substantiate that carcinoma in situ, or hyperplasia with atypia, represents a progression from benign hyperplasias. This issue is considered in the following section.

The Borderline Between Normality and Abnormality

The basic question has to be asked, What determines whether a clinical condition is normal or abnormal? In the past, the presentation of a lump—whether it be a fibroadenoma or an area of cyclic nodularity—was combined with a histologic picture, which was considered to be abnormal, to provide a definition of disease. In fact, normality and abnormality are best defined in pragmatic terms, taking into account factors such as incidence, clinical impact, and histology.

Incidence is important because if a condition is present in everyone, it must be regarded as normal. As an example of the importance of incidence, macrocysts are very common and commonly multiple, whereas microcysts are found in almost all breasts if looked for carefully on histologic examination. Clearly, microcysts must be regarded as normal, and macrocysts are at most an aberration of normality and cannot be considered disease.

Clinical impact is also important, as can be illustrated by the example of breast pain. A very large proportion of women experience premenstrual discomfort for a few days. This causes little interference with quality of life and, thus, must be regarded as normal. However, when pain persists for 3 of the 4 weeks of the menstrual cycle and is of great severity, it should be approached differently. Such pain is quite uncommon, and its impact in some patients can be severe—for example, in relation to such factors as physical work and family relationships with children or husbands. Hence, pain of increasing severity could be regarded as an aberration from normality or, perhaps with the most extreme cases, as disease.

The significance of histologic findings has given rise to more confusion about what is normal or abnormal than have the impact of other aspects of BBDs. Not long ago, even more benign degrees of hyperplasia were often considered as representing a cancer risk. However, a number of specialists have shown that simple hyperplasia is common in the perimenopausal period (Parks, 1959; and Sloss et al., 1957), and Dupont and Page (1985) have defined histologic patterns precisely. It is now recognized that a spectrum exists from the normal apocrine change through the development of simple hyperplasias to the formation of atypical hyperplasias and carcinoma in situ.

The ANDI Concept Relates to All Aspects: Signs and Symptoms, Histology, and Physiology

The confusion that has surrounded the fibrocystic disease concept has arisen from the consideration of clinical features (pain and nodularity) along with histologic features (e.g., fibrosis and adenosis) and building the combination into a disease. The recognition that the clinical features cannot be regarded as disease because of their high incidence and that the histologic features cannot be regarded as disease because of their lack of specificity has resulted in rejection of the clinical significance of BBD in favor of a concept of nondisease (Love et al., 1982). Although there is an element of truth in this concept, it is not helpful in understanding the basic processes and the problems of patients. The situation can be resolved by considering each aspect separately, whether it be clinical, radiologic, histologic, or physiologic, without trying to correlate each with the others artificially. The ANDI framework, and particularly the spectrum concept, allows for this.

THE ANDI FRAMEWORK

Thus, the ANDI classification can be characterized as a two-dimensional framework that involves the reproductive periods as its vertical element and the spectrum from normality through aberration to disease as its horizontal ele-

Table 6–5. THE BASIC ANDI FRAMEWORK

Reproductive Period	Spectrum			
	Normal	*Aberration*	*Clinical Presentation*	*Disease*
Early (15–25 y)				
Mature (25–45 y)				
Involutional (35–55 y)				

ment (Table 6–5). An additional column—clinical presentation—is included to clarify the fact that clinical presentation should only be correlated with histologic or physiologic changes when such a correlation can be shown to be valid.

This basic framework can then be filled in to give the complete ANDI classification (Table 6–6).

Early Reproductive Life

Fibroadenoma

Since there is a spectrum from normal lobule to fibroadenoma, it is not surprising that fibroadenomas are seen predominantly in the period of lobular development, even though they may not be diagnosed until later, when postpregnancy or involutional changes facilitate palpation. The factors supporting the view that fibroadenoma should be considered part of the ANDI concept rather than as a benign neoplasm have been discussed earlier. Particularly important is the fact that fibroadenomas rarely grow beyond 1 or 2 cm in size and thereafter remain static.

What about continuing growth beyond the 1- to 2-cm limit? Growth to greater than 5 cm is sufficiently uncommon in Western populations (and continued growth can represent a significant clinical problem) to be classified as a disease—giant fibroadenoma. Similarly, whereas two or three fibroadenomas are relatively common, more than five in one breast is rare and causes sufficient management problems to be regarded as disease.

Juvenile Hypertrophy

This condition is associated with gross stromal hyperplasia at the time of breast development. Since so little is known about the control of breast stromal growth, it is not surprising that the cause of juvenile hypertrophy is unknown. It is likely that the condition has a hormonal basis, a view supported by reports that danazol may have a beneficial effect in patients with the condition. The continuous spectrum from the presence of small breasts to the manifestation of massive hyperplasia justifies this classification within the ANDI concept; unilateral hypoplasia and breast asymmetry presumably have a related pathogenesis.

Mature Reproductive Period

Mastalgia and Nodularity

Premenstrual enlargement and postmenstrual involution of the breast that occur with each cycle are so commonly associated with discomfort and nodularity that they are regarded as normal. In more severe cases, they cause sufficient trouble to the patient to be moved into the aberration category of cyclic mastalgia and cyclic nodularity. In a few patients, the clinical impact is so severe that this condition might be classified as a disease; however, clinical experience shows that such disease (and particularly that resistant to standard treatments) is likely to have a more complex basis than the simple exaggeration of hormonal effects.

Table 6–6. THE ANDI CLASSIFICATION

Stage (Peak Age)	Normal Process	Aberration		Disease State
		Underlying Condition	*Clinical Presentation*	
Early reproductive period (15–25 y)	Lobule formation Stroma formation	Fibroadenoma Juvenile hypertrophy	Discrete lump Excessive breast development	Giant fibroadenoma Multiple fibroadenomas
Mature reproductive period (25–40 y)	Cyclic hormonal effects on glandular tissue and stroma	Exaggerated cyclic effects	Cyclic mastalgia and nodularity generalized or discrete	
Involution (35–55 y)	Lobular involution (including microcysts, apocrine change, fibrosis, and adenosis)	Macrocysts Sclerosing lesions	Discrete lumps X-ray abnormalities (mastalgia, lumps)	
	Ductal involution (including periductal round cell infiltrates)	Duct dilatation Periductal fibrosis	Nipple discharge Nipple retraction	Periductal mastitis with bacterial infection and abscess formation
	Epithelial turnover	Mild epithelial hyperplasia	Histologic report	Epithelial hyperplasia with atypia

Involutional Reproductive Period

Cyst Formation

The desirable integrated involution of lobular stroma and epithelium is not always seen, and it is not surprising that minor aberrations of the process are common during a period of fluctuating involution that extends over 20 years. Although the mechanism of this involution is far from completely understood, the normal variant of microcystic involution clearly sets the scene for macrocyst development. This concept of the macrocyst as an involutional aberration (and, hence, part of the ANDI concept) rather than as a disease is consistent with its high frequency of occurrence and with the fact that it is so often found to be multiple and subclinical.

The observation that macrocysts appear to develop by two different pathways (apocrine and nonapocrine) is still poorly understood, but the evidence is strong that both develop from a common origin of microcystic involution (Dixon et al., 1985).

Sclerosing Adenosis

This condition may be considered an aberration of either the cyclic or the involutional phase of breast activity, since it can show histologic changes that are both proliferative and involutional. This illustrates the complexity, on the one hand, but the simplicity of concept, on the other, of regarding these as aberrations of so many interacting normal processes. When one considers the complex interrelationship of stromal fibrosis and epithelial regression that occurs during involution and that this is superimposed on cyclic changes of ductal sprouting, it is not surprising that this complex picture, in which epithelial acini are strangulated and distorted by fibrous tissue, should arise. Perhaps it is surprising that it does not occur more commonly. Although predominantly a histologic lesion presenting as a radiologic finding, sclerosing adenosis may also present as pain or a lump, allowing a more complete description within the ANDI concept.

Duct Ectasia and Periductal Mastitis

The second major group of BBDs are those associated with duct ectasia and periductal mastitis. The pathogenesis of these disorders is obscure and has been blurred by the confusion between the involutional changes of ectasia and the periductal inflammatory change occurring with the syndrome of mammary duct fistula (associated particularly with inverted nipple in the early reproductive period). Ectasia is very common both subclinically and clinically in the menopausal period and appears to be related to the ductal involutional process. In subclinical form, it is so common as to be regarded as a variant of normality; when it is complicated by nipple discharge, it moves into the aberration range of the spectrum. The development of gross bacterial sepsis has sufficient clinical impact to be regarded as disease.

Although the origin of benign menopausal nipple retraction is not clear, it seems likely that it arises as a variant of normal ductal involution subsequent to excessive periductal fibrosis and fibrous tissue contraction.

Epithelial Hyperplasia

Epithelial hyperplasia has given rise to the greatest confusion and problems with regard to management. Many clinicians would consider this entity as a disease rather than as a disorder, but a number of studies have shown that this classification is not so easily made with simple hyperplasia. Parks (1959) showed that lobular and intraductal papillary hyperplasia is common in the premenopausal period and that it tends to regress spontaneously after the menopause; hence, it should be regarded as a variant of normal involution (Parks, 1959). Other studies have confirmed this (Sloss et al., 1957). Hence, simple epithelial hyperplasias may be categorized firmly within the concept of BBD; some are a variant of normality, and the more active forms can perhaps be moved into the aberration column. However, epithelial hyperplasias with atypia are associated with malignancy sufficiently often to be regarded as an associated or premalignant condition, and these forms belong under the disease column (Dupont and Page, 1985; and Wellings et al., 1975). However, the spectrum from normality to disease is broad enough to allow the pathologist, using the criteria of Dupont and Page, to separate the more serious variants from those that are better regarded as normal or as carrying only a very small increase in cancer risk.

ABERRATION TO DISEASE?

The ANDI concept is based on the progression of a normal process to aberration to disease. Solid evidence for the direct progression from normality to aberration does exist, as was discussed earlier in the section on fibroadenoma. However, no evidence exists for or against the supposition that giant fibroadenomas develop from the continued growth of simple, small fibroadenomas. It seems more likely that giant fibroadenoma is a separate condition.

Likewise, it is likely that epithelial and apocrine changes form a continuum with simple hyperplasias, but there is less evidence to support the direct progression from the latter to atypical hyperplasias or to carcinoma in situ. Thus, on the basis of the present evidence, we must accept that we do not know whether "disease" in this case is a progression from aberration or whether disease and aberration are two separate entities.

However, this is one of the most interesting areas of the study of BBDs, and recent evidence is beginning to provide answers to some of the questions that exist. For instance, simple fibroadenoma is classified in the aberration column, but multiple fibroadenomas (>5 per breast) are sufficiently rare to be classified as disease. Recent evidence shows that patients undergoing kidney transplantation have an increased incidence of multiple fibroadenomas, which are an otherwise extremely rare condition. Whether this finding is linked to the immunosuppression associated with transplantation or to a specific drug treatment, such as the use of cyclosporin, it gives a new insight into the question of progression from aberration to disease.

Likewise, the increasing recognition that severe periductal mastitis is strongly correlated with cigarette smoking gives another possible mechanism whereby aberration (duct ectasia) progresses to disease (abscess formation). It is likely that in the near future, various factors that lead to the development of atypical hyperplasias will also become elucidated on the basis of genetics and molecular biology.

The time is approaching when we may be able to answer with much greater insight the question of progression from aberration to disease. Meanwhile, this question does not compromise the utility of the ANDI classification in helping us to understand BBDs, and the ANDI concept is sufficiently flexible to be able to incorporate new information as it becomes available.

IMPLICATIONS FOR MANAGEMENT

Whereas the main benefits from the ANDI concept arise from its providing a greater understanding of the spectrum of BBDs and its facilitating the teaching of students and physicians, the concept also has significant implications for management.

A most important element is the implication that every patient should be assessed individually in relation to the point on the spectrum where her condition lies. This approach is more than an intellectual exercise, for it allows the patient to understand the implications of the condition and permits the clinician to decide how aggressive the treatment plan should be. For instance, a patient's mastalgia may be quantified through the use of a pain chart, and the patient then can be told how her symptoms relate to normality. Epithelial hyperplasia can be categorized by the pathologist on the basis of the criteria laid down by Dupont and Page (1985), and an appropriate course of action can then be taken. Some of the implications inherent in this classification have already been borne out by changes in clinical practice.

Fibroadenoma

Since fibroadenoma is a benign and self-limited condition in the vast majority of patients, the idea of its being a part of the ANDI concept changes the emphasis of management from treating of a disease to clarifying a problem of diagnosis and to reassuring the patient. Diagnosis can be made confidently in a patient under the age of 25 years, and the patient can safely remain untreated. I have observed many such patients without cause for regret, and the case for this policy is strengthened by the high incidence of hypertrophic scars found in young girls. Many are now extending the conservative approach to diagnosis of fibroadenoma to patients over the age of 25 years in whom a policy of conservative treatment may still be appropriate; however, the diagnostic implications for leaving a mass in the breasts of such women need to be given full consideration. This approach is a marked policy change from that followed 10

years ago, when most authorities considered it mandatory to remove all fibroadenomas as neoplasms.

In contrast to simple fibroadenoma, a giant fibroadenoma (i.e., one >5 cm in diameter) is unlikely to regress or remain static; thus, the clinical problem of continuing growth demands an active treatment policy.

Pain and Nodularity

Pain and nodularity are so common that their management is very important. It is unhelpful to tell a patient that she has a nondisease when she has a symptom that both worries her and that may interfere with her quality of life. The ANDI concept that her status is most commonly normal but may be severe enough to represent aberration and, very rarely, a disease demands that the patient's symptoms be assessed in order to place them individually along the spectrum. This determines appropriate treatment: reassurance, if status is normal; hormonal or other therapy, if status indicates an aberration; and consideration that some other underlying condition (such as a psychologic disturbance) may be present if symptoms seem to be so severe or are so resistant to treatment that they suggest classification of the condition in the disease category. The fact that severe pain and nodularity have an association with excessive stimulated prolactin release suggests that the appropriate method of treatment in cases of sufficient severity is hormonal manipulation; this approach has proved to be the most effective method in clinical practice (Kumar et al., 1985; and Hughes et al., 1989).

Whenever nodularity is predominantly focal, diagnostic implications take precedence in determining management.

Cysts

Macrocysts and microcysts are so common that patients with them require no active treatment other than the allaying of their concerns. It is now well established that cysts are managed satisfactorily in many patients by aspiration, if necessary. Since the condition is a minor aberration of a normal process, no excisional procedure is required for multiple or recurrent cysts, provided that the aspirated fluid is not blood-stained (blood implies concomitant epithelial hyperplasia) and no residual mass is present (a residual mass implies associated disease).

Menopausal Nipple Retraction

The only importance of this condition is that it may be caused by the simple involutional process of periductal fibrosis. It requires no active management if the presence of cancer has been excluded, and, fortunately, its diagnosis is easily made because the postmenopausal breast lends itself to accurate mammography. However, it is important to recognize that nipple retraction can be a benign variant of a normal process.

Duct Ectasia/Periductal Mastitis Complex

Those symptoms of this condition that can be categorized under the aberration column cause little clinical upset and require no therapy other than reassurance of the patient if the nipple discharge is creamy and opaque (which is typically the case). Very rarely, the discharge itself may be so excessive as to be a source of social embarrassment to the patient. In this case, after the presence of a pituitary adenoma has been excluded, the patient may be treated in a mechanical fashion by major duct excision. This approach is a rare necessity, but it again demonstrates the value of assessing the patient in relation to impact of symptoms on quality of life. When suppuration supervenes (as occurs particularly in cigarette smokers), therapy appropriate for a disease state is indicated—that is, drainage, administration of antibiotics, and eradication of the underlying cause (usually by major duct excision).

Epithelial Hyperplasia

Epithelial hyperplasias without atypia, which are usually found as a chance histologic picture, fall into the ANDI category somewhere between normality and aberration. They carry no significant cancer risk and require no specific management. With atypical hyperplasias, the emphasis moves along the spectrum toward the disease state, and special consideration must be given to assessment of cancer risk as defined in particular by Dupont and Page (1985).

CONCLUSION

Confusion and concern that relate to the management of BBDs can best be resolved through the use of a clear classification that allows precise definition of these conditions from the pathogenetic, histologic, and clinical perspectives. In general, careful assessment allows conditions to be divided into those that may be regarded as normal, those that may be regarded as minor aberrations of normal processes, and those that should be regarded as disease. Consideration of where an individual patient with a clinical or histologic problem lies within the ANDI framework and within the spectrum from normality to aberration to disease should aid understanding and help to define appropriate management.

References

Azzopardi, J. G.: Problems in Breast Pathology. Philadelphia, W. B. Saunders, 1979, p. 57.

Davies, J. D.: Inflammatory damage to ducts in mammary dysplasia: A cause of duct obliteration. J. Pathol., *117*:47–54, 1975.

Dixon, J. M., Scott, W. N., and Miller, R. W.: An analysis of the content and morphology of human breast microcysts. Eur. J. Surg. Oncol., *ii*:151–154, 1985.

Dupont, W. D., and Page, D. L.: Risk factors for breast cancer in women with proliferative disease. N. Engl. J. Med., 312:146–151, 1985.

Hayward, J. L., and Parks, A. G.: Alterations in the microanatomy of the breast as a result of changes in the hormonal environment. *In* Currie, A. R. (Ed.): Endocrine Aspects of Breast Cancer. Edinburgh, E & S Livingstone, 1958, pp 133–134.

Hughes, L. E., Mansel, R. E., and Webster, D. J. T.: Aberrations of normal development and involution (ANDI): A new perspective on pathogenesis and nomenclature of benign breast disorders. Lancet, *ii*:1316–1319, 1987.

Hughes, L. E., Mansel, R. E., and Webster, D. J. T.: Benign Disorders and Diseases of the Breast: Concepts and Clinical Management. London, Bailliere Tindall, 1989.

Hughes, L. E., Smallwood, J., and Dixon, J. M.: Nomenclature of benign breast disorders: Report of a working party on the rationalisation of concepts and terminology of benign breast conditions. Breast, *1*:15–17, 1992.

Kumar, S., Mansel, R. E., Hughes, L. E., et al.: Prolactin response to thyrotropin-releasing hormone stimulation and dopaminergic inhibition in benign breast disease. Cancer, *53*:1311–1315, 1984.

Kumar, S., Mansel, R. E., Hughes, L. E., et al.: Prediction of response to endocrine therapy in pronounced cyclical mastalgia using dynamic tests of prolactin release. Clin. Endocrinol., *23*:699–704, 1985.

Love, S. M., Gelman, R. S., and Silen, W.: Fibrocystic 'disease' of the breast: A non-disease. N. Engl. J. Med., *307*:1010–1014, 1982.

Parks, A. G.: The microanatomy of the breast. Ann. R. Coll. Surg., *25*:295–311, 1959.

Preece, P. E., Richards, A. R., Owen, G. M., and Hughes, L. E.: Mastalgia and total body water. Br. Med. J., *iv*:498–500, 1975.

Sandison, A. T.: An autopsy study of the human breast. National Cancer Institute Monograph No. 8, U.S. Department of Health, Education and Welfare, 1962.

Sloss, P. T., Bennett, W. A., and Calyden, O. J.: Incidence in normal breasts of features associated with chronic cystic mastitis. Am. J. Pathol., *33*:1181–1191, 1957.

Vorherr, H.: The Breast: Morphology, Physiology and Lactation. New York, Academic Press, 1974.

Wellings, S. R., Jensen, H. M., and Marcus, R. E.: An atlas of subgross pathology of the human breast with special reference to precancerous lesions. J. Natl. Cancer Inst., *55*:231–273, 1975.

7

Common Benign Conditions of the Breast

William L. Donegan

Nonmalignant conditions of the breast occur far more frequently than do malignant disorders of the breast. Few nonmalignant disorders are life-threatening, but they produce considerable misery and can mimic the symptoms and signs of cancer. Approximately 70% of all minor breast operations, the majority of which are biopsies, are conducted for benign disorders, principally because they cannot otherwise be distinguished from cancer.

The frequency of benign disorders begins to rise steeply during the second decade of life (Wang and Fentiman, 1985). The incidence is greatest in patients 40 years of age; the incidence declines over the following two decades and reaches a low level thereafter.

Noteworthy is the gamut of pathology that occurs; in some cases the problems can be traced clearly to misadventures of development, to infections, or to neoplasia, but in others the causes remain obscure. Table 7–1 shows the variety of benign diagnoses made subsequent to a series of consecutive breast biopsies. Even this fails to convey the spectrum of problems encountered in a general breast clinic or in a hospital (Wang and Fentiman, 1985; Hughes et al., 1989; Smallwood and Taylor, 1990; and Souba, 1991). The following sections address some of the more frequently encountered problems.

DISORDERS OF DEVELOPMENT

Ectopic breasts and absent breasts (amastia) are anomalies of embryonic development. During the sixth week of fetal development, two streaks of ectodermal thickening—the milk lines—appear on the ventral side of the human embryo, each of which extends from the axilla to the groin (Arey, 1966). Normally, the lines disappear by the eighth week, except in the pectoral region, where they persist and develop rudimentary ducts at the site of the future breasts.

Failure of portions of the milk line to disappear accounts for the occurrence of extra nipples (polythelia), ectopic breast tissue, and fully formed accessory breasts (polymastia). Although ectopic mammary tissue is customarily found in the axilla, along the abdomen, and in the groin, the occasional reports of breast tissue in scapular areas and on the lateral side of the thigh suggest some variation in the course of embryonic milk lines (Cohen et al., 1986; and Johnson et al., 1986). Ectopic tissue in the axilla is often mistaken for folds of fat (Fig. 7–1), and accessory nipples

are easily mistaken for nevi (Fig. 7–2). Fully formed ectopic breasts are rare (Fig. 7–3).

Ectopia is more frequent in females than in males and is perhaps more frequent among Asian than among European women. An estimated 1% to 2% of white women are affected versus 5.19% of Japanese women (Iwai, 1907; and Parikh and Singer, 1983). Ectopia may be hereditary, as it has been noted in four generations of one family (Klinkerfuss, 1924) and in twins (DeCholnoky, 1929).

Ectopic breast tissue has been reported in conjunction with vertebral anomalies, multiple endocrine neoplasia, and aberrant ventricular conduction defects; however, whether the manifestation of ectopia is related to these disorders or is coincidental is uncertain (Mehes, 1979). A high frequency of renal defects and pyloric stenosis was found by Mehes and associates among infants and children with po-

Table 7–1. BENIGN TISSUE DIAGNOSES IN 883 CONSECUTIVE BREAST BIOPSIES

Diagnosis	No. of Biopsies (%)
Fibrocystic changes	413 (47%)
Fibroadenoma	220 (25%)
Duct papilloma	30 (3%)
Cyst	28 (3%)
Sclerosis	23 (3%)
Intramammary lymph node	22 (2%)
Lipoma	19 (2%)
Fat necrosis	17 (2%)
Papillomatosis	17 (2%)
Duct hyperplasia	14 (2%)
Duct ectasia	13 (1%)
Atypical duct hyperplasia	11 (1%)
Lactating adenoma	11 (1%)
Gynecomastia	10 (1%)
Squamous metaplasia	6 (<1%)
Calcification	6 (<1%)
Chronic mastitis	4 (<1%)
Adenolipoma	3 (<1%)
Nipple adenoma	3 (<1%)
Abscess wall	2 (<1%)
Foreign body reaction	2
Granular cell tumor	2
Fistula	1
Lipoblastomatosis	1
Sarcoidosis	1
Infarction	1
Myofibroblastoma	1
Hemangioma	1
Adenoma	1

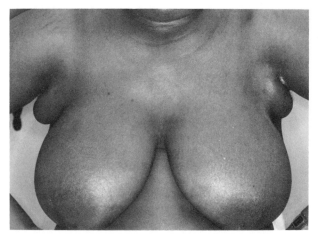

Figure 7–1. Ectopic breast tissue presenting as prominent axillary folds. Axillary breast tissue may be noticed for the first time when it enlarges during pregnancy.

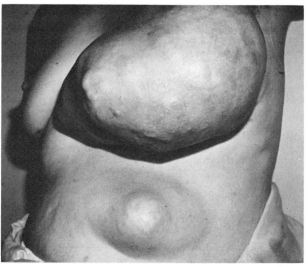

Figure 7–3. This patient, who has a large phylloides tumor of the left breast, demonstrates a prominent ectopic breast on the abdomen that is complete with areola. (Photograph courtesy of Radmilo Tomin, M.D.)

lythelia (Mehes, 1979; and Meggyessy and Mehes, 1987). Goedert and coworkers (1981) reported a greater-than-expected frequency of polythelia among adults with adenocarcinoma of the kidney. At puberty, ectopic breast tissue may become prominent along with the developing breasts and may be mistaken for lipomas or other soft tissue tumors. Unrecognized ectopic tissue can also be expected to hypertrophy with pregnancy; this frequently leads gravid women to seek medical attention because of the presence of enlarging "tumors" in their axillae. Ectopic tissues are susceptible to pathologic conditions found in the normally situated breasts, including carcinoma (Parikh and Singer, 1983; Simon et al., 1988; and Siegel et al., 1990). If recognized for what it is, accessory breast tissue is usually accepted by the patient; however, it may be removed, either for cosmetic reasons or for diagnostic purposes if pathology is suspected.

Congenital Absence of the Breasts

Total absence of the breasts (amastia) probably does not occur, but partial or nearly complete unilateral absence (hypoplasia) does, most often as a component of Poland's syndrome (Ravitch, 1987; and Seyfer et al., 1988). Alfred Poland described this congenital defect in 1841 while a student at Guy's Hospital in London. The essential element of the abnormality is absence of the pectoralis major muscle (Fig. 7–4). The deformity can involve variable loss of the breast and of the muscles of the upper limb girdle and ribs as well as deformity of the upper extremity, including brachysyndactyly (the "mitten hand"). The only vestige of the breast may be a hypoplastic nipple (Fig. 7–5). The anomaly

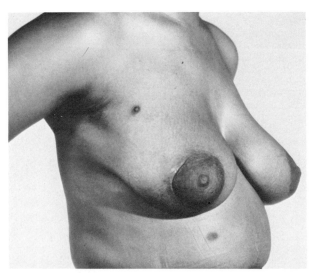

Figure 7–2. Multiple ectopic nipples (polythelia). This patient had two extra nipples symmetrically located in the milk line on each side. Polythelia may be associated with congenital renal abnormalities.

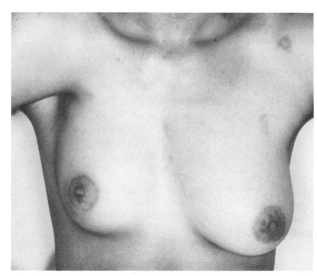

Figure 7–4. This patient with Poland's syndrome shows absence of the right pectoralis major muscle associated with mild hypoplasia of the breast.

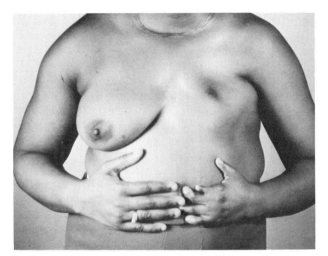

Figure 7-5. This patient with Poland's syndrome shows absence of the pectoralis major muscle and almost complete amastia. She also has deformity of the upper extremity as well as bone abnormalities of the ribs, forearm, and hand.

is invariably unilateral, predominantly affects males (75% of patients), occurs most often on the right side, and has an estimated frequency of 1 in 30,000 infants. It tends to be familial and is probably hereditary. The cause is apparently a defect in the developing limb bud. Associated conditions include Möbius's syndrome (facial and abducens nerve paralysis), and patients have a greater-than-usual risk of leukemia.

Treatment of Poland's syndrome is for cosmetic improvement. The operation often used for women involves transferring the latissimus dorsi muscle to replace the pectoralis major muscle and reconstruction of the breast with a prosthetic implant (Seyfer et al., 1988). For men, improvement can be obtained with latissimus dorsi muscle transfer and rib grafts (if necessary) to repair chest wall defects.

ABNORMAL DEVELOPMENT

In the United States, the breasts of girls begin to enlarge at approximately the age of 10.5 years (on the average at 2.3 years before menarche), and development is complete within 4 to 6 years (Drife, 1986; and Goldsmith and Weiss, 1986). Development sometimes begins unilaterally (with "false starts") before it becomes established. Haagensen warns against mistaking this process for pathology, as removal of the nodule will result in failure of breast development (Haagensen, 1971a). Growth of one of a young woman's breasts may outpace that of the other for a period before she reaches maturity; this should not be a source of concern. At maturity, the size of the left breast averages slightly larger than that of the right, but differences in size and symmetry can be considerable (Smith et al., 1986).

Problems of puberty include precocious breast development, failure of breasts to enlarge, and excessive breast enlargement. Bilateral involvement suggests a systemic disorder; unilateral involvement implies an aberrant end-organ response. Precocious puberty may be constitutional, but

possible manifestation of hormone-secreting granulosa cells or of lutein cysts of the ovary should be considered. Failure of breast development can result from pituitary failure (e.g., in the presence of craniopharyngioma), from ovarian dysgenesis (Turner's syndrome), and, more rarely, from masculinizing adrenal hyperplasia. Unilateral hypomastia can result from exposure of the prepubertal breast to ionizing radiation; alternatively, it may present without obvious cause (Fig. 7–6) (Kolar et al., 1967). For individuals with unilateral hypomastia, breast reconstruction is an option.

Excessive breast enlargement—so-called "adolescent" or "virginal hypertrophy"—may affect one or both breasts. Hormone suppression in young patients with this disorder may have undesirable consequences. Reduction mammoplasty is the mainstay of treatment for breasts that reach great size and is best performed after breast growth has stabilized. Continued enlargement may require removal of all breast tissue (Ship and Shulman, 1971; and Bauer et al., 1987).

NEOPLASMS

Fibroadenomas

Whether fibroadenomas are neoplasms or are aberrations of lobular development is an unsettled issue (Hughes et al., 1989a). In either case, they are the most frequent benign tumor of the breast in black women and in adolescent white females. (Gogas, 1979; and Oluwole and Freeman, 1979). Fibroadenomas are composed of fibrous stromal tissue that surrounds tissue clefts lined with epithelium, which is sometimes hyperplastic. The histologic appearance suggests stromal proliferation that has displaced, stretched, and distorted the normal ductal system of the breast. Fibroadenomas in which the clefts are narrow and linear have been described as "pericanalicular," whereas those in which the clefts are characterized by elaborate infolding have been called "intracanalicular"; however, this distinction has no

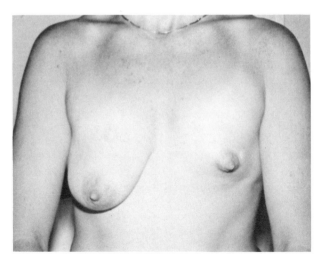

Figure 7-6. Unilateral failure of breast development. The cause was unknown. The areola was mature, and the patient was otherwise normal and healthy.

clinical relevance. Gross fibroadenomas are well circumscribed and separate easily from surrounding tissues, but some surfaces can blend intimately with the surrounding breast tissue. The cut surfaces are homogeneous, with multiple fine clefts (Fig. 7–7).

Clinically, fibroadenomas present as firm, discrete, round or lobulated masses that are nontender and highly mobile. They are found most often in young women, and they are multiple in some cases. Haagensen (1971*b*) called these tumors "adenofibromas" and found that most patients were in their early twenties. In the author's patients, the median age was 37 years, and no patient was younger than 12 years of age (Fig. 7–8). The tumors appeared shortly after puberty and predominated during reproductive life. In 17.5% of the patients, fibroadenomas were multiple, presenting in both breasts in 8.8% of patients and in one breast in 8.2%. Four patients (2.3%) subsequently developed additional fibroadenomas; more patients may have done so if the period of follow-up had been protracted. Women who had multiple tumors initially were younger than the others (median age = 27.5 years) and were more likely to develop future tumors than were women with single tumors (10.3% of the former versus only 0.7% of the latter). Fibroadenomas range widely in size (Fig. 7–9). Most are 1 to 3 cm in diameter. Occasionally, they reach a large size in young women and are distinguished as "giant" fibroadenomas or as "juvenile" fibroadenomas. The author has removed one such tumor that measured 10 cm in diameter from the breast of a 15-year-old girl. Fibroadenomas respond to hormonal influences; lactation may be found within them in postpartum women (see Fig. 7–7). Occasionally, fibrocystic changes, infarction, or carcinoma is found within a fibroadenoma. These associations have no special significance. The presence of fibroadenomas does not increase a woman's risk of future breast carcinoma. Carney and Toorkey (1991) described a familial syndrome in which myxomatous change in fibroadenomas was associated with cardiac myxomas. Other manifestations included spotty cutaneous pigmentation, endocrine overactivity, and melanotic schwannomas. Breast tumors tended to be multiple and

bilateral and were the presenting manifestation of this syndrome in 23% of patients. Recognition is important, since cardiac myxomas can cause sudden death.

The needle aspirates from fibroadenomas typically contain normal ductal and stromal cells, often present in large numbers. On mammography, fibroadenomas are either not seen in the dense breast tissue of young patients or appear as well-marginated densities against a radiolucent background. Cysts, lymph nodes, phylloides tumors, and some cancers (e.g., medullary carcinomas) have a similar radiographic appearance. Often, a thin radiolucent halo of compressed fat surrounds the tumor. In elderly women, fibroad-

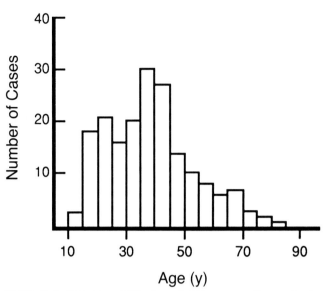

Figure 7–8. The age distribution of 186 consecutive patients with fibroadenomas (1982–1991). The majority of patients (73%) were from 15 to 45 years of age. (From author's personal series.)

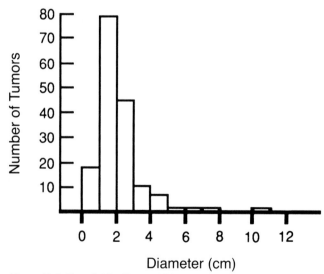

Figure 7–9. Size distribution of 170 fibroadenomas. Most tumors were 1.0 to 2.0 cm in diameter and rarely exceeded 5.0 cm. (From author's personal series.)

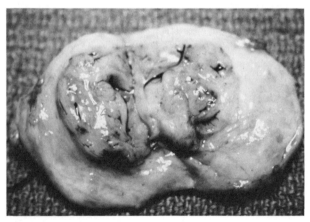

Figure 7–7. Fibroadenoma. This tumor, surrounded by breast tissue, displays characteristic discrete margins and a cut surface with clefts. The patient was lactating, and the tumor showed signs of lactation.

enomas may contain deposits of coarse ''popcorn''-like calcification. Sonography helps to distinguish fibroadenomas from cysts by the internal echoes they produce, but some fibroadenomas are sufficiently homogeneous that they produce no internal echoes and have the sonographic appearance of a cyst. Conversely, cysts with thick contents may produce internal echoes and thus mimic fibroadenomas.

A diagnosis of fibroadenoma can be made with considerable confidence when a solid tumor with typical clinical features is found in the breast of a teenager. It is also highly accurate in the elderly woman whose mammogram shows a small, spherical density with typical gross calcifications. Observation may be justified in some circumstances, but ordinarily fibroadenomas are removed for definitive diagnosis or for esthetic reasons, or to prevent continued enlargement.

Surgical removal is the only form of definitive treatment and can be accomplished with local anesthesia except when the tumor is unusually large or when the patient is very young or unable to cooperate. A common surgical mistake is beginning the excision of breast tissue before the tumor is reached, the consequence of which is the needless removal of normal tissue. Instead, the incision should be deepened until the tumor capsule clearly bulges into the field; the tumor is then removed discretely but in its entirety, and no attempt is made to remove a margin of normal tissue. Placement of a suture into the tumor for use as a tenaculum facilitates this process. No attempt is made to close the defect in the breast parenchyma. If left unsutured, it will close most naturally. Only the subcutaneous tissues and the skin are closed, and the latter with the use of buried sutures. Multiple tumors are excised as are subsequent tumors. The treatment of one woman in the author's series illustrated the hazards of presumption. Previously and on separate occasions, she had three fibroadenomas removed from her right breast. Later, she returned with what appeared to be a fourth fibroadenoma. It proved to be a malignant phylloides tumor. Local recurrence of a fibroadenoma is rare. It has happened only once in this author's experience. For cosmetic reasons, subsequent tumors should be removed through previous scars whenever feasible. Subcutaneous mastectomy is rarely if ever indicated.

Lipoma

Lipomas are composed of mature fat cells. They are single or multiple and arise in subcutaneous fatty tissues. Location on the breast is incidental, and lipomas have no particular affinity for the right or left breast or for any particular quadrant. Clinically, they present as well-marginated, smooth or lobulated masses that are soft and have some mobility. Small lipomas may be semifirm. They are usually nontender but may be mildly so. Their growth is slow, so enlargement can be appreciated only over extended periods; rapid enlargement is uncharacteristic. Long duration, multiplicity, and typical physical signs strongly support the diagnosis. On aspiration, the needle passes through lipomas without resistance; fine-needle aspiration produces typical fat cells. When the tumors are large, mammography shows

characteristic radiolucency and compression of adjacent breast tissue (Fig. 7–10). When the tumors are small, mammograms are usually normal. On sonography, lipomas appear as solid masses. These harmless tumors are removed only if the diagnosis is uncertain, if they create a cosmetic problem, or if they show rapid growth. Removal without excision of a margin of normal tissue is the customary procedure, but lipomas can recur if incompletely excised.

The last 11 lipomas removed by the author (white women aged 30–82 years; average age = 49 years) were all excised for diagnostic purposes. Ten of the eleven presented as masses measuring 1 cm to 5 cm in diameter (average = 2.4 cm). One patient had observed her lipoma's presence for 12 months; the remainder of the patients had noted theirs for shorter periods. Sixty per cent of the lipomas were located in the lower hemisphere of the breast. One lipoma presented as a nonpalpable density on mammography.

Hamartomas

Hamartomas are encapsulated tumors composed of abnormal mixtures of normal mammary tissues. Jones and col-

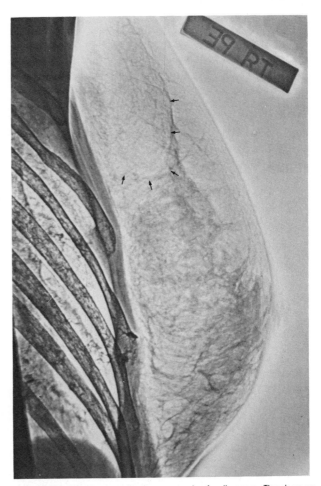

Figure 7–10. Mammogram (xerogram) of a lipoma. The tumor is radiolucent (*arrows*) and displaces the adjacent breast tissue.

leagues (1991) found 17 cases of hamartoma among the files of the Armed Forces Institute of Pathology; they described four varieties on the basis of composition: (1) fibrocystic changes; (2) fibroadenoma with glandular tissue and mature fat (and, in one instance, with cartilage); (3) typical fibroadenoma containing normal lobules; and (4) adenolipoma with adipose tissue, ducts, and lobules. The patients' ages ranged from 13 to 65 years, and the tumors varied in size from 1 to 13.5 cm. Clinically, hamartomas present as discrete, mobile, and encapsulated masses. Mammographically, they appear smooth and margined and delimited from the surrounding breast by a lucent halo. Their appearance has been described as a "breast within a breast" (Riveros et al., 1989). Generally, they are single, but they can be multiple. They are invariably benign, and treatment is by excision. Figure 7–11 shows the gross and mammographic appearances of an adenolipoma removed from the breast of a 26-year-old woman.

Adenomas

Adenomas are pure epithelial tumors of the breast. Hertel and colleagues (1976) distinguished them from fibroadenomas and adenomas of the nipple by the presence of only scant stroma. Their histology is homogeneous, and they are discretely separated from the surrounding breast tissue. Several types are recognized, including tubular adenoma, lactating adenoma, and sweat gland tumors. Lactating adenomas are the most frequent benign tumor found during pregnancy and lactation (Fig. 7–12). Pleomorphic adenomas (mixed tumor) of the breast have also been described and are histologically identical to those found in the salivary glands. Their clinical and mammographic features can closely mimic those of cancer, and recurrence has occurred after incomplete excision (Sheth et al., 1978; and Soreide et al., 1988).

Adenoma of the nipple was described originally in 1955 by Jones as florid papillomatosis and later in 1962 by Handley and Thackray as adenoma of the nipple. It is a benign lesion that clinically mimics Paget's disease of the nipple and that histologically suggests invasive carcinoma. It is to be differentiated from syringomatous adenoma of the nipple, which is derived from the skin. Adenoma of the nipple affects primarily adult females. Less than 5% of cases occur in males. It has been reported in an accessory nipple (Doctor and Sirsat, 1971; and Rosen and Caicco, 1986).

Typically, this lesion presents as a discrete, firm tumor of the papilla of the nipple. It is sometimes associated with pruritus but rarely with pain. Often, a serous or bloody discharge is noted, and excoriation or ulceration is observed (Fig. 7–13). The tumors are usually diagnosed at 1 cm or

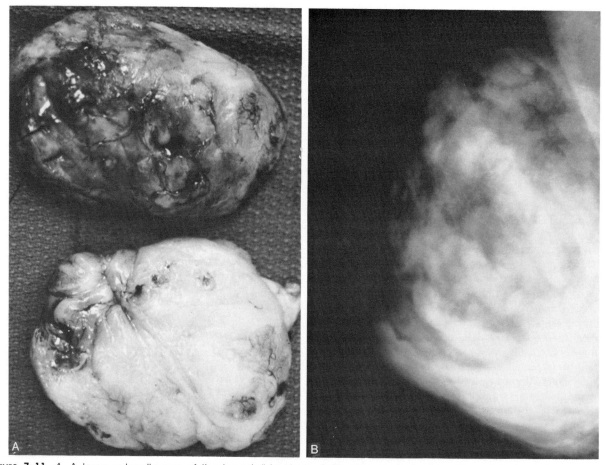

Figure 7–11. *A,* A large adenolipoma of the breast (bisected). *B,* The tumor produced a flocculated appearance on a mammogram.

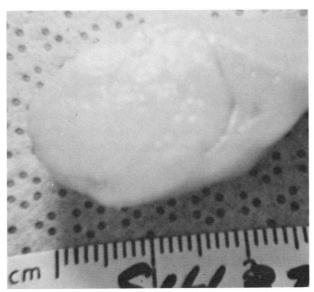

Figure 7-12. Lactating adenoma from the breast of a nursing mother.

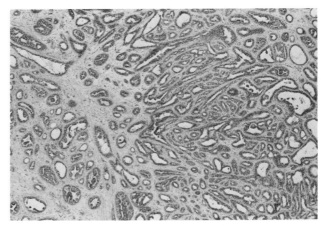

Figure 7-14. This histologic section of a nipple adenoma shows proliferation of glandular elements within a fibrous stroma.

more in size and, when sectioned, are homogeneous and gray with poorly defined margins. Histologically, a tubular or a papillomatous pattern is seen with a fibrous stroma (Fig. 7–14). Doctor and Sirsat (1971) felt that serosanguineous discharge was more often associated with the papillomatous type and nipple enlargement with the adenomatous (tubular) pattern. A biopsy is necessary for diagnosis. Complete excision of the tumor is adequate treatment. Usually, the tumor occupies only the papilla, and it is not necessary to routinely remove the entire areola.

Sclerosing papillary proliferations that may be related to adenoma of the nipple have been described in the subareolar area (Rosen, 1987) and at other locations in the breast (Fenoglio and Lattes, 1974). In some instances, dense fibrosis is associated with centrifugal dispersion of epithelium and is described as a "radial scar" (Fig. 7–15). These lesions present as palpable lumps or as spiculated densities on mammograms, and they can be adherent to the skin, suggesting the presence of cancer. When the papillary component is not prominent, the small glands seem to be infiltrating a desmoplastic stroma and suggest tubular carcinoma. It was suspected that radial scars might be premalignant, but their benign nature seems confirmed, and complete excision is definitive (Andersen and Gram, 1984; and Nielsen et al., 1987).

Granular Cell Tumor (Previously Granular Cell Myoblastoma)

Originally described by Abrikossoff in 1926, this tumor is of uncertain origin. A primitive myoblast was originally suspected as its source, but more recent evidence favors the Schwann cell (Sobel et al., 1972). The tumor stains positive for S-100 protein and negative for keratin, myoglobin, and gross cystic disease fluid protein (Damiani et al., 1992). The granules may result from intracellular myelin forma-

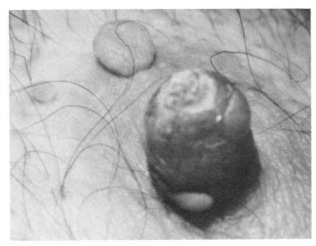

Figure 7-13. Adenoma of the nipple. This benign tumor typically involves the papilla and presents as a discrete, firm mass. It may be seen in men (as in this case) as well as in women and is adequately treated by local excision.

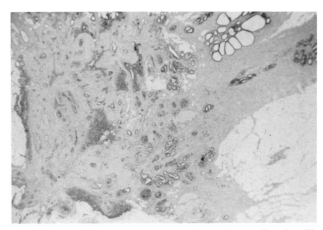

Figure 7-15. This radial scar shows focal dense fibrosis with radial dispersion of glandular elements.

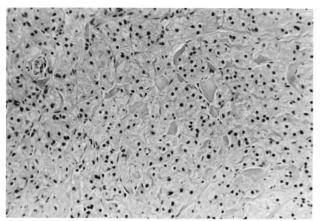

Figure 7–16. Histologic view of a granular cell tumor of the breast.

tion (Mittal and True, 1988). Six per cent of granular cell tumors occur in the breast (Bassett and Cove, 1979). These tumors can be infiltrative, recur after incomplete excision, and rarely metastasize. Granular cell tumors occur in both men and women between the ages of 15 and 73 years. Weitzner and coworkers (1979) reviewed 52 previously documented cases of mammary granular cell tumors and reported that the youngest patient to date was a 15-year-old girl. The right and left breasts are involved with equal frequency.

A solitary, painless lump with progressive increase in size is the usual presentation. Fixation of the skin or underlying fascia as well as ulceration of the skin or adjacent nodules of similar histologic nature (thus mimicking satellites) can be highly suggestive of carcinoma (McCracken et al., 1979). For unknown reasons, the upper inner quadrant of the breast is the most frequent location of the tumor. The tumors measure from 1 to 10 cm in diameter at the time they are diagnosed, and edema of the skin, dimpling, retraction, and pigmentation may be present. Mammographically, the tumor presents as a density with sharp margins except for the tendonlike extensions into adjacent breast tissue that suggest carcinoma. Aspiration cytology and even frozen sections can be misleading; therefore, local excision and analysis of permanent sections constitute the proper method of diagnosis. The cut surface is white and hard, and in 9 of 34 cases in which frozen section was used, the tumor was initially thought to be malignant. Microscopic examination revealing the characteristic plump cells with granular inclusions permits the correct diagnosis (Fig. 7–16).

Wide local excision is the treatment of choice (Townsend and Stellato, 1985). Irradiation is not effective. As the tumor infiltrates freely into surrounding tissues, complete removal may require inclusion of muscle and other adjacent structures, and histologic evaluation is advisable to be certain that the surgical margins are free of tumor. After adequate removal, recurrence is unusual. None of Umansky and Bullock's 19 patients (1968) had recurrence after from 4 months to 12.5 years of observation. The rare malignant behavior of this tumor is evidenced by the case of Crawford and DeBakey (1953), in which widespread involvement of the lungs, liver, and retroperitoneal tissues was associated

with a 4-cm mass in the upper outer quadrant of the left breast that was presumed to represent the primary tumor. Spread to regional lymph nodes has been reported (Chetty and Kalan, 1992).

The author has discovered two granular cell tumors in 644 consecutive breast biopsies for palpable masses—a frequency of 0.3%. Since one was in a man, the frequency among women who had breast biopsies for masses was 1:634, or 0.16%. The first presented as a 1.5-cm firm, discrete nodule in the lower midline of the left breast of an 18-year-old white female. After local excision with tumor-free margins, she was free of recurrence at her last follow-up examination 13 months later. The second presented as a 7-mm firm nodule in the breast of a 58-year-old black man who also had a carcinoma of the stomach.

Miscellaneous Benign Tumors

A variety of other benign tumors arise in the breast. They are described according to their composition—for example, benign spindle-cell tumor (Toker et al., 1981), myofibroblastoma (Wargotz et al., 1987), spindle-cell adenomyoepithelioma (Weidner and Levine, 1988), neurilemmoma (Harrison and Elliott, 1989), and chondrolipoma (Kaplan and Walts, 1977). Benign vascular tumors are particularly rare, usually affect young women, and must be carefully distinguished from angiosarcomas. They can enlarge during pregnancy (Morrow et al., 1988). Complete excision is adequate treatment.

INFECTIONS AND ABSCESSES

Abscesses of Inclusion Cysts

Epidermal inclusion cysts occur in the skin of the breast at any site and occasionally become infected with abscess formation. They are identified as discrete, subcutaneous masses attached to the dermis and marked by an overlying pore. Keratinaceous material can sometimes be expressed from the pore. A cyst visualizes on mammography as a discrete density within the breast (Fig. 7–17). Repeat mam-

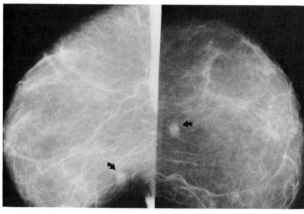

Figure 7–17. A cutaneous inclusion cyst creates a mammographic density that suggests a breast tumor (*arrows*).

mography with a lead spot on the cyst, or removal of the cyst, serves to identify it as the source of the density.

When infection supervenes, the responsible organism is typically a staphylococcus. The cyst becomes tender, warm, swollen, and red. Eventually, an abscess forms and drains spontaneously; however, the epidermal lining of the cyst persists, and resolution is usually accompanied by a small scar with underlying induration that is subject to repeated cycles of inflammation.

If patients present with inflammation alone, warm soaks and administration of oral antibiotics targeted at cutaneous pathogens are appropriate. When pus is present, incision and drainage are indicated. The pasty contents are evacuated. When healing is complete, local excision of the cyst prevents future problems.

Subareolar Abscesses (Chronic Recurrent Subareolar Abscess, Mammary Duct Fistula, and Duct Ectasia)

Subareolar abscesses represent a complex problem with a disputed pathogenesis. Clinical features include recurrent episodes of mastitis and abscess formation as well as the presence of thick nipple discharge, subareolar masses, chronic nonhealing fistulas at the areolar margin, and inverted nipples. Four pathologic processes form the basis of this clinical complex, but the origin and sequence of events remain uncertain. These processes are duct ectasia, periductal inflammation, fibrosis, and squamous metaplasia.

Duct ectasia may be the initial change and is caused possibly by ductal obstruction, inflammatory destruction of the muscle wall, hormonal influences, or failure to absorb secretions. Ectatic ducts are frequently limited to the subareolar area, but they may extend more deeply into the breast. Periductal inflammation can be attributed initially to chemical inflammation from erosion of retained secretions. Plasma cell mastitis probably has its origin in this process. It has been suggested that periductal inflammation is an autoimmune process, but blood sometimes seen in the thick nipple discharge suggests erosion (Hughes et al., 1989*b*). Ultimately, bacterial inflammation supervenes with abscess and fistula formation. Cultures produce a mixed bacterial flora, and anaerobic bacteria are regularly found (particularly peptostreptococci) (Walker et al., 1988). Other isolates include bacteroides, diphtheroids, *Staphylococcus epidermidis*, protei, lactobacilli, and *Streptococcus viridans*.

Squamous epithelium normally extends into the lactiferous ducts only 1 to 2 mm from the surface of the nipple; however, in patients with subareolar abscess, it extends far more deeply (Fig. 7–18). What remains uncertain is whether this is a congenital change or a result of chronic infection. Habif and associates (1970) found progression of squamous epithelium to an ''abnormal'' depth in 17% of nipples from 83 breasts that had been removed owing to cancer. As a result of squamous metaplasia, keratin plugs that block the elimination of normal secretions are produced; furthermore, desquamation contributes to the volume of intraluminal debris. In some patients, a pasty mate-

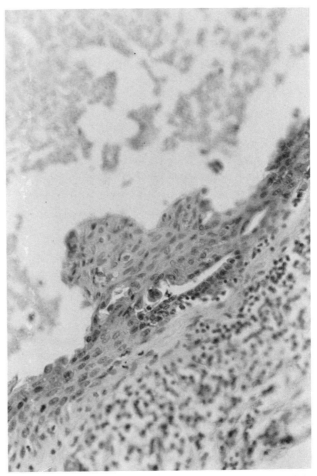

Figure 7–18. Squamous metaplasia lines ectatic major ducts in a patient with recurrent subareolar abscesses.

rial can be expressed from the ducts (Fig. 7–19*A* & *B*). The histologic changes are remarkably similar to those of acne (i.e., the presence of keratin plugs, inspissation of secretions, and inflammation). Failure of fistulas to heal, recurrence of abscesses, and a foreign body giant cell reaction in the tissues can be attributed to retained squamous epithelium and keratin debris. Nipple inversion is often a part of the clinical complex, but it is not regularly present at the outset and is not likely an essential element of the pathologic process. Fixed nipple retraction ultimately results from periductal inflammation and fibrosis.

Patients with subareolar abscesses are predominantly premenopausal. Twenty-six patients who were treated by the author had an average age of 41 years. Ages ranged from 21 to 73 years, but 81% of the patients were younger than 50 years of age. Both white and black patients were affected, and the right and left breasts were affected with equal frequency. Thirty-one per cent of patients presented with bilateral involvement. Some cases were associated with acne, hidradenitis suppurativa, and perineal inclusion cysts, suggesting a more general problem involving cutaneous glands. A strong association with cigarette smoking has been reported in a number of works (Schäfer et al., 1988; and Bundred et al., 1992).

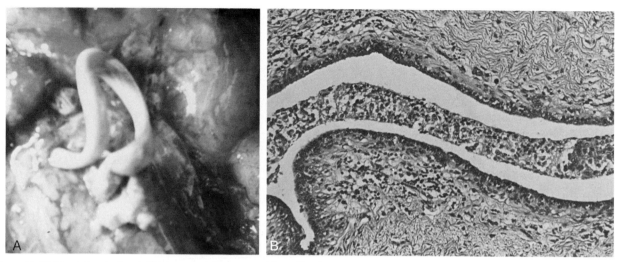

Figure 7–19. Ductal ectasia. *A,* Thick material expressed from the tissues of a patient with duct ectasia. *B,* This histologic section shows a dilated duct with periductal inflammation and luminal debris.

The typical history includes recurrent mastitis and the presence of abscesses centered under the nipple. Patients often note that flare-ups occur premenstrually, suggesting a hormonal influence. The problem continues for months to years, and the management record typically includes repeated administration of antibiotics and incisions for drainage. Chronic fistulas appear characteristically at the margin of the areola (Fig. 7–20A). The nipple is flattened or inverted and is usually displaced toward the fistula. A probe confirms a communication between the fistula and the ductal system (see Fig. 7–20B). Women suffer considerable distress from the inconvenience and embarrassment caused by this condition. Mammography is not helpful except to exclude unrelated lesions not appreciated on the physical examination. It should be kept in mind that some cancers present as subareolar abscesses (Ferrara et al., 1990).

Antibiotics are required if a patient presents with acute infection. Abscesses are drained and cultured, and acute

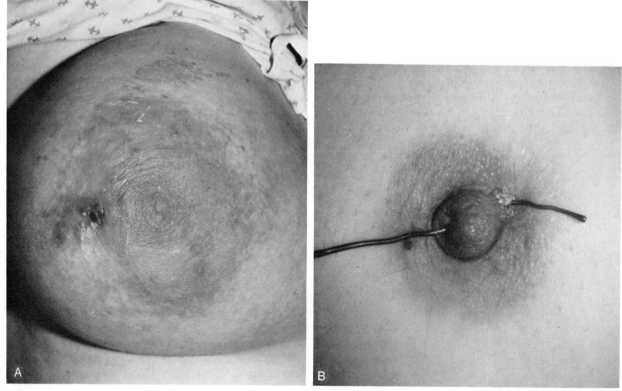

Figure 7–20. *A,* A chronic mammary fistula located typically at the areolar margin. *B,* A probe demonstrates communication between a chronic fistula and a nipple duct.

infection is treated with broad-spectrum antibiotics chosen to address both aerobes and anaerobes. Cephalexin and metronidazole or ampicillin with sulbactam are effective. Ferrara and coworkers (1990) had a 47% success rate with antibiotics and simple aspiration of subareolar abscesses in 19 cases. To rule out cancer, these authors recommend biopsy of the abscess wall when open drainage is necessary or when the abscess is produced by gram-negative organisms. Recurrent abscess or fistula formation after initial treatment establishes the pattern associated with this clinical entity.

For patients who present with an established fistula, limited fistulectomy and fistulotomy have met with variable success. Either procedure can only be expected to succeed when a single duct is involved. A single fistulectomy was successful in 7 of 14 patients (50%) reported by Abramson (1969); the remainder required multiple operations. Resection of the major subareolar ducts en bloc as definitive treatment was developed by Urban (1963) and by Hadfield (1960). Major duct resection involves elevation of the areola by means of a periareolar incision and meticulous excision of all of the major ducts (Fig. 7–21). The specimen

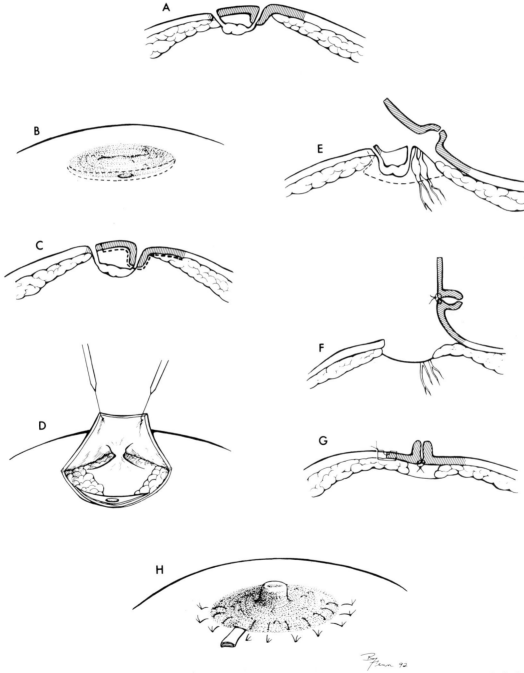

Figure 7–21. The technique of major duct resection for treatment of chronic recurring subareolar abscess. *A, B,* A periareolar incision that encompasses the fistula is used. *C, D,* The areola is completely elevated in the subdermal plane, and the ducts are transected near the apex of the papilla. *E,* The major ducts and fistula are excised as a cone of tissue. *F–H,* An absorbable pursestring suture at the base of the papilla is used to maintain eversion, and the incision is closed around a drain.

Table 7–2. RESULTS WITH MAJOR DUCT RESECTION FOR RECURRENT SUBAREOLAR ABSCESS AND CHRONIC MAMMARY FISTULA

Reference	No. of Cases	Success	Duration	Subsequent Mastectomy
Kilgore and Flemming, 1952	64	52%	?	9
Hadfield, 1968	30	100%	12–84 mo	
Abramson, 1969	4	75%	12–72 mo	
Habif et al., 1970*	14	100%	?	
Urban, 1987	42	100%	?	0
Thomas et al., 1982	40	83%	?	2
Hughes, 1989e	122	84%	12–120 mo	2
Hartley et al., 1991	46	74%	?	

*All patients were treated with removal of major ducts and the nipple.

is a cone of tissue as broad as the areola, and excision includes all tissues from the base of the dermis to as deep as necessary to eliminate dilated ducts and other abnormal tissues. It includes removal of existing fistulas. An eversion of the nipple is performed at the same time. The incision is closed around a small drain, and prophylactic antibiotics are used for several days. Reports of successful major duct resection often include short or uncertain follow-up periods (Table 7–2). The operation is also more effective in uncomplicated cases. Hartley and associates (1991) had failures in 6 of 33 patients who presented without abscess and in 6 of 13 who presented with abscess. The results of 26 major duct resections performed by the author for recurrent subareolar abscesses and fistulas deteriorated with time (Fig. 7–22). Fifty-five per cent of the patients were free of recurrent infections at 1 year and 40% at 7 years postoperatively. Repeat major duct resection for recurrences on the presumption that ducts were missed or that more had become affected has not always been successful. The tissues from such a resection suggest that squamous epithelium from ducts of the retained nipple proliferate downward to line cavities and perpetuate the process. In fact, in the author's experience, if a major duct resection is left open to heal by secondary intention, the rapid downward growth of this epithelium will line the wound and eventually reconstitute a fistula.

When major duct resection fails, complete removal of the nipple is curative in the experience of the author. In sections of excised nipples, histologic changes often suggest that the areola itself participated in the disease process. Mastectomy is rarely necessary for this condition, as removal of the nipple and the involved underlying ducts regularly results in permanent cure. After healing is secure, nipple reconstruction can be offered to the patient.

Puerperal (Lactational) Abscess

Abscesses associated with lactation are less common than in the past, probably owing to better hygiene and prompt use of antibiotics. They accounted for only 30% of all breast abscesses in a report by Bundred and coworkers (1992). Acute mastitis develops in about 2.5% of nursing mothers, and no more than 1 in 15 of these women develops abscesses (Olsen and Gordon, 1990). The onset is at one to several weeks postpartum, with symptoms that include redness, swelling, tenderness, chills, and fever. The predominant causative organism is *Staphylococcus aureus*, but coagulase-negative staphylococci, beta-hemolytic streptococci, *Streptococcus faecalis*, *Escherichia coli*, and diphtheroids are also cultured from infected patients (Olsen and Gordon, 1990). Gram-negative bacilli are infrequently the source of infection. Cracked nipples may be the portal of entry for bacteria, and the colonized mouth of an infant tends to spread the infection from one breast of the mother to the other. Toxic shock syndrome has resulted from postpartum staphylococcal mastitis (Demey et al., 1989). Epidemic puerperal mastitis due to virulent hospital-acquired

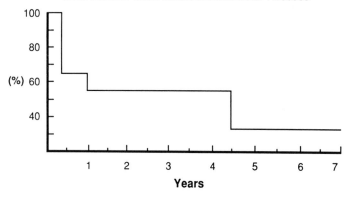

Freedom from Recurrent Infection after Major Duct Resection of 26 Breasts with Recurrent Subareolar Abscess

Figure 7–22. Results of major duct resection for chronic recurrent subareolar abscess.

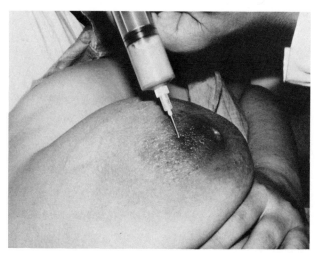

Figure 7–23. Aspiration of a breast abscess. Aspiration serves to confirm the presence of pus and to provide material for immediate culture prior to surgical drainage.

strains of *S. aureus* has become unusual with current nursery practices.

Warm compresses, gentle expression of milk, and prompt treatment with administration of appropriate antibiotics generally results in prompt resolution (Bertrand and Rosenblood, 1991). The majority of women who present with lactational abscesses can be treated as outpatients. Antibiotics of choice are broad-spectrum and focus on gram-positive, penicillinase-resistant cocci. First-generation cephalosporins (cephalexin or cephradine), intravenous amoxicillin–clavulanate potassium, or oral ampicillin–sulbactam sodium are suitable. Culture of the mother's milk or purulent nipple discharge serves to confirm the initial choice of antibiotics or to guide a change. Most practitioners feel that it is not necessary to interrupt lactation or breast feeding if the infection is minor.

If abscess is suspected, needle aspiration serves to confirm the presence of pus and to provide a sample for smear and culture (Fig. 7–23). Ultrasound study can be useful for identifying abscess formation (Hayes et al., 1991). Some success has been reported with repeated aspiration of abscesses combined with antibiotic therapy as an alternative to open drainage (Dixon, 1988; Tam and Brooks, 1988; and Nash and Powles, 1989). Dixon (1988) treated six postpartum abscesses by this method with resolution of all, and Karstrup and coworkers (1990) reported on the successful treatment of four abscesses. This approach has the advantage of avoiding of the use of a general anesthetic and the inconvenience of an open wound; however, it is probably most likely to be successful for the management of small unilocular abscesses. The author has found aspiration definitive for breast abscesses in a few instances.

The most dependable management of breast abscesses is open drainage. Administration of antibiotics is begun preoperatively, and the operation is performed with the patient under general anesthesia (local anesthetics are not effective in the presence of inflammation). The incision is made where the skin over the abscess is thinnest so as to minimize the disruption of normal tissues. Cultures are taken if

this has not been done preoperatively. Any loculations are gently disrupted with the finger, and the abscess cavity is irrigated with saline. Although cancer is rarely associated with puerperal abscesses, it is routine to take a biopsy from the abscess wall. The wound is filled loosely with gauze, or a rubber drain is left in the wound; the wound is then allowed to heal by secondary intention. Antibiotic administration is continued until the patient has been afebrile for 3 consecutive days. Lactation is suppressed with the administration of bromocriptine mesylate (Parlodel). Benson (1989) and Khanna and associates (1989) reported rapid healing after management of lactational abscesses with curettement of the abscess wall and primary closure. Although the failure rate was a low 6%, this technique may sacrifice more tissue than is necessary and requires close observation of the patient. It has not gained widespread acceptance.

Occasionally, virulent infections result in severe sepsis and extensive necrosis of the breast (Fig. 7–24). Administration of antibiotics and prompt débridement of all necrotic tissue are necessary in these cases. Even when most of the breast is involved, the results of débridement are preferable to those of mastectomy.

Granulomatous Mastitis

Granulomatous mastitis has numerous origins, including sarcoidosis, tuberculosis, leprosy, and typhoid infection, as well as fungi, metazoa, and foreign material (Gansler and Wheeler, 1984). All may present as a mass, and, fortunately, all are rare. A biopsy is usually necessary for diagnostic evaluation as are appropriate stains and cultures.

Sarcoidosis of the breast is most often found in conjunction with involvement of the lungs and other organs but is sometimes found incidentally in breast tissues. Typical of sarcoidosis are epithelioid granulomas and giant cells with no central necrosis. The diagnosis is one of exclusion and is justified only when the histology is characteristic, no organisms are found histologically, and cultures are nonproductive. Involvement of the breast is unusual, even in the presence of disseminated sarcoidosis.

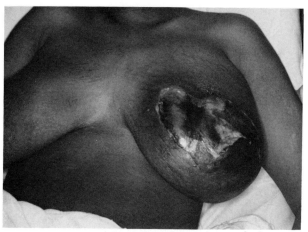

Figure 7–24. Postpartum mastitis. This patient developed a severe necrotizing infection in the left breast while nursing her newborn infant. Extensive surgical débridement was required.

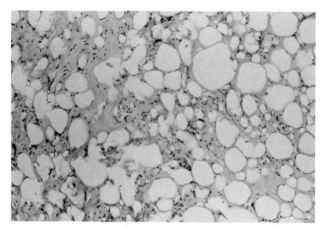

Figure 7–25. Histologic section of tissue reaction to leakage from a silicone gel–filled breast prosthesis. Silicone droplets are dispersed in a dense fibrous reaction that features chronic inflammation and foreign body giant cells.

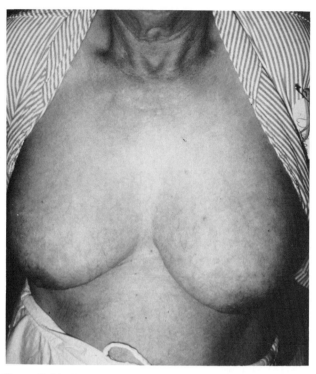

Figure 7–26. Prominent bilateral gynecomastia in an adult male. The causes of gynecomastia are multiple and, as in this case, sometimes obscure.

Tuberculosis of the breast, which is now very rare, presents as an abscess or a mass (Hale et al., 1985; and Wapnir et al., 1985). Usually, the disease is already evident in other organs, but it can involve the breast alone. The presence of acid-fast bacteria in special stains and their growth in cultures confirm the diagnosis.

Foreign bodies in the breast can produce chronic granulomas. Injection of paraffin, a waxy petroleum distillate previously used for augmentation, results in hard masses and chronically draining sinuses (Alagaratnam and Ong, 1983). Silicone gel from modern prostheses also produces a foreign body reaction if it leaks into the tissues (Mason and Apisarnthanarax, 1981). The result is hard masses that migrate toward the axilla (Fig. 7–25).

Nonspecific granulomatous mastitis features granulomas, giant cells, and chronic inflammation as well as fat necrosis, necrosis of ductal epithelium, and microabscess formation.

result from any condition that causes the circulating ratio of estradiol to testosterone to exceed the norm of 1:100. In some cases, however, the stimulus to breast development is not clear. In one series of 351 cases, one-third (103) had no obvious cause, 18% were due to medications, 15% were due to malignancies, 14% were associated with puberty, 14% were related to endocrine problems, and the remainder were associated with chronic illness and metabolic diseases (Bannayan and Hajdu, 1972) (Figs. 7–26 and 7–27).

GYNECOMASTIA

Gynecomastia, which literally means "female breasts," refers to enlargement of the male breast due to growth of ductal tissue and stroma. Lobules are rarely found (Donegan, 1991). Pseudogynecomastia refers to breast enlargement due to other causes, such as fat accumulation or tumors.

Gynecomastia was first described in detail by Basedow in 1848 (Basedow, 1848). It is a symptom rather than a disease entity and results from physiologic changes, drug effects, tumors, and diseases. The basic mechanism is excess estrogen stimulation. Estrogens are produced in males in small amounts by the testes and in larger amounts by peripheral aromatization of androgens to estrogens in muscles, fat, and skin. Testosterone from the testes is metabolized to estradiol, and androstenedione from the adrenal glands is metabolized to estrone. Wilson and colleagues (1980) indicated that feminization and gynecomastia can

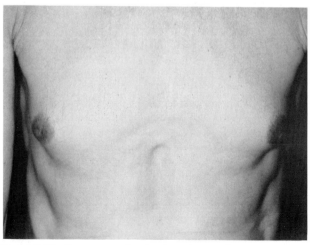

Figure 7–27. Gynecomastia due to estrogen therapy for prostate cancer. The nipples are darkened by the hormone.

Physiologic Gynecomastia

Breast enlargement in newborns presumably results from exposure to circulating maternal estrogens. Normally, it disappears after a few weeks. A case of infantile gynecomastia with bloody nipple discharge was reported by Olcay and Gokoz (1992).

Temporary physiologic gynecomastia is common at puberty when production of testicular estrogens precedes the increase of androgen levels. Mahoney attributed this to increased conversion of adrenal androgens to estrogens in peripheral sites and in the breast while testosterone production was still low (Mahoney, 1990). A firm button of tender tissue appears beneath one or both nipples of adolescent boys but almost always disappears spontaneously within 3 years as androgen levels increase (Nuttall, 1979). The peak incidence (65%) is at age 14 years and declines thereafter; however, in some cases, gynecomastia persists into early adult life (Nydick et al., 1961). Breast development associated with precocious puberty before the age of 10 years suggests the possible presence of an endocrine tumor.

Gynecomastia is also seen in elderly men, in whom testicular function declines. Surveys indicate that breast tissue can be found on physical examination surprisingly often in apparently healthy adult males, and the incidence increases with age. Nuttall (1979) found palpable breast tissue in 36% of 306 army personnel and recruits who were from 17 to 58 years of age. The frequency rose to 57% in 28 men who were older than 44 years of age. In most patients, gynecomastia was bilateral and rarely exceeded 5 cm in diameter.

Gynecomastia Due to Drugs

A number of commonly used medications produce gynecomastia by means of their estrogenic activity, inhibition of testosterone, or stimulation of estrogen synthesis. The mechanism is not always known (Table 7–3).

Gynecomastia Due to Neoplasms

Hormone-secreting neoplasms can cause gynecomastia. These include tumors of the lung, testicle, liver, pituitary gland, hypothalamus, and adrenal gland. All types of primary carcinomas of the lung are potential sources of ectopic hormone production and can produce gynecomastia through elaboration of human chorionic gonadotropin. Germ cell tumors of the testicle also secrete human chorionic gonadotropin (Cantwell et al., 1991). Granulosa cell (Matoska et al., 1992), interstitial (Leydig) cell (Kuhn et al., 1989), and Sertoli cell tumors of the testicle can produce estrogens or human chorionic gonadotropin. Most pituitary neoplasms associated with gynecomastia secrete luteinizing hormone (LH). They can also interfere with secretion of LH, with resultant reduction in testicular androgen levels. Pituitary tumors that secrete prolactin may cause lactation. Primary carcinomas of the liver that stimulate breast development do so by converting androgen precursors to estrogen (Kew et al., 1977). Gynecomastia associated with adrenal neoplasms or hyperplasia results from

Table 7–3. MEDICATIONS ASSOCIATED WITH THE DEVELOPMENT OF GYNECOMASTIA

Estrogenic Activity
Diethylstilbestrol (Kosuda et al., 1990)
Testosterone cypionate
Digitalis
Heroin
Oral contraceptives
Marijuana? (Harmon and Aliapoulios, 1972; Cates and Pope, 1977)
Clomiphene citrate
Vaginal estrogen cream exposure (DiRaimondo et al., 1980)
Inhibition of Testosterone Synthesis or Blockage of Its Action
Cimetidine (Tagamet)
Cyproterone acetate
Penicillamine (Cuprimine)
Diazepam (Valium)
Flutamide (Eulexin)
Ketoconazole (Nizoral)
Spironolactone (Aldactone)
Phenytoin (Dilantin)
Medroxyprogesterone acetate (Provera)
Stimulation of Estrogen Synthesis
Human chorionic gonadotropin
Testicular Damage
Busulfan
Vincristine
Nitrosoureas
Procarbazine
Methotrexate
Cyclophosphamide
Chlorambucil
Unknown Mechanism
Antituberculous Drugs
  Ethionamide
  Isoniazid
Cardiovascular Drugs
  Methyldopa
  Verapamil
  Clonidine (Catapres) (Weiss, 1991)
  Captopril (Capoten) (Murray and Daly, 1991; Nakamura et al., 1990)
  Reserpine (Serpasil)
  Nifedipine (Procardia)
Diuretics
  Furosemide (Lasix) (Murray and Daly, 1991)
  Amiloride (Midamor)
Psychotropic Drugs
  Tricyclic antidepressants (e.g., amitriptyline (Elavil))
  Phenothiazines (e.g., Thorazine, Compazine)
Antinausea Drugs
  Domperidone (Motilium) (Keating and Rees, 1991)
  Metoclopramide (Reglan)
Other Drugs
  Ibuprofen (e.g., Motrin)
  Theophylline (Theo-Dur)
  Omeprazole (Convens et al., 1991)
  Metronidazole (Fagan et al., 1985)

production of estrogens or increased production of androstenedione, which is converted to estrogens (Wilson et al., 1980).

Medical Conditions Associated with Gynecomastia

Medical conditions associated with gynecomastia are diverse. Those associated with liver damage, such as cirrhosis, chronic ulcerative colitis, and starvation with refeeding, produce gynecomastia by reducing the liver's ability to degrade estrogens (Klatskin, 1947; and Mahoney, 1990). The mechanism by which thyrotoxicosis causes the problem is apparently the increased production of androstenedione by the adrenal glands (Ashkar et al., 1970). Testicular failure from viral infections (e.g., mumps-related orchitis) or granulomatous infections (e.g., tuberculosis and lepromatous leprosy) is associated with gynecomastia, as is castration, congenital anorchia, and true hermaphroditism. Chronic renal failure causes testicular damage; breast development in these patients is associated with reduced androgen and elevated gonadotropin levels (Nagel et al., 1973). Other conditions that sometimes produce breast development include chest wall injury, paraplegia, and acquired immunodeficiency syndrome (AIDS) (Mahoney, 1990). Gynecomastia in a prepubertal boy due to a marked increase in aromatase activity was described by Hemsell and coworkers (1977).

A number of hypogonadal syndromes include gynecomastia as a feature. Kleinfelter's syndrome is the most widely known of these syndromes (Klinefelter et al., 1942). Men with Kleinfelter's syndrome demonstrate hypogonadism, azoospermia, and a 47,XXY karyotype. They are also believed to have an increased risk of breast cancer, although this conjecture has not been well substantiated (Evans and Crichlow, 1991). Hypogonadal states usually result in high LH levels, since the negative feedback of testosterone to the pituitary gland is lacking or reduced. Reifenstein's syndrome (Reifenstein, 1947) is a form of familial hypogonadism that features hypospadias and arrest of spermatogenesis. Patients have high levels of LH and estrogens but do not have reduced concentrations of androgens. They have a form of androgen resistance that is due to deficiency of cytoplasmic androgen receptors. Bland and Page (1991) describe a number of rare and often genetic syndromes that are characterized by gynecomastia, including Rosewater-Gwinlup-Hamwi familial gynecomastia, Kallmann's syndrome (multiple congenital anomalies and anosmia), and Kennedy's disease (fasciculations, muscle weakness, and atrophy of limb girdles). Wilson and associates (1991) described an X-linked familial syndrome of mental retardation, obesity, speech difficulties, emotional lability, tapering fingers, and small feet that is associated with gynecomastia.

Evaluation

Breast tissue on one or both sides may be apparent as diffuse glandular tissue or as a firm subareolar nodule. One side is often more prominent than the other. It is said that unilateral gynecomastia will ultimately become bilateral. The tissue is typically centered under the nipple but rarely is eccentric. The nipple may be inverted. In an adult, a unilateral, firm mass raises the possibility of carcinoma of the breast.

A complete history and physical examination are necessary. A patient's drug history and family history are particularly important. Signs of malnutrition, renal failure, hypogonadism, hyperthyroidism, or liver disease should be sought. A careful examination of the testes for evidence of

hypogonadism or tumor should be made. If the examination suggests Kleinfelter's syndrome, karyotype determination is appropriate. A mammogram (Fig. 7–28) serves to document the presence of breast tissue and to detect radiologic signs of cancer (Dershaw, 1986; and Rissanen et al., 1992). Radiography of the chest, particularly in smokers, is needed to determine whether lung cancer is present. Liver function tests are appropriate. If the clinical presentation includes signs of hyperthyroidism, assays of thyroid function should be performed. Serum prolactin levels should be determined if lactation is present. The basic endocrine work-up suggested by Wilson and colleagues (1980) includes determination of (1) urinary 17-ketosteroids (elevation indicates the presence excess androgen substrates from the adrenal glands or elsewhere); (2) plasma estradiol; (3) plasma LH; and (4) plasma testosterone. High LH and testosterone levels suggest androgen resistance or the presence of a gonadotropin-secreting tumor. If both LH and testosterone levels are low, an estrogen-secreting tumor is possible. A high LH level and a low or normal testosterone level are consistent with testicular failure or with an LH-secreting tumor.

Cantwell and coworkers (1991) recommended routine measurement of beta–human chorionic gonadotropin and alpha-fetoprotein in young men to detect germ cell tumors of the testicle. In addition to this, Mahoney (1990) recommends determination of follicle-stimulating hormone and dehydroepiandrosterone sulfate. If the concentration of the latter is elevated, imaging of the adrenal glands is necessary. An elevated estradiol concentration leads to sonographic evaluation of the testes, adrenal glands, and liver,

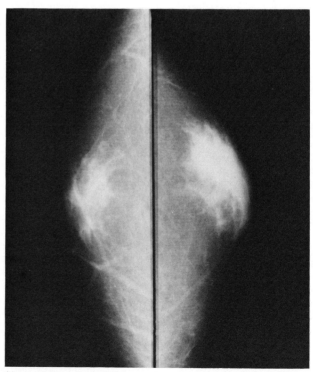

Figure 7–28. A mammogram of gynecomastia shows dense breast tissue beneath each areola and no sign of cancer (craniocaudal views of both breasts).

and an elevated human chorionic gonadotropin level requires imaging of the chest, abdomen, brain, and testes.

Treatment

The objectives of management are an accurate diagnosis and elimination of the predisposing condition. When the cause cannot be determined or cannot be eliminated, treatment depends on the severity of the problem and may be medical or surgical.

Gynecomastia in newborns can be expected to resolve and requires no treatment. In children under the age of 10 years, gynecomastia with or without signs of precocious puberty suggests a neoplasm and should prompt an endocrine evaluation (Mahoney, 1990). In otherwise healthy pubertal boys, gynecomastia can be managed by observation and by reassuring patients that the signs of its manifestation should disappear within 2 to 3 years. Only occasionally is gynecomastia severe enough to require treatment. In adults, the objective is to identify and treat the underlying cause. When gynecomastia is drug-induced, discontinuation or a change of medication may be all that is necessary. If no cause is found, it is important to appreciate that gynecomastia is not premalignant and that mastectomy is not necessary to prevent breast cancer. Also, excision for diagnosis is not routinely necessary.

Indications for operation are twofold: (1) for diagnosis, and (2) for cosmetic improvement. If carcinoma of the breast is suspected, biopsy or excision is necessary for diagnosis. Adult males with a firm unilateral nodule or suspicious mammograms are most likely to be affected, and firmness with fixation or bloody nipple discharge reinforces suspicion. Fine-needle aspiration cytology (FNAC) as a means to confirm the diagnosis of gynecomastia and assess the possibility of breast cancer may be useful, but experience with it is still limited. Russin and associates (1989) described the cytologic features of aspirates from the breasts of 50 men with gynecomastia and felt that they were distinctive. Only seven patients underwent biopsy for confirmation. Bhagat and Kline (1990) reported on 14 cases of malignant breast masses in males evaluated with FNAC and recommended its routine use. Gupta and coworkers (1988) performed FNAC on the breast masses of 44 men and diagnosed 1 carcinoma. Four gynecomastias judged cytologically suspicious were biopsied and found to be benign. The remaining 39 patients had lesions that were consistent cytologically with gynecomastia and were observed from 6 months to 3 years with no development of cancer. FNAC may well support a clinical diagnosis of gynecomastia and enable open biopsy to be used more selectively.

Reduction of obviously enlarged breasts may be necessary to avoid embarrassment to the male patient. Removal of the sensitive tissues is occasionally desired for comfort. In most cases, the breast tissue can be removed cosmetically through a para-areolar incision as described by von Kessel and colleagues (1963), employing when necessary a small lateral extension. Since the nipple is not removed by this operation, recurrent breast enlargement can occur if the stimulus to breast tissue continues. Among nine patients treated in this manner by the author, one had recurrent

gynecomastia; within 3 months, the breast of the 50-year-old man had again become prominent. In severe cases, a more extensive operation is required. Recent publications describe liposuction as an option, usually in combination with a limited operation to remove glandular tissue (Dolsky, 1990; Mladick, 1991; and Rigg, 1991).

In selected patients, the use of antiestrogens is useful. Jacobs (1991) reported a good response of gynecomastia to tamoxifen (Nolvadex) in a patient with cirrhosis of the liver. Men with recurrent gynecomastia after excision might also be candidates for treatment with tamoxifen. The side effects in men are generally limited to mild nausea and abdominal discomfort (Mahoney, 1990). The use of danazol (Danocrine), a suppressor of gonadotropin, has had some success in treatment of idiopathic, thyrotoxic, and drug-induced gynecomastia, with improvement occurring in 83% of patients (Buckle, 1980).

FIBROCYSTIC CHANGES

''Fibrocystic changes'' undoubtedly constitute the most frequent benign disorder of the breast, affecting an estimated 50% to 90% of women (Hutter, 1985). The term designates a spectrum of apparently related symptomatic and histologic conditions of uncertain cause that are also known as fibrocystic disease, cystic mastopathy, chronic cystic disease, chronic cystic mastitis, Schimmelbusch's disease, mazoplasia, Cooper's disease, Reclus's disease, fibroadenomatosis, and cystic mastopathy in addition to a number of other uninformative and even misleading terms. The problem is not inflammatory, as the term ''mastitis'' would imply, and it probably is not a ''disease'' in the usual sense. A hormonal basis is presumed because the problem is most evident during the reproductive period of life (Devitt, 1986): the symptoms are often cyclic and most severe immediately preceding menstruation; and cyst formation is often initiated by the approach of menopause, when hormonal fluctuations are pronounced. Nevertheless, no definite hormonal abnormality has been identified in affected women. Reviews of the subject have found intriguing but inconclusive evidence for theories of unopposed estrogen stimulation, progesterone deficiency, and excess prolactin production (Fentiman and Wang, 1986; Vorherr, 1986; and Dogliotti et al., 1989). No consistent abnormalities have been found in androgen metabolism, gonadotropin levels, or thyroid function. Alcohol consumption is unrelated to the condition (Rohan and Cook, 1989). Some evidence suggests that excess dietary fat contributes to the problem (Lubin et al., 1989). The association of severe fibrocystic changes with the familial syndrome known as ''Cowden's disease'' raises the possibility of a genetic influence (Lloyd and Dennis, 1963). Minton and Abou-Issa (1989) postulated a genetic predisposition for increased activity of the beta-adrenergic/adenylate cyclase system found in the breasts of these patients.

Painful and tender breasts and nodularity are the signs of fibrocystic changes (Schwartz, 1983). Pain and tenderness varied in the Canadian Benign Breast Disease Study reported by Deschamps and colleagues (1986). In this study, 26% of 736 women were asymptomatic, 37% had tenderness alone, 3% had pain alone, and 20% had both pain and tenderness. Three patterns of onset were recognized. Tenderness appeared about age 25 years and remained premenstrual in the majority; it sometimes radiated to the axilla or the back and rarely was associated with weakness of the arm. Breast pain described at a later age (40 years) was noncyclic but had a similar pattern of radiation. The combination of pain and tenderness appeared in the early thirties and was either noncyclic from the onset or soon became so. This third pattern was the most distressing and was the one most likely to be associated with nodularity.

Nodularity may not be accompanied by symptoms; alternatively, it may be absent in women with symptoms. If the normal breast can be described as soft or softly glandular, the changes associated with fibrocystic breasts vary and can be described as diffuse firmness, fine granularity, coarse granularity, nodular, irregular patterns of firmness, or as a single mass. Nipple discharge can often be expressed from multiple ducts of one or both breasts. The discharge is thin but can be of any color (including blue) and either clear or opaque. A thick discharge suggests duct ectasia. In severe cases, axillary lymph nodes are enlarged and tender.

Changes in the tissues are both cystic and solid. Cysts are found in as many as one-third of women 35 to 50 years of age on ultrasound examination (Leis, 1991). Most are subclinical "microcysts." Others are easily palpable as masses and may reach great size (Fig. 7–29) (England et al., 1989). The age distribution of women with gross cysts (Fig. 7–30) suggests that the occurrence of cysts increases in frequency as the menopause approaches. Most patients are 40 to 55 years of age, and few are postmenopausal (Leis, 1991; and Sterns, 1992). Only 5% of cysts are found

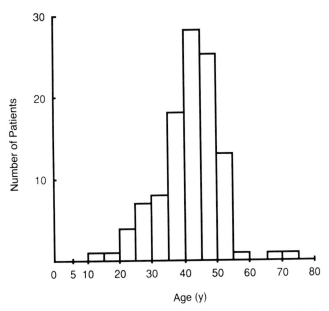

Figure 7–30. Age distribution of 108 women at first diagnosis of a palpable breast cyst. Cysts predominated in the upper outer quadrant of the breast. When multiple cysts occurred, they were bilateral in 53% of patients. (From author's personal series.)

in women over 60 years of age, and one-half of these are associated with the use of replacement estrogens. According to Sterns (1992), palpable cysts accounted for 4% of all visits to a breast clinic. Forty per cent recurred two to five times after aspiration, and 4% recurred more than five times. Hughes and Bundred (1989) reported a much lower rate of recurrence (10%) after aspiration. More than one-half of women with cysts will eventually have more than one cyst (Hughes and Bundred, 1989). Most cysts have no true lining. The small fraction of cysts that are lined by apocrine epithelium and that contain fluid with a high ratio of potassium to sodium may be more often multiple and more likely to recur than unlined cysts. Some clinicians suspect that they are also associated with an increased risk of cancer (Leis, 1991; and Naldone et al., 1992).

Solid elements include a variety of epithelial and stromal changes. Adenosis, papillomatosis, sclerosis, apocrine metaplasia, and epithelial hyperplasia are terms often used to describe these changes (Page and Anderson, 1987a). Adenosis (blunt duct adenosis) refers to the presence of an increased number of glandular elements. It features mildly increased cellularity of lobules and dilatation of lumina. Sclerosing adenosis includes proliferation of the intralobular stroma and dispersion of the glandular elements (Fig. 7–31). The lobule is enlarged, but the general lobular configuration is maintained. Sclerosing adenosis can result in discrete palpable masses (Silverman et al., 1989). Microglandular adenosis is similar to sclerosing adenosis but lacks a lobular configuration and can be mistaken for tubular carcinoma. However, a myoepithelial cell layer is maintained.

Apocrine metaplasia may be seen lining cysts or within lobules. These large, pink cells, which resemble the cells of apocrine glands, can become heaped up or assume papillary configurations. They are easily recognizable and have no

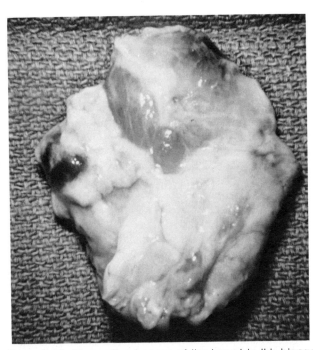

Figure 7–29. Fibrocystic changes of the breast in this biopsy specimen include irregular firm tissues and multiple gross cysts that contain thin fluid. Simple cysts do not require excision, and their presence implies no increased risk for breast carcinoma.

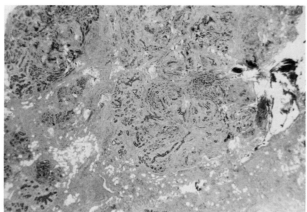

Figure 7–31. Sclerosing adenosis. Terminal ducts within the lobules are separated by a sclerotic reaction, but the lobular configuration is maintained.

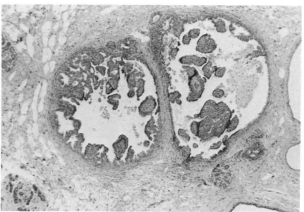

Figure 7–33. Papillomatosis of mammary ducts. The papillomas have fibrovascular cores and diffusely involve the ductal wall.

special significance. Squamous metaplasia of ductal epithelium can also be found.

Hyperplasia represents an increase in the layers of the cells lining the ducts of the breast with no increase in the number of ducts or glands (Fig. 7–32). "Epitheliosis" is a term that also is used to describe this proliferative change, which was found in 12.9% of breasts in Sandison's autopsy series (Sandison, 1962). Normally no more than two cell layers in thickness, the epithelium of the duct increases to five or more cell layers. The changes can be focal or diffuse; hyperplasia can also be found in lobules in the form of increased cellularity and crowding of cells. The hyperplasia sometimes assumes an exuberant branching configuration that is designated as "papillomatosis" (Fig. 7–33). Papillomatosis has received special attention in young women when it presents as a mass in an otherwise normal breast (Rosen et al., 1985; and Bazzocchi et al., 1986). This so-called "juvenile papillomatosis" is associated with a family history of breast cancer and probably with an increased risk for breast cancer. Juvenile papillomatosis has also been described in young males (Sund et al., 1992).

Atypia in hyperplastic tissues is an ominous change. Atypical ductal hyperplasia and atypical lobular hyperplasia

occupy the spectrum between hyperplasia and carcinoma in situ. Disturbing features include poor cell differentiation, nuclear hyperchromatism, and other marks of carcinoma in situ; however, these features are not sufficient to permit a diagnosis of malignancy with confidence (Fig. 7–34). It is not unusual for pathologists to differ in opinion regarding whether the changes in a particular patient represent atypical hyperplasia or carcinoma in situ. Page and Dupont (1988) estimated that 25% of women with surgical biopsies demonstrate hyperplasia, but fewer than 5% have atypia. A diagnosis of atypical ductal hyperplasia or atypical lobular hyperplasia is associated with a fourfold to fivefold increase in a patient's risk for future breast cancer compared with that of women in the general population (Page et al., 1987). This risk is doubled if the patient has a mother, sister, or daughter who has breast cancer (Page et al., 1985).

Duct papillomas represent focal hyperplastic changes that are supported by a well-developed fibrovascular core (Fig. 7–35). Their presence is usually signaled by a persistent nipple discharge. When they reach sufficient size, they present a characteristic clinical picture of spontaneous bloody or serosanguineous nipple discharge associated with a pal-

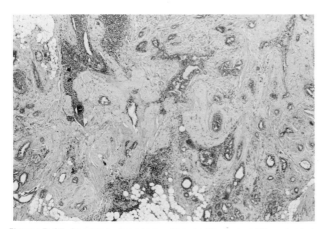

Figure 7–32. Ductal hyperplasia. The epithelium of the ducts is cytologically normal but has become multilayered.

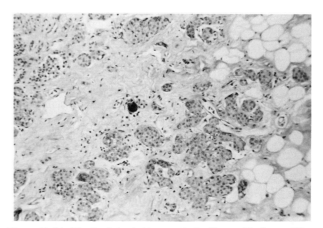

Figure 7–34. Atypical ductal hyperplasia. The epithelium of the ducts fills the lumen and suggests ductal carcinoma in situ but does not meet all criteria. This change is associated with an increased risk of breast carcinoma.

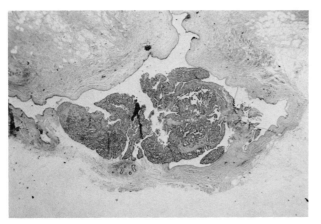

Figure 7–35. Histologic section of a duct papilloma. The tumor arises from a single site and distends the duct.

pable mass, the application of pressure to which produces the discharge. Murad and coworkers (1981) reviewed 158 papillary tumors of the breast and found that 47% were benign solitary papillomas, 13% were benign and multiple, and 40% were papillary carcinomas. Spontaneous nipple discharge was associated with 88%, 48%, and 23% of these tumors, respectively. Solitary duct papillomas occur in large ducts and within a short radius around the areola. Histologically, benign duct papillomas do not carry a risk for breast cancer beyond that inferred by the presence of hyperplasia or atypia. Multiple papillomas tend to be bilateral, smaller, and more peripherally placed than single ones and possibly confer a higher risk of cancer to the patient (Carter, 1977). Abe (1990) illustrated an effective technique for discretely removing solitary duct papillomas.

Proliferation of stromal elements can produce a palpable mass. Focal hyperplasia of fibrous connective tissue has been termed "fibrous disease of the breast" (Haagensen, 1971c), "fibrous tumor" (Puente and Potel, 1974), "focal fibrous disease" (Rivera-Pomar et al., 1980), and "fibrous mastopathy" (Page and Anderson, 1987b). These localized but poorly marginated mass-forming lesions occur in young women and are characterized by dense fibrosis with scant evidence of ducts or lobules. It is not unusual for them to recur after excision: 3 of 13 lesions reviewed by Gump and coworkers (1981) did so. A patient of the author required re-excision for recurrence of the lesion at the same location.

Fibrosis of the breast with vasculitis is a complication of insulin-dependent diabetes mellitus (Byrd et al., 1987). Vuitch and associates (1986) described nine cases of pseudoangiomatous hyperplasia of mammary stroma that presented as a painless mass; in two cases, re-excision was required.

Fibrocystic Changes, and Risk for Breast Carcinoma

Fibrocystic change has long been suspected of placing a woman at increased risk for breast cancer (Veronesi and Pizzocaro, 1968; Haagensen, 1974; Donnelly et al., 1975; and Hans-Beat et al., 1988). Webber and Boyd (1986) crit-

ically analyzed 36 reports and concluded that the weight of evidence supported this conclusion. Among the histologic changes most closely associated with risk were epithelial proliferation and atypia. Dupont and Page (1985) reviewed 10,366 breast biopsies for benign lesions to identify 3303 women who had a median follow-up of 17 years. Compared with women without proliferative changes, the relative risk of subsequent breast cancer was 1.9 among those with proliferative changes and 5.3 among those with atypical hyperplasia. A family history of breast cancer (mother, sister, or daughter) elevated the relative risk to 11 in women with atypical hyperplasia. Only 60% of women with this combination were free of invasive breast cancer after 25 years. Carter and coworkers (1988) reviewed the experience with 16,692 women with biopsy-diagnosed benign breast disease from the Breast Cancer Detection Demonstration Projects conducted in the United States from 1973 to 1978. Among these women, 485 cases of cancer were diagnosed subsequently. They concluded that risk was associated with degree of epithelial atypia. The relative risks (RRs) for developing breast cancer in increasing order of magnitude were as follows: nonproliferative disease (RR = 1.5), proliferative disease without atypia (RR = 1.9), and atypical hyperplasia (RR = 3.0). A consensus meeting in 1985 chaired by the College of American Pathologists and supported by the American Cancer Society produced a statement on the cancer risk associated with specific histologic components of benign breast disease. The categories agreed upon are shown in Table 7–4 (Consensus Statement, 1986). Well-developed sclerosing adenosis was subsequently added to the original category of Slightly Increased Risk (Jensen et al., 1989; and Page and Dupont, 1991).

It is now appreciated that only some women with fibrocystic changes are at increased risk for breast cancer. The risk for women with symptoms but without histologic diagnoses is unknown. Although it is now possible to more

Table 7–4. RISK OF FUTURE INVASIVE BREAST CARCINOMA BASED ON HISTOLOGIC DIAGNOSIS FROM BREAST BIOPSIES*

I. No Increase
Adenosis
Apocrine metaplasia
Cysts, small or large
Mild hyperplasia (>2 but <5 cells deep)
Duct ectasia
Fibroadenoma
Fibrosis
Mastitis, inflammatory
Periductal mastitis
Squamous metaplasia
II. Slightly Increased (Relative Risk = 1.5–2)
Moderate or florid hyperplasia, solid or papillary
Duct papilloma with fibrovascular core
Sclerosing adenosis, well-developed
III. Moderately Increased (Relative Risk = 4-5)
Atypical hyperplasia, ductal or lobular

(Data from Page, D. L., and Dupont, W. D.: Histologic indicators of breast cancer risk. Am. Coll. Surg. Bull., 76:16–23, 1991, and Jensen, R. A., Page, D. L., Dupont, W. D., et al.: Invasive breast cancer risk in women with sclerosing adenosis. Cancer, 64:1977–1983, 1989.)
*Compared with women with no breast biopsy.

precisely define the risk of individual patients with histology, the consensus committee made clear that the guidelines were not intended to justify breast biopsy simply for the determination of risk. Because histologic criteria do provide a useful assessment of risk, pathologists should report precisely the changes present in biopsies rather than simply reporting "fibrocystic changes." Finally, the committee encouraged use of the term fibrocystic "changes" rather than fibrocystic "disease" as a more appropriate description of this condition.

Medical Treatment

The most important objective of management is to determine at the outset and on a continuing basis that a more serious problem (i.e., cancer) is not present. Many women are adequately relieved simply upon receiving this information. A careful physical examination, aspiration of cysts, and biopsy of suspicious masses or suspicious lesions found on mammography serve this end.

Treatment has been directed at the relief of symptoms and the reduction of cysts and nodularity. Nonspecific measures for symptomatic relief have traditionally included reduction of the motion of the breasts with firm brassiere support, local heat application, and administration of mild analgesics (e.g., aspirin, ibuprofen, or acetaminophen) as needed. Diuretics reduce fluid accumulation late in the menstrual cycle, but they have no selective effect on the breasts.

Strategies for specific medical treatment have been guided by theories of causation. Hormonal imbalances (Sitruk-Ware et al., 1979), thyroid dysfunction (Adamopoulos et al., 1986), and dietary influences (Minton and Abou-Issa, 1989) are among the bases of these theories, but all remain unproved. Reduced estrogen stimulation of the breasts is the goal of most hormonal therapy. Although hormone therapy often provides relief, unwanted side effects limit its acceptability; in addition, the effects are usually temporary.

Efforts to evaluate therapy are hampered by the difficulty encountered in measuring success objectively and by the inconsistent correlation between symptoms and physical findings. Since symptoms normally "wax and wane," strictly controlled studies are necessary; however, such studies are few and involve relatively small numbers of patients and limited follow-up.

Danazol alone has Food and Drug Administration's approval for use in the treatment of "fibrocystic breast disease." This synthetic androgen suppresses gonadotropin output by the pituitary gland (both follicle-stimulating hormone and LH) and, hence, decreases ovarian function. Gorins and associates (1984) reported on a double-blind placebo-controlled trial involving patients with "severe benign mastopathy." At a dosage of 400 mg/d, symptomatic improvement was obtained in 32 of 38 patients. Brookshaw (1979) reviewed the experience with the treatment of 514 patients who were included in a multicenter study in the United States. At doses of 50 to 400 mg/d, more than 90% of women had decreased pain, tenderness, and nodularity (Brookshaw, 1979). Both postmenopausal women and premenopausal women benefited. Nodularity responded less

often and more slowly than did pain and tenderness. Treatment with danazol is initiated during menstruation, and patients taking it must avoid pregnancy. Bothersome side effects include weight gain, acne, and oiliness of hair. Amenorrhea or irregular menses are common as is a reduction of breast size (Dhont et al., 1979). Danazol also has weak androgenic effects that may not be reversible. Unfortunately, symptoms often recur when treatment is discontinued.

Progesterone has been used to correct a perceived luteal deficiency. Sitruk-Ware and colleagues (1979) found a lower ratio of estrogen to progesterone during the luteal phase of the ovarian cycle in women with fibrocystic changes compared with normal women. Kuttenn and coworkers (1983) treated 249 cases of benign breast disease with daily application of a progesterone-containing alcohol-water gel to the skin of the breasts in addition to the oral administration of progestin (lynestrenol) at a dosage of 10 mg/d from days 10 to 25 of the menstrual cycle. With this regimen, 96% of patients with mastodynia had relief, and 85% with nodularity experienced improvement. Side effects were "minor." However, only 10% of patients with chronic fibrocystic disease derived benefit, and cyst formation was not often affected. Others have found progestogens to be effective (von Fournier et al., 1989). The balanced estrogen and progestogen oral contraceptive Enovid, 5–10 mg three times daily, provides subjective and objective relief to about 50% of women but at the cost of weight gain and frequent gastrointestinal upset (Ariel, 1973).

The synthetic antiestrogen tamoxifen produces clinical improvement in two-thirds of women with symptoms (Fentiman et al., 1986; and von Fournier et al., 1989). Ricciardi and Ianniruberto (1979) reported that 71.4% of 63 women were symptom-free and that physical findings were improved after treatment with 10 mg of tamoxifen on days 5 to 25 of the menstrual cycle for 4 months. This study included patients with fibroadenomas, and only 41 women had tissue diagnoses. The principal side effects of tamoxifen are hot flushes, nausea, and dizziness. Risk for thrombophlebitis and for endometrial cancer are also increased by this drug.

Bromocriptine, a long-acting dopaminergic drug that suppresses prolactin, has been approved in Great Britain for the treatment of cyclic mastalgia (Scott, 1987). Bromocriptine at a dosage of 7.5 mg/d for 3 months reduced breast pain, tension, nodularity, and tenderness in 90% of 120 patients treated by Dogliotti and coworkers (1983); the benefits of treatment persisted in most patients after treatment stopped. In a study by Raso and colleagues (1986) of 15 patients, bromocriptine (5 mg/d) more effectively reduced pain and engorgement than did treatment with cutaneous progesterone. In a small study of 40 randomized patients, Sandrucci and coworkers (1986) found bromocriptine (7.5 mg/d) and tamoxifen (10 mg/d) to be equally effective for reducing symptoms and nodularity. The mechanism by which prolactin inhibition produces benefit is unknown (Dogliotti et al., 1986). Prolactin levels of patients with symptomatic fibrocystic changes are normal but are reduced by bromocriptine (Dogliotti et al., 1986). Nausea and vomiting, headache, and symptomatic hypotension are disturbing side effects of bromocriptine and are severe enough to prevent continued treatment with the drug in about 12% of patients.

Abstinence from caffeine as a method of management is based on the work of Minton and associates (1979). These researchers found methylxanthine consumption to be associated with elevated levels of cyclic adenosine monophosphate and cyclic guanosine monophosphate in breasts with fibrocystic changes compared with normal breasts. They postulated that breast tissues were excessively stimulated by these hormone mediators. Catecholamines were believed to exaggerate the effect. Patients with large intakes of methylxanthines (caffeine, theophylline, theobromine) and tyramines often experienced relief by eliminating them from the diet. The most common sources of caffeine are coffee, tea, caffeinated soft drinks, and chocolate. Sources of tyramines include nuts, wine, avocadoes, and cheese. Smoking cessation is also recommended to reduce catecholamine release. In individual patients, the results of these restrictions can be convincing; however, in critical evaluations, they have remained controversial (Ernster et al., 1982; Lubin et al., 1985; and Parazzini et al., 1986). All sufferers are not heavy caffeine users, and this places a limit on the treatment's application. The appeal of this theory lies in the biochemical evidence that supports it and the innocuous and healthful nature of the recommendations. It is often given an initial trial by the author.

Thyroid hormone or iodine deficiency is the rationale of some therapies. Administration of diatomic iodine reduced the pain and fibrosis of fibrocystic changes in an uncontrolled study by Ghent and Eskin (1986). These investigators theorized that cells in terminal ducts of the breast lose their ability to use iodine complexes. Ghent reported that almost three-quarters of 253 women treated with diatomic iodine (3–6 mg/d) were returned to health (Ghent, 1986). Complications included acne and a transient increase in breast pain. According to Estes (1981), treatment with levothyroxine, 0.1 mg/d, lowered prolactin levels and provided complete relief of mastodynia in 47% of 19 patients.

Use of evening primrose oil is advocated by Hughes and associates (1989c) for treating mild cyclic mastalgia. The rationale is that it replenishes a deficiency of essential fatty acids. This natural substance is one of the richest known sources of essential fatty acids, and it has no side effects.

In uncontrolled studies, vitamin E (alpha-tocopherol) had initial success that was attributed to restoration of hormonal balance. Ultimately, it was found in double-blind randomized controlled trials that treatment with vitamin E of up to 3 months duration had no significant effect on physical findings (London et al., 1985) nor on mammographic findings (Meyer et al., 1990).

Surgical Treatment

Mastectomy is rarely necessary for treatment of symptomatic fibrocystic changes. It is employed in only the most extreme cases—that is, in women with intractable, incapacitating symptoms or with an unacceptably high risk of breast cancer based on histologic findings and other factors. It is prudent to seek additional supporting opinions before proceeding with mastectomy. Total mastectomy is preferable to subcutaneous mastectomy. Although the latter provides a better cosmetic result, it does not remove all breast tissue; only complete removal of breast tissue eliminates future risk of breast cancer (Prpic et al., 1983; Goodnight et al., 1984; and Hughes et al., 1989d).

COUMARIN NECROSIS

A rare complication of anticoagulation therapy with coumarin is hemorrhagic necrosis of the skin and soft tissues (Cole, 1988). An estimated 200 cases of coumarin-associated necrosis of the breast have been reported. The complication was described by Flood in 1943 and was first related to coumarin by Verhagen in 1954 (Verhagen, 1954). The lesion typically develops after 3 to 4 days of therapy as ecchymotic areas that enlarge and darken and become painful on palpation. Bullae appear, and the lesion progresses to full-thickness skin necrosis. The entire breast may be lost, and the involvement may be bilateral. This dangerous complication has been attributed to large loading doses of coumarin, which act to reduce protein C more rapidly than other vitamin K–dependent clotting factors. The restraining effect of protein C on thrombin formation at the epithelial surface is lost, resulting in progressive local thrombosis in venules. Treatment requires discontinuation of coumarin use and administration of vitamin K. Heparin administration is also begun to prevent further clotting and is continued at therapeutic doses if prolonged anticoagulation is needed. Areas of necrosis are treated with débridement or excision as necessary.

FAT NECROSIS

Traumatic fat necrosis is not infrequent in the breast. It received attention originally because it so closely mimicked the clinical signs of cancer (Lee and Adair, 1920) (Fig. 7–36). Fat necrosis accounted for 2.5% of breast masses in an

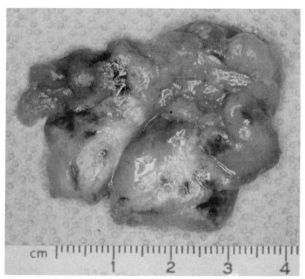

Figure 7–36. A focus of fat necrosis within breast tissue creates a pale, firm, irregular mass.

early review (Adair and Munzer, 1947). It is seen as the sequela to blunt injury (Fig. 7–37), a blow to the breast, vigorous exercise, or operations on the breast such as biopsy or breast reduction. However, a traumatic event is not always recalled. It may also occur with therapeutic irradiation and injection of foreign substances (Stefanik et al., 1982).

Fat necrosis presents clinically as a palpable mass and may cause skin or nipple retraction. Discoloration of the skin and tenderness are often absent. The mammographic features are varied, including a spiculated mass, suspicious rodlike or branching microcalcifications, skin thickening and deformity, or radiolucent lipid-filled cysts with calcified walls (Fig. 7–38). These signs occur singly or in combination and can strongly suggest malignancy (Bassett et al., 1978). A spiculated mass with a radiolucent center is suggestive of fat necrosis. Grossly, the tissues show dense fibrosis and often a necrotic, oily central cavity. Histologically, they consist of oily debris, fibrous connective tissue, foamy macrophages, and giant cells. Fine-needle aspiration of the palpable mass is seldom conclusive. Although a history of trauma is suggestive of fat necrosis, cancer is more frequently the cause of a breast mass than is fat necrosis, and differentiation from cancer in the adult female usually requires biopsy.

Poorly understood processes of progressive focal liponecrosis involve the breast. An example is Weber-Christian disease (chronic relapsing febrile nodular nonsuppurative panniculitis). Fever is not essential, however; furthermore, suppuration sometimes occurs, and the process can involve intra-abdominal as well as subcutaneous fat (Kaufman, 1960). Two of 15 cases reported by Panush and coworkers (1985) involved the breast but were not confined to it. The onset is characterized by the development of tender subcutaneous nodules with or without systemic symptoms. Biopsies show inflammation, necrosis, and fibrosis. A mammogram may feature calcifications (Bernstein, 1977). Figure 7–39 shows a case of panniculitis involving the right breast that resulted in scarring and retraction. Laboratory results often suggest an autoimmune process, and therapy has been

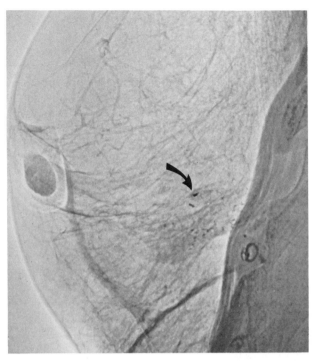

Figure 7–38. Fat necrosis after surgical reduction of the breast. In this mammogram, fat necrosis produces a focal density that contains microcalcifications *(arrow)*—signs that mimic carcinoma.

varied and has included the use of nonsteroidal anti-inflammatory drugs, antimalarials, corticosteroids, and immunosuppressives (Panush et al., 1985). Systemic or discoid lupus erythematosus can produce a panniculitis of the breast with subcutaneous nodules that progress to ulcers (Harris and Winkelmann, 1978).

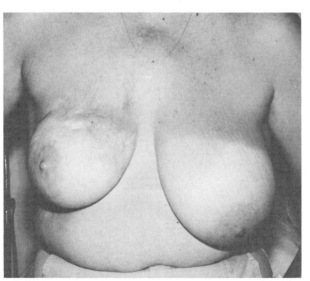

Figure 7–39. Chronic progressive panniculitis of the right breast. This process caused discomfort to the patient and contraction of the breast. The tissues showed chronic inflammation, fat necrosis, and fibrosis.

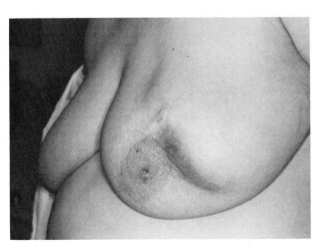

Figure 7–37. Retraction of the breast due to traumatic fat necrosis that resulted from injury in an automobile accident.

MONDOR'S DISEASE (THORACOEPIGASTRIC THROMBOPHLEBITIS)

Henri Mondor described thrombophlebitis of the thoraco-epigastric vein in 1939, but this disease had been identified earlier in 1870 by Fagge at Guy's Hospital (Mondor, 1939; and Fagge, 1870). Thrombophlebitis of this vein, which courses across the breast, presents as mild tenderness and the development of a firm, subcutaneous cord. The cord produces a groove on the breast or a "bowstring" across the axilla or inframammary fold (Figs. 7–40 and 7–41). Tenderness is temporary and may go unnoticed, but the cord persists for weeks.

Mondor's disease has been associated with trauma, infections, physical activity, rheumatoid arthritis, intravenous drug abuse, and, occasionally, cancer of the breast (Chiedozi and Aghahowa, 1988; and Cooper, 1990). The author has seen it most often after breast biopsies, when the thoracoepigastric vein was apparently interrupted. A similar condition is frequent in the arm after mastectomy or axillary dissection due to thrombosis of superficial afferent veins (Fig. 7–42). These long, tight, subcutaneous cords

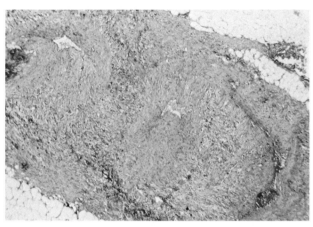

Figure 7–41. Histologic section from a patient with Mondor's disease shows an organizing clot within a vein.

cross the antecubital space and course toward the axilla. They are often noticed by patients and may hamper the process of shoulder mobilization.

The correct diagnosis is usually apparent on physical examination. In spontaneous cases, mammography is prudent, since cancer has been reported with Mondor's disease. Biopsy is indicated only if the diagnosis is uncertain or if cancer is suspected. Anticoagulation is not necessary. Treatment is generally with local heat application (to speed resolution) and nonsteroidal anti-inflammatory drugs (e.g., ibuprofen). The cords in the arm seen after axillary dissection stretch and disappear with continued arm exercise.

HEART FAILURE AND BREAST EDEMA

Unilateral breast enlargement with edema and nipple retraction mimicking carcinoma can be a manifestation of congestive heart failure. McElligott and Harrington (1986) reported two cases and mentioned other reports. The right

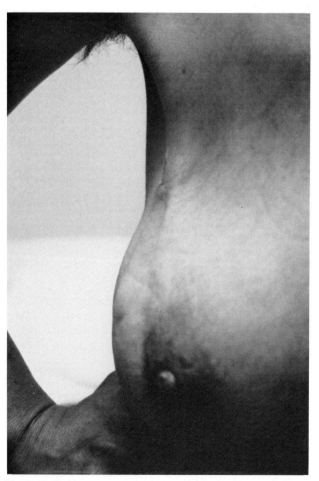

Figure 7–40. Mondor's disease (thrombophlebitis of the thoracoepigastric vein) presents as a firm, subcutaneous cord on the breast.

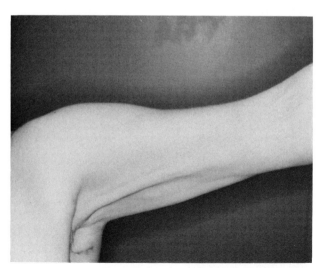

Figure 7–42. A process similar to Mondor's disease produces subcutaneous cords in the axilla and upper arm after axillary dissection.

breast was involved in both of the former cases and was associated with edema of the right arm in one. The patients were elderly, and obvious signs of heart failure were present, including cardiomegaly and pleural effusions. Unilateral edema was attributed to the gravitational effect of lying on one side. The breast returned to normal after effective treatment for cardiac failure. The author has seen several cases of unexplained unilateral breast edema that suggested inflammatory carcinoma but that resolved spontaneously. Heart failure was not involved.

INFARCTION ASSOCIATED WITH PREGNANCY

Localized infarction of breast tissue associated with pregnancy and lactation has been recognized since 1961 (Hasson and Pope, 1961). The report of Jimenez and associates (1986) brought the total number of cases to 28. Relative vascular insufficiency imposed by increased metabolic demands is presumably responsible. The lesion presents as a palpable mass late in pregnancy or in the early postpartum period. Its size averages 3 cm; mobility is usual, although skin fixation may be present; and the mass may be tender. Multiple and bilateral masses have been reported. Mammograms show a circumscribed density. Grossly, the lesion is a yellow-gray, firm, discrete nodule. Histologically, the tissues show coagulative necrosis and, in various reports, suggest infarction of hyperplastic breast tissue, a lactating adenoma, or a pre-existing fibroadenoma. Fibroadenomas occasionally undergo infarction in the absence of pregnancy (Robitaille et al., 1974). Excision is necessary for diagnosis and is sufficient treatment, but it may be followed by formation of a temporary milk fistula.

ECZEMA OF THE NIPPLE

Chronic dermatitis of the nipple (eczematous dermatitis) is a nonspecific inflammatory response to endogenous or exogenous agents. It is often an allergic reaction and responds to removal of a contact irritant and to the topical application of hydrocortisone. Hughes and associates (1989*b*) suggest that eczema might in some cases develop as an allergic response to nipple discharge. The important differential diagnosis is with Paget's disease of the breast. Haagensen (1986) suggested that eczema of the nipple is less frequent than Paget's disease and noted that it develops more rapidly and does not destroy the nipple. He also pointed out that since Paget's disease emerges from the central ducts of the papilla and then spreads to involve the areola and finally the skin, a lesion that involves the areola and not the papilla is unlikely to be Paget's disease. Figure 7–43 is a case in point. This clinical guide may not be dependable, since carcinoma can arise in the mammary ducts that connect with the tubercles of Montgomery. To avoid mistakes, any questionable dermatitis of the nipple is biopsied for diagnosis. Punch biopsy serves well for this purpose and is performed as an office procedure with the use of local anesthesia.

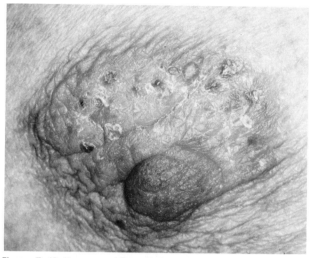

Figure 7–43. Eczema of the nipple. This lesion developed over the course of 1 month in an 85-year-old woman and was confined to the areola of the right nipple. A mammogram showed edema of the nipple.

MUCOCELE-LIKE TUMOR OF THE BREAST

A mucocele-like tumor, which is analogous to mucoceles found in the minor salivary glands, is occasionally found in the breast. Clinically, the tumor presents as a mass, and histologically it shows multiple segregated cysts filled with mucin and lined with low epithelium manifesting a focal tendency to hyperplasia. The pathogenesis of these lesions is uncertain, but they are benign and should not be confused with mucinous carcinoma. Local excision is adequate therapy. Rosen (1986) reported six patients whose ages ranged from 25 to 61 years. The author has had one case in an 81-year-old white woman. The tumor presented as a nonpalpable, 11-mm spiculated mass on a routine mammogram that was highly suggestive of carcinoma.

References

Abe, R.: The operative management of intraductal papilloma of the breast. Jpn. J. Surg., *20*:240–245, 1990.

Abramson, D. J.: Mammary duct ectasia, mammillary fistula and subareolar sinuses. Ann. Surg., *169*:217–226, 1969.

Abrikossoff, A. J.: Über Myome, Ausgehend von der quergestreiften willwerklichen Musklature. Arch. Pathol. Anat., *260*:215, 1926.

Adair, F. E., and Munzer, J. T.: Fat necrosis of the female breast: Report of 110 cases. Am. J. Surg., *74*:117–128, 1947.

Adamopoulos, D. A., Vassilaros, S., Kapolla, N., et al.: Thyroid disease in patients with benign and malignant mastopathy. Cancer, *57*:125–128, 1986.

Alagaratnam, T. T., Ong, G. B.: Paraffinoma of the breast. J. R. Coll. Surg. Edinb., *28*:260–263, 1983.

Andersen, J. A., and Gram, J. B.: Radial scar in the female breast. Cancer, *53*:2557–2560, 1984.

Arey, L. B.: Developmental Anatomy. 7th ed. Philadelphia, W. B. Saunders, 1966, p. 449.

Ariel, I. M.: Enovidu therapy (norethynodrel with mestranol) for fibrocystic disease. Am. J. Obstet. Gynecol., *117*:453–459, 1973.

Ashkar, F. S., Smoak, W. M., Gilson, A. J., and Miller, R.: Gynecomastia and mastoplasia in Graves' disease. Metabolism, *19*:946, 1970.

Bannayan, G. A., and Hajdu, S. I.: Gynecomastia: Clinicopathologic study of 351 cases. Am. J. Clin. Pathol., *57*:431–437, 1972.

Basedow, K. A.: Die Glotzaugen. Wochenschr. Gesellsch. Heilkunde, *49*:769, 1848.

Bassett, L. W., Gold, R. H., and Cove, H. C.: Mammographic spectrum of traumatic fat necrosis: The fallibility of ''pathognomonic'' signs of carcinoma. Am. J. Roentgenol., *130*:119–122, 1978.

Bassett, L. W., and Cove, H. C.: Myoblastoma of the breast. J. Radiol., *132*:122, 1979.

Bauer, B. S., Jones, K. M., and Talbot, C. W.: Mammary masses in the adolescent female. Surg. Gynecol. Obstet., *165*:63–65, 1987.

Bazzocchi, F., Santini, D., Martinelli, G., et al.: Juvenile papillomatosis (epitheliosis) of the breast. Am. J. Clin. Pathol., *86*:745–748, 1986.

Benson, E. A.: Management of breast abscesses. World J. Surg., *13*:753–756, 1989.

Bernstein, J. R.: Nonsuppurative nodular panniculitis (Weber-Christian disease): An unusual cause of mammary calcifications. J.A.M.A., *238*:1942–1943, 1977.

Bertrand, H., and Rosenblood, I. K.: Stripping out pus in lactational mastitis: A means of preventing breast abscess. Can. Med. Assoc. J., *145*:299–306, 1991.

Bhagat, P., and Kline, T. S.: The male breast and malignant neoplasms: Diagnosis by aspiration biopsy cytology. Cancer, *65*:2338–2341, 1990.

Bland, K. I., and Page, D. L.: Gynecomastia. *In* Bland, K. I., and Copeland, E. M. (Eds.): The Breast. Philadelphia, W. B. Saunders, 1991, pp. 150–151.

Brookshaw, J. D.: Danazol treatment of benign breast disease: A survey of USA multi-centre studies. Postgrad. Med. J., *55*(Suppl. 5):52-58, 1979.

Buckle, R.: Danazol in the treatment of gynaecomastia. Drugs, *19*:356–361, 1980.

Bundred, N. J., Dover, M. S., Coley, S., and Morrison, J. M.: Breast abscesses and cigarette smoking. Br. J. Surg., *79*:58-59, 1992.

Byrd, B. E., Hartmann, W. J., Graham, L. S., and Hogle, H. H.: Mastopathy in insulin-dependent diabetics. Ann. Surg., *205*:529–532, 1987.

Cantwell, B. M., Richardson, P. G., and Campbell, S. J.: Gynaecomastia and extragonadal symptoms leading to diagnosis delay of germ cell tumours in young men. Postgrad. Med. J., *67*:675–677, 1991.

Carney, J. A., and Toorkey, B. C.: Myxoid fibroadenoma and allied conditions (myxomatosis) of the breast: A heritable disorder with special associations including cardiac and cutaneous myxomas. Am. J. Surg. Pathol., *15*:713–721, 1991.

Carter, C. L., Corle, D. K., Micozzi, M. S., et al.: A prospective study of 16,692 women with benign breast disease. Am. J. Epidemiol., *128*:467–477, 1988.

Carter, D.: Intraductal papillary tumors of the breast: A study of 78 cases. Cancer, *39*:1689–1692, 1977.

Cates, W. Jr., and Pope, J. N.: Gynecomastia and cannabis smoking: A nonassociation among US army soldiers. Am. J. Surg., *134*:613–615, 1977.

Chetty, R., and Kalan, M. R.: Malignant granular cell tumor of the breast. J. Surg. Oncol., *49*:135–137, 1992.

Chiedozi, L. C., and Aghahowa, J. A.: Mondor's disease associated with breast cancer. Surgery, *103*:438–439, 1988.

Cohen, N., Modai, D., Pik, A., et al.: Coexistence of sporadic multiple endocrine neoplasia and scapular ectopic breast: Coincidence or biologically associated? Arch. Intern. Med., *146*:1822–1823, 1986.

Cole, M. S., Minifee, P. K., and Wolma, F. J.: Coumarin necrosis: A review of the literature. Surgery, *103*:271–277, 1988.

Consensus Statement: ''Is 'Fibrocystic Disease' of the Breast Precancerous?'' Arch. Pathol. Lab. Med., *110*:172–173, 1986.

Convens, C., Verhelst, J., and Mahler, C.: Painful gynaecomastia during omeprazole therapy (Letter). Lancet, *338*:1153, 1991.

Cooper, R. A.: Mondor's disease secondary to intravenous drug abuse. Arch. Surg., *125*:807–808, 1990.

Crawford, E. S., and DeBakey, M. E.: Granular-cell myoblastoma: Two unusual cases. Cancer, *6*:786, 1953.

Damiani, S., Koerner, F. C., Dickersin, G. R., et al.: Granular cell tumour of the breast. Virchows Arch. A. Pathol. Anat. Histopathol., *420*:219–226, 1992.

DeCholnoky, T.: Supernumerary breast. Arch. Surg., *39*:926–941, 1929.

Demey, H. E., Hautekeete, M. L., Buylaert, P. L., and Bossaert, L. L.: Mastitis and toxic shock syndrome. Acta Obstet. Gynecol. Scand., *68*:87–88, 1989.

Dershaw, D. D.: Male mammography. A.J.R., *146*:127–131,1986.

Deschamps, M., Hislop, T. G., Band, P. R., and Coldman, A. J.: Study of benign breast disease in a population screened for breast cancer. Cancer Detect. Prev., *9*:151–156, 1986.

Devitt, J. E.: Benign disorders of the breast in older women. Surg. Gynecol. Obstet., *162*:340–342, 1986.

Dhont, M., van Eyck, J., Delbeke, L., and Voorhoof, L.: Danazol treatment of chronic cystic mastopathy: A clinical and hormonal evaluation. Postgrad. Med. J., *55*(Suppl. 5):66–70, 1979.

DiRaimondo, C. V., Roach, A. C., and Meador, C. K.: Gynecomastia from exposure to vaginal estrogen cream. N. Engl. J. Med., *302*:1089–1090, 1980.

Dixon, J. M.: Repeated aspiration of breast abscesses in lactating women. Br. Med. J., *297*:1517–1518, 1988.

Doctor, V. M., and Sirsat, M. V.: Florid papillomatosis (adenoma) and other benign tumours of the nipple and areola. Br. J. Cancer, *25*:1–9, 1971.

Dogliotti, L., Mussa, A., and Sandrucci, S.: Prolactin and benign breast disease with special emphasis to bromocriptine therapy. *In* Angeli, A., Bradlow, H. L., and Dogliotti, L. (Eds.): Endrocrinology of Cystic Breast Disease. New York, Raven Press, 1983, pp. 273–284.

Dogliotti, L., Orlandi, F., and Angeli, A.: The endocrine basis of benign breast disorders. World J. Surg., *13*:674–679, 1989.

Dogliotti, L., Fikoretti, P., Melis, G. B., et al.: Current status of hormonal therapy of fibrocystic breast disease. Ann. N. Y. Acad. Sci., *464*:350–363, 1986.

Dolsky, R. L: Gynecomastia: Treatment by liposuction subcutaneous mastectomy. Dermatol. Clin., *8*:469-479, 1990.

Donegan, W. L.: Cancer of the breast in men. C. A. Cancer J. Clin., *41*:339–354, 1991.

Donnelly, P. K., Baker, K. W., Carney, J. A., and D'Fallon, W. M.: Benign breast lesions and subsequent breast carcinoma in Rochester, Minnesota. Mayo Clin. Proc., *50*:650–656, 1975.

Drife, J. O.: Breast development in puberty. Ann. N. Y. Acad. Sci., *464*:58–65, 1986.

Dupont, W. K., and Page, D. L.: Risk factors for breast cancer in women with proliferative breast disease. N. Engl. J. Med., *312*:146–151, 1985.

England, M. D., Bundy, C., and Sarr, M. G.: Giant cyst of the breast. Surgery *106*:578, 1989.

Ernster, V. L., Mason, L., Goodson, W. J. III, et al.: Effects of caffeine-free diet on benign breast disease: A randomized trial. Surgery *91*:263–267, 1982.

Estes, N. C.: Mastodynia due to fibrocystic disease of the breast controlled with thyroid hormone. Am. J. Surg., *142*:764–766, 1981.

Evans, D. B., and Crichlow, R. W.: Carcinoma of the male breast and Klinefelter's syndrome: Is there an association? C. A. Cancer J. Clin., *37*:246–251, 1991.

Fagan, T. C., Johnson, D. G., and Grosso, D. S.: Metronidazole-induced gynecomastia. J.A.M.A., *254*:3217, 1985.

Fagge, C. H.: Remarks on certain cutaneous affections. Guy's Hosp. Rep., *15*:302, 1870.

Fenoglio, C., and Lattes, R.: Sclerosing papillary proliferations in the female breast: A benign lesion often mistaken for carcinoma. Cancer, *33*:691–700, 1974.

Fentiman, I. S., Caleffi, M., Brame, K., et al.: Double blind controlled trial of tamoxifen therapy for mastalgia. Lancet, *i*:287–288, 1986.

Fentiman, I. S., and Wang, D. Y.: Hormonal background of benign breast disease. Rev. Endocrin. Cancer, *24*:11–15, 1986.

Ferrara, J. J., Leveque, J., Dyess, D. L., and Lorino, C. O.: Nonsurgical management of breast infections in nonlactating women: A word of caution. Am. Surg., *56*:668–671, 1990.

Gansler, T. S., and Wheeler, J. E.: Mammary sarcoidosis: Two cases and literature review. Arch. Pathol. Lab. Med., *108*:673–675, 1984.

Ghent, W. R.: Elemental iodine in clinical breast dysplasia. Report presented to the American Association for Cancer Research, Los Angeles, CA, May 1986.

Ghent, W. R., and Eskin, B. A.: Elemental iodine supplementation in clinical breast displasia (Abstract). Presented at the meeting of the American Association for Cancer Research, Los Angeles, May 7, 1986, vol. 27, p. 189.

Goedert, J. J., McKeen, E. A., and Fraumen, J. F. Jr.: Polymastia and renal adenocarcinoma. Ann. Intern. Med., *95*:182–184, 1981.

Gogas, J., Sechas, M., and Skalkeas, G.: Surgical management of diseases of the adolescent female breast. Am J. Surg., *137*:634–637, 1979.

Goldsmith, L. T., Weiss, G.: Puberty, adolescence and the clinical aspects of normal menstruation. *In* Danforth, D. N., and Scott, J. R. (Eds.):

Obstetrics and Gynecology. Philadelphia, J. B. Lippincott, 1986, pp. 148–162.

Goodnight, J. E. Jr., Quaghana, J. M., and Morton, D. L.: Failure of subcutaneous mastectomy to prevent the development of breast cancer. J. Surg. Oncol., 26:198–201, 1984.

Gorins, A., Perret, F., Tournant, B., et al.: A French double-blind cross-over study (danazol versus placebo) in the treatment of severe fibrocystic breast disease. Eur. J. Gynaecol. Oncol., 2:85–89, 1984.

Gump, F. E., Sternschein, M. J., and Wolff, M.: Fibromatosis of the breast. Surg. Gynecol. Obstet., 153:57–60, 1981.

Gupta, R. K., Naran, S., and Simpson, J.: The role of fine needle aspiration cytology (FNAC) in the diagnosis of breast masses in males. Eur. J. Surg. Oncol., 14:317–320, 1988.

Haagensen, C. D.: Diseases of the Breast. 2nd ed. Philadelphia, W. B. Saunders, 1971a, p. 72.

Haagensen, C. D.: Diseases of the Breast. 2nd ed. Philadelphia, W. B. Saunders, 1971b, p. 214.

Haagensen, C. D.: Diseases of the Breast. 2nd ed. Philadelphia, W. B. Saunders, 1971c, pp. 185–189.

Haagensen, C. D.: Diseases of the Breast. 3rd ed. Philadelphia, W. B. Saunders, 1986, p. 776.

Haagensen, C. D.: Management of benign lesions related to the diagnosis of early breast cancer. In Reid, D. E., and Christian, C. D. (Eds.): Controversies in Obstetrics and Gynecology II. Philadelphia, W.B. Saunders, 1974, pp. 467–488.

Habif, D. V., Perzin, K. H., Lipton, R., and Lattes, R.: Subareolar abscess associated with squamous metaplasia of lactiferous ducts. Am. J. Surg., 119:523–526, 1970.

Hadfield, G. J.: Excision of the major duct system for benign disease of the breast. Br. J. Surg., 47:472–477, 1960.

Hadfield, G. J.: Further experience of the operation for excision of the major duct system of the breast. Br. J. Surg., 55:530–535, 1968.

Hale, J. A., Peters, G. N., and Cheek, J. H.: Tuberculosis of the breast: Rare but still extant. Review of the literature and report of an additional case. Am. J. Surg., 150:620–623, 1985.

Handley, R. S., and Thackray, A. C.: Adenoma of nipple. Br. J. Cancer, 16:187–194, 1962.

Hans-Beat, R., Niederer, U., Stirnemann, H., et al.: Long-term follow-up of patients with biopsy-proven benign breast disease. Ann. Surg., 207:404–409, 1988.

Harmon, J., and Aliapoulios, M. A.: Gynecomastia in marijuana users. N. Engl. J. Med., 287:938, 1972.

Harris, R. B., and Winkelmann, R. K.: Lupus mastitis. Arch. Dermatol., 114:410–412, 1978.

Harrison, G. O., and Elliott, R. L.: Neurilemoma presenting as a breast lump. Surgical Rounds, October 1989, pp. 77–79.

Hartley, M. H., Stewart, J., and Benson, E. A.: Subareolar dissection for duct ectasia and periareolar sepsis. Br. J. Surg., 178:1187–1188, 1991.

Hasson, J., and Pope, C.: Mammary infarcts associated with pregnancy presenting as breast tumors. Surgery, 49:313–316, 1961.

Hayes, R., Michell, M., and Nunnerley, H. B.: Acute inflammation of the breast: The role of breast ultrasound in diagnosis and management. Clin. Radiol., 44:253–256, 1991.

Hemsell, D. L., Edman, C. D., Marks, J. F., et al.: Massive extraglandular aromatization of plasma androstenedione resulting in feminization of a prepubertal boy. J. Clin. Invest., 60:455, 1977.

Hertel, V. F., Zaloudek, C. Z., and Kempson, R. I.: Breast adenomas. Cancer, 37:2891–2905, 1976.

Hughes, L. E., and Bundred, N. J.: Breast macrocysts. World J. Surg., 13:711–714, 1989.

Hughes, L. E., Mansel, R. E., and Webster, D. J. T.: Benign Disorders and Diseases of the Breast. Philadelphia, Bailliere-Tindall, 1989.

Hughes, L. E., Mansel, R. E., and Webster, D. J. T.: Benign Disorders and Diseases of the Breast. Philadelphia, Bailliere-Tindall, 1989a, p. 61.

Hughes, L. E., Mansel, R. E., and Webster, D. J. T.: Benign Disorders and Diseases of the Breast. Philadelphia, Bailliere-Tindall, 1989b, p. 120.

Hughes, L. E., Mansel, R. E., and Webster, D. J. T.: Benign Disorders and Diseases of the Breast. Philadelphia, Bailliere-Tindall, 1989c, pp. 85, 88.

Hughes, L. E., Mansel, R. E., and Webster, D. J. T.: Benign Disorders and Diseases of the Breast. Philadelphia, Bailliere-Tindall, 1989d, pp. 203–204.

Hughes, L. E., Mansel, R. E., and Webster, D. J. T.: Benign Disorders and Diseases of the Breast. Philadelphia, Bailliere-Tindall, 1989e, p 127.

Hutter, R. V.: Goodbye to "fibrocystic disease." N. Engl. J. Med., 312:179-181, 1985a.

Iwai, T.: A statistical study on the polymastia of the Japanese. Lancet, ii:753, 1907.

Jacobs, M. B.: Gynecomastia: A bothersome but readily treatable problem. Postgrad. Med., 89:191–193, 1991.

Jensen, R. A., Page, D. L., Dupont, W. D., and Rogers, L. W.: Invasive breast cancer risk in women with sclerosing adenosis. Cancer, 64:1974–1983, 1989.

Jimenez, J. F., Ryals, R. O., and Cohen, C.: Spontaneous breast infarction associated with pregnancy presenting as a palpable mass. J. Surg. Oncol., 32:174–178, 1986.

Johnson, C. A. C., Felson, B., and Jolles, H.: Polythelia (supernumerary nipple): An update. South. Med. J., 79:1106–1112, 1986.

Jones, D. B.: Florid papillomatosis of the nipple ducts. Cancer, 8:315–319, 1955.

Jones, M. W., Norris, H. J., and Wargotz, E. S.: Hamartomas of the breast. Surg. Gynecol. Obstet., 173:54–56, 1991.

Kaplan, L., and Walts, A. E.: Benign chondrolipomatous tumor of the human female breast. Arch. Pathol. Lab. Med., 101:149–151, 1977.

Karstrup, S., Holste, C., Brabrand, K., and Nielsen, K. R.: Ultrasonically guided percutaneous drainage of breast abscesses. Acta Radiol., 31:157–159, 1990.

Kaufman, P. A.: Relapsing focal liponecrosis (Weber-Christian syndrome) of the breast. Arch. Surg., 80:219–223, 1960.

Keating, J. P., and Rees, M.: Gynaecomastia after long-term administration of domperidone (Letter). Postgrad. Med. J., 67:401–402, 1991.

Kew, M. C., Kirschner, M. A., Abrahams, G. E., and Katz, M.: Mechanism of feminization in primary liver cancer. N. Engl. J. Med., 296:1084, 1977.

Khanna, Y. K., Khanna, A., Aroora, T. K., et al.: Primary closure of lactational breast abscess. J. Indian Med. Assoc., 87:118–120, 1989.

Kilgore, A. R., and Flemming, R.: Abscesses of the breast: Recurring lesions in the areolar area. Calif. Med., 77:190–191, 1952.

Klatskin, G., Saltin, W. T., and Jumm, F. D.: Gynecomastia due to malnutrition. Am. J. Med. Sci., 213:19, 1947.

Klinefelter, H. F. Jr., Reifenstein, E. C., and Albright, F.: Syndrome characterized by gynecomastia, aspermatogenesis without A-Leydigism, and increased excretion of follicle-stimulating hormone. J. Clin. Endocrinol., 2:615–627, 1942.

Klinkerfuss, G. H.: Four generations of polymastia. J.A.M.A., 82:1247–1249, 1924.

Kolar, J., Bek, V., and Vrabeck, R.: Hypoplasia of the growing breast after contact x-ray therapy for cutaneous angiomas. Arch. Dermatol., 96:427, 1967.

Kosuda, S., Kawahara, S., Tamura, K., et al.: Ga-67 uptake in diethylstilbestrol-induced gynecomastia: Experience with six patients. Clin. Nucl. Med., 15:879–882, 1990.

Kuhn, J. M., Reznik, Y., Mahoudeau, J. A., et al.: hCG Test in gynaecomastia: Further study. Clin. Endocrinol., 31:581–590, 1989.

Kuttenn, F., Fournier, S., Sitruk-Ware, R., et al.: Progesterone insufficiency in benign breast disease. In Angeli, A., Bradlow, H. L., and Dogliotti, L. (Eds.): Endocrinology of Cystic Breast Disease. New York, Raven Press, 1983, pp. 231–252.

Lee, C. F., and Adair, F. E.: Traumatic fat necrosis of the female breast and its differentiation from carcinoma. Ann. Surg., 72:188–195, 1920.

Leis, H. P. Jr.: Gross breast cysts: Significance and management. Contemp. Surg., 39:1320, 1991.

Lloyd, K. M., and Dennis, M.: Cowden's disease: A possible new symptom complex with multiple system involvement. Ann. Intern. Med., 58:136–142, 1963.

London, R. S., Sundaram, G. S., Murphy, L., et al. The effect of vitamin E on mammary dysplasia: A double-blind study. Obstet. Gynecol., 65:104–106, 1985.

Lubin, F., Ron, E., Was, Y., et al.: A case-control study of caffeine and methylxanthines in benign breast disease. J.A.M.A., 253:2388–2391, 1985.

Lubin, F., Wax, Y., Ron, E., et al.: Nutritional factors associated with benign breast disease etiology: A case-control study. Am. J. Clin. Nutr., 50:551–556, 1989.

Mahoney, C. P.: Adolescent gynecomastia: Differential diagnosis and management. Pediatr. Clin. North Am., 37:1389–1404, 1990.

Mason, J., and Apisarnthanarax, P.: Migratory silicone granuloma. Arch. Dermatol., 117:366–367, 1981.

Matoska, J., Ondrus, D., and Talerman, A.: Malignant granulosa cell tumor of the testis associated with gynecomastia and long survival. Cancer, *69*:1769–1772, 1992.

McCracken, M., Hamal, P. B., and Benson, E. A.: Granular cell myoblastoma of the breast: A report of 2 cases. Br. J. Surg., *66*:819, 1979.

McElligott, G., and Harrington, M. G.: Heart failure and breast enlargement suggesting cancer. Br. Med. J., *292*:446, 1986.

Meggyessy, V., and Mehes, K.: Association of supernumerary nipples with renal anomalies. J. Pediatr., *111*:412–413, 1987.

Mehes, K.: Association of supernumerary nipples with other anomalies. J. Pediatr., *95*:274–275, 1979.

Meyer, E. C., Sommers, D. K., Reitz, C. J., and Mentis, H.: Vitamin E and benign breast disease. Surgery, *107*:549–551, 1990.

Minton, J. P., and Abou-Issa, H.: Nonendocrine theories of the etiology of benign breast disease. World J. Surg., *13*:680–684, 1989.

Minton, J. P., Foecking, M. K., Webster, D. J. T., and Mathews, R. H.: Caffeine, cyclic nucleotides, and breast disease. Surgery, *86*:105–109, 1979.

Mittal, K. R., and True, L. D.: Origin of granules in granular cell tumor: Intracellular myelin formation with autodigestion. Arch. Pathol. Lab. Med., *112*:302–303, 1988.

Mladick, R. A.: Gynecomastia, liposuction and excision. Clin. Plast. Surg., *18*:815–822, 1991.

Mondor, H.: Tronculite sous-cutanée subaiguë de la paroi thoracique antéro-latérale. Mém. Acad. Chir., *65*:1271–1278, 1939.

Morrow, M., Verger, D., and Thelmo, W.: Diffuse cystic angiomatosis of the breast. Cancer, *62*:2392–2396, 1988.

Murad, T. M., Contesso, G., and Mouriesse, H.: Papillary tumors of large lactiferous ducts. Cancer, *48*:122–133, 1981.

Murray, N. P., and Daly, M. J.: Gynaecomastia and heart failure: Adverse drug reaction or disease process? J. Clin. Pharm. Ther., *16*:275–279, 1991.

Nagel, T. C., Freinkel, N., Bell, R. H., et al.: Gynecomastia, prolactin and other peptide hormones in patients undergoing chronic hemodialysis. J. Clin. Endocrinol. Metab., *36*:428, 1973.

Nakamura, Y., Yoshimoto, K., and Saima, S.: Gynaecomastia induced by angiotensin converting enzyme inhibitor. Br. Med. J., *300*:541, 1990.

Naldone, C., Costantini, M., Dogliotti, L., et al.: Association of cyst type with risk factors for breast cancer and relapse rate in women with gross cystic disease of the breast. Cancer Res., *52*:1791–1795, 1992.

Nash, A. G., and Powles, T.: Review of a hospital experience of breast abscesses. Br. J. Surg., *76*:103, 1989.

Nielsen, M., Christensen, L., and Andersen, J.: Radial scars in women with breast cancer. Cancer, *59*:1019–1025, 1987.

Nuttall, F. Q.: Gynecomastia as a physical finding in normal men. J. Clin. Endocrinol. Metab., *48*:338–340, 1979.

Nydick, M., Bustos, J., Dale, J. H., and Rawson, R. W.: Gynaecomastia in adolescent boys. J.A.M.A., *178*:449–457, 1961.

Olcay, I., and Gokoz, A.: Infantile gynecomastia with bloody nipple discharge. J. Pediatr. Surg., *27*:103–104, 1992.

Olsen, C., and Gordon, R. E. Jr.: Breast disorders in nursing mothers. Am. Fam. Physician, *41*:1509–1516, 1990.

Oluwole, S. F., and Freeman, H. P.: Analysis of benign breast lesions in blacks. Am. J. Surg., *137*:786–789, 1979.

Page, D. L., and Anderson, T. J.: Diagnostic Histopathology of the Breast. New York, Churchill Livingstone, 1987a, p. 51.

Page, D. L., and Anderson, T. J.: Diagnostic Histopathology of the Breast. New York, Churchill Livingstone, 1987b, p. 66.

Page, D. L., Anderson, T. J., and Rogers, L. W.: Epithelial hyperplasia. *In* Page, D. L., and Anderson, T. J. (Eds.): Diagnostic Histopathology of the Breast. Churchill Livingstone, New York, 1987, pp. 143.

Page, D. L., and Dupont, W. D.: Histopathologic risk factors for breast cancer in women with benign breast disease. Semin. Surg. Oncol., *4*:213–217, 1988.

Page, D. L., and Dupont, W. D.: Histologic indicators of breast cancer risk. Am. Coll. Surg. Bull., *76*:16–23, 1991.

Page, D. L., Dupont, W. D., Rogers, L. W., and Rados, M. S.: Atypical hyperplastic lesions of the female breast. Cancer, *55*:2698–2708, 1985.

Panush, R. S., Yonker, R. A., Dlesk, A., et al.: Wever-Christian disease. Medicine, *64*:181–191, 1985.

Parazzini, F., Vecchia, C. L., Riundi, R., et al. Methylxanthine, alcohol-free diet and fibrocystic breast disease: A factorial clinical trial. Surgery, *99*:576–581, 1986.

Parikh, K. J., and Singer, J. A.: Pathologic ectopic breast tissue. Dis. Breast, *9*:16–17, 1983.

Prpic, I., Montani, D., Marinac, P., et al.: Surgical management of fibrocystic disease of the breast. *In* Angeli, A., Bradlow, H. L., and Dogliotti, L. (Eds.): Endocrinology of Cystic Breast Disease. New York, Raven Press, 1983, pp. 297–301.

Puente, J. L., and Potel, J.: Fibrous tumor of the breast. Arch. Surg., *109*:391–394, 1974.

Raso, A. F., Ibanez, M. J., Viralto, M. P., et al.: Relative efficacy of bromocriptine and progesterone per cutem in treating fibrocystic breast disease. Ann. N. Y. Acad. Sci., *464*:617–619, 1986.

Ravitch, M. M.: Poland's syndrome. Surgical Rounds, July 1987, pp. 17–26.

Reifenstein, E. C. Jr.: Hereditary familial hypogonadism. Proc. Am. Fed. Clin. Res., *3*:86, 1947.

Ricciardi, I., and Ianniruberto, A.: Tamoxifen-induced regression of benign breast lesions. Obstet. Gynecol., *54*:80–84, 1979.

Rigg, B. M.: Morselization suction: A modified technique for gynecomastia. Plast. Reconstr. Surg., *88*:159–160, 1991.

Rissanen, T. J., Makarainen, H. P., Kiviniemi, H. O., and Salemla, P. I.: Radiography of the male breast in gynecomastia. Acta Radiol., *33*:110–114, 1992.

Rivera-Pomar, J. M., Vilanova, J. R., Burgos-Bretones, J. J., and Arocena, G.: Focal fibrous disease of breast: A common entity in young women. Virchows Arch. A Pathol. Anat. Histopathol., *386*:59–64, 1980.

Riveros, M., Cubilla, A., Perotta, F., and Solalinde, V.: Hamartoma of the breast. J. Surg. Oncol., *42*:197–200, 1989.

Robitaille, Y., Seemayer, T. A., Thelmo, W. L., and Cumberlidge, M. C.: Infarction of the mammary region mimicking carcinoma of the breast. Cancer, *33*:1183–1189, 1974.

Rohan, T. E., and Cook, M. G.: Alcohol consumption and risk of benign proliferative epithelial disorders of the breast in women. Int. J. Cancer, *43*:631–636, 1989.

Rosen P. P., Holmen, G., Lesser, M. L., et al.: Juvenile papillomatosis and breast carcinoma. Cancer, *55*:1345–1352, 1985.

Rosen, P. P.: Subareolar sclerosing duct hyperplasia of the breast. Cancer, *59*:1927–1930, 1987.

Rosen, P. P., and Caicco, J. A.: Florid papillomatosis of the nipple: A study of 51 patients, including nine with mammary carcinoma. Am. J. Surg. Pathol., *10*:87–101, 1986.

Rowen, P. P.: Mucocele-like tumors of the breast. Am. J. Surg. Pathol., *10*:464–469, 1986.

Russin, V. L., Lachowicz, C., and Kline, T. S.: Male breast lesions: Gynecomastia and its distinction from carcinoma by aspiration biopsy cytology. Diagn. Cytopathol., *5*:243–247, 1989.

Sandison, A. T.: Autopsy Study of Adult Human Breast. Monogr. Natl. Cancer Inst., *4*:31–44, 1962.

Sandrucci, S., Mussa, A., Festa, V., et al.: Comparison of tamoxifen and bromocriptine in management of fibrocystic breast disease: A randomized blind study. Ann. N. Y. Acad. Sci., *464*:626–628, 1986.

Schäfer, P., Fürrer, C., and Mermillod, B.: An association of cigarette smoking with recurrent subareolar breast abscess. Int. J. Epidemiol., *17*:810–813, 1988.

Schwartz, G. F.: Cystic disease: A definition. *In* Angeli, A., Bradlow, H. L., and Dogliotti, L. (Eds.): Endocrinology of Cystic Breast Disease. New York, Raven Press, 1983, pp. 1–6.

Scott, E. B.: Fibrocystic breast disease. Am. Fam. Physician, *36*:119–126, 1987.

Seyfer, A. E., Icochea, R., and Graeber, G. M.: Poland's Anomaly: Natural history and long-term results of chest wall reconstruction in 33 patients. Ann. Surg., *208*:776–782, 1988.

Sheth, M. T., Hathway, D., and Petrelli, M.: Pleomorphic adenoma ("mixed" tumor) of human female breast mimicking carcinoma clinico-radiologically. Cancer, *41*:659–665, 1978.

Ship, A. G., and Shulman, J.: Virginal and gravid mammary gigantism: Recurrence after reduction mammoplasty. Br. J. Plast. Surg., *24*:396, 1971.

Siegel, B. M., Tahan, S. R., Mayzel, K. A., and Love, S. M.: Carcinoma of aberrant breast tissue. Contemp. Surg., *36*:42–44, 1990.

Silverman, J. F., Dabbs, K. J., and Filbert, C. F.: Fine needle aspiration cytology of adenosis tumor of the breast. Acta Cytol., *33*:181–187, 1989.

Simon, K. E., Dutcher, J. P., Runowicz, C. D., and Wiernik, P. H.: Adenocarcinoma arising in vulvar breast tissue. Cancer, *62*:2234–2238, 1988.

Sitruk-Ware, R., Sterkers, N., and Mauvais-Jarvis, P.: Benign breast disease: I. Hormonal investigation. Obstet. Gynecol., *53*:457–460, 1979.

Smallwood, J. A., and Taylor, I.: Benign Breast Disease. Baltimore, Urban & Schwarzenberg, 1990.

Smith, D. J., Palin, W. E., Katch, V. L., and Bennett, J. E.: Breast volume and anthropomorphic measurements: Normal values. Plast. Reconstr. Surg., *78*:331–335, 1986.

Sobel, H. J., Schwartz, R., and Marguet, E.: Light- and electron-microscope study of the origin of granular-cell myoblastoma. J. Pathol., *109*:101, 1972.

Soreide, J. A., Anda, O., Eriksen, L., et al.: Pleomorphic adenoma of the human breast with local recurrence. Cancer, *61*:997–1001, 1988.

Souba, W. W.: Evaluation and treatment of benign breast disorders. *In* Haagenson, C. D., Bodian, C., and Haagenson, D. E. (Eds.): Diseases of the Breast. 3rd ed. Philadelphia, W. B. Saunders, 1991, pp. 715–729.

Stefanik, D. E., Brereton, H. D., Lee, T. C., et al.: Fat necrosis following breast irradiation for carcinoma: Clinical presentation and diagnosis. Dis. Breast, 8:4–6, 1982.

Sterns, E. E.: The natural history of macroscopic cysts in the breast. Surg. Gynecol. Obstet., *174*:35–40, 1992.

Sund, B. S., Topstad, T. K., and Nesland, J. M.: A case of juvenile papillomatosis of the male breast. Cancer, *70*:126–128, 1992.

Tam, P. K., and Brooks, P.: Review of a hospital experience of breast abscesses. Br. J. Surg., *75*:190, 1988.

Thomas, W. G., Williamson, R. C. N., Davies, J. D., and Webb, A. J.: The clinical syndrome of mammary duct ectasia. Br. J. Surg., *69*:423–425, 1982.

Toker, C., Tang, C., Whitely, J. F., et al.: Benign spindle cell breast tumor. Cancer, *48*:1613–1622, 1981.

Townsend, M. C., and Stellato, T. A.: Granular cell myoblastoma of the breast: A report of five cases and a review. Breast, *11*:12, 1985.

Umansky, C., and Bullock, W. K.: Granular cell myoblastoma of the breast. Ann. Surg., *168*:810, 1968.

Urban, J. A.: Excision of the major duct system of the breast. Cancer, *16*:516–520, 1963.

Urban, J. A.: Non-lactational nipple discharge. C. A. Cancer J. Clin., *28*:130–140, 1978.

Verhagen, H.: Local hemorrhage and necrosis of the skin and underlying tissues during anti-coagulant therapy with dicumarol or dicumacyl. Acta Med. Scand., *145*:453–462, 1954.

Veronesi, U., and Pizzocaro, G.: Breast cancer in women subsequent to cystic disease of the breast. Surg. Gynecol. Obstet., *126*:529–532, 1968.

von Fournier, D., Junkermann, H., Stolz, W., et al.: Hormonal and non-hormonal medical therapy of benign breast disease. Horm. Res., *32*(Suppl. 1):28–31, 1989.

von Kessel, F., Pickrell, K. L., Huger, W. E., and Matton, G.: Surgical treatment of gynecomastia: An analysis of 275 cases. Ann. Surg., *157*:142–150, 1963.

Vorherr, H.: Fibrocystic breast disease: Pathophysiology, pathomorphology, clinical picture, and management. Am. J. Obstet. Gynecol., *154*:161–178, 1986.

Vuitch, M. F., Rosen, P. P., and Erlandson, R. A.: Pseudoangiomatous hyperplasia of mammary stroma. Hum. Pathol., *17*:185–191, 1986.

Walker, A. P., Edmiston, C. E., Krepel, C. J., and Condon, R. E.: A prospective study of the microflora of nonpuerperal breast abscess. Arch. Surg., *133*:908–911, 1988.

Wang, D. Y., and Fentiman, I. S.: Epidemiology and endocrinology of benign breast disease. Breast Cancer Res. Treat., *6*:5–36, 1985.

Wapnir, I. L., Pallan, T. M., Faudino, J., and Stahl, W. M.: Latent mammary tuberculosis: A case report. Surgery, *98*:976–978, 1985.

Wargotz, E. S., Weiss, S. W., and Norris, H. J.: Myofibroblastoma of the breast. Am J. Surg. Pathol., *11*:2493–2502, 1987.

Webber, W., and Boyd, N.: A critique of the methodology of studies of benign breast disease and breast cancer risk. J. Natl. Cancer Inst., *77*:397–403, 1986.

Weidner, N., and Levine, J. D.: Spindle-cell adenomyoepithelioma of the breast. Cancer, *62*:1561–1567, 1988.

Weiss, R. J.: Effects of antihypertensive agents on sexual function. Am. Fam. Physician, *44*:2075–2082, 1991.

Weitzner, S., Nascimento, A. G., and Scanlon, L. J.: Intramammary granular cell myoblastoma. Am. Surg., *45*:34, 1979.

Wilson, J. D., Aiman, J., and Macdonald, P. C.: The pathogenesis of gynecomastia. Adv. Intern. Med., *25*:1–32, 1980.

Wilson, M., Mulley, J., Gedeon, A., et al.: New X-linked syndrome of mental retardation, gynecomastia, and obesity is linked to DXS255. Am. J. Med. Genet., *40*:406–413, 1991.

8 Epidemiology and Etiology

John S. Spratt
William L. Donegan
Curtis P. Sigdestad

Cancer of the breast occurs most frequently in mice, rats, dogs, and humans and almost exclusively affects the females of the species. Among humans, it is widely disseminated throughout the world. Few diseases have had the intense epidemiologic study that has been accorded breast cancer; as a result, much information about breast cancer is available in the United States as well as from numerous other countries. Beyond simply defining the magnitude and course of the breast cancer problem, epidemiologic studies determine characteristics to identify individuals at high risk for this cancer and provide clues to its causes.

Information on mortality from breast cancer in the United States is derived from causes of death reported by the U.S. Division of Vital Statistics. They are standardized to the age distribution of the 1970 population. Estimates for 1993 are based on the extrapolation of data from 1983 through 1989. As no nationwide cancer registry currently exists in the United States, incidence data are derived from the Surveillance, Epidemiology and End Results program of The National Cancer Institute begun in 1973. The Surveillance, Epidemiology and End Results program collects information on cancer from state and regional tumor registries, covering about 10% of the United States' population. The World Health Organization provides data on mortality throughout the world (Guinee, 1985; and Boring et al., 1993).

MORTALITY

In the United States, deaths from cancer of the breast surpassed deaths from cancer at any other site in women from 1948 until 1985, when breast cancer deaths were exceeded by deaths from cancer of the lung. It is now the third leading cause of death from cancer overall and is exceeded only by cancer of the lung and of the colorectum. The number of deaths attributable to breast cancer in the United States in 1993 was 46,300 (300 males and 46,000 females [Cancer Facts and Figures—1993]). This correlates to an age-adjusted death rate of 22.4 per 100,000 women (Fig. 8–1). Almost one-third (32%) of all new cancer cases and 18% of cancer deaths in women were related to breast cancer (Boring et al., 1993).

Age-specific and ethnicity-specific age-adjusted annual death rates from breast cancer for women by decades of life are shown in Table 8–1. Beginning in the third decade of life, they show a steep rise during the premenopausal years

and continue to rise after menopause, although at a diminished rate. For age 80 years, 150.5 breast cancer deaths are recorded annually per 100,000 white females and 135.3 per 100,000 black females. Mortality rates in the nonwhite population are similar to those for the white population. Ninety-two per cent of the nonwhite population is black. Statistics for 1991 reflect a death rate of 26 per 100,000, with little difference in mortality rates between white and nonwhite women. The gap that had previously existed, which was due to low cancer rates in the nonwhite population, has closed, probably as a result of more complete reporting. In view of the low breast cancer mortality rates generally reported from black nations and of the association of breast cancer with high socioeconomic status, one may speculate that some of the increase in mortality reflects environmental influences or increasing affluence of the black population in the United States. The increase occurred in almost all age groups. Table 8–2 provides an estimation of the number of woman-years of life lost per 100,000 women as a result of breast cancer. By relating census tract data indicators of education and income to stage of cancer at diagnosis, Wells and Horm (1992) concluded that both blacks and whites with lower median education and income have cancers diagnosed at later stages compared with patients with greater education and income. The disadvantage of blacks with respect to stage at diagnosis and mortality disappeared at upper education and income levels.

The annual death rate for women, adjusted based on the 1970 census population, has risen slightly since 1930 from

Table 8–1. ANNUAL DEATH RATES FOR MALIGNANT NEOPLASMS OF THE BREAST, ACCORDING TO RACE AND AGE, 1989, PER 100,000 WOMEN

Age	White Female	Black Female
All ages, adjusted	22.9	26.0
All ages, crude	35.6	27.3
Under 25 years	0.0*	0.1*
25–34 years	2.7	5.1
35–44 years	17.0	25.4
45–54 years	43.6	59.2
55–64 years	79.5	82.2
65–74 years	113.2	106.9
75–84 years	150.5	135.3
85 years and over	188.9	170.9

(Adapted from National Center for Health Statistics: Health, United States, 1991. Hyattsville, MD, Public Health Service, 1992, p. 171.)
*Based on fewer than 20 deaths.

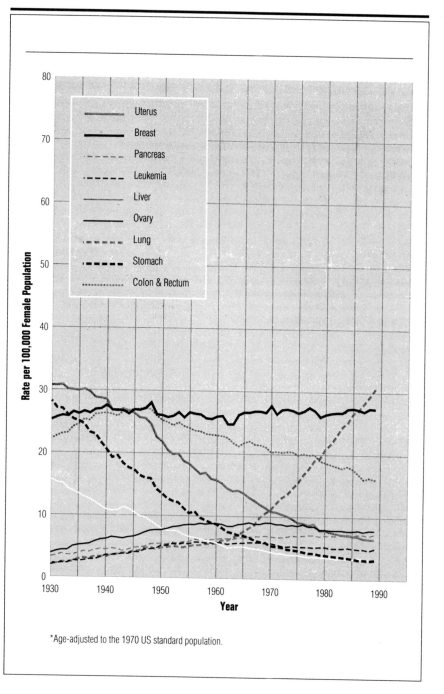

Figure 8–1. Age-adjusted death rates for cancer of the breast and other common cancers. No significant decline is seen in the death rate from breast cancer since 1930. (Reprinted from Boring, C. C., Squires, T. S., and Tong, T.: Cancer Statistics 1993. CA Cancer J. Clin., *43:7–26,* 1993.)

*Age-adjusted to the 1970 US standard population.

25 to 27.1 deaths per 100,000 women. Except at the extremes of age, it maintains pre-eminence, surpassed in females under 15 years of age only by leukemia, in women 55 to 74 years of age by lung cancer, and in women over 74 years by colorectal cancer. Its ravages are such that among women 40 to 44 years of age it exceeds all other causes of death, interrupting many otherwise vigorous and healthy lives.

In 1975, the Epidemiology Branch of the National Cancer Institute published an atlas of death rates from breast cancer for the white population by county of residence for the continental United States. It clearly demonstrated a remarkable concentration of mortality in the northeastern part of the country, particularly in urban industrial areas. The

geographic pattern suggests environmental influences on mortality. Although exposure to carcinogens might be inferred from the association, it should be noted that Japan is also a highly urban and industrialized nation, but its death rate for breast cancer is one-fifth that of the United States. Nevertheless, men and women are increasingly exposed to a wide range of environmental pollutants (Epstein, 1994). These include contaminants in the food chain, most of which are fat-soluble, have long biologic half-lives, and induce breast cancers in animals. Most are organochlorine carcinogens, such as chlorophenothane dichlorodiphenyltrichloroethane (DDT).

Striking differences are evident in international breast cancer death rates. Figure 8–2 shows death rates for 50

Table 8–2. YEARS OF POTENTIAL LIFE LOST BEFORE AGE 65 YEARS PER 100,000 FROM BREAST CANCER, 1989

White female	215.3
Black female	253.5

(Adapted from National Center for Health Statistics: Health, United States, 1991. Hyattsville, MD, Public Health Service, 1992, p. 162.)

countries. The United States ranks 16th. Notable are the highest rate, found in England and Wales, and the low rates, found in Japan and Thailand (which are only one-fifth and one-thirtieth that of England and Wales, respectively). Mortality rates are steady or rising in most countries. Changing mortality in migrant populations strengthens the inferences that environments or lifestyles are important determinants of breast cancer risk. Japanese living in the continental United States or Hawaii have higher mortality rates from breast cancer than do Japanese living in Japan, and the rates are higher for Japanese born in the United States (Nisei) than for immigrants who were born in Japan (Issei) (Seidman et al., 1976) (Fig. 8–3).

INCIDENCE

In 1993, an estimated 183,000 new cases of breast cancer occurred in the United States. Only 1000 of these were in males. New cases of breast cancers are exceeded in number only by cases of cancers of the skin. Women accounted for 182,000 of new cases, for an annual rate of 100.2 cases per 100,000 white females. Since 1973, the incidence has increased at an average of 1.8% per year for white females and 2.0% per year for black females (Table 8–3). The estimated lifelong probability for developing a breast cancer among females born in 1987 was 10% and that for eventually dying from breast cancer was 3% (Cancer Facts and Figures—1993). Over a lifespan of 85 years, currently about 1 in 9 women would be expected to develop breast cancer. The risk varies with age, sex, and race. A more meaningful figure for each woman is the residual lifetime probability of being diagnosed with breast cancer after she attains a specific age (Fig. 8–4).

Risk for the disease is strongly age-related (Fig. 8–5A). The age-specific incidence (i.e., the number of cases per year per 100,000 women in each age group) displays a progressive rise with increasing age. The characteristic curve displays a rapid climb during reproductive years after the age of 30, a slight dip at the time of menopause (Clemmesen's hook), and a slower continued rise during the postmenopausal years. The change in the slope of the curve at menopause suggests an underlying age-related incidence on which is superimposed an accelerated rate during the hormonally active reproductive years. DeWaard (1969) interpreted the peculiarities of the curve as evidence of a bimodal age distribution caused by a change from ovarian to adrenal hormonal predominance at menopause. One might speculate that keeping women "premenopausal" with hormone replacement therapy would extend the early rapid rise and result in an overall increase in incidence.

The observation that most patients with cancer of the

breast are in the sixth and seventh decades of life is consistent with the progressive rise in the annual incidence with aging. The elderly represent a relatively small segment of the total population, with the result that younger age groups contribute the majority of cases. During the years from 1967 to 1979 and from 1982 to 1993, 67.5% of 1381 breast cancer patients who received care at the Medical College of Wisconsin–affiliated hospitals were between 40 and 70 years of age. Women between the ages of 41 and 50 years accounted for 21%, and those over 80 years of age represented 6% of the total. The average age was 59.8 years (Fig. 8–5B).

The major differences in international incidence and death rates occur in postmenopausal women (Fig. 8–6). Little difference is seen in premenopausal rates. In the United States, the age-specific mortality continues to rise after menopause, whereas that in the former Yugoslavia becomes flat. In Japan, the rate declines after menopause and continues to do so as age advances. The reason for this is unknown. Major differences in the incidence of breast cancer are found among racial and ethnic groups living in the United States (Fig. 8–7). As no genetic basis for breast cancer is known, these differences have been attributed to environmental factors, differences in lifestyle, and socioeconomic status (Freeman, 1989).

Fox (1979) observed that the incidence of breast cancer increased by 18% between 1935 and 1965 but increased by 50% between 1965 and 1975. During this period, the mortality rate remained unchanged. He observed that only 40% of the women afflicted with breast cancer had a fatal illness. The other 60% had more benign disease with a relative mortality rate that was only moderately different from that for women of the same age without cancer. The incidence of breast cancer has increased dramatically since 1981 and has coincided with an increase in the screening of asymptomatic women (Fig. 8–8). A sharp rise in 1974 was followed by a lesser increase in subsequent years (Bailar and Smith, 1986). The 1974 spike coincided with the public disclosure that the wives of the President and Vice President of the United States both had breast cancer. This promoted a major public effort to screen women for breast

Table 8–3. AGE-ADJUSTED ANNUAL INCIDENCE RATES FOR BREAST CANCER, PER 100,000 WOMEN

Year	White Female	Black Female
1973	84.0	68.0
1975	89.5	77.5
1980	87.4	74.4
1984	100.0	84.0
1985	106.4	92.9
1986	109.0	94.1
1987	117.0	90.8
1988	113.5	97.4
1989	108.2	87.6
Estimated annual percentage change*	1.8	2.0

(Adapted from National Center for Health Statistics: Health, United States, 1991. Hyattsville, MD, Public Health Service, 1992, p. 198.)
*The estimated annual percentage change was calculated by fitting a linear regression model to the natural logarithm of the yearly rates from 1973 to 1989.

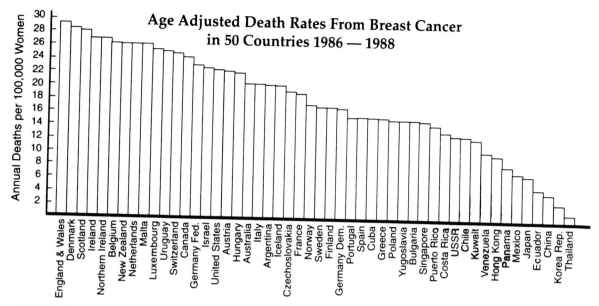

Figure 8–2. Death rates from breast cancer in 50 countries show wide variation. Death rates are much higher in European than in Asian countries. (Adapted from Boring, C. C., Squires, T. S., and Tong, T.: Cancer Statistics 1993. CA Cancer J. Clin., *43*:7–26, 1993.)

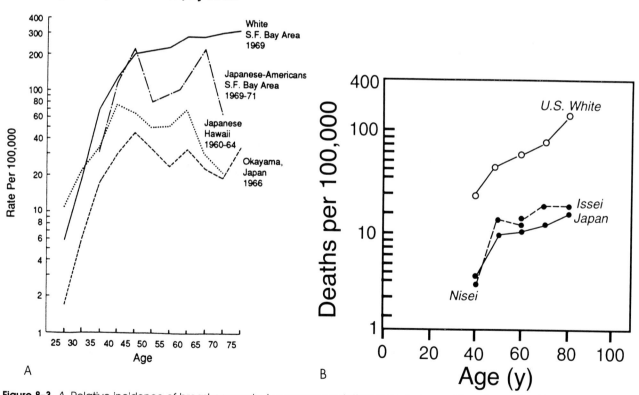

Figure 8–3. *A,* Relative incidence of breast cancer in Japanese populations living in Japan, Hawaii, and the San Francisco Bay area of the United States, respectively, compared with the incidence of breast cancer in the white female population in the San Francisco Bay area. (From Buell, P.: Changing incidence of breast cancer in Japanese-American women. J. Natl. Cancer Inst., *51*:1479–1483, 1973.) *B,* Age-specific death rates from breast cancer are higher in Japanese who immigrate to the United States than in Japanese who remain in Japan. This is seen in both first-generation (Nisei) and second-generation (Issei) immigrants and infers an environmental influence on the frequency of the disease. (From Haenszel, W., and Kurihara, M.: Studies of Japanese migrants: 1. Mortality from cancer and other diseases among Japanese in the United States. J. Natl. Cancer Inst., *40*:43–68, 1968.)

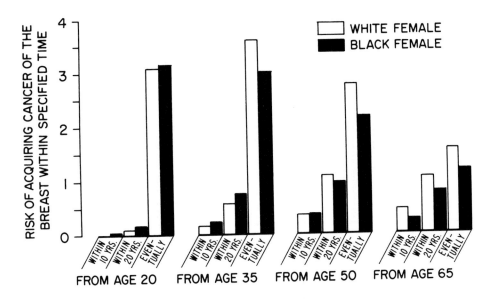

Figure 8–4. The risk for breast cancer is both age- and time-dependent. It increases with time but decreases with decline in remaining lifetime. Hence, although the age-specific incidence of breast cancer rises with age, the residual lifetime risk of developing it declines. (From Spratt, J. S., Greenburg, R. A., Kuhns, J. G., and Amin, E. A.: Breast cancer risk: a review of definitions and assessments of risks. J. Surg. Oncol., *41*:42, 1989. Copyright © 1989. Printed by permission of Wiley-Liss, a division of John Wiley and Sons, Inc.)

cancer. The Surveillance, Epidemiology and End Results program data show a rise in annual incidence between 1980 and 1989 from 85 per 100,000 to 105 per 100,000 and an increase in overall 5-year survival; however, no decline in mortality was demonstrated (Boring et al., 1993). An increase in in situ and localized cases was consistent with an increase in early detection. Miller and colleagues (1991) also confirmed that the incidence of in situ and localized cancers has increased, whereas that of cancers with regional and distant metastases has remained stable. Increased detection accounts for some but not all of the increasing incidence. The detection of asymptomatic cancers accounts for only 40% of the increase in whites and 25% of the increase in blacks (Liff et al., 1991). The overall increase in the two groups rose 29% and 41%, respectively.

Considerable controversy surrounds the interpretation of a rising incidence of breast cancer in the presence of stable mortality. Since the recent increase in incidence is at least partially attributable to widespread screening, these controversies pertain to both screening and diagnosis. The most favorable interpretation is that increased curability of the cancers has kept mortality from showing a similar rise. This is a tribute to earlier diagnosis with screening or to increasingly effective treatment, and if this is true, mortality might be expected eventually to decline. While no decline is evident overall, there is some evidence of decreased mortality in young women (Blot et al., 1987). Furthermore, some increase in survival is seen in recent statistics (Table 8–4). Alternative interpretations are also possible. One is that the additional cancers are not those likely to progress and cause death. In this case the cancers that were formerly lethal continue to be so either because they are not being diagnosed earlier or they remain lethal despite earlier diagnosis. It is possible that in vigorous pursuit of earlier diagnosis subtle changes have occurred in diagnostic criteria. Some lesions formerly considered benign may currently be diagnosed as cancer. Adding lesions of low level or of questionable malignancy to the total would leave death rates undisturbed.

ETIOLOGY AND RISK

The cause of breast cancer in humans is not known. In animals, certain chemicals (e.g., dimethylbenz[*a*]anthracine), ionizing radiation, and viruses can cause breast cancers. All of these agents are mutagenic, and mutagenesis is

Table 8–4. FIVE-YEAR RELATIVE CANCER SURVIVAL RATES FOR BREAST CANCER, ACCORDING TO RACE AND PERIOD

Period	White Female	Black Female
1974–1976	74.8	62.9
1977–1979	75.1	62.5
1980–1982	76.7	65.6
1983–1988	79.3	62.1

(Adapted from National Center for Health Statistics: Health, United States, 1991. Hyattsville, MD, Public Health Service, 1992, p. 199.)

Table 8–5. ASSOCIATIONS WITH HIGH RISK OF BREAST CANCER

Fixed
Being female
Aging
Western European origin
Family history of breast cancer
Previous cancer in one breast
Epithelial hyperplasia of breast tissues
Flexible (able to be modified)
Nulliparity
Late first full-term pregnancy (after age 30)
Early menarche (less than 12 years old)
Late menopause (age 55 or after)
Exposure to ionizing irradiation
High fat diet and obesity
Exogenous estrogen use
Urban environment
Alcoholic drinks

Age Specific Incidence of Invasive Breast Cancer in the United States-SEER Cancer Statistics Review 1973-1990

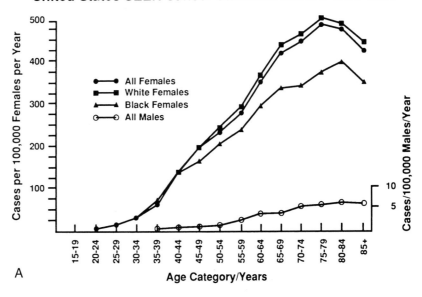

Figure 8–5. *A*, The age-specific incidence of breast cancer in the United States shows progressive rise with age but with a slight decline after the age of 75 years. After age 45 years, the age-specific incidence in white women exceeds that in black women. (From Seer Cancer Statistics Review, 1973–1990. Section IV: Breast. Miller, B. A., Gloeckler Ries, L. A., Hankey, B. F., et al. (Eds.): U. S. Department of Health and Human Services, Public Health Service, National Institutes of Health, National Cancer Institute, Bethesda, MD, 20892-9903, NIH publication No. 93–2789, p. IV.6.) *B*, The model age of women with breast cancer is between 61 and 65 years. Twenty-one per cent are younger than 50 years of age.

Age Distribution of 1381 Cases of Breast Carcinoma Milwaukee, WI 1967-79 and 1982-93

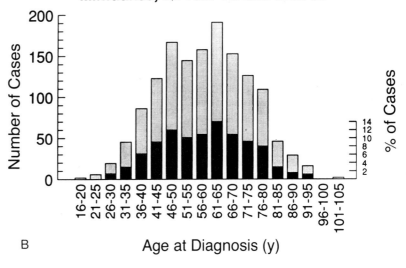

apparently the common mechanism of action. Chromosomal mutations are also closely associated with the origin and progression of cancer in humans and are apparently fundamental to the process of carcinogenesis (Tannock and Hill, 1992). Knowledge about oncogenes, the mutant forms of genes normally concerned with regulation of cell growth and differentiation, produce the phenotype and cellular behavior recognizable as cancer. Genetic mutation is also the mechanism for hereditary susceptibility to cancer, which is so evident in the genealogies of some patients with breast cancer.

Although the deliberate exposure of humans to suspected mammary carcinogens is not feasible, the identification of populations at high risk for breast cancer serves as a means of obtaining insights about causation. This information is also valuable for counseling individuals at high risk and for identifying potential means of prevention. The fact that most women with breast cancer have no features that identify them as being at special risk illustrates the current limits of this endeavor. Table 8–5 summarizes the major factors that place an individual at a higher-than-average risk for breast cancer. They are divided into those that are fixed

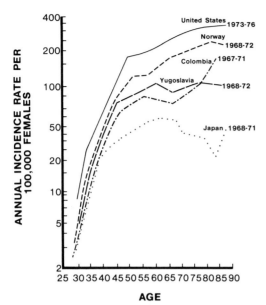

Figure 8–6. International breast cancer incidence rates by age. Differences are primarily in the postmenopausal population. (Modified from Seidman, H., and Mushinski, M. H.: In Feig, S. A., and McLelland, R. (Eds.): Breast Carcinoma: Current Diagnosis and Treatment. New York, Masson, 1983, p. 9. Used with permission.)

and those that are potentially subject to manipulation. The following sections address some of these factors.

Assessment of Risk

Identifying women with a high risk for developing breast cancer is a considerable challenge. The ultimate intent of quantifying risk is to test interventions that have the potential for reducing risk and to implement those interventional strategies that are of proven value. Concise definition for different types of risk were adopted by the International Epidemiological Association (Last, 1988).

Average lifetime risk indicates the probability of developing breast cancer over the period from birth to a final age, assuming that no individuals are lost from other causes before the final age is attained. Reports from current vital statistics are classified by age and ethnicity. The lifelong risk for white females of developing breast cancer through age 110 years is 10.2%, and that of dying from breast cancer is 3.0%.

Relative risk (RR) refers to the relative frequency of an event (breast cancer) occurring in a test population compared with a control population with subjects of similar age during a similar period. If 10 breast cancers develop in 80 women with a certain exposure and 1 breast cancer develops in 80 women without the exposure, the RR would be 10/80 divided by 1/80. Hence, 10/80 × 80/1 = 800/80, or a RR of 10. The RR of the exposed women is 10 for that age group *over the specified interval*. A 10-fold increase in risk does not mean that a woman's actual risk is 10 times greater than the average lifetime risk (i.e., it is not 10 × 10 = 100%). The 10% value refers to a woman's *cumulative risk* to 110 years of age. The risk to women ages 35 to 45 years is only 1%, and an eightfold increase in risk is only 8% (8 × 1%); 92% of the population (100 − 8 = 92) would be at no increased risk.

Projected probability for developing breast cancer can be estimated for an individual of a specific age through a defined interval. One tool for estimation is the Gail formula, which uses family history, age at menarche, age at first birth, the number of breast biopsies, and the presence of epithelial hyperplasia in the breast (Gail et al., 1989) (Fig. 8–9). This formula was used to determine the eligibility of women for the National Breast Cancer Prevention Trial that was initiated in 1992.

Berg (1984) pointed out that even women in the United States with the lowest risk for developing breast cancer still had a lifetime risk of 1:40, which is substantially higher than for most other forms of cancer. No subset of adult women has a risk so low as to permit their exclusion from an effective breast cancer control program. The hazard is that targeting ''high-risk'' groups might lead to these groups' experiencing a high level of anxiety, whereas the ''low-risk'' groups acquire an unjustified sense of security. Even when high-risk groups are identified, controlled clinical trials confirming that a particular intervention strategy reduces the risk are scant.

Breast Cancer Incidence in U.S.A. by Racial and Ethnic Groups

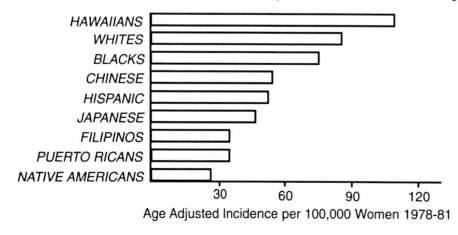

Figure 8–7. Breast cancer incidence varies considerably among racial and ethnic groups residing in the United States. (Adapted from Freeman, H. P.: Cancer in the socioeconomically disadvantaged. CA Cancer J. Clin., *39:*267–287, 1989.)

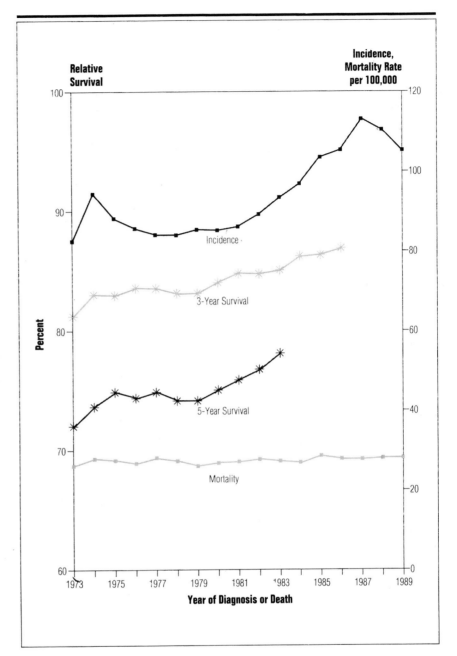

Figure 8–8. The incidence of breast cancer has increased in the United States since 1973; survival also has increased, probably owing to earlier detection. Despite the increasing incidence, mortality has remained unchanged. (From Miller, B. A., Feuer, A. J., and Hankey, B. F.: Recent influence trends for breast cancer in women and the relevance of early detection: An update. CA Cancer J. Clin., *43*:27–41, 1993.)

Genetic and Familial Aspects

Indications that breast cancer risk is genetically influenced are found in its association with racial predispositions, genetically determined traits and medical conditions, and familial tendencies. Steel and associates (1991) provided a review of the subject, and Lynch (1981) has written an entire volume on cancer-prone families.

The wide disparity in international breast cancer mortality rates, particularly that between Asian and Western women, suggests a role for genetically determined racial differences in susceptibility. If genetic factors are involved, it is necessary to postulate environmental influences that explain the changes that occur in immigrant populations. The issue of greatest clinical relevance involves the accurate estimation of individual risk based on family history.

A number of familial syndromes are associated with increased frequency of breast cancer. These include multiple cancer families, such as Lynch Type II, Li-Fraumeni syndrome (*S*arcoma, *B*reast cancer, and brain cancer, *L*ung and laryngeal cancer and leukemia, and *A*drenal cortical carcinoma, or SBLA syndrome), Cowden's disease, nevoid basal cell cancers (Gorlin's syndrome), and ataxia-telangiectasia. The high frequency of breast cancer in men with Klinefelter's syndrome (eunuchoidism, gynecomastia, testicular atrophy, and aspermia) is associated with an extra X chromosome that characterizes these individuals (i.e., XXY). Rather than a marker for breast cancer, however, the extra X chromosome probably serves only to increase the risk of female-related diseases in these men.

Breast cancer appears as one component of Cowden's syndrome, a symptom complex associated with an autoso-

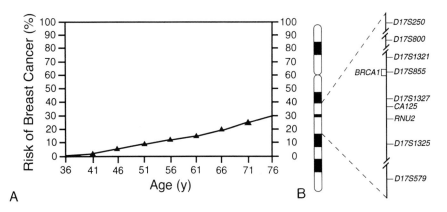

Figure 8–9. *A,* This projected lifetime risk of breast cancer for a 36 year old woman is based upon the Gail formula. It indicates a 30% chance of developing cancer of the breast by age 76. (From Gail, M. H., Brinton, L. A., Byar, D. P., et al.: Projecting individualized probabilities of developing breast cancer for white females who are being examined annually. J. Natl. Cancer Inst., *81:*1979–1986, 1989.) *B,* Schematic drawing of human chromosome 17. The region containing the breast cancer susceptibility gene, *BRCA1,* is expanded to show the relative positions of various linkage markers. (From Miki, Y., Swensen, J., Shattuck-Eidens, D., et al.: A strong candidate for the breast and ovarian cancer susceptibility gene *BRCA1.* Science, *266:*67, 1994. Copyright 1994 by the AAAS.)

mal dominant, single-gene trait. Also known as the "multiple hamartoma syndrome" and as "Cowden's disease," this syndrome is characterized by lipomas, fibromas, angiomas, gastrointestinal polyps, thyroid tumors, fibrocystic changes of the breast, nervous system abnormalities, and mucocutaneous warts (trichilemmomas). Both men and women are affected by Cowden's syndrome (Gentry et al., 1974). About 50% of women with Cowden's disease have developed breast cancer. Willard and colleagues (1992) confirmed the high risk of bilateral breast cancer associated with Cowden's disease and recommended prophylactic bilateral total mastectomies. Alternatively, frequent breast examinations for life with biopsy of all suspicious lesions are required.

Families with ataxia-telangiectasia have reduced capacity to repair deoxyribonucleic acid (DNA) that has been damaged by ionizing radiation and have an increased susceptibility to breast cancer (Swift et al., 1991). The susceptibility of DNA to breaks from toxic, environmental, and metabolic causes and the incompleteness of repair of certain breaks provides an explanation for the ecogenic causes of cancer. Many anticancer agents are associated with DNA breaks. The inherent instability of DNA sequences is such that with no exogenous agent at all, the spontaneous disintegration of DNA is estimated to proceed at over 100,000 bases per cell per day. Spontaneous depurination or deamination of DNA and damage by free radicals go on continuously and are normally countered by DNA repair. The process of DNA repair contributes to the ineffectiveness of many chemotherapeutic agents (Eastman and Barry, 1992).

Certain metabolic processes that characterize women with breast cancer or those who are at high risk for it may have a genetic basis. Low estriol excretion rates and low renal clearances of estriol as well as deficiencies of estradiol hydroxylating activity in leukocytes are found in 58% of women with breast cancer (Lemon, 1974). Lemon postulated a genetic impairment of 16-alphahydroxylase (which converts estradiol to estriol), possibly expression of a mutant allele. Women with familial risk have lower urinary estrone and estradiol levels than do matched controls (Fish-

man et al., 1979). Lynch and coworkers (1981) reported consistently lower levels of plasma prolactin, gonadotropin, estrone, and estradiol for familial high-risk groups, but the differences were not significant.

Repeated demonstrations of strong familial tendencies for mammary cancer suggest the existence of an inherited factor. The majority of investigations on this subject show that female relatives of women with cancer of the breast have a higher rate of the disease than is expected among women in the general population. Jacobsen (1946) reviewed early reports; among these was the personal genealogy of Paul Broca in 1866, in which 10 of 24 female relatives died of breast cancer. Subsequent studies indicated that the probability of breast cancer for mothers of probands is approximately double that of the general population, and for sisters it was almost 2.5 times the expected risk. Not only mothers and sisters, but also grandmothers, female cousins, and aunts of probands manifested an increased risk, which was present in both the maternal and paternal lines (Macklin, 1959). The risk was significantly greater than in relatives of individuals without cancer or in those of patients with cancer of other sites.

Risk among relatives is not uniform. The study of Anderson and Badzioch (1985) confirmed a breast cancer frequency that was twice as high in first-degree relatives of probands as it was in relatives of controls with other types of cancer. Risk was highest for mothers (RR = 8.8), sisters (RR = 2.7), and daughters (RR = 4.6). Risk was not increased in relatives of postmenopausal patients but rose to 3.1 for relatives of premenopausal patients. A fivefold excess was observed in families of patients with bilateral disease, and a ninefold excess was seen if the disease occurred both premenopausally and bilaterally. If the proband's cancer was bilateral, first-degree relatives had a risk of bilateral cancer that was nine times higher than would be expected. A young woman whose mother and sister had premenopausal breast cancer (bilateral in either case) had an estimated 50% lifetime risk of developing breast cancer. Patients with family histories of breast cancer tend to be younger and to have a higher frequency of bilaterality than those without (Anderson, 1974). Studies have shown a tendency for earlier development of the disease in patients whose mothers were affected (Busk and Clemmeson, 1947; and Bucalossi and Veronesi, 1957). Haagensen (1971) found that daughters developed breast cancer an average of 12 years earlier than did their mothers and maternal aunts. A practical guide for estimating familial risk based on the publications of Ottman and coworkers (1983) and Anderson and Badzioch (1985) is shown in Figure 8–10.

Knudsen's model for heritable and nonheritable tumors provides a logical explanation for some observations that implicate inheritance in breast cancer (Knudsen et al., 1976). It presumes that tumors are derived from a single cell and are the product of two mutations. The first mutation may be either prezygotic or postzygotic. The second is always postzygotic. Two prezygotic events would likely be lethal and not transferred. When the first event is prezygotic, it will be inherited and conferred to every cell. Subsequently, since all cells are potentiated and may be triggered by only one additional mutation, tumors would be expected to be multiple and to occur early in life. If both mutations were postzygotic, convergence in the same cell would be required. Such a convergence would be relatively unlikely and, as a consequence, noninherited tumors would tend to be single and occur later in life. On the basis of this model, the age distribution and bilaterality of breast cancer suggest that 30% of cases are of an inherited type.

The extent of linkage between genetic factors and the development of breast cancer remains incompletely defined. The high incidence of breast cancer often creates difficulty in differentiating between environmental and genetic associations. If a cancer is genetically predisposed to occur, biomarkers consistent with genetic aberration should be discoverable. Lynch and colleagues (1984) analyzed the pedigrees of breast cancer patients and concluded that only 5% of the patients reported family pedigrees compatible with hereditary (autosomal dominant) breast cancer syndromes. An additional 13% reported family aggregations

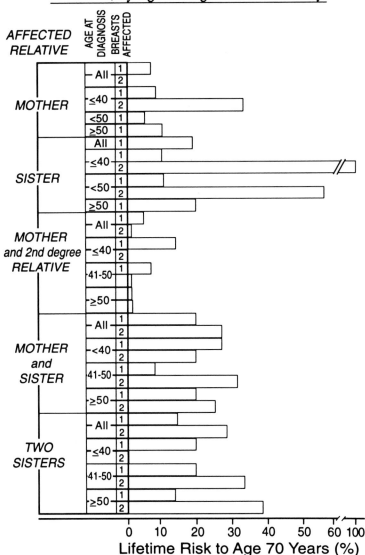

Figure 8–10. The lifetime risk of developing breast cancer (to age 70 years) is shown relative to family history. The age at which the relative was diagnosed and whether the relative had involvement of one or both breasts are important. For example, a woman who had two sisters with breast cancer, both of whom developed the disease before age 50 years and for whom it was bilateral in at least one of the two sisters, has a 38% chance of developing breast cancer before she is 70 years of age. (Based on data from Ottman, R., King, M., Pike, M. C., et al.: Practical guide for estimating risk for familial breast cancer. Lancet, *ii*:556, 1983.) Projected lifetime risk is a better basis for counseling women than relative risk.

that failed to meet the criteria for being hereditary. They concluded that among 112,000 new breast cancers occurring in the United States in 1982, between 2410 and 8790 patients (95% confidence limits) would have met the criteria for hereditary associations. Associated factors included young age at onset, bilaterality, vertical transmission, and specific tumor associations consistent with genetic heterogeneity. Lynch and colleagues observed that monolayer tissue cultures of dermal biopsy specimens from patients and high-risk relatives were associated with hyperdiploidy. The enzyme glutamate pyruvate transaminase was associated with a "breast cancer susceptibility gene." Both low urinary estrone and estradiol glucuronide levels were associated with hereditary breast cancer. Phenotypes of hereditary breast cancer were not found. The prognosis for hereditary breast cancer was better than that for breast cancer in general (Albano et al., 1982).

Using data from the Danish Twin Register, Holm and colleagues (1980) observed that the number of breast cancers that develop in twins after the first breast cancer diagnosis was increased by a factor of nearly six in monozygotic twins and was a factor in dizygotic twins. For cancers at other sites, the observed and expected numbers of cancers were similar in both groups. No significant difference was observed in the mean age at diagnosis. Among 40 monozygotic twins with only one twin affected, a greater association with breast cancer was seen in unmarried and nulliparous women. No tendency was found for a twin with cancer to have her first child at a later age than did her twin sister.

In comprehensive reviews of factors associated with breast cancer, including heritage, menses, marital state, parity, nursing, contraceptive use, benign epithelial disorders of the breast, hormonal factors, cancer, iatrogenic factors, and immunologic factors, a major difficulty is the stratification of the degree of relevance (Moore et al., 1983). Relationships are often synergistic, and no single item is of great importance. Predisposition, carcinogens, promoters, and inhibitors all interact in the individual in unique ways and begin to assume importance in the early years of life. Claus and associates (1990) reported a large case-control study conducted on 4730 women between the ages of 20 and 54 years with histologically confirmed breast cancer and 4688 matched controls. They concluded that in addition to family history, younger age at onset proved to be the strongest indicator of a possible genetic association of breast cancer. The highest hazard ratio, 17.1 (95% confidence interval [CI] = 9.4–31.3), was for a sister of a breast cancer patient with both an affected mother and one affected sister. When the case was diagnosed at 50 and 30 years of age, the hazard ratios reached 27.5 (95% CI = 15.0–50.3) and 44.2 (95% CI = 23.5–83.2), respectively. Such a combination is infrequent, and the hazard ratio falls to 1.7 for the mother of a patient with breast cancer diagnosed by age 50 years. Menopausal status and bilaterality were not significant contributors to the hazard.

A careful family history of breast cancer documented through as many family generations as possible is necessary to identify the existence of hereditary breast cancer and cancer family syndromes (Lynch et al., 1990). Hereditary breast cancer should be suspected in young women with bilateral cancers and multiple primary cancers. By chance alone, common cancers may be found among members of the same family. Lynch and associates restrict the term to families in which there exists a mendelian distribution of breast cancer. Patient anxiety with even an unconfirmed family history can reach serious states, and caution has to be exercised in concluding that a particular woman is at high risk for genetically familial breast cancer.

The problems with putting familial information to practical use are multiple. Distinguishing between environmental and genetic influences is difficult. Identification of cases can be tenuous or faulty (Lynch et al., 1978), and no controlled data exist to show that prophylactic intervention enhances survivorship. Controls are essential, as survivorship is greater with genetically familial breast cancers. The most virulent and lethal breast cancers tend to occur in young women with negative family histories (Spratt et al., 1983).

The genetic basis of familial breast cancer is becoming increasingly clear. An inherited gene designated *BRCA1*, which is linked to increased risk for breast and ovarian cancer, was isolated and cloned by researchers in 1994 (Futreal et al., 1994, and Miki et al., 1994). The gene is located on the long (q) arm of chromosome 17 in region 21 (see Fig. 8–9*B*). Increased risk is conferred by the mutated form of this gene. Carriers need only lose or sustain damage to the second copy of the gene to develop breast cancer. Estimates are that women who inherit the mutated form of *BRCA1* have an 85% chance of developing breast cancer by the age of 70 years and a 40% chance of developing ovarian cancer. Whereas only 1 in 200 women in the United States may have the mutated form, approximately 45% of families with a high rate of breast cancer and 80% with a high rate of both breast and ovarian cancer carry the mutated gene. The role of *BRCA1* in nonfamilial breast cancer is not clear. A clinical test to identify individuals with the mutated form of *BRCA1* is under development. However, other genetic determinants of high risk appear to exist. A second gene known as *BRCA2,* which is believed to convey susceptibility to breast cancer but not to ovarian cancer, is located on chromosome 13, but it has yet to be isolated (Reynolds, 1994).

Viruses

Viruses cause a number of benign and malignant neoplasms in animals and are strongly associated with several cancers in humans (Benchimol, 1992). Examples are the human T-cell leukemia virus type 1 (HTLV-1), which is associated with adult T-cell leukemia, and hepatitis B virus (HBV), which is linked to hepatocellular carcinoma. Retroviruses—so called because their genetic information is in the form of ribonucleic acid (RNA)—are the best known. The study of these cancer-causing viruses (oncoviruses) led to the discovery that they contained genes (oncogenes) that, in the presence of a second helper virus, quickly transformed normal cells and caused tumor formation. Subsequently, similar but structurally somewhat different oncogenes were identified in human cancer cells. These oncogenes represented mutated or amplified forms of genes (proto-oncogenes) whose normal function was to regulate cell growth and differentiation.

After an oncovirus penetrates a cell, its RNA core is

converted in the cytoplasm into DNA with the enzyme reverse transcriptase. This DNA is then integrated randomly into the chromosomal DNA of the cell as a "provirus." Viruses can cause transformation of normal cells either by introducing an oncogene into the cellular DNA or by inserting viral DNA into the chromosome adjacent to a proto-oncogene, thereby causing its malfunction. A number of oncogenes have been identified in the genetic material of breast cancers, among which are *erb* B, *neu*, and p53, which are generally on chromosome 17 (Minden and Pawson, 1992).

Of particular interest with regard to the possible viral cause of human breast cancer is the mouse mammary tumor virus (MMTV). The observations by Bittner in 1936 that mice with a high incidence of spontaneous mammary cancer passed the disease to their offspring through nursing led to the identification of a MMTV that has an RNA core and a Type B virion morphology. The virus is transmitted not only in milk but also in tissues and in gametes at the time of fertilization. The oncogenic potential of the virus is modified by genetic as well as by hormonal influences. The MMTV has proved a promising model for investigation. The case for a viral role in human mammary cancer may be summarized as follows:

1. Type B particles morphologically similar to MMTV, as well as particles of other types, can often be found in human breast milk and in some human mammary cancers.

2. RNA-directed DNA polymerase, an enzyme characteristic of RNA-type oncogenic viruses, can be found in human milk and is associated with particles having the same density as MMTV.

3. On migration inhibition testing, human leukocytes that are immunologically sensitive to human in situ breast cancer are also sensitive to MMTV.

4. The sera of some patients with breast cancer react immunologically with both MMTV virions and with mouse tumors rich in MMTV.

5. Molecular hybridization studies using MMTV-generated DNA probes demonstrate a relationship between the RNA in human breast cancers and the RNA of MMTV. Thus, oncogenic virus-related information can be found in human breast cancer.

6. Based on viral dynamics associated with high and low cancer strains, the mouse model suggests that viral expression in humans would be expected late in life and could be variable, an expectation consistent with human experience.

The evidence suggests that MMTV or a similar virus may be instrumental in the genesis of human breast cancer, but infectivity and oncogenicity of the particles found in human breast milk are not demonstrated. Furthermore, mouse mammary cancer, which seldom metastasizes and is promoted rather than reduced by early pregnancy, is less akin to the human form than is mammary cancer in the rat, in which evidence for a viral cause is tenuous. The mode by which a human virus might be transmitted remains obscure; in the United States, where breast feeding has declined, the incidence of breast cancer has risen. Despite these inconsistencies, the example of a viral agent in the mouse keeps open the possibility of a viral etiology.

Endocrine Factors

As mammary cancers arise in an endocrine-dependent organ and are responsive to hormones, it is tempting to link their genesis with disturbed hormone metabolism. Among the possibilities are excessive estrogen production, subnormal androgen production, and prolactin abnormalities.

Estrogens

As a secondary sex organ, the breast responds to the body's hormonal milieu throughout life. Estrogens stimulate the growth of both normal and neoplastic breast tissue but are primarily promotional and not causative (Miller, 1990). However, replicating cells are more sensitive to alterations by carcinogens, and mutagenesis is more likely to occur.

Endogenous estrogens come from many sources other than the ovaries and the adrenal cortex. Androgens produced by the adrenal glands serve as a substrate for estrogen production on a variety of tissues, including fat tissue, brain tissue, breast tissue, and some breast cancers. Estrogen has direct effects on tumor cells. It stimulates the release of mitogenic growth factors and the release of proteases that degrade extracellular matrix, facilitating tumor invasion and metastasis. When breast tumors are deprived of estrogen, they develop estrogen independence, most likely owing to adaptive changes.

Patients with breast cancer tend to excrete a smaller portion of estriol (E_3) in the urine compared with two other major estrogen fractions, estrone (E_1) and estradiol (E_2). The significance of this observation lies in the fact that E_2 and E_1 are carcinogens for mice and rats, whereas E_3 shares little of this activity. E_3 impedes the action of some mammary carcinogens (e.g., dimethylbenz[*a*]anthracene) and may inhibit the other two estrogens (Villee and Hagerman, 1957; and Pullinger, 1961). Subnormal production of E_3 could create a carcinogenic environment as a result of the relatively unantagonized remaining estrogens. Lemon (1974) found an E_3 quotient, expressed as (E_3) mg/24 h/(E_1) + (E_2) mg/24 h, low in 71% of patients with breast cancer but in only 30% of controls. The quotient tends to decline as risk rises for Asians when they migrate to Hawaii (Dickinson et al., 1974). However, the quotient is not uniformly decreased in patients with breast cancer, is not correlated with circulating levels of E_3, and may not differ in women with high and low urinary fractions (Zumoff et al., 1975). E_1 and E_2 are interconvertible, but E_3 is formed irreversibly from E_2. If an abnormality of estrogen metabolism is involved in the genesis of breast cancer, its locus might be in processes controlling the conversion of E_2 to E_3.

Androgens

Etiocholanolone and its precursor dehydroepiandrosterone are products of androgen metabolism. Low levels of etiocholanolone could result from subnormal androgen production and have the same effect as overstimulation from estrogen. To clarify whether an unfavorable excretion pattern found in patients preceded or resulted from the disease, Bulbrook (1973) studied urine specimens from 5000 normal women between the ages of 25 and 55 years on the island of Guernsey in the English Channel. The result was that women who developed carcinoma of the breast had lower levels of etiocholanolone compared with controls. Etiocholanolone has no known biologic function, however, and Japanese women have a low (rather than the expected high) excretion of the hormone (Cole, 1974).

It has been proposed that production of dehydroepiandrosterone and dehydroepiandrosterone sulfate by the adrenal cortex contributes to the development of breast cancer. Gordon and coworkers (1990) found a significant increase in serum levels in women who developed postmenopausal breast cancer compared with controls. Also, cigarette use increased concentrations, whereas increasing age was associated with a decrease in levels.

Prolactin

A number of observations suggest that prolactin, the pituitary hormone important for milk production, has a role in the genesis of human breast cancer (Wilson et al., 1973). Prolactin stimulates the growth of dimethylbenz[a]anthracene-induced breast cancer in rodents. Hypophysectomy, which eliminates the source of prolactin, not only prevents normal breast development but also often causes regression of both rodent and human mammary cancers. In tissue culture, 31% of human breast cancers are prolactin-dependent (Hobbs et al., 1973). Patients with painful osseous metastases may experience marked transient reduction of bone pain after prolactin suppression (Minton and Dickey, 1973; and Sasaki et al., 1976). Nevertheless, significant elevation of serum prolactin levels have not been demonstrated in breast cancer patients, and prolactin suppression has proved of little therapeutic value in treatment of the human disease (Wilson et al., 1973; and Kwa et al., 1974).

Reproductive Function

In 1700, Ramazinni of Padua noted that breast cancer was frequent among nuns and attributed their susceptibility to a celibate lifestyle. More than a century later, in 1844, Rigoni-Stern in Verona associated the disease with aging, noting—as did Ramazinni—the high frequency among single women in addition to observing four cases in priests and, thus, he advocated an investigation of religious orders (Shimkin, 1973). Links between breast cancer and reproductive functions are well established. Compared with controls, women with breast cancer are more likely to be unmarried, to have married later in life, to have become pregnant for the first time at an older age, and to have fewer children. Furthermore, they are less likely to have had an artificial menopause and more likely to have had a late menopause.

Shapiro and associates (1968) analyzed risk factors in 20,211 women interviewed at the initial visit to a breast screening project in New York City. In this population, 111 cancers were diagnosed during a mean follow-up period of 1.5 years. The ratio of observed to expected cancers was computed for various characteristics (Table 8–6). An excess

Table 8–6. COMPARISON OF RELATIVE RISKS FOR BREAST CANCER AND SELECTED CHARACTERISTICS

Characteristics	Relative Risk
Never married versus married	2.3*
1 or 2 pregnancies versus 3 or more pregnancies	2.0*
Age at menarche, under 12 versus 15 or older	1.7
Aggregate years menstrual activity, 30 years or more versus less than 30 years	1.4
Breast conditions, 1 or more versus none	3.1*
Sisters, 1 or more with breast cancer versus none	1.9

(Adapted from Shapiro, S., Strax, P., Venet, L., et al.: The search for risk factors in breast cancer. Am. J. Public Health, *58*:820, 1968. Used with permission.)
*Statistically significant increase.

of breast cancers occurred in women who had never been married, those who had no more than two pregnancies, those with an early menarche, and those with 30 or more aggregate years of menstrual activity. In addition, high risks were confirmed in connection with benign breast disease and a family history of breast cancer. A minor increase was associated with high educational attainment, and Jewish women were more susceptible than non-Jewish women. A protective effect of breast feeding and prolonged lactation was not found. A case control study from Australia performed between 1981 and 1985 suggested that breast feeding may modestly reduce the risk of breast cancer (Siskind et al., 1989).

A factor of considerable importance is the reduced risk that accrues from full-term pregnancy at an early age (Fig. 8–11). Women who give birth to their first child at or after the age of 35 years have a twofold higher risk of developing breast cancer than do women who have their first child when younger than 20 years of age. A pregnancy late in life increases the risk above that of nulliparous women. This observation explains the association of reduced risk with early marriage and multiparity. Early marriage provides no protection to nonparous women, and multiparity is less important if the first full-term pregnancy fails to occur at an early age. The importance of early first birth suggests that early maturation of mammary epithelium makes it less susceptible to carcinogens. It also suggests that carcinogenic exposure occurs early in life. Similarity is seen with pregnancy in the rat, which protects against a mammary carcinogen if it precedes exposure but promotes cancer formation if it follows exposure. The protective effect of early pregnancy in humans suggests that carcinogen exposure occurs in the second or third decade of life.

A population-based study in Norway considered the relationship between childbearing and the development of cancers of the breast and uterus (Tretli and Haldorsen, 1990). The authors concluded that changes in childbearing patterns may account for part of the observed increase in both breast and uterine cancer in Norway but did not account for most of the increase. A significant inverse correlation was found with the number of children born to women between ages 20 and 29 years. Births to women under the age of 20 years and between ages 30 and 39

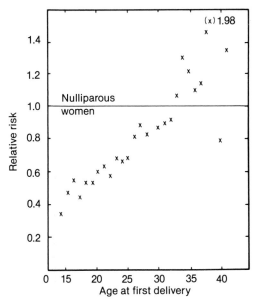

Figure 8–11. Relative risk of breast cancer related to age at first delivery. (From MacMahon, B., et al.: Etiology of human breast cancer: A review. J. Natl. Cancer. Inst., *50*:21, 1980. Used with permission.)

showed no significant association. The Norwegian data again showed Clemmesen's hook. In a second study using Nordic data, Lund (1990) found a reduction in mortality from breast cancer of 7.2% for each child borne. In a cohort of 14,421 Danish women, the RR of breast cancer was lowest among women whose first pregnancy occurred before the age of 25 years and decreased with increasing numbers of pregnancies, reaching the lowest RR (0.7) for 6 or more pregnancies (Mellemgaard et al., 1990). In a meta-analysis of numerous studies on age at first birth and on parity related to breast cancer that in total included 5508 patients (Ewertz et al., 1990), low parity and late age at first birth were independent determinants of breast cancer risk. For every two births, the risk dropped by 16%. Women with a first birth after the age of 35 years were at a 40% greater risk than those with a first birth before the age of 20 years. Cohen (1990) supported hormonal simulation of pregnancy early in life as a preventive measure against breast cancer. He estimated that breast cancer risk could be reduced by as much as 33% with this intervention.

Ovarian Function

The predilection of females for breast cancer relates it to ovarian function, and interruption of ovarian activity markedly reduces risk. Bilateral oophorectomy before the age of 40 years reduces the incidence of breast cancer by 75% in both parous and nulliparous women (Feinleib, 1968). After the fourth decade of life surgical castration provides no protection. Pelvic irradiation sufficient to produce artificial menopause similarly protects against the disease. Hysterectomy or tubal ligation alone has no influence on risk. Irwin and associates (1988) found that when performed before 55 years of age, hysterectomy in combination with bilateral

oophorectomy decreased the RR of breast cancer; however, hysterectomy alone or tubal ligation did not.

Abortions exert no influence on breast cancer risk. In a case control study, Rosenberg and colleagues (1988) determined that 1.3 was the RR for breast cancer in nulliparous women who had induced abortions compared with women who had no abortions. For spontaneous abortions, the estimate was 0.9 (95% CI = 0.5–1.5). Among parous women, the comparable risk was 1.2 (95% CI = 0.8–1.0), and for women who had spontaneous abortions, the estimate was 0.9 (95% CI = 0.8–1.0). Neither the time of the abortion nor the age of the woman had an effect on the RR for breast cancer. Among 49,000 women who had legal abortions in Sweden before the age of 30 years, no increase in breast cancer incidence was found through 5 years of follow-up (Harris et al., 1989).

Estrogen Replacement and Oral Contraceptives

Physiologic effects of estrogens on the breast include stimulation of ductal growth, promotion of stromal development, accretion of fat, and pigmentation of the areola. It is uncertain whether estrogens can cause cancer of mammary tissues. Concern stems from the fact that estrogens can stimulate the development of cancer in strains of mice predisposed to this disease and can stimulate, as well as retard, the growth of breast cancer in humans (Kennedy, 1962). Both synthetic and natural estrogens are widely consumed by women in the United States for the prevention of postmenopausal changes and for contraception; for this reason, evidence of carcinogenicity is of considerable importance.

Mammary parenchyma removed in biopsies of women on estrogen replacement or oral contraceptive therapy displays no distinctive changes when compared with tissues from other women not taking these hormones; likewise, the nature of the lesions found at biopsy do not differ between the two groups (Vessey et al., 1971; Fechner, 1972; and Ariel, 1973). In an unpublished review by Pakalns at the Medical College of Wisconsin, 75% of benign tumors removed from the breasts of 28 users of oral contraceptives proved to be fibroadenomas; this frequency was no greater than that in age-matched controls not taking oral contraceptives.

Estrogen Replacement

Studies of estrogen replacement provide mixed results but suggest that some increased risk of breast cancer is related to this therapy. Burch and Byrd (1971) reported a follow-up of 511 women treated with estrogens (usually Premarin) for prolonged periods after hysterectomy. During a total of 5441 patient-years of observation, 45 benign breast tumors and 9 mammary carcinomas were diagnosed. No bilateral or inflammatory cancers were observed, and the frequency of cancers did not exceed the expected age-specific incidence. Arthes and associates (1971) could not document a higher frequency of estrogen use among women with breast cancer than in controls matched for age, race, marital status, hospital, and time of hospital admission. However, Hoover and associates (1976) found evidence for delayed risk. Excess risk of breast cancer among 1891 women given conjugated estrogens for natural or surgical menopause was found only after 10 years of observation; this risk increased thereafter to twice the expected risk at 15 years. Risk increased with cyclic use, and the expected protection afforded by castration and multiparity was not evident.

Steinberg and coworkers (1991) combined 16 studies to produce dose-response slopes of the RR of breast cancer with the duration of estrogen use. Among women undergoing any type of menopause, the RR did not increase until after 5 years of estrogen use, when a 30% increase in risk was shown. After 15 years of use, most of the increase occurred in women using estradiol with or without progestin. The risk was significantly higher among users with a positive family history (3.4 compared with 1.5). In a prospective study accessioning 356,187 person-years of observation, long-term use of estrogen replacement was not related to the risk of developing breast cancer (Colditz et al., 1990). However, among current users, an increase was observed (RR = 2.36, 95% CI = 1.11–1.67). A stronger relationship was seen at increased age. Ross and colleagues (1979) also reported a significant increase in risk among women who had received more than 1500 mg of lifetime conjugated estrogen (3 years at 1.25 mg daily). Bergkvist and associates (1989b) reported the observations of a prospective study of 23,244 women, aged 35 years and older, who had received prescriptions for estrogen replacement. The RR for breast cancer increased with the duration of replacement therapy, reaching an RR of 4.4 (95% CI = 0.9–22.4) among women who used a combination of estrogen and progestin for extended periods. No increase was found with the use of conjugated estrogens. Evidence that the use of estrogen and progesterone combinations in postmenopausal women might reduce the risk of breast cancer was found by Gambrell and coworkers (1983) in a prospective study of 5563 postmenopausal women. After 37,236 patient-years of follow-up, the frequency of breast cancer in estrogen-progesterone users was significantly lower than in the untreated group (67.3 per 100,000 per year versus 342.3 per 100,000 per year) and lower than would be expected based on data from the National Cancer Institute Surveillance, Epidemiology and End Results program. Dupont and associates (1989) reported on the longitudinal follow-up of 3303 women who had undergone breast biopsy and who were followed for a median duration of 17 years. With the use of exogenous estrogens, the RR of breast cancer in women whose biopsies had shown atypical hyperplasia ranged from 1.8 to 0.98. No increase in risk was found with the use of birth control pills, cigarette smoking, or alcohol consumption. They concluded that a prior history of benign breast disorders without further definition did not contraindicate estrogen replacement therapy.

The literature contains results both confirming and denying that there is an increased risk of breast cancer with estrogen replacement (Henderson, 1990). Clearly, no indication exists for the use of progestins to protect against endometrial cancer in women who have undergone hysterectomy. One of the authors (J. S. Spratt) sees a number of postmenopausal women whose breasts are either overstimulated by an inappropriately high dosage of estrogens or whose breasts are overly sensitive to the usual dose. The breasts become congested and painful, and cysts form. The most frequent error made by clinicians is to place women on continuous daily estrogen therapy. Whether progestins are used or not, a break of 5 to 10 days each month is needed to reduce mammary stimulation. The dosage should be titrated until a level is obtained that is sufficiently high to avoid hot flashes, mucosal dryness, and osteoporosis, but that does not bring about breast discomfort. In the postmenopausal woman, calcium supplementation is uniformly added. Henderson (1990) concluded that the possible slight increase in the incidence of breast cancer with estrogen replacement is not associated with an increased risk of dying from breast cancer. In fact, breast cancers diagnosed in women on replacement therapy are as curable as those in women who are not (Bergkvist et al., 1989a). Whether the use of oral contraceptives in youth followed by postmenopausal use of estrogens increases the risk of breast cancer is not known.

An unresolved issue is whether postmenopausal women who have been treated for breast cancer and are disease-free can take hormone replacement therapy to relieve hot flashes and vaginal dryness and to prevent osteoporosis. Marchant (1994) provided a review of this question, and the answer does not exist. The concern is that estrogens might stimulate growth of any residual cancer and invite recurrence, but it has been argued that benefit may exceed this risk. No controlled clinical trial has been conducted to establish safety. Hormone replacement therapy in this circumstance probably should not be given unless menopausal symptoms are severe and cannot be relieved by other measures, and unless patients understand the potential risks.

Oral Contraceptives

Oral contraceptives ordinarily contain both estrogen and progesterone. In a case control study, Vessey and associates (1971) found more users among matched controls than among 220 breast cancer patients, suggesting that any influence may be a protective one. Paffenbarger and colleagues (1975) also found no greater frequency of use overall among 425 breast cancer patients than among 872 controls, but a significantly higher use was observed among the former before first childbirth. Delay of first full-term pregnancy by oral contraceptives, or perhaps by other means, increases breast cancer risk. Further analyses of these data for RR revealed that whereas use of oral contraceptives in general did not increase risk, long-term use (2–4 years) was associated with a significantly increased RR (1.9) of breast cancer (Fasal and Paffenbarger, 1975). The risk reached 11-fold among long-term users with previous benign disease.

Two extensive studies, one in England by the Royal College of General Practitioners (1981) and another in the United States by the Centers for Disease Control (CDC) (1983) found no increased risk associated with the use of oral contraceptives, either overall or within high-risk subgroups. The CDC report involved a case control study of 689 breast cancers in women from 20 to 54 years of age and in 1077 controls. RR was 0.9 between users and those who had never used oral contraceptives, and use of oral contraceptives did not increase risk in women with benign breast disease or a family history of breast cancer or in those who used oral contraceptives before their first pregnancy. The Royal College of General Practitioners observed 23,000 users and a similar number of non-users entered in 1968. No significant increase of breast cancer was found in users.

A meta-analysis of studies on oral contraceptives was performed by Romieu and coworkers (1990). In general, the authors found no increased association except in premenopausal women who used oral contraceptives for at least 4 years before their first pregnancy (RR = 7.72, CI = 1.36–2.19). The authors concluded that this subgroup required further study before final conclusions could be drawn.

The potentially long latency periods between exposure to oral contraceptives and the appearance of cancers may well bias conclusions in studies of oral contraceptives (McPherson and Doll, 1990). This possibility cannot yet be excluded. Early oral contraceptive use may be associated with a worse prognosis when breast cancer does occur. Olsson and associates (1988) carried out a study to ascertain whether proliferation (S-phase fraction) and DNA ploidy differed in breast cancer patients with early oral contraceptive use and in women with breast cancer but no history of early contraceptive use. The data indicated a higher S-phase fraction and a greater prevalence of aneuploid cancers in women with a history of oral contraceptive use before age 20 years compared with women without such a history.

Whether a causative or aggravating association exists between the use of oral contraceptives and fibrocystic changes has been the subject of a number of studies with contradictory results. The contradictions are easily attributable to the hospital-based nature of most studies, the relatively small number of cases that they include, and follow-up for inadequate time periods. If a relationship does exist, it is not a strong one. Two recent studies found no reduction in fibrocystic changes by oral contraceptives (Francheschi et al., 1984). Berkowitz and colleagues (1984) reported an increase in fibrocystic changes in postmenopausal women who had been oral contraceptive users. However, even a strong association would not establish cause and effect; numerous covariables would have to be considered before the existence of a causative relationship could be implied.

Ionizing Radiation

It was only 7 years after the discovery of x-rays by Röntgen in 1895 that the first radiogenic cancer of the skin was observed. Subsequently, many pioneering investigators of ionizing radiation died prematurely of skin cancer or leukemia. Cancers in these individuals, animal studies, and epidemiologic studies of human exposure provide the bases of our knowledge of radiation injury.

The effects of ionizing radiation on tissue are both immediate and delayed. Late effects are either somatic (i.e., affecting the irradiated individual) or genetic (i.e., affecting future generations). Induction of cancer is the most serious late somatic effect of irradiation. The capacity of ionizing

radiation to produce breast cancer has been repeatedly confirmed.

The immature breast is highly sensitive to irradiation, and exposure results in growth disturbance as well as breast cancer. Classic studies describing the sensitivity of the developing breast were performed by Cluzet at the turn of the century (1908, 1909, 1910). Early rabbit studies showed that estrogen stimulation of virginal breasts resulted in an increase in radiation sensitivity by 30% to 50% (Turner and Gomez, 1936). The first report of breast growth disturbance was by Underwood and Gaul (1948), who described a patient treated with radium therapy for a cavernous angioma of the left breast. Similar results were observed in children irradiated for mammary hemangiomas (Martin, 1954). Modern radiation therapy to the immature female breast and chest wall with doses less than 3 Gy produce no clinical retardation in breast development (Kolar et al., 1967). Doses greater than this likely produce hypoplasia (Fig. 8–12). The risk of inducing breast cancer is also increased. Hildreth and coworkers (1989) examined breast cancer induction in 1201 women who received radiation treatment in infancy for an enlarged thymus. The results were compared with the incidence of breast cancer in their 2469 unirradiated sisters. The irradiated group showed an increase in the induction rate by a factor of 3.6. They further described a linear dose-response relationship and a latency period of about 28 years. These authors concluded that exposure of the breast to ionizing radiation in infancy increased the risk of breast cancer later in life. The radiation sensitivity of the developing female breast should be kept in mind when chest wall irradiation is used for the treatment of metastatic Wilm's tumor or other pediatric neoplasms.

In 1950, Lorenz and associates were able to demonstrate that mice and guinea pigs subjected to chronic whole-body gamma irradiation developed many breast cancers compared with controls. Later, Mackenzie (1965) reported an increased incidence of breast cancer in women who received high doses of radiation to the anterior chest during

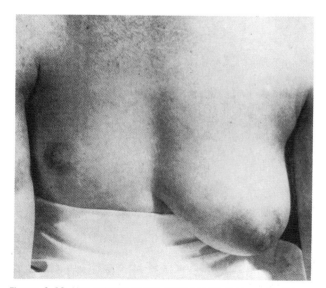

Figure 8–12. Hypoplasia of the right breast that resulted from radiation exposure of the breast at a young age. (From Martin, J. A.: Treatment of cystic hygroma. Tex. J. Med., *50:*217–220, 1954. Used with permission of the Texas Medical Association.)

repeated fluoroscopic procedures in conjunction with the treatment of pulmonary tuberculosis. The excess of breast cancers began to appear after an average latency period of 16 years, at an earlier age than would be expected in the general population, and in the areas of the breast most heavily irradiated (Mackenzie, 1965; Myrden and Hiltz, 1969; Boice and Monson, 1977; Boice et al., 1978; and Boice et al., 1991). A similar effect was found in patients who were irradiated for postpartum mastitis (Shore et al., 1977; Prince and Hildreth, 1986; and Shore et al., 1986). A survey of 606 such women who received doses ranging from 75 to 1000 rad (cGy) had more than twice the expected number of breast cancers, and these cancers were invariably located in the treated breast (Mettler et al., 1969). This hazard was confirmed by others (Lowell et al., 1968; Logan et al., 1979; Dvoretsky et al., 1980; and Howe et al., 1982). Baral and colleagues (1977) reviewed the experience with 1115 women treated for benign breast disease with ionizing radiation. After an average follow-up of 31.5 years, the number of breast cancers was four times that expected, and this finding was independent of the age at exposure. Perhaps the most important studies are those of the Atomic Bomb Casualty Commission that involved women exposed to whole-body irradiation as a result of the bombings of Hiroshima and Nagasaki (Wanebo et al., 1968; Tokunaga et al., 1986; and Tokunaga et al., 1987). The most recent include a reassessment of dose using the Dosimetry System 1986 (DS86) (Shimizu et al., 1989 and 1990). Exposure to 0.9 cGy (90 rad) or more was followed by development of breast cancers at a two- to fourfold greater rate than that in comparison groups after a mean latency period of 15 years. The increase was most evident in women who had been exposed at an early age.

Human data were compiled into a comprehensive model for radiation-induced cancers in the BEIR V Report (BIER V, 1990) and the UNSCEAR Report (United Nations, 1986 and 1988). The data suggest the following generalizations:

1. Radiation-induced cancers appear in almost every tissue of the body. Sensitivity to radiation carcinogenesis differs in various tissues and organs. The highest sensitivity is found in the female breast, thyroid gland, and myelogenous tissues.

2. Radiation-induced cancers are indistinguishable from naturally occurring cancers. For the breast, this finding was confirmed by a pathologic review of breast cancers that occurred in atomic bomb survivors (Tokuoka et al., 1984).

3. Risk estimates for cancer are based largely on high dose data. The reason for this is that the smaller numbers of cancers induced by lower doses of radiation lead to statistical uncertainty. The dose-response model and the threshold dose are estimated by extrapolating dose-response curves derived from higher doses.

4. The dose-response relationships are different for different cancers. Breast cancer seems to fit a linear (no threshold) dose-response model (Boice et al., 1978; Tokunaga et al., 1986; and BEIR V, 1990). Figure 8–13 shows the age-adjusted breast cancer rate in the survivors of Hiroshima and Nagasaki as a function of breast dose (Tokunaga et al., 1986). Similar results were observed in the studies of multiple fluoroscopic examinations of the chest and of irradiation for postpartum mastitis.

5. Cancer induction by radiation has a long latency pe-

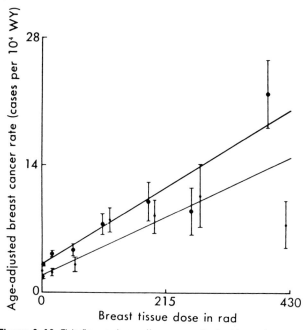

Figure 8–13. This figure shows the age-adjusted breast cancer rate in the female survivors of whole-body radiation at Hiroshima and Nagasaki as a function of breast dose. The linear relationship suggests the absence of a threshold. (Reprinted with permission from Tokunaga, M., Tokuoka, S., and Land, C. E.: Breast cancer in atomic bomb survivors. Jpn. J. Cancer Res., Monograph No. 32, 1986, pp. 167–177.)

riod. Whether this latency period is a result of induction time or a result of slow subclinical progression is uncertain. For breast neoplasms, the latency period may range from 20 to 30 years (Figs. 8–14 to 8–17).

6. Age, sex, and other factors influence cancer induction. Radiation carcinogenesis in the breast is critically dependent on the hormonal status of the target cells.

In the BEIR V report, the preferred model indicates high risk for patients irradiated at or before the age of 15 years (see Figs. 8–14 and 8–15). The risk declines dramatically with increasing age and is barely detectable in patients 40 years of age or older. The risk appears to peak at the age of 20 years after irradiation, with a dramatic decline thereafter. Excess mortality (see Figs. 8–16 and 8–17) from breast cancer is also highest in the younger age groups. Patients irradiated at 5 to 15 years of age show increasing excess mortality with age that peaks at 40 years and remains high for the rest of their lives (BEIR V, 1990). The consensus is that 50 to 200 excess breast cancers occur per 1 million persons per lifetime exposure per centigray (rad) of radiation, and 10 to 60 excess deaths occur from breast cancer under the same parameters (UNSCEAR, 1988). Based on modern low-dose techniques in which the mean breast dose for a two-view study is 1.7 mGy (0.17 rad), Feig (1983) estimated that one mammogram theoretically would cause one excess breast cancer per 2 million women per year after a latency period of 10 years.

The potential danger from irradiation to the whole body or breast seems clear. The fact that a threshold dose below which danger is nonexistent is not acknowledged justifies concern about cumulative exposures for diagnostic purposes as well as for therapy. Perhaps the single greatest

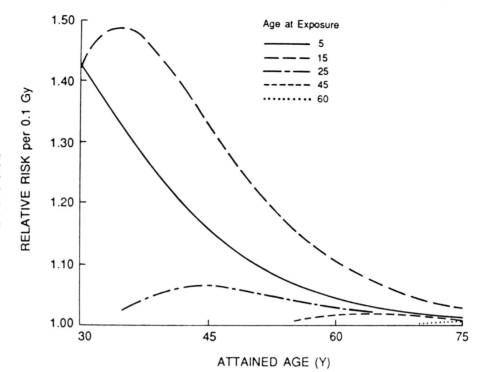

Figure 8–14. This figure shows the relative risk of breast cancer per unit of radiation exposure for women exposed at different ages. Relative risk is higher if the breasts are exposed during development (i.e., 15 years of age).

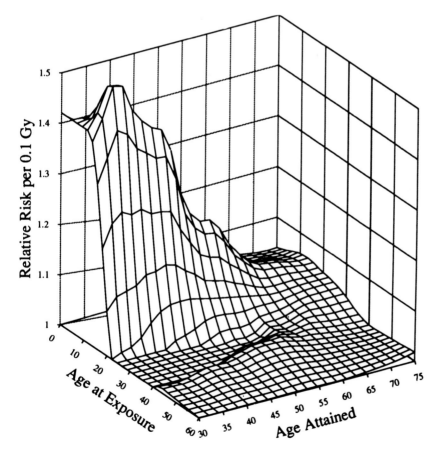

Figure 8–15. Relative risk of women for breast cancer based on age at radiation exposure and attained age. The greatest increase in risk is for women younger than age 20 years. As age advances, the relative risk for those who remain well declines.

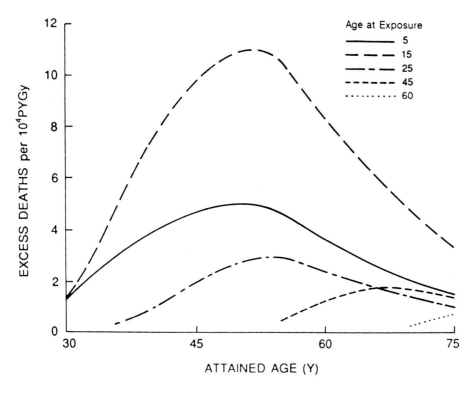

Figure 8–16. Excess death from breast cancer is greatest for women exposed to radiation during the period of breast development. Excess deaths may be delayed for 30 years.

source of breast irradiation at present is mammography, which is used to detect small breast cancers. With poor technique, poorly calibrated equipment, and repetitive examinations without clear indications, this valuable diagnostic tool may enhance the problem it was designed to address. Midbreast exposure per examination is now as low as 1 mGy per view (100 mrad) (Law, 1991). With proper technique and indications and with dose-reducing techno-

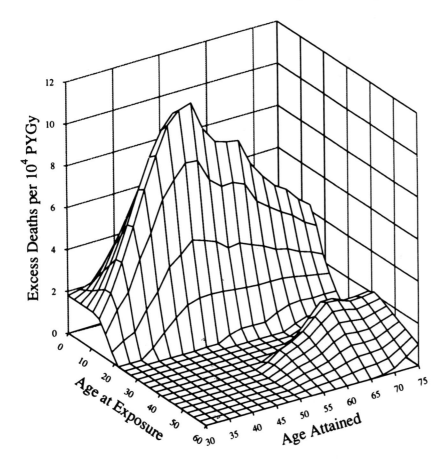

Figure 8–17. The greatest rise in excess deaths from breast cancer is seen 30 to 40 years after the age of exposure to ionizing radiation. (Adapted with permission from Health Effects of Exposure to Low Levels of Ionizing Radiation: BEIR V. © 1990 by the National Academy of Sciences. Courtesy of National Academy Press, Washington, D.C.)

logic improvements, the biologic price of mammography can be kept low. Nevertheless, the small risk should be paid only by those who can be expected to obtain a net benefit. In view of the long latency of radiation carcinogenesis, the ultimate consequences of both diagnostic and therapeutic irradiation of the breast must remain under continuing evaluation.

Various populations are exposed to nonionizing radiations, such as electromagnetic fields. Reports of increased breast cancer in exposed groups require further study (Demers et al., 1990; and Matanoski et al., 1991).

Diet and Obesity

Considerable laboratory and epidemiologic evidence links breast cancer risk to diet and body habitus. These two factors are of special interest, since they are subject to modification and potentially have other health benefits. Both diets high in animal fats and obesity have been linked to increased cancer risk by circumstantial evidence (such as that shown in Figure 8–18), but controlled clinical studies in this area are difficult to perform and data from such studies are virtually nonexistent. The critical elements involved are currently unknown. A diet reduced in fat content is one component of a population-based controlled clinical trial implemented in the United States known as the Woman's Health Initiative (Palca, 1991; and Cummings, 1993). A separate chapter is devoted to the subjects of nutrition and breast disease owing to the interest in these issues and to their complexity.

Trauma

The appearance of malignant neoplasms at the site of burn scars (Marjolin's ulcer), chronic osteomyelitic sinuses, and chronic anal fistulas suggests that chronic trauma is a factor in carcinogenesis. Two patients who developed mammary carcinoma in burn scars on the breast were reported by Peden in 1947. The authors are aware of a 56-year-old man who developed adenocarcinoma of the breast in a chronic

scar that resulted from total avulsion of the areola at 16 years of age and of a 63-year-old woman who developed breast cancer in a burn scar involving the breast and axilla.

Patients often trace the onset of cancer to a recent injury, raising the question of whether acute trauma is an initiating factor. It is generally believed that this association represents a need to find an explanation for illness. More likely, the trauma served to draw the individual's attention to a pre-existent lesion. Eleven per cent of 2529 patients at the Ellis Fischel State Cancer Hospital (EFSCH), Columbia, Missouri, related antecedent trauma to their breast cancer. Wynder and coworkers (1976) produced a similar figure (9.0%) in 632 patients.

The induction of neoplasia by acute mechanical trauma is an extremely unlikely event; however, it should be noted that the work of Klamer, Donegan, and Max (1983) and that of Jackson and colleagues (1984) provide some evidence that direct trauma may promote mammary tumor development in certain circumstances. Rats were exposed to the carcinogen dimethylbenz[*a*]anthracene, and breast tissue was surgically resected to various extents (up to 75%). Animals with resections developed as many tumors as did intact animals with a full complement of breast tissue, suggesting that carcinogenesis was promoted by partial removal of the breast. Whether an enhancement secondary to ablative trauma occurred in residual breast tissue remains to be resolved.

Implanted Foreign Material

Carcinoma of the breast has developed adjacent to implanted cardiac pacemakers (Biran et al., 1979). The observations of two such cancers led the authors to change the placement of pacemakers to a position not likely to be in the breast tissue. Mastitis induced by leaking silicone prostheses and injected silicone interferes with an accurate physical and mammographic examination and can obscure early cancers. Morgenstern and coworkers (1985) reported a series of 12 women with silicone-associated cancers. Causation was not implied but could not be excluded. Inflammatory breast cancer has been reported in breasts in-

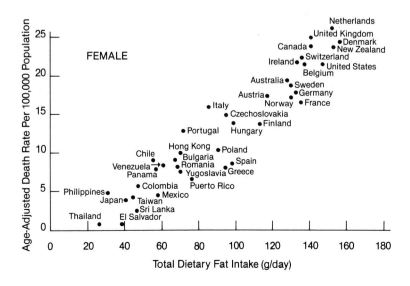

Figure 8–18. Correlation between per capita consumption of dietary fat and age-adjusted mortality from breast cancer in different countries. (From Carroll, K. K.: Experimental evidence of dietary factors and hormone-dependent cancers. Cancer Res., 35:3374, 1975. Used with permission.)

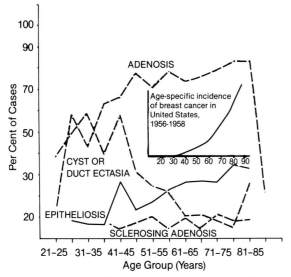

Figure 8–19. Age-specific incidence of various manifestations of fibrocystic changes in breasts of 800 females at autopsy. (Chart compiled based on data from Sandison, A. T.: Autopsy study of adult human breast. National Cancer Institute Monograph No. 8. U.S. Department of Health, Education and Welfare, 1962.)

jected with silicone. Patients with inflammatory cancer have often been misdiagnosed as having "silicone mastitis" (Lewis, 1980). Whether any breast implants used for augmentation mammoplasties have a carcinogenic potential is an incompletely resolved issue. An estimated 1 million women in the United States have implants for breast augmentation. If their average age were 30 years, about 130 of these women could be expected to develop an associated breast cancer each year purely by chance.

Fibrocystic Changes

Symptomatic fibrocystic changes, also known as "fibrocystic disease," "chronic cystic mastopathy," "cystic disease," "chronic cystic disease," "chronic cystic mastitis," "Schimmelbusch's disease," "Reclus's disease," and a number of other synonyms, is an affliction of women in their reproductive years. Of the types of fibrocystic changes known, proliferative changes have constituted the major risk for development of breast cancer. Sandison's (1962) examination of 1300 breasts at autopsy permits construction of age-specific prevalences of various cystic and proliferative changes that associate epithelial proliferation, or "epitheliosis," with mammary cancer (Fig. 8–19). Pathologists report the association of duct hyperplasia and infiltrative cancer in the same breast, suggesting an evolution from hyperplasia to cancer. Gallagher and Martin (1969) postulated induction and promotion phases in this transition, the first being a reversible change from normal ductal epithelium to hyperplasia, and the second being an irreversible change to carcinoma or permanent hyperplasia. Foote and Stewart (1945) implicated atypical ductal papillomatosis as leading to cancer of the breast. In a large study, an equal incidence of ductal papillomatosis was found in carcinomatous and noncarcinomatous breasts, but atypical cellular

changes were evident five times more frequently in the former. Solid hyperplasia may be even more dangerous than papillomatosis. Davis and associates (1964) reported that 6.2% of women with solid hyperplasia subsequently developed breast cancer compared with only 3.8% of those with papillomatosis. Fully 50% of carcinomas developed in the breast opposite that in which the diagnosis of cystic change was established, an observation in support of the "field" theory of mammary carcinogenesis and one that illustrates the futility of ipsilateral mastectomy for this condition as a prophylactic measure against cancer. Solid hyperplasia in large ducts is possibly more dangerous than similar changes in small ducts. In one study, carcinoma developed in 6 of 18 patients with large duct hyperplasia within 1 to 13 years of diagnosis (Humphrey and Swerdlow, 1968). Cancer developed under skin flaps in residual breast tissue in 2 of these 18 patients after simple mastectomy, emphasizing that operations that fail to remove all breast tissue do not provide effective prophylaxis against mammary cancer.

In a longitudinal study, Spratt and coworkers (1985) reported the experience with fibrocystic changes confirmed by biopsy in a breast screening program for 10,128 women between 35 and 74 years of age in the Breast Cancer Detection Demonstration Project at the University of Louisville in Kentucky. In this period, 1936 breast biopsies were recommended, with results as shown in Figure 8–20. After 6 to 10 years of follow-up, only four cancers developed during 2443.5 woman-years of follow-up, yielding an incidence of 0.00164 per woman-year; this value is entirely within the expected range. Both cases in which some type of fibrocystic change was found to be synchronous with a cancer and cases in which only fibrocystic changes and no synchronous cancer were found were sorted in matrices. Tables 8–7 and 8–8 show the association of this histologic type of fibrocystic changes, Wolfe's parenchymal mammographic patterns, and cancers diagnosed in follow-up. There is no clustering in the matrices, implicating neither a xeromammographic pattern nor a histologic type of fibrocystic change as being precancerous. As the authors note, a much larger series with patients followed for longer periods of time might produce different results. The majority of women develop fibrocystic changes with no strongly cancerous predisposition. These women need reassurance to alleviate their anxiety.

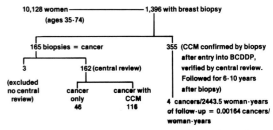

Figure 8–20. Stratification flow diagram for patients on whom biopsy was performed as a result of recommendations originating from screening in the Breast Cancer Demonstration and Detection Project, University of Louisville (BCDDP), according to histopathologic diagnoses. CCM = chronic cystic mastopathy. (From Spratt, J. S., Alagia, D. P., Greenberg, R. A., et al.: Association of chronic cystic mastopathy, xeromammographic patterns and cancer. Cancer, 55:1372, 1985. Used with permission.)

Table 8–7. MATRIX ASSOCIATION OF TYPES OF CHRONIC CYSTIC MASTOPATHY (CCM), WOLFE'S PARENCHYMAL MAMMOGRAPHIC PATTERNS (XM), AND CANCERS DIAGNOSED IN FOLLOW-UP AFTER DIAGNOSIS OF CCM AND XM

Type of Chronic Cystic Mastopathy	Wolfe's Parenchymal Patterns						Cancers/ Category
	D_y	N_1	P_1	P_2C	P_2L	P_2N	
Lobular hyperplasia	10	12	15	26	66*	27	1/156
Sclerosing adenosis	7	11	15	17*	45	22*	2/117
Ductal papillary hyperplasia	13	16	19	26*	60	25*	2/159
Ductal papillary hyperplasia with apocrine metaplasia	3	9	6	8	26	8	0/60
Ductal nonpapillary hyperplasia	2	1	11	5	9	4	0/32
Ductal nonpapillary hyperplasia with apocrine metaplasia	1	0	0	1	1	4*	1/7
Cyst, epithelial	12*	14	37	45*	90*	38	3/246
Cyst, epithelial, with apocrine metaplasia	13	21	21	34*	79*	30	2/198
Lobular hyperplasia with atypia	0	0	0	0	1	1	0/2
Ductal hyperplasia with atypia	2	2	4	4*	8	2	1/22
Cancers/category	1/63	0/06	0/178	1/166	1/385	1/161	4/355

(From Spratt, J. S. Alagia, D. P., Greenberg, R. A., et al.: Association of chronic cystic mastopathy, xeromammographic patterns and cancer. Cancer, *55*:1372, 1985. Reprinted with permission.)

*Cancer (1) in subset.

Two studies with long-term follow-up have given better definition to what might and might not be histologically precancerous. Dupont and Page (1985) followed 10,366 women undergoing breast biopsies consecutively in a hospital in Nashville, Tennessee. Among 3303 patients selected for follow-up, the median duration of follow-up was 17 years. These authors observed that women with proliferative disease but without atypical hyperplasia had a risk of cancer that was 1.9 times the risk of women with nonproliferative lesions. In women with atypical hyperplasia, this risk rose to 5.3 times (3.1 to 8.8 = 95% CI). Family history associated with nonproliferative changes imposed little risk. When family history was combined with atypia, the breast cancer risk was 11-fold greater (5.5 to 24 = 95% CI) than the risk of cancer in women with nonproliferative lesions and a negative family history. The presence of calcification in association with proliferative changes increased the cancer risk. Benign cysts alone did not increase

cancer risk. However, when their presence was combined with a family history of cancer, the risk rose to 2.7 times greater than that in women without these factors. Of great significance was the observation that the majority (70%) of all women who undergo breast biopsy are not at increased risk for the development of cancer. The authors suggested that breast biopsies might be considered in women with family histories of breast cancer to ascertain the degree of hyperplasia with atypia. Women with no proliferative histologic changes in the breast could be reassured that their risk for breast cancer was not excessive for their age. More effective surveillance might then be justified for women with a combination of family history of breast cancer and atypia.

Dupont and Page (1985) evaluated the RR associated with a combination of histopathologic variables and selected clinical and epidemiologic factors. They confirmed that the risk of breast cancer associated with different sub-

Table 8–8. ASSOCIATION OF CANCERS CONFIRMED AT FIRST BIOPSY WITH CHRONIC CYSTIC MASTOPATHY

Type of Chronic Cystic Mastopathy	Number with Cancer at First Biopsy	umber with No Cancer at First Biopsy	Number with No Cancer at First Biopsy in Whom Cancer Developed During Follow-up
Lobular hyperplasia	29	156	1
Sclerosing adenosis	43	117	2
Ductal papillary hyperplasia	63	159	2
Ductal papillary hyperplasia with apocrine metaplasia	23	60	0
Ductal nonpapillary hyperplasia	22	32	0
Ductal nonpapillary hyperplasia with apocrine metaplasia	5	7	1
Cyst, epithelial	72	246	3
Epithelial cyst with apocrine metaplasia	41	198	2
Lobular hyperplasia with atypia	10	2	0
Ductal hyperplasia with atypia	35	22	1
Total number of patients	116	355	4

(From Spratt, J. S., Alagia, D. P., Greenberg, R. A., et al.: Association of chronic cystic mastopathy, xeromammographic patterns and cancer. Cancer, *55*:1372, 1985. Reprinted with permission.)

sets of benign breast disease could be influenced by nonhistopathologic risk factors. Age at first birth and nulliparity increased the risk of breast cancer in patients with both atypical hyperplasia and a family history of breast cancer. In the absence of proliferative changes, no enhancement of risk was observed. Large breasts were associated with increased risk in association with either a family history or minimal proliferative disease. Thus, multiple factors are associated with risk of breast cancer. The need to categorize histopathologically benign changes in the breast in order to refine the study of risk led to a consensus conference in New York in October 1985. The first conclusion made at this conference was to recommend discontinuation of the term ''fibrocystic disease,'' substituting for it either the term ''fibrocystic changes'' or the term ''fibrocystic condition.'' The participants limited the consensus statement to only those risk factors derived from the pathologic examination of benign breast tissue. When any of the diagnostic terms describing fibrocystic change is used, the component lesions should be specified. Then, by evaluating the lesions in combination with other relevant epidemiologic data, the RR for subsequent invasive cancer can be estimated. By way of example, epithelial hyperplasias were assigned to risk categories. Ducts or ductules (lobules) with an epithelial lining of no more than two cells' depth were considered normal. Mild hyperplasia exists when the epithelium has a depth of greater than two but not more than four cells. Moderate and florid hyperplasia refers to more extensive degrees of epithelial proliferation. In the absence of atypical hyperplasia, mild hyperplasia is not associated with increased risk for invasive carcinoma. Moderate or florid hyperplasia without atypical hyperplasia is associated with slightly increased RR (1.5- to 2-fold) for invasive carcinoma. Atypical hyperplasia (ductal or lobular) was used to refer to lesions that have some features of carcinoma in situ but not enough to make an unequivocal diagnosis of carcinoma in situ, the so-called ''borderline lesion.'' Whereas women with atypical hyperplasia have moderately increased risk for invasive cancer (approximately fivefold the risk of control populations), the RR of lesser degrees of atypia (mild, moderate) has not been established. Carcinoma in situ was considered during the discussion only to establish the endpoint for atypical hyperplasia. Women diagnosed with carcinoma in situ (ductal or lobular) on breast biopsy who have no further treatment are at high risk for invasive carcinoma (8- to 10-fold) relative to comparable women who have had no breast biopsy. This is about the same degree of risk found in women with a first-degree family history of breast cancer and atypical duct or lobular hyperplasia (Dupont and Page, 1985). The radial scar and the lactiferous sinus solitary papilloma were not included in the risk categories because of the lack of specific data on these lesions. Until data are available for these entities, they should be categorized based on the characteristics of their epithelial components.

The use of variable nomenclature to indicate the precancerous potential of various types of mastopathy has caused confusion. A consensus conference sponsored by the College of American Pathologists recommended a simplification of nomenclature (1986). Slightly increased cancer risk (1.5- to 2-fold) was considered to exist with moderate to florid hyperplasia (either solid or papillary) and with papillomas with a fibrovascular core. A moderately increased risk (fivefold) was considered to exist in patients with atypical hyperplasia (either duct or lobular). Other histopathologic patterns were not considered to pose an increased risk of cancer.

Cystosarcoma Phyllodes

The epidemiologic aspects of cystosarcoma phyllodes have been incompletely studied but do seem to be different from those of breast carcinomas (Bernstein et al., 1993). Women born in Mexico and Central American are at significantly greater risk for cystosarcomas than are Latinos born in the United States. No cause for cystosarcoma phyllodes has been identified.

EPIDEMIOLOGY OF MALE BREAST CANCER

Breast cancer in males is infrequent but not rare. The Third National Cancer Survey for 1969–1971 placed the annual incidence at 0.6 per 100,000 men. Breast carcinoma accounts for 0.17% of all cancers in males. The 1000 cases that occur in the United States each year constitute 0.55% of total newly diagnosed breast cancers (Cancer Facts and Figures—1993).

It is tempting to relate the comparatively low risk of breast cancer in males to the obvious difference in breast size between the sexes. This comparison was made by LeDran in the eighteenth century (LeDran, 1757). Otherwise, the epidemiologic features of male breast cancers are similar to those of breast cancers in women. The incidence increases with age, but onset is generally later in life (male patients are on average 5 to 10 years older than women at onset). Occasional cases occur as early as in the third decade of life. No hormonal abnormality is regularly identified in men with breast cancer. Some aspects of the disease are reminiscent of the rat model. In high incidence rat lines, males share little of the risk unless they are feminized with exogenous estrogens, in which case breast development occurs and breast cancers appear. Similarly, signs of feminization may be present in men with breast cancer. Gynecomastia is associated in 5% to 18% of cases, and duct hyperplasia is seen. Men with Klinefelter's syndrome, which includes breast development among its features, have an increased risk. Breast cancer has also been reported in male transsexuals who take maintenance estrogens (Symmers, 1968). Hypogonadism may be a predisposing factor. A high incidence of past orchitis and previous orchiectomy has been found in some studies (Schottenfeld et al., 1963). Associations are also found with prior exposure to x-rays and with familial susceptibility. The RR for men is greater when a first-degree relative develops breast cancer before the age of 45 years. The risk also increases as the number of relatives with breast cancer increases. The odds are similar whether relatives with breast cancer are paternal or maternal (Rosenblatt et al., 1991).

The risk of cancer after breast irradiation is not restricted to females. Cancer of the male breast was reported in one patient 35 years after irradiation for prepubertal gynecomastia (Lowell et al., 1968). Eldar and colleagues (1989) described a similar patient and compared the results with those of 10 other cases reported previously.

SUMMARY

The cause of mammary cancer in humans still remains obscure, but insights continue to be obtained through epidemiologic and genetic studies and through work with animal models. The patterns of risk are complex and suggest that both heredity and environment are influential.

References

Albano, W. A., Recabaren, J. A., and Lynch, H. T.: Natural history of hereditary cancer of the breast and colon. Cancer, *50*:360, 1982.

Anderson, D. E.: Genetic study of breast cancer: Identification of a high risk group. Cancer, *34*:1090, 1974.

Anderson, D. E., and Badzioch, M. D.: Risk of familial breast cancer. Cancer, *56*:383, 1985.

Ariel, I. M.: Enovid therapy (norethynodrel with Mestranol) for fibrocystic disease. Am. J. Obstet. Gynecol., *117*:453, 1973.

Arthes, F. G., Sartwell, P. E., and Lewison, E. F.: The pill, estrogens, and the breast. Cancer, *28*:1391, 1971.

Bailar, J. C., and Smith, E. M.: Progess against cancer? N. Engl. J. Med., *314*:1226–1232, 1986.

Baral, E., Larsson, L. E., and Mattsson, B.: Breast cancer following irradiation of the breast. Cancer, *40*:2905, 1977.

BEIR V Report, Health Effects of Exposure to Low Levels of Ionizing Radiation. Advisory Committee on the Biological Effects of Ionizing Radiation: Washington, D.C., Division of Medical Sciences, National Research Council, National Academy of Science Press, 1990.

Benchimol, S.: Viruses and cancer. *In* Tannock, I.F., and Hill, R.P. (Eds.): The Basic Science of Oncology. 2nd ed. New York, McGraw-Hill, 1992, pp. 88–101.

Berg, J. W.: Clinical implications of risk factors for breast cancer. Cancer, *53*:589, 1984.

Bergkvist, L., Adami, H. O., Persson, I., et al.: Prognosis after breast cancer diagnosis in women exposed to estrogen and estrogen-progestogen replacement therapy. Am. J. Epidemiol., *130*:221–228, 1989a.

Bergkvist, L., Adami, H. O., Persson, I., et al.: The risk of breast cancer after estrogen and estrogen-progestin replacement. N. Engl. J. Med., *321*:293–297, 1989b.

Berkowitz, G. S., Kelsey, J. L., LiVoisi, V. A., et al.: Oral contraceptive use among pre- and postmenopausal women. Am. J. Epidemiol., *120*:82, 1984.

Bernstein, L., Deapen, D., and Ross, R. K.: The descriptive epidemiology of malignant cystosarcoma phyllodes tumors of the breast. Cancer, *71*:3020–3024, 1993.

Biran, S., Keren, A., Farkas, T., et al: Development of carcinoma of the breast at the site of implanted pacemakers in two patients. J. Surg. Oncol., *11*:7, 1979.

Bittner, J. J.: Some possible effects of nursing on the mammary gland tumor incidence in mice. Science, *84*:162, 1936.

Blot, W. J., Devesa, S. S., and Fraumeni, J. F. Jr: Declining breast cancer mortality among young American women. J. Natl. Cancer Inst., *78*:451–454, 1987.

Boice, J. D., Jr., and Monson, R. R.: Breast cancer in women after repeated fluoroscopic examinations of the chest. J. Natl. Cancer Inst., *59*:823–832, 1977.

Boice, J. D., Preston, D., Davis, F. G., and Monson, R. R.: Frequent chest x-ray fluoroscopy and breast cancer incidence among tuberculosis patients in Massachusetts. Radiat. Res., *125*:214–222, 1991.

Boice, J. D., Rosenstein, M., and Trout, E. D.: Estimation of breast doses and breast cancer risk associated with repeated fluoroscopic chest examinations of women with tuberculosis. Radiat. Res., *73*:373, 1978.

Boring, C. C., Squires, T. S., and Tong, T.: Cancer Statistics 1993. C. A. Cancer J. Clin., *43*:7–26, 1993.

Bucalossi, P., and Veronesi, U.: Some observations on cancer of the breast in mothers and daughters. Br. J. Cancer, *11*:337, 1957.

Buell, P.: Changing incidence of breast cancer in Japanese women. J. Natl. Cancer Inst., *51*:1479–1483, 1973.

Bulbrook, R. D.: Prediction of response of breast cancer treatment. *In* Holland, J. F., and Frei, E. (Eds.): Cancer Medicine. Philadelphia, Lea & Febiger, 1973, p. 907.

Burch, J. C., and Byrd, B. F.: Effects of long-term adminstration of estrogen on the occurrence of mammary cancer in women. Ann. Surg., *174*:414, 1971.

Busk, T., and Clemmesen, J.: Frequencies of left and right sided breast cancer. Br. J. Cancer, *1*:345 1947.

Cairns, J.: The origin of human cancers. Nature, *289*:353, 1981.

Cancer Facts and Figures—1993. American Cancer Society, Inc., 1599 Clifton Road, NE, Atlanta, GA. 30329-4251.

Carroll, K. K.: Experimental evidence of dietary factors and hormone-dependent cancers. Cancer Res., *35*:3374, 1975.

Centers for Disease Control: Cancer and hormone study: Long-term oral contraceptive use and the risk of breast cancer. J.A.M.A., *249*:1951, 1983.

Claus, E. B., Risch, N. J., and Thompson, W. D.: Age at onset as an indicator of familial risk of breast cancer. Am. J. Epidemiol., *131*:961, 1990.

Cluzet, J.: De l'action des rayons X sur la glande mammaire. Lyon Med., *112*:1076, 1909.

Cluzet, J.: Action des rayons X sur le développement du cal. Lyon Med., *42*:22, 1910.

Cluzet, J.: De l'action des rayons X sur l'évolution de la mammelle pendant la gestation. Arch. Electric. Med., *16*:959, 1908.

Cohen, P.: Host heterogeneity in female breast cancer: Possible significance for pathophysiology, therapy and prevention. Breast Cancer Res. Treat., *15*:205, 1990.

Colditz, G. A., Stampfer, M. J., Willett, W. C., et al.: Prospective study of estrogen replacement therapy and risk of breast cancer in post-menopausal women. J.A.M.A., *264*:2648, 1990.

Cole, P.: Epidemiology of breast cancer: An overview. Report to the Profession, Breast Cancer. U.S. Department of Health, Education and Welfare, September 30, 1974, p. 11.

Godfrey, S. E.: Is "fibrocystic disease" of the breast precancerous (Letter)? Arch. Pathol. Lab. Med., *110*:171–173, 1986.

Cook, G. B.: A comparison of single and multiple primary cancers. Cancer, *19*:959, 1966.

Cummings, N. B.: Women's health and nutrition research: U.S. governmental concerns. J. Am. Coll. Nutr. *12*:329–336, 1993.

Davis, H. H., Simons, M., and Davis, J. B.: Cystic disease of the breast: Relationship to carcinoma. Cancer, *17*:957, 1964.

Demers, P. A., Thomas, D. B., Rosenblatt, K. A., et al.: Occupational exposure to electromagnetic radiation and breast cancer in males. Am. J. Epidemiol., *132*:775–776, 1990.

de Waard, F.: The epidemiology of breast cancer: Review and projects. Int. J. Cancer, *4*:577, 1969.

Dickinson, L. E., MacMahon, B., Cole, P., et al.: Estrogen profiles of Oriental and Caucasian women in Hawaii. N. Engl. J. Med., *291*:1211, 1974.

Dupont, W. D., and Page, D. L.: Risk factors for breast cancer in women with proliferative breast disease. N. Engl. J. Med., *312*;146, 1985.

Dupont, W. D., Page, D., Rogers, L. W., et al.: Influence of exogenous estrogens, proliferative breast disease, and other variables on breast cancer risk. Cancer, *63*:948–957, 1989.

Dvoretsky, P. M., Woodard, E., Bonfiglio, T. A., et al.: The pathology of breast cancer in women irradiated for acute postpartum mastitis. Cancer, *46*:2257, 1980.

Eastman, A., and Barry, N.: The origins of DNA breaks: A consequence of DNA damage, DNA repair, or apoptosis. Cancer Invest., *10*:229, 1992.

Eldar, S., Nash, E., and Abrahamson, J.: Radiation carcinogenesis in the male breast. Eur. J. Surg. Oncol., *15*:274–278, 1989.

Epstein, S. S.: Environmental pollutants as unrecognized causes of breast cancer. Int. J. Health Serv., *24(1)*:145–150, 1994.

Ewertz, M., Duffy, S. W., Adami, H.-O., et al.: Age at first birth, parity and risk of breast cancer: A meta-analysis of 8 studies from the Nordic countries. Int. J. Cancer, *46*:597, 1990.

Fasal, E., and Paffenbarger, R. S. Jr.: Oral contraceptives as related to cancer and benign lesions of the breast. J. Natl. Cancer Inst., *55*:767, 1975.

Fechner, R. E.: Benign breast disease in women on estrogen therapy. Cancer, *29*:273, 1972.

Feig, S. A.: Low dose mammography: assessment of theoretical risk. *In* Feig, S. A., and McLelland, R. (Eds.): Breast Carcinoma, Current Diagnosis and Treatment. New York, Masson, 1983, pp. 69–76.

Feinleib, M.: Breast cancer and artificial menopause: A cohort study. J. Natl. Cancer Inst., *41*:315, 1968.

Fishman, J., Fukushima, D., O'Connor, J., et al.: Low urinary estrogen glucuronides in women at risk for familial breast cancer. Science, *204*:1089, 1979.

Foote, F. W., and Stewart, F. W.: Comparative studies of cancerous versus noncancerous breasts. Ann. Surg., *121*:197, 1945.

Fox, M. S.: On the diagnosis and treatment of breast cancer. J.A.M.A., *241*:489, 1979.

Francheschi, S., La Vecchia, C., Parazzini, F., et al.: Oral contraceptives and benign breast disease: A case control study. Am. J. Obstet. Gynecol., *149*:602, 1984.

Freeman, H. P.: Cancer in the socioeconomically disadvantaged. C. A. Cancer J. Clin., *39*:267–287, 1989.

Futreal, P. A., Liu, Q., Shattuck-Eidens, D., et al.: *BRCA1* mutations in primary breast and ovarian carcinomas. Science, *266*:120–122, 1994.

Gail, M. H., Brinton, L. A., Byar, D. P., et al.: Projecting individualized probabilities of developing breast cancer for white females who are being examined annually. J. Natl. Cancer Inst., *81*:1979–1986, 1989.

Gallagher, H. S., and Martin, J. E.: Early phases in the development of breast cancer. Cancer, *24*:1170, 1969.

Gambrell, R. D., Jr., Maier, R. C., and Sanders, B. I.: Decreased incidence of breast cancer in post-menopausal estrogen-progesterone users. Obstet. Gynecol., *62*:435, 1983.

Gentry, W. C. Jr., Eskrit, N. R., and Gorland, R. J.: Multiple hamartoma syndrome (Cowden's disease). Arch. Dermatol., *109*:521, 1974.

Gordon, G. B., Bush, T. L., Helzlsouer, J., et al.: Relationship of serum levels of dehydroepiandrosterone and dehydroepiandrosterone sulfate to the risk of developing postmenopausal breast cancer. Cancer Res., *50*:3859, 1990.

Guinee, V.: Cancer data systems. Curr. Probl. Cancer, *9*:1, 1985.

Haagensen, C. D.: Diseases of the Breast. Philadelphia, W.B. Saunders, 1971, p. 364.

Haenszel, W., and Kurihara, M.: Studies of Japanese migrants: 1. Mortality from cancer and other diseases among Japanese in the United States. J. Natl. Cancer Inst., *40*:43–68, 1968.

Harris, B.-M. L., Eklund, G., Meirik, O., et al.: Risk of cancer after legal abortion during first trimester: A Swedish register study. Br. Med. J., *199*:1430, 1989.

Henderson, I. C.: What can a woman do about her risk of dying of breast cancer? Curr. Probl. Cancer, *14*:163, 1990.

Hildreth, N. G., Shore, R. E., and Dvoretsky, P. M.: The risk of breast cancer after irradiation of the thymus in infancy. N. Engl. J. Med., *321*:1281–1284, 1989.

Hobbs, J. R., Salih, H., Flax, H., et al.: Prolactin dependence in human breast cancer. Proc. R. Soc. Med., *66*:866, 1973.

Holm, N. V., Hauge, M., and Harvald, B.: Etiologic factors of breast cancer elucidated by a study of unselected twins. J. Natl. Cancer Inst., *65*:285, 1980.

Hoover, R., Gray, L. A. Sr., Cole, P., et al.: Menopausal estrogens and breast cancer. N. Engl. J. Med., *295*:401, 1976.

Howe, G. R., Miller, A. B., and Sherman, G. J.: Breast cancer mortality following fluoroscopic irradiation in a cohort of tuberculosis patients. Cancer Detect. Prev., *5*:175, 1982.

Humphrey, L. J., and Swerdlow, M. A.: A large duct epithelial hyperplasia and carcinoma of the breast. Arch. Surg., *97*:592, 1968.

Irwin, K. L., Lee, N. C., Peterson, H. B., et al.: Hysterectomy, tubal sterilization, and the risk of breast cancer. Am. J. Epidemiol., *127*:1192, 1988.

Jackson, C. F., Palmquist, M., Swanson, J., et al.: Effectiveness of prophylactic subcutaneous mastectomy in Spague-Dawley rats induced with 7,12-dimethylbenzanthracene. Plast. Reconstr. Surg., *73*:249, 1984.

Jacobsen, C. O.: Heredity in Breast Cancer: A Genetic and Clinical Study of 200 Probands. Copenhagen, NyT Nordirk Forlag, 1946.

Kennedy, B. J.: Massive estrogen administration in premenopausal women with metastatic breast cancer. Cancer, *5*:641, 1962.

Klamer, T. W., Donegan, W. L., and Max, M. H.: Breast tumor incidence in rats after partial mammary resection. Arch. Surg., *118*:933, 1983.

Knudsen, A. G., Strong, L. C., and Anderson, D. E.: Heredity and cancer in man. Prog. Med. Genet., *9*:113, 1976.

Kolar, J., Bek, V., and Vrabeck, R.: Hypoplasia of the growing breast after contact x-ray therapy for cutaneous angiomas. Arch. Dermatol., *96*:427, 1967.

Kwa, H. G., Engelsman, E., De Jong-Bakker, M., et al.: Plasma-prolactin in human breast cancer. Lancet, *i*:433, 1974.

Last, J. M.: A Dictionary of Epidemiology. 1st ed. New York, Oxford University Press, 1983, and 2nd ed., 1988.

Law, J.: Patient dose and risk in mammography. Br. J. Radiol., *64*:360–365, 1991.

LeDran, H. F.: Memoire avec un précis de plusieurs observations sur le cancer. Mem. Acad. Roy. Chir., *3*:1, 1757.

Lemon, H. M.: Estrogens. *In* Holland, J.F., and Frei, E. III (Eds.): Cancer Medicine. Philadelphia, Lea & Febiger, 1974, p. 911.

Lewis, C. M.: Inflammatory carcinoma of the beast following silicone injections. Plast. Reconstr. Surg., *66*:134, 1980.

Liff, J. M., Sung, J. F. C., Chu, W.-H., et al.: Does increased detection account for the rising incidence of breast cancer? Am. J. Public Health, *81*:462, 1991.

Logan, W. W., Plansur, P. S., Cullinan, A., et al.: Increased incidence of breast carcinoma in patients with irradiation for postpartum mastitis: A screening situation. J. Surg. Oncol., *11*:239, 1979.

Lorenz, E.: Some biologic effects of long continued irradiation. Am. J. Roentgenol., *63*:176, 1950.

Lowell, D. M., Martineau, R. G., and Luria, S. B.: Carcinoma of the male breast following radiation: Report of a case occurring 35 years after radiation therapy of unilateral prepubertal gynecomastia. Cancer, *22*:581, 1968.

Lund, E.: Number of children and death from hormone dependent cancers. Int. J. Cancer., *46*:998, 1990.

Lynch, H. T., Harris, R. E., Organ, C. H. Jr., et al.: Management of familial breast cancer: I. Biostatistical genetic aspects and their limitations as derived from a familial breast cancer resource. Arch. Surg., *113*:1053, 1978.

Lynch, H. T., Albano, W. A., Danes, B. S., et al.: Genetic predisposition to breast cancer. Cancer, *53*:612, 1984.

Lynch, H. T., Albano, W. A., Organ, C. H. Jr., et al.: Surveillance and management of hereditary breast cancer. Breast, *7*:2, 1981.

Lynch, H. T., Watson, P., Conway, T. A., and Lynch, J. F.: Clinical/genetic features in hereditary breast cancer. Breast Cancer Res. Treat., *15*:63, 1990.

Lynch, H. T.: Genetics and Breast Cancer. New York, Van Nostrand Reinhold, 1981.

Mackenzie, I.: Breast cancer following multiple fluoroscopies. Br. J. Cancer, *19*:1, 1965.

Macklin, M. T.: Comparison of the number of breast cancer deaths observed in relatives of patients and the number expected on the basis of mortality rates. J. Natl. Cancer Inst., *22*:927, 1959.

MacMahon, B., Cole, P., and Brown, J.: Etiology of human breast cancer: A review. J. Natl. Cancer Inst., *50*:21, 1980.

Marchant, D. J.: Supplemental estrogen replacement. Cancer, *74*(Suppl):512–517, 1994.

Martin, J. A.: Treatment of cystic hygroma. Tex. J. Med., *50*:217–220, 1954.

Matanoski, G. M., Breysse, P. N., and Elliot, E. A.: Electromagnetic field exposure and male breast cancer. Lancet, *337*:737, 1991.

McPherson, K., and Doll, H.: Oestrogens and breast cancer: Exogenous hormones. Br. Med. Bull., *47*:484, 1990.

Mellemgaard, A., Ewertz, M., and Lynge, E.: The association between a risk of breast cancer and age at first pregnancy and parity in Maribo County, Denmark. Acta Oncol., *29*:705, 1990.

Mettler, F. A., Hempelmann, L. H., Outton, A. M., et al.: Breast neoplasms in women treated with x-rays for acute postpartum mastitis: A pilot study. J. Natl. Cancer Inst., *43*:803–811, 1969.

Miki, Y., Swensen, J., Shattuck-Eidens, D., et al.: A strong candidate for the breast and ovarian cancer susceptibility gene *BRCA1*. Science, *266*:66–71, 1994.

Miller, B. A., Feuer, E. J., and Hankey, B. F.: Recent incidence trends for breast cancer in women and the relevance of early detection: An update. C. A. Cancer J. Clin., *43*:27–41, 1993.

Miller, B. A., Feuer, E. J., and Hankey, B. F.: The increasing incidence of breast cancer since 1982: Relevance of early detection. Cancer Causes Control, *2*:67, 1991.

Miller, W. R.: Oestrogens and breast cancer: Biological considerations. Br. Med. Bull., *47*:470, 1990.

Minden, M. D., and Pawson, A. J.: Oncogenes. *In* Tannock, I.F., and Hill, R.P. (Eds.): The Basic Science of Oncology. 2nd ed. New York, McGraw-Hill, 1992, pp. 61–87.

Minton, J. P., and Dickey, R. P.: Levodopa test to predict response of carcinoma of the breast to surgical ablation of endocrine glands. Surg. Gynecol. Obstet., *136*:971, 1973.

Moore, D. H., Moore, D. H. II, and Moore, C. T.: Breast carcinoma etiological factors. Adv. Cancer Res. *40*:189, 1983.

Morgenstern, L., Gleischman, S. H., Michel, S. L., et al.: Relation of free silicone to human breast carcinoma. Arch. Surg., *120*:573, 1985.

Myrden, J. A., and Hiltz, J. E.: Breast cancer following multiple fluoroscopies during artificial pneumothorax treatment of pulmonary tuberculosis. Can. Med. Assoc. J., *100*:1032, 1969.

National Center for Health Statistics: Health, United States, 1991. Hyattsville, MD, Public Health Service, 1992.

Olsson, H., Moller, T. R., Ranstam, J., et al.: Early oral contraceptive use as a prognostic factor in breast cancer. Anticancer Res., *8*:29, 1988.

Ottman, R., King, M., Pike, M. C., et al.: Practical guide for estimating risk for familial breast cancer. Lancet, *ii*:556, 1983.

Paffenbarger, R. S. Jr., Fasal, E., Simmons, M. E., et al.: Cancer risk as related to use of oral contraceptives during fertile years. Report presented at the symposium on Cancer Epidemiology and the Clinician, Boston, MA, October 23–25, 1975.

Palca, J.: NIH unveils plan for women's health project. Science, *254*:792, 1991.

Peden, J. G. Jr.: Carcinoma of the breast following burn. Am. J. Surg., *73*:519, 1947.

Prince, M. M., and Hildreth, N. G.: The influence of potential biases on the risk of breast tumors among women who received radiotherapy for acute postpartum mastitis. J. Chron. Dis., *39*:553–560, 1986.

Pullinger, B. D.: Increase in mammary carcinoma and adenoma and incidences of other tumors in C_3HF females after oophorectomy and high dosages with some estrogens. Br. J. Cancer, *15*:574, 1961.

Reynolds, T.: Questions and answers: The *BRCA1* breast cancer susceptibility gene. Bethesda, MD, National Cancer Institute Office of Cancer Communications, National Institutes of Health, September 28, 1994.

Romieu, I., Berlin, J. A., and Colditz, G.: Oral contraceptives and breast cancer: Review and meta-analysis. Cancer, *66*:2253, 1990.

Rosenberg, L., Palmer, J. R., Kaufman, D. W., et al.: Breast cancer in relation to the occurrence and time of induced abortion. Am. J. Epidemiol., *127*:981, 1988.

Rosenblatt, K. A., Thomas, D. B., McTiernan, A., et al.: Breast cancer in men: Aspects of familial aggregation. J. Natl. Cancer Inst., *83*:849, 1991.

Ross, R. K, Gerkins, V. R., Paganini-Hill, A., et al.: Menopausal estrogen use and breast cancer. Cancer Treat. Res., *63*:1209, 1979.

Royal College of General Practitioners: Breast cancer and oral contraceptives: Findings of the Royal College of General Practitioners study. Br. Med. J., *282*:208, 1981.

Sasaki, G. H., Leung, B. S., and Fletcher, W. S.: Levodopa test and estrogen receptor assay in prognosticating response of patients with advanced cancer of the breast to endocrine therapy. Ann. Surg., *183*:341, 1976.

Sandison, A. T.: Autopsy study of the adult human breast. National Cancer Institute Monograph No. 8, U.S. Department of Health, Education and Welfare, 1962.

Schottenfield, D., Lilienfeld, A. M., and Diamond, H.: Some observations on the epidemiology of breast cancer among males. Am. J. Public Health, *53*:890, 1963.

Seidman, H., Silverberg, E., and Helleb, A.: Cancer Statistics, 1976: A Comparison of White and Black Populations. New York, American Cancer Society, 1976.

Seidman, H., Mushinski, M. H., Gelb, S. K., and Silverberg, E.: Probabilities of eventually developing or dying of cancer—United States 1985. Cancer, *35*:36–56, 1985.

Seidman, H., and Mushinski, M. H.: Breast cancer: Incidence, mortality, survival, and prognosis. *In* Feig, S. A., and McLelland, R. (Eds.): Breast Carcinoma—Current Diagnosis and Treatment. New York, Masson Publishing, 1983, p. 9.

Shapiro, S., Strax, P., Venet, L., et al.: The search for risk factors in breast cancer. Am. J. Public Health, *58*:820, 1968.

Shimkin, M. B.: Epidemiology of breast cancer in recent results of cancer research. New York, Springer-Verlag, 1973, p. 6.

Shimizu, Y., Kato, H., Schull, W. J., et al.: Studies of the mortality of A-bomb survivors. 9. Mortality, 1950–1985: Part 1. Comparison of risk coefficients for site-specific cancer mortality based on the DS86 and T65DR shielded kerma and organ doses. Radiat. Res., *118*:502–524, 1989.

Shimizu, Y., Kato, H., and Schull, W. J.: Studies of the mortality of A-bomb survivors. 9. Mortality, 1950–1985: Part 2. Cancer mortality based on the recently revised doses (DS86). Radiat. Res., *121*:120–141, 1990.

Shore, R. E., Hempelmann, L. H., Kowaluk, E., et al.: Breast neoplasms in women treated with x-rays for acute postpartum mastitis. J. Natl. Cancer Inst., *59*:813–822, 1977.

Shore, R. E., Hildreth, N., Woodard, E., et al.: Breast cancer among women given x-ray therapy for acute postpartum mastitis. J. Natl. Cancer Inst., *77*:689–696, 1986.

Siskind, V., Schofield, F., Rice, D., and Bain, C.: Breast cancer and breast feeding: Results from an Australian case-control study. Am. J. Epidemiol., *130*:119–236, 1989.

Spratt, J. S., Alagia, D. P., Greenberg, R. A., et al.: Association of chronic cystic mastopathy, xeromammographic patterns and cancer. Cancer, *55*:1372, 1985.

Spratt, J. S., Chang, A. F.-C., Heuser, L. S., et al.: Acute carcinoma of the breast. Cancer, *157*:220, 1983.

Spratt, J. S., Greenberg, R. A., Kuhns, J. G., and Amin, E. A.: Breast cancer risk: A review of definitions and assessments of risk. J. Surg. Oncol., *41*:42, 1989.

Steel, M., Thomson, A., and Clayton, J.: Genetic aspects of breast cancer. Br. Med. Bull., *47*:504, 1991.

Steinberg, K. K., Thacker, S. B., Smith, S. J., et al.: A meta analysis of the effect of estrogen replacement therapy on the risk of breast cancer. J.A.M.A., *265*:1985, 1991.

Swift, M., Morrell, D., Massey, R. B., and Chase, C. L.: Incidence of cancer in 161 families affected by ataxia-talengiectasia. N. Engl. J. Med., *325*:1831, 1991.

Symmers, W.: Carcinoma of breast in transsexual individuals after surgical and hormonal interference with primary and secondary sex characteristics. Br. Med. J., *2*:83, 1968.

Tannock, I. F., and Hill, R. P. (Eds.): The Basic Science of Oncology. 2nd ed. New York, McGraw-Hill, 1992.

Tokuoka, S., Asano, M., Yamamoto, T., et al.: Histologic review of breast cancer cases in survivors of atomic bombs in Hiroshima and Nagasaki, Japan. Cancer, *54*:849, 1984.

Tokunaga, M., Land, C. E., Yamamoto, T., et al.: Incidence of female breast cancer among atomic bomb survivors, Hiroshima and Nagasaki, 1950–1980. Radiat. Res., *112*:243–272, 1987.

Tokunaga, M., Toduoka, S., and Land, C. E.: Breast cancer in atomic bomb survivors. Jpn. J. Cancer Res. Monograph No. 32, 1986, pp. 167–177.

Tretli, S., and Haldorsen, T.: A cohort analysis of breast cancer, uterine corpus cancer, and childbearing pattern in Norwegian women. J. Epidemiol. Community Health, *44*:215, 1990.

Turner, C. W., and Gomez, E. T.: The radiosensitivity of the cells of the mammary gland. Am. J. Roentgenol., *36*:79, 1936.

Underwood, G. B., and Gaul, L. E.: Disfiguring sequelae from radium therapy: Results of treatment of birthmark adjacent to breast in female infant. Arch. Dermatol. & Syph., *57*:918, 1948.

UNSCEAR (United Nations Scientific Committee on the Effects of Atomic Radiation): 1986 Report to the General Assembly, Annex B. Dose-response relationships for radiation-induced cancer. New York, United Nations, 1986 and 1988.

UNSCEAR (United Nations Scientific Committee on the Effects of Atomic Radiation): Sources, effects and risks of ionizing radiation. 1988 Report to the General Assembly, with Annexes. New York, United Nations, 1988.

Vessey, M. P., Doll, R., and Sutton, P. M.: Investigation of the possible relationship between oral contraceptives and benign and malignant breast disease. Cancer, *28*:1395, 1971.

Villee, C. A., and Hagerman, D. D.: Compounds with antiestrogenic activity in vivo. Endocrinology, *60*:552, 1957.

Wanebo, C. K., Johnson, K. G., Sato, K., et al.: Breast cancer after exposure to the atomic bombings of Hiroshima and Nagasaki. N. Engl. J. Med., *279*:667, 1968.

Wells, B. L., and Horm, J. W.: Stage in diagnosis in breast cancer: Race and socioeconomic factors. Am. J. Public Health, *82*:1383, 1992.

Willard, W., Borgen, P., Bol, R., et al.: Cowden's disease: A case report with analyses at the molecular level. Cancer, *69*:2969, 1992.

Wilson, R. G., Buchan, R., Roberts, M. M., et al.: Prolactin and breast cancer. Proc. R. Soc. Med., *66*:865, 1973.

Wynder, E. L., Kajatani, T., and Kuno, J.: Comparison of survival between American and Japanese patients with breast cancer. Surg. Gynecol. Obstet., *117*:196, 1976.

Zumoff, B., Fishman, J., Bradlow, H. L., et al.: Hormone profiles in hormone-dependent cancers. Cancer Res., *35*:3365, 1975.

9

Prevention of Breast Cancer

Richard R. Love
Polly A. Newcomb

While LaCassagne, in 1936, had the prescience to envision the day when an intervention would "prevent ... the congestion of oestrone in the breast" (LaCassagne, 1936), it is only during the last decade that primary prevention of human breast cancer has been discussed as a practical possibility and only currently that the first breast cancer prevention clinical trials are in their early stages. Apparent continuing increases in the incidence of breast cancer have added an urgency to investigations of prevention. Primary prevention entails prevention of clinically recognized breast cancer—that is, a reduction in the incidence of diagnosed cases of invasive disease. This may be achieved by preventing disease from ever beginning or by suppression or fostering regression of "preclinical" disease. As is discussed here, prospects for prevention through the latter process—modification of promotion—seem more promising. Although preventive interventions may act also to reduce the occurrence of noninvasive breast cancers and other presumed obligate precursor conditions for invasive breast cancer, the focus of attention here is on prevention of invasive cancers. Considerable attention is being directed toward prevention of excess morbidity and mortality from breast cancer by increasing use of early detection or screening tests, particularly mammography, in postmenopausal women. This so-called secondary prevention is not the subject of this chapter. Animal models and experimental data are not addressed. The goal of this chapter is to define some rational approaches for individuals.

DEFINITIONS AND MODELS OF BREAST CANCER

Although there is a wealth of epidemiologic data on breast cancer, currently these data appear fragmented to many investigators because they do not appear to fit well together in a rational model of development of breast cancer. Current models are incomplete or do not explain some identified risk factors. For example, it is evident that ovarian function is important in breast cancer development, but which hormones are most critical, and in particular, what the effects of progestogens are on the breast, are unknown. Additionally, too little is known about the multisystem effects of hormones at different times in a woman's life. Finally, the preponderance of breast cancers occur in women without attributable risk factors (Seidman et al., 1982). Nevertheless, some models are well enough substantiated to provide bases for testing of interventions, and

some practical interventions worthy of evaluation on multiple grounds are available.

Certain important and evolving concepts in cancer biology form the scientific basis for breast cancer prevention. First, the development of malignancies is characterized by step-by-step progression. Although a well-developed model of the steps in breast cancer is not yet available, the recent creation of experimental and data-supported models for other common cancers (e.g., colorectal cancer) strongly suggest that such a framework is applicable to breast cancer (Vogelstein et al., 1988). A second idea is that cancers take many years to evolve to an invasive process. For breast cancer, this concept is best supported by data showing that radiation exposure is associated with an increase in invasive disease 10 to 15 years later (Tokunaga et al., 1987). A third concept is that during a prolonged period in cancer development, the process is reversible. The dramatic reduction in incidence of tobacco-related cancers following smoking cessation illustrates the reversibility of this promotional phase in cancer development. Finally, the development of cancers is a multiple-factor process: both host and environmental exposure factors are critical, but most significantly more than one of each usually appears to play important roles.

These concepts are critical to the emerging picture of cancers as chronic processes before, as well as after, their usual clinical diagnosis. Acute disease models under which many biologic processes are categorized, have single, rapidly acting, irreversible causes. Prevention of pneumococcal pneumonia by vaccination is a logical, highly efficacious strategy for one such acute disease. The characteristics of preclinical chronic diseases present both challenges and unique opportunities for prevention, both at the biologic level and in the clinical practice of preventive medicine.

INTERVENTIONS

Despite an absence of complete models that embrace all risk factors for breast cancer development, several interventions likely to prevent clinical breast cancer are defined and others are under evaluation. In this discussion, we have grouped some specific risk factors under general mechanisms and consider these according to the phase of cancer development in which they are likely to operate (Tables 9–1, 9–2, and 9–3).

Table 9-1. INITIATING PHASE FACTORS IMPORTANT IN DEVELOPMENT OF BREAST CANCER, AND POSSIBLE ASSOCIATED ACTIONS TO PREVENT INVASIVE DISEASE

Factor	Possible Preventive Action
Genetic constitution*	Modification of gene function
Breast irradiation†	Avoidance, particularly in young, possibly susceptible women‡
Cigarette smoking, active or passive§	Avoidance, particularly in adolescence‖
Each of the above and other unknowns	Early first full-term pregnancy or pseudopregnancy to render quiescent proliferating cells of breast¶

*Ottman, 1990.
†Tokunaga et al., 1984; Tokunaga et al., 1987; and Committee on the Biological Effects of Ionizing Radiations, 1990.
‡Swift et al., 1991.
§Hirayama, 1988.
‖Palmer et al., 1991.
¶Ciocca et al., 1982; and Key and Pike, 1988.

Prevention of Initiation

For breast cancer, this phase of cancer development is the least understood but most readily observed in familial aggregations (see Table 9–1). Because of the clustering of breast cancers in some families, affecting multiple individuals in successive generations, usually at early ages and occasionally bilaterally, it is widely believed that familial breast cancer is a proxy for genetic susceptibility (Ottman, 1990). Intensive efforts are ongoing in search of a gene or genes that may predispose women to breast cancer. Recent evidence linking early breast cancer to a marker on the long arm of chromosome 17 (Hall et al., 1990; and Narod et al., 1991), as well as findings regarding the p53 gene on the short arm of chromosome 17, suggest that a gene or genes predisposing to breast cancer may soon be found (Maklin et al., 1990). Identification of the specific genetic change in some individuals and families will allow for careful study of the critical gene. It is possible that preventive actions discussed here, may in other contexts also be directed at modifying consequences of genetic changes. Most cases of breast cancer, however, do not fit readily into the profile of families carrying an autosomal dominant allele.

The strongest evidence for a particular initiating factor in breast cancer is that for irradiation (Tokunaga et al., 1984 and 1987; Committee on the Biological Effects of Ionizing Radiations, 1990). The practical conclusion is that breast irradiation should be avoided, particularly by young women and children. In the past chest radiation was given as treatment for thymus enlargement, acne, and asthma. The difficulty is in knowing how much to be concerned about low-dose diagnostic exposures. With mammography, the best estimate of risk to women exposed after age 20 is 6.6 excess cancers per million woman-years per centigray (Boyce et al., 1979). The uncertainty is accentuated by the studies of families with ataxia-telangiectasia. Heterozygotes for this genetic disorder, apparently otherwise normal, have increased risk for breast cancer and may constitute 9% to

18% of all persons with breast cancer in the United States (Swift et al., 1986; Barresen et al., 1990; and Swift et al., 1991). The ataxia telangiectasia gene is associated with increased sensitivity to ionizing radiation; it is estimated that heterozygotes for this gene constitute 1.4% of the American population (Swift et al., 1986). In a study by Swift and associates, heterozygotes for the ataxia telangiectasia gene were found to be at greater risk for breast cancer if they had diagnostic or therapeutic radiation to the chest (Swift et al., 1991). This result and the demonstration of a two-fold increase in breast cancer in women exposed during scalp radiotherapy have led to a vigorous debate about study methods and consistency of observations in studies of low-dose radiation effects (Modan et al., 1989; and Correspondents, 1992). This debate is not germane for women older than 50 years of age for whom screening mammography is of certain benefit (Screening for breast cancer, 1989). For younger women, however, further rigorous studies are needed. Whether other familial and chromosome breakage syndromes, which occur with frequencies similar to that of ataxia telangiectasia in the American population, are also associated with radiation sensitivity is unknown at present.

Evidence that other carcinogens initiate breast cancer development is extremely limited. A suspected initiator of breast cancer is cigarette smoking, either active or passive. Here the evidence is weak, but the hypothesis is rational and appealing and data from Hirayama cannot be ignored (Hirayama, 1988). Although data are not consistent, this relationship may reflect an unstable balance between opposing direct (carcinogenic) and indirect (hormonal) effects (Rohan et al., 1989). Palmer and associates have presented data supporting the hypothesis that smoking during adolescence may increase breast cancer risk (Palmer et al., 1991). Adolescent cigarette smoking may offer a credible explanation for some increase in breast cancer. Clearly, if this hypothesis is supported by further evidence, particular attention to smoking in young women is needed.

Any initiating factor may have a greater chance of causing a breast cancer to develop if the number of target cells in the breast at the time of exposure is also greater. There is ample evidence that hormonal effects mediate sensitivity to breast radiation carcinogenesis (Tokunaga et al., 1984; and Committee on the Biological Effects of Ionizing Radiations, 1990). An epidemiologic observation is that early first full-term pregnancy in humans or pseudopregnancy, evaluated in elegant animal experiments (Key et al., 1988), protects against breast cancer. This appears to be a result of the fact that these events render quiescent the proliferating cells of the breast (Ciocca et al., 1982). These observations suggest that hormonal intervention to cause pseudopregnancy would have a preventive effect.

Prevention or Modification of Promotion

The prolonged and reversible promotional phase of cancer development is an optimal target for breast cancer prevention (see Table 9–2). A well-supported general conclusion is that since the longer the time of regular ovulation and

Table 9–2. PROMOTION PHASE FACTORS IMPORTANT IN DEVELOPMENT OF BREAST CANCER, AND POSSIBLE PREVENTIVE ACTIONS

Factor	Possible Preventive Action
Prolonged duration of ovulation (Key and Pike, 1988)	Delay of onset of menarche • Avoidance of overnutrition (?) (Frisch and McArthur, 1974) • Increase physical activity (Bernstein et al., 1992)
	Initiate menopause at earlier age • Surgical or radiation oophorectomy (Trichopoulos et al., 1968) • Hormonal oophorectomy with luteinizing hormone–releasing hormone agonist treatment (Pike et al., 1989; and Bernstein et al., 1992)
	Prolong total lifetime duration of lactation (Luan et al., 1988)
Hormone exposure (Key and Pike, 1988)	Modification of estrogen metabolism • Increase physical activity (Bernstein et al., 1992) • Weight loss (Grodin et al., 1973) • Low-fat diet (Prentice et al., 1990) • Pharmacologic modification (Michnovicz and Bradlow, 1990)
	Abolition of ovarian activity (premenopausal women) • Oral contraceptive use (Pike et al., 1983)
	Hormone replacement therapy (postmenopausal women) • Proscription (Bergvist et al., 1989; Mills et al., 1989; Colditz et al., 1990; and Hulka, 1990) • Prescription: antiestrogens, progestogens
Ornithine decarboxylase induction (Boutwell, 1974)	Suppression of ornithine decarboxylase induction with • Specific inhibitors, such as difluoromethyl ornithine (Thompson et al., 1984) • Retinoid (Verna, 1992)
Growth factor exposure (McCarty, 1989)	Manipulation of breast growth factor effects
Uncertain	Modify exposures to: • Alcohol (Longnecker et al., 1988) • Vitamin A and its analogues (Katsouyanni et al., 1988) • Other vitamins (Wlad et al., 1984) • Selenium (Schamberger et al., 1976) • Limonene (Elegbede et al., 1984) • Exogenous food estrogens, such as soy (Messina and Barnes, 1991)

menstrual cycling the greater the risk of breast cancer (Key et al., 1988), a reduced lifetime exposure to ovarian hormones will decrease risk. Delaying the onset of menarche or causing menopause to occur earlier should be associated

Table 9–3. PROGRESSION PHASE FACTORS IMPORTANT IN THE DEVELOPMENT OF BREAST CANCER, AND POSSIBLE ACTIONS TO PREVENT INVASIVE DISEASE

Factor	Preventive Action
Tumor clinical growth*	Treatment with cytostatic agent • Antiestrogen†,‡ • Retinoid§
Absence of tumor cell differentiation§	Treatment with differentiating agent • Retinoid ‖, ¶

*Moolgavkar and Knudson, 1981.
†Love, 1990a.
‡Nayfield et al., 1991.
§Astrup and Paulsen, 1982.
‖Moon et al., 1976.
¶Moon et al., 1977.

with a lowered risk (MacMahon et al., 1982). Age at menarche is related to the balance between energy intake and energy expenditure (Frisch et al., 1974). Means for delaying menarche are poorly defined and understood. Avoidance of overnutrition in preadolescence is one strategy, but this risks caloric restriction with attendant harmful effects on growth. Increased physical activity in adolescence may also be effective, but untoward consequences are also possible and inadequately studied (Bernstein et al., 1992). Each of these interventions, however, deserves careful study because of its practical character.

For many years it has been known that surgical or radiation oophorectomy is associated with subsequent decreased risk of breast cancer (Trichopoulos et al., 1968). Apart from the lifestyle and fiscal costs, the adverse consequences for the cardiovascular and skeletal systems have discouraged this intervention (Ettinger et al., 1985; Stampfer et al., 1985). It is possible that the reduced risk of breast cancer with oophorectomy persists despite hormone replacement therapy to prevent the cardiovascular and skeletal problems (Weiss et al., 1980; Stampfer et al., 1991). Pike and Bernstein advocated hormonal oophorectomy with a luteinizing hormone-releasing hormone agonist and low-dose estrogen hormone replacement therapy as a rational approach to breast cancer prevention. This follows logically from epidemiologic observations (Pike et al., 1989; and Bernstein et al., 1992).

An additional method for decreasing the total cumulative number of regular ovulatory cycles is to prolong the duration of lactation (which delays the re-establishment of ovulation). The effect of lactation may be mediated, however, through changes in prolactin levels or through physical changes in the breasts (Musey et al., 1987). Long total lifetime lactation periods are unusual in Western countries. For some years lactation has been uncommon, numbers of children are small, and study of this factor has been constrained. In Asian populations, however, the opposites are true and a protective effect has been demonstrated (Luan et al., 1988).

More specific strategies to alter hormone exposure of the breasts are known. A variety of interventions modify estrogen metabolism. Increased physical activity can suppress ovarian activity and disrupt menstrual cycling (Bernstein et al., 1992). Major weight loss, particularly in obese postmenopausal women, may reverse the peripheral fat metabolism of androgens to estrogens and modestly reduce the risk of obese women (Grodin et al., 1973). This effect may be limited to women with a specific "apple" distribution of body fat (a high waist : hip ratio) (Folsom et al., 1990). The effect of this type of obesity appears to be greatest in women with a family history of breast cancer; thus these women might benefit from weight reduction (Sellers et al., 1992). Some direct evidence does suggest that a low-fat diet lowers estrogen (Prentice et al., 1990) and is adequate to explain the differences in Western and Asian rates of breast cancer (Prentice et al., 1989). However, large population-based studies have been remarkably consistent in failing to provide evidence of a positive association between dietary lipid intake and breast cancer risk (Willet et al., 1991). Finally, detailed studies of estrogen metabolism suggest ways of intervening pharmacologically to achieve alteration in hormone levels that may be protective (Michnovicz et al., 1990).

Another method of limiting the total duration of normal ovarian activity is through use of oral contraceptives (OCs). To date OCs have not been shown to either increase or decrease risk of breast cancer, although there is a suggestion of increased risk in younger long-term users. The ability of OCs to suppress ovarian activity and the ability of some OC hormones to decrease breast mitotic activity suggests that an OC could be developed that decreases breast cancer risk (Pike et al., 1983).

Strategies to limit or alter breast hormonal exposure are more immediately applicable and relevant for postmenopausal women, who have more preclinical tumors later in promotion. The preponderance of evidence suggests that there is a modestly increased risk associated with estrogen hormone replacement therapy (HRT) and possibly a greater risk associated with combination replacement therapy (Berquist et al., 1989; Mills et al., 1989; Colditz et al., 1990; and Hulka, 1990). Two findings from the Nurses' Health Study are particularly noteworthy. First, there appears to be a risk-increasing interactive effect of hormone replacement therapy with alcohol, and second, the risk associated with

HRT disappears rapidly with cessation of therapy (Colditz et al., 1990). Nonetheless, the protection that HRT provides against heart disease and osteoporosis is believed to outweigh any risks.

A national randomized intervention study of hormone replacement therapies is under discussion. Such a study is necessary to resolve questions concerning risks and benefits of different hormone replacement therapies.

The pioneering studies of Boutwell suggested that the enzyme ornithine decarboxylase (ODC) is an appropriate target for modification of promotion (Boutwell, 1974). This enzyme catalyzes the synthesis of putrescine from ornithine, which is the first and rate-controlling step in the synthesis of polyamines (Pegg et al., 1982). The precise cellular functions of polyamines are incompletely understood, but they play a major role in growth regulation (Pegg, 1986). Suppression of ODC may be integral to reversing tumor promotion. In animals, specific irreversible inhibitors of ODC, such as difluoromethyl ornithine (DFMO), are potent inhibitors of mammary tumor development (Thompson et al., 1984). While of limited efficacy in the treatment of established breast tumors, DFMO given at a dose that exhibits no discernible toxicity in humans can inhibit the inducting effects of ODC on the skin (Love et al., 1993) and at slightly higher doses suppress the effects of polyamines on rectal mucosa (Boyle et al., 1992). Other ODC-suppressing agents such as retinoids and nonsteroidal anti-inflammatory drugs may also have potential (Verma, 1992). At present, a study of 4-hydroxyphenylretinamide (4HPR) for prevention of second primary breast cancer is completing accrual in Italy.

Growth factors other than polyamines (e.g., transforming growth factors α and β) are of interest in breast cancer research (McCarty, 1989). Manipulation of the local effects of these proteins, through a variety of means, holds promise for both therapy and prevention. A number of exposures may act to promote breast cancer through mechanisms that are poorly defined (see Table 9–2). Moderate alcohol consumption has the most consistent and modifiable relationship to increased risk (Longnecker et al., 1988). For none of these is there yet adequate data to provide the basis for rational interventions.

Prevention or Modification of Progression

Any cytostatic therapy will prevent production of tumor cells that have acquired the properties of progression (Moolgaukar et al., 1981) (see Table 9–3). Through a variety of mechanisms tamoxifen and retinoids appear to act as anti-proliferative agents (Moon et al., 1976 and 1977; and Astrup et al., 1982). Certain retinoids are particularly intriguing because they appear to control differentiation (Moo et al., 1979); the optimum timing for retinoids may be in the progression or the immediate preprogression phase. In an animal model, the combination of retinoid and tamoxifen (antiestrogen) is a very potent preventive measure for mammary cancer (McCormick et al., 1986).

Tamoxifen

The first clinical trials of breast cancer prevention are testing the hypothesis that the synthetic antiestrogen, tamoxifen, can reduce the incidence of invasive breast cancer in healthy women. Since the suggestions by Gazet and Cuzick that the biologic rationale for prevention with tamoxifen was adequately developed (Gazet, 1985; and Cuzick et al., 1986), considerable attention has been given to toxicities of tamoxifen and, more recently, to designing and conducting a prevention trial (Costa et al., 1990; and Love, 1990a). Major differences exist between cancer prevention and treatment trials. In treatment trials, toxicity is secondary because the primary goal, which is important to *all* patients, is cure. In prevention trials, only a few "patients"—actually healthy subjects—will benefit if the treatment is successful, whereas the majority are affected by toxicity. Of critical importance in prevention trials are population size, which is usually much greater than in treatment trials, and subject compliance over a long period. These are of limited concern with highly motivated patients in treatment trials, which are usually of limited duration.

Reviews are available pertaining to the use of tamoxifen to prevent breast cancer, particularly emphasizing the biologic rationale. Here will be highlighted details of major clinical importance in the use of tamoxifen as a preventive measure (Jordan, 1990; Kiang, 1991; Love, 1991a; and Nayfield et al., 1991).

Tamoxifen Pharmacology and Mechanisms of Action (Jordan, 1984; Jordan et al., 1990). After oral administration, maximal blood levels of tamoxifen are reached in 4 to 7 hours, which appears to coincide with the time of maximal vasomotor side effects in some patients. A steady state of drug levels in the blood is achieved after daily administration for 4 weeks, and it takes 6 to 8 weeks for all serologic evidence of drug and metabolites to disappear. This presents an important problem in premenopausal women who become pregnant, because if tamoxifen is a human teratogen, the fetus is likely to receive continuous exposure to the drug during the entire first trimester, even if the drug is stopped as soon as pregnancy is recognized. Tamoxifen is metabolized by the liver, excreted in bile, and eliminated from the body in the feces.

The major cellular effects of tamoxifen are shown in Figure 9–1. Tamoxifen is predominantly a tumorstatic agent (as opposed to a tumoricidal agent) and thus, to derive maximal benefit, prolonged therapy is optimal. This concept is supported by data from meta-analysis of adjuvant therapy trials with tamoxifen (Early Breast Cancer Trialists' Collaborative Group, 1992). A prolonged effect clinically is seen with therapy of 2 years' duration (Baum et al., 1988), and a modeling study suggests that even therapy of limited duration might have prolonged benefits (Trock, 1991). Tamoxifen doubles levels of sex hormone–binding globulin (SHBG) and may therefore exert its antiestrogen effects by making it unavailable to breast cancer cells (see Fig. 9–1) (Love et al., 1990a). The major mechanism of action, however, is thought to be the combination of tamoxifen with nuclear estrogen receptor protein (ERP), which produces a G1 block (see Fig. 9–1). Decreased production of growth-stimulating proteins, such as transforming

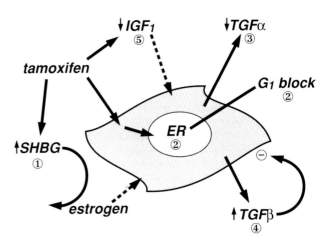

Figure 9–1. Major effects of tamoxifen on breast cancer cells. SHBG = sex hormone–binding globulin; ER = estrogen receptor; TGFα = transforming growth factor alpha; TGFβ = transforming growth factor beta; IGF₁ = insulin-like growth factor 1.

growth factor (TGF)-alpha, and stimulation of growth-inhibiting proteins like TGF-beta (which may be through an effect on stromal cells) may be the main consequence of combining with ERP (see Fig. 9–1). These changes in cell regulatory proteins may explain the favorable effects of tamoxifen on women with ERP-negative tumors (Early Breast Cancer Trialists' Collaborative Group, 1992). Biologic effects of tamoxifen on the immune system and consequent to binding to cytoplasmic antiestrogen binding sites are not well understood. The reductions in insulin-like growth factor (IGF₁) seen with tamoxifen therapy (Pollak, 1990) are presumably a hepatic effect (see Fig. 9–1).

The hormonal pharmacology of tamoxifen is complex. Species-specific differences prevent extrapolation of hormonal effects in animals to humans (Jordan, 1990). Changes in hormones seen in humans are summarized in Table 9–4. The most important are the observations in premenopausal women. Increases in circulating estrogen and progesterone levels are seen in healthy women who are given tamoxifen to treat their infertility (Groom et al., 1976; and Senior et al., 1978). Similar changes are seen in women treated for breast cancer as is enlargement of the ovaries (Jordan et al., 1991). The consequences of these changes are unknown.

Most data on clinical effects of tamoxifen are from studies using a dose of 10 mg bid or 20 mg/d (Early Breast Cancer Trialists' Collaborative Group, 1992). Whether toxicities are greater with the 30 and 40 mg/d doses used in some studies, or are less with a lower dose is unknown.

Animal carcinogenicity experiments with tamoxifen are remarkable in three respects. First, significant suppression of tumors occurs when tamoxifen is given continuously after exposure to a mammary carcinogen such as dimethylbenz[a]anthracine (DMBA) (Jordan, 1976; and Gottardis et al., 1987). Second, if tamoxifen is stopped, most of the animals develop the expected tumors. Third, tumors that develop during tamoxifen treatment are hormone independent, aggressive malignancies that are resistant to treatment (Fendl, 1992).

Clinical Effects of Tamoxifen Important in Preven-

Table 9-4. HORMONAL EFFECTS OF TAMOXIFEN IN PREMENOPAUSAL AND POSTMENOPAUSAL WOMEN

Hormone	Premenopausal Levels*	Postmenopausal Levels†
Total estrogens	Large increases in some women	No change
Estradiol	Large increases in some women	No change
Follicle-stimulating hormone	No changes	Decreases
Luteinizing hormone	No changes	Decreases
Progesterone	Increases in some women	No change
Prolactin	No change	No change

*Groom and Griffiths, 1976.
†Jordan, 1990.

tion. The preponderance of data about tamoxifen have come from adjuvant treatment trials mostly in postmenopausal women (Early Breast Cancer Trialists' Collaborative Group, 1992). These data show that tamoxifen has a greater beneficial effect on postmenopausal women than on premenopausal women, an observation consistent with laboratory studies suggesting that the drug works most effectively in a low estrogen environment (Gibson et al., 1990). The most persuasive case for prevention of preclinical breast cancer by tamoxifen is made by the data from trials that show reductions of contralateral breast cancers by 40% (Table 9–5). Consistent with laboratory data is the evidence that longer therapy is more effective (Early Breast Cancer Trialists' Collaborative Group; and Fisher et al., 1989). It may be critical that these data are mostly from studies in postmenopausal women. The Cancer Research Campaign (CRC) data show an *increased* frequency of contralateral breast cancer in premenopausal women after tamoxifen therapy was stopped (Baum, in press). It should be noted that the demonstration of these contralateral cancers has been retrospective, and while the data are from randomized trials, biases may have operated to produce the findings (see Table 9–4). Similar to the findings in animals (Fendl, 1992), one study team reported that the frequency of hormone receptor-positive, contralateral tumors was lower than expected (Rutqvist et al., 1991).

In considering the clinical effects of tamoxifen, it should be kept in mind that tamoxifen is target site–specific in its actions, having antiestrogenic effects in some tissues, estrogen effects in others, and sometimes different effects in the same tissues of the same groups of women (Jordan, 1990). For example, estrogenic and antiestrogenic effects of tamoxifen on vaginal epithelium are seen clinically in postmenopausal women. Second, most of the data on clinical effects of tamoxifen have been obtained in adjuvant therapy trials, in which concerns have been to prevent life-threatening disease. The way the data were obtained may significantly influence what data were developed and their interpretation. Low frequency adverse effects of major concern in a healthy population may not be fully appreciated in therapy-related trials.

Effects of tamoxifen that are important when considering its use as a preventive measure are summarized in Table 9–6. Comprehensive data are for postmenopausal women

Table 9-5. CONTRALATERAL BREAST CANCERS IN CONTROLLED CLINICAL TRIALS WITH ADJUVANT TAMOXIFEN THERAPY*

Clinical Trial	No. of Contralateral Breast Cancers	
	With Tamoxifen	**Controls**
CRC†	13 Premenopausal	8
	8 Postmenopausal	16
NATO‡	11	21
Scottish§	9	12
Stockholm‖	18	32
NSABPB14¶	13	29
Meta-analysis**	122	184

*There are comparable numbers of women at risk in each group in each trial.
†Baum (in press).
‡Baum et al., 1988.
§Breast Cancer Trials Committee, 1987.
‖Fornander et al., 1989.
¶Fisher et al., 1989.
**Early Breast Cancer Trialists' Collaborative Group, 1992.

Table 9-6. MAJOR EFFECTS OF TAMOXIFEN RELEVANT TO ITS USE AS A PREVENTIVE AGENT IN POSTMENOPAUSAL WOMEN

Changes in cardiovascular disease risk factors	↓ total cholesterol 12%* ↓ low-density lipoprotein cholesterol 20%* ↓ fibrinogen 15%† Blood pressure, glucose level, weight: no change*
Cardiovascular deaths in adjuvant trials	↓ 27‡
Change in osteoporosis risk factors	↑ bone mineral density in lumbar spine (with likely decreased risk for osteoporotic fracture)§
Incidence of thrombophlebitis	↑ by 1/800 woman treatment years ‖
Incidence of endometrial cancer	↑ ¶
Incidence of ovarian cancer	↓ ?¶
Incidence of hepatocellular cancer	? **
Incidence of depression	↑ by 1–5%¶
Incidence of retinal and other eye changes	↑ ?††
Vasomotor and gynecologic symptoms	↑ significantly in 50% of treated women‡‡

*Love et al., 1991b.
†Love et al., 1992a.
‡Early Breast Cancer Trialists' Collaborative Group, 1992.
§Love et al., 1992b.
‖Fisher et al., 1989.
¶Nayfield et al., 1991.
**Rutqvist et al., 1991.
††Longstaff et al., 1989.
‡‡Love et al., 1991c.

only. The likelihood of each and the fraction of healthy treated women who might be affected deserve careful consideration. After 60 years of age coronary heart disease becomes the most frequent cause of death in women. In postmenopausal women tamoxifen lowers lipids, lipoproteins, and fibrinogen, and has no effect on blood pressure, glucose metabolism, or weight (Love et al., 1991*b* and 1992*a*) (Fig. 9–2). The effect of tamoxifen on high-density lipoprotein (HDL) cholesterol is uncertain. Data from cholesterol-lowering trials in men suggest that a decrease in cardiovascular events of 20% to 30% might follow the changes produced by tamoxifen (Love, 1991*b*). Meta-analysis of adjuvant trials suggests a 27% decrease in cardiovascular deaths (Early Breast Cancer Trialists' Collaborative Group, 1992). In one careful study an even greater reduction of myocardial infarction was found (McDonald et al., 1991).

In castrated female rats tamoxifen has a bone-preserving effect, whereas in intact rats it has the opposite effect (Kalu et al., 1991). Data are available that show preservation of bone mineral density in the lumbar spine of postmenopausal women (Love et al., 1992*b*) (Fig. 9–3). This might also be expected in the hip, the most frequent fracture site in women.

Small increases in thrombophlebitis and pulmonary embolism have now been confirmed in one adjuvant study (Fisher et al., 1989). The mechanism for this is unknown; decreases in antithrombin III do occur with tamoxifen therapy, but decreases in fibrinogen and platelet numbers also occur (Love et al., 1992*a*).

Although definitive data are not yet available, it does appear that the incidence of endometrial cancer is increased with long-term tamoxifen therapy (Nayfield et al., 1991). High dose and previous estrogen therapy may be additional risk factors (NSABP Protocol Pl, 1992). In a proposed Italian chemoprevention study, concern about this has been great enough that a hysterectomy is a requirement for participation. Detailed data concerning the frequency, stage, and grade of endometrial cancers associated with tamoxifen are awaited. The role of endometrial sampling for monitoring women is poorly defined. As a result of the reduction of gonadotropins in postmenopausal women on tamoxifen treatment (see Table 9–3), a reduction in ovarian malignancies has been suggested (Nayfield et al., 1991).

Animal data have raised concern about the possibility of hepatocellular malignancy due to tamoxifen (Jordan, 1990; and Nayfield et al., 1991). Careful animal studies suggest that tamoxifen, like other steroid hormones, is a weak promoter of hepatocellular tumors, and at the usual doses does not exceed a threshold for promotion in humans (Maltoni et al., 1988; and Dragan et al., 1991). One adjuvant trial has reported liver cancers in 2 treated patients out of 931 (Rutquist et al., 1991). No other clinical reports of liver cancers are available, although concern has been raised that some lesions in the liver may be attributed incorrectly to metastatic breast cancer.

Depression was associated with tamoxifen treatment in the NATO Adjuvant and Wisconsin Tamoxifen toxicity studies (Baum et al., 1988; Love et al., 1991*c*). Failure to measure depression and an assumption that depression was consequent to the disease may be responsible for missing this problem in other studies.

Amphophilic compounds like tamoxifen might be expected to have an effect on the retina, and higher than usual doses of tamoxifen have produced a spectrum of eye changes apparently as a result of treatment (Kaiser-Kupfer et al., 1978). However, it appears that at recommended doses ocular toxicity, if a real occurrence at all, must occur at low frequency (Longstaff et al., 1989).

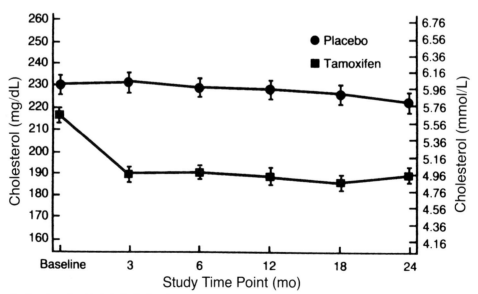

Figure 9–2. Mean fasting levels of total cholesterol over time in patients receiving tamoxifen or placebo. ● = Control patients; *n* = 70 at baseline, and *n* = 70, 68, 67, 64, and 62 patients at 3, 6, 12, 18, and 24 months, respectively. ■ = Patients receiving tamoxifen; *n* = 70 at baseline, and *n* = 66, 66, 65, 64, and 64 patients at 3, 6, 12, 18, and 24 months, respectively. *Bars* indicate 95% confidence intervals (CIs). Cholesterol levels decreased significantly at all time points in patients receiving tamoxifen ($P <$ 0.001). (From Love, R. R., Wiebe, D. A., Newcomb, P. A.: Effects of tamoxifen on cardiovascular risk factors in postmenopausal women. Ann. Intern. Med., *115*:860–864, 1991*b*. Used with permission.)

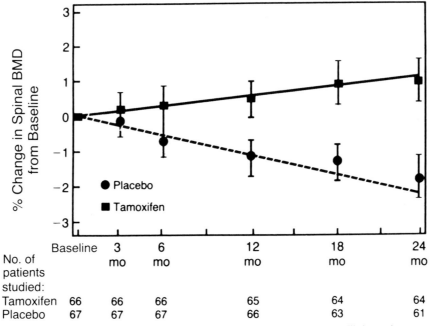

Figure 9-3. Change in mean (± SE) lumbar spine bone mineral density (BMD) in women with breast cancer given tamoxifen or placebo for 2 years. The *solid* and *dashed lines* represent the mean regression lines for the tamoxifen and placebo groups, respectively, as determined from the individual regression lines for each woman (only women with ≥3 data points were included in this analysis). (From Love, R. R., Mazess, R. B., Barden, H. S., et al.: Effects of tamoxifen on bone mineral density in postmenopausal women with breast cancer. N. Engl. J. Med., *326*:852–856, 1992c. Reprinted by permission of the New England Journal of Medicine.)

The toxicity profile of tamoxifen may be influenced by circumstances of those receiving the drug and particularly by the way in which questions are framed. Data from the Wisconsin Tamoxifen Study are shown in Table 9-7. Two results from this study are particularly salient to the use of tamoxifen in healthy women. First, almost half of women treated with tamoxifen in this study had toxicity that they attributed to the drug compared with 20% of placebo subjects (Love et al., 1991c). Second, distressing gynecologic symptoms were increased with tamoxifen (see Table 9-7) (Love et al., 1991c). These symptoms would be expected to compromise compliance of healthy women with long-term therapy.

Other possible effects of tamoxifen have been suggested. Swedish investigators have noted a modest increase in gastrointestinal cancers (Arriagada et al., 1992), and a decrease in hospitalization for immunologic diseases (Fornander et al., 1991). Headache has been less frequent in tamoxifen recipients (Love et al., 1991c). Finally, given the increased incidence of cholelithiasis with estrogen therapy (Boston Collaborative Drug Surveillance Program, 1978), and the excretion route of tamoxifen, an increase in cholelithiasis might be expected.

As Table 9-6 makes clear, there are major benefits and risks with tamoxifen treatment for postmenopausal women, but there are many questions about premenopausal women,

Table 9-7. VASOMOTOR AND GYNECOLOGIC SYMPTOMS IN ONE STUDY OF TAMOXIFEN TOXICITY IN POSTMENOPAUSAL WOMEN

	Proportion of Subjects Reporting Severe Hot Flashes			
	Baseline, n (%)	*At 3 Months, n (%)*	*At 6 Months, n (%)*	*At 12 Months, n (%)*
Placebo subjects	0/70 (0.0)	2/69 (3.0)	5/66 (7.6)	2/64 (3.1)
Tamoxifen subjects	0/70 (0.0)	13/66 (20.0)	13/64 (20.3)	8/60 (13.3)
P	—	< .01	< .04	< .04
	Proportion of Subjects Reporting Gynecologic Symptoms			
	Baseline, n (%)	*At 3 Months, n (%)*	*At 6 Months, n (%)*	*At 12 Months, n (%)*
Placebo subjects	5/70 (7.1)	7/69 (10.1)	10/66 (15.1)	9/64 (14.1)
Tamoxifen subjects	7/70 (10.0)	14/66 (21.2)	19/64 (29.7)	16/60 (26.7)
P	< .55	< .08	< .05	< .08

(Modified from Love, R. R., Cameron, L., Connell, B., and Leventhal, H.: Symptoms associated with tamoxifen treatment in postmenopausal women. Arch. Intern. Med., *151*:1843–1844, 1991c. Copyright 1991, American Medical Association.)

in whom changes may be different (see Table 9–4). In postmenopausal women, carefully monitored prevention studies seem justified because overall benefits may exceed the risks. Whether the data developed from patients with breast cancer will be similar in healthy women is uncertain. Additionally, whether excluding selected individuals will decrease the likelihood of adverse effects needs to be determined.

Clinical trials to address major hypotheses about the effects of tamoxifen in healthy, particularly postmenopausal women are justified. Two hypotheses are of interest:

1. Is the incidence of primary breast cancer reduced with tamoxifen treatment?
2. Is the overall health of tamoxifen-treated women improved, and what precisely are the benefits and costs?

Given the possibility that less favorable breast cancers develop during tamoxifen treatment, it can be argued that breast cancer *mortality* and not incidence should be the endpoint.

It is logical to expect that a healthy woman would want to know that her overall health would improve consequent to tamoxifen treatment. She would also want to know the precise benefits and costs. Theoretical risks inhibit individuals from taking particular actions even when overall benefits are assured. If tamoxifen proves to have overall benefits, women will want to know the precise risks even if they are low.

The challenge in addressing hypothesis 2 is how prevention trials can obtain adequate data on *all* desired endpoints. A trial will reach one major endpoint *first,* at which time a decision must be made about continuing the trial. This first endpoint may *not* be the one of most interest. There is no completely satisfying resolution to such dilemmas. It should be clear that tamoxifen chemoprevention of breast cancer is a promising but complex undertaking. Until the clinical trials of tamoxifen now beginning are completed, this hormone should not be routinely administered to healthy women.

PROPHYLACTIC MASTECTOMY

As a strategy for preventing invasive and possibly lethal breast cancer, prophylactic mastectomy has an uncertain role because at present it is difficult to quantify precisely a woman's risk and because the extent of benefit from this operation is not known. There is some agreement about how risk may be calculated, however, and about what surgical procedure should be performed.

Indications

The multiple costs of prophylactic mastectomy mandate that physicians, and patients have accurate estimates of risk so that benefits can be compared with costs. Decisions for prophylactic mastectomy should not be based on unsupported assumptions or misunderstandings about magnitudes of risk. In the absence of comprehensive risk models for individual patients, indications for prophylactic mastectomy must be specific and strong. Four separate indications are worthy of discussion (Table 9–8). Confirmation of each indication in the medical record is the first step in management. In 6% of cases, documentation of invasive breast cancer in first-degree family members will be absent (Love et al., 1985). Additionally, review of the pathology of existent lesions is an appropriate step.

Diagnosis of unilateral invasive breast cancer, particularly in a premenopausal woman is seen as an indication for prophylactic mastectomy of the unafflicted breast. From cooperative group adjuvant studies and other sources have come data suggesting that the risk for a second breast cancer is slightly under 1% per year, significantly greater than for the general population (Prior et al., 1978). Whether and under what particular conditions this risk diminishes over time are poorly defined. Three observations are confirmed: (1) The presence of lobular carcinoma-in-situ, a family history of breast cancer and multiple foci of disease each increases the risk for contralateral breast cancer (Robbins et

Table 9–8. POSSIBLE INDICATIONS FOR PROPHYLACTIC MASTECTOMY AND ASSOCIATED RANGES OF RISK FOR DEVELOPING BREAST CANCER IN THE NEXT 20 YEARS FOR A 30- TO 40-YEAR-OLD WOMAN

Indication	Relative Risk	Range of Absolute Risk for Developing Breast Cancer over the Next 20 Years (Either Breast)	References
None	1.0	3–4% (either breast)	
Invasive breast cancer in one breast	2–3	10–16% (in one unaffected breast)	Prior and Waterhouse, 1978
Carcinoma in situ in one breast		(in one unaffected breast)	
Ductal carcinoma in situ	1–2	4–7%	Frazier et al., 1977
Lobular carcinoma in situ	4.5	15%	Hutter, 1984; Haagensen, 1986
Breast biopsy with atypical hyperplasia	3.5	(either breast) 11–14%	Dupont and Page, 1985
Family history of breast cancer		(either breast)	
Mother and sister	8	32%	Anderson and Badzioch, 1985
Mother only	2–2.5	8–10%	Anderson and Badzioch, 1985
Sister only (Premenopausal)	1.8	7%	Schwartz et al., 1985

al., 1964); (2) radiation therapy to the chest wall and regional lymph nodes, or to the remaining breast tissue in cases in which partial mastectomy has been performed, is not associated with additional increased risk to the contralateral breast (Boice, 1992); (3) adjuvant tamoxifen therapy is associated with a 40% reduction in risk of contralateral breast cancer (Early Breast Cancer Trialists' Collaborative Group, 1992). Whether a diagnosis of invasive lobular carcinoma in one breast carries a greater-than-average risk of contralateral breast cancer is uncertain. Contralateral breast biopsy without specific physical or mammographic indications ("blind" or "mirror image" biopsy) remains controversial. Many academic surgeons have abandoned this practice, but some believe that the threat posed by contralateral breast cancers justifies this aggressive approach (Wanebo et al., 1984). A series from the NSABP failed to demonstrate any difference in survival between women with unilateral and bilateral cancers (Fisher et al., 1984). If prophylactic surgery is considered, postponement until after treatment of the known invasive cancer may avoid delays in beginning adjuvant therapy.

A second possible indication for prophylactic mastectomy is a diagnosis of carcinoma in situ of ductal or lobular type in one breast. Whether a patient with carcinoma in situ of either type in one breast is more likely than a patient with invasive cancer to have simultaneous contralateral invasive breast cancer is uncertain. The patient with unilateral ductal carcinoma in situ appears to have a risk of contralateral invasive cancer that is less than that of women with an invasive cancer (Frazier et al., 1977). In contrast, the individual with unilateral lobular carcinoma in situ does appear to be at modestly increased risk for invasive cancer in the contralateral breast, but this increased risk is not significantly greater than that for women with unilateral invasive disease generally and is expressed over many years (Hutter, 1984; and Haagensen, 1986). Increasingly, these considerations have led to conservative management with careful observation of patients with carcinoma in situ instead of prophylactic mastectomy.

There are data to suggest that the presence of atypical hyperplasia in the breast indicates increased risk for invasive breast cancer (Dupont and Page, 1985; and Page et al., 1985). Agreement among pathologists on this has been only recent. Although increased risk for invasive disease appears to characterize women with this diagnosis, it is not clear whether atypical hyperplasia is an obligate precursor or simply a marker of risk. Only a minority of benign breast biopsies (3%) result in this diagnosis. With atypical hyperplasia the estimated risk figures are for the development of breast cancer in *either* breast during the next 20 years (see Table 9–8), and for a 30- to 40-year-old woman these are 11% to 14%.

The most commonly discussed indication for prophylactic mastectomy is a history of breast cancer in first-degree relatives. This is presumed to indicate possible genetic predisposition. While greater risk for invasive breast cancer appears to characterize families in which cancers have been diagnosed in premenopausal women, or bilaterally (Ottman, 1990), clinicians are often confronted by women with small families in which some of the cancers have occurred postmenopausally and in which some women at risk have already had prophylactic mastectomies. Breast cancer is a common malignancy, and in the absence of a specific genetic marker, it is often impossible to distinguish whether families that seek counseling have had clustering of breast cancer on the basis of chance or because of exposure to causative factors. Anderson (Anderson et al., 1985), Ottman (Ottman et al., 1983), and Schwartz (Schwartz et al., 1985) developed useful data for estimating empirical risk. In practice the woman's age is important in developing a specific empiric risk estimate. Because familial cancer is characterized by the occurrence of malignancies at young ages, the older an individual becomes without developing a cancer, the less likely it is that she is at "genetic" risk, and the lower is her risk for development of breast cancer before 55 years of age.

Very uncommon genetic syndromes (e.g., Cowden's disease, Li-Fraumeni syndrome, and Muir's syndrome) and more common adenocarcinoma family syndromes described by Lynch, require careful evaluation by genetic specialists (Lynch, 1981).

The data in Table 9–8 provide partial guidance for the clinician regarding prophylactic mastectomy. Clearly more than one indication may coexist. Some data suggest that atypical hyperplasia, nulliparity, and family history operate independently as risk factors. The woman with these is at greater empiric risk than suggested by any single factor (Dupont and Page, 1987). These data are limited and must be viewed as preliminary.

A risk factor recently identified is breast density (Brisson et al., 1988). Whether increased density is independent of proliferative changes such as atypical hyperplasia, is uncertain. For the present it should be considered primarily a characteristic likely to prevent mammographic identification of small malignancies.

The foregoing discussion has been of risks for *developing* breast cancer, not risks of dying of this cancer. The detection of breast cancers at early stages and the favorable impact of adjuvant therapies have resulted in long-term survival for the majority of women with breast cancer. These points should be made with women considering prophylactic mastectomy, who may inappropriately equate developing breast cancer with dying from it or who may conclude that the fate of family members with breast cancer would also be true for them.

Finally, in discussing indications for prophylactic mastectomy, alternative strategies must be considered. Small breast size and soft, nonglandular breast texture are characteristics that may allow more successful monitoring and greater chances of "early" diagnosis of breast cancers. In contrast, mammographic breast density may be associated with less successful monitoring. Mammography as a strategy for early detection in premenopausal women at increased risk is unproven, and repeated mammography could be harmful to women with a genetic predisposition (Swift et al., 1991). At present the risks and benefits of screening women at increased risk for breast cancer are incompletely defined.

Procedure

Subcutaneous mastectomy, in which the majority of glandular breast tissue is removed but some is retained with the nipple-areolar complex, was formerly a common choice for prophylactic surgery (Goldman et al., 1973; and Snyderman, 1984). Reports of breast cancer developing in residual breast tissue, however, and laboratory experiments demonstrating less reduction in risk than reduction in breast tissue, have lessened enthusiasm for this procedure (Eldar et al., 1984; Goodnight et al., 1984; and Wong et al., 1986). Total mastectomy is now the procedure of choice for prophylactic mastectomy. It is important for the surgeon to evaluate the patient for cancer prior to surgery and to obtain intraoperative pathologic evaluation of the breast tissue. If invasive breast cancer is discovered an extension of the operation would be necessary.

In conclusion, prophylactic mastectomy (i.e., total mastectomy) is an option for women at risk for breast cancer, but defining precisely the extent of risk for individual women is imprecise and the magnitude of benefit with this procedure remains undocumented.

PRACTICAL ADVICE

Women are told that their risk of developing breast cancer is high. Recently this risk estimate has been adjusted upwards to state that the chance a woman will develop breast cancer is 1 in 9 (American Cancer Society, 1993). This popular presentation has motivated many women to seek counsel from their physicians on methods to reduce their risk of breast cancer.

Certain behaviors may reduce the risk of breast cancer. It is perhaps most important that any advice be preceded by an explanation of age-specific risk of both developing breast cancer and dying of breast cancer. Since this probability as generally presented is the cumulative lifetime risk calculated through age 110 years (Table 9–9), it is frequently misunderstood by women. The average woman's lifetime risk of *dying* of breast cancer is much lower than the estimated risk of *developing* cancer that has alarmed many women. Women should also be reassured that the majority of increase in incidence is an artifact of increased screening (White et al., 1990; and Lantz et al., 1991). The incidence for the majority of women has not changed.

However, since most cancers occur in women without recognized risk factors (Seidman et al., 1982), specific recommendations are limited.

First, for postmenopausal women the behavior with the greatest certainty of reducing the risk of dying from breast cancer is regular screening mammography (Screening for Breast Cancer, 1989).

Irradiation should be avoided, particularly by young women. Avoiding childhood obesity and having regular physical activity may reduce risk (Frisch et al., 1974). Earlier childbearing and lactation should be encouraged. Reduced consumption of alcoholic beverages is advisable. Reducing intake of animal fat and consuming five servings or more of fruits or vegetables per day are sensible whether or not they influence the occurrence of breast cancer (Willet et al., 1991). Exposure to endogenous hormones should be reduced by regular physical activity and avoiding obesity.

Ovariectomy to produce early menopause is effective but is not justified for breast cancer prevention alone. This benefit should be considered, however, when deciding whether to remove the ovaries at the time of hysterectomy for other reasons.

Finally, exposure to exogenous hormones may increase the risk of breast cancer. Decisions to use oral contraceptives at early ages for long duration or to use estrogen replacement therapy for long periods with progestin components should weigh the benefits against suspected risks.

COUNSELING

The previous section summarized practical advice about prevention of breast cancer. A framework is suggested for giving this advice within the context of medical visits. The suggestions are based on the author's personal experience with 200 families over a decade as well as on experience reported in the medical literature (Josten et al., 1985; Love, 1990a; Stefanek, 1990; and Kelly, 1991). An ideal counseling service might have all the elements presented, and such services are increasingly available at major centers (Stefanek, 1990). To some extent, however, the issues as pre-

Table 9–9. PROBABILITY OF EVENTUALLY DEVELOPING AND DYING OF BREAST CANCER*

Age Interval (y)	Risk of Developing Breast Cancer (%)	Risk of Developing Invasive Breast Cancer (%)	Risk of Dying of Breast Cancer (%)
Birth–110	10.2	9.8	3.6
20–30	0.04	0.04	0.00
20–40	0.49	0.42	0.09
20–110	10.34	9.94	3.05
35–45	0.88	0.83	0.14
35–55	2.53	2.37	0.56
35–110	10.27	9.82	3.56
50–60	1.95	1.86	0.33
50–70	4.67	4.48	1.04
50–110	8.96	8.66	2.75
65–75	3.17	3.08	0.43
65–85	5.48	5.29	1.01
65–110	6.53	6.29	1.53

(From Seidman, H., Mushinski, M. H., Gelb, S. K., and Silverberg, E.: Probabilities of eventually developing or dying of cancer—United States, 1985. C.A. Cancer J. Clin., *35*:36–56, 1985. Used by permission.)

sented above should be useful to any prepared clinician and support staff who wish to assist concerned women.

Some Preparation Before a Prevention Counseling Visit

More so than in many medical encounters, the content of a counseling visit depends on analysis of outside information. Specifically, the following data should be sought: (1) medical records to allow preparation of a family pedigree (Love et al., 1985) and to confirm important medical history; (2) pathology reports, and slides of breast biopsies, to determine if risk-increasing benign conditions, such as atypical hyperplasia, are present (Dupont and Page, 1985); and (3) mammogram reports and the films themselves to assess breast density (Brisson et al., 1988). The reasons for a counseling visit can influence the preparation and timing of a visit, so prior discussion can be helpful. Women are often encouraged to seek counseling for themselves at a time of crisis, for example, when a sister or mother is diagnosed with or is dying of breast cancer. The major goals of a visit are sharing information and preparation for behavioral changes. Grieving can interfere with these, and women often want instead to discuss details of their relative's course. We have found that postponing visits in this situation is helpful.

Prevention Counseling Visit

Counseling for prevention is accomplished best in a quiet, relaxed setting where charts and blackboards are available. An increasing body of literature points to the importance of the environment for supporting the reassurance that should characterize these visits. The parts of a visit are suggested in Table 9–10.

1. Present an overview. This should include some discussion of the long natural history of preclinical disease, the interactions of causes, and the favorable impact of early detection and treatment. The true age-specific risk of developing and dying of breast cancer should be presented.

2. Present an opinion on modifiable risk factors and an analysis of the client's diet. The data about diet and its role in causation are controversial, but women want to know specific actions to take, and if this is not discussed, the counselor will be unprepared for inquiries that are frequent.

3. Conduct a careful breast examination and teach breast self-examination. These need to be done prior to counseling because they will provide information and will reassure the woman that the counselor understands her personal needs.

4. Provide an objective assessment of risk. The parameters of risk have been discussed previously and in articles by Stefanek and Love (Love, 1990*a*; and Stefanek, 1990). These should be addressed in general terms first. Then careful review of the woman's pedigree and personal information about breast biopsies, reproductive risk factors, and mammograms should be made. Absolute risk assessment is a difficult exercise. The data of Anderson (Anderson et al., 1985), Ottman (Ottman et al., 1983), and Schwartz

Table 9–10. MAJOR ELEMENTS OF A PROGRAM FOR COUNSELING INDIVIDUAL WOMEN REGARDING BREAST CANCER PREVENTION

Precounseling Visit
1. Obtain a. medical records of woman and first degree relatives to construct pedigree
   b. pathology reports and slides of any breast biopsies
   c. mammography reports and films
2. Ascertain reasons for the counseling visit

Visit
1. Provide general information on breast cancer's natural history, causes, diagnosis, and treatment
2. Provide specific information on diet (optional)
3. Conduct a careful breast examination and teach breast self-examination if the client is comfortable with procedure
4. Provide an objective assessment of risk
5. Provide specific information on personal prevention options
6. Provide specific information on screening options
7. Counsel on psychologic reactions to risk

Postcounseling Visit
1. Provide a written summary to the client and to all relevant health care personnel (with the client's permission)
2. Make a follow-up telephone call to the client to review the written summary

(Schwartz et al., 1985) are useful when family history is an operative risk factor. How to use additional information from biopsies, parity, and mammographic breast density is uncertain. In reviewing the woman's pedigree it is important to be clear about conclusions that can and cannot be drawn. For example, whether for each stage survival is better or worse in familial breast cancer is uncertain. It is important to talk about the difference between absolute risk for developing breast cancer and risk of dying of this disease. Estimates of absolute risk should be offered to women, but not forced upon them.

5. Provide personal directives on options for prevention. Genetic counseling is a nondirective activity whereas clinical medicine is usually directive. The spectrum of interventions should be addressed, including prophylactic mastectomy. Any ongoing research should be mentioned and the future possibility of identifying susceptibility genes. Whenever possible, concrete recommendations and specific action plans should be made.

6. Provide specific directives about screening. Such counseling is appropriate for specific discussions about mammography.

7. Finally, time should be devoted to the psychologic reactions women have to being at risk for a terrifying and mutilating disease. Fear, denial, guilt, anger, and grief are all common in women at risk for breast cancer (Josten et al., 1985). These reactions need to be inquired about and explored. Three other subjects are often important. First, women have major concerns about loss of personal control, which being at risk entails. The self-directed nature of visits and options are important for restoring women's sense of personal control. Second, women often want to review the courses and treatment of relatives. While counselors must be nonjudgmental, they can often address, helpfully, specific concerns about events. Finally, women often use visits to discuss problems that they perceive in dealing with the medical system.

Follow-up After a Prevention Counseling Visit

1. A summary report should be prepared. In our experience the women themselves are the most appropriate recipients of these reports, but they are also sent to other health care providers as directed by the woman.

2. A follow-up telephone call to the woman after she receives the summary report is worthwhile. This is well received and allows further counseling as well as an opportunity to correct misinformation or misunderstandings.

References

American Cancer Society: Cancer Facts and Figures 1993. Atlanta, GA, American Cancer Society, 1993.

Anderson, D. E., and Badzioch, M. D.: Risk of familial breast cancer. Cancer, 56:383–387, 1985.

Arriagada, R., and Rutquist, L. E.: Adjuvant systemic therapy in early breast cancer and incidence of new primary malignancies (Abstract 34). Proc. Am. Soc. Clin. Oncol., 11:52, 1992.

Astrup, E. G., and Paulsen, J. E.: Effect of retinoic acid pretreatment on 12-0-tetradecanoylphorbol-13-acetate-induced cell population kinetics and polyamine biosynthesis in hairless mouse epidermis. Carcinogenesis (London), 3:312–320, 1982.

Barresen, A-L., Andersen, T. I., Treti, S., et al.: Breast cancer and other cancers in Norwegian families with ataxia-telangiectasia. Genes Chromosom Cancer, 2:339–340, 1990.

Baum, M.: The NATO and CRC trials of adjuvant tamoxifen therapy. In Jordan, V. C. (Ed.): Long-term Tamoxifen Treatment for Breast Cancer. Madison, WI, University of Wisconsin Press (in press).

Baum, M., et al.: Controlled trial of tamoxifen as a single adjuvant agent in management of early breast cancer. Br. J. Cancer, 57:608–611, 1988.

Bernstein, L., Ross, R. C., and Hendersen, B. E.: Prospects for primary prevention of breast cancer. Am. J. Epidemiol., 135:142–152, 1992.

Berquist, L., Adami, H. O., Persson, I., et al.: The risk of breast cancer after estrogen and estrogen-progestin replacement. N. Engl. J. Med., 321:293–297, 1989.

Boice, J. D. Jr.: Cancer in the contralateral breast after radiotherapy for breast cancer. N. Engl. J. Med., 326:781–785, 1992.

Boice, J. D. Jr., Land, C. E., Shore, R. E., et al.: Risk of breast cancer following low-dose radiation exposure. Radiology, 131:589–597, 1979.

Boston Collaborative Drug Surveillance Program: Surgical confirmed gallbladder disease, venous thromboembolism, and breast tumors in postmenopausal women with estrogen treatment. N. Engl. J. Med., 290:15–19, 1974.

Boutwell, R. K.: The function and mechanisms of promoters of carcinogenesis. Crit. Rev. Toxicol., 2:419–443, 1974.

Boyle, P., Meykens, F. L. Jr., Gareiwal, H. S., et al.: Polyamine contents in rectal and buccal mucosae in humans treated with oral α-difluoromethylornithine. Ca Epidemiol. Biomed. Prev., 1(2):131–136, 1992.

Breast Cancer Trials Committee: Adjuvant tamoxifen in the management of operable breast cancer: The Scottish Trial. Lancet, 2:171–175, 1987.

Brisson, J., Morrison, A. S., and Khalid, N.: Mammographic parenchymal features and breast cancer in the Breast Cancer Detection Demonstration Project. J. Natl. Cancer Inst., 80:1534–1540, 1988.

Ciocca, D. R., Parente, A., and Russo, J.: Endocrinologic milieu and susceptibility of the rat mammary gland to carcinogenesis. Am. J. Pathol., 109:47–56, 1982.

Colditz, G., Stampfer, M. J., Willett, W. C., et al.: Prospective study of estrogen replacement therapy and risk of breast cancer in postmenopausal women. J.A.M.A., 264:2648–2653, 1990.

Committee on the Biological Effects of Ionizing Radiations: Health Effects of Exposure to Low Levels of Ionizing Radiation: BEIR V. Washington, DC, National Academy Press, 1990, pp. 253–267.

Correspondents: Risk of breast cancer in ataxia-telangiectasia. N. Engl. J. Med., 326:1357–1360, 1992.

Costa, A., and Love, R. R.: Breast cancer prevention with tamoxifen. Eur J Cancer, 26:655–657, 1990.

Cuzick, J., and Baum, M.: Tamoxifen and contralateral breast cancer. Lancet, 2:282, 1985.

Cuzick, J., Wong, D. Y., and Bellbrook, R. V.: The prevention of breast cancer. Lancet, 1:83–86, 1986.

Dragan, Y. P., Xu, Y., and Pitot, H. C.: Tumor promotion as a target for estrogen–antiestrogen effects in rat hepatocarcinogenesis. Prev. Med., 20(1):15–26, 1991.

Dupont, W. D., and Page, D. L.: Breast cancer risk associated with proliferative disease, age at first birth, and family history of breast cancer. Am. J. Epidemiol., 125:769–779, 1987.

Dupont, W. D., and Page, D. L.: Risk factors for breast cancer in women with proliferative breast disease. N. Engl. J. Med., 312:146–151, 1985.

Early Breast Cancer Trialists' Collaborative Group: Systemic treatment of early breast cancer by hormonal, cytotoxic or immune therapy: 133 randomized trials involving 31,000 recurrences and 24,000 deaths among 75,000 women. Lancet, 339:1–15, 1992.

Eldar, S., Meguid, M. M., and Beatty, J. D.: Cancer of the breast after prophylactic subcutaneous mastectomy. Am. J. Surg. 148:692–693, 1984.

Elegbede, J. A., Elson, C. E., Qureshi, A., et al.: Inhibition of DMBA-induced mammary cancer by the monoterpene d-limonene. Carcinogenesis, 5:661–664, 1984.

Ettinger, B., Genant, H. K., and Cann, C. E.: Long-term estrogen replacement therapy prevents bone loss and fractures. Ann. Intern. Med., 102:319–324, 1985.

Fendl, K.: Role of tamoxifen in the induction of hormone-independent rat mammary tumors. Cancer Res., 52:235–237, 1992.

Fisher, B., Constantino, J., Redmon, C., et al.: A randomized clinical trial evaluation of tamoxifen in the treatment of patients with node negative breast cancer who have estrogen receptor positive tumors. N. Engl. J. Med., 32:479–484, 1989.

Fisher, E. R., Fisher, B., Sass, R., et al.: Pathologic findings from the National Surgical Adjuvant Breast Project (protocol no. 4). XI: Bilateral breast cancer. Cancer, 54:3002–3011, 1984.

Folsom, A. R., Kay, S. A., Prineas, R. J., et al.: Increased incidence of carcinoma of the breast associated with abdominal adiposity in postmenopausal women. Am. J. Epidemiol., 131:794–803, 1990.

Fornander, T., Cedarmark, B., Mattson, A., et al.: Adjuvant tamoxifen in early breast cancer: Occurrence of new primary cancers. Lancet, 1:117–119, 1989.

Fornander, T., Rutquist, L. E., Cedarmark, B., et al.: Adjuvant tamoxifen in early stage breast cancer: Effects on intercurrent morbidity and mortality. J. Clin. Oncol., 9:1740–1748, 1991.

Frazier, T. G., Copeland, E. M., Gallager, H. S., et al.: Prognosis and treatment in minimal breast cancer. Am. J. Surg., 133:607–701, 1977.

Frisch, R. E., and McArthur, J. W.: Menstrual cycles: Fatness as a determinant of minimum weight for height necessary for their maintenance or onset. Science, 185:949–951, 1974.

Gazet, J. C.: Tamoxifen prophylaxis for women at high risk of breast cancer (Letter). Lancet, 2:1119, 1985.

Gibson, D. F. C., Gottardis, M. M., and Jordan, V. C.: Sensitivity and insensitivity of breast cancer to tamoxifen. J. Steroid. Biochem. Mol. Biol., 37:765–770, 1990.

Goldman, L. D., and Goldwyn, R. M.: Some anatomical considerations of subcutaneous mastectomy. Plast. Reconstr. Surg., 51:501–503, 1973.

Goodnight, J. E. Jr., Quagliana, J. M., and Morton, D. L.: Failure of subcutaneous mastectomy to prevent the development of breast cancer. J. Surg. Oncol., 26:198–201, 1984.

Gottardis, M. M., and Jordan, V. C.: Antitumor actions of keoxifene and tamoxifen in the N-nitrosomethylurea-induced rat mammary carcinoma mode. Cancer Res., 47:4020, 1987.

Grodin, J. M., Siiteri, P. K., and MacDonald, P. C.: Source of estrogen production in postmenopausal women. J. Clin. Endocrinol. Metab., 36:207–214, 1973.

Groom, G. V., and Griffiths, K.: Effect of the antioestrogen tamoxifen on plasma levels of luteinizing hormone, follicle stimulating hormone, prolactin, oestradiol, and progesterone in normal premenopausal women. J. Endocrinol., 70:421, 1976.

Haagensen, C. D.: Lobular neoplasia (lobular carcinoma in situ). In Haagensen, C. D. (Ed.): Diseases of the Breast. Philadelphia, W. B. Saunders, 1986, pp. 192–241.

Hall, J. M., Lee, M. K., Newman, B., et al.: Linkage of early-onset familial breast cancer to chromosome 17q21. Science, 250:1648–1649, 1990.

Hirayama, T.: Health effects of active and passive smoking. In Aoki, M., Hisamian, S., and Taminoga, S. (Eds.): Smoking and Health 1987. Amsterdam, Elsevier, 1988, pp. 75–86.

Hulka, B. S.: Hormone replacement therapy and the risk of breast cancer. CA Cancer J. Clin., *40*:289–296, 1990.

Hutter, R. V. P.: The management of patients with lobular carcinoma in situ of the breast. Cancer, *53*:798–802, 1984.

Jordan, V. C.: Biochemical pharmacology of antiestrogen action. Pharmacol. Rev., *36*:245–276, 1984.

Jordan, V. C.: Effect of tamoxifen (ICI46,474) on initiation and growth of DMBA-induced rat mammary carcinoma. Eur. J. Cancer, *12*:419–424, 1976.

Jordan, V. C.: Tamoxifen for the prevention of breast cancer. *In* De Vita, V. T., Hellman, S., and Rosenberg, S. A. (Eds.): Cancer Prevention. Philadelphia, J. B. Lippincott, 1990, pp. 1–12.

Jordan, V. C., Fritz, N. F., Langan-Fahey, S., et al.: Alteration of endocrine parameters in premenopausal women with breast cancer during long-term adjuvant treatment with tamoxifen as the single agent. J. Natl. Cancer Inst., *83*:1488–1491, 1991.

Jordan, V. C., and Murphy, C. S.: Endocrine pharmacology of antiestrogens as antitumor agents. Endocr. Rev. *11*:578–610, 1990.

Josten, D. M., Evans, A., and Love, R. R.: The cancer prevention clinic: A service program for cancer prone families. J. Psychosoc. Oncol., *3*:5–20, 1985.

Kaiser-Kupfer, M. I., and Lippman, M. E.: Tamoxifen retinopathy. Cancer Treat. Rep., *62*:315–320, 1978.

Kalu, D. N., Salerno, E., Liu, C. C., et al.: A comparative study of the actions of tamoxifen, estrogen and progesterone in the ovariectomized rat. Bone Miner., *15*:109–124, 1991.

Katsouyanni, K., Willett, W., Trichopoulou, A., et al.: Risk of breast cancer among Greek women in relation to nutrient intake. Cancer, *181*:61, 1991.

Kelly, P. T.: Understanding Breast Cancer Risk. Philadelphia, Temple University Press, 1991.

Key, T. J. A., and Pike, M. C.: The role of estrogens and proestrogens in epidemiology and prevention of breast cancer. Eur. J. Cancer Clin. Oncol., *24*:29–43, 1988.

Kiang, D.: Chemoprevention for breast cancer: Are we ready? (Editorial) J. Natl. Cancer Inst., *83*:462–463, 1991.

LaCassagne, A.: Hormonal pathogenesis of adenocarcinoma of breast. Am. J. Cancer, *27*:217–228, 1936.

Lantz, P. M., Remmington, P. L., and Newcomb, P. A.: Mammography screening and increased incidence of breast cancer. J. Natl. Cancer Inst., *83*:1540–1547, 1991.

Longnecker, M. P., Berlin, J. A., Orza, M. J., et al.: A meta-analysis of alcohol consumption in relation to risk of breast cancer. J.A.M.A., *652*:260, 1988.

Longstaff, S., Sigurdsson, H., O'Keefe, M., et al.: A controlled study of the ocular effects of tamoxifen in usual dosage in the treatment of breast carcinoma. Eur. J. Cancer Clin. Oncol., *25*:1805–1808, 1989.

Love, R. R.: Antiestrogen chemoprevention of breast cancer: Critical issues and research. Prev. Med., *20*:64–78, 1991*a*.

Love, R. R.: Commentary: Prospects for antiestrogen chemoprevention of breast cancer. J. Natl. Cancer Inst., *82*:18–21, 1990*a*.

Love, R. R.: The article reviewed (Stefanek). Oncology, *4*(1):37–38, 1990.

Love, R. R., Cameron, L., Connell, B., et al.: Symptoms associated with tamoxifen treatment in postmenopausal women. Arch. Intern. Med., *151*:1842–1847, 1991*c*.

Love, R. R., Carbone, P. P., Verma, A. K., et al.: A randomized phase 1 chemoprevention dose-seeking study of α-difluoromethylornithine. J. Natl. Cancer Inst., *85*:732–737, 1993.

Love, R. R., Evans, A., and Josten, D.: The accuracy of patient reports of a family history of cancer. J. Chron. Dis., *38*:289–293, 1985.

Love, R. R., Mazess, R. B., Barden, H. S., et al.: Effects of tamoxifen on bone mineral density in postmenopausal women with breast cancer. N. Engl. J. Med., *326*:852–856, 1992*b*.

Love, R. R., Newcomb, P. A., Wiebe, D. L., et al.: Lipid and lipoprotein effects of tamoxifen therapy in postmenopausal women with node negative breast cancer. J. Natl. Cancer Inst., *82*:1327–1332, 1990*b*.

Love, R. R., Surawicz, T. S., and Williams, E. C.: Antithrombin III, fibrinogen and platelet changes with adjuvant tamoxifen therapy. Arch. Intern. Med., *152*:317–320, 1992*a*.

Love, R. R., Wiebe, D. L., Newcomb, P. A., et al.: Effects of tamoxifen on cardiovascular risk factors in postmenopausal women. Arch. Intern. Med., *115*:860–864, 1991*b*.

Luan, J. M., Yu, M. C., Ross, R. K., et al.: Risk factors for breast cancer in Chinese women in Shanghai. Cancer Res., *48*:1949–1953, 1988.

Lynch, H. T.: Genetics and Breast Cancer. New York, Van Nostrand Reinhold, 1981.

MacMahon, B., Trihopoulos, D., Brown, J., et al.: Age at menarche, probability of ovulation and breast cancer risk. Int. J. Can., *29*:13–16, 1982.

Maklin, D., Li, F. P., Strong, L. C., et al.: Germ line p53 mutations in a familial syndrome of breast cancer, sarcomas, and other neoplasms. Science, *250*:1233–1238, 1990.

Maltoni, C., Pinto, C., and Paladini, C.: Project of experimental bioassays on chemoprevention agents performed at the Bologna Institute on Oncology: Report on tamoxifen control of spontaneous mammary tumors on Sprague-Dawley rats. Cancer Invest., *6*:643–658, 1988.

McCarty, K. S. Jr.: Proliferative stimuli in the normal breast: Estrogens or progestins. Human Pathol., *20*(12):1137–1138, 1989.

McCormick, D. L., and Moon, R. C.: Retinoid-tamoxifen interaction in mammary cancer chemoprevention. Carcinogenesis, *7*:193–196, 1986.

McDonald, C. C., and Stewart, H. J.: Fatal myocardial infarction in the Scottish adjuvant tamoxifen trial. B.M.J., *303*:435–437, 1991.

Messina, M., and Barnes, S.: The role of soy products in reducing risk of cancer. J. Natl. Cancer Inst., *83*:541–546, 1991.

Michnovicz, J. J., and Bradlow, H. L.: Dietary and pharmacological control of estradiol metabolism in humans. Ann. N.Y. Acad. Sci., *595*:291–299, 1990.

Mills, P. K., Beeson, W. L., Phillips, R. L., et al.: Prospective study of exogenous hormone use and breast cancer in Seventh Day Adventists. Cancer, *64*:591–597, 1989.

Modan, B., Chetrit, A., Afandary, E., et al.: Increased risk of breast cancer after low-dose irradiation. Lancet, *1*:629–631, 1989.

Moo, R. C., Thompson, H. J., Becci, P. J., et al.: *N*-(4-hydroxyphenyl) retinamide: A new retinoid for prevention of breast cancer in the rat. Cancer Res., *39*:1339–1346, 1979.

Moolgavkar, S. H., and Knudson, A. G.: Mutation and cancer: A model for human carcinogenesis. J. Natl. Cancer Inst., *66*:1037–1052, 1981.

Moon, R., Grubbs, C., and Sporn, M.: Inhibition of 7,12-dimethylbenz-*a*-anthracene induced mammary carcinogenesis by retinyl acetate. Cancer Res., *36*:2626–2630, 1976.

Moon, R., Grubbs, C., Sporn, M., et al.: Retinyl acetate inhibits mammary carcinogenesis induced by *N*-methyl-*N*-nitrosourea. Nature, *267*:620–621, 1977.

Musey, V. C., Collins, D. C., Musey, P. I., et al.: Long-term effect of a first pregnancy on the secretion of prolactin. N. Engl. J. Med., *316*:229–234, 1987.

Narod, S. A., Feunteum, J., Lynch, H. T., et al.: Familial breast-ovarian cancer locus on chromosome 17q21-q23. Lancet, *338*:82–83, 1991.

Nayfield, S. G., Karp, J. E., Ford, L. G., et al.: Potential role of tamoxifen in prevention of breast cancer. J. Natl. Cancer Inst., *83*:1450–1459, 1991.

NSABP Protocol P1: A clinical trial to determine the worth of tamoxifen for prevention of breast cancer. Pittsburgh, PA, NSABP Operations Office, 1992, p. 12.

Ottman, R.: An epidemiologic approach to gene-environment interaction. Genet. Epidemiol., *7*:177–185, 1990.

Ottman, R., Pike, M. C., King, M. C., et al.: Practical guide for estimating risk for familial breast cancer. Lancet, *2*:556–558, 1983.

Page, D. L., Dupont, W. D., Rogers, L. W., et al.: Atypical hyperplastic lesions of the female breast: A long-term follow-up study. Cancer, *55*:2698–2708, 1985.

Palmer, J. R., Rosenberg, L., Clarke, E. A., et al.: Breast cancer and cigarette smoking: An hypothesis. Am. J. Epidemiol., *134*:1–13, 1991.

Pegg, A. E.: Recent advances in the biochemistry of polyamines in eukaryotes. Biochem. J., *234*:249–262, 1986.

Pegg, A. E., and McCann, P. P.: Polyamine metabolism and function. Am. J. Physiol., *243*:c212–c221, 1982.

Pike, M. C., Henderson, B. E., Krailo, M. D., et al.: Breast cancer in young women and use of oral contraceptives: Possible modifying effects of formulation and age. Lancet, *2*:926–930, 1983.

Pike, M. C., Ross, R. K., Lobo, R. A., et al.: LHRH agonists and the prevention of breast and ovarian cancer. Br. J. Cancer, *60*:142–148, 1989.

Pollak, M.: Effect of tamoxifen on serum insulin like growth factor I levels in stage I breast cancer patients. J. Natl. Cancer Inst., *82*:1693–1697, 1990.

Prentice, R., Thompson, D., Clifford, D., et al.: Dietary fat reduction and plasma estradiol concentration in healthy postmenopausal women. J. Natl. Cancer Inst., *82*:129–134, 1990.

Prentice, R. L., Pepe, M., and Self, S. G.: Dietary fat and breast cancer: A quantitative assessment of the epidemiological literature and a discussion of methodological issues. Cancer Res., *49*:3147–3156, 1989.

Prior, P., and Waterhouse, J. A. H.: Incidence of bilateral tumors in a population-based series of breast cancer patients. I: Two approaches to an epidemiological analysis. Br. J. Cancer, *37*:620–634, 1978.

Robbins, G. F., and Berg, J. W.: Bilateral primary breast cancers: A prospective clinicopathological study. Cancer, *17*:1501–1527, 1964.

Rohan, T. E., and Baron, J. A.: Cigarette smoking and breast cancer. Am. J. Epidemiol., *129*:36–42, 1989.

Rutquist, L. E., Cedermark, B., Glas, U., et al.: Contralateral primary tumors in breast cancer patients in a randomized trial of adjuvant tamoxifen. J. Natl. Cancer Inst., *83*:1299–1306, 1991.

Schwartz, A. G., King, M-C., Belle, S. H., et al.: Risk of cancer to relatives of young breast cancer patients. J. Natl. Cancer Inst., *75*:665–668, 1985.

Screening for breast cancer. *In* Guide to Clinical Preventive Services: Report of the U.S. Preventive Services Task Force. Baltimore, Williams & Wilkins, 1989, pp. 39–46.

Seidman, H., Stellman, S. D., and Mushinski, M. H.: A different perspective on breast cancer risk factors: Some implications of the nonattributable risk. CA Cancer J. Clin., *32*:301–313, 1982.

Sellers, T. A., Kushi, L. H., Potter, J. D., et al.: Effect of family history, body fat distribution, and reproductive factors on the risk of postmenopausal breast cancer. N. Engl. J. Med., *326*:1323–1329, 1992.

Senior, B. E., Cawood, M. L., Oakey, R. E., et al.: A comparison of the effects of clomiphene and tamoxifen treatment on the concentration of oestradiol and progesterone in peripheral plasma of infertile women. Clin. Endocrinol. (Oxf), *8*:381, 1978.

Shamberger, R. J., Tytko, S. A., and Willis, C. E.: Antioxidants and cancer. Part VI. Selenium and age-adjusted human cancer mortality. Arch. Environ. Health, *231*:31, 1976.

Snyderman, R. K.: Prophylactic mastectomy: Pros and cons. Cancer, *53*:803–808, 1984.

Stampfer, M., and Colditz, G.: Estrogen replacement therapy and coronary heart disease: A quantitative assessment of epidemiologic evidence. Prev. Med., *1*(20):47–63, 1991.

Stampfer, M. J., Willett, W. C., Colditz, G. A., et al.: A prospective study of postmenopausal estrogen therapy and coronary heart disease. N. Engl. J. Med., *313*:1044–1049, 1985.

Stefanek, M. E.: Counselling women at high risk for breast cancer. Oncology, *4*(1):27–33, 1990.

Swift, M., Morrell, D., Cromarche, E., et al.: The incidence and gene frequency of ataxia telangiectasia in the United States. Am. J. Hum. Genet., *39*:573–583, 1986.

Swift, M., Morrell, D., Massey, R. B., et al.: Incidence of cancer in 161 families affected by ataxia telangiectasia. N. Engl. J. Med., *325*:1831–1836, 1991.

Swift, M., Reitnauer, P. J., Morrell, D., and Chase, C. L.: Breast and other cancers in families with ataxia-telangiectasia. N. Engl. J. Med., *316*:1289–1294, 1986.

Thompson, H. J., Herbst, E. J., Meeker, L. D., et al.: Effect of D,L-alpha-difluoromethyl-ornithine on murine mammary carcinogenesis. Carcinogenesis, *5*:1649–1651, 1984.

Tokunaga, M., Land, C. E., Tamamora, T., et al.: Incidence of female breast cancer among atomic bomb survivors. Hiroshima and Nagasaki. Radiat. Res., *11*(2):243–272, 1987.

Tokunaga, M., Land, C. E., Yamamoto, T., et al.: Breast cancer among atomic bomb survivors. *In* Boice, J. D. Jr., and Fraumeni, J. F. Jr. (Eds.): Radiation Carcinogenesis: Epidemiology and Biological Significance. New York, Raven Press, 1984, pp. 45–55.

Trichopoulos, D., MacMahon, B., and Cole, P.: Menopause and breast cancer risk. J. Natl. Cancer Inst., *41*:315–329, 1968.

Trock, B.: A mathematical model to predict the effect of tamoxifen chemoprevention: Poster at 15th Annual Meeting of the American Society of Preventive Oncology, Seattle, WA, April 1991.

Verma, A. K.: Ornithine decarboxylase: A possible target for human cancer prevention. *In* Steele, V. E., Stoner, G. D., Boone, C. W. et al. (Eds.): Cellular and Molecular Targets for Chemoprevention. Chicago, CRC Press, 1992, pp. 207–224.

Vogelstein, B., Fearon, E. R., Hamilton, S. R., et al.: Genetic alterations during colorectal tumor development. N. Engl. J. Med., *319*:525–532, 1988.

Wald, N. J., Boreham, J., Hayward, J. L., et al.: Plasma retinol, β-carotene and vitamin E levels in relation to the future risk of breast cancer. Br. J. Cancer, *49*:321–324, 1984.

Wanebo, H. J., Senofsky, G. M., Fechner, R. E., et al.: Bilateral breast cancer: Risk reduction by contralateral biopsy. Trans. South Surg. Assoc., *96*:131–141, 1984.

Weiss, N. J., Ure, C. L., Ballard, J. H., et al.: Decreased risk of fractures of the hip and lower forearm with postmenopausal use of estrogen. N. Engl. J. Med., *303*:1195–1198, 1980.

White, E., Lee, C. Y., and Kristal, A. R.: Evaluation of the increase in breast cancer in relation to mammography use. J. Natl. Cancer Inst., *82*:1546–1552, 1990.

Willet, W., and London, S. J.: Dietary factors and the etiology of breast cancer. *In* Harris, J. R., Hellman, S., and Henderson, I. G. (Eds.): Breast Diseases. Philadelphia, J. B. Lippincott, 1991, pp. 136–142.

Wong, J. H., Jackson, C. F., Swanson, J. S., et al.: Analysis of the risk reduction of prophylactic partial mastectomy in Sprague-Daley rats with 7,12-dimethylbenzanthracene-induced breast cancer. Surgery, *99*:67–71, 1986.

10

Diagnosis

William L. Donegan

There is but one method of making a definitive diagnosis of breast cancer. It is histologic examination—that is, the microscopic study of tissue. By contrast, there are many ways of suspecting it. These include medical history, physical examination, mammography, ultrasonography, and cytologic examination of needle aspirates and nipple discharges. Thermography and transillumination are techniques that now are largely of historical interest. The utility of computed tomography (CT) and magnetic resonance imaging (MRI) is under evaluation. The accuracy and usefulness of each of these techniques is ultimately determined by comparison with the results of histologic analysis of relevant tissues. A definitive diagnosis is essential for appropriate staging and treatment.

Most patient complaints referred to the breasts are not cancer-related. Benign conditions are far more frequent than cancer (Table 10–1). Unfortunately, the signs and symptoms of cancer are not unique and not easily distinguished from those of benign conditions. They are also extraordinarily varied. For this reason, and because cancer poses the most serious threat to a patient's well-being, any symptom related to the breast must raise the possibility of cancer. As Haagensen said, ''The price of skill in the diagnosis of breast carcinoma is a kind of eternal vigilance based upon an awareness that any indication of disease in the breast may be due to carcinoma'' (Haagensen, 1971*b*). One might also observe, in view of the frequency of this malignancy and its capacity to spread, that *any* metastatic adenocarcinoma without an obvious source in a woman should suggest the breast as its source.

Physicians should be aware that failure to diagnose breast cancer has become a source of serious professional liability. It is the second most frequent cause of legal action against physicians and the most expensive (Physician Insurers Association of America, 1990). The problem most often is failure of the physician to be sufficiently impressed by the presence of a breast mass, particularly in young women and in women who have normal mammograms.

Breast cancer is almost exclusively a disease of women. Although men are not exempt, women account for more than 99% of all cases. It is unusual for breast cancer to occur in patients under the age of 30 years and is a medical curiosity in children. Especially susceptible are the aged, women with a strong family history of breast cancer, nulliparous women, and those women with an initial full-term pregnancy after the age of 30 years. A previous breast biopsy showing atypical ductal or lobular hyperplasia also places a woman at high risk. However, most people who develop breast cancer are not unique; only a minority have a family history of the disease or would be considered

otherwise at high risk (Table 10–2). A substantial number of new cases are asymptomatic and are detected by mammography alone (Table 10–3).

Cancers occur in the breast in a predictable pattern, and this pattern is similar for both invasive and in situ carcinomas. The upper hemispheres of the breasts are involved more often than the lower, and the lateral hemispheres more often than the medial. In terms of quadrants, the upper outer quadrant of the breast is most frequently involved (Table 10–4). The lower inner quadrant is the least frequent location, with the central (subareolar and periareolar) breast and the remaining quadrants intermediate with respect to frequency of cancer occurrence. If the breasts are each likened to the face of a clock, breast cancers predominate in the regions between 12 and 3 o'clock in the left breast and between 12 and 9 o'clock in the right breast. The distribution corresponds generally to the distribution of breast parenchyma and suggests a tissue volume–related risk. This may account for a slight predominance of cancers in the left breast, as its volume averages slightly greater than that of the right breast (Smith et al., 1986). The difference between the two breasts is only 2% or 3% and is not always seen. In the author's most recent 407 cases, cancers were located in the left breast in 45.9% and in the right breast in 51.0%, with 3.1% being bilateral. Rarely, cancers arise in ectopic mammary tissue along the axillary or abdominal portions of the primitive milk lines, and even in the vulva (Nicolesco and Velciu, 1968; and Parikh and Singer, 1983).

Table 10–1. BREAST CLINIC CASES, MEDICAL COLLEGE OF WISCONSIN

Fibrocystic changes	197
Fibroadenoma	72
Infections	41
Carcinoma	37
Gynecomastia	16
Lipoma	6
Fat necrosis	5
Duct ectasia	3
Inappropriate lactation	3
Fibrosis	2
Intraductal papilloma	2
Superficial thrombophlebitis (Mondor's disease)	2
Amastia	2
Polymastia	1

Normal examination, 195; unexplained breast pain, 50; mass, 15; nipple discharge, 23; enlarged axillary node, 4.

Note: Benign disorders far outrank carcinoma as causes of complaints related to the breast.

Table 10–2. PROFILE OF 385 CONSECUTIVE CASES OF BREAST CANCER*

Item	Total	Invasive Cancer	In Situ Cancer
Total No. of patients	385	329	56
Female (%)	99.2	99.1	97.8
Average age (y)	55.6	56.2	52.1
Age range (y)	26–102	26–102	30–80
Bilateral carcinoma (%)	3.1	2.4	7.1
Left breast (%)	45.9	47.1	39.2
Right breast (%)	51.0	50.4	53.6
Weight (lb)	152.4	152.9	150.0
Height (inches)	63.7	63.8	63.1
Race, white	93.9	93.1	97.7
Family history† (%)	21.0	18.2	34.6
Average age at menarche (y)	12.7	12.7	12.6
Hysterectomy (%)	25.5	26.1	21.4
Pregnant or lactating (%)	2.6	2.5	3.4
Pregnancies (average No.)	2.1	2.7	2.4
Live births (average No.)	2.0	2.1	1.9
Diabetes mellitus (%)	7.0	5.2	16.7
Hypertension (%)	19.7	19.0	22.2
Average age at first pregnancy (y)	24.6	24.4	25.6
Average age at first live birth (y)	26.5	24.4	35.5

*Author's personal series. Complete data were not available for all items.
†Breast cancer in a mother, sister, or daughter.

SIGNS AND SYMPTOMS

The initial signs and symptoms of mammary carcinoma are varied and may be multiple at the time of presentation.

Mass

The most common physical sign of breast cancer is a mass (Fig. 10–1). The mass is discovered in 73% of cases by women themselves, either accidentally or on self-examination (Nemoto et al., 1982). Less often, it is discovered by a physician on routine physical examination (23% of cases) and, occasionally, by a woman's husband or a male friend. The mass may be tender, but it is more often painless. Sometimes a spontaneous sensation of "drawing," vague

discomfort, or a blow to the breast leads to its discovery. The fact that almost 15% of palpable cancers are accompanied by discomfort emphasizes that pain or tenderness, usually associated with benign conditions, is no guarantee of innocence. Unfortunately, the age distributions of various mass-forming lesions of the breast have considerable overlap. Figure 10–2 diagrams the age distribution for the three most common lesions. Occasionally, breast cancers present as more than one mass.

Nipple Discharge

Nipple discharge is not a frequent complaint nor a frequent sign of mammary carcinoma. Only 3% to 5% of consultations (Murad et al., 1982) and 7.4% of breast operations

Table 10–3. METHOD OF DISCOVERY OF 402 CONSECUTIVE BREAST CANCERS*

	No. of Patients	Per Cent
Physical Examination	284	70.6
Palpable mass +/− other signs	264	65.7
Nipple discharge	12	3.0
Nipple lesion	5	1.2
Skin edema +/− redness	2	0.4
Axillary adenopathy	1	0.2
Mammography Only	118	29.4
Microcalcifications	61	15.2
Mass	44	10.9
Mass with microcalcifications	12	3.0
Architectural change	1	0.2
Other	1	
Unknown	3	

*Invasive and in situ cancers, author's personal series (1982–1993).

Table 10–4. LOCATION OF PRIMARY CANCERS IN THE BREAST*

Location	Author's Cases (n/(%))	NCDB† (%)
Upper outer quadrant	59 (40.0)	35.7
Upper inner quadrant	25 (17.4)	8.0
Central	18 (12.5)	5.2
Upper midline	13 (9.0)	
Lower outer quadrant	13 (9.0)	5.8
Lower inner quadrant	8 (5.6)	4.6
Midlateral	4 (2.8)	
Lower midline	3 (2.0)	
Undetermined	1 (0.6)	18.1
Nipple		2.1
Axillary tail		0.7
Overlapping		19.8

*One hundred forty-four consecutive cases.
†National Cancer Data Base (64,780 cases reported in 1990).

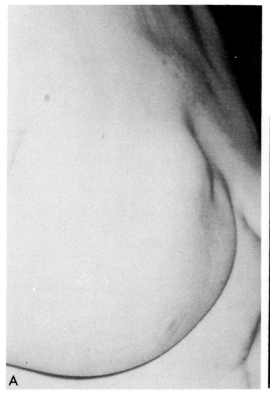
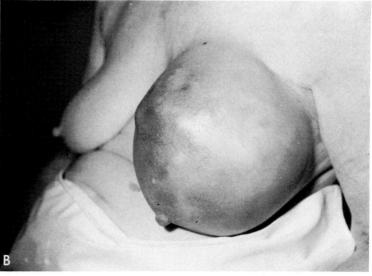

Figure 10–1. A palpable, and sometimes visible, mass is the most frequent presenting sign of mammary carcinoma. *A,* The frequency of metastasis increases progressively with size, emphasizing the importance of prompt detection, but some less frequent histologic types, such as mucinous carcinoma *(B),* may reach impressive size without metastasizing or becoming incurable.

(Leis et al., 1985) are in response to such discharge. No more than 2% of cancers were associated with discharge in Devitt's series (1985); most that were (80%) also appeared with a mass. Twelve to 20% of cancer-associated discharges occur without a mass, and 10.4% appear without mammographic evidence of abnormality (Leis et al., 1985). In the author's series, 3% of patients' cancers presented initially with nipple discharge, but in 86% of these cases, a mass or an abnormality was also found on mammography or ductography.

Figure 10–2. The age distributions of the three most common mass-producing breast lesions demonstrate considerable overlap in women in the 35 to 55 year age range. Although fibroadenomas predominate in the younger groups, carcinomas in the older ones, and fibrocystic disease during reproductive years, the range for each is wide. (Data from Haagensen, C. D.: Diseases of the Breast. 3rd ed. W. B. Saunders, Philadelphia, 1981, p. 256, *and* Seidman, H.: Cancer of the Breast. American Cancer Society Professional Education Publication, New York, 1972, p. 28).

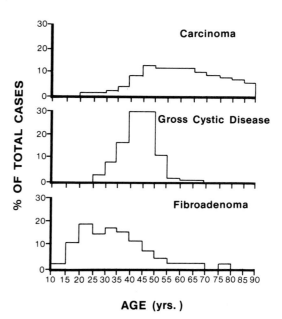

Discharge from multiple ducts of both breasts is generally endocrine in nature, drug-induced, or due to diffuse fibrocystic changes. Inappropriate lactation with hyperprolactinemia suggests the presence of lactogenic medications such as tricyclic antidepressants, hypothyroidism (elevated levels of thyrotropin-releasing hormone stimulate prolactin secretion from the pituitary gland), or a prolactinoma in the pituitary gland (Table 10–5). Appropriate tests on breast milk (fat stain or assay for alpha-lactalbumin) and a serum prolactin determination confirm the problem. The careful taking of a drug history, determination of serum TSH, triiodothyronine, and thyroxine, and a CT scan of the head can all be helpful in evaluating the possibilities. It should

be noted that multiparous women can have a small amount of milky discharge for years without obvious cause. A thin, bloody discharge from both breasts late in pregnancy in the absence of other abnormalities is ordinarily of no consequence. It is likely due to epithelial hyperplasia, and it ceases after parturition (Haagensen, 1971a; and Lafreniere, 1990).

Discharges that are spontaneous, from one breast only, and confined to one duct suggest the presence of a local lesion and raise the possibility of cancer. Persistent unilateral discharge is due to cancer in 4% to 21% of cases. In the remainder, its origin is a duct papilloma, papillomatosis, fibrocystic changes, or duct ectasia. In the absence of a

Table 10–5. CAUSES OF CHRONIC HYPERPROLACTINEMIA WITH INAPPROPRIATE LACTATION

Mechanisms	Causes		Diagnosis
Physiologic	Excessive breast manipulation		Discontinue stimulation
Pharmacologic		BRAND OR GENERIC NAMES	Discontinue medication if appropriate
	reserpine, methyldopa	Aldomet	
	chronic opiate use	Morphine, methadone, heroin	
	phenothiazines, chlorpromazine	Thorazine	
	perphenazine	Trilafon	
	thioridazine	Mellaril	
	prochlorperazine	Compazine, Chlorazine	
	fluphenazine	Permitil, Prolixin	
	trifluoperazine	Stelazine	
	thioxanthenes	Taractan	
	butyrophenones	Haldol	
	pimozide	Orap	
	metoclopramide	Reglan	
	dibenzoxazepine antidepressants	Amoxapine (Asendin)	
	cimetidine	Tagamet	
	tricyclic antidepressants	Imipramine, desipramine (Norpramin, Pertofran), amitriptyline, nortriptyline (Aventyl, Pamelor)	
	papaverine derivatives	Verapamil (Calan, Isoptin)	
Pathologic	Primary hypothyroidism		Thyroid function tests
	Hypothalamic disorders (e.g., neoplastic, infectious, vascular, degenerative or granulomatous)		
	Pseudocyesis		Pregnancy test
	Pituitary stalk section		History
	Prolactin-secreting adenoma of pituitary gland		Serum prolactin; CT scan
	Acromegaly		Growth hormone; CT scan
	Cushing's disease		Urinary cortisol measurement; dexamethasone suppression test
	Ectopic production of prolactin (bronchogenic carcinoma, hypernephroma)		Chest radiograph; CT scans
	Chronic renal failure (decreased prolactin clearance)		Renal function tests
	Chest wall lesions (e.g., surgical scars, neoplasms, herpes zoster)		Physical examination
Functional	Undiagnosed cases		

(Modified with permission from Adashi, E. Y.: Diagnostic evaluation of hyperprolactinemia. Resident & Staff Physician, *31*:16PC, 1985.)
Abbreviation: CT = computed tomography.

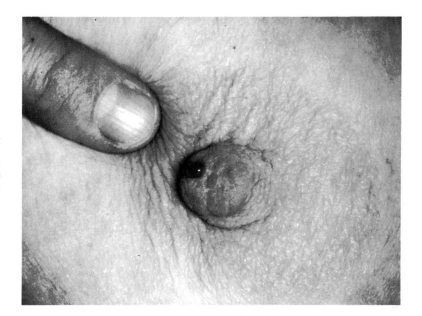

Figure 10-3. Serosanguineous discharge expressed with point pressure from a nonlactating breast. Note that the location of the discharging duct on the nipple corresponds to the involved quadrant of the breast. Palpation with one finger in this manner can localize the diseased duct in the absence of a mass.

palpable mass or an abnormality on mammography, a nipple discharge of this type was due to cancer in 8% of cases in the series of Chaudary and coworkers (1982). The author has found only one cancer, a ductal carcinoma in situ, among 36 such cases of persistent unilateral discharge—a frequency of only 2.8%. A papilloma or papillomatosis was responsible in more than one-half of the cases.

Discharges may be of almost any color (e.g., red, green, brown, blue, gray, white, or colorless), thin or thick, and clear or opaque. The nature of the discharge is suggestive of its cause: that from a papilloma is usually serous or bloody; in contrast, a thick, pasty discharge suggests duct ectasia. Discharges associated with cancer can be of any type. Leis and associates (1985) found the following types of discharge to be associated with cancer: watery (45%); sanguinous (24%); serosanguinous (11.9%); and serous (6.3%). Discharges that accompany cancer usually contain gross or occult blood. Two-thirds of the women with cancer-associated nipple discharges at Ellis Fischer State Cancer Hospital (EFSCH), Columbia, Missouri, reported that they were bloody. Chaudary and colleagues (1982) obtained positive results on a test for hemoglobin on all discharges associated with cancer. Cytologic examination of nipple discharge is often performed but is unreliable for detecting cancer (Knight et al., 1986; and Johnson and Kini, 1991).

Both advanced age and the presence of an accompanying mass increase the probability of a diagnosis of cancer (Seltzer et al., 1970; and Murad et al., 1982) A serosanguinous or bloody discharge is more likely to indicate a benign than a malignant lesion in women younger than 50 years of age, but the reverse is true for women over the age of 50 years (Copeland and Higgins, 1960). In the absence of a mass, Seltzer and associates (1970) found cancer in 12% of patients with discharges; however, the frequency rose to 32% in those over 60 years of age. When a palpable mass was present, the overall incidence of cancer was 31%; this incidence rose to 65% in those older than 60 years of age.

If a mass is not palpable and mammography reveals no lesion, several means are available to locate the source of discharge. The position of the discharging orifice on the nipple generally corresponds to the quadrant of the breast in which the lesion is located. Often, careful palpation with one finger identifies a site at which pressure produces the discharge (Fig. 10–3). A ductogram sometimes demonstrates a filling defect, but ductograms are not performed routinely (Fig. 10–4). As pointed out by Devitt (1985), nipple discharge is not often due to cancer. When it is, a

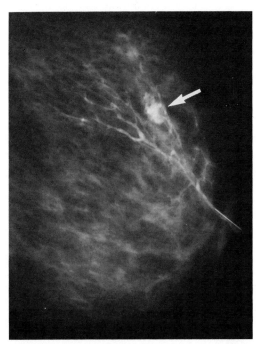

Figure 10-4. A galactogram (or ductogram) on a patient with bloody nipple discharge demonstrates an upper ductal system in which a cystic structure *(arrow)* with a filling defect is seen, representing a papilloma. An injection of the offending duct immediately prior to biopsy with a vital dye (methylene blue) is useful for identifying the tissues to be removed.

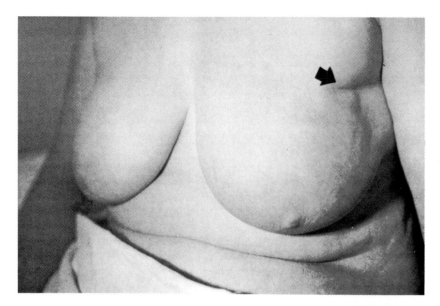

Figure 10–5. Skin dimpling caused by attachment of an underlying carcinoma.

tumor is usually palpable. When cancer is present but not palpable, it is almost always in an early, noninvasive form.

Skin Changes

Dimpling or retraction of the skin by cancer is produced by the shortening of Cooper's ligaments owing to infiltration (Fig. 10–5). Dimpling may be fixed or evident only when the breast is in certain positions. Skin retraction is not pathognomonic of cancer. Scars, fat necrosis, plasma cell mastitis, and Mondor's disease can all produce skin retraction. Mondor's disease is a thrombophlebitis of the thoracoepigastric vein and occurs spontaneously or after breast biopsy (Mondor, 1939). It can involve arteries and lymphatics and produces a characteristic subcutaneous band or groove in the skin (Hatteland and Kluge, 1965).

Rather than producing dimpling, attachment of cancers to the overlying dermis may only alter the normal contours of the breast. Deviation of the nipple or of the entire affected breast disturbs the usual symmetry, and flattening of the skin disrupts the normal curvature (Fig. 10–6).

Direct infiltration of the skin presents as a firm dermal plaque that eventually ulcerates (Fig. 10–7). Prominent subcutaneous veins may be seen on the affected breast (Fig. 10–8). Marked firmness and retraction of the entire breast is seen in some advanced cases (Fig. 10–9). Dermal satellite nodules are also a characteristic of advanced disease (Fig. 10–10).

Edema of the skin of the breast with characteristic peau d'orange changes is an ominous sign. Edema in association with redness, heat, and tenderness is the hallmark of inflammatory cancer of the breast (Fig. 10–11). The gravity of inflammatory changes was recognized in 1814 by Bell, and

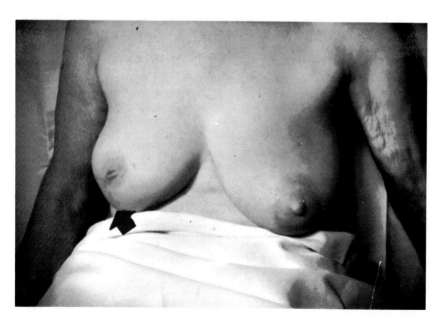

Figure 10–6. A carcinoma of the right breast producing nipple inversion and a flattened contour.

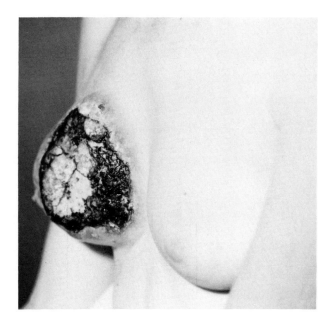

Figure 10–7. Ulceration of the skin in a young woman with locally advanced carcinoma of the right breast. A black, malodorous inflammatory membrane occupies most of the ulcer base.

a classic report on the subject by Lee and Tannenbaum in 1924 was responsible for establishing ''inflammatory carcinoma'' as a clinical entity. Signs of inflammation may herald the disease (primary inflammatory carcinoma) or may appear later in its course (secondary inflammatory carcinoma). The latter case is less frequent, but both carry the same grave implications. This dramatic and aggressive variant so closely mimics mastitis that the unwary physician is led to prescribe prolonged treatment with antibiotics or to perform an incision and drainage for a suspected abscess. Antibiotic administration with or without an attempt at drainage was the initial therapy of 10.5% of 38 consecutive patients with inflammatory carcinomas reviewed at EFSCH. Fortunately, this form of breast cancer constitutes only 1.5% to 4% of all cases (Taylor and Meltzer, 1938; Donnelly, 1948; Barber et al., 1961; Richards and Lewison,

1961; Byrd and Stephenson, 1962; Wang and Griscom, 1964; and Donegan et al., 1990). Although patients with this variant tend to be younger than the average breast cancer patient, no special association with pregnancy or lactation has been confirmed. A palpable tumor may precede or follow the manifestation of the inflammatory signs, but typically the breast is swollen and indurated without a discrete palpable mass. Despite tenderness and redness and the presence of local heat, systemic signs of infection are infrequent. Only 21% of patients with this presentation at EFSCH had an elevated white blood cell count (the highest was 13,900/per cubic millimeter), and fever was documented in only two patients (5.2%). Metastasis to axillary nodes is early and extensive. Seventy-nine per cent of cases at EFSCH had clinically involved axillary nodes, 47% had involved supraclavicular nodes, and 13% had evidence of

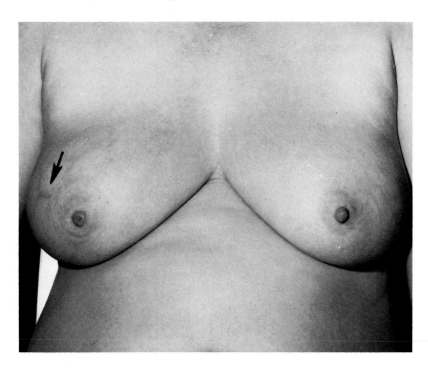

Figure 10–8. Prominent veins associated with a carcinoma within the right breast.

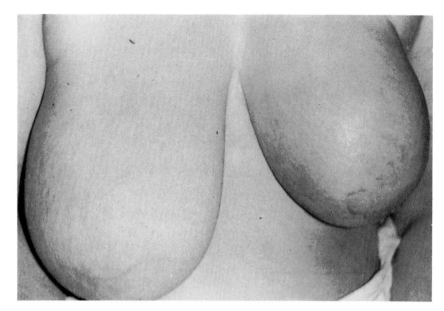

Figure 10–9. Marked retraction of the left breast caused by a large neglected carcinoma.

distant metastases. The tumor has no distinguishing histologic characteristics other than extensive involvement of lymphatics within the breast and in the dermis. Tumor within dermal lymphatics was once considered the sine qua non of this entity, but it is not always demonstrable (Ellis and Teitelbaum, 1974). It was found in 62.5% of skin biopsies in cases reviewed by the author. Saltzstein (1974) found dermal lymphatic invasion to be a sign of poor prognosis in cases of breast cancer that lacked typical inflammatory signs, and as a result suggested the concept of "occult" inflammatory carcinoma. Lucas and Perez-Mesa (1978) found that both dermal lymphatic invasion and signs of inflammation were dire developments; patients with signs of inflammation combined with dermal lymphatic invasion; those with dermal lymphatic invasion without inflammatory signs; and those with both had equally poor prognoses. Inflammatory carcinoma has been defined by the

American Joint Committee on Cancer as "a clinicopathologic entity characterized by diffuse brawny induration of the skin of the breast with an erysipeloid edge, usually without an underlying palpable mass" (American Joint Committee on Cancer, 1992). It should be suspected in any case of mastitis, particularly in one not associated with parturition.

Nipple Changes

Breasts removed owing to cancer often show extension of tumor to the nipple (Smith et al., 1976; and Morimoto et al., 1993). Up to 31% of nipples in patients with breast cancer show histologic involvement, and this involvement is more likely if primary tumors are within 2.5 cm of the nipple or are larger than 2.0 cm in diameter (Lagios et al.,

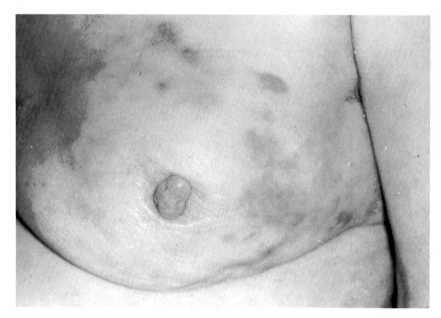

Figure 10–10. Multiple pink satellite nodules in the skin around a locally advanced mammary carcinoma.

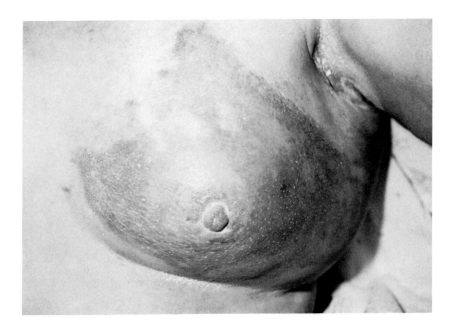

Figure 10-11. An inflammatory carcinoma of the breast demonstrating erythema and edema of the dermis with a peau d'orange appearance. Invasion of dermal lymphatics is a histologic hallmark of this lesion.

1979). In one-half of patients with nipple involvement, its presence is not suspected clinically.

Two clinical changes are noteworthy: nipple inversion and Paget's disease of the nipple. Normally, inverted nipples are pliable and can be temporarily everted. When cancer is the cause, the inversion is fixed, and even temporary eversion is not possible. On closer examination, thickened subareolar ducts or an underlying mass may be detected (Fig. 10–12).

The changes known as *Paget's disease of the nipple* were described as a sign of breast cancer by Sir James Paget in 1874. He warned that cancer within the breast followed within 1 to 2 years after detection of the changes (Paget, 1874). The cutaneous changes vary from moist and eczematoid to dry and psoriatic. The nipple may display a red granular erosion or simply subtle thickening (Fig. 10–13).

Often, no change is evident. In only one of seven mastectomy specimens with histologically confirmed Paget's disease examined by Lagios and colleagues (1979) was a nipple lesion noted clinically. Symptoms include itching, burning, or a sensation of sharp sticking of the nipple and can include an exudate that may be interpreted by the patient as a discharge. Spread of Paget's disease is centrifugal from ductal orifices; the expanding lesion progressively involves the nipple, the areola, and even the adjacent skin. Large tumor cells with pale cytoplasm and large nuclei found within the epidermis of the nipple (Paget's cells) were described by Darrier in 1889 (Fig. 10–14). The most widely held interpretation is that they represent intraepithelial migration of carcinoma through ducts from a primary tumor within the breast (Jacobaeus, 1904). Rarely, Paget's disease is found in isolation or associated solely with intra-

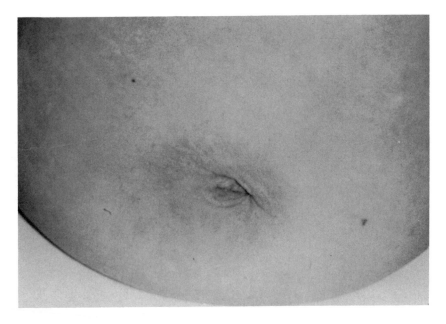

Figure 10-12. Nipple retraction is the only outward sign of this large carcinoma in the adjacent portion of the breast.

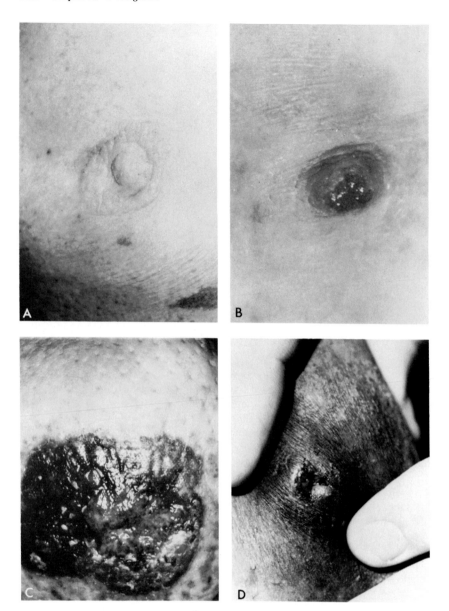

Figure 10–13. Four cases of Paget's disease illustrate its clinical variations. *A,* The nipple is thickened, but the epithelium is intact and the appearance mimics a chronic eczema. *B,* A small, moist area of granulation is confined to the papilla of the nipple. *C,* Paget's disease destroys the entire nipple-areolar complex and is associated with edema of the surrounding skin. *D,* Minimal changes produced only a spot of moisture and were largely hidden within an inverted nipple.

epithelial carcinoma that is confined to the ducts of the nipple.

Paget's disease is not confined to the breast. Extramammary Paget's disease can appear on the skin wherever apocrine glands are found—primarily in the anogenital and axillary areas, but also in the ear canals and on the eyelids (Helwig and Graham, 1963; and Kawatsu and Miki, 1971). It has also been observed to involve the epidermis superficial to cutaneous metastases of breast cancer (Greenwood and Minkowitz, 1971).

Resembling a benign dermatitis and not always associated with a palpable tumor, Paget's disease is sometimes treated for prolonged periods inappropriately with topical medications by unsuspecting physicians. Whenever Paget's disease is suspected, or whenever a benign-appearing nipple lesion does not respond to a brief period of topical therapy, a biopsy of the lesion is indicated. Histologic confirmation of the disease is proof of mammary cancer and an indication for the initiation of cancer therapy.

Axillary Adenopathy

In 1907, Halsted pointed out that enlarged axillary lymph nodes could be the only sign of occult cancer in the breast, but fewer than 1% of cases are discovered based on their presence (see Table 10–3). The Yorkshire Breast Cancer Group (1983) documented 15 such presentations among 1205 cases of breast cancer. Merson and colleagues (1992) studied 60 cases of axillary lymph node enlargement at the National Cancer Institute in Milan and, noting a relatively favorable prognosis (58% survival at 10 years), suggested that the occurrence of this peculiar circumstance represents a strong immunologic control over the primary tumor.

Pierce and coworkers (1957) reviewed 222 biopsies of clinically enlarged axillary nodes and found that 6.9% of them contained metastatic adenocarcinoma. The possible origins of metastatic adenocarcinoma are many and include the breast, lungs, ovaries, liver, kidney, stomach, pancreas, and colon. With breast cancer being the most frequent ma-

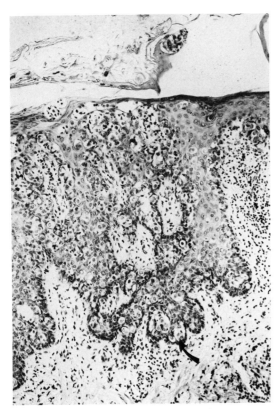

Figure 10-14. Paget's disease of the breast in a histologic section. Characteristic large cells with clear cytoplasm (Paget's cells) representing intraepithelial carcinoma replace and distort the epidermis of the nipple.

still first detected on physical examination performed either by the physician or, more often, by the patient herself. A survey by the American College of Surgeons showed that prior to 1982, 73% of breast cancers were found by patients; 23% during physician examinations; and only 4% on mammography (Nemoto et al., 1982). These proportions have changed with the increase in screening with mammography. Approximately 30% of tumors among the author's last 402 patients with breast cancer were discovered with mammography alone (in asymptomatic women) (see Table 10–3). Of the 70% of patients who were symptomatic, a palpable mass was the complaint of almost all of them (93%). Among symptomatic women, mammography detected an abnormality in 78.2% of them. Hence, in 11.8% of patients with a complaint related to the breast, the cancer was detected on physical examination alone. Almost 50% of tumors that are 0.6 to 1.0 cm in diameter are detectable on physical examination (Wolfe, 1974). Detectability increases with increased tumor size and with greater examination duration (Fletcher et al., 1985; and Campbell et al., 1991). The technique is not self-evident; both training and experience contribute to a skilled examination (Hall et al., 1977). Premenopausal women are best examined 1 week after the onset of their last menstrual period. At this time, engorgement of the breast is least and any masses are most evident (Fig. 10–15).

The limitations of physical examination must be appreciated, both when determining whether an abnormality or a mass is present and when deciding whether a mass is benign or malignant. Considerable subjectivity is involved,

lignancy among women and lung cancer being the most likely cause of death from cancer among women, the lungs and the breasts are highly suspect, particularly if the gastrointestinal and other systems are asymptomatic (Copeland and McBride, 1973). A mammogram reveals a primary carcinoma in 12% to 50% of cases, but a normal mammogram does not rule out the presence of a primary cancer in the breast (Ashikari et al., 1976). The presence of estrogen and progesterone receptors in nodal metastases is highly suggestive of the presence of a primary tumor in the breast. Pathologists find a small, occult primary carcinoma in about two-thirds of clinically normal resected breasts, usually in the upper outer quadrant (Feuerman et al., 1962; Westbrook and Gallager, 1971; and Ashikari et al., 1976). Breast-conserving treatment rather than mastectomy is being used with increasing frequency to treat women who present with axillary metastases and no apparent primary tumor in the breast, and results are comparable with those of mastectomy (Vilcoq et al., 1982; Kemeny et al., 1986; and Merson et al., 1992).

CLINICAL EVALUATION OF THE BREAST

A carefully recorded history and a physical examination are fundamental to the evaluation of breast disease, and they remain indispensable for the detection and clinical staging of mammary carcinoma. The majority of breast cancers are

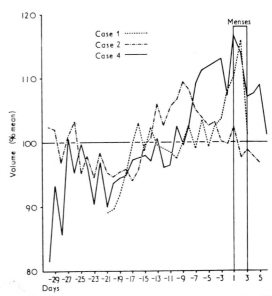

Figure 10–15. Volumetric measurements of the breasts of three premenopausal women during a complete menstrual cycle show that breast volume is least approximately 21 days before onset of the next menses and, therefore, approximately 7 days after onset of the menstrual flow. Volume changes in all normal cycles were expressed as percentages of mean volume for each cycle and plotted backward from the first day of menses. (From Milligan, D., Drife, J. O., and Short, R. V.: Changes in breast volume during normal menstrual cycle and after oral contraceptives. Br. Med. J., *29*:494, 1975. Reprinted with permission.)

and the results of physical examination are not completely reproducible. In clinical practice, related information, such as a patient's age and family history, influence judgments about the probable nature of a mass. Advanced cancers are easily recognizable, but otherwise, the distinction between benign and malignant lesions is blurred. Despite these problems, the opinion of an experienced examiner that a breast mass represents cancer is correct in 70% to 90% of cases and that it is benign is correct in 90% of cases (Rimsten et al., 1975). Boyd and coworkers (1981) reported a study in which four surgeons examined 100 patients. Forty-one of the patients had been admitted for a breast biopsy, and the remaining 59 for other problems, (i.e., without known breast disease). Fifteen of the first 41 patients (37%) proved to have cancer on subsequent biopsy. The individual opinions that an abnormality was present varied among the four surgeons from 37% to 74%, with agreement occurring in only 25% of cases. The opinion that a mass was present varied from 32% to 42%, but agreement was reached in only 16% of cases. The abnormalities were considered malignant in 13% to 19% of cases, but the four surgeons concurred on this in only 5% of cases. Examiners correctly recommended biopsies for 80% to 93% of the 15 cancers. Of concern was that no recommendation for biopsy would have been made for 7% to 20% of the patients with cancers. In another study of 201 women with palpable solid breast masses who were examined by gynecologists prior to biopsy, 12% of 95 cancers were considered clinically benign (van Dam et al., 1988). The overall accuracy of physical examination was 81%, the positive predictive value 73%, and the negative predictive value 87%. Breast cancers less than 1.0 cm in diameter are not often palpable, and in screening examinations, only an estimated 45% of cancers are detected on physical examination (Baker, 1982).

Medical History

The taking of a medical history is directed toward defining and evaluating symptoms related to the breasts and toward establishing risk. The location, character, and duration of pain or tenderness and whether it is related to the menstrual cycle are important. The location of lumps and their size, duration, and change is also elicited from a patient. Nipple discharge is defined with respect to its location, quantity, and color and whether it occurs spontaneously or only when the nipple is squeezed. Inquiry is made about skin changes and about changes in the size of the breasts. Also of importance are the results of previous mammographic studies, ultrasound examinations, aspirations, biopsies, and operations on the breasts as well as other consultations about the current problem. Whether a patient uses hormone drugs (e.g., oral contraceptives or replacement hormones) and the date of her last menstrual period are recorded. Inquiry should be made about whether the patient practices breast self-examination (BSE) regularly. A patient's menopausal status is also important (if a patient has experienced menopause, whether it was natural or artificial should be ascertained). Whether a previous pelvic operation or hysterectomy included removal of the ovaries should be recorded for patients who have undergone such a procedure. It is

surprising how often patients are unclear when questioned on this point. Previous records may be needed for clarification.

For establishing risk, additional information is obtained—in particular, a patient's age at menarche and at menopause as well as the number of pregnancies she has experienced, number of live childbirths she has had, and the earliest age at which she experienced each. A carefully recorded family history of cancer is essential and should specifically include which family members have had cancer of the breast, their ages at diagnosis (premenopausal or postmenopausal), and whether their cancer was unilateral or bilateral. Asking about other cancers in close relatives serves to detect family cancer syndromes. An outline that has served well for recording information at an initial patient visit is shown in Figure 10–16.

Physical Examination

Physical examination of the breasts includes inspection and palpation of the breasts and of the regional lymph nodes.

Inspection

The breasts are inspected in a well-lit room with the patient seated, unclothed to the waist, and facing the examiner (Fig. 10–17). The breasts should generally be symmetric and have smooth outlines. It is not unusual for one breast to be noticably larger. A particularly small breast may be a sign of Poland's syndrome. The breasts can be widely separated or synthesized in the midline. Observable striae may have resulted from previous pregnancies. Fullness in the axillary areas is far more often because of the presence of ectopic breast tissue than due to adenopathy. The presence of accessory nipples is noted as is that of any scars from previous operations and recent incisions. The nipples should have similar directionality; they are inspected for deviation or inversion as well as for any change suggestive of Paget's disease. An increased venous pattern may be a sign of pathology. Any dimpling, retraction, ecchymosis, or localized flattening of the skin is recorded.

Inspection should be performed first with the patient's arms at her side and then with them extended above her head (Fig. 10–18). The patient is then directed to place her hands on her hips and press inward to tense the pectoralis major muscles (Fig. 10–19). Some physicians find it useful to have their patients lean forward. These maneuvers serve to elicit retraction of the skin or deviation of the breasts due to tumors.

Palpation

Examination of regional lymph nodes precedes palpation of the breasts and is performed while the patient is still seated. The examination should include the axillary, supraclavicular, and infraclavicular nodes; the internal mammary nodes are not normally palpable. Normal axillary nodes are soft, mobile, and no greater than 1 cm in diameter. Supraclavicular nodes, when palpable at all, are soft and less than 0.5 cm in diameter. Infraclavicular nodes are actually nodes at the apex of the axilla and can be felt in the deltopectoral triangle only when they are enlarged. In thin individuals, the coracoid process can be felt at this site and should not be mistaken for adenopathy. The supraclavicular and infraclavicular nodes can be examined from the front or from behind the patient (Figs. 10–20 and 10–21). The axillae are best examined with a patient's arms loosely at her sides, a position that relaxes the axillary fascia. To examine the left axilla, the physician's left hand steadies the patient's shoulder to keep it from rising while the right hand palpates (Fig. 10–22). Slight inward pressure applied with the heel of the left hand serves to keep nodes centralized in the axilla. The fingers of the right hand are cupped slightly and inserted high into the axilla before they are approximated to the chest wall. In so doing, nodes are trapped rather than pushed away. As the fingers are then drawn inferiorly along the chest wall, nodes can be felt to escape, characteristically "popping" away from beneath the fingers. Several passes are made to deliberately examine the anterior, medial, and posterior regions of the left axilla. The right axilla is examined in similar fashion, with the position of the physician's hands reversed. The size, number, consistency, and mobility or fixation of nodes to the skin or deep fascia are noted as is the presence or absence of tenderness. The axillae frequently contain extensions of breast tissue, which is recognizable by its characteristic glandular consistency and mild tethering to the skin. In obese individuals, the axillae and supraclavicular areas may contain a soft fat pad that interferes with the examination. This fat pad should not be mistaken for adenopathy, and nodes may be felt within it.

If the patient seeks consultation because of a lump, it is useful to have her indicate the location. The examiner can then give careful attention to this site. Palpation of the breast with the patient in the upright position and with the breast pendulous and folded upon itself can be misleading. More accurate information is obtained with the patient in the supine position (Fig. 10–23). In this position, the breast is flattened and thinned on the chest wall. Since the breast tends to fall laterally, further advantage may be gained by elevating the side to be examined with the placement of a pad or pillow beneath the patient's back; however, the author has not found this essential. The breast can simply be displaced more medially with the hands during palpation. The ipsilateral arm is abducted with the patient's hand placed comfortably behind her head. The contralateral hand is positioned at her side or on her abdomen.

The entire breast is gently and thoroughly examined with the flats of the fingertips. It must be kept in mind that glandular tissue potentially extends into the axilla, to the clavicle, to the anterior midline of the chest, laterally to the midaxillary line, and to the epigastrium (Hicken, 1940); these are the boundaries of the examination. For orientation, the breast is conceptualized either as comprising four quadrants and a central subareolar area or as a clock centered at the nipple. To ensure that the entire breast is palpated, it may be considered a wheel with the nipple as its hub. Each spoke is examined in turn. Alternatively, a pinwheel pattern of palpation can be used either beginning at the hub and working outward in a spiral fashion, or beginning peripherally and progressing inward. Most glandular tissue is normally in the upper outer quadrant. Here tissues are thicker and more difficult to examine, but it is here also that most cancers arise. The best examination of each breast is obtained if the examiner stands on the side of the table opposite to the breast to be examined so that the fingers are directed toward the lateral quadrants of the breast and the axilla. A circular motion of the fingers or a kneading motion that causes the breast tissue to move back and forth beneath the skin is used. By this means, the consistency of the tissue can be appreciated. Terms such as "soft," "dense," "lobular or glandular," "firm," "irregular," "granular," "finely nodular," or "coarsely nodular" often seem appropriate to describe the consistency of breast tissue. Sometimes, the firmness of the tissue is such that the breast can be displaced laterally to allow palpation of the deep side. Vacancies of tissue are often found beneath the areola or beneath the scars of previous biopsies. Normal breast tissue may be configured as scattered large islands of tissue or as a large "doughnut" around the areola. Tissues in the upper outer quadrant are usually more dense than those in the remainder of the breast and may feature a peninsular extension toward the axilla. Firm transverse ridges of tissue are often present near the inframammary folds. In patients who have undergone breast reduction, one often finds the breast tissue in irregular aggregates and a vacancy beneath the scar that extends from the nipple to the inframammary fold.

A mass may be defined as three-dimensional, distinct from the surrounding tissues, having a definable periphery, and asymmetric with respect to the other breast. Other clinicians have defined a mass as "any area that is palpably distinct or different from the surrounding tissue" (Masur, 1983). Several items may be mistaken for a mass. These include a prominent rib or costochondral junction; a firm inframammary ridge; dense tissue in the upper outer quadrant; the fill valve on a prosthesis; and a firm, irregular border of tissue at a previous biopsy site, at the edge of the areola, or at the peripheral terminus of the breast tissue. Simultaneous palpation of both breasts can help determine if asymmetry exists (Fig. 10–24). In equivocal cases, an acceptable practice in premenopausal women is to repeat the examination 1 week after onset of the next menstrual period. If hormonal stimulation was responsible, it may have resolved. Interruption of the use of oral contraceptives or replacement hormones may also help in the formulation of a diagnosis.

The importance of determining whether a mass is present cannot be overemphasized, for masses require a definitive diagnosis. The presence of a dominant nodule has the same importance. A *dominant nodule* is one that is larger, firmer, or otherwise obviously different from the rest. Masses are carefully described with respect to size (in centimeters), shape, mobility, attachment to skin or deep fascia, tenderness, consistency, and location (Fig. 10–25). A useful mnemonic is to describe each MASS with Tender Loving Care (M for *mobility*, A for *attachments*, S for *shape*, S for *size*, T for *tenderness*, L for *location*, and C for *consistency*). Failure of the skin to move independently of the mass establishes the presence of attachment. Complete immobil-

Text continued on page 176

BREAST INITIAL EXAMINATION FORM

Date: _____ Age: _____ Race: _____ Sex: _____ Height: _____ Weight: _____

CHIEF COMPLAINT:

PRESENT ILLNESS:

PAST HISTORY:
  Illnesses: _____

  Operations: _____

  Allergies: _____

  Meds, Hormones, and OCS: _____

  _____

  Irradiation: _____

REVIEW OF SYSTEMS:
  Gravida: _____ Para: _____ L.M.P.: _____ Menarche: _____

  Age at 1st Pregnancy: _____ Age at 1st Childbirth: _____

  Other: _____

  _____

FAMILY HISTORY:
  Breast cancer: _____

  Other cancer: _____

X-RAY/SLIDES: _____

  _____

  _____

PATIENT'S NAME _____

Figure 10–16. Outline used by the author for initial evaluation of patients with a complaint related to the breast.[5] It is supplemented as needed.

PHYSICAL EXAMINATION

GENERAL: _____

Height:	Weight:	Blood Pressure:	Pulse:

LYMPH NODES:

	AXILLARY		SUPRACLAVICULAR			INFRACLAVICULAR	
	RT	LT	RT	LT		RT	LT
Present	( )	( )	( )	( )		( )	( )
Absent	( )	( )	( )	( )		( )	( )

BREASTS:

RT	LT		RT	LT	
( )	( )	Normal	( )	( )	Redness
( )	( )	Fine nodularity	( )	( )	Ulcerations
( )	( )	Coarse nodularity	( )	( )	Mass(es)
( )	( )	Skin edema	( )	( )	Nipple change
( )	( )	Tenderness	( )	( )	Surgically absent
( )	( )	Nipple discharge (describe) _____			

INDICATE SKIN CHANGES AND LOCATION, SIZE, SHAPE, AND MOBILITY
OF MASSES AND NODES

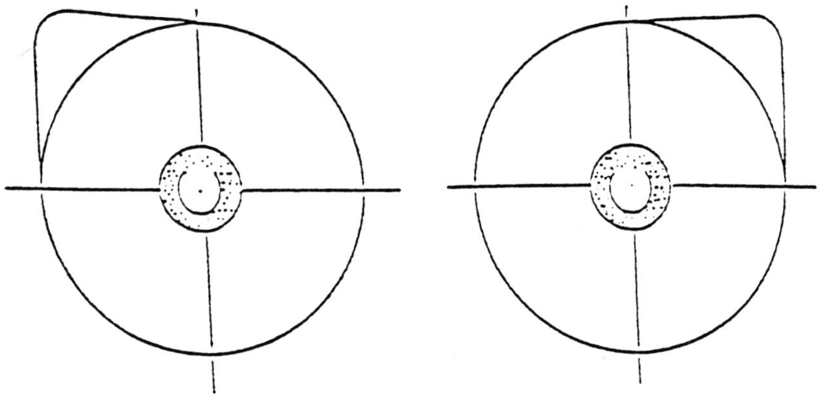

BREAST ASPIRATION: _____
HEAD AND NECK: _____ LUNGS: _____
HEART: _____ ABD: _____ EXTR: _____

IMPRESSION: _____
DISPOSITION: _____
_____
_____
_____

SIGNED: _____ , M.D.

Figure 10–16 *Continued*

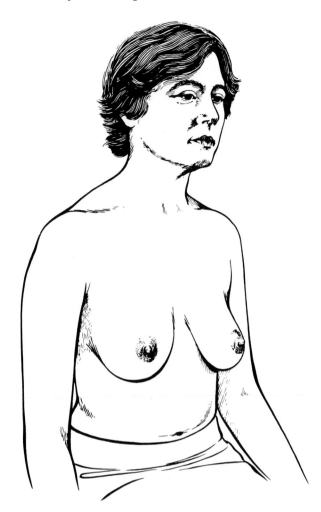

Figure 10–17. The breasts are inspected with the patient seated and facing the examiner. Asymmetry, changes in the nipple or skin, and prominent veins are signs that may be due to the presence of cancer. (From Donegan, W. L.: Diseases of the breast. *In* Danforth, D. N., and Scott, J. R. (Eds.): Obstetrics and Gynecology. 5th ed. Philadelphia, J. B. Lippincott, 1986, p. 1165. Reprinted with permission.)

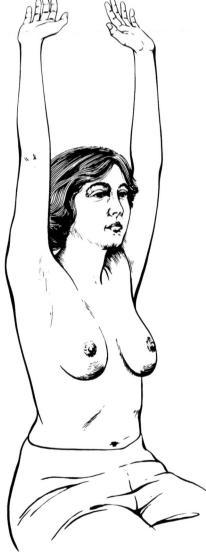

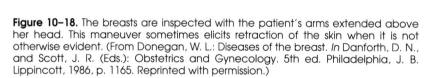

Figure 10–18. The breasts are inspected with the patient's arms extended above her head. This maneuver sometimes elicits retraction of the skin when it is not otherwise evident. (From Donegan, W. L.: Diseases of the breast. *In* Danforth, D. N., and Scott, J. R. (Eds.): Obstetrics and Gynecology. 5th ed. Philadelphia, J. B. Lippincott, 1986, p. 1165. Reprinted with permission.)

Figure 10–19. Inspection with the patient's hands pressed against her hips fixes the pectoralis major muscle and its fascia. Attachment of the breast to the skin and fascia produces skin retraction or deviation of the breast during this maneuver. (From Donegan, W. L.: Diseases of the breast. *In* Danforth, D. N., and Scott, J. R. (Eds.): Obstetrics and Gynecology. 5th ed. Philadelphia, J. B. Lippincott, 1986, p. 1165. Reprinted with permission.)

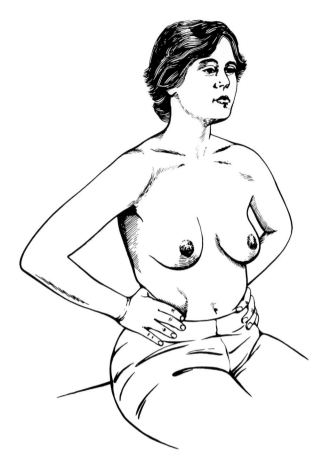

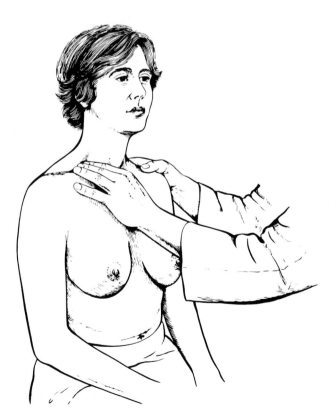

Figure 10–20. Palpation of supraclavicular nodes is performed while the patient is seated. Attention is also given to the pre-scalene nodes located behind the lower end of the sterno-cleidomastoid muscle. (From Donegan, W. L.: Diseases of the breast. *In* Danforth, D. N., and Scott, J. R. (Eds.): Obstetrics and Gynecology. 5th ed. Philadelphia, J. B. Lippincott, 1986, p. 1165. Reprinted with permission.)

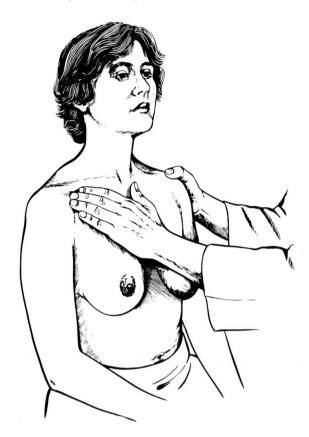

Figure 10–21. An attempt is made to detect enlargement of infra-clavicular nodes located in the deltopectoral groove. These are, in fact, apical axillary nodes. A prominent coracoid process should not be mistaken for adenopathy. (From Donegan, W. L.: Diseases of the breast. *In* Danforth, D. N., and Scott, J. R. (Eds.): Obstetrics and Gynecology. 5th ed. Philadelphia, J. B. Lippincott, 1986, p. 1165. Reprinted with permission.)

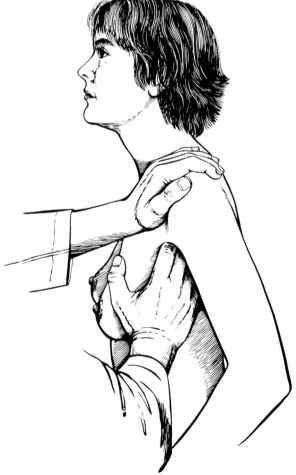

Figure 10–22. The technique is shown for palpating axillary lymph nodes. The fingers of the examining hand are cupped and inserted high into the axilla before being drawn down to trap nodes against the chest wall. Pressure with the other hand keeps the shoulder from moving upward and moves anterior nodes into the center of the axilla, where they are more easily felt. (From Donegan, W. L.: Diseases of the breast. *In* Danforth, D. N., and Scott, J. R. (Eds.): Obstetrics and Gynecology. 5th ed. Philadelphia, J. B. Lippincott, 1986, p. 1165. Reprinted with permission.)

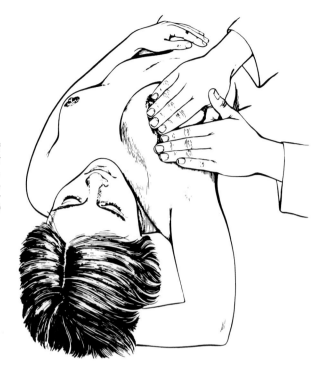

Figure 10-23. Palpation of the breast is performed with the flats of the fingertips. The patient is in a supine position with the side that is being examined slightly elevated and the arm abducted. (From Donegan, W. L.: Diseases of the breast. *In* Danforth, D. N., and Scott, J. R. (Eds.): Obstetrics and Gynecology. 5th ed. Philadelphia, J. B. Lippincott, 1986, p. 1165. Reprinted with permission.)

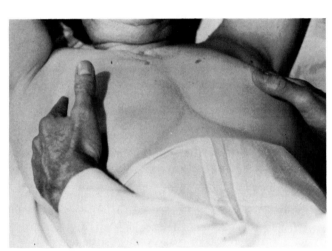

Figure 10-24. Bilateral simultaneous palpation of the breasts is sometimes useful to determine whether asymmetry is present.

Figure 10-25. Attachment of a mass to the overlying skin can be demonstrated by squeezing the skin as shown. The skin remains fixed and creates a furrow over the mass, the ``plateau'' sign.

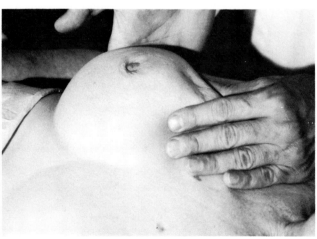

ity indicates that a mass is fixed to the chest wall (i.e., to the ribs and intercostal muscles). Fixation of a mobile mass when a patient presses her hand against her hip establishes the presence of attachment to the deep pectoral fascia or pectoral muscle.

Examination of the Nipple

The nipples are inspected for signs of asymmetry, retraction, dermatitis, or edema. An attempt is made to determine whether inverted nipples can be everted. The depressions created by chronically inverted nipples tend to collect cutaneous debris; this debris should be cleaned away so that the surface of the nipple can be inspected. This debris should not be mistaken for discharge. The ducts ascending through the nipple can be palpated for thickness and nodulation by rolling them between the index finger and thumb (Fig. 10–26). The nipple is gently squeezed to elicit nipple discharge. This is more effective if compression of the breast is begun

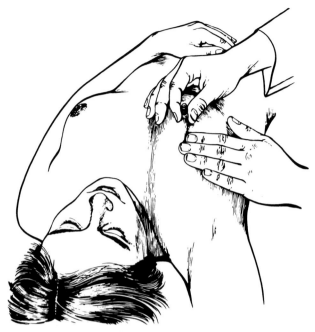

Figure 10–27. Compression of the nipple and adjacent breast to elicit nipple discharge. (From Donegan, W. L.: Diseases of the breast. *In* Danforth, D. N., and Scott, J. R. (Eds.): Obstetrics and Gynecology. 5th ed. Philadelphia, J. B. Lippincott, 1986, p. 1165. Reprinted with permission.)

far out and moved toward the nipple (Fig. 10–27). Patients are often more successful in demonstrating discharge than is the physician, and if they can they should be requested to do so. It is noteworthy that patients usually prefer a sitting position and that they compress the breast bimanually. This probably explains why the most copious discharge is sometimes seen during compression of the breast for mammography. The location of the discharging orifice or orifices is noted as is the character of the discharge. Any discharge is collected and tested for occult blood. If blood is present, if the discharge is spontaneously released, if it originates from only a single duct, or if it is associated with a mass, it is also collected for cytologic examination.

FINE-NEEDLE ASPIRATION

Fine-needle aspiration of palpable masses is a convenient and expeditious means of differentiating cysts from solid tumors. Cysts cannot be distinguished from solid tumors reliably by palpation alone (Rosner and Blaird, 1985). Aspiration at the time of the physical examination is convenient and does not interfere with the interpretation of a subsequent mammogram if care is taken to avoid causing a hematoma.

The procedure is performed with a 21-gauge needle and a 10-mL syringe, and it usually causes less discomfort to the patient than a routine venipuncture. The patient is placed in the supine position described for palpation of the breast. A local anesthetic can be used if the patient prefers. The skin is wiped with alcohol, and sterile technique is observed. The mass is steadied with the fingers of one hand

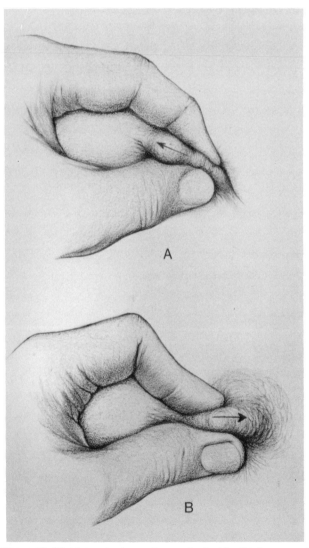

Figure 10–26. Major ducts can be evaluated for thickness and nodularity by rolling the nipple between the fingers as shown.

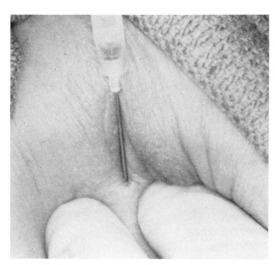

Figure 10–28. Aspiration of palpable masses can be performed as an office procedure to rapidly distinguish cystic from solid lesions. The patient can be assured that there is minimal discomfort. The skin is prepared with an alcohol wipe. Drapes and gloves are not necessary, although they are shown here: a small needle (21-gauge) and syringe are suitable equipment. One pass generally is sufficient to determine the nature of the lesion; if fluid is encountered, it is aspirated entirely.

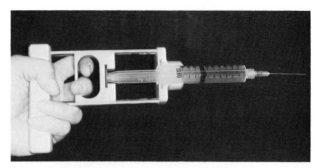

Figure 10–29. A pistol-grip instrument for aspiration of breast masses.

while the needle is directed into the mass at an angle to the chest wall that is sufficient to reduce the risk of pneumothorax (Fig. 10–28). Pistol-grip instruments that hold the syringe and make aspiration easier are available, but the author has not found them to be necessary (Fig. 10–29). If fluid is obtained, it is evacuated totally. Complete disappearance of the mass and removal of nonbloody (hemoccult-negative) fluid is indicative of a simple cyst. The routine cytologic examination of fluid from cysts is not recommended, as the yield of unsuspected carcinoma is negligible (McSwain et al., 1978; and Ciatto et al., 1987). If the fluid contains blood, if the mass does not completely disappear, or if the cyst recurs after a short interval, the aspirated fluid is examined cytologically. Less than half of all fluid specimens from cystic carcinomas are cytologically positive for cancer, but a positive or suspicious cytologic result should expedite investigation (Devitt, 1988). Intracystic carcinomas are rare (Table 10–6). According to Goode and associates (1955), only 2 were found among 281 carcinomas of the breast in their series. Rosemond and colleagues (1969) found only 3 such carcinomas among 3000 cyst aspirations (Fig. 10–30). Devitt (1988) reported that 8 of 11 cystic carcinomas yielded bloody fluid, 7 left a

residual mass, and 1 was detected because of rapid fluid reaccumulation. Hamed and coworkers (1989) found two cancers among six biopsies performed because of a finding of bloody fluid or residual mass, and the two cancers showed both of these signs. These authors emphasized the importance of scheduling a follow-up visit for patients 6 to 8 weeks after aspiration of what appears to be a simple cyst. In a study of 315 patients who returned for such follow-up, 20 patients had a mass at the site of the previous cyst, 44 had a recurrence of the cyst, and 22 had a new cyst. After repeat aspiration, 20 patients had biopsies on the basis of bloodstained fluid, residual mass, or recurrent cyst, and two cancers were found, both of which were in patients with a residual mass. Carcinoma should be considered if needle aspiration (1) produces no fluid, (2) produces fluid that is bloody, (3) leaves a residual mass, or (4) is required repeatedly to drain the same cyst.

Confirmation that a nonpalpable mammographic density is cystic rather than solid can be obtained with ultrasound or with mammographically guided needle aspiration. The latter technique is simple to perform and can reduce the need for biopsy. Meyer and associates (1992) described the indications as (1) a mammographic mass that is either invisible on ultrasound or has features atypical for a cyst, (2) an enlarging mass on mammography with sonographic features of a cyst, and (3) confirmation of a suspected cyst. Of the 183 occult, solitary breast masses that these clinicians studied, 83% proved to be cysts. Since palpation for a residual mass is not possible, the collected fluid is usually examined cytologically; a pneumocystogram can provide further evidence that no intracystic lesion is present (Fig. 10–31). A repeat mammogram should demonstrate a return to normality after the procedure, and follow-up mammography several months later is prudent to confirm the absence of recurrence.

Table 10–6. INTRACYSTIC BREAST CARCINOMA

	Number	Cystic Carcinomas	Per Cent
Abramson (1974)	3000 cysts	3	0.1
Gatchell et al. (1958)	9000 carcinomas	48	0.5
Czernobilsky (1967)	2500 carcinomas	14	0.5
Rosemond et al. (1969)	1275 cysts	1	0.1

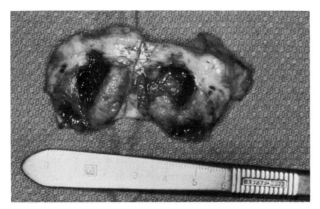

Figure 10–30. A carcinoma of the breast with a cystic center. Bloody fluid returned on aspiration, and a palpable mass remained.

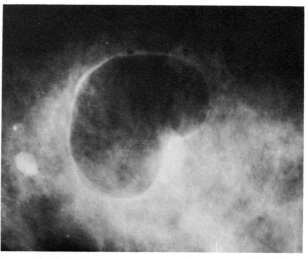

Figure 10–31. A pneumocystogram of a benign cyst. Following aspiration of all fluid, the needle is left in place and an equal amount of air is injected. This creates a radiolucent image against the denser breast tissue. The cyst wall is thin and smooth, indicating that no intracystic lesion is present.

MAMMOGRAPHY

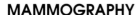

Mammography has an indispensable role in the detection of breast cancer. Many cancers can be discovered at a smaller size by mammography than by physical examination alone. It is an essential complement to the physical examination for the complete evaluation of symptomatic adults and for the screening of asymptomatic women at risk for breast cancer or for those who have undergone treatment for breast cancer. It has also helped to demonstrate the natural history of breast cancer (Fig. 10–32). Mammography is used to direct the aspiration or core needle biopsy of nonpalpable lesions and to localize such lesions for surgical excision. Specimen radiographs serve to confirm that the appropriate site was removed for diagnosis.

The development of mammography can be traced to 1913, when Salomon correlated the clinical, pathologic, and roentgenologic characteristics of 3000 amputated breasts and noted many of the radiologic features of breast tumors. By the 1920s, several workers were investigating mammography's clinical application, and in 1929, Warren achieved an 85% to 95% diagnostic accuracy in 119 cases of breast disease (Warren, 1930; and Egan, 1972). The results, however, were inconsistent, and over the next two and a half decades only a few clinicians continued to investigate the modality's possibilities (Leborgne, 1953; and Gershon-Cohen et al., 1962). In 1960, Egan improved breast imaging by using a high-milliamperage, low-kilovoltage technique and standardized views. The reproducibility of his method and of the interpretation of its results led to widespread use.

At present, two views of each breast are standard: the

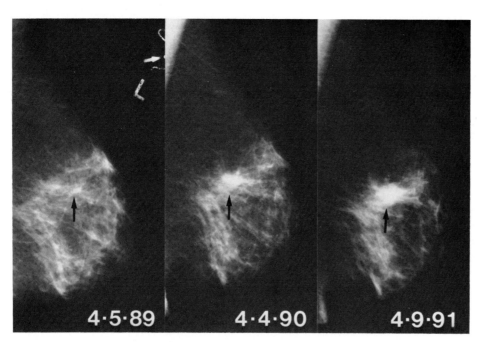

Figure 10–32. The growth of this 40-year-old woman's breast cancer during the course of 2 years is seen on serial mammograms. Originally, the tumor measured 0.3 cm in diameter. One year later, it measured 0.7 cm in diameter, and on the final radiograph, it measured 1.4 cm in diameter. Using these measurements to calculate the volume of a sphere, it was estimated that the tumor had a net doubling time of 2.5 months.

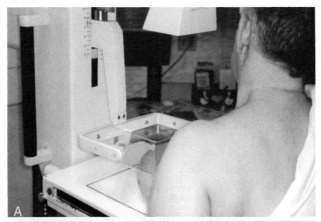

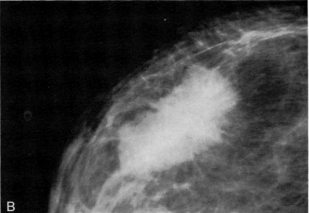

Figure 10-33. Typically, cancer appears as a spiculated density on a mammogram. *A,* Breast compressed in mammography unit for CC view. *B,* Mammographic image of a typical cancer.

mediolateral oblique (MLO) view and the *craniocaudal* (CC) view. With the former, the x-rays pass through the breast from the upper inner quadrant to the lower outer quadrant, including much of the axillary extension; with the latter view, the x-rays pass through vertically, from the upper hemisphere to the lower hemisphere. Special views include the mediolateral (ML); an exaggerated CC view that includes more of the lateral breast (XCCL); focal compression views; and magnification views. Compression of the breast during the examination reduces the amount of tissue that must be penetrated and produces better images. In this way, calcifications are seen more clearly; the same is true for tumors, which are not as compressible as breast tissue.

Mammography exposes the breast to ionizing radiation, but the dose of this radiation is small. The estimated dose to the midbreast for each view is less than 40 mrad. For comparison, a single posteroanterior view chest radiograph involves an average of 10 mrad of exposure (add another 15 mrad for the lateral view), and a CT scan more than 1000 mrad (National Council on Radiation Protection and Measurements, 1989). Digital mammography is a more recent innovation that reproduces the mammographic image on a computer screen. The image can then be manipulated

to advantage with magnification and contrast. Hence, less radiation exposure is needed to evaluate some patients.

The images of the two breasts of a patient should be compared for symmetry, and current mammograms should always be compared with previous ones in an effort to detect evolving signs that are too subtle to be detected on a single examination. The most frequent signs of cancer on mammograms are masses (Fig. 10–33), clustered microcalcifications (Fig. 10–34), architectural distortions, and asymmetries. Suspicious masses are typically dense and spiculated or have irregular borders. New or obviously enlarging masses are also suspect. Some benign masses with typical features are easily recognizable. These include intramammary lymph nodes, which are bean-shaped and have hilar notches; multiple round discrete cysts; and degenerating fibroadenomas, with their well-defined borders and gross inner calcifications. Suspicious calcifications are pinpoint, linear, or branched in character. Ordinarily, five or more calcifications clustered within a 1-cm^2 area is considered a threshold for suspicion, and the risk of cancer increases with increases in the number of calcium specks in a cluster (Erickson et al., 1990; Franceschi et al., 1990; and Roses et al., 1991). Benign calcifications include large "popcorn" calcium aggregates, the distinctive streaked calcifications of secretory disease, the tortuous parallel lines typical of calcified vessel walls, and the circular calcifications associated with oil cysts. With close attention to suspicious signs, cancers as small as 2 to 3 mm in diameter can be discovered. Failure of a mammographic mass to enlarge between examinations or of suspicious microcalcifications to increase in number provides no proof of the absence of cancer (Berend et al., 1992; and Lev-Toaff and Feig, 1992) (Fig. 10–35).

Silicone implants used for breast augmentation can hide occult cancers that would be otherwise visible on a mammogram and delay their detection (Silverstein et al., 1990;

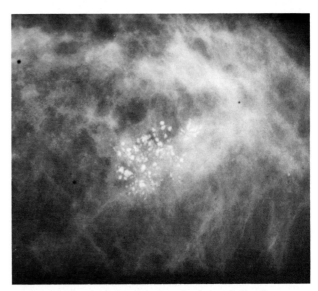

Figure 10-34. Suspicious, clustered microcalcifications on a mammogram betray the presence of a nonpalpable carcinoma.

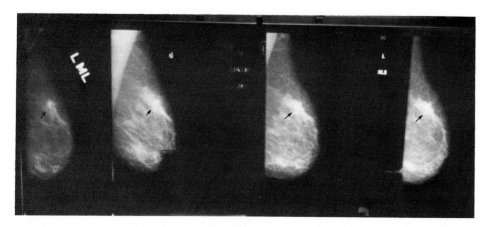

Figure 10–35. Stability of a mammographic density is not inconsistent with the presence of cancer. After its appearance in 1989 (left), this cancer showed no sign of enlargement during the 3 years between 1990 and 1993 (next three images to the right). After it was removed, its S-phase fraction was calculated to be an exceptionally low 0.1%.

and Clark et al., 1993). A special technique that involves displacement of the prosthesis backward away from breast tissue during the examination (the ''pinch'' technique) helps to reduce this problem (Fig. 10–36).

When cancers are large enough to be palpable or are manifest by other clinical signs, they are visible on a mammogram in about 80% to 90% of cases. Of 205 patients with cancers that presented as palpable masses reviewed by the author, mammography showed an abnormality in 169 (82%); this represents the sensitivity of the examination (Table 10–7). The relatively high false-negative rate (18%) seems a paradox until it is appreciated that the detection of mammographic signs of cancer is largely dependent on the visualization of contrast between the lesion and its background. As cancers tend to be radiodense, the fatty radio-lucent breasts of postmenopausal women provide the best background against which to detect tumors. Mammograms of the dense breasts of younger women are less revealing (Fig. 10–37). Consequently, mammography fails to image cancers much more often in women younger than 50 years of age than in older women (Lesnick, 1977; Egeli and Urban, 1979; Niloff and Sheiner, 1981; and Baker, 1982). Cancers are not seen on the mammograms of up to 58% of premenopausal women (Lesnick, 1977). The reasons for the false-negative results include high breast density, failure of the cancer to be included in the standard views, interposition of breast implants, and special clinical presentations, such as Paget's disease of the nipple or small intraductal cancers that present as bloody nipple discharge (Martin et al., 1979). Twenty per cent of missed cancers can be seen on mammograms in retrospect but are simply missed by the radiologist who originally reads the films (Fig. 10–38) (Reintgen et al., 1993). The substantial rate of false-negative results with mammography means that its use must be supplemented with physical examination if optimal detection of breast cancers is to be achieved. It also means that a normal mammogram is of no consequence when signs of cancer are present on physical examination.

Figure 10–36. Breast implants can hide carcinomas unless the proper mammographic technique is used. A breast implant obscured this carcinoma (right). Displacing the implant backward with a ''pinch'' technique permitted its visualization (left).

Table 10–7. MAMMOGRAPHIC DIAGNOSIS OF PALPABLE BREAST MASSES*

Mammographic Diagnosis	Biopsy Diagnosis		
	Cancer	Benign	Total
All Cases			
Normal	36 (18%)	151	187
Mass	150	96	246
Abnormal	19	15	34
Total	205	262	467
<50 Years of Age			
Normal	21 (29%)	122	143
Mass	42	72	114
Abnormal	10	11	21
Total	73	205	278
≥50 Years of Age			
Normal	15 (11%)	29	44
Mass	108	24	132
Abnormal	9	4	13
Total	132	57	189

*Author's personal series (1982–1991).

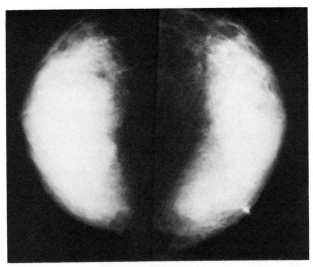

Figure 10–37. This mammogram (craniocaudal views of the right and left breasts) shows the extreme density of the breasts of a premenopausal woman. Breast density such as this often hampers cancer detection in young women.

Since the radiologic signs of cancer are not unique, mammography is an inexact means of evaluating a palpable mass. Considerable variation exists among radiologists with respect to the interpretation of mammograms (Choucair et al., 1988), and it is difficult to document the assumption that accuracy is improved by experience. Masses considered suspicious on physical examination but benign on mammography prove to be cancers in up to 6% of cases (Lewis et al., 1976). This fact makes it difficult to exclude the presence of cancer when a palpable mass either cannot be visualized or when such a mass has benign radiologic characteristics.

In the absence of clinical abnormalities, mammography is invaluable for detecting small, early cancers, which are infrequently associated with axillary metastases and are highly curable (Fig. 10–39A). Presently, most cancers smaller than 2.0 cm in diameter are detected only with mammography (see Fig. 10–39B). Since the introduction of widespread screening with mammography, breast biopsies are increasingly being performed solely for the assessment of mammographically detected abnormalities (Fig. 10–40). The detection of these cancers, however, is obtained with a high rate of false-positive results. In the author's series, cancers were found in 16.1% of 631 biopsies performed to assess mammographically detected lesions, which is equivalent to a false-positive rate of 83.9% (see Table 10–15).

Mammography is indicated as part of the basic diagnostic examination of all symptomatic adult females over 20 years of age. Younger women are excluded because their breasts are sensitive to the mutagenic effects of ionizing radiation, the incidence of cancer among them is negligible, and the probability of obtaining any useful information from mammography is remote. When the results of physical examination of the breasts are normal, a normal mammogram provides additional assurance that a lesion has not been missed. Mammography is of less value for evaluating the nature of a palpable mass than it is for detecting additional lesions in the same or opposite breast that may also need

attention. Mammography is also indicated in women who are to undergo any surgical procedure involving the breast, such as open biopsy, breast reduction, or implantation of prostheses. It is a useful means of evaluating the breasts as a potential site of an occult primary tumor when metastatic adenocarcinoma is found in axillary lymph nodes. Mammography's use in screening is discussed elsewhere.

ULTRASOUND EXAMINATION

Ultrasound is often a valuable complement to physical examination and mammography. It is noninvasive and involves no radiation exposure. According to Kobayashi (1982), the early development of ultrasonic detection began in 1951 with Wild's unidimensional A-mode display, which rapidly evolved into the two-dimensional "echograph" (Wild and Neal, 1951). In 1954, Howry and coworkers reported the first echographic demonstration of a scirrhous carcinoma with a two-dimensional B-mode radioscanner (Kobayashi, 1982). At present, ultrasound is used for the evaluation of breast lesions and, in some cases, for guiding aspiration (Ciatto et al., 1993).

Two techniques for examination of the breast are in use. One involves the use of a hand-held real-time scanner. Direct contact is made between the scanner and the skin of the breast, and a lubricant is used to eliminate the air-tissue interface (Fig. 10–41). A two-dimensional, gray-scale image is produced. The second technique is a dedicated, whole-breast, computed ultrasonic examination that uses multiple step images. The air-surface interface is eliminated either by supporting the patient in the prone position, with the dependent breast immersed in a tank of water, or, more conveniently, by placing a bag of degassed water on the breast with the patient in a supine position. The hand-held unit may yield more accurate results than the automated scanner (Bassett et al., 1987). On an echogram, echogenic structures appear bright, and nonechogenic structures appear dark. Three features of a structure are notable: (1) its boundaries and shape; (2) its internal echoes; and (3) its posterior shadowing. Benign masses tend to have a regular, smooth, and round or oval boundary. They either are free of internal echoes, as are cysts (Fig. 10–42), or have

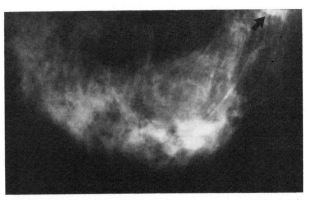

Figure 10–38. The misreading of mammograms contributes to false-negative results. The cancer in this breast is located on the extreme posterolateral side but was not noticed (arrow).

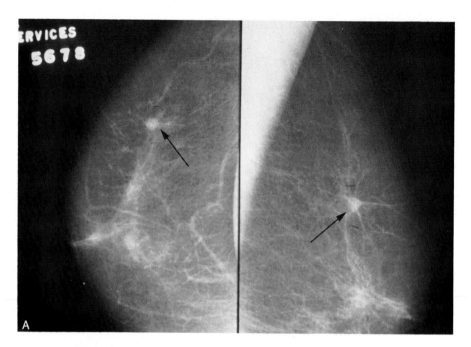

Method of Detection of 242 Breast Cancers by Size from 1982 to 1989

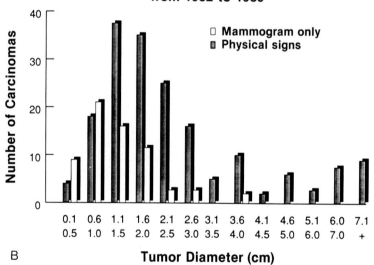

Figure 10–39. *A,* The occult cancer detected in the craniocaudal and mediolateral oblique views of this mammogram is less than 1 cm in diameter. At this size, axillary metastases are unlikely, and cancers are highly curable. *B,* Most cancers smaller than 1.0 cm in diameter are detected only with mammography. The exceptions are those in small breasts, those situated superficially, or those that present as Paget's disease or nipple discharge (author's cases).

Changing Indications for Breast Biopsy
(722 Consecutive Biopsies)

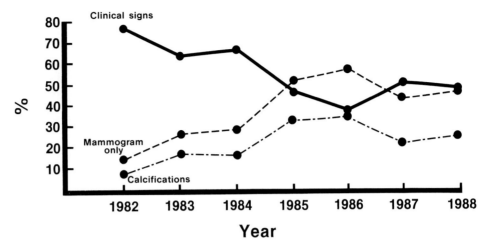

Figure 10–40. An increasing proportion of all breast biopsies are performed for abnormalities detected by mammography alone (author's cases).

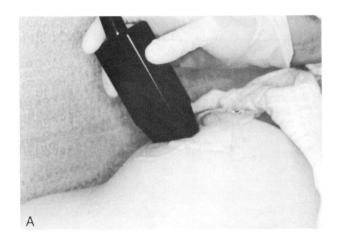

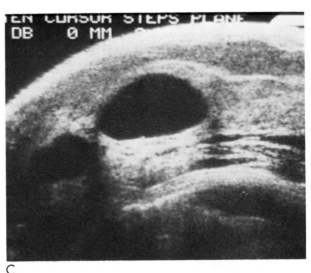

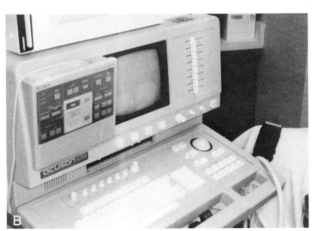

Figure 10–41. Hand-held ultrasonography of the breast. The transducer (A) is moved in contact with the skin over the area of interest with an interface of lubricating jelly. The image is produced on the console (B). C, Ultrasound image of a cyst showing smooth margins, dark center, edge shadows, and a bright posterior wall.

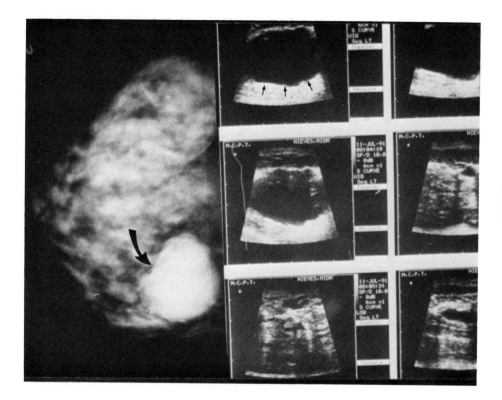

Figure 10–42. Mammographic *(left)* and ultrasonic *(right)* images of a typical cyst.

homogeneous, uniformly sized internal echoes, such as are seen with fibroadenomas (Fig. 10–43). Lateral shadow signs may be present; these are anechoic, distal projections from the borders of the lesion. The deep margin is characteristically bright and echogenic, projecting posteriorly as a "tadpole sign." By contrast, boundary echoes of typical maligant masses are irregular and jagged. The internal echoes are nonhomogeneous, and the posterior margin is obscure, with a dark, anechoic shadow projecting posteriorly (the middle shadow sign; Fig. 10–44). Cancers may have variable features (Fig. 10–45), as described by Maturo and colleagues (1982): (1) a hypoechoic mass with uneven, discontinuous boundaries, nonuniform internal echoes, and a poorly defined back wall with variable posterior sonic attenuation; (2) a hyperechoic focus appearing as a bright mass with a discrete posterior shadow; (3) a disrupted mammary parenchyma with an irregular echogenic zone and a discrete distal acoustic shadow; or (4) an atypical,

cystic mass with an anechoic center, poorly defined edges, and posterior bright sonic enhancement.

With ultrasound, it is possible to confuse small cancers with fibroadenomas, miss diffusely infiltrating cancers, and either miss or fail to discern the pattern of calcifications (Guyer, 1989). Although ultrasound can suggest the nature of a solid mass, the sonographic characteristics of cancers are not sufficiently unique for them to be considered definitive for distinguishing benign tumors from malignant ones. Ultrasound is least accurate in detecting cancers in the fatty, postmenopausal breast and poor in detecting microcalcifications. Also, small cancers often escape detection (McSweeney and Murphy, 1985). The accuracy of ultrasound in detecting cancers smaller than 2 cm in diameter is no greater than 57% and only 23% of minimal cancers are detected (Rosner and Blaird, 1985). It is unusual for ultrasound to detect cancers not already evident on physical examination or a mammogram (Bassett et al., 1987). For

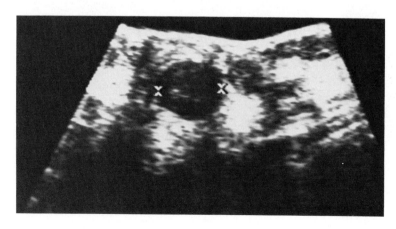

Figure 10–43. Ultrasonic image of a fibroadenoma, which appears dark and with a smooth outline. Echoes from its homogeneous interior are relatively few but appear as bright spots (variable shadowing projects posteriorly). Boundaries are marked by **X** for measuring purposes. (Courtesy of John R. Milbrath, M.D.)

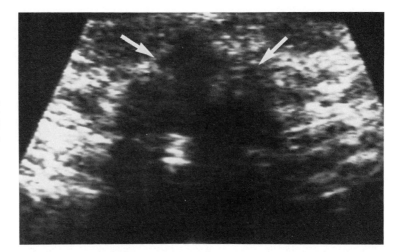

Figure 10–44. Ultrasonic image of a carcinoma, which appears as a dark area with irregular borders and internal echoes. A large, dark shadow projects posteriorly. (Courtesy of John R. Milbrath, M.D.)

these reasons, ultrasound is not an effective modality for screening.

Ultrasound excels, however, in the identification of lesions in radiologically dense breasts and in the differentiation of cysts from solid tumors. Occasional errors in interpretation are caused by cysts that contain thick fluid or fluid-containing particulate matter (such fluid creates internal echoes, making the cysts appear solid) and by homogenous tumors, such as some fibroadenomas (these reflect few internal echoes and can appear cystic) (Boyd et al., 1981). Among the author's cases, 3 (6%) of 84 mammographic densities that were considered solid on ultrasound proved to be cysts when they were removed. At least two fibroadenomas had the sonographic characteristics of cysts. Cysts that lack the classic characteristics (e.g., a thin, smooth wall, a round or ovoid shape, and an absence of internal echoes) are worthy of suspicion. Despite its limitations, ultrasound is a useful complement to mammography for

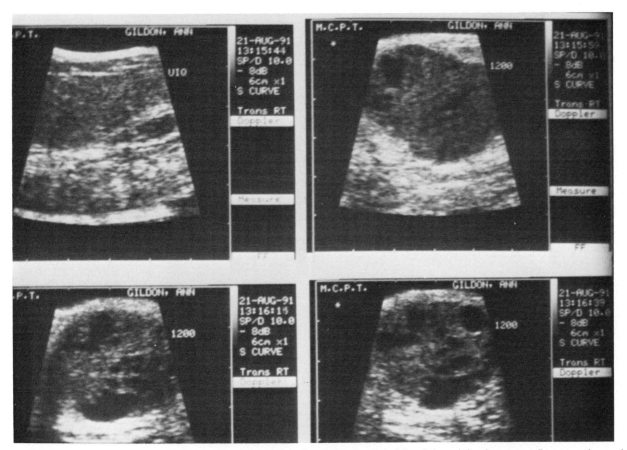

Figure 10–45. An invasive papillary carcinoma shows mixed ultrasonic characteristics: internal shadows as well as an echogenic posterior wall.

evaluating the dense breast and can provide additional information when the results of physical examination and mammography are equivocal. Rubin and colleagues (1985) found ultrasound to be a useful adjunct to mammography in three groups of patients: (1) those with dense breasts and localized symptoms, or with a suspicious area detected on mammography; (2) those with nonpalpable abnormalities discovered on mammograms; and (3) those with palpable masses considered indeterminant on a mammogram. The author has found ultrasound most useful for evaluating symptomatic dense breasts, nonpalpable densities found on mammograms that suggest cysts, and equivocal physical findings when the mammogram is normal. It is also useful as a method to guide aspiration of nonpalpable cystic structures. When a mass is palpable, fine-needle aspiration of the mass is a quick and inexpensive means of determining whether it is cystic or solid. If it is a cyst, aspiration is therapeutic as well. Ultrasound can be employed for the assessment of palpable masses when a patient does not permit aspiration or if a mass is too small and deep to serve as a reliable target.

COMPUTED TOMOGRAPHY OF THE BREAST

CT of the breast has attributes that make it valuable for evaluating breast lesions in special situations, and it can detect breast cancers that are overlooked by other methods. CT body scanners have performed as well in this respect as have dedicated CT mammographic units. CT permits visualization of both the axillary and the internal mammary lymph nodes and provides excellent delineation of the deep mammary and retromammary tissues. Detection is facilitated by asymmetry in the architecture of the breast tissue

and by the fact that breast cancers concentrate intravenous iodinated contrast media, as do some benign lesions, with marked contrast enhancement on postinjection scans (Fig. 10–46). Tumors as small as 2 mm in diameter have been detected with CT; however, no definite relationship exists between tumor size and contrast enhancement. Chang and associates (1982) suggested several situations in which CT imaging of the breast may be of value. These include (1) the detection of cancers in dense breasts when mammography is of limited value owing to lack of tissue contrast, (2) the detection of mammographically and physically unsuspected small breast cancers, and (3) the detection of breast cancer when axillary lymph node biopsy results are positive for carcinoma and when mammograms fail to demonstrate the presence of a primary tumor. The detection of unsuspected primary tumors in the contralateral breast is also possible with CT. Occasionally, CT can localize a tumor that is seen in only one mammographic view.

The limitations of CT prevent it from achieving widespread use and from replacing conventional mammography. These limitations are several. A high dose of radiation is involved; this dose may vary between 3.2 and 1.2 rads to the skin per examination, depending on the number of images obtained (Doust et al., 1981). This is approximately 15 times the dose received with low-dose film mammography and is high enough to exclude CT as a screening method. Other disadvantages include the unnecessary irradiation of other parts of the thorax during examination, the need to use intravenous contrast media to optimize the results, the high cost of examination, and the excessive duration of the procedure. Finally, microcalcifications without an associated mass cannot be identified owing to the averaging effect of the CT computer matrix. This is a serious limitation, as not only the presence of calcifications but also their pattern is important in deciding for or against the need for biopsy.

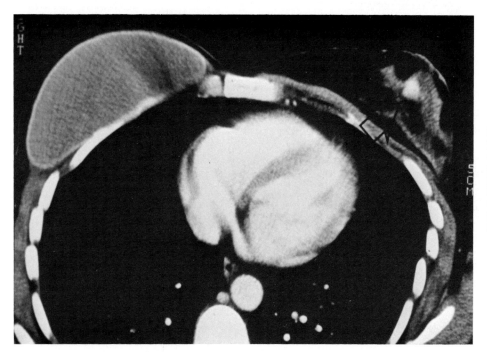

Figure 10–46. Both cancers and benign tumors can become enhanced on CT scans. This patient has a reconstructed right breast and a bright focus in the left breast. The latter was proved to be attributable to the presence of a fibroadenoma *(arrow).*

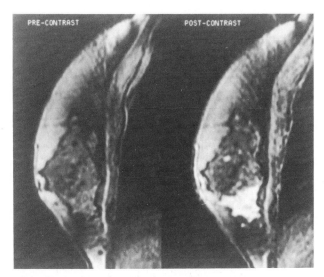

Figure 10–47. MRI scan with enhancement showing a carcinoma in the lower portion of the breast. The unenhanced scan *(left)* shows the tumor only vaguely. The enhanced scan *(right)* provides vivid contrast between the cancer and normal tissues and a more accurate representation of its true extent. (Courtesy of Steven E. Harms, M.D., Director of Magnetic Resonance at Baylor University Medical Center, Houston, TX.)

MAGNETIC RESONANCE IMAGING

MRI is under evaluation as a means for the detection and diagnosis of breast lesions. It does not involve the exposure of patients to ionizing radiation, but the method is cumbersome and expensive. The image is produced by energy released from the motion of atoms subjected to a powerful magnetic field. With MRI, cysts are easily distinguished from solid tumors, and masses as small as 2 mm in diameter can be detected (Powell and Stelling, 1988). It is particularly useful in the examination of the breasts of women with silicone prostheses and in the detection of leaks from prostheses (silicone can be subtracted from the image and made to appear black). However, microcalcifications are not well visualized with MRI, and the morphologic characteristics of cancers do not readily distinguish them from benign masses (Sickles, 1990). These limitations make MRI unsuited for screening, but the modality may prove useful for the evaluation of lesions detected by other means and for the staging of cancers. With the use of special coils designed for the breast, fat-suppressed chemical-shift imaging, and enhancement with the intravenous administration of gadopentetate dimeglumine, cancers can often be distinguished from benign changes both by their degree of enhancement and their temporal pattern (Fig. 10–47) (Rubens et al., 1991; and Porter and Smith, 1993). Cancers also may be detected in regional nodes. The true sensitivity and specificity of MRI for the evaluation of breast cancers remains uncertain.

FINE-NEEDLE ASPIRATION CYTOLOGY

Fine-needle aspiration of a breast mass provides an opportunity not only to determine whether the mass is cystic or solid but also to obtain a specimen for cytologic examina-

tion, which can provide a strong indication of whether cancer is present. A result on fine-needle aspiration cytology (FNAC) that is positive for carcinoma serves to prepare a patient for a probable diagnosis of cancer, to justify a staging evaluation, and, since the probability of error is small, to offer the convenience of biopsy and treatment in one step (Lannin et al., 1986). FNAC is a safe procedure, and if its limitations are recognized, it is a useful adjunct to the clinical examination (Robbins et al., 1954).

When no free fluid is found on aspiration of a palpable mass, a specimen for cytology is always obtained. The needle is moved back and forth within the mass several times while suction is continually applied (Fig. 10–48). When a small amount of tissue fluid appears in the hub of the needle, the suction is discontinued, and the needle is removed from the breast. The specimen is prepared for cytologic examination by disengaging the needle from the syringe, drawing some air into the syringe, reconnecting the syringe to the needle, and ejecting the material in the needle onto a slide. The specimen is smeared using a second slide and quickly fixated using a 95% alcohol solution or other fixative. Careful execution of the technique and access to an experienced cytopathologist provide optimum results (Fig. 10–49). Accuracy increases with experience, and

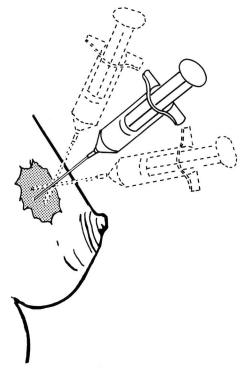

Figure 10–48. The technique for FNAC of solid breast tumors is shown. A 21-gauge needle and a small syringe are used. After engaging the mass, suction is applied to the syringe while the needle is passed back and forth through the tumor at several angles. Suction is released before the needle is withdrawn to avoid aspirating normal tissues. The entire specimen is contained within the needle; it is expelled onto a glass slide by first disconnecting the needle from the syringe, drawing air into the syringe, reconnecting the needle, and blowing the specimen out onto a glass slide. To avoid air drying, the specimen is smeared immediately with another glass slide, and both slides are dropped into 95% alcohol solution.

Table 10–8. FINE-NEEDLE ASPIRATION CYTOLOGY (FNAC) OF SOLID BREAST MASSES[*]

	Total FNACs (n)	Sensitivity +/CAs (%)	Specificity −/Benign (%)	False-Positive[†] (%)	False-Negative (%)	Accuracy (%)
Abele et al. (1983)	92	88	97	0	13	93
Bell et al. (1983)	583	69	67	0	17	68
Kaufman et al. (1983)	163	90	97	2	12	93
Frable and Frable (1982)	588	91	98	2	9	95
Malberger et al. (1981)	206	92	95	0	8	94
Kher et al. (1981)	80	94	93	0	6	94
Kline et al. (1979)	3545	66	98	0	10	95
Zajdela et al. (1975)	2772	88	89	0.3	12	89
Rosen et al. (1972)	206	82	100	0	18	84
Franzen and Stenkvist (1968)	1713	76	93	0.1	24	92
Total	9948	82	94	0.2	18	89

[*]Confirmed histologically.
[†]Total = 13.
This table shows the correlation of 9948 fine-needle aspiration cytologies of breast masses with biopsies that were read as either positive or negative for malignancy. The procedure is highly accurate in practiced hands, and false-positive results are unusual.

false-negative and false-positive results are unique to specific users.

FNAC is a highly operator-dependent technique, and one finds considerable variation in the experience reported with its use for the diagnosis of breast masses (Giard and Hermans, 1992). Several extensive reviews on the subject are available (Grant et al., 1986; Hammond et al., 1987; Layfield et al., 1989; and Kline, 1990) (Table 10–8). From 32% to 99% of specimens are satisfactory for analysis. Overall accuracy of analysis varies from 89% to 99%. When the cytologic preparation is considered definitely indicative of cancer by an experienced cytopathologist, the opinion is seldom incorrect. The rate of false-positive results ranges as high as 18%, but the median is closer to 1% or 2%. False-negative rates reach levels of 35% and have been associated with the presence of small tumors, a scanty number of cells collected, and special histologic types of cancers for example, infiltrating lobular, tubular and mucinous carcinomas (O'Malley et al., 1993). In the opinion of some physicians, a positive diagnosis of cancer on FNAC obviates the need for biopsy and histologic diagnosis prior to

the initiation of treatment (Sheikh et al., 1988; Watson et al., 1987; Smith et al., 1988; Nicastri et al., 1991; and Saunders et al., 1991). Others advise that caution be exercised with its use (Bell et al., 1983; and Kahky et al., 1988). The author's experience with 153 FNACs of breast masses has indicated that FNAC is not sufficiently accurate either to rule out the presence of cancer or to guarantee its presence (Table 10–9). Misinterpretation of atypical hyperplasias, fat necrosis, duct papillomas, and even fibroadenomas can cause false-positive diagnoses. Also, with FNAC, one is incapable of making the important distinction between in situ and invasive carcinoma or between lymphoma and undifferentiated carcinoma. The inherent limitations of FNAC are also encountered with stereotactic guided fine-needle aspiration cytology of nonpalpable breast lesions found on mammography (Kopans, 1989). Dowlatshahi and associates (1989) reported a sensitivity of 95% and a specificity of 91% for 528 guided FNACs.

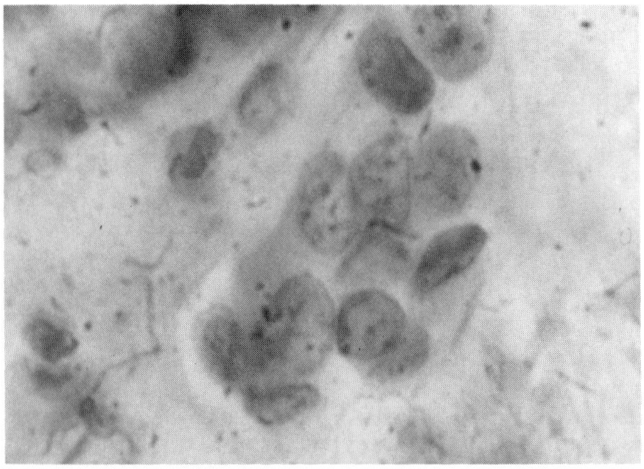

TRIPLE DIAGNOSIS

The combination of FNAC, mammography, and physical examination—often referred to as "triple diagnosis"—may be more reliable than cytology alone. When the results of all three are indicative of cancer, open biopsies confirm cancer in 99.4% of cases. Conversely, when the results of

Figure 10–49. This specimen was positive for cancer on cytologic examination. The sample was obtained from a breast mass with fine-needle aspiration.

Table 10–9. AUTHOR'S PERSONAL EXPERIENCE WITH CYTOLOGIC DIAGNOSIS OF 153 PALPABLE BREAST MASSES BY FINE-NEEDLE ASPIRATION (FNAC)

	Result on Cytologic Diagnosis		
Histologic Diagnosis	Negative*	Suspicious	Positive[†]
Carcinoma	18	22	41
Benign	64	5	3[‡]

Accuracy (based on negative or positive cytology results) = 83.3%.
*False-negative = 22.0%.
[†]False-positive = 6.89%; positive predictive value = 93%.
[‡]Fibrocystic changes, duct papilloma, and fat necrosis.

Table 10–10. PROBABILITY OF CANCER IN PATIENTS WITH PALPABLE BREAST MASSES ACCORDING TO RESULTS OF "TRIPLE DIAGNOSIS"

	Result on FNAC, Probability of Cancer (%)		
	Benign	*Suspicious*	*Positive*
Result on Physical Examination—Benign			
Results of Mammography:			
Benign	0.6	16.0	100
Suspicious	4.1	32.4	100
Positive	5.7	55.7	100
Result on Physical Examination—Suspicious or Positive			
Results of Mammography:			
Benign	7.1	43.8	94.7
Suspicious	6.9	62.5	96.6
Positive	35.7	91.4	99.4

(From Donegan, W. L.: Current concepts: Evaluation of a palpable breast mass. N. Engl. J. Med., *327:*937–942, 1992, by permission of the New England Journal of Medicine.)

all three suggest a benign lesion, cancer is found in only 0.4% of cases (Donegan, 1992). Some physicians feel that observation is justified if the results of all three tests are negative for cancer (Butler et al., 1990; and Somers et al., 1992). Impressions are not uniform, however, and concurrence is not regularly obtained. When the results of either physical examination or mammography suggest cancer, a negative result on FNAC is not reliable. The probabilities of cancer being present when varying results are obtained from these three modalities are shown in Table 10–10. The data in Table 10–10 were obtained from one institution. Results tend to vary between institutions and should be determined in each case.

BIOPSY

The diagnosis of cancer is based on histology, and this fundamental axiom is not safely ignored. Only with biopsy—that is, the removal of a sample of tissue sufficient for histologic examination—can a diagnosis of breast cancer be made with ultimate confidence. The accuracy of the information obtained from a biopsy specimen is limited only by the accuracy of the sampling and of the histologic interpretation. Since a negative result on biopsy analysis can be due to sampling error, cancer cannot be excluded unless all pathologic tissue is removed and examined. Therapy for cancer should be predicated on histologic verification. Pertinent issues are the need for frozen sections, the indications for biopsy, and the results of various methods. Techniques of biopsy are discussed more fully in Chapter 18.

Permanent Versus Frozen Sections

The most accurate method for histologic examination of tissues is with stained paraffin (permanent) sections; the only disadvantage of this method is the 24 to 48 hours it requires for preparation. Preparation involves the fixing of

tissue in a preservative, encasing it in paraffin blocks, the sectioning and mounting of sections of the blocks onto glass slides, the staining of the slides, and, finally, interpretation of the slides. At the turn of the century, the theoretical risk of spreading cancer with a biopsy spurred the development of frozen sectioning by Welch (Sparkman, 1962) and by Wilson (1905); this technique permits diagnosis and treatment to be performed at the same operation. With frozen sectioning, tissues are quickly frozen, sectioned, mounted on slides, stained, and interpreted within a few minutes of the time that they were obtained. Permanent sections are also routinely prepared at the same time, and a final diagnosis follows at a later date. Incorrect diagnoses that result from interpretation of frozen sections are rare if decisions are deferred in the event of any uncertainty. In a review by Rosen (1978) of 556 consecutive breast biopsy specimens examined with frozen sections, no false-positive reports attended the diagnosis of cancer in 145 cases. Because of doubt, a diagnosis was deferred until paraffin sections could be prepared in 5.4% of the biopsies, and 8 of 381 biopsies (2.1%) initially considered benign proved to contain carcinoma after examination with permanent sections. Lesions that can cause problems on frozen sectioning are papillary lesions, sclerosing adenosis, florid adenosis, atypical duct hyperplasia, fat necrosis, and lobular carcinoma in situ (Kagali, 1983). These lesions are best diagnosed with permanent sections. Layfield and coworkers (1989) collected from the literature 15,867 reports of diagnoses based on the evaluation of frozen sections compared with diagnoses based on the study of permanent sections. They found 155 false-negative and 3 (0.019%) false-positive diagnoses. False-positive diagnoses are rare but are potentially tragic; for greatest accuracy, treatment decisions are based on the evaluation of permanent sections.

Numerous studies fail to substantiate a prognostic advantage for diagnosis and treatment of breast cancer in one step (Table 10–11). A delay of several days or longer between biopsy and treatment appears to have no adverse effect on prognosis, an observation supported with this author's personal data (Table 10–12). For the most part, these studies are faulty owing to the small numbers of specimens studied, biased case selection and inadequate controls. However, Fisher and colleagues (1985) found no adverse effect of delay on the survival of 1640 patients—regardless of whether residual cancer was found at the site of biopsy and with delays of up to 14 days between biopsy and mastectomy—when compared with 510 concomitant but nonrandomized controls who had undergone one-step diagnosis and treatment. It would appear that any risk inherent in the trauma of biopsy and of the modest delay of treatment is too small to measure easily or is inconsequential with respect to the prospects for cure. Protracted delays attended by clinical tumor progression may be associated with less favorable prospects for cure (Charlson, 1985). In 1979, a "two-step" procedure (i.e., diagnosis and treatment at separate times) was recommended by the National Cancer Institute, the rationale for which was to permit an interval for staging, for considering treatment alternatives, and for thorough pathologic consultation prior to the initiation of treatment. With the safety of a two-step approach to diagnosis and treatment reasonably established, the necessity for di-

Table 10–11. BIOPSY WITH DELAYED MASTECTOMY*

	No. of Cases	Duration of Delay	5-Year Survival	Controls and 5-Year Survival	Conclusion
Nohrman (1949)	91	0–3 d 4–14 d 15+ d	81% 74% 71%	Own, historical (78%)	3 days' delay OK
Pierce et al. (1956)	96	6 mo	61.1% 44% Ax + 75% Ax −	Own, historical (60%), 554 cases	No harm
Jackson and Pitts (1959)	51	2–145 d	62.7%	Others, historical	No harm
Sayago and Sirebrenik (1959)	40		14% Ax +	Own, historical (82%), Ax+	30 days' delay OK
Prechtel and Hallbauer (1979)	64	7 d		Own, historical Worse if > 3 cm diameter and Ax+ 15 cases	7 days' delay OK
Knapp and Mullen (1976)	58	0–46 d	72.4%	Own, historical, 48% (31 cases)	No harm
Abramson (1976)	41	1–30 d	79.5% 44.5% Ax + 90% Ax −	Others, historical	No harm
Fisher (1985)	164	27 d	Stages I and II 59%	Own, concomitant (52%), 510 cases	14 days' delay OK; no information on longer delay

*A number of studies have failed to demonstrate an adverse effect of delay between biopsy and mastectomy. Almost all, however, have included inadequate numbers of cases or lacked randomized concomitant controls, permitting small differences to be missed. In general, no adverse effect on survival has been demonstrated by modest delays in treatment.

agnosis of breast lesions based on frozen sections has largely disappeared (Oberman, 1993). Frozen section is still useful during biopsy for the immediate relief of a patient's anxiety, to identify cancers for tests that require viable tissues, and to ensure that a tissue sample has provided a secure diagnosis of cancer. It is useful when cancer is highly likely and the patient prefers a one-step procedure, and it is helpful for the evaluation of questionable surgical margins during treatment with segmental mastectomy.

Outpatient biopsy of the breast under local anesthesia is routine practice both for patients with clinically and mammographically discovered lesions (Stein, 1982; Bertario et al., 1985; and Charlson, 1985). The benefits of this procedure include convenience and economy. If a lesion is benign, and most lesions are, uncertainty is quickly resolved; if a lesion is malignant, treatment can be discussed and planned based on a secure diagnosis.

Indications for Biopsy

Indications for biopsy are generally derived from the results of physical examination or mammography. On physical examination, they are the presence of

1. a persistent mass or dominant nodule;
2. a persistently discharging nipple duct;
3. an abscess or unexplained inflammation;
4. unexplained changes in the nipple;
5. undiagnosed cutaneous nodules or ulcerations;
6. exaggerated firmness of the entire breast.

On mammography, the indications are the presence of

1. a suspicious mass;
2. suspicious microcalcifications;
3. architectural distortion;
4. suspicious or evolving asymmetry.

Table 10–12. SURVIVAL VERSUS DURATION OF DELAY BETWEEN BIOPSY AND RADICAL MASTECTOMY IN CLINICALLY LOCALIZED CASES (ELLIS FISCHER STATE CANCER HOSPITAL, 1940 TO 1958)*

Delay (d)	Total No. of Cases	5-Year Survival (%)	Median Tumor Diameter (cm)
No biopsy	49	57.1	3.0
Biopsy at surgery	133	70.7	2.0
1–7	51	64.7	3.0
8–14	36	63.9	2.8
15–21	17	47.1	3.3
22–28	13	61.5	2.3
29–35	11	90.9	1.5
36–42	7	85.7	1.8
>42	15	60.0	1.5

*The duration of delay between biopsy and radical surgery is not correlated with the per cent 5-year postoperative survival. Patients with a prolonged delay, however, had smaller tumors and a disproportionate number of less aggressive histologic types. No deleterious effect of biopsy or of a delay before mastectomy of up to 42 days can be shown on prognosis.

Table 10–13. CORE NEEDLE BIOPSY

	Number	Sensitivity	Accuracy	False-Negative Results	False-Positive Results
Tru-Cut					
Foster (1982)	30 carcinomas	90%		10%	0
Roberts et al. 1975	87 carcinomas	67%			0
Blamey (1982)	932 carcinomas	76%		19%	
Drill					
Meyerowitz (1976)	135 carcinomas		99%	1.6%	0
Sieninski and Dabska (1976)	600 carcinomas	87%	94%		0

Any one of these indices may substantiate the need for biopsy. A suspicious mass detected with ultrasound alone is unusual, but it too might be an indication for biopsy (Fornage, 1992). Elective biopsy of the normal breast is discussed in the chapter on second primary tumors (Chapter 27).

Essentially, two techniques are available for obtaining tissue suitable for histologic evaluation: core needle biopsy and open biopsy. Either can be performed with local anesthesia; the important difference between the two methods is that core needle biopsy obtains a sample of a lesion, which may or may not be representative, whereas open biopsy provides an opportunity for complete removal of the lesion. Both palpable and clinically occult lesions can be addressed with either technique.

Biopsy Procedures

Core Needle Biopsy

Since core needle biopsy is an office procedure, it is a swift and convenient means of confirming that cancer is present. It can be performed through a small puncture wound and provides a slender core of tissue that is 1 to 2 cm in length (Fig. 10–50). For the biopsy of palpable masses, a hand-held disposable needle is available (the Tru-Cut needle Baxter Health Care, Valencia, CA). Minkowitz and associates (1986) reported a sensitivity of 80% and no false-positive results for 146 core needle biopsies. Accuracy is

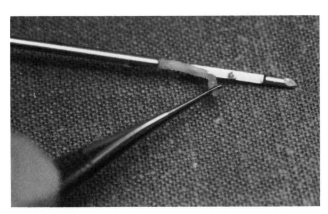

Figure 10–50. A specimen from core needle biopsy of the breast.

directly related to the size of the palpable mass that is biopsied. Nonpalpable lesions that are visualized on mammography can be sampled with stereotactic guided needle biopsy—that is, the application of dedicated equipment that uses mammography to guide the needle (Parker et al., 1991). With the guided needle biopsy, very small targets can be sampled accurately. No false-positive diagnoses with core needle biopsy have been reported (Table 10–13). The rate of false-negative diagnoses with hand-held needle biopsy varies from 1.6% to 19%. The false-negative rate with stereotactic needle biopsy is very low but measurable (4.3%) (Parker et al., 1991). The possibility of sampling error continues to make open biopsy prudent whenever core needle biopsy evaluation of a suspicious lesion fails to reveal cancer.

Open Biopsy

Open biopsy requires an incision and is performed in an operating room. As the analysis of only one of every three biopsies of palpable masses reveals cancer, care is taken to ensure cosmetic healing. Whenever feasible, incisions are made in the lines of cutaneous tension of the breast (Fig. 10–51). Incisions should be made directly over lesions and, whenever possible, within the bounds of a future mastectomy in the event that one proves necessary. Incisions at the periphery of the breast pose no problem when a lumpectomy is used for treatment. When a mastectomy is planned, they can be circumscribed and left in continuity with the specimen, and thus avoid gerrymandering the mastectomy incision (Scanlon, 1989). Since circumareolar incisions are maximally cosmetic, they are often used for central lesions, even when a short flap is necessary if the lesion is likely to be benign. Sometimes, incisions can be made through old scars to avoid making new ones.

Surgical biopsies may be either *incisional* (removal of only a part of a tumor) or *excisional* (removal of the entire lesion). Small tumors are best excised completely with minimal disturbance to them. This provides optimal tissues for the pathologist, and, if the tumor proves to be benign, it serves as adequate treatment. If the surgical margins are normal, excision can also serve as a satisfactory lumpectomy for cancer in preparation for treatment with primary irradiation. Removal of a small sample of large masses is usually sufficient for diagnostic purposes and is preferable to a wide dissection. If a diagnosis of cancer is not forthcoming on frozen section, the remaining abnormal tissue is

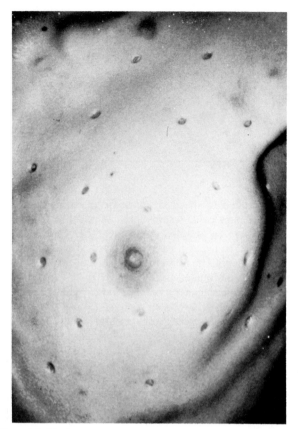

Figure 10–51. An example of Langer's technique used to study lines of skin tension on the female breast (autopsy case). The distortion of circular skin defects makes a pattern concentric with the nipple.

removed for examination. Biopsy incisions should be closed only after meticulous hemostasis, and on closure no drains should be used. Only the subcutaneous fat and the skin are closed. No attempt is made to suture the parenchyma of the breast because it can reconstitute itself in a more natural way than the surgeon can contrive (Fisher, 1985). Having a patient wear a brassiere for support during the first few days after surgery improves her comfort, and the incision is kept dry until it has healed.

Determination of estrogen and progesterone receptors is routine on cancers. Biochemical determination of receptors requires living tissue, and when such determination is desired, the tissue is transported in ice and quickly frozen. More recently, it has become possible to perform immunocytochemical assays for receptors (estrogen receptor–immunocytochemical assay [ER-ICA]) and cell kinetic studies (S-Phase fraction, DNA index, and ploidy determinations) on fixed tissue. Receptor values obtained on tumors from mastectomy specimens are not appreciably different from those on tumors from biopsies; the additional ischemic time that occurs during mastectomy is of no importance (Rodier et al., 1993).

Skin Biopsy

In two instances, biopsy of the skin of the breast is important for diagnosis: when Paget's disease of the nipple is present, and when inflammatory carcinoma is suspected. A full-thickness punch biopsy of the areola can establish whether Paget's disease is present, and this technique requires only local anesthesia for the patient. In the absence of a palpable mass or mammographic lesion, a punch biopsy diagnosis of Paget's disease is sufficient to justify treatment. Skin biopsy is also useful to confirm inflammatory carcinoma as it can demonstrate invasion of dermal lymphatics. The biopsy specimen should be from areas of reddened and edematous skin; a biopsy specimen of the underlying breast tissue or a subjacent mass should also be taken.

In many instances, a locally advanced, ulcerated carcinoma can be diagnosed easily with a small wedge of tissue excised from the infiltrated cutaneous margin. The area may already be rendered insensitive by the cancer and little or no local anesthesia is required.

Open Biopsy of Nonpalpable Lesions

With current emphasis on early diagnosis, surgeons are increasingly confronted with the need to biopsy nonpalpable lesions found on mammography (Fig. 10–40). The problem of removing the suspicious site without causing undue morbidity and sacrifice of breast tissue requires that localizing techniques be used in conjunction with biopsy (Schwartz and Feig, 1991). These are performed immediately prior to biopsy and permit biopsies to be performed accurately on an outpatient basis with a patient under local anesthesia (Smith-Behn and Ghani, 1987). The two most widely used techniques are *hooked-wire localization* and *spot localization*. Both require introduction of a needle into the breast using mammographic guidance and placement of the tip into or through the lesion. An approach tangential to the chest wall is used to avoid causing a pneumothorax. With hooked-wire localization, a fine wire with a barb is introduced through the needle and left in the breast to guide the surgeon; with spot localization, a dye is injected through the needle as it is withdrawn, providing a visible tract to the lesion. Teamwork between the radiologist, the surgeon, and the pathologist is essential. The hooked-wire technique was introduced by Funderburk and Flax in 1976 but has seen many changes with respect to approach and needle configuration. Currently, the following technique is used: The shortest approach to the lesion is determined based on evaluation of previous mammograms. The breast is then positioned in the mammography unit with a perforated plastic compressor on the side of the breast that is closest to the lesion (Fig. 10–52A). A mammogram is taken to determine which perforation the lesion is under, and with the patient still in position, a sterile needle is introduced into the breast through this perforation so that it passes through the lesion. The breast is then repositioned in the unit, and another mammogram is taken at 90° to the previous view. This permits the needle to be withdrawn sufficiently so that its tip lies within or close to the target. With the position confirmed, a fine wire is introduced through the needle; the needle is then removed, leaving the wire in place. Injecting a small amount of visible dye into the needle prior to introduction of the wire is a precaution that serves to stain the lesion for identification in case the wire is dislocated

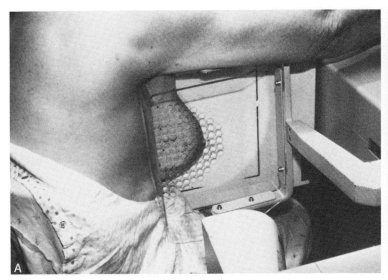

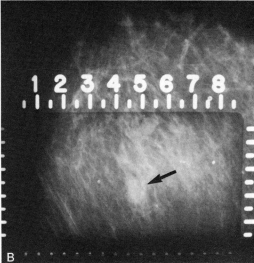

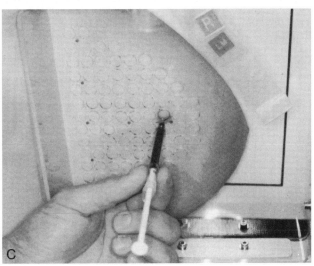

Figure 10–52. *A,* A perforated compressor used for wire localization of mammographic lesions prior to biopsy. *B,* An alternative compressor with a calibrated window. *C,* Localization can be performed by inserting a wire or by injecting a streak of visible and radiopaque dye. Here, a needle has been inserted into the breast through the aperture under which the lesion lies. For "streak" localization, dye is injected as the needle is withdrawn. ML and CC mammographic views are obtained to confirm that the dye passed through the target.

during biopsy. An alternative to the perforated compressor is a compressor with a window that is calibrated along its margin (see Fig. 10–52*B*). A mammogram obtained with the lesion located within the window allows mobile cross-hairs to be positioned so that their junction marks the site of the lesion. The needle is introduced at this point. At the end of the procedure, the projecting wire is covered with sterile gauze, and the patient is taken to the operating room with the mammograms. If the surgeon did not participate in the localization, the radiologist communicates the results of the procedure to the surgeon. Complications of hooked-wire localization are unusual, but they include migration of the wire into the chest, transection of the wire during biopsy with the resultant loss of a fragment, and dislocation of the wire during biopsy (Bronstein et al., 1988).

The spot technique is preferred by the author because of its simplicity (Simon et al., 1972). Again, the breast is compressed either in the craniocaudal or mediolateral position with the perforated compressor on the side closest to the lesion. After a mammogram has been taken to locate the lesion, a 1.5-inch, 25-gauge needle is passed into the breast through the appropriate perforation to a depth that ensures passage through the target. Using a tuberculin (1.0-

mL) syringe, approximately 0.8 mL of a solution of methylene blue (0.3 mL) and water-soluble contrast medium (0.5 mL of Reno-M-60 [Squibb]) is injected continuously as the needle is withdrawn. A small amount is also injected into the skin to mark the site of the needle puncture. A two-view mammogram (CC and ML views) is obtained immediately to confirm that the dye has accurately penetrated the lesion. At the time of biopsy, the location of the lesion with respect to the nipple is used as a guide to estimate the length of the dye tract to be excised (Fig. 10–53).

The specimen is taken immediately for specimen radiography to confirm that the lesion is included (Fig. 10–54). This is useful for confirmation of both microcalcifications and masses. The radiologist identifies the site of interest with a pin and transfers the specimen to the pathologist. Since lesions are small and the important diagnostic material is scant, frozen sections are generally not performed. This avoids the risk of losing diagnostic material. All of the specimen is saved for the preparation of paraffin sections. In cases in whom no cancer is found, a mammogram of the biopsied breast is repeated within 3 months to confirm that the area in question was removed and to provide a new baseline for future reference. Compared with postbiopsy

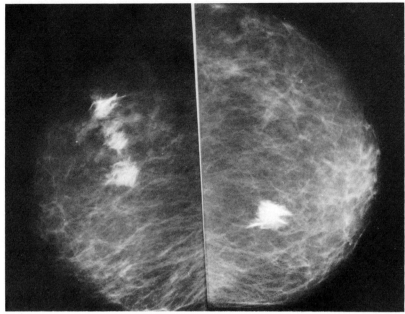

A

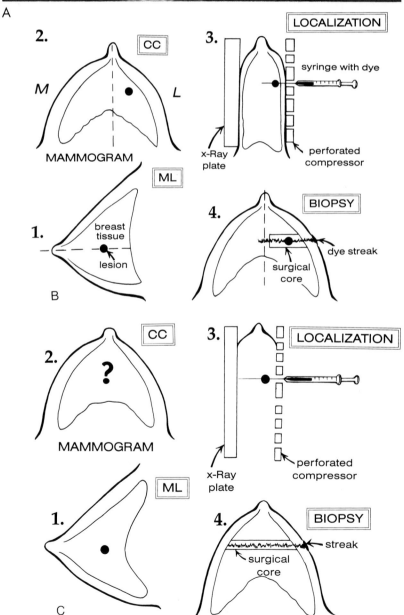

Figure 10–53. *A,* A dye tract in the breast after spot localization accurately penetrates the target lesion and provides a guide for excision. *Left,* The linear tract. *Right,* The tract end-on. *B,* The "streak" localization procedure. In this illustration, the ML mammographic view shows that the lesion *(dark circle)* lies in the plane of the nipple (1). The CC view shows that it is lateral to the nipple (2). The perforated compressor is positioned laterally, as this is the shortest distance to the lesion (3). After an ML view is taken, a fine needle is inserted through the appropriate aperture in the compressor, and dye is injected. At the time of biopsy (4), the surgeon removes a cylinder of tissue around the dye streak staying lateral to the nipple; no skin or subcutaneous tissue is removed. A specimen radiograph is obtained to confirm that the lesion is in the surgical specimen. *C,* The "streak" localization procedure used for a lesion seen in only one mammographic view. In this illustration, the lesion *(dark circle)* can be seen in the ML view *(lower left)* but not the CC view *(upper left),* so it is uncertain whether it lies medially or laterally in the breast. An ML view is taken with the perforated compressor in place; the compressor is placed laterally, since most lesions are lateral. Injection is made through the appropriate aperture and through the entire thickness of the breast *(upper right).* The surgeon chooses a cosmetic incision that intercepts the dye streak, and the path of the streak through the entire parenchyma is removed, sparing the subcutaneous tissue.

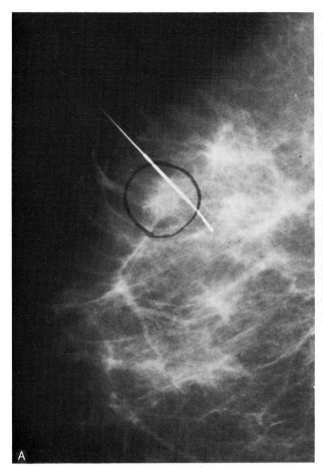

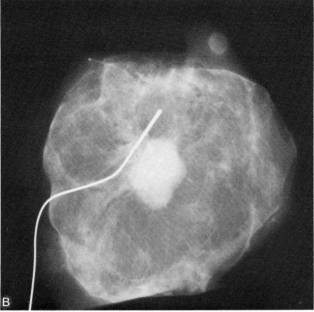

Figure 10-54. *A,* Localizing wire in place in the breast prior to biopsy. *B,* Specimen radiography performed with the localizing wire in place shows that the lesion (mass) is contained in the specimen.

mammograms, Hasselgren and colleagues (1993) found the sensitivity, specificity, and accuracy of specimen radiographs in 192 cases to be 96%, 28%, and 89%, respectively.

Core Needle Biopsy of Nonpalpable Lesions

Special dedicated equipment is available to permit histologic diagnosis of nonpalpable lesions using mammographically guided core needle biopsy. The technique has the advantage of involving only a small puncture wound rather than an incision, and thus it may reduce the number of open biopsies necessary for diagnosis. The unit consists of a table, a mammography unit on a swinging arm, and a securely mounted, 14-gauge core biopsy needle that can be advanced with precision. The patient lies in the prone position on the table with the relevant breast positioned through an aperture in the table and compressed with a fenestrated plate. Mammograms are taken 15° to the right and left of the midline at established distances from the target. Using the trigonometry of right triangles, a computer program determines the distance the core needle located in the midline must be advanced into the breast to engage the target. With the needle in place, a spring-loaded ''gun'' advances the cutter, and a core of tissue is obtained. Parker and coworkers (1991) compared the results of automated core needle biopsies with those of open surgical biopsies in 102 cases. Core needle biopsy identified 22 of 23 cancers (sensitivity = 96.7%), and as a result the authors believed

that it could be an acceptable alternative to surgical biopsy. However, some lesions do not lend themselves to this technique, and the necessary equipment is expensive and not widely available. Owing to core needle biopsy's 4.3% false-negative rate, a core biopsy that does not show cancer may not be definitive (Meyer, 1992).

Biopsy of the Discharging Duct

Cytologic examination of fluid from a persistently discharging duct is generally not reliable; however, it does serve to expedite diagnostic intervention when suspicious cells are found. The rate of false-negative cytologic results was 16.4%, and that of false-positive results was 2% in Leis's review of 560 cases of nipple discharge (Leis et al., 1985). Mammography following injection of radiocontrast material into the duct (ductography) does not provide a definitive diagnosis but can serve to identify filling defects as definite targets for biopsy (see Fig. 10–4). When no other abnormality is found on physical examination or on a mammogram, removal of the offending duct (microdochectomy) is required for diagnosis and to eliminate the discharge. The technique of microdochectomy is described in Chapter 18. In the absence of a mass, Chaudary and colleagues (1982) found cancer in 5.9% of 254 explorations. In most instances, the lesion was a duct papilloma (45%), duct ectasia (31%), or fibrocystic changes (9.5%). In 22 cases in which no lesion was found, 2 patients later developed carcinoma in the breast—a morbidity rate similar to the 2% to 7%

Table 10–14. RESULTS OF MICRODOCHECTOMY FOR NIPPLE DISCHARGE WITHOUT MASS OR ABNORMAL MAMMOGRAM IN 36 CASES*

Diagnosis	No. of Patients	Per Cent
Duct papilloma	16	44.4
Fibrocystic changes	12	33.3
Papillomatosis	3	8.3
Duct hyperplasia	2	5.6
Atypical duct hyperplasia	1	2.8
Ductal carcinoma in situ	1	2.8
Fat necrosis	1	2.8

*Author's personal series.

observed in other series. Thus, microdochectomies must be accurate and thorough, and when a lesion is not found, the patient should remain under periodic surveillance. Cancer was found in 13.0% of the author's cases of nipple discharge but in only 2.8% of cases without other physical or mammographic abnormalities (Table 10–14).

Results of Breast Biopsies

The results of a personal series of 1347 breast biopsies are shown in Table 10–15 along with their indications. A palpable mass was the single most frequent indication (47.5%); clinically occult lesions accounted for 46.8% of all biopsies. Among the latter, clustered microcalcifications predominated, accounting for 51.2% of all biopsies performed for mammographic abnormalities. Nearly one-quarter of all biopsies (23.5%) resulted in a diagnosis of cancer, as did one-third (32.3%) of biopsies for palpable masses. Palpable masses associated with microcalcifications on mammography had a higher rate of malignancy than did

any other combination of features. The low rate of malignancy when mammography was not performed is owing to the fact that it was not done on the youngest patients. Cancers were the cause of nipple discharges in 13% of cases.

Clinically occult mammographic lesions were cancers in 15.5 per cent of cases. The positive rate in reports ranges from 10 to 37 per cent, reflecting considerable diversity in case selection for biopsy (Table 10–16). In two large series, Alexander and associates (1990) found carcinoma in 29% of 531 biopsies, and Franceschi and colleagues (1991) reported cancer in 24% of 1144 biopsies. As indicated by others, the most ominous mammographic finding was a density that contained fine microcalcifications; these proved to be malignant in 30.6% of biopsies. Masses without suspicious calcifications are substantially less often cancerous, particularly those with a round, oval, or lobulated outline; Baute and coworkers (1992) found cancer in only 2% of the latter. Biopsies for microcalcifications alone revealed cancer in 13.9% of the author's cases. As few as three microcalcifications were biopsied if they were particularly suspect, and in one such case biopsy yielded an invasive carcinoma. Other reports indicate cancer in 17% to 49% of biopsies performed for microcalcifications. Roses and associates (1991) found cancer in 53% of biopsies performed for suspicious calcifications with or without an associated mass. When the number of linear calcifications exceeded 10, cancer was found in 16 of 17 cases. Table 10–15 shows no cancers in biopsies of architectural distortions, but Baute and coworkers (1992) found cancers in 50% of such cases.

Patients with cancers discovered with mammography before they have become clinically detectable have a relatively good prognosis (Fig. 10–55*A* and *B*). These cancers are small and often noninvasive, and they have a low frequency (usually <20%) of nodal metastases (Purdue et al., 1992). In this series, 23.5% were noninvasive cancers; the

Table 10–15. RESULTS OF BREAST BIOPSIES FOR PHYSICAL AND MAMMOGRAPHIC ABNORMALITIES

	No. of Total Biopsies	No. of Total Cancers (%)		No. of In Situ Cancers (%)	
Physical Examination					
Palpable mass*	640	207	(32.3)	9	(1.4)
Nipple discharge	54	7	(13.0)	1	(1.9)
Nipple changes	12	4	(33.3)	1	(8.3)
Edema +/− Erythema	10	1	(10.0)		
Subtotal	716	219	(30.6)	11	(1.5)
Mammogram Only (Normal Results on Physical Examination)					
Mass	261	42	(16.1)	3	(1.1)
Microcalcifications	323	45	(13.9)	19	(5.9)
Mass + calcifications	36	11	(30.6)	1	(2.8)
Asymmetry	8	0	(0.0)		
Architectural distortion	3	0	(0.0)		
Subtotal	631	98	(15.5)	23	(3.6)
Total	1347	317	(23.5)	34	(2.5)

*Presence of palpable mass in addition to the following on mammogram (No. of patients with carcinoma/Total No. of patients with feature (%)):
  Microcalcifications 17/20 (85.0)
  Microcalcifications in a mass 13/23 (56.5)
  Mass 135/256 (52.7)
  Architectural distortion 2/5 (40.0)
  No abnormalities 29/233 (12.4)
  No mammogram performed 14/75 (8.0)

Breast Cancers Found with Physical Examination Versus Mammography Only from 1982 to 1988

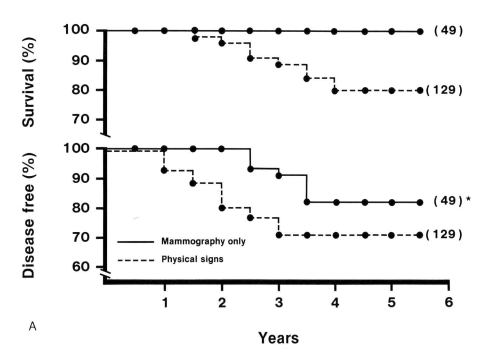

A

Figure 10–55. *A* and *B*, Patients with cancers discovered on mammography have a better prognosis than do those whose cancers are clinically evident. *Top*, All cancers, both invasive and noninvasive. *Bottom*, Invasive cancers alone, showing that the improved survival is not simply due to the inclusion of noninvasive cancers.

Survival: Invasive Breast Cancer Detected by Physical Examination or by Mammography Only from 1982 to 1988

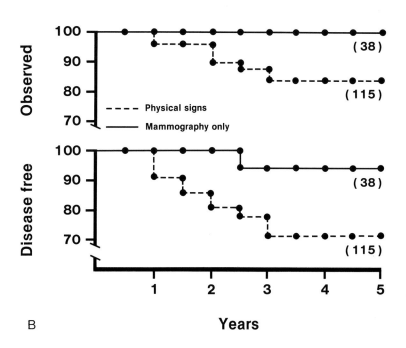

B

Table 10-16. RESULTS OF MAMMOGRAPHY-ASSISTED BIOPSY OF NONPALPABLE BREAST LESIONS CATEGORIZED ACCORDING TO INDICATION

Reference	No. of Biopsies	Cancers (%)					
		Mass	Calcifications	Architectural Distortion	Asymmetry	Mass and Calcifications	Total
Baute et al. (1992)	200	56	31	50		54	37
McManus et al. (1992)	289	10	10	13		21	10
McCreery et al. (1991)	358	45	49		6	52	27
Hasselgren et al. (1991)	350	17	22	24	0		19
Franceschi et al. (1991)	1144						24
Silverstein et al. (1987)	653	19	25	10		31	23
Landercasper et al. (1987)	203	17	22			30	22
Bigelow et al. (1985)	150	7	24			33	16

reported frequency ranges widely from 9% to 40%. Noninvasive carcinomas are found more often in microcalcifications than in mass lesions. Efforts are being made to increase the true-positive rate of mammography and thereby reduce the number of negative biopsy results, but increasing selectivity has been attended by the delayed diagnosis of some cancers (up to 12%), with uncertain economic, emotional, and ethical implications (McCreery et al., 1991; Baute et al., 1992; and McManus et al., 1992).

As shown in Figure 10–56, the probability of a biopsy diagnosis of cancer increases with patient age. In patients under the age of 30 years, the frequency was 2.8%; this is similar to the 2.5% frequency found by Palmer and Tsangaris (1993). The probability reached 41% for women aged 70 to 79 years. Noteworthy is that 34% of cancers were found in women younger than 50 years of age. For patients with palpable masses or clinically occult lesions, advancing age was still related to increasing probability of cancer (Figs. 10–57 and 10–58). The author's data indicate that a strong family history of breast cancer increases the chances that a patient's palpable breast mass will prove to be cancer (Table 10–17).

A SYSTEM OF DIAGNOSIS

Tools for detection and diagnosis of breast cancer should be used in a systematic fashion with due regard for the virtues and limitations of each and for the importance of accurate diagnosis without needless testing. This is not an

Table 10-17. FAMILY HISTORY OF BREAST CANCER VERSUS INCIDENCE OF CANCER IN BIOPSIES FROM 341 PATIENTS WITH PALPABLE BREAST MASSES*

Family Member Involved	Total No. of Masses Biopsied	Total No. of Cancers (%)
First Degree†	50	24 (48.0‡)
Second Degree	38	7 (18.4)
None	230	62 (27.0‡)
Unknown	19	3 (15.8)
Personal History	4	2 (50.0)

*Author's personal series.
†Mother, sister or daughter.
‡Significant difference between these two values: *P* < .05.

Results of 1393 Breast Biopsies by Decade of Age

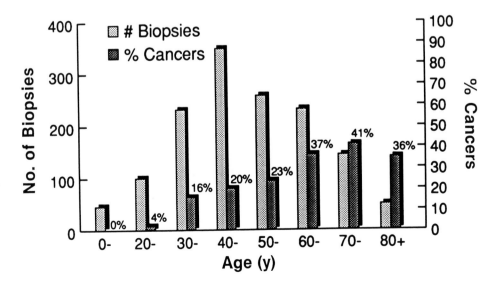

Figure 10–56. The probability that a breast biopsy will reveal cancer increases with patient age (author's cases).

Results of 681 Breast Biopsies for Palpable Masses by Age

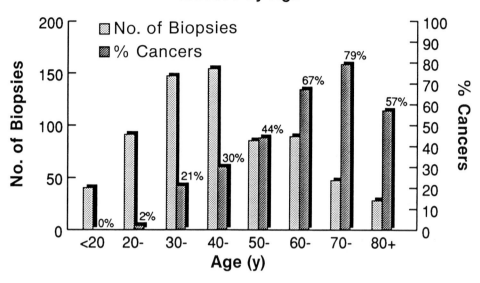

Figure 10–57. Breast biopsies performed for analysis of palpable masses show a direct correlation between patient age and the presence of cancer (author's cases).

Breast Biopsies for Nonpalpable Mammographic Lesions

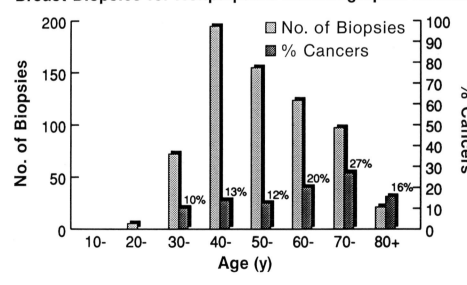

Figure 10–58. Six hundred sixty open biopsies of the breast performed for subclinical lesions detected on mammography demonstrate that the probability of cancer increases with patient age (author's cases).

Table 10-18. AN ALGORITHM FOR THE DIAGNOSIS OF BREAST CANCER

Finding	Evaluation	Action
Presence of Palpable Mass →	Aspirate; if fluid obtained, no blood, mass disappears, and results on mammography are normal, then ⟶	Re-examine patient in 4–8 wk
	If no fluid obtained, or blood in fluid, or residual mass, or results on mammography suspicious, and results on cytology are positive, then ⟶	Staging, intraoperative biopsy, and treatment
	or results on cytology are negative, then ⟶	Biopsy
Presence of Persistent Focal Nipple Discharge →	If results of physical examination and mammography are normal, and test results for blood are positive or negative, and results on cytology are positive or negative, then ⟶	Perform microdochectomy for diagnosis and therapy
	If results of physical examination or mammography are suspicious, then ⟶	Biopsy abnormality and remove discharging duct
Presence of Surface Nipple Lesion →	If results on mammography are normal, then ⟶	Perform punch biopsy of nipple
	If results on mammography are abnormal, then ⟶	Biopsy nipple and abnormality
Presence of Mammographic Lesion →	If results of physical examination are normal and suspicious microcalcification or mass (spiculated), then ⟶	Biopsy
	If mass not spiculated: Perform ultrasound; if a cyst, then ⟶	Observe or perform guided aspiration
	Perform ultrasound; if normal or a solid mass, then ⟶	Biopsy
	Architectural distortion, then ⟶	Biopsy
	Asymmetry (evolving), then ⟶	Biopsy
	Asymmetry (stable), then ⟶	Observe
	Equivocal findings, perform special views: If resolves, then ⟶	Repeat mammogram in 4–6 mo
	If suspicious, then ⟶	Biopsy

easy task. A basic algorithm for diagnosis is proposed in Table 10–18.

The value of early diagnosis is most evident in terms of stage and tumor size rather than of the duration of symptoms; the latter does not correlate well with curability (Table 10–19). The reason for this seems to be that symptoms occur late in the natural history of breast cancer, and the symptomatic interval between discovery and treatment is only a small segment of the overall course of the disease. The diverse biologic behavior of this disease and the human reaction to it conspire to prevent a reliable relationship between prompt consultation and a good prognosis. Sometimes, patients report that they have discovered large and obvious tumors only a week earlier. Rapidly growing, aggressive breast cancers are likely to cause alarm and to be brought quickly to the attention of a physician; more slowly growing and indolent ones with relatively good prognoses often are tolerated for longer periods. Provided that primary tumors do not increase in size or advance in stage, delay may have little effect on prognosis (Philipshen et al., 1984); however, spontaneous regressions are rare (Lewison, 1976), and breast cancers do progress with time. Data support a correlation between tumor size, adenopathy, and symptom duration (Fig. 10–59). At some point, distant metastases occur, and the tumor becomes incurable. Whether dissemination has already occurred remains unclear in most cases, but avoidance of unnecessary or protracted delay in diagnosis and treatment should minimize the proportion of cases that have passed this critical point.

Despite the evidence to support prompt consultation, delay is still too often the rule. Contributing to delay are ignorance of the signs of breast cancer, hope that the signs will go away, fear of the diagnosis, and the expense of treatment. Unfortunately, physicians sometimes contribute to further delay by ''watching'' breast masses, by having unjustified confidence in their ability to distinguish clini-

Mean Tumor Diameter Versus Symptomatic Interval

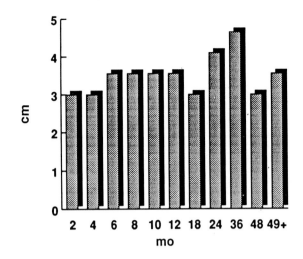

Axillary Involvement Versus Symptomatic Interval

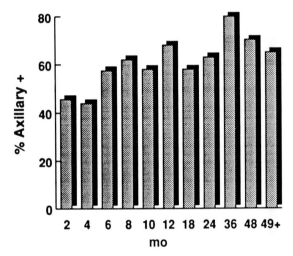

Figure 10–59. Size of tumor and probability of occurrence of nodal metastases are related to the length of symptomatic interval in 700 patients with breast cancer treated with radical mastectomy at Ellis Fischel State Cancer Hospital from 1940 to 1958.

cally between benign and malignant masses, and by placing too much credence in a normal mammogram when physical signs indicate disease. Progress is being made, but the need for public and professional education about breast cancer continues to exist. Women should understand the importance of regular breast self-examinations and learn the proper technique. Established guidelines for screening examinations should be followed. The public should be aware that most breast cancers can be cured if found while they are small or before they have become invasive and, ideally, before their symptoms appear. This knowledge will reduce unwarranted despair among susceptible individuals about the diagnosis of breast cancer. Also, physicians need to be suspicious of changes in a woman's breasts and must not miss opportunities for prompt diagnosis.

The National Cancer Data Base provides an overview of

Table 10–19. DURATION OF SYMPTOMS CORRELATED WITH 5-YEAR SURVIVAL AFTER RADICAL MASTECTOMY (700 CASES AT ELLIS FISCHER STATE CANCER HOSPITAL, 1940 to JUNE 1958)

Duration of Symptoms (mo)	Total No. of Cases	5-Year Survivors	
		No.	*Per Cent of Total**
1	58	38	65.0
2	65	35	53.8
3	68	38	55.9
4	49	30	61.2
5	33	13	39.4
6	67	38	56.7
7	21	8	38.1
8	30	16	53.3
9	14	8	57.1
10–12	92	40	43.5
13–24	102	58	56.9
25–36	33	15	45.5
37–48	23	16	69.6
≥49	45	24	53.3

*A chi square test fails to show a significant difference in 5-year survival for the 14 categories. Chi square = 17.2763, df = 13, P > .20.

the current status of the diagnosis of breast cancer in the United States (Steele et al., 1993). Based on 143,051 cases reported in 1985, 1988, and 1990, it reflected that almost 72% of patients were high-income, nonhispanic whites and that 78.4% of patients were diagnosed and treated in the same hospital. In 1990, 11% of the cancers were noninvasive, and over half (50.3%) were staged as being either in situ or localized. Fewer than 1 in 20 tumors (4.2%) were overtly disseminated at diagnosis.

References

Abele, J. S., Miller, T. R., Goodson, W. H. III, et al.: Fine-needle aspiration of palpable breast masses. A program for staged implementation. Arch. Surg., *118*:859, 1983.

Abramson, D. J.: A clinical evaluation of aspiration of cysts of the breast. Surg. Gynecol. Obstet., *139*:531, 1974.

Abramson, D. J.: Delayed mastectomy after outpatient breast biopsy. Long-term survival study. Am. J. Surg., *132*:596, 1976.

Alexander, H. R., Candela, F. C., Dershaw, D., and Linne, D. W.: Needle-localized mammographic lesions. Arch. Surg., *125*:1441–1444, 1990.

American Joint Committee on Cancer: Manual for Staging of Cancer. 3rd ed. Philadelphia, J. B. Lippincott, 1992, p. 150.

Ashikari, R., Rosen, P. P., Urban, J. A., et al.: Breast cancer presenting as an axillary mass. Ann. Surg., *183*:415, 1976.

Baker, L. H.: Breast cancer detection demonstration project five-year summary report. C. A. Cancer J. Clin., *32*:194–225, 1982.

Barber, K. W. Jr., Dockerty, M. B., and Clagett, O. T.: Inflammatory carcinoma of the breast. Surg. Gynecol. Obstet., *112*:406, 1961.

Bassett, L. W., Kimme-Smith, C., Sutherland, L. K., et al.: Automated and hand-held breast US: Effect on patient management. Radiology, *165*:103–108, 1987.

Baute, P. B., Thibodeau, M., and Newstead, G.: Improving the yield of biopsy for nonpalpable lesions of the breast. Surg. Gynecol. Obstet., *174*:93–96, 1992.

Bell, C. A.: A System of Operative Surgery. Vol. ii. 1814, p. 136, cited in Lee, B. J., and Tannenbaum, N. E. Inflammatory carcinoma of the breast. Surg. Gynecol. Obstet., *39*:580, 1924.

Bell, D. A., Hajdu, S. I., Urban, J. A., et al.: Role of aspiration cytology in the diagnosis and management of mammary lesions in office practice. Cancer, *51*:1182, 1983.

Berend, M. E., Sullivan, D. C., Koraguth, P. J., et al.: The natural history of mammographic calcification subjected to interval follow-up. Arch. Surg., *127*:1309–1313, 1992.

Bertario, L., Reduzzi, D., Piromalli, D., et al.: Outpatient biopsy of breast cancer: Influence on survival. Ann. Surg., *201*:64, 1985.

Bigelow, R., Smith, R., Goodman, P. A., and Wilson, G. S.: Needle localization of nonpalpable breast masses. Arch. Surg., *120*:565–569, 1985.

Blamey, R. W.: The diagnosis and prognosis of breast cancer. Practitioner, *226*:1385, 1982.

Blichert-Toft, M., Dyreborg, U., Bogh, L., et al.: Nonpalpable breast lesions: Mammographic wire-guided biopsy and radiologic-histologic correlation. World J. Surg., *6*:119, 1982.

Boyd, N. F., Sutherland, H. J., Fish, E. B., et al.: Prospective evaluation of physical examination of the breast. Am. J. Surg., *142*:331–337, 1981.

Bronstein, A. D., Kilcoyne, R. F., and Moe, R. E.: Complications of needle localization of foreign bodies and nonpalpable breast lesions. Arch. Surg., *123*:775–779, 1988.

Butler, J. A., Vargas, H. I., Worthen, N., and Wilson, S. E.: Accuracy of combined clinical mammographic-cytologic diagnosis of dominant breast masses. Arch. Surg., *125*:893–896, 1990.

Byrd, B. F. Jr., and Stephenson, S. E. Jr.: Inflamed or inflammatory carcinoma of the breast. Am. Surg., *28*:303, 1962.

Campbell, H. S., Fletcher, S. W., and Lin, S.: Improving physicians' and nurses' clinical breast examination: A randomized controlled trial. Am. J. Prev. Med., *7*:1–8, 1991.

Chang, C. H. J., Nesbit, D. E., Fisher, D. R., et al.: Computed tomographic mammography using a conventional body scanner. Am. J. Radiol., *38*:553, 1982.

Charlson, M. E.: Delay in the treatment of carcinoma of the breast. Surg. Gynecol. Obstet., *160*:393, 1985.

Chaudary, M. A., Millis, R. R., Davies, G. C., et al.: Nipple discharge: The diagnostic value of testing for occult blood. Ann. Surg., *196*:651, 1982.

Cheek, J. H., and Sears, A. D.: Results of breast biopsies for mammographic findings. Am. J. Surg., *136*:726, 1978.

Choucair, R. J., Holcomb, M. B., Mathews, H., et al.: Biopsy of nonpalpable breast lesions. Am. J. Surg., *156*:453–456, 1988.

Ciatto, S., Calarzi, S., Morrone, D., and De Turco, M. R.: Fine-needle aspiration cytology of nonpalpable breast lesions: US versus stereotaxic guidance. Radiology, *188*:195–198, 1993.

Ciatto, S., Cariaggi, P., and Bulgaresi, P.: The value of routine cytologic examination of breast cyst fluids. Acta Cytol., *31*:301–304, 1987.

Clark, C. P., Peters, G. N., and O'Brien, K. M.: Cancer in the augmented breast. Cancer, *72*:2170–2174, 1993.

Copeland, E. M., and McBride, C. M.: Axillary metastases from unknown primary sites. Ann. Surg., *178*:25, 1973.

Copeland, M. M., and Higgins, T. G.: Significance of discharge from the nipple in nonpuerperal mammary conditions. Ann. Surg., *151*:638, 1960.

Czernobilsky, B.: Intracystic carcinoma of the female breast. Surg. Gynecol. Obstet., *124*:1, 1967.

Darrier, M. J.: La maladie de Paget du mamelon. Soc. de Biol. Ser., *9*:294, 1889.

Devitt, J. E.: Management of nipple discharge by clinical findings. Am. J. Surg., *149*:789, 1985.

Devitt, J. E.: Association of breast cysts and breast cancer. Can. J. Surg., *31*:356–358, 1988.

Donegan, W. L.: Evaluation of a palpable breast mass. N. Engl. J. Med., *327*:937–942, 1992.

Donegan, W. L., and Padrta, B.: Combined therapy for inflammatory breast cancer. Arch. Surg., *125*:578–582, 1990.

Donnelly, B. A.: Primary "inflammatory" carcinoma of the breast: A report of five cases and a review of the literature. Ann. Surg., *128*:918, 1948.

Doust, B. D., Milbrath, J. R., and Doust, V. L.: CT scanning of the breast using a conventional CT scanner. J. Comput. Assist. Tomogr., *5*:296, 1981.

Dowlatshahi, K., Gent, H. J., Schmidt, R., et al.: Nonpalpable breast tumors: Diagnosis with stereotaxic localization and fine-needle aspiration. Radiology, *170*:427–433, 1989.

Egan, R. L.: Mammography. 2nd ed. Springfield, Charles C. Thomas, 1972, p. 5.

Egan, R. L., McSweeney, M. B., and Sewell, C. W.: Intramammary calcifications without an associated mass in benign and malignant diseases. Radiology, *137*:1, 1980.

Egeli, R. A., and Urban, J. A.: Mammography in symptomatic women 50 years of age and under, and those over 50. Cancer, *43*:878, 1979.

Ellis, D. L., and Teitelbaum, S. L.: Inflammatory carcinoma of the breast: A pathologic definition. Cancer, *33*:1045, 1974.

Erickson, E. J., McFreevy, J. M., and Muskett, A.: Selective nonoperative management of patients referred with abnormal mammograms. Am. J. Surg., *160*:659–664, 1990.

Feuerman, L., Attie, J. N., and Rosenberg, B.: Carcinoma in axillary lymph nodes as an indicator of breast cancer. Surg. Gynecol. Obstet., *114*:5, 1962.

Fisher, B.: Reappraisal of breast biopsy prompted by the use of lumpectomy: Surgical strategy. J.A.M.A., *253*:3585, 1985.

Fisher, E. R., Sass, R., and Fisher, B.: Biologic considerations regarding the one- and two-step procedures in the management of patients with invasive carcinoma of the breast. Surg. Gynecol. Obstet., *161*:245, 1985.

Fletcher, S. W., O'Malley, M. S., and Bunce, L. A.: Physicians' abilities to detect lumps in silicone breast models. J.A.M.A., *253*:2224, 1985.

Fornage, B. D.: Ultrasound-guided needle biopsy of the breast and other interventional procedures. Radiol. Clin. North Am., *30*:167–185, 1992.

Foster, R. S. Jr.: Core-cutting needle biopsy for the diagnosis of breast cancer. Am. J. Surg., *143*:622, 1982.

Frable, M. A., and Frable, W. J.: Fine-needle aspiration biopsy revisited. Laryngoscope, *92*:1414, 1982.

Franceschi, D., Crowe, J. P., Lie, S., et al.: Not all nonpalpable breast cancers are alike. Arch. Surg., *126*:967–971, 1991.

Franceschi, D., Crowe, J., Zollinger, R., et al.: Biopsy of the breast for mammographically detected lesions. Surg. Gynecol. Obstet., *171*:449–455, 1990.

Franzen, S., and Stenkvist, B.: Diagnosis of granular cell myoblastoma by fine-needle aspiration biopsy. Acta Pathol. Microbiol. Scand., *72*:391, 1968.

Funderburk, W. S., and Flax, R. L.: Localization of nonpalpable carcinoma of the breast utilizing xeromammography: Technique A. Breast, *2*:28, 1976.

Gatchell, F. G., Dockerty, M. B., and Clagett, O. T.: Intracystic carcinoma of the breast. Surg. Gynecol. Obstet., *106*:347, 1958.

Gershon-Cohen, J., Yiu, L. S., and Berger, S. M.: The diagnostic importance of calcereous patterns in roentgenography of breast cancer. A.J.R. Am. J. Roentgenol., *88*:1117, 1962.

Giard, R. W. M., and Hermans, J.: The value of aspiration cytologic examination of the breast. Cancer, *69*:2104–2110, 1992.

Goode, J. V., McNeill, J. P., and Gordon, C. E.: Routine aspiration of discrete breast cysts: Report of 267 breast aspirations. Arch. Surg., *70*:686, 1955.

Grant, C. S., Goeliner, J. R., Welch, J. S., et al.: Fine-needle aspiration of the breast. Mayo Clin. Proc., *61*:377, 1986.

Greenwood, S. M., and Minkowitz, S.: Paget's disease in metastatic breast carcinoma. Arch. Dermatol., *104*:312, 1971.

Guyer, P. B.: The use of ultrasound in benign breast disorders. World J. Surg., *13*:692–698, 1989.

Haagensen, C. D.: Diseases of the Breast. Philadelphia, W. B. Saunders, 1971*a*, p. 74.

Haagensen, C. D.: Diseases of the Breast. Philadelphia, W. B. Saunders, 1971*b*, p. 501.

Hall, D. C., Goldstein, M. K., and Stein, G. H.: Progress in manual breast examination. Cancer, *40*:364, 1977.

Halsted, W. S.: The results of radical operations for the cure of carcinoma of the breast. Ann. Surg., *46*:1–19, 1907.

Hamed, H., Coady, A., Chaudary, M. A., and Fintiman, I. S.: Follow-up of patients with aspirated breast cysts is necessary. Arch. Surg., *124*:253–255, 1989.

Hammond, S., Keyhani-Rofagha, S., and O'Toole, R. V.: Statistical analysis of fine-needle aspiration cytology of the breast: A review of 678 cases plus 4265 cases from the literature. Acta Cytol., *131*:276–280, 1987.

Hasselgren, P., Hummel, R. P., and Fieler, M. A.: Breast biopsy with needle localization: Influence of age and mammographic feature on the rate of malignancy in 350 nonpalpable breast lesions. Surgery, *110*:623–628, 1991.

Hasselgren, P., Hummel, R. P., Georgian-Smith, D., and Fieler, M.: Breast biopsy with needle localization: Accuracy of specimen x-ray and management of missed lesions. Surgery, *114*:836–842, 1993.

Hatteland, K., and Kluge, T.: Mondor's disease: A subcutaneous form of periarteritis nodosa? Acta. Chir. Scand., *129*:67, 1965.

Helwig, E. B., and Graham, J. H.: Anogenital (extramammary) Paget's disease. Cancer, *16*:387, 1963.

Hicken, N. F.: Mastectomy: A clinical pathologic study demonstrating why most mastectomies result in incomplete removal of the mammary gland. Arch. Surg., *40*:6, 1940.

Jackson, P. P., and Pitts, H. H.: Biopsy with delayed radical mastectomy for carcinoma of the breast. Am. J. Surg., *98*:184, 1959.

Jacobaeus, H. C.: Paget's disease und sein Verhältnis zum Milchdrüsenkarzinom. Virchows Arch. Anat., *178*:124, 1904.

Johnson, T. L., and Kini, S. R.: Cytologic and clinicopathologic features of abnormal nipple secretions: 225 cases. Diagn. Cytopathol., *7*:17–22, 1991.

Kagali, V. A.: The role and limitations of frozen section diagnosis of a palpable mass in the breast. Surg. Gynecol. Obstet., *156*:168, 1983.

Kahky, M. P., Rone, V. R., Duncan, D. L., et al.: Needle aspiration biopsy of palpable breast masses. Am. J. Surg., *156*:450–452, 1988.

Kaufman, M., Bider, D., and Weissberg, D.: Diagnosis of breast lesions by needle aspiration biopsy. Am. Surg., *49*:558, 1983.

Kawatsu, T., and Miki, T.: Triple extramammary Paget's disease. Arch. Dermatol., *104*:316, 1971.

Kemeny, M. M., Rivera, D. E., Terz, J. J., and Benfield, J. R.: Occult primary adenocarcinoma with axillary metastases. Am. J. Surg., *152*:43, 1986.

Kher, A. V., Marwar, A. W., and Raichur, B. S.: Evaluation of fine needle aspiration biopsy in the diagnosis of breast lesions. Indian J. Pathol. Microbiol., *24*:100, 1981.

Kline, T. S.: Survey of aspiration biopsy cytology of the breast. Diagn. Cytopathol., *7*:948–1005, 1990.

Kline, T. S., Joshi, L. P., and Neal, H. S.: Fine-needle aspiration of the

breast: Diagnoses and pitfalls. A review of 3545 cases. Cancer, *44*:1458, 1979.

Knapp, R. W., and Mullen, J. T.: Triage for the breast biopsy. Am. J. Surg., *131*:626, 1976.

Knight, D. C., Lowell, D. M., Heimann, A., and Dunn, E.: Aspiration of the breast and nipple discharge cytology. Surg. Gynecol. Obstet., *163*:415–419, 1986.

Kobayashi, T.: Ultrasonic detection of breast cancer. Clin. Obstet. Gynecol., *25*:409, 1982.

Kopans, C. B.: Fine-needle aspiration of clinically occult breast lesions. Radiology, *170*:313–314, 1989.

Lafreniere, R.: Bloody nipple discharge during pregnancy: A rationale for conservative treatment. J. Surg. Oncol., *43*:228–230, 1990.

Lagios, M. D., Gates, E. A., Westdahl, P. R., et al.: A guide to the frequency of nipple involvement in breast cancer: A study of 149 consecutive mastectomies using a serial subgross and correlated radiographic technique. Am. J. Surg., *138*:135, 1979.

Landercasper, J., Gundersen, S. B., Gundersen, A. L., et al.: Needle localization and biopsy of nonpalpable lesions of the breast. Surg. Gynecol. Obstet., *164*:399–403, 1987.

Lannin, D. R., Silverman, J. F., Pores, W. J., et al.: Cost-effectiveness of fine-needle biopsy of the breast. Ann. Surg., *203*:474, 1986.

Layfield, L. J., Glasgow, B. J., and Cramer, H.: Fine-needle aspiration in the management of breast masses. Pathol. Annu., *24*:23–62, 1989.

Leborgne, R. A.: The Breast in Roentgen Diagnosis. Montevideo, Uruguay, Impresora Uruguaya S.A. 1953.

Lee, B. J., and Tannenbaum, N. E.: Inflammatory carcinoma of the breast. Surg. Gynecol. Obstet., *39*:580, 1924.

Lefor, A. T., Numann, P. J., and Levinsohn, E. M.: Needle localization of occult breast lesions. Am. J. Surg., *148*:270, 1984.

Leis, H. P. Jr., Cammarata, A., and LaRaja, R. D.: Nipple discharge: Significance and treatment. Breast, *11*:6, 1985.

Lesnick, G. J.: Detection of breast cancer in young women. J.A.M.A., *237*:967, 1977.

Lev-Toaff, A. S., and Feig, S. A.: Stability of malignant breast microcalcifications. Presented at the 92nd annual meeting of the American Roentgen Ray Society, Orlando, FL, May 10–15, 1992.

Lewis, J. D., Milbrath, J. R., Shaffer, K. A., et al.: Which breast to biopsy: An expanding dilemma. Ann. Surg., *184*:253, 1976.

Lewison, E. F.: Spontaneous regression of breast cancer. Natl. Cancer Inst. Monogr., *44*:23–26, 1976.

Lucas, F. V., and Perez-Mesa, C.: Inflammatory carcinoma of the breast. Cancer, *41*:1595, 1978.

Malberger, E., Toledano, C., Barzilai, A., et al.: The decisive role of fine needle aspiration cytology in the preoperative work-up of breast cancer. Isr. J. Med. Sci., *17*:899, 1981.

Martin, J. E., Moskowitz, M., and Milbrath, J. R.: Breast cancer missed by mammography. A.J.R. Am. J. Roentgenol., *132*:737–739, 1979.

Masur, R. W.: Management of the solitary breast mass. Postgrad. Med., *73*:73, 1983.

Maturo, V. G., Zusmer, N. R., Gilso, A. J., et al.: Ultrasonic appearance of mammary carcinoma with a dedicated whole-breast scanner. Radiology, *142*:713, 1982.

McCreery, B. R., Frankl, G., and Frost, D. B.: An analysis of the results of mammographically guided biopsies of the breast. Surg. Gynecol. Obstet., *178*:223–226, 1991.

McManus, V., Desautels, J. E. L., Benediktsson, H., et al.: Enhancement of true-positive rates for nonpalpable carcinoma of the breast through mammographic selection. Surg. Gynecol. Obstet., *175*:212–218, 1992.

McSwain, G. R., Valicenti, J. F. Jr., and O'Brien, P. H.: Cytologic evaluation of breast cysts. Surg. Gynecol. Obstet., *146*:921, 1978.

McSweeney, M. B., and Murphy, C. H.: Whole-breast sonography. Radiol. Clin. North Am., *23*:157, 1985.

Merson, M., Andreola, S., Galimberti, V., et al.: Breast carcinoma presenting as axillary metastases without evidence of a primary tumor. Cancer, *70*:504–508, 1992.

Meyer, J. E.: Value of large-core biopsy of occult breast lesions. A.J.R. Am. J. Roentgenol., *158*:991–992, 1992.

Meyer, J. E., Christian, R. L., Frenna, T. H., et al.: Image-guided aspiration of solitary occult breast "cysts." Arch. Surg., *127*:433–435, 1992.

Meyerowitz, B. R.: Drill biopsy confirmation of breast cancer. Arch. Surg., *111*:826, 1976.

Minkowitz, S., Moskowitz, R., Khafif, R. A., and Alderete, M. N.: TRU-CUT needle biopsy of the breast. Cancer, *57*:320–323, 1986.

Mondor, H.: Tronculite sous-cutanée subaiguë de la paroi thoracique an-téro-latérale. Mém. Acad. Chir. (Paris), *65*:1271, 1939.

Morimoto, T., Okazaki, K. K., Komaki, K., et al.: Cancerous residue in breast-conserving surgery. J. Surg. Oncol., *52*:71–76, 1993.

Murad, T. M., Contesso, G., and Mouriesse, H.: Nipple discharge from the breast. Ann. Surg., *195*:259–264, 1982.

National Council on Radiation Protection and Measurements: Radiation protection for medical and allied health personnel. N.C.R.P.M. Report No. 105. Bethesda, MD, N.C.R.P.M., 1989, p. 7.

Nehme, A. E., and Macksood, M. J.: Nonpalpable breast lesions: Diagnosis and management. Breast, *16*:19, 1984.

Nemoto, T., Natarajan, N., Smart, C. R., et al.: Patterns of breast cancer detection in the United States. J. Surg. Oncol., *21*:183, 1982.

Nicastri, G. R., Reed, W. P., and Dziura, B. R.: The accuracy of malignant diagnoses established by fine-needle aspiration cytologic procedures of mammary mass. Surg. Gynecol. Obstet., *172*:457–460, 1991.

Nicolesco, S., and Velciu, V.: Tumors arising from heterotopic mammary rudiments. Gynecol. Obstet., *67*:241, 1968.

Niloff, P. H., and Sheiner, N. M.: False-negative mammograms in patients with breast cancer. Can. J. Surg., *24*:50, 1981.

1989 Survey of Physician's Attitudes and Practices in Early Cancer Detection. C.A. Cancer J. Clin., *40*:77–101, 1990.

Nohrman, B. A.: Cancer of the breast. Clinical study of 1,042 cases treated at Radiumhemmet 1936–41. Acta Radiol., *77*(Suppl):1, 1949.

Oberman, H.: Frozen-section diagnosis of breast biopsy specimens: A necessary procedure? Arch. Surg., *128*:955–956, 1993.

O'Malley, F., Casey, T. T., Winfield, A. C., et al.: Clinical correlates of false-negative fine-needle aspirations of the breast in a consecutive series of 1005 patients. Surg. Gynecol. Obstet., *176*:360–364, 1993.

Paget, J.: On the disease of the mammary areola preceding cancer of the mammary gland. St. Bartholomew's Hospital Reports, *10*:87, 1874.

Palmer, M. L., and Tsangaris, T. N.: Breast biopsy in women 30 years old or less. Am. J. Surg., *165*:708–712, 1993.

Parikh, K. J., and Singer, J. A.: Pathologic ectopic breast tissue. Breast, *9*:16, 1983.

Parker, S. H., Lovin, J. D., Jobe, W. E., et al.: Nonpalpable breast lesions: stereotactic automated large-core biopsies. Radiology, *180*:403–407, 1991.

Philipshen, S. J., Gerardi, J., Brefsky, S., and Robbins, G. E.: The significance of delay in treating patients with potentially curable breast cancer. Breast, *10*:16–23, 1984.

Physician Insurers Association of America: Breast Cancer Study. March 1990. Pennington, N.J., Physician Insurers Association of America, 1990.

Pierce, E. H., Clagett, O. T., McDonald, J. R., et al.: Biopsy of the breast followed by delayed radical mastectomy. Surg. Gynecol. Obstet., *103*:559, 1956.

Pierce, E. H., Gray, H. K., and Dockerty, M. B.: Surgical significance of isolated axillary adenopathy. Ann. Surg., *145*:104, 1957.

Porter, B. A., and Smith, J. P.: MRI enhances breast cancer detection and staging. Diagnostic Imaging, September-October 1993, pp. 18–26.

Powell, D. E., and Stelling, C. B.: Magnetic resonance imaging of the human female breast: Current status and pathologic correlation. Pathol. Annu., *23*:159–194, 1988.

Powell, R. W., McSweeney, M. B., and Wilson, C. E.: X-ray calcifications as the only basis for breast biopsy. Ann. Surg., *197*:555, 1983.

Prechtel, K., and Hallbauer, M.: Ein Beitrag zur Prognose des Mamma-karzinoma nach zweizeitigem Operations-verfahren. Geburtshilfe. Frauenheilkd., *39*:187, 1979.

Purdue, P., Page, D., Nellestein, M., et al.: Early detection of breast carcinoma: A comparison of palpable and nonpalpable lesions. Surgery, *111*:656–659, 1992.

Reintgen, D., Berman, C., Cox, C., et al.: The anatomy of missed breast cancers. Surg. Oncol., *2*:65–75, 1993.

Richards, G. J. Jr., and Lewison, E. F.: Inflammatory carcinoma of the breast. Surg. Gynecol. Obstet., *113*:729, 1961.

Rimsten, A., Stenkvist, B., Johanson, H., et al.: The diagnostic accuracy of palpation and fine-needle biopsy and an evaluation of their combined use in the diagnosis of breast lesions: Report on a prospective study in 1244 women with symptoms. Ann. Surg., *182*:1, 1975.

Robbins, F. F., Brothers, G. H., Eberhardt, W. F., and Quan, S.: Is aspiration biopsy of breast cancer dangerous to the patient? Cancer, *7*:774, 1954.

Roberts, J. G., Preece, P. E., Bolton, P. M., et al.: The "tru-cut" biopsy in breast cancer. Clin. Oncol., *1*:297, 1975.

Rodier, J. F., Millon, R., Janser, J. C., et al.: Influence of mastectomy techniques on estrogen and progesterone receptor analysis in carcinoma of the breast. Surg. Gynecol. Obstet., *177*:352–356, 1993.

Rosemond, G. P., Maier, W. P., and Brobyn, T. J.: Needle aspiration of breast cysts. Surg. Gynecol. Obstet., *128*:351, 1969.

Rosen, P., Hajda, S. I., Robbins, G., et al.: Diagnosis of carcinoma of the breast by aspiration biopsy. Surg. Gynecol. Obstet., *134*:837, 1972.

Rosen, P. P.: Frozen section diagnosis of breast lesions: Recent experience with 556 consecutive biopsies. Ann. Surg., *187*:17, 1978.

Roses, D. F., Mitnick, J., Harris, M. N., et al.: The risk of carcinoma in wire localization biopsies for mammographically detected clustered microcalcifications. Surgery, *110*:877–886, 1991.

Rosner, D., and Blaird, D.: What ultrasonography can tell in breast masses that mammography and physical examination cannot. J. Surg. Oncol., *28*:308, 1985.

Rubens, D., Totterman, S., Chacko, A. K., et al.: Gadopentetate dimeglumine–enhanced chemical-shift MR imaging of the breast. A.J.R. Am. J. Roentgenol., *157*:267–270, 1991.

Rubin, E., Miller, V. E., Berland, L. L., et al.: Hand-held real-time breast sonography. A.J.R. Am. J. Roentgenol., *144*:623, 1985.

Salomon, A.: Beitrage zur Pathologie und Klinik der Mammacarcinoma. Arch. Klin. Chir., *101*:573, 1913.

Saltzstein, S. L.: Clinically occult inflammatory carcinoma of the breast. Cancer, *34*:382, 1974.

Saunders, G., Lakra, Y., and Libcke, J.: Comparison of needle aspiration cytologic diagnosis with excisional biopsy tissue diagnosis of palpable tumors of the breast in a community hospital. Surg. Gynecol. Obstet., *172*:437–440, 1991.

Sayago, C., and Sirebrenik, D.: Surgical biopsy as a disseminating factor in breast cancer. Acta Un. Int. Canc., *15*:1161, 1959.

Scanlon, E. F.: The breast biopsy. Cancer, *64*:2671–2673, 1989.

Schwartz, G. F., and Feig, S. A.: Management of patients with nonpalpable breast lesions. Oncology, *5*:39–63, 1991.

Seltzer, M. H., Perloff, L. J., Kelley, R. I., et al.: The significance of age in patients with nipple discharge. Surg. Gynecol. Obstet., *131*:519, 1970.

Sheikh, F. A., Tinkoff, G. H., Kline, T. S., and Neal, H. S.: Final diagnosis by fine-needle aspiration biopsy for definitive operation in breast cancer. Am. J. Surg., *154*:470–575, 1988.

Sickles, E. A.: Imaging techniques other than mammography for the detection and diagnosis of breast cancer. Recent Results Cancer Res., *119*:127–135, 1990.

Sieninski, W., and Dabska, M.: Usefulness of drill biopsy in the diagnosis of breast tumors. Cancer, *38*:2567, 1976.

Silverstein, M. J., Gamagami, P., Rosser, R. J., et al.: Hooked-wire–directed breast biopsy and overpenetrated mammography. Cancer, *59*:715–722, 1987.

Silverstein, M. J., Gierson, E. D., Gamagami, P., et al.: Breast cancer diagnosis and prognosis in women augmented with silicone gel–filled implants. Cancer, *66*:97–101, 1990.

Simon, N., Lesnick, G. J., Lerer, W. N., et al.: Roentgenographic localization of small lesions of the breast by the spot method. Surg. Gynecol. Obstet., *134*:572, 1972.

Smith, C., Butler, J., Cobb, C., and State, D.: Fine-needle aspiration cytology in the diagnosis of primary breast cancer. Surgery, *103*:178–183, 1988.

Smith, D. J., Palin, W. E., Katch, V. L., and Bennet, J. E.: Breast volume and anthropomorphic measurements: Normal values. Plast. Reconstr. Surg., *78*:331, 1986.

Smith, J., Payne, W. S., and Carney, J. A.: Involvement of the nipple and areola in carcinoma of the breast. Surg. Gynecol. Obstet., *143*:546, 1976.

Smith-Behn, J., and Ghani, A.: Non-palpable breast lesions: Out-patient needle localization and biopsy. Postgrad. Med. J., *63*:17–18, 1987.

Somers, R. G., Sandler, G. L., Kaplan, M. J., et al.: Palpable abnormalities of the breast not requiring excisional biopsy. Surg. Gynecol. Obstet., *175*:325–328, 1992.

Sparkman, R. S.: Reliability of frozen sections in the diagnosis of breast lesions. Ann. Surg., *155*:924, 1962.

Steele, G. D. Jr., Winchester, D. P., Menck, H. R., and Murphy, G. P.: National Cancer Data Base—Annual Review of Patient Care, 1993. Atlanta, American Cancer Society, Inc., 1993, pp. 10–19.

Stein, H. D.: Ambulatory breast biopsies: The patient's choice. Am. Surg., *48*:221, 1982.

Taylor, G. W., and Meltzer, A.: "Inflammatory carcinoma" of the breast. Am. J. Cancer, *33*:33, 1938.

Van Dam, P. A., Van Goethem, M. L. A., Kersschot, E., et al.: Palpable solid breast masses: Retrospective single- and multimodality evaluation of 201 lesions. Radiology, *166*:435–439, 1988.

Vilcoq, J. R., Caloe, R., Ferme, F., et al.: Conservative treatment of axillary adenopathy due to probable subclinical breast cancer. Arch. Surg., *117*:1136, 1982.

Wang, C. C., and Griscom, N. T.: Inflammatory carcinoma of the breast: Results following orthovoltage and supervoltage radiation therapy. Clin. Radiol., *15*:167, 1964.

Warren, S. L.: Roentgenologic study of the breast. A.J.R., *24*:113–124, 1930.

Watson, D. P. H., McGuire, M., Nicholson, F., and Given, H. F.: Aspiration cytology and its relevance to the diagnosis of solid tumors of the breast. Surg. Gynecol. Obstet., *165*:435–441, 1987.

Westbrook, K. C., and Gallager, H. S.: Breast carcinoma presenting as an axillary mass. Am. J. Surg., *122*:607, 1971.

Wild, J. N., Neal, D.: The use of high frequency ultrasonic waves for detecting changes of living tissues. Lancet, *i*:655, 1951.

Wilson, L. B.: A method for the rapid preparation of fresh tissues for the microscope. J.A.M.A., *45*:1737, 1905.

Wolfe, J. N.: Analysis of 462 breast carcinomas. A.J.R. Am. J. Roentgenol., *121*:846, 1974.

Yorkshire Breast Cancer Group: Symptoms and signs of operable breast cancer, 1976–1981. Br. J. Surg., *70*:350, 1983.

Zajdela, A., Ghossein, N. A., Pillerow, J. P., et al.: The value of aspiration cytology in the diagnosis of breast cancer: Experience at the Foundation Curie. Cancer, *35*:499, 1975.

11

Breast Imaging

Myron Moskowitz

In the past, the role of breast imaging—specifically mammography—was poorly understood and little appreciated by some members of the surgical community (Lesnick, 1977; Devitt, 1979; and Mahoney et al., 1979). This was provoked in part by failure of imaging specialists to acknowledge the limitations as well as the benefits of this clinical aid.

Reduction of disease-specific population mortality by screening has far reaching implications for our understanding of the natural history of breast cancer. It also allows us to ratify or reject many of our current concepts of treatment. A well-known example is the *lead time bias* concept. Patients who are treated for "localized" disease, for small tumors, or for tumors with few positive nodes survive longer than do patients who have evidence of disseminated disease. Is this longer survival for a given patient the result of treatment, or are we simply watching her disease unfold before us for a longer period without extending the patient's lifespan?

If a properly controlled and performed screening trial can demonstrate that a disease-specific mortality reduction among those screened does indeed occur, then the lead time bias effect, along with certain other biases, has been removed. Therefore, the longer survival that is seen can be translated into a longer lifespan for the affected patient. The Health Insurance Plan of Greater New York Trial (HIP) clearly showed that this could be achieved for women ages 40 to 69 years who are screened annually with two-view mammography and clinical examination and are given breast self-examination instruction (Shapiro et al., 1982). A curious observation was made: women between 40 and 49 years of age required a longer time to see this mortality reduction than did women aged 50 years and older. An analysis by Chu and Connor (1991) strongly indicates that the reason for the delay among women ages 40 to 49 years in that study was due to a shift in the detection of earlier Stage I cancers *(internal shift)* rather than a shift in the reduction of cancers Stage II or higher compared with controls. For older women, however, a remarkable reduction occurred in the detection of cancers of Stage II or higher compared with controls *(external shift)*. Therefore, for the younger women, until the patients in the study group with cancers of Stage II or higher had died, the net beneficial effect of the internal shift was obscured and delayed. On the other hand, for the older women, since the external shift resulted in early downstaging compared with the controls, the decrease in mortality could be seen earlier. It is intuitively apparent to almost all clinicians that not all cancers grow at the same rate. It is also apparent to almost all clinicians that all patients with Stage I disease do not progress at the same rate. The explanation of Chu and Connor

is entirely clinically consistent with the observed results and with the model to evaluate the effects of altering screening strategies proposed by Pelikan and Moskowitz (1993).

Thus, the benefit of screening is not necessarily equal among patients with detected tumors. Some tumors detected in screening, whether large or small, will have an indolent course, and the patient, if left untreated, would go on to die of intercurrent disease. Indeed, we do know that all large cancers were at one time small; we do not know whether all small cancers will become big. However, a "positive" study means that in the context of a specific trial, sufficient numbers of affectable cancers were detected and these cancers had their courses altered favorably. For the HIP trial, it has been estimated that 3.5 years were added to the lifespans of women who were destined to die of breast cancer. Since the data collected included those for women who refused screening as well as those for screened women, and since the positive mortality reduction seen in the whole population resulted only from the cases detected at screening, this author has estimated that, on average, 8 years were added to the lifespan of each woman whose cancer was detected by screening.

It would be naive to argue that screening is the ultimate means for the control of breast cancer. Even if screening is biologically effective, the cost in terms of both financial and time expenditures and the sensitivity and the specificity of screening might render it of marginal value as a public health policy tool. The decision as to whether it should be implemented is politicoeconomic, not medical. Generally speaking, it would be preferable to have available a tool of primary prevention. For the patient with breast cancer, nondeforming, low-morbidity, curative treatment for any stage of the disease would be ideal. Unfortunately, at the time of this writing, the first condition does not exist, and the therapeutic options that are available are most effective for the treatment of small lesions, which are best detected when the patient is asymptomatic. A "Catch-22"!

There is a clear-cut separation between using imaging techniques for diagnosis and using them for detection or screening (Moskowitz, 1979; and Kopans et al., 1984*a*). In the former circumstance, the clinician needs to answer a specific, clinical question. On the other hand, for screening the objective is to detect the suspected disease in an asymptomatic population when the cancer is small and most amenable to therapy. In this circumstance, the test needs to "cull out" abnormals from the large number of normals. To impose the experience gained from one of these situations onto the other results in confusion.

Regarding breast disease, the problem is compounded by the fact that over the millennia breast cancers have been classically discovered either by the patient or by clinical palpation. Out of this experience has arisen a great body of expertise. Generally, this expertise is such that the predictive value, or positive biopsy rate, ranges from 20% to 33%. Advocates for a new technique may claim a 97% "accuracy" (often undefined) rate, a 98% sensitivity rate, and a 99% specificity rate. Unfortunately, these unrealistic claims may be derived from studies that are poorly controlled, based on series of cases selected because of clinically suspicious, large cancers, and interpreted after the results of palpation, and occasionally biopsy, are known.

It is doubtful that there is, or ever will be, a breast imaging method that, by itself, can be expected to be 97% to 100% sensitive. It would appear that the sensitivity of mammography is on the order of 80% to 90% (Baker, 1982). If a surgeon requests imaging consultations for palpable masses and receives reports that miss these palpable cancers 20% of the time, his or her natural reaction is to reject the method as useless (Lesnick, 1977; Devitt, 1979; Mahoney et al., 1979; and Mahoney and Csima, 1983).

For example, in Mahoney and coworkers' study (1979), a classic example of tautology in action, a population of women were screened with clinical examination, and mammography was reserved for those women in whom clinical examination was abnormal or questionable. The reader will recall that mammography will not find about 20% of palpable cancers. When palpable lesions were missed by mammography, the impression was gained that screening mammography was unnecessary, as all the cancers in this series were picked up clinically. Because preclinical detection virtually could not exist in this circumstance, the tautology was fulfilled.

On the basis of data from the Breast Cancer Detection Demonstration Projects (BCDDPs) (Baker, 1982), if this same experiment were performed with mammography as the primary examination and clinical examination reserved for abnormal or suspicious cases, only 30% to 60% of cases could be expected to be detected by clinical methods. The impression would then follow that clinical examination is worthless as a screening tool.

These extremes are both fallacious and totally disregard the fact that each method contributes independently to detection of cancer (Baker, 1982; Moskowitz, 1983*c;* and Strax, 1984). Failure to appreciate this point can contribute to delay in diagnosis and may be associated with clinically significant upstaging of the disease. The diagnosis of breast cancer should be based on histologic evaluation.

If biopsy is necessary to make the diagnosis of cancer, of what value are imaging studies? In this chapter, the answers to this question are explored for the imaging modalities currently available.

Sensitivity, specificity, accuracy, and predictive values are measures used to evaluate diagnostic tests. To avoid semantic confusion, the following definitions are used for each of these parameters in this chapter:

1. Sensitivity (True-Positive [TP] Rate): The ratio of the number of cancers correctly identified to the number of all cancers currently detectable by either clinical breast examination, mammography, or both.

2. Specificity (True-Negative Rate): The portion of normal examinations correctly called negative.

3. False-Positive (FP) Rate: The fraction of normal examinations incorrectly called positive, expressed as a percentage. In this chapter, the term "false-positive" (FP) rate is often be used in lieu of specificity.

4. Positive Predictive Value (PPV): The ratio of the number of correct positive diagnoses to the number of all tests called positive. In the case of breast cancer, if correctly calculated, this should equal the percentage yield of cancers among patients who are biopsied.

Positive predictive value depends on the disease frequency in the examined population as well as on the sensitivity and specificity of the test. The lower the incidence (or prior probability) of disease, the lower the PPV, even if the sensitivity and specificity are held constant. As Swets and associates (1991) have shown, a group of expert mammography readers all read along the same *receiver operating curve*. This author has noted findings identical to those of Swets and associates in receiver operating curve analyses for mammograms in general and for microcalcifications in particular (Moskowitz, 1992). Recent clinical reports by Haiart and Henderson (1991), Monostori and colleagues (1991), and Morrone and coworkers (1991) support the same observations. Thus, in a blinded reading test, each reader has the same FP and TP rates. No one reader's interpretations varied significantly from those of the others. Although there are several who would be quick to adopt the mantle of "mammographic Messiah," there is no scientific reason to believe that there exists one person whose reading curve would be significantly better than the curves of the other readers tested (there certainly could be and, undoubtedly, are [Swets et al., 1991] readers who perform significantly worse). Therefore, if the expert readers all recognize the same findings and all quantify malignant potential similarly, given the same screened population, then the PPVs for each reader should be the same. Yet, they are not.

Why not? Because biopsy decisions, particularly in low probability situations, are often based on perceived risks, stop loss, or prior perceptions of "cost effectiveness," or any combination of these. A simple example demonstrates this point. For women aged 40 to 49 years, assume that the age-specific incidence rate is 1.5/1000. Assume further that 10,000 women are screened, the sensitivity is 0.85 (a realistic number), and the specificity is 0.99 (FP rate = 0.01). The PPV would equal 0.114. Next, assume that all remains the same except that the situation demands that the specificity be 95%. This may lower the sensitivity to 70%, and the PPV approaches 20%. The resultant cost is obvious.

It must be recognized that demanding a PPV that is higher than that which the test can deliver is feasible only at the cost of the TP rate. Unfortunately, in the case of breast cancer screening, it is the small and most curable lesions that will be lost. For the women between 40 and 49 years of age referred to earlier, if one demands a PPV of 0.5, the FP rate must be kept at 0.0013 if the TP rate of 0.85 is to be maintained (as to the achievability of this preposterous figure, editorial comment is reserved). If one demands a PPV of 0.3, an FP rate of 0.003 must be maintained. For women of ages 50 to 59 years, a prior requirement for a PPV of 0.3 would mean that an FP rate of 0.005 must be maintained. Although this begins to approach achievability, its attainment still remains wishful thinking given the current technology. PPVs must not be allowed to become the sole driving force behind breast cancer screening.

One can only recognize the missed cases by following the whole population of women screened for a minimum of 10 years after their entry into the study and by quantifying interval cancer rates, the stage of detection of all cases, and the disease-specific mortality. In this author's own screening, in which a very aggressive approach was pursued with regard to mammographic and clinical examination screening, only 5% of positive cases occurred within the 1 to 11 months after completely negative screening results were obtained. The Falun (Sweden), Malmö (Sweden), and Edinburgh studies, among others, report rates that are four- to fivefold higher (Stomper and Gelman, 1989).

5. Accuracy: This term is perhaps misused more than any of the others. It represents the ratio of all correct diagnoses (positive and negative) to all outcomes. This category is of little relevance, particularly in screening situations in which the frequency of disease is expressed as a few cases per 1000. For example, if an investigator were to screen a population of 10,000 asymptomatic volunteers in which there resided as many as 100 with cancers and arbitrarily, without reference to the test itself, were to diagnose all tested women as normal or free of cancer, the "accuracy" of the test would be 0.99, and yet every cancer would have been misdiagnosed!

It is also possible to have an acceptable PPV and yet be operating close to, or even at, random chance levels. For example, let us assume that a population of 400 patients were referred for imaging. Furthermore, assume that the subsequent course of clinical events demonstrated 100 cancer cases in that population. Let us say that the test identified 50 of the cancers correctly. In addition, 200 normal patients were incorrectly called positive. The predictive value, or expected biopsy yield, would be 20%, an acceptable clinical level. However, a moment's reflection reveals that 50% of normal persons were called abnormal (FP) and that 50% of persons with cancer were called abnormal (TP). In point of fact, this test was operating on a random chance level.

In a representative sample of the literature, sensitivity rates for mammography (TP) ranging from 65% to 97% have been reported (Moskowitz, 1983*b*). The mean TP rate in these series was 84%. The FP rate was reported to range from 1% to a high of 48%, with a mean of 9%. Even in the worst case situation (48% FP), the TP-FP ratio was better than chance alone. Generally speaking, the articles reporting higher sensitivities resulted from diagnostic situations in which masses tended to be larger. In the BCDDPs, the TP rate for mammography was a little better than 80% if cases occurring within 12 months of a negative screen are considered.

In the author's center, about 7% to 9% of cases were missed by both clinical examination and mammography. Forty-six per cent of all cases were identified by mammography alone. Physical examination alone was responsible for the detection of 16% of cases not detected by mammography, and the remainder were found by both.

Data reported by Sickles (1984*b*) show that in his re-

ferred practice, 64% of cases were detected by clinical examination and the remainder by mammography alone.

Taken as a whole, these data would indicate that it is most reasonable to expect that the TP rate for mammography is in the range of 80% to 85%; its FP rate may be as high as 13% in diagnostic situations and about 5% in screening situations. Clearly, mammography and clinical examination contribute different cases to detection or screening. It is painfully clear that no test that will miss or misdiagnose up to 20% of cancers can be used to exclude cancer when a dominant palpable mass is present. However, given a suspicious mammographic finding and a negative result on clinical examination, the surgeon who ignores the mammographic report does so at his or her, and at the patient's, peril.

X-RAY MAMMOGRAPHY

It is tempting to suggest that x-ray mammography is the oldest of techniques for imaging the breast. However, it was probably long preceded by simple light transillumination. Nevertheless, radiographic mammography has been in clinical use for over 30 years. The radiographic parameters for differentiating benign and malignant masses are well known. A relationship between microcalcifications and breast cancer is recognized. Although it is apparent that the calcifications are not so specific as originally thought, the presence of calcifications remains an invaluable clue to the diagnosis and, perhaps, to the prognosis of tiny carcinomas (Galkin et al., 1977; Snyder, 1980; Hajek et al., 1983; Moskowitz, 1983*c;* Paterok et al., 1983; Prorok et al., 1983; Anastassiades et al., 1984; LeGal et al., 1984; Meyer et al., 1984; and Kopans et al., 1985*b*).

Strax and coworkers (Shapiro, et al., 1982; and Strax, 1984) demonstrated that the combination of mammography and clinical examination, when applied to an asymptomatic population, could help lower mortality rates from this disease. The results of the Swedish trial (Tabar et al., 1985) and Dutch studies (de Waard et al., 1984; Verbeek et al., 1984; and Verbeek, 1985) not only demonstrate that mammographic screening alone can contribute to the detection of cancers 5 mm and smaller in screened women of all ages, but also reproduce the earlier findings of the HIP study regarding mortality reduction almost exactly.

The HIP of New York study was a prospective, matched cohort study; the Swedish trial (Tabar et al., 1985) a population-based, controlled trial; the Nijmegen study (Verbeek et al., 1984; and Verbeek, 1985) a case control study; and the BCDDPs (Baker, 1982) were simply what their names implied.

The results from the first three controlled studies have surprisingly similar results—namely, that screening for breast cancer can reduce breast cancer mortality by one-third in the intermediate term (i.e., 4–6 years post-screening) and that this benefit appears to be limited to women over the age of 50 years at entry. In the HIP study (Shapiro et al., 1982), long-term follow-up shows a later (7–15-year) mortality reduction for both older and younger women. In the HIP study, this was accomplished with annual mammography and clinical examination, whereas in the Swedish

Table 11-1. AGE-SPECIFIC LEAD TIME GAINED BY SCREENING*

	(1) Fox et al. (1978)	(2) BCDDP Calculated	(3) BCDDP Observed	(4) BCDDP Calculated
35–49	2 ± 0.5 y	2 y	>2 y	1.6 y
>50	3.5 ± 0.5 y	2.9 y	≅ 4 y	2.5 y

*This table shows the age-specific projected lead time gained by screening over the nonscreened setting for the Cincinnati BCDDP and all other BCDDPs. The actual, or observed, lead time for the Cincinnati BCDDP is shown in column 3.

and Dutch studies, only single, mediolateral oblique–view mammography was used.

As indicated earlier, for women 40 to 49 years old, an early mortality reduction was not shown in the HIP study, perhaps owing to a high detection threshold in this age group. For example, in the HIP study, mammography alone was responsible for the detection of about 42% of cancers in women 50 years of age and older. In the BCDDPs (performed about 12 years later), it was also noted that in this age group mammography alone detected 42% of cancers. However, in women 40 to 49 years old in the HIP study, only 19% of cases were detected by mammography alone, whereas in the BCDDPs about 35% were detected only by mammography. This is important because in the HIP study survival was best for those patients whose cancers were detected by mammography alone. Furthermore, about 40% of cancers in the BCDDPs were less than 1 cm in size, whereas very few such cancers were detected in the HIP study. Thus, it appears that for younger women the threshold size of detection was relatively high in the HIP screen. Despite this threshold, however, 7 years after the beginning of the screening, a reduction in mortality rate developed.

Whereas HIP women of all ages were screened annually, in both the Swedish and Dutch studies, women over the age of 50 years were examined at 3-year intervals. Screening for women aged 40 to 49 years was performed at 2-year intervals. If these intervals were beyond the lead time gained by screening, even though threshold sensitivity was lowered meaningfully, the following might have occurred: an excess number of cancers would be expected to occur between screens; the proportion of Stage II or higher disease would be excessive; and a large portion of the cases detected at the second screen would already have passed beyond the threshold of curability, despite being screen detected.

In an earlier model, Fox and coworkers (1978) (Table 11–1) predicted that for a randomly selected, asymptomatic population, the mean detection lead time gained by the screening of women aged 35 to 49 years would be about 2 ± 0.5 years. For older women, the estimates were 3.5 ± 0.5 years. Key to that model was the ability to project the detectable prevalence of cancer by age. The model correctly predicted the age-specific, detectable prevalence subsequently found in both the Swedish and Dutch trials. Therefore, there is reason to believe that the lead time predictions are reasonably close to correct.

After 10 complete years of follow-up of the author's own cohort of 6000 younger women and 4500 older women (Fig. 11–1; see also Table 11–1), the actual observed lead time for younger women is less than 2 years, and for older women it appears to be about 4.0 years.

If correct, these figures would suggest that the lead times chosen for the Dutch and Swedish screens are inappropriate for maximum effect, particularly in younger women. This is further attested to in the Dutch data (de Waard et al., 1984; Verbeek et al., 1984; and Verbeek, 1985) (Table 11–2), which show that, in younger women, 56% of cases occurred in the 2-year interval between screens, whereas in older women screened at 3-year intervals, only 28% occurred between screens. Thus, even within the Dutch data, the interval cancer rate for older women is less than that for younger women despite the longer time between screens in older women.

Within the data from the BCDDPs, it can be seen (Table 11–3) that for women screened annually the interval rate is inversely related to the lead time gained.

Another bit of supporting evidence for the effect of lengthening screen intervals is the increasing percentage of Stage II cancers by age in the Nijmegen cohorts (Verbeek et al., 1984; and Verbeek, 1985) (see Table 11–2). In older women, 36% of cancers (excluding noninvasive cancers) were Stage II or higher. This includes interval cases, cases detected at screening, and cases detected in women who did not return for their second appointment. In younger women, on the other hand, 49% of cases were Stage II. Unfortunately, the numbers are too small for statistical significance, but the age-specific parallelism is striking.

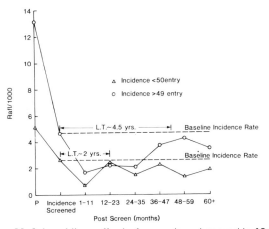

Figure 11-1. Lead time effect of screening observed in 10,500 volunteers. As expected, a high prevalence rate of breast cancer is observed in the initial pass. During the 5-year period that screening was offered, the incidence screened rate per 1000 person-years is about 4.5 for women over the age of 49 years at entry and about 2.5 for women 35 to 49 years of age. When screening is discontinued, a sharp drop in incidence occurs in both age groups. The effect lasts for about 2 years in younger women and longer than 4 years in older women.

Table 11–2. SCREEN SENSITIVITY BY AGE IN NIJMEGEN, NETHERLANDS*

	Number of TP	TP Rate	FP Rate	Per Cent of Stage II +
Birth cohort 1925–1939	42/96	44%	56%	49%
Birth cohort 1910–1924	100/138	72%	28%	36%

*Note that in younger women, 56% of cases occurred between screens (interval cancers), whereas in older women, this rate was halved.

However, both of these effects (enhanced interval rate and more advanced staging) may well be the result of iatrogenic enhancement of length bias sampling effect.

Length bias sampling can be enhanced in several ways. Some number of rapidly growing tumors will always occur between screens. If the size threshold of detection is changed, more cases will be seen as interval cancers (Moskowitz, 1983c). If a low threshold is maintained but the interval between screens is extended to the end of lead time or beyond, not only the number of cases of intermediate growth rate that occur between screens, but also the number of advanced cases that will be detected at the screen but whose course will not be altered by it, will be increased.

This clearly happened in the Nijmegen studies, in which a long screen interval was selected. Although the best survival was, as expected, in prevalence cases, screened detected cases experienced the poorest outlook, probably because a larger pool of more advanced disease was being created artificially. Interval cases survived at a better rate than expected, and even better than incidence cases. This is probably because a greater number of more slowly growing tumors were allowed to reach clinical threshold at the end of the lead time but before the next screen.

The data suggest that inappropriate screening intervals may prove to be a more fatal flaw than a less sensitive screen. If intervals are unduly lengthened, only the most slowly growing tumors will be detected by the screen. Therefore, short-term and intermediate-term mortality rates will not be reduced. The number of years required to observe any long-term effect may be exceedingly long. A less sensitive screen performed yearly may also not affect short-term mortality because it did not catch the rapidly growing tumors while they were small enough and most amenable to treatment. However, it may detect sufficient numbers of tumors of slower to more moderate growth, perhaps not in a completely curable stage, but at a time when the course

Table 11–3. AGE-SPECIFIC LEAD TIME VERSUS INTERVAL RATES*

	All BCDDPs	Interval Cancers (%)
35–39	1	33
40–44	1.5	23
45–49	1.8	18
50–54	2.4	17
55–59	2.25	13
60–64	2.6	14
65–69	2.6	12
70–74	2.6	8

*The relation of lead time gained by annual screening and interval cancer rates. As the lead time increases, the interval rates decrease.

is still alterable, so that an intermediate and long-term effect can be achieved.

For younger women, the screening sensitivity for all cancers, even the smallest, is improved by the combined use of aggressive clinical screening and mammography. In the author's series, 17% of the minimal cancers found (i.e., ductal carcinoma in situ and invasive carcinomas less than 5 mm in maximum diameter) were detected by clinical examination alone (Moskowitz, 1983c). In the Swedish and Dutch trials, clinical examination was omitted. This omission may be an important contributing factor in failure to find a mortality decrease in the younger women.

If some proportion of cancers in young women is not found when they are minimal, they will be detected later, when they are more advanced. For example, in the author's program in the post-screening period, failure to detect a significant portion of minimal cancers (5 mm or smaller) was accompanied by an excess rate of Stage II cancers (Table 11–4).

In the author's experience with screening older women (Table 11–5), the 10-year cumulative survival for all invasive cancers occurring during screening (incidence, interval, and prevalent) is 71%. In the case of invasive cancers, this represents an improvement of 29 percentage points in 10-year survival over breast cancer survival in the United States (Axtell et al., 1976). These data would lead us to believe that the benefit the author obtained for older women is at least comparable with the results obtained in Falun, Nijmegen, and New York. Because it may be argued that in older women small noninvasive cancers may never present as clinical tumors, they are not considered here in this analysis. If they were included, survival at 10 years would be 81%.

It is only the results with younger women that appear anomalous. For young women, after 10 years of follow-up (see Table 11–5), the survival rate (including prevalence, incidence, and interval cases) is 95%. If noninvasive cancer is excluded, the overall survival is 88%. Correcting for a 3.0-year lead time gained over clinical detection, the 10-year survival is projected to be 79%. Thus, a 30–percentage point gain is seen by screening in this age group. (If a 2-year lead time was used, the gain would be more striking.) However, these women were screened annually, and a particularly vigorous and successful effort was made to detect noninvasive and minimal cancers. Given these considerations, there is every reason to believe that the survival rate noted represents a true alteration in the natural history of this disease in younger women.

In both the Malmö trial and the Canadian National Breast Screening Study (NBSS), a trend toward mortality reduction for women over the age of 50 years is observed. For women aged 40 to 49 years at entry, both of these trials

Table 11–4. INCIDENCE OF CANCERS BY YEAR (AGE <50 YEARS AT ENTRY)*

| | Prevalence | Screened | Months After Last Screen | | | | | Total Number Stage II Cancers | |
			1–11	12–23	24–35	36–47	48–59	Screened	Postscreen
Number of persons	6000	12,600	6000	6000	6000	6000	6000	24,600	24,00
Number of cancers	31	32	5	16	9	13	8	18	28
Rate per 1000	5.2	2.5	0.83	2.77	1.5	2.2	1.3	0.73/1000	1.15/1000
Invasive cancer only	15	18	4	12	7	13	7	NA	NA
Rate per 1000	2.5	1.43	0.6	2.0	1.16	2.2	1.16		

*Note that in younger women, the lead time is short, although a rebound occurs shortly after cessation of screening. The average incidence for 4 years after screening is about 2 per 1000, or 22% less than screened incidence. This may be the long-term effect of removing minimal cancers, or the result of excess ''nonkilling cancers'' found at screening.
NA = Not applicable.

show a statistically nonsignificant excess mortality among screened women compared with controls (Stomper and Gelman, 1989).

In the Malmö trial, the subjects initially underwent two-view mammography. Subsequent single-view mammograms were obtained at 20-month intervals. Women with mammographically dense breasts at the time of the first study underwent two-view mammography. Clinical examination was not offered, and breast self-examination was not stressed. The interval chosen for screening younger women was essentially at the end of the lead time gained by screening. Lack of clinical examination reduces screen sensitivity by about 15%, and single-view mammography reduces the sensitivity for minimal cancer by about 20% (Moskowitz and Libshitz, 1977). In the Malmö trial, 33% of cases occurred between screens (Stomper and Gelman, 1989); of these, one-third were present on the preceding screen (although about 20% of these were subtle findings).

The interval cancers grew the fastest, particularly in younger women; furthermore, women with interval cancers died at a rate greater than that of the controls.

In the author's experience, in younger women the combination of annual clinical examination and two-view mammography resulted in the detection of only 5% of cases that occurred earlier than 12 months after a completely negative screen. None of these interval case patients died of breast cancer for 5 to 14 years after detection (average = 9.2 years). It should be borne in mind that extending the interscreen interval tends to bias the screen to detect the more slowly growing tumors. Thus, the results of the Malmö trial are predictable.

In the Canadian NBSS, the experimental design varied

by age group. For the purposes of the present discussion, it is sufficient to state that the study was performed on self-selected women and with self-selected women acting as the controls. Screening was done at annual intervals, and both the younger and older women underwent clinical breast examination. Baines and coworkers (1990a) have reported the results of an external review of the technical quality of the images obtained during the NBSS. The results showed clearly that mammographic quality improved substantially over time. However, during the early years of the study, only 60% of the images obtained were satisfactory. By 1985 to 1987, about 85% of the images were satisfactory. However, owing to the pattern of enrollment over time, only 68% of the women received satisfactory breast imaging. In addition to the usual causes of poor technical quality, failure to use the Lundgren mediolateral oblique view resulted in exclusion of the tail of Spence and of much of the upper outer quadrant in many of the subjects screened. Since the majority of breast cancers occur in these areas, this circumstance was particularly unfortunate.

Baines and associates (1990b) have additionally reported the interobserver agreement and potential delay in diagnosis in the NBSS. After review of approximately 5000 mammograms by the reference radiologist for the trial, the following was noted: (1) of the 102 cases that were detected within 11 months of a negative screening visit, 43 were clearly present at the time of the prior visit; (2) of the 575 cases that were detected during a screening visit, 100 could have been detected 1 or more years earlier; and (3) 40 cases that were detected at a screening visit could have been detected mammographically at that visit but were found only on physical examination. Another 28 cases could be

Table 11–5. CINCINNATI BCDDP SURVIVAL RATES*

Months	1–11	12–23	24–35	36–47	48–59	60–71	72–83	84–95	96–107	108+
				Age >50 Years at Entry						
All	100%	100%	99%	99%	98%	98%	95%	95%	95%	95%
Invasive	100%	100%	97%	97%	94%	94%	88%	88%	88%	88%
				Age <49 Years at Entry						
All	100%	96%	94%	93%	93%	90%	87%	85%	83%	81%
Invasive	100%	94%	91%	90%	90%	85%	81%	78%	74%	71%

*Survival of breast cancer cases, younger and older women. This includes all cases found at initial (prevalence) screening, incidence (1-year intervals) screening, and cases occurring between screens (1–11 months). Includes cases found by mammography, clinical examination, by both methods, and those detected between screens by the patient herself.

identified as having been missed owing to technical problems. Therefore, among the 677 evaluated cancers, 40% were not detected by the screen. Of the 168 cases that were missed, 143 (85%) could have been found 1 or more years prior to detection; 211 (31%) represent frank mammographic failures due either to faulty technique or interpretation.

It is intuitive that the screens discussed can be expected to have limited impact upon mortality. It is likewise easily understandable how they might produce no mortality reduction. Is it equally comprehensible how some excess mortality might come about? Diagnostic delay has been shown to result in more advanced disease (Walker et al., 1989) and in a shortened 3-year rate of survival (Rossi et al., 1990). Screening studies have proved that time is added to lifespan by earlier detection and treatment. Therefore, delay in diagnosis should result in the cancer being found at a point further along the natural history curve, and less time is added to lifespan (i.e., a patient with a delayed diagnosis will die sooner than if her cancer were detected earlier, the lead time bias notwithstanding). If told that the mammography results are negative, many women will accept this information, even if they have palpable lumps. This "false-negative reassurance" can be expected to result in up to 35% to 40% of interval cancers. Compared with non-screened controls, diagnosis will be delayed for these women, and an earlier demise will probably ensue. For populations with a significant number of slowly growing tumors, the effect can be expected to be less; for populations with a significant number of rapidly growing tumors, the effect can be expected to be accentuated. It has been shown (Pelikan and Moskowitz, 1993) that altering screen intervals or screen sensitivities, or both (as occurred in the referenced trials) could produce excess mortalities in younger women if as few as 30% of interval cases receive an unfounded sense of confidence in the effectiveness of screening. The extent of the excess mortality is determined by the number of missed cases and by the pervasiveness of the negative reassurance. The interval cancer rate is profoundly affected by the screen threshold sensitivity, the age of the subjects in the examined population, and the interval between screens. Therefore, some of the results of screening follow from the tautology of study design.

Risks of Screening Mammography

Ionizing radiation is carcinogenic. At high levels, the breast carcinogenic effect over time is linearly related to dose. The effect of each dose of radiation is assumed to be cumulative to every preceding dose. This effect can be demonstrated in women exposed to the atomic detonation in Japan (Committee on the Biological Effect of Ionizing Radiation, 1980), in patients irradiated during pneumothorax therapy for tuberculosis in Canada (Myrden and Hiltz, 1969; and Howe et al., 1982), in those irradiated for postpartum mastitis in the United States (Committee on the Biological Effect of Ionizing Radiation, 1980), and patients irradiated for treatment of benign conditions in Sweden (Baral et al., 1977).

All of these studies demonstrate that the carcinogenic

effect is clearly related to age at time of initial exposure to radiation. The greatest effect is seen in childhood, adolescence, and early adulthood (ages 10–19 years). However, there is *no* important detectable effect on breast cancer incidence for exposure beginning at about the age of 40 years (Feig, 1983, 1984*a,* 1984*b;* and Miller, 1985).

At levels of radiation in the diagnostic range, it is doubtful that the effect is linear. Theoretically, it could be linear, sublinear, or even supralinear. However, Miller (1985) and Howe and colleagues (1982), in their reanalysis of the Canadian fluoroscopy series, find strong evidence that the dose response seems to be quadratic-linear at the low levels. This is extremely important in that it means there is effectively a threshold effect. Miller and Howe and coworkers have estimated this to be at the 50- to 75-rad level. Modern mammography can deliver as little as 0.060 to 0.500 rad for a two-view examination. Digital mammography is on the horizon, and doses as low as 0.003 to 0.004 rad per examination may be possible.

The native cumulative risk for development of breast cancer is about 8%, assuming no threshold. If a population of women were assumed to receive 1 rad per year to the breasts beginning at age 35 years, lifetime cumulative risk would be increased to about 8.3%. If the annual dose is only 0.1 rad, the cumulative effect would be 8.03%.

At 1 rad per year, if there is a threshold effect at 50 rad, the population would have to reach age 90 years before the linear phase would be entered. At 0.1 rad per examination, the population would have to reach age 900 years. In either case, no effect could be seen for another 10 to 35 years. In this phase, note that the maximum risk is estimated to be 6 cases per rad per 10^6 women, and that this is for women aged 10 to 19 years.

Because the target population is 40 years of age and older, the risk associated with modern mammography is essentially negligible (Feig, 1983, 1984*a,* 1984*b;* and Miller, 1985).

It would appear to this observer that, at this time and for at least the next 5 years, good high-quality mammography will be the mainstay of early breast cancer detection.

Screening Recommendations

As a result of the data generated from the HIP study and the BCDDPs, the following guidelines for screening asymptomatic women have been suggested:

1. For women over the age of 50 years, annual mammographic and clinical examination should be performed.
2. For women aged 40 to 49 years, a baseline screening mammogram should be done with annual or biennial examinations thereafter, as indicated by risk factors or other considerations. A clinical examination should be performed annually.

The author would suggest that, in view of the results of the Swedish and Dutch studies already cited and of the lead time estimates and effects noted in this chapter, it would be rational to change these guidelines as follows:

1. Women over the age of 50 years can be screened at

least every 2 years, and mammography alone seems to be sufficient.

2. Because no mortality reduction was shown in the controlled trials, it might be argued that no screening is required for women in the 40- to 49-year age group. However, for three reasons—the serious flaws in the design of those studies for younger women (already pointed out), the high yield of small cancers and low yield of large cancers in the BCDDPs in younger women, and the fact that at this time there is no viable alternative—the author believes that it is neither wise nor prudent to deny these women the potential benefit of early detection.

3. It is necessary to shorten the interval between screens to 12 months for this age group.

4. For these younger women, clinical examination should be offered.

Mammographic Technique

It might be said that of all noncontrast, nondigital, radiologic procedures, mammography requires the greatest attention to meticulous detail. From the training of technologists to the selection of film, the constant monitoring of processing, the choosing of equipment, and the positioning of the patient, this requirement must be constantly emphasized. The author has heard it said by Sir John Price that mammography requires dedicated equipment, a dedicated room, and dedicated film and that it must be performed and interpreted by dedicated people. It is not a procedure to be performed by the untutored.

The clinician should be certain that the facility to which he or she refers patients has been accredited by the American College of Radiology or has received an equivalent rating as required by the state of residence. Film screen mammography has regained predominance in the field, and currently few xeromammography units remain in operation. Those that are operational should be shown to generate dosages in the same range as can be achieved with the film screen technique (i.e., 150 mrad or less per exposure).

Two views per breast are necessary for routine screening. This requirement can occasionally be reduced to one view under certain limited circumstances and only under the supervision of a board-certified radiologist with training in mammography. For film screen procedures, one of the two views must be a Swedish mediolateral oblique view and the other a craniocaudal view. Because of the limitations imposed by the screen film technique, a horizontal beam mediolateral projection gives an excellent picture of the ventral portion of the breast but excludes the axillary tail. Additional views may be obtained as indicated. For women with breast prostheses, "pinch" views are used to displace the prostheses back toward the chest. They are often effective in allowing more of the breast tissue to be displayed than was previously thought possible in women with such prostheses.

Technical Features

Xeroradiography uses the photoconductive principle, wherein a precharged selenium-coated plate is exposed to incoming x-rays. A residual charge proportional to the photon bombardment remains on the plate. Bipolar-charged particulate dust is sprayed onto the plate; this dust adheres to the charged surface and, in turn, is printed onto an opaque paper.

Gas electron radiography is a variant of the photostatic principle that uses a sealed chamber of xenon gas as the ionizable material and a thin Mylar sheet on which the charge and powder are collected. This process is said to preserve the edge-enhancing effect of xerography and the visual effect of film at a significantly lower dose.

Film screen, on the other hand, simply represents the classic light photon interaction with film, the light being generated by bombardment of x-ray photons of the screen within the cassette.

The xeroradiographic process produces a low-contrast, flat image. Because of the edge-enhancement effect, anatomic changes with relatively sharp borders stand out boldly. It is generally accepted that microcalcifications are readily demonstrated owing to this edge-enhancement effect.

The film screen image, on the other hand, is a high-contrast image with a wide array of densities from white to black. It tends to favor the display of small, subtle areas of asymmetric density. For women with dense fibrous breasts, the image may be difficult to evaluate. Otherwise, in high-quality film images, microcalcifications can usually be demonstrated, but a careful search pattern is important, backlighting must be diminished, and coning of extraneous light is very helpful. Although dense breasts render microcalcifications difficult to detect, use of a moving grid reduces scatter and greatly improves image quality.

Xeroradiography, because of its inherently low contrast, may lead the examiner to believe that dense breasts may be better visualized than with film. However, in the author's experience, it is very doubtful that lesions are routinely seen better with xeroradiography than they are on film.

An advantage that film offers that is not available with xeromammography is that the examiner can cone to an area of suspicious density for better detail. Owing to the toner-robbing effect with xeroradiography, severe coning is difficult. Magnification, however, can be performed with both. Magnification may be used as an alternative to coning, but it requires a somewhat greater exposure dose.

For the average 6-cm-thick breast, the generally accepted range for midbreast absorbed dose with xerography systems is about 0.27 to 0.34 rad per exposure. Newer developments may reduce this level further. For film screen systems, doses as low as 0.03 rad have been noted, but generally, the midbreast dose ranges from 0.09 to 0.15 rad per exposure.

Xeroradiography is more forgiving of exposure error than is film mammography. In film mammography systems, exposure latitude is not as wide as it is in xeroradiography. This can be overcome to a great degree through the use of phototiming devices. In both systems, positioning and adequate compression are important.

Clinical Utility of Mammographic Signs in Screening

Generally speaking, the mammographic signs of breast cancer can be divided into the *direct* signs and the *indirect*

Table 11–6. THE UNIQUE VALUE OF CERTAIN MAMMOGRAPHIC SIGNS IN THE PRESENCE OF A *POSITIVE CLINICAL EXAMINATION** OF THE BREASTS

Mammographic Sign	Number of Cancers Found by This Sign Alone		Percentage of Minimal Cancers			False-Positive Rate of This Sign (%)	Percentage of All Cancers Detected (%)†	Predictive Value for Cancer Given This Sign	
	n	SE	%	n	SE			P	SE
Punctate calcification	8	(± 2.8)	38.0	3	(± 1.7)	0.38	3.90	5.16	(± 1.8)
Mass, possibly malignant	13	(±3.6)	15.4	2	(± 1.4)	0.30	6.30	10.65	(± 2.8)
Mass, definitely malignant	7	(± 0.0)	14.0	1		0.01	3.40	100.00	(± 0)
Mass, benign	6	(± 2.4)	33.0	2	(± 1.4)	0.79	2.90	1.86	(± 0.8)
Mass, questionable	4	(± 2.0)	0.0	0		0.25	1.90	3.88	(±1.9)
Vein dilation	1		100.0	1		0.02	0.48	9.00	
Skin thickening	0		0.0	0		0.00	0.00	0	
Nipple retraction	2	(± 1.4)	50.0	1		0.05	0.90	9.09	(± 8.6)
Duct dilation	1		0.0	0		0.22	0.45	1.08	(± 1.0)

(From Moskowitz, M.: The predictive value of certain mammographic signs in screening for breast cancer. Cancer, *51*:1007, 1983. Reprinted with permission.)
SE = Standard error; *n* = number.
*Any localized abnormality.
†Percentage of 205 potentially detectable cancers identified by this sign alone.

signs. The direct signs can be further subdivided into primary signs and secondary signs.

The direct signs are those that reflect the radiographic shadow of the cancerous mass itself. This shadow has certain features that can be used to quantitate the probability of malignancy being present. These are the *primary* direct signs. *Secondary* direct signs are those that result directly from the presence of the cancer itself but that usually produce changes at some distance. In this latter category, for example, are skin thickening as a result of lymphatic permeation, skin or nipple retraction, and even cicatricial contraction of the whole breast.

When direct signs of breast cancer are present (whether primary or secondary), the lesion is usually well established, and the PPV for mammography is usually reasonably high (Tables 11–6 and 11–7).

The indirect signs of breast cancer are those that reflect changes within the breast that often occur in benign processes and, occasionally, in cancerous ones. As a result (when cancer is detected by these signs), the tumor is more often minimal (5 mm or less, or wholly noninvasive by

light microscopy) than when direct signs are present. The PPV of the secondary signs is, however, distinctly less than that of the primary signs (Moskowitz, 1979, 1983*a,b,c;* and Sickles, 1984*b*). Even in these cases, however, the PPV is greater than chance alone.

To bring some degree of quantification to mammographic interpretation, the author and colleagues have evaluated certain radiographic signs and diagnoses as they were used by them over a 5-year period of screening from 1973 to 1979 (see Tables 11–6 and 11–7) in asymptomatic, self-selected women over the age of 35 years (average age at entry = 42.5 years). These signs are discussed in some detail because they impinge heavily on clinical decision-making.

Smoothly Contoured, Solitary, Round Mass Larger Than 1 cm. When such a mass was present with margins visible in their entirety, whether clinically palpable or not, the PPV for cancer was about 2% (±0.8). Of the 12 cancers detected by pursuing this sign, one-half were minimal. These were either small cancers intimately attached to or within fibroadenomas or intracystic papillary carcinomas.

Table 11–7. THE UNIQUE VALUE OF CERTAIN MAMMOGRAPHIC SIGNS IN THE PRESENCE OF A *NEGATIVE CLINICAL EXAMINATION* OF THE BREASTS

Mammographic Sign	Number of Cancers Found by This Sign Alone		Percentage of Minimal Cancers			False-Positive Rate of This Sign (%)	Percentage of All Cancers Detected (%)*	Predictive Value for Cancer Given This Sign	
	n	SE	%	n	SE			P	SE
Punctate calcification	41	(± 6.4)	71	29	(± 5.4)	88.0	20.5	11.50	(± 1.7)
Mass, possibly malignant	15	(± 3.9)	33	5	(± 2.2)	68.0	7.3	5.43	(± 1.3)
Mass, definitely malignant	14	(± 3.7)	14	2	(± 1.4)	4.0	6.8	73.68	(± 10.7)
Mass, benign	6	(± 2.4)	67	4	(± 2.0)	67.0	2.9	2.20	(± 0.8)
Mass, questionable	0		0			10.0	0	0	
Vein dilation	0		0			0.0	0	0	
Skin thickening	0		0			0.0	0	0	
Nipple retraction	0		0			3.0†	0	0	
Duct dilation	0		0			6.0‡	0	0	

(From Moskowitz, M.: The predictive value of certain mammographic signs in screening for breast cancer. Cancer, *51*:1007, 1983. Reprinted with permission.)
*Percentage of 205 potentially detectable cancers identified by this sign alone.
†N = 13.
‡N = 26.

Spiculated, Stellate, or Knobby Mass. When this finding was present and the results of clinical examination were negative, the PPV for cancer was 74% (±10.7). If clinical examination revealed *any* positive finding, ranging from minimal thickening to a fixed mass, the PPV of these signs was 100%. Only 14% of the cancers detected by these findings were minimal; these minimal cancers constitute about 4% of all the minimal cancers found during screening. Most cancers with this finding were present in the *first* year, and they accounted for 6% of all the cancers of the author's group. Therefore, this sign is highly specific but very insensitive to minimal cancers and, when present, unequivocally requires biopsy. Fat necrosis and sclerosing duct proliferation (indurative mastopathy) may mimic this kind of cancer very closely. Occasionally, certain features may be present that allow reasonably reliable differentiation from cancer.

Relatively Well-Circumscribed Mass with Partial Loss of Border or That Is Too Dense for Size. When results on clinical examination were negative, the PPV for this constellation of findings was about 5% (±1.3) (Fig. 11–2). When results on clinical examination were positive, the PPV was about 11% (±2.8). Combined, the PPV of this sign was about 7%. However, about 25% of cancers detected as a result of this finding represented minimal cancers. The FP rate for this sign approached 1%. Twenty per cent of cancers with these findings were minimal, and they represented 13% of all minimal cancers that occurred in this population. Today, biopsy may be avoided in many of these cases if ultrasonography is available. However, for ultrasonography to be as reliable as aspiration in the diagnosis of cysts, strict criteria must be followed, and the possible presence of a number of different cysts must still be explored (Boon and deGraaf Guillond, 1981; Sickles, 1984*a;* and Sickles et al., 1984). If the lesion is solid on ultrasonography (in the cancer age group), excisional biopsy or aspiration cytology should be considered.

Microcalcifications

The reported positive predictive value of detecting microcalcifications varies widely in the literature (Paterok et al., 1983; Prorok et al., 1983; Anastassiades et al., 1984; Kopans, 1984; Kopans et al., 1984*a;* LeGal et al., 1984; Rasmussen, 1984; and Dupont and Page, 1985). It has long been empirically recognized that certain kinds of microcalcifications are associated with a high probability of cancer (Snyder, 1980; Stamp et al., 1983; Boisselier et al., 1983; Anastassiades et al., 1984; and Dupont and Page, 1985). Most early workers in mammography described these calcifications in association with soft tissue densities that often had radiographic features of malignancy.

As the use of mammography matured, it became apparent that breast microcalcifications were not so specific as was initially hoped. Often, cancer-associated calcifications do not reside within the malignancy but may be regional to it in as many as 60% of the cases.

It is reasonable to divide microcalcifications into five categories, namely (1) clearly benign, (2) probably benign, (3) possibly cancer, (4) probably cancer, and (5) cancer.

Categories 3, 4, and 5 encompass most cancer-associated calcifications and keep a reasonably low and manageable FP rate and a satisfactory PPV.

It must be recognized that all calcifications within the breast are not equally predictive. Some calcifications do not enter into the differential diagnosis of malignancy and can be confidently excluded from biopsy. These calcifications are usually larger than 200 to 250 mm, often coarse, and not usually clustered or lined up in a duct; or, if smaller, they are round and smooth and are often hollow. On occasion, a calcified blood vessel wall may mimic microcalcifications, but close inspection usually permits a firm diagnosis. The large, coarse, linear ductal calcifications of secretory disease are not usually a problem of differential diagnosis.

Skin calcifications may be mistaken for intramammary calcium. If the characteristic lobulated, hollow appearance of cutaneous calcium is not present or if the calcifications do not project on the skin surface tangential to the x-ray beam, they may be difficult to distinguish from significant microcalcifications. Also, the soft tissue detail is such with modern mammography that care must be taken not to confuse the shadows of deodorant or talcum powder with breast microcalcifications.

Although microcalcifications have long been recognized to have an association with cancer and benign disease, it is only within the last 15 to 20 years that an interest in the biochemical makeup of these radiographic shadows has appeared in the literature (Galkin et al., 1977; Anastassiades et al., 1984; and Fandos-Morera et al., 1988). Galkin and associates' work suggests that there is indeed a biochemical difference between the tiny microcalcifications associated with cancer and those microcalcifications associated with bland, benign pathologic findings. It is intriguing that, on the basis of electron microscope spectroscopy, Galkin and associates suggest that some of these tiny particles are not calcium at all. They have reported the appearance of such metals as gold, lithium, zinc, and tin in the small, dense spots seen in biopsy specimens.

The chief value of microcalcifications is that they are markers that permit the earlier detection of some breast cancers in asymptomatic women when the cancer is still wholly intraductal or, if invasive, is often less than 5 mm in size. For example, in the author's own series, 42% of all minimal cancers were detected based on this radiographic sign.

In the author's screening program, when the only sign of suspicion was microcalcification, the positive predictive value was about 12%; 71% of these cancers were minimal. Given that in nonscreened women in the United States about 20% to 25% of all biopsies are cancerous and 45% to 50% are Stage II and higher disease, this appears to be an acceptable trade-off. Although this approach has been unpopular in the past among radiologists as well as surgeons, there is a growing awareness that mass screening and detection of minimal cancer by indirect signs almost mandates a lower PPV (Moskowitz, 1979, 1983*a,c,* 1984; and Sickles, 1984*b*). This approach is only justifiable if the yield of minimal cancer can be increased and if the absolute incidence of far advanced disease can be decreased. That it can do so has been established (deWaard et al., 1984; and Tabar et al., 1985).

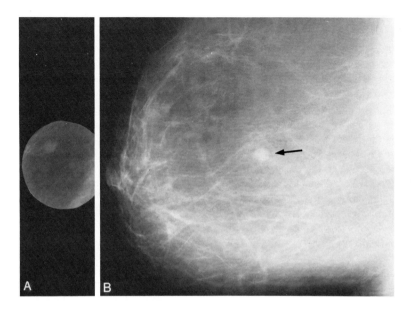

Figure 11–2. Note the small, relatively well-cir-cumscribed mass *(B)*. It is of relatively low den-sity, but the coned view *(A)* demonstrates an undulating border, betraying its solid nature. The partial loss of border and faint fibrillary retrac-tions strongly suggest cancer. Pathologic diag-nosis: 8-mm colloid carcinoma of the breast.

The author's group tends to be more aggressive concerning biopsy in younger women when it is known that the yield per biopsy will be less but that the potential gain is greatest. As has been shown by postmortem studies of coroner's cases (Sandison, 1962; and Pollei et al., 1987), no intraductal or minimal cancers are present in asymptomatic women below the age of 40 years, and few are present at the ages of 40 to 70 years. Therefore, those that are present should be sought out vigorously.

For older women with microcalcifications, the author's group tends to be less aggressive; this is because as the population ages, many more subclinical, and probably indolent, cancers may be present (Sandison, 1962; and Pollei, 1987). Therefore, the examination often is repeated in 3 months, and if no change is seen, the assumption is made that the disease, if present, is not growing rapidly. Another examination is performed in 6 to 9 months, with monthly breast self-examination and appropriately timed interval clinical examinations. If all remains stable, annual mammography is again advised. If the calcium has developed as an interval finding and the woman is in otherwise good general health, performance of a biopsy is usually the most prudent course.

Sign of Asymmetry

The breasts are said to be "optical isomers," and any asymmetry is highly suspicious. It is self-evident that a cancer casting an image on one side is an asymmetric density. Martin and colleagues (1979), in reviewing interval cases in several of the BCDDPs, determined that an asymmetric density was the most frequently overlooked sign of cancer. However, nonspecific asymmetric areas of fibrosis occur frequently in the general population, and these, too, are "asymmetric densities."

In the author's experience, if obvious carcinomas or masses, areas of architectural distortion, or calcifications are excluded, asymmetry alone has been a very low-yield sign. In the absence of a palpable abnormality in the author's screened population, no cancer was found by this sign alone. When accompanied by an area of clinical thickening or by a mass, the PPV for cancer was 3% to 4%. Currently, given asymmetric shadowing and no clinical finding, the patient may be asked to return for a recheck mammogram examination in 6 months. Monthly breast self-examination is encouraged, and a clinical examination at 3 to 6 months is suggested. If any change occurs, clinically or mammographically, biopsy is urged.

Cost-Effectiveness of Mammographic Screening

Whether mammographic screening is cost-effective depends on the viewpoint of the observer and on the context in which the question is being posed (Moskowitz, 1979; Turnbull et al., 1979; Eddy, 1981, 1985; Mooney, 1981, 1982; Friedlander and Tattersall, 1982; Kays, 1983; Evans, 1984; O'Conner et al., 1985; and Ward, 1985). However, the actual costs and some associated comparisons are measurable.

Screening mammography as covered by Medicare can be performed at $50 per examination, including interpretation fee, if (1) the volume of cases is sufficiently high, (2) highly skilled technologists are available, (3) images are developed in batches, (4) current images and old images are mounted on a multiviewer by a clerk, and (5) they are batch-read by a skilled, experienced mammographer.

If 20,000 self-selected women aged 40 to 49 years were screened annually at a cost of $50 per screen, with an average annual incidence rate of 2.5 per 1000, 50 women would probably be found to have cancer (see Table 11–4), and the cost per case detected would be $20,000. If 10 biopsies were performed for every cancer detected, at $1200 per outpatient biopsy, another $600,000 is added to the cost. Therefore, including biopsy, the total cost per cancer found, excluding prevalence cases, is $32,000. If prevalence cases were included, the cost per case detected would drop (Moskowitz, 1979).

If 35% of the cancers found were less than 5 mm in diameter, then 16 more cases found would be at this stage than in the nonscreened situation. The cost of each added case of cancer found at this stage would be $100,000. Instead of 25 of the 50 women dying by the 10th year, only 3 to 10 would die (see Table 11–5). Therefore, the cost per death averted at 10 years would range from $34,000 to $107,000.

These costs can be compared with reported costs (Turnbull et al., 1979; Boon and deGraaf Guillond, 1981; Schroeder et al., 1981; Friedlander and Tattersall, 1982; Lansky et al., 1983; Blommers, 1984; Long et al., 1984; and Kelly et al., 1985) for other medical procedures, as follows: (1) cost per cervical cancer detected, $17,000; (2) cost for 10 years of renal dialysis, $230,000 to $320,000; (3) cost for first year of coronary bypass surgery, $13,500; and (4) $1200 to $1500 per day for the last month of life of terminal cancer patients. The costs for cardiac and hepatic transplant and use of artificial hearts are not considered here.

If prices are contained to reasonable levels, if high-quality mammography can be ensured, and if the limitations of screening are recognized, a significant impact on breast cancer management can be achieved.

Needle Localization

It is self-evident that some means of assisting the surgeon in localizing nonpalpable lesions is necessary. To attempt blind resection or unaided quadrantectomy results not only in unnecessary deformity to the patient but also in an unacceptably high level of unresected lesions.

The technique for needle localization is limited only by the capabilities of the equipment available (Chang et al., 1980; Snyder, 1980; Kopans et al., 1984*b;* and El Yousef et al., 1985). It may vary from a simple method of estimating skin entry points from mammograms to the use of highly sophisticated computerized equipment costing many thousands of dollars. Either a simple grid system or a coordinate system is highly satisfactory, and one of these is usually available with modern mammography units (Figs. 11–3 and 11–4). A satisfactory level of skill is achievable in a very short time.

Is it necessary to use special needles and wires? Certainly, a wide variety of localizing trocars are available, ranging from variants of miniharpoons to crimped wires passed into the breast through a needle trocar (Meyer et al., 1984; Rasmussen and Serrup, 1984; Homer, 1985; and Kopans et al., 1985*b*). Generally speaking, the author has not found these to be necessary if the lesion is within 5 cm (2 inches) of the breast surface. Special instruments are of most help when the breast is very large and the lesion is deeply seated (i.e., central). In general, if a 22- to 25-gauge needle of the appropriate length is selected for the estimated depth of the suspicious area (when the breast is noncompressed) and the full length of the needle is inserted up to the hub, the needles will usually stay in place for several hours or until they are removed by operating room personnel. The author has occasionally used collodion to hold the

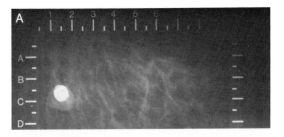
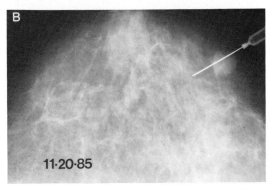

Figure 11–3. Needle localization coordinate system. A needle has been placed into a soft, circumscribed mass. Note that right angle films are used to verify that the lesion has been transfixed.

needles in place, and this seems to offer some measure of added protection.

It may be useful to insert more than one needle into the area of the abnormality (Fig. 11–5). This seems to be of

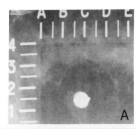
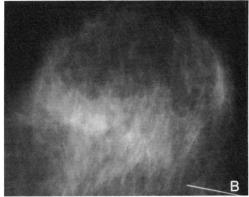

Figure 11–4. Coordinate system localization from the inferior approach. In this case, the lesion was close to the chest wall and near the inframammary fold. This image was achieved with the x-ray apparatus inverted for the caudal view. This can also be done with a BB placed on the skin and multiple film localization.

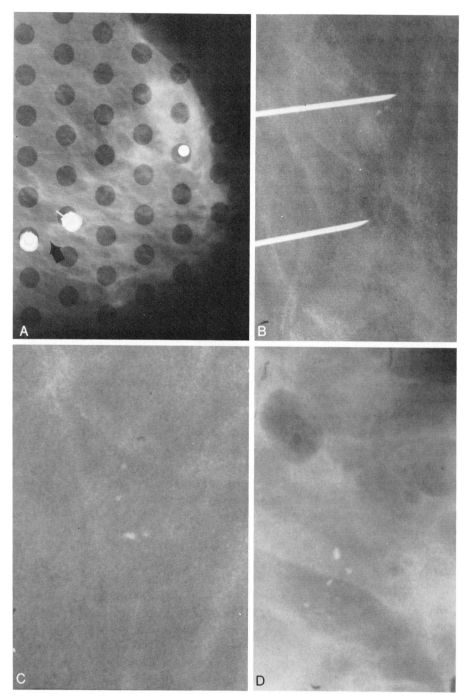

Figure 11–5. *A,* Needle localization from the lateral aspect of the breast using the perforated compression grid and multiple needles. *B,* Caudal view demonstrating the needle tips relative to the calcifications. *C,* Close-up view of calcifications as seen on the mammogram. *D,* Close-up view of calcifications seen on the specimen radiograph. The pathologic diagnosis was intraductal carcinoma.

more help when the calcifications are strung out in a fairly long linear array or cover a slightly larger area. The author tries to encompass the area of interest or the central area and an outer margin. Methylene blue or radiopaque contrast agent, or both, may be injected as an option

Surgeons who review the position of the needles with the radiologist just before surgery are more successful in removing the suspected area at the first pass. Those who depend on the localization films alone or on a map seem to have more difficulty.

No matter how the procedure is performed, certain principles are straightforward and important:

1. After preliminary localizing films are obtained, a needle of the appropriate length is inserted at the site of the shortest distance from skin to lesion. The length of the

needle is based on the estimated depth of the lesion in the noncompressed breast.

2. Confirmatory films, at right angles to one another, must be obtained (Fig. 11–6). Any necessary adjustment to positioning requires a new set of films at right angles.

3. The localization is discussed and, ideally, reviewed directly with the operating surgeon in the physical presence of the patient. As experience is gained by the biopsy team,

this becomes less necessary. However, until a good three-dimensional reconstruction is established in the mind of the operating surgeon, this step is very useful. A map localizing the needle placement in reference to the lesion may be of help in the operating room.

4. If the biopsy is performed for microcalcifications, the specimen should be radiographed (Fig. 11–7). This only adds a few minutes to the biopsy procedure. If, in the course of evaluating the biopsy specimen, an obvious cancer is encountered, specimen radiography may be less important. Sectioning the specimen and tagging and radiographing it is helpful to the pathologist in narrowing the search for calcifications. It is obvious, however, that the pathologist needs to evaluate the total specimen provided.

If the biopsy was done not for calcifications but for the study of some other radiographic sign, specimen radiography, in the author's experience, has been of less help. In this circumstance, it is valuable for the radiologist to be present in the pathology laboratory when the biopsy specimen is macrosectioned. He or she can recognize if the gross lesion for which biopsy was recommended has been removed.

For a number of years we have recommended a single-view mammogram of the biopsied breast 2 months after the operation to verify that the suspicious tissues have been removed and to serve as a new baseline for future screening.

Failure to follow this course of action increases the probability that cancers will be left in place, and some of these tumors are of considerable size. On occasion, even following this course, the area of abnormality may remain in the patient (Fig. 11–8).

Mammographic Patterns and Breast Cancer Risk

Wolfe (1976*b*) introduced a classification system of four groups with increasing risk for breast cancer: N1 and P1 breasts are composed chiefly of fat; P2 breasts have severe involvement with a prominent duct pattern; DY describes breasts that have severe involvement with dysplasia that often obscures the prominent duct pattern. Since Wolfe (1976*a,b*) first described this relationship between mammographic patterns and the risk of developing breast cancer, many reports have appeared, some supporting and some rejecting his thesis (Egan and Mosteller, 1977; Mendell et al., 1977; Moskowitz et al., 1980*a;* Moskowitz, 1982; Tabar and Dean, 1982; Chaudary et al., 1983; Danes, 1983; Witt et al., 1983; Boyd et al., 1984; Brisson et al., 1984; Verbeek et al., 1984; Witt et al., 1984; Horwitz et al., 1984; Kojima et al., 1984; Carlile et al., 1985; Spratt et al., 1985; and Whitehead et al., 1985). Wolfe (1976*a,b*) originally estimated the highest risk pattern to be on the order of 30:1. Subsequently, his estimates were reduced considerably, although his group estimated a relative risk of 10:1 (Wolfe et al., 1985).

In a blinded prospective study testing Wolfe's patterns, Moskowitz and coworkers (1980*a*) found a statistically significant correlation between Wolfe's high-risk patterns and severe hyperplastic breast disease demonstrated by histology, but this could only be demonstrated if the two high-

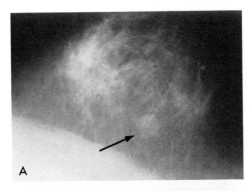

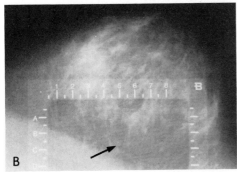

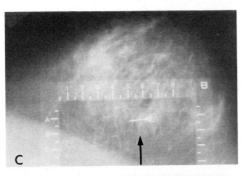

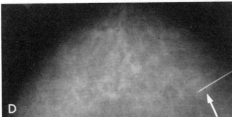

Figure 11–6. A well-circumscribed lesion localized by coordinates. *A,* The lesion seen in the mediolateral view. *B,* The lesion seen in the mediolateral view with a calibrated compressor in place. *C,* The localizing needle is approximately 3 mm superior to the lesion. *D,* In the craniocaudal view, the lesion appears transfixed by the needle.

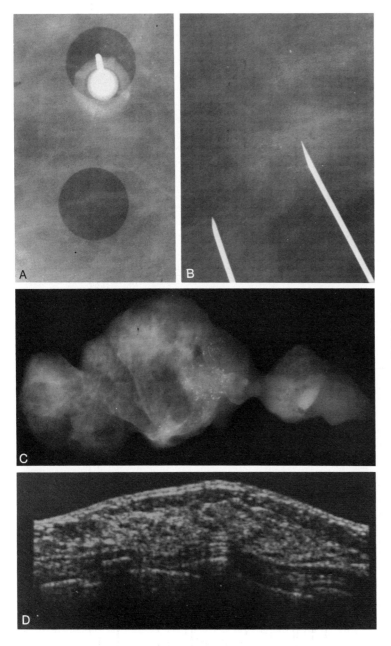

Figure 11-7. *A and B,* Needle localization in an area of clustered calcification surrounded by a poorly defined mass. No lesion was palpable. *C,* Specimen radiograph of the same lesion. *D,* A negative ultrasonographic examination.

risk groups were consolidated. Although the risk was statistically significant, it was only about 1.67 times the risk of the lower risk patterns. However, when the authors tested their interpretation of patterns against Wolfe's interpretation of the same cases, only a 50% agreement rate was achieved.

Wellings and Wolf (1978) and Wilkinson and colleagues (1977) presented data supporting Wolfe's observations. In that same time period, Egan and Mosteller (1977), Mendell and colleagues (1977), Rideout and Poor (1977), and Peyster and coworkers (1977) found only weak support or no support for a mammographic pattern and risk relationship.

Horwitz and colleagues (1984) reported the results of a case control study wherein women were classified into high-risk and low-risk categories, according to Wolfe's cri-

teria. This study failed to show any significant difference in the proportion of high-risk parenchymal patterns among patients who either were clinically normal or had clinical "fibrocystic disease" versus those with histologically confirmed breast cancer. It was believed that Wolfe's patterns could not be used to select women for breast screening.

Spratt and coworkers (1985) report no significant difference in the distribution of incidence cancers according to Wolfe's parenchymal pattern. However, only 4 patients with cancer were observed in 355 patients followed. The numbers are too small to draw a meaningful conclusion, as these authors pointed out. Similarly, they found no relation between various types of pathologic proliferative disorders and the distribution among Wolfe's parenchymal patterns. It must be noted, however, that these same authors did not

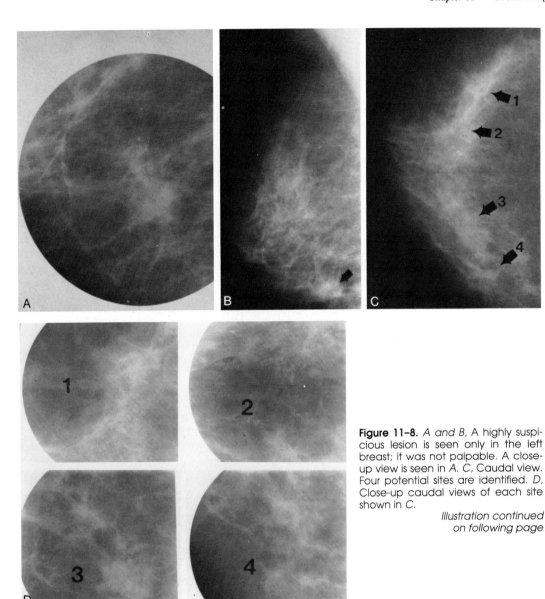

Figure 11–8. *A and B,* A highly suspicious lesion is seen only in the left breast; it was not palpable. A close-up view is seen in *A. C,* Caudal view. Four potential sites are identified. *D,* Close-up caudal views of each site shown in *C.*

Illustration continued on following page

find any significant excess risk of breast cancer among *any* of the various forms of "chronic cystic mastopathy." This is in stark contradistinction to the prospective long-term study reported by Dupont and Page (1985), who found a significant excess of cancers appearing in patients with atypical hyperplasia. Others (Black et al., 1972; Ashikari et al., 1974; Page et al., 1978; Moskowitz et al., 1980b; and Boisselier et al., 1983) also found a consistent relationship between subsequent breast cancer risk and hyperplastic epithelial breast disease. As Spratt and colleagues pointed out, the failure to establish an association between patterns and subsequent risk may be a function of the small sample size.

Witt and associates (1984) and Ward (1985) reported that they reviewed the mammograms of 597 women whose images were obtained during the years 1971 to 1975. This was done prospectively and blindly, and 18 patients were excluded because of technically inadequate imaging. Subsequently, during the period of follow-up, which ranged from 5 to 9 years, 12 cases of breast cancer developed, and

they occurred with equal frequency in the low-risk and high-risk patterns. Again, however, the sample size is very small. Chaudary and colleagues (1983), in a matched study of about 1000 women over the age of 30 years, failed to demonstrate an association between the P2 mammographic pattern and breast cancer. Verbeek and coworkers (1984) reported the results of a prospective study based on the Nijmegen screening program. Patients were followed for 6 years; the authors demonstrated a relative risk for women with P2 and DY breasts of 0.7, with 95% confidence limits of 0.2 and 2.4.

On the other hand, a prospective case control study involving several of the BCDDPs' investigations has resulted in several supportive reports (Carlile et al., 1985; and Whitehead et al., 1985). In these studies, intensive training in patterns was given to the radiologists, and it was required that a satisfactory interobserver agreement rate with Wolfe's readings be achieved. Rates of agreement of 95% were reported. To keep agreement high, atlas material was

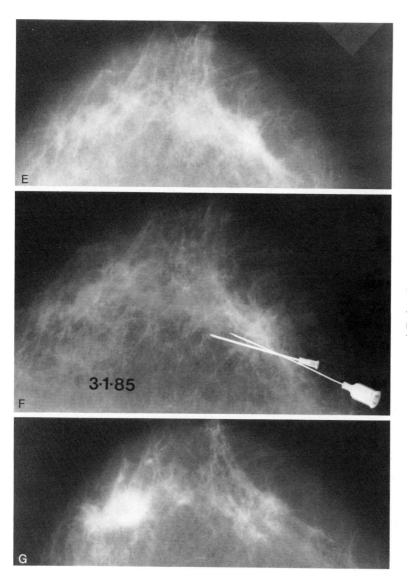

Figure 11–8 *Continued E,* One month later (2–18–85), the lateral site (4 in *D*) seems to have increased in density. *F,* Two weeks after *E* (3–1–85), needle localization at the lateral site revealed marked atypical hyperplasia. *G,* Seven months after *F,* an obvious cancer is present at the medial site.

prepared and kept available at each institution. An excess risk on the order of 3.5:1 was noted, and mammographic patterns were found to be risk factors independent of other common epidemiologic risk factors. These authors conclude that whereas risk estimates are statistically demonstrable, they are not of sufficient order of magnitude to use for management decisions for the individual woman, nor for selecting populations for screening.

In a subanalysis of this study, Whitehead and colleagues (1985) evaluated the possibility that dense breasts simply "mask" the presence of cancers, and that subsequent appearance of "new" lesions is not a risk marker but an artifact of density. Their analysis shows some masking effect, but Whitehead and colleagues believe there is an excess risk that is not accounted for by so-called masking.

Brisson and colleagues (1984) reported the results of a case control study of 362 women with newly diagnosed breast cancers identified in 1978–1979 and controls selected from 686 women referred for a "routine" mammogram. In this study, breast cancer was first confirmed histologically

in the month preceding or in the 12 months following their examination, and, thus, the study essentially represents the results of a prevalence trial rather than a long-term incidence or prospective study. They found that an increase in body weight was associated with a marked reduction of the P2 or DY pattern, so that 94% of tall and thin women had a P2 or DY pattern, whereas only 19% of short, stocky, and heavy women had a P2 or DY pattern. They also found that the concentration of nodular densities was inversely related to body weight but varied little with body height. When these authors did not adjust for body weight and height, they found that the P2 pattern had an excess relative risk compared with the N1 pattern's risk of 2.0. When adjustments were made, a relative risk of 2.6 was found, with a range of 1.7 to 4.1 at the 95% confidence level.

These authors also estimated the relative risk to be 4.4 (2.5–7.9), with correction for body weight and height based on the percentage of the breast affected by nodular densities and involvement of over 60% of the breast. When the densities were homogeneous, the maximum relative risk was 2.0. It should be noted here that Myers and coworkers (1983) reported that volumetric estimates of the percentage of breast involved by a given pattern are *not* highly reliable and reproducible.

Nevertheless, Brisson and colleagues concluded that the data showed a strong inverse association between mammographic features of breast tissue and body weight. They believe that the strength of the associations of mammographic features of breast cancer risk is underestimated in other studies in which body size was not taken into account. It should be pointed out, however, that their study is essentially a study of prevalence cases, and prevalence studies have almost uniformly shown an excess risk as compared with incidence studies (Moskowitz, 1982). Furthermore, although a twofold to threefold excess relative risk may be large in epidemiologic terms, in practical terms for patient management or planning for screening it has little value. More specifically, selections of populations of women for screening based on all known risk factors will exclude 75% of women who will subsequently develop breast cancer (Seidman, 1977).

Although these authors are able to increase the relative risk by adjusting for body height and weight, the differences observed between the uncorrected and corrected ranges fall well within the 95% confidence interval for either. In addition, the ranges given for the confidence intervals of relative risk include the risk ranges presented by Moskowitz and colleagues (1980a), even though the latter group did not take into account body size.

Boyd and coworkers (1984) have reported the results of a literature review of 17 selected studies. They critically analyzed the methodologic standards that each of the studies reported. They concluded that ''a large part of the controversy on this subject arises from the methodologic differences among the studies.'' Boyd and coworkers calculated the relative risks from the reported data and tabulated it in relation to the number of acceptable scientific methodologic criteria that they judged to be present.

Of seven *prevalence* surveys analyzed, only a maximum of four criteria of a possible nine were met by any study, and the relative risk ranged from 0.24 to 1.60. Of five evaluable *cohort* studies, two met seven of the criteria; one met five (although the authors credited it with only four); one met four; and one met three. In the two studies scoring seven criteria (both reported by the same author on the same database), a relative risk of 7 to 8 was reported. The highest risk of 8 was reported by a study meeting only four of the standards set by Boyd and coworkers. Of the eight cohort studies, a relative risk exceeding 2 was found in two studies with a score of four, and in one study with a score of six.

These authors concluded that studies that follow the usual scientific methods employed in the epidemiologic evaluation of risk generally have confirmed an association between mammographic pattern and breast cancer risk.

The data overall suggest that some slight excess risk of breast cancer is present in patients with a P2 or DY pattern compared with a parenchymal pattern composed mostly of fat and that this is somehow related to body habitus. At present, the magnitude of the excess risk does not seem to be strong, and the uncertainty associated with its level precludes it from being clinically useful.

An interesting application of the use of parenchymal patterns was suggested by Hinton and colleagues (Hinton et al., 1985), who reported that parenchymal patterns correlate relatively well with estrogen receptor content of tumors and prognosis. On the other hand, Nielsen and Poulsen (1985) found no correlation between parenchymal pattern and estrogen receptor content of tumors. They did find that high estrogen receptor levels were present in spiculated masses. Well-defined masses or cancers found by calcification alone, or mammographically negative cancers, had a low estrogen receptor level. The numbers are small but tend to follow the pattern previously reported by Broberg and colleagues (1983).

Mammography for Purposes Other Than Screening

For patients with symptoms, mammography may provide support for a clinical impression of malignant disease. However, if the clinical impression is strong and mammography results are negative, delay in biopsy should not be allowed to occur.

Used preoperatively, mammography may help to stage and evaluate the extent of the disease. Magnification views, in particular, may show unsuspected foci of microcalcifications in addition to the major primary lesion. This is of great help in selecting patients for breast conserving surgery.

Mammography is important as a clinical adjunct in following the residual breast in patients with unilateral mastectomy (Schalldach and Schumann, 1982) and is helpful in following the breasts of patients who have had breast preserving procedures (Dodd, 1984; and Paulus, 1984).

Mammography can also occasionally be useful in defining early recurrences in the site of mastectomy or in the ipsilateral axilla if the patient has sufficient tissue remaining on the chest wall to make radiography possible.

When axillary nodes are large and dense or, on rare occasions, contain spiculated microcalcifications in the presence of a known breast neoplasm, the PPV for metastatic cancer is on the order of 90% to 95%. However, these findings identify only about 40% of the patients who subsequently are shown to have lymph node involvement by axillary dissection (Kalisher et al., 1976; and Coopmans de Yoldi et al., 1983).

In patients with breast prostheses, mammography and ultrasonography have limitations insofar as preclinical detection is concerned. Jensen and Mackey (1985) reported, however, that xeromammography is very useful in clarifying the nature of palpable masses under this circumstance. In their series, the mammogram proved that about 50% of such palpable masses were prosthesis related.

In the author's opinion, the most important function of mammography lies in earlier detection (Shapiro et al., 1974; Fox et al., 1978; Andersson et al., 1979; Andersson, 1980; Baker, 1982; Shapiro et al., 1982; Council on Scientific Affairs, 1984; deWaard et al., 1984; Gad et al., 1984; Hebert et al., 1984; Kambouris et al., 1984; Kopans et al., 1984a; Moskowitz, 1984; Rasanen et al., 1984; Verbeek et al., 1984; Watanabe, 1984; Editorial, 1985; Fox et al.,

1985; Tabar et al., 1985; and Verbeek, 1985). To date, no other method, including breast self-examination or clinical examination, has proved capable of reducing mortality in screened populations.

NEEDLE BIOPSY OR ASPIRATION CYTOLOGY UNDER MAMMOGRAPHIC CONTROL

These remarks are directed at the concept of establishing definitive diagnoses by mammographically guided needle techniques for nonpalpable abnormalities found on the mammograms of asymptomatic women. In terms of mass screening, these techniques can only be acceptable if they do not decrease the sensitivity of the primary screen while increasing the specificity of the primary screen. As the author and associates have shown (Pelikan and Moskowitz, 1993), the case for mass screening of young women is particularly sensitive with regard to this point. Delay in diagnosis of even a relatively small portion of the patients in this age group can result in failure of a screen to reduce mortality and has the potential to create an excess disease-specific mortality among those screened. Therefore, any diagnostic test that is to be applied to a screened population must take into consideration (1) patient age, (2) the differentiation of women with screen-detected lesions from symptomatic women, (3) the absence of known risk factors that increase incidence of cancer, (4) careful and specific delineation and description of the mammographic signs that prompted biopsy, (5) careful comparison of results with those of the usual diagnostic test (in this case, open surgical biopsy), (6) a number of subjects sufficient to give the test statistical power, and (7) that appropriate care in designing the test is taken so that clinical validity is ensured.

The history of medicine in general, and that of radiology in particular, is replete with examples of poorly designed studies. (This author does not exempt himself from performing well-intentioned medical error). As a result, many procedures become incorporated into routine practice because we can do them. How does this apply to the discussion of screening? The role of screening is to detect abnormalities and to quantify degree of suspicion as to the possible presence of malignancy. All expert readers follow the same receiver operating characteristic curve, and the most reasonable operating point is at about the sensitivity level of 0.85. Above this point, the role of chance is increased. There may be situations in which this is desirable, and in the assessment of certain microcalcifications, it can be cogently argued that this is the case. However, this approach can be justified only if the total biopsy rate is reasonable and if the yield of minimal breast cancers (smaller than 5 mm or wholly intraductal) is acceptable. The author suggests that a 10% PPV would be acceptable if the per cent of minimal breast cancers were 35% to 40% or greater.

The role of consultative (problem-solving?) breast imaging in the screening situation is to winnow out the lesions having a very high probability of being benign that are detected on mammographic screening from the others and

to select those lesions for which a more definitive diagnosis is required. (It cannot be expected to do this with sufficient reliability for palpable lesions not demonstrated on a mammogram; such lesions must be handled based on the clinical suspicion of their presence.)

The role of a diagnostic test is to establish the definitive diagnosis so that therapy can be planned and instituted. If negative diagnoses cannot be relied upon to exclude minimal breast cancer, then they only add cost, time, and increased morbidity to the screening procedure. If operative morbidity is markedly reduced, perhaps the argument that some reduction in sensitivity is acceptable could be made. However, considering that we are dealing with the potentially most curable lesions, this decision should be weighed very carefully before this argument is accepted. It is this author's opinion that the entire thrust of the screening process in younger women rests on this decision.

If a lesion is deemed sufficiently suspicious to require biopsy for diagnosis, can a stereotactically guided core needle biopsy or fine-needle aspiration cytology reliably replace open biopsy? An open surgical biopsy is not perfect, even with the assistance of needle localization. In this author's experience, about 3% to 5% of cases are not removed at the initial biopsy. Miss rates for open biopsies performed with local anesthesia as high as 20% have been reported (Norton, 1988). Recently, Campbell and associates (1991) reported results similar to this author's findings.

Parker and associates addressed the validity of stereotactic core needle biopsy (1990, 1991). Initially, they performed stereotactic biopsy using 18-, 16-, or 14-gauge biopsy needles. Later, they reported on 102 additional patients in whom they used 14-gauge needles. The findings of all cases were compared with the results of surgical biopsy.

Although a protocol "approved by the human use committee" was followed, no details of patient selection were given. In this study, 34 of 36 cancers (excluding one lobular carcinoma) verified at surgical biopsy were identified by the needle procedure. There were no FP results. In another study (Dowlatshahi et al., 1991), 63 of 76 cancers were equal to or less than 1 cm in size; in addition, 31 (41%) were detected by stereotactic core biopsy alone, and 24 (32%) were detected by stereotactically guided fine-needle aspiration alone.

Modern stereotactic devices make needle placement close to or within a radiographic lesion a reasonable probability. However, even biopsy with 14-gauge needles requires three or more passes if a reliable diagnosis is to be obtained (Parker et al., 1991). Considering the size of the needles, the frequency of the "passes," and the use of local anesthetic, the morbidity may not be significantly less than that with open biopsy for an outpatient under local anesthesia. If a malignant diagnosis is established by needle biopsy it cannot be assumed that excision for treatment planning is unnecessary.

It is entirely possible that a core, highly localized biopsy is perfectly satisfactory for small masses or even for high-yield, specific microcalcifications as long as a specific tissue diagnosis that is compatible with the presumptive radiographic diagnosis is obtained. However, in screening (particularly in younger women), most small cancers are detected based on indirect signs of breast cancer. These signs have little to do with cancer per se: they indicate the presence of a local abnormality in a region and are more frequently seen in benign than malignant disease. For example, the author has asked ''expert'' radiologists to classify 200 consecutive radiographs of biopsy specimens that contain microcalcifications on a scale from 1 to 5 (1 = benign; 2 = probably benign; 3 = suspicious; 4 = probably malignant; 5 = malignant). When a specimen was classified in Categories 4 and 5, the PPV for malignancy was 75% to 100%. For Category 1 lesions, the PPV approached 100%. For Category 3 specimens, the PPV was 38%. Unfortunately, when the diagnosis was ''malignancy'' or ''probably malignancy,'' fewer than one-half of the cancers present in the sample were detected. When Category 3 lesions were added, 12% of cancers were still missed. If Category 2 lesions were added, all of the cancers were detected, and the PPV was approximately 20%.

Some microcalcifications are clearly produced by cancer and have a specific pattern. These calcifications are within the cancer, and a biopsy specimen (core or open) that contains these calcifications can be expected to lead to correct diagnosis. However, the other calcifications (those of Category 3, in particular) are nonspecific and are often not within the cancer but rather regional to it; thus, a negative result on core biopsy cannot be expected to exclude neoplasm as a diagnosis.

As pointed out in a summary report of a National Cancer Institute workshop on state-of-the-art and new technologies held in the fall of 1991 in Bethesda, Maryland (Gohagan and Shterm, 1992), ''well designed studies comparing cost effectiveness and morbidity of this technique [to open surgical biopsy] are required.'' As of this writing, stereotactic core biopsy is an immature technology with important potential.

In the future, it is possible that definitive diagnosis and possibly even treatment can be achieved with needle techniques (perhaps coupled with laser energy methods and fiberoptics).

Galactography

Galactography is simply retrograde injection of a radiographic contrast medium into a lactiferous duct, followed by appropriate radiographic imaging. The injection usually is accompanied by minimal discomfort unless the duct is ruptured. If a duct's discharge has been of long duration, the duct usually is relatively ectatic, and cannulation is accomplished easily. If it is difficult to express a discharge, the procedure becomes, pari passu, similarly difficult to perform.

The author employs iothalamate meglumine (Conray 60) for this purpose and, generally, no more than 2 mL is necessary.

Galactography should not be done in the absence of a demonstrable discharge on the day of the examination, not only because of the difficulty involved in cannulating a nondischarging duct, but also because, if the duct is cannulated, it might be the wrong one. Indeed, the author has had the experience of initially cannulating a duct from which a

small amount of serous fluid was expressed, and finding the underlying system to be perfectly normal. Further milking of the breast demonstrated a small bloody effluent from another site nearby; and galactography of this duct demonstrated an intraductal papillary lesion.

Some authors have gone so far as to call galactography the most important examination in the diagnosis of the secreting breast, and that it is indicated in all patients with spontaneous bloody or serous discharge (Kindermann et al., 1979; Peyster and Kalisher, 1979; Alberti and Troiso, 1982; and Tabar et al., 1983). However, what can realistically be expected of this study is an excellent retrograde delineation of the anatomy of the duct injected. Ectasias, strictures, intraluminal filling defects, cut-offs, and duct displacement can be discerned. Multiple papillomas can be diagnosed confidently, but the cause of a larger, solitary mass (Fig. 11–9) cannot be determined without biopsy. Unfortunately, as with most imaging procedures, a firm diagnosis of cancer can be rendered only occasionally. As DiPietro and coworkers (1979) point out, ''in practice it should be the type of discharge that indicates surgery rather than the galactographic data.''

In the author's experience, the major value of this procedure has been to locate the site of the abnormality or abnormalities, often reducing the magnitude of the surgical procedure necessary to ensure resection of the papillary growth. If performed just prior to surgery, 0.1 mL of methylene blue may be mixed with the radiographic contrast medium. After injection for this purpose, the author puts a drop or two of collodion on the surface of the nipple to temporarily occlude the duct. If the duct has not been ruptured by the pressure of the injection, the contrast material will remain confined to the duct system.

In the presence of a spontaneous bloody or serous discharge, galactography may be helpful for further evaluation. In the author's opinion, other types of nipple discharge are even weaker relative indications for the study. The only absolute contraindication is known hypersensitivity to the contrast medium.

Although this author does not believe that galactography is the most useful test in the imaging armamentarium, and certainly it is not absolutely necessary in all cases of discharge, bloody or otherwise, it does appear that the method is probably being relatively underutilized, considering the information that might be gained from it.

Ultrasonography

Ultrasonography is an important complementary breast imaging tool. It can do what no other imaging test can do: make possible differentiation between cystic and solid masses (Jellins et al., 1977; Kobayashi, 1977; Harper and Kelly-Fry, 1980; Fleischer et al., 1983; Dempsey and Wilson, 1984; Egan and Egan, 1984; and Rubin et al., 1985). In fact, Sickles and coworkers (Sickles, 1984a; and Sickles et al., 1984) have clearly shown that when the ultrasonographic criteria for a cyst have been scrupulously observed, the predictive value for cysts is equal to that of needle aspiration. This is of extreme importance in evaluating certain mammographic findings that may be nonpalpable.

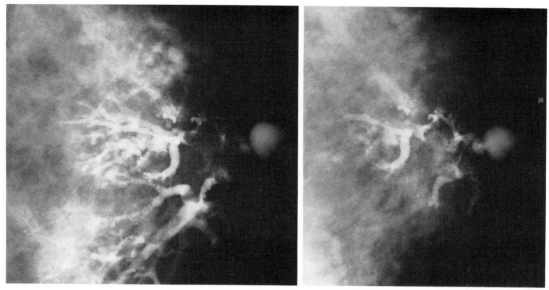

Figure 11–9. Ductogram. This is a large drop of contrast medium hanging from the nipple. About 1.5 cm deep to the nipple is a large filling defect. Pathologic examination proved this to be an intraductal papilloma. Note also the diffuse duct ectasia and an incidental stricture of a side duct just distal to the papilloma, about halfway between it and the nipple.

On the other hand, in the presence of an easily palpable mass, the diagnosis of cyst can be quickly established by needle aspiration. If the cyst is benign, this procedure has the added advantage of often being curative. In older women, however, intracystic papillary neoplasms are not uncommon, and ultrasonography, or pneumocytography at the time of aspiration, should be strongly considered. In patients with cysts that tend to recur, pneumocystography not only is useful for diagnosis but has also been reported to prevent benign cysts from refilling (Tabar et al., 1981b).

Although it was initially thought that ultrasonography could ultimately substitute for screening mammography, the technique currently possesses neither the threshold sensitivity nor the specificity to make it a viable screening option. Stated another way, minimal cancer cannot yet be detected with sufficient frequency to justify its use for screening asymptomatic women (Sickles et al., 1983; Dempsey and Moskowitz, 1987; Egan and Egan, 1984; Kopans et al., 1984a, 1985a; Sickles, 1984a; and Sickles et al., 1984).

Wagai (1983) used ultrasonography as part of a screening program in the Tokyo Prefecture from 1975 to 1981. It is worth critiqueing this study in some detail as it repeats some classic errors of study design. Primary screening was performed with physical examination, and mammography and ultrasonography were reserved for evaluation of suspicious areas. Thus, the most sensitive detection tool (mammography) was relegated to diagnostic status, and ultrasonography was used for its diagnostic capabilities. In this study, 30,000 women were screened, and only 20 cancers were found. As expected, all 20 cancers were detected by ultrasonography and clinical examination. The stage distribution of cancers found was as follows: T0 = 0, T1 = 20% and T2+ = 80%. Considering that in the BCDDPs, the Swedish trial, and the Dutch study, only 20% to 30% of cases were Stage II, and 30% to 40% were less than 5

mm in size, this distribution, reported by Wagai, represents a major step backward.

Kopans and associates (1985a) reported the results of a prospective study involving xeromammography, whole-breast waterpath ultrasonography, and clinical examination. The images were interpreted independently, and the population was a referred one. There were 125 cancers, of which 91% were detected by clinical examination and 94% by mammography. Eight clinical lesions were missed by mammography, and 12 mammographic lesions were missed by clinical examination. Ultrasonography detected 64% of the cancers, and all of these were palpable. To determine if cancers were present in the group of "false" positives noted by ultrasonography but possibly missed by the other methods, long-term follow-up (4 years) was carried out. No case of cancer has yet occurred in 255 women who had lesions identified as suspicious by ultrasonography.

Therefore, in general, ultrasonography should not be used as a primary breast imaging tool but should probably be reserved to answer specific clinical questions or problems (Harper and Kelly-Fry, 1980; Fleischer et al., 1983; Harper et al., 1983; and Kopans et al., 1984a, 1984b). In this way, it can be clinically useful and reasonably cost-effective.

For example, in the presence of a palpable abnormality not clearly diagnosable on x-ray mammography, ultrasonography may be particularly helpful (Harper and Kelly-Fry, 1980; and Fleischer et al., 1983) (Fig. 11–10). In 186 malignancies demonstrated on sonography (Dempsey and Moskowitz, 1987), 14 were not noted on mammography.

The author found that when a small, nonpalpable malignancy is seen only on one mammographic projection, an ultrasonographic examination may be a useful adjunct for three-dimensional spatial localization (Fig. 11–11).

Although most carcinomas are hypoechoic and some may cause acoustic shadowing (Kobayshi, 1977, 1979; Har-

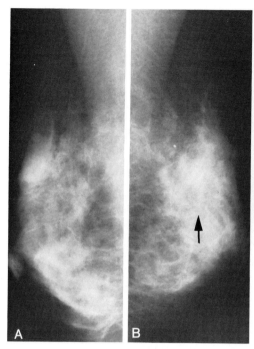

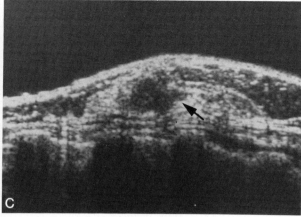

Figure 11–10. *A and B,* A dense breast pattern with a mass superior to the nipple is seen on the left side *(arrow).* Owing to the surrounding density, a firm diagnosis cannot be made, but the findings favor benignity. *C,* Ultrasonography of the mass clearly reveals malignant characteristics *(arrow).*

per and Kelly-Fry, 1980; and Harper et al., 1983), about 2% mimic a cyst. Close inspection may reveal some wall irregularity. Increasing the gain usually demonstrates some increase in irregular central echoes, indicating its solid nature.

Fibroadenomas may present as ovoid, solid masses with well-circumscribed borders, regular internal echoes, and, perhaps, some increased through-transmission. Such a sonographic abnormality in a woman aged 14 to 25 years has a very high probability of being a fibroadenoma (Harper et al., 1983). Cystosarcoma phylloides, benign or malignant, may have an identical sonographic picture. With the patient's increasing age, given these sonographic criteria, cancer cannot be excluded.

Twenty-five per cent of 130 cancers reported by Kopans and associates (1982, 1985a) were solid and sharply defined (i.e., benign), solid masses by ultrasonographic criteria, and 12% of cancers had retrotumoral enhancement rather than shadowing. Kasumi and coworkers (1982) report that about 20% of 743 cancers they examined were circumscribed lesions. In the author's experience, malignant lesions with these characteristics are often medullary carcinomas, occasionally lymphomas, and less frequently invasive necrotic ductal carcinomas.

As in other areas of the body, masses with mixed cystic and solid features could be the result of abscess, cyst with hemorrhagic debris, resolving hematoma, necrotic ductal cancer, medullary cancer, or lymphoma.

Decreased through-transmission (shadowing) seems to be related to fibrosis (Kobayashi, 1979; and Harper et al., 1983) or dense calcifications (Fig. 11–12). Shadowing in the breast can be seen in the absence of malignancy or frank mass and may result from beam attenuation owing to intramammary fibrosis, fat necrosis, or normal breast structure. The nipple-areola complex regularly produces shadowing.

A problem with breast sonographic imaging that is not

to be taken lightly is the fact that fat lobules may present as hypoechoic demarcated lesions and lead to FP diagnoses. Although with experience this problem tends to diminish (Fig. 11–13), it does not completely disappear.

In patients with the clinical features of diffuse nodularity, mammography may show a dense breast with multiple nodular shadows or, surprisingly, a fatty, "clear" breast. On the other hand, it has been somewhat surprising to the author to find that sonography of the mammographically dense, nodular breast in some women demonstrates that many "nodules" are not cysts but cannot be differentiated from normal glandular tissue. In other women, multiple cysts of varying size may be seen. Routine whole-breast, or large-segment, ultrasonographic evaluation of these women in the author's experience has produced many solid or shadowing foci, resulting in a high FP rate and a very low TP yield. If there is an area of clinical suspicion in such breasts, restricting the examination to that area may prove diagnostically rewarding. Therefore, the author currently does not recommend routine whole-breast or large-segment breast ultrasonography for dense or nodular breasts in the absence of a local area of clinical or mammographic suspicion.

In women with breast prostheses, the prone whole-breast scanners may offer some help in evaluation of the "rind" of residual breast tissue (Cole-Beauglet et al., 1983), but the specificity, sensitivity, and PPV relative to tumor size still remain to be established.

In Egan and coworkers' study (Egan et al., 1984), ultrasonography alone identified 15 of 31 (48%) of cancers, and mammography identified 24 (77%). When positive for cancer, however, the PPV of ultrasonography was 83%. Generally, it is the smallest lesions that can be detected by mammography that are missed by ultrasonography.

It is abundantly clear that ultrasonography can distinguish cysts from solid lesions, and in many cases it has performed as well as mammography in symptomatic

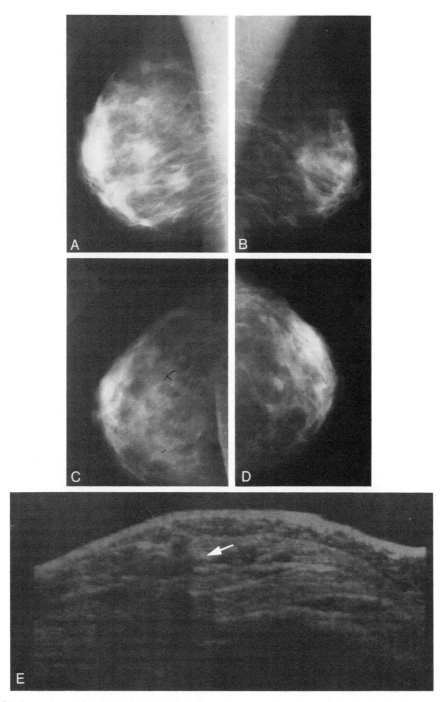

Figure 11-11. *A–D,* Obvious cancer is present in the upper aspect of the left breast in the mediolateral oblique view *(upper left)* but is not seen in the craniocaudal view *(lower left). E,* Transverse ultrasonography shows the location to be slightly medial *(arrow).*

women with local findings (Texidor and Kazam, 1977; Kasumi et al., 1982; and Harper et al., 1983); however, it is not a screening tool. Perhaps improvements in technology will change its status in the future.

Diaphanography

In years gone by, when a physician desired to distinguish between a solid or cystic mass, he or she might have retired into a dark closet with the patient and a flashlight. After an appropriate period of dark adaptation, the flashlight was lit and applied to the suspect area. Some cysts would transilluminate, and solid lesions often would not, depending on size and proximity to the skin. The total cost of equipment involved was about 50¢. Today, the light-tight closet is larger, a technologist often performs the examination, and the equipment consists of a light source, a television (TV) receptor, a computer, and color TV display. In addition, the

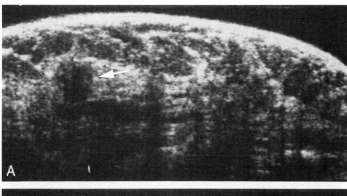

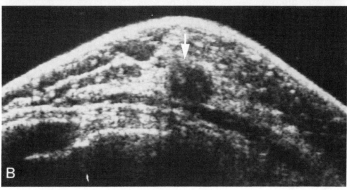

Figure 11-12. Note the irregular, hypoechoic mass without shadowing *(arrows)*. The patient was a 31-year-old pregnant woman with a palpable mass. The histologic diagnosis was medullary carcinoma.

procedure has acquired a new name. Instead of transillumination, it has acquired the title *diaphanography.* The cost of the equipment alone is many thousands of dollars. It must be asked if this marvelous technologic wonder contributes more information than a good flashlight and an attentive doctor.

Diaphanography is thought to depend in great part on the proclivity of some tissues to differentially absorb energy in the visible and near-infrared portions of the electromagnetic spectrum. The TV recording device usually is sensitive to the shorter, near-infrared range. In at least one popular instrument, the light source output varies rapidly between

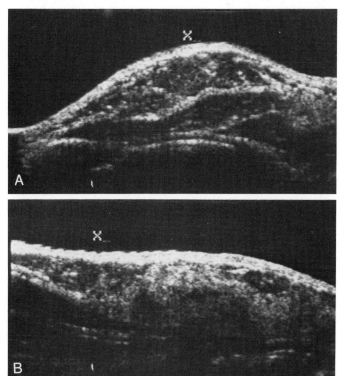

Figure 11-13. This patient is a young woman with a palpable lump. Mammograms were not obtained. Ultrasonographic examination was interpreted as lipoma. Pathologic diagnosis was "fatty tissue consistent with lipoma." The x's are located over the palpable mass.

visible red and near-infrared. The intensity of the source can be varied. The relative absorption of these two spectra is digitized, expressed as a ratio of absorption, and a color display corresponding to the absorption ratios is demonstrated on a TV screen.

As of this writing, active research programs are under way to determine rationales for differential absorption (Key et al., 1991*a*; Key et al., 1991*b*; Jarlman et al., 1992*a*; Jarlman et al., 1992*b*; Jarlman et al., 1992*c*; Seltzer et al., 1992; Orel et al., 1993; and de Haller et al., 1993). It is clear that hemoglobin can absorb strongly in the near-infrared range, but it is unclear if this is the sole cause of the image or abnormalities that may be seen.

The role of diaphanography has not yet been clearly elucidated. It still is in a state of Phase I clinical experimental evaluation. Wallberg (1984) reported the results of a retrospective review of 116 patients with breast cancer and 167 patients with benign disease. Eighty-four per cent of the cancer patients were examined because of the presence of a palpable mass, axillary node involvement, or retraction of the skin or nipple. Wallberg reports that mammography sensitivity was 88%, that of diaphanography was 85%, and together a TP rate of 95% was achieved. In nine patients in whom calcifications were the sole sign of suspicion, diaphanography was positive in seven. A disturbing note, however, is that in 12% of patients with benign disease who had mammographically suspicious calcifications, biopsy was not done because the results on diaphanography were negative. Given mammography's proven track record, this seems a rather bold move and may alter the sensitivity significantly after a longer period of observation.

Muirhead and Seright (1984) missed only 2 of 11 cancers with diaphanography, one being a 5-mm lesion detected by mammography. Sickles (1984*a*) reported a stepwise increase in detection with increasing lesion size. Twenty per cent of cancers less than 1 cm were detected, and 76% of cancers 2 cm and larger were found.

Marshall and colleagues (1984) reported results in a population of 1000 women in whom 33 cancers were present. (The prevalence indicates quite clearly that the population is heavily skewed in favor of symptomatic women.) There was one in situ cancer in this group that went undetected, but 79% of the invasive lesions were found. The sensitivity achieved by Marshall and colleagues was essentially the same for mammography as for diaphanography.

Geslien and coworkers (1985) in a nonblinded, Phase I study, found that 6 of 11 nonpalpable cases were detected by light scanning. Only 3 of 10 tumors less than 1 cm in size were found by this technique, however. These investigators did find one case that presented only as mammographic microcalcifications. The larger the tumor, the more likely it was to be found. These authors were unable to determine a definitive adjunctive role for light scanning at this time, and they also did not note a role for screening.

Angquist and coworkers (1981) and Thomas (1981) report sensitivities of 38% and 20%, respectively, whereas Bartrum and Crow (1984) and Merritt and colleagues (Merritt et al., 1984; and Merritt and Dempsey, 1985) report sensitivity on the order of 75%.

Drexler and colleagues (1985) in a prospective, nonblinded study found that diaphanography detected only 58% of the 26 cancers present in their series, did not pick up the two noninvasive ductal cancers, did identify two of three 5-mm cancers, and missed eight cancers less than 2 cm in size. From testing a physical model that they developed, they determined that diaphanography detection is a function of both size of lesion and its depth in the breast. They also pointed out that the FP rate was three times higher than that of mammography.

To date, these data can not justify the use of diaphanography as a primary screening device. It is unclear to this observer that the data, overall, indicate that it is a useful diagnostic device. The Phase I studies cited suggest some potential advantages, several major pitfalls, and areas in which technical development may be needed.

In the author's opinion, this technique has not matured sufficiently to deserve widespread, general use in a nonexperimental setting. Certainly, in its current state of development, it should not be used to deter biopsy of suspicious areas identified by standard tests.

Thermography*

At this point, it is tempting to state that thermography has no proven role in breast cancer detection. However, so that the reader might better appreciate the problems associated with thermography and, perhaps more specifically, with the means by which the technique is evaluated, a detailed review is undertaken in this section.

As pointed out earlier, the HIP study demonstrated a decreased mortality rate for a population screened for breast cancer compared with nonscreened controls. In that study, about 40% of the cancers in the control population were Stage I or smaller, compared with 56% for those in the study group.

Today in the United States, in the absence of widespread screening, about 55% of cancers are Stage I or less. If mortality rates are to be decreased by screening, the stage of detection must be lowered below 55% Stage I. There is simply no evidence in the literature reviewed that thermography can contribute to lowering the stage at detection in any meaningful way. In fact, a body of data suggests that the converse is the case.

Wenth and Stein (1983) reviewed data presented by 26 investigators from the early 1960s into the mid-1970s; most were obtained prior to 1970. Their review showed that the combined data for 32,972 women (including 1998 women with breast cancer) yielded a sensitivity for thermography of 83.4%, a specificity of 85.9%, and a receiver operating characteristic detectability index of 2.04. From these data, the authors concluded that thermography is a viable screening tool for breast cancer that should be restored to its "rightful" place. On the basis of these very data, rediscovered by Wenth and Stein, thermography was introduced into the Breast Cancer Detection Demonstration Projects (BCDDPs).

The major problem with these data is that the studies that generated them failed to take into account the size and stage of tumors detected versus the size and stage of tumors that

---

*Much of this section is reproduced with permission from Moskowitz, M.: Journal of Reproductive Medicine, *30*:451, 1985.

would become detectable by current mass screening methods. A related and not necessarily separate problem is that many of the reported data were derived from symptomatic patients, and the results were extrapolated to the screening situation. This is simply not acceptable. Also, few if any of the studies were blinded, and, as a result, the independent value of a nonlocalizing screening test (particularly one which alone cannot generate a biopsy) is almost impossible to resolve.

That large tumors can be detected by thermography, clinical examination, breast self-examination, and simple inspection is not in question. That these methods can lower the stage of detection significantly is, indeed, in question. No statistical manipulation of data, despite its elegance and sophistication, can overcome the elementary failure of experimental design, beginning with the failure to ask the right question.

As indicated earlier, thermography was introduced into the BCDDPs' studies. Contrary to some reports (Haberman et al., 1980; and Nyirjesy, 1982), most of the investigators in the BCDDPs did undergo a period of training, and the equipment used was state-of-the-art for the time. The method was not considered a diagnostic tool but was used as a risk indicator requiring short-term (6 months) follow-up of all patients with positive results on thermography and negative results on testing with all other techniques. It soon became apparent that the FP rate was so high that short-term recall was not a viable, practical option. Worse yet was the fact that the sensitivity of thermography for the cancers being found in the BCDDPs was very low. Because of its low TP rate, thermography was dropped from the screening program.

Prior to this, a blinded, prospective study to evaluate the efficacy of thermography in detecting minimal and Stage I breast cancers was performed by Moskowitz and coworkers (1976a). It was found that these small cancers could not be identified by expert observers at any rate greater than that of chance alone. In fact, totally naive observers did as well as the experts. This observation caused a furor in the thermographic community, but only Threatt and colleagues (1980) repeated the study. Their investigation was not limited to minimal cancers, however. For in situ carcinomas, the same results were obtained. For all cancers, the overall detection rate could be pushed relatively little above the random chance line.

Haberman and coworkers (1979) reported on the development of a computer-based interpretation of thermograms that was obtained under highly controlled environmental conditions. Although advanced cancers were found at a rate greater than that of chance, this was not found to be the case for cancers less than 5 mm in size, intraductal cancers, or in situ lobular cancers. Perhaps thermographic monitoring to reflect circadian rhythm changes may be of help in the future to identify women at risk.

Reader Agreement

Even among expert thermographers, extreme interobserver disagreement exists in the interpretation of thermograms (Moskowitz et al., 1976a; Threatt et al., 1980; and Stern et al., 1982). In all three series just cited, it is quite apparent that agreement on what constitutes a thermogram with a positive result simply did not exist. In the study of Stern and coworkers, the readers had been especially trained and tested, and still agreement was elusive.

Gautherie (1982a) developed a computer-assisted interpretation schema that is said to eliminate this problem. Although computer-assisted interpretation should ensure greater consistency among observers, it is not obvious yet whether it will affect risk prediction, cancer detection, or other variables. This must await the results of blinded prospective trials.

Thermography as a Screening Tool

An earlier critical review of the thermographic literature (Moskowitz, 1982) indicated that thermography offered little benefit as a screening device, even in the hands of its advocates. At that time, the data suggested that thermography simply could not detect the smaller cancers. The data from Jones and colleagues (1975), for example, showed that thermography correctly identified 77% of *clinical* lesions. However, only 10% of 300 cancers in this study were undetectable clinically. Today, in mass screening centers, 40% to 60% of cancers are undetectable clinically.

In Feig and coworkers' study (1977), only 31% of cancers less than 1 cm in size were found by thermography, and 32% of those between 1 cm and 2 cm were found. Sixty-two per cent of cancers larger than 2 cm were identified correctly. The thermograms were interpreted by thermographers with a long history of experience and interest in clinical thermography.

Clark and associates (1978) had a TP rate of 84% for thermography, but only 5% of 170 cancers were in situ at the time of detection. This represents no increase in yield of small cancers over that for nonscreening.

Rodes and colleagues (1977) state that ''30 per cent of the early cancers found with mass screening will not be detected by infrared scanning, and the bulk of false negatives occur in those patients most amenable to therapy.'' Significantly, this indictment of thermography as a screening device comes from proponents—not opponents—of the art.

The data obtained by Stark and coworkers (Stark and Way, 1974; and Stark, 1976) suggest that reliance on thermography may be responsible for a significant delay in detection of cancers that could be found earlier by a different approach to screening (Moskowitz, 1982). Revesz (1978), in a model suggesting strategies for screening, simply failed to take into account stage at detection.

Haberman and colleagues (1980) published results of a large-scale screening effort. They examined 31,322 screenees, who received a total of 47,155 examinations. Ten per cent of these women were under the age of 40 years, and 14% were at high risk. Mammography was not part of the screening examination. Seventy-one cancers were found: 56 were screen-detected; 10 within 12 months of a negative result on screening; and 5 more than 12 months later. The prevalence rate, therefore, was 2.1 per 1000 (66 in 31,322).

This prevalence rate for this age population is, quite simply, low (vide infra).

Prevalence rates should reflect cancers that would normally "surface" during the initial year, some slowly growing cancers that might never surface, and some "dip" into future incidence, depending on the threshold sensitivity of the screen. For this age population, it may be estimated that detectable breast cancer prevalence should be about three to four times the annual incidence. Prevalence of morphologically recognizable, but not detectable, cancers seems to be about 20 to 22 per 1000 (Moskowitz et al., 1976*b;* and Pollei et al., 1987). Indeed, the population-based trials in Sweden and Holland are yielding prevalence rates of 6 to 7 per 1000 (Moskowitz, 1983*a*). The BCDDPs, a nonrandomized nonpopulation-based screen, also yielded rates of this order (Baker, 1982). Although the HIP screen (Shapiro et al., 1973) in the 1960s found a prevalence rate of 2.73 per 1000, it is probable that the lead time gained was only 6 months to 9 months over the nonscreened population, in contrast with an estimated 2.0 to 3.5 years (depending on age) gained today. Remember that even though the HIP study gained 6 to 9 months of lead time, about 5.5 years were added to the life of each woman with breast cancer on average.

It is difficult to determine stage distribution of the detected cancers from the data provided by Haberman and colleagues (1980), but approximately 60% of the patients were free of axillary lymph node involvement. Although the 56% Stage I disease in the HIP screen represented an improvement over the 40% Stage I found in their control group, neither the HIP 56% nor the 60% Stage I found by Haberman and colleagues represents a clinically significant improvement over the 55% Stage I distribution found in nonscreened populations in the United States (Moskowitz et al., 1975; Third National Cancer Survey, 1975; and Axtell et al., 1976). Furthermore, on the basis of the BCDDPs' data (Baker, 1982) and data presented by Andersson and colleagues (1979), Tabar and Gad (1981*a*), and Rombach (1980), an adequate screen can find up to 40% of the cases while still less than 5 mm in size or wholly in situ, and up to 80% of cancers while they are Stage I or less.

These data would suggest that Haberman and colleagues' reported screen was not sensitive to the detection of small tumors and, in fact, was not doing any more than could be achieved by physical examination alone.

Rosselli del Turco and coworkers (1983) stated that their own results "confirm that thermography cannot play a primary role in breast cancer diagnosis, because of its high proportion of false negatives and false positives; its sensitivity is significantly affected by the tumor size and its specificity by age."

Siu and colleagues (1982) examined 300 women aged 19 to 79 years referred for evaluation of symptoms of breast disease; 22 cases of cancer were found. Clinical examination *guided by thermography* had a reported sensitivity of 71% and a specificity of 98%. A statistical equation for "screening" was then derived from the information generated by these patients. Data derived from a high-risk, symptomatic population in which relatively large cancers exist in profusion simply cannot be extrapolated to a low-risk, large population of asymptomatic women in whom just the opposite is the case.

Gohagan and coworkers (1980) reported that in their BCDDPs' study, 16.5% of the cancers they detected were less than 5 mm in size, and 27.8% were 5 mm to 1 cm in size; 44% were less than 1 cm in diameter. Of all cases in which lymph nodes were *not* involved, 42% were detected by thermography. When lymph nodes were positive for cancer, thermography correctly identified 41.7% of the cases. The FP rates for thermography were estimated to range from 6% to 21%.

Nyirjesy (1982) states, "We are aware of the fact that minimal or subclinical carcinomas can only be detected by mammograms and that thermograms are normal in many of these early tumors." Despite the statement, he believes that in his hands thermography is an important tool and goes on to buttress his argument with the following data:

1. 6459 thermograms were obtained in 2799 patients.
2. In this population were found 34 cancers, 8 of which were less than 1 cm in size and 10 of which were between 1 cm and 2 cm in size.
3. The 6459 thermograms were read as:
    a. Th1 or Th2 (normal) = 63.5%
    b. Th3 (atypical or doubtful) = 21.5%
    c. Th4, Th5 (abnormal) = 15%
4. TP rate = 79%. (It is not stated what fraction of the small cancers were detected.)

From these data, if it is assumed that all of the detected cancers occurred only in the Th4 and Th5 groups, the PPV of thermography would be 2.7%. If, as seems more likely, some cancers occurred in the Th3 group, the PPV for cancer would be 1.1%. From these data, it is not clear to this observer how thermography was helpful.

Graphic stress thermography (GST) has been proposed as an effective modification of thermography that is applicable to screening. Snyder and colleagues (1979) have shown in a group of patients already scheduled for biopsy at Memorial Hospital (New York, NY) that GST had a sensitivity for cancer of approximately 90%. In that same series, about 89% of the patients with benign lesions were also considered positive for cancer.

Brooks and coworkers (1983) reported on 1030 patients who received 2012 thermographic studies using computerized evaluation after stress (GST). Of these, 289 patients were selected for mammography; from this group were distilled 61 patients for surgical consultation, and 31 of these were selected for biopsy. It is unclear from the report how the initial selection was made and even less clear how subsequent dichotomies were determined. In this group, six cancers were detected, five of which were detected by GST. The average size of the lesions was 1.1 cm. Sufficient information was not presented to allow determination of the actual PPV. It can only be estimated from the presented data. Assuming that all five detected cancers occurred in those patients with only a Class 3 examination, the PPV of a positive test result would be 1.3%. Assuming that some cancers occurred in Class 2 as well as Class 3 GST scores, the PPV of a positive test result would equal 0.3%.

Gautherie and colleagues (Gautherie and Gros, 1980; Gautherie, 1982*a,b*, 1983; Gautherie et al., 1982, 1983; and personal communication) have presented extensive clinical and laboratory data to support all of the various claimed uses of thermography.

It would appear that neoplasms of some bulk and relatively advanced state can produce sufficient heat under laboratory conditions that it can be measured and quantified. It is unclear, however, that in situ and 5-mm carcinomas can produce sufficient heat to be detected clinically at a significant rate. As fat is a very efficient thermal insulator, and since minimal amounts of heat at a depth would not reach the surface unless "piped" there by blood vessels, frequent detection of these lesions seems unlikely. It is tempting to postulate that capillary angiogenesis factor or elaboration of local tumoral effects induces sufficient blood flow when the cancers are tiny to allow measurable surface shunting to occur, but this is only speculation at this point.

However, at a meeting in Liege, Gautherie and coworkers (1985) presented preliminary data that suggest, for the first time, that thermography might be able to detect minimal cancers. They attribute this to improvements in thermographic technology and to the development of specific and objective interpretation criteria. As they point out, however (1985), the small amount of heat produced by a minimal cancer "would exclude all possibility of detecting the tumor, whatever its depth may be." Gautherie and coworkers believe rather that the thermal abnormalities at the surface reflect local vascular changes accompanying the development of early cancer. The bulk of Gautherie and colleagues' reported work would suggest that such is not the case (Gautherie et al., 1982). For example, of 637 cancers occurring in a referral symptomatic population (1970–1980), only 13% were in situ or nonpalpable, or both. Only 27% were less than 2 cm in size, including the 13% already noted.

In Cincinnati, a study of the tumor registry since 1950 (Moskowitz et al., 1975) revealed that 55% of the cases detected were Stage I or less. This rate is significantly greater than the 27% reported by Gautherie and colleagues.

In a group of 106 cancer patients selected from a screening population by thermography, 69.5% of the clinically palpable cancers were Stage II at detection, and by histologic criteria, 97.5% were Stage II or higher. Of the total 106 cancers, only 27% were Stage I or less, including 13.2% minimal breast cancer (as defined by Gautherie) and 4% in situ disease. In the author's screened population, approximately 20% of cases are Stage II or higher; 80% are Stage I or less, including 50% less than 1 cm; 40% are less than 5 mm; and 20% are noninvasive. The author's figures generally are reflected in the BCDDPs as a whole (Baker, 1982). Thus, in the hands of Gautherie and coworkers there was no difference in stage at detection whether patients were referred for evaluation of a mass or were screened. Needless to say, at this junction of knowledge, this is not the goal of a screening process.

Overall, the data strongly suggest that small, deep-seated cancers do not emit sufficient thermal signals to be detected at the surface of the breast. Larger cancers, which are more peripherally located and usually palpable, may be detected.

Thermography as Risk Indicator

It has been postulated that thermography is a risk indicator for subsequent development of breast cancer (Gautherie and

Gros, 1980; Almaric et al., 1983; and Hobbins, 1983). It is probably most difficult to design an adequate, nonbiased, prospective trial to measure this parameter among all the aspects discussed. Unless the study is performed in a blinded fashion on an asymptomatic population with adequate controls, a sufficient number of screenees, and long-term follow-up, and unless it is associated with an independent, highly sensitive screening process, a self-fulfilling tautology will ensue; each observation will feed and flow into the other.

Moskowitz and colleagues (1981) performed a blinded prospective study comparing liquid crystal thermography to generally accepted histopathologic parameters of high risk prediction. An international expert in thermography taught the technical performance, critiqued and rejected technical failures, and interpreted the study images without knowledge of the clinical, historical, or mammographic information. Cases with high-risk histopathologic findings were not detected at a rate greater than that of chance alone.

Gautherie and Gros (1980) reported on 740 patients who met their criteria for isolated, suspicious thermographic findings. Within 10 years, approximately 40% of these patients developed a breast cancer. Compared with women with thermographically negative results, in the study, this represents a 10-fold increase in risk. However, most of the subsequently detected carcinomas that occurred within the group with suspected lesions occurred within *18 months* of a previous clinical and mammographic examination with negative results. Rather than thermography representing an excess risk indicator, perhaps in light of the data reviewed earlier concerning size and threshold of Gautherie and coworkers' primary detecting method, an alternative explanation might prevail:

1. On the basis of the data of Gautherie and colleagues, the threshold sensitivity of the clinical and mammographic evaluation at their institution is between Stage I and Stage II or higher (predominantly Stage II).
2. There are undoubtedly cancers that are Stage I or borderline Stage II that are currently not being detected by the relatively insensitive physical examination and mammography performed at Gautherie's center. (Such a high threshold level of detection for their clinical and mammographic tests suggests that early detection is being sacrificed for a high PPV.)
3. The missed lesions subsequently reach the unusually high threshold of detectability achieved by their clinicians and radiologists in 12 to 18 months.
4. By this time, the lesions are mostly Stage II or higher.
5. As a result of being found at an advanced state, the cancers generally have a poor prognosis.

Gautherie and coworkers (1982) published an interesting descriptive chapter of their methodology. To a major degree, this can explain some of the apparent discrepancies in their data (Gautherie and Gros, 1980; and Gautherie, 1982b, 1983) and in those generated by other prospective studies (Moskowitz et al., 1976a; Threatt et al., 1980; Moskowitz et al., 1981; Baker, 1982; Stern et al., 1982; and Moskowitz, 1983b). First, their case material is derived from evaluation of symptomatic, referred patients. For reasons discussed earlier, extrapolation of these data to an asymptomatic, self-selected population is, to say the least, dangerous. The thermograms were analyzed by a preliminary "blind" reading. This preliminary blind study was then followed by "a careful comparison of the distinct thermal signs with regard to the physical findings in order to eliminate those signs that become less significant than would have appeared to be the case if the thermograms were considered by themselves" (Gautherie et al., 1982). Already a potentially major bias has been introduced.

As noted earlier, 73% of the 637 cancers found in this population were clinical Stage II or higher. Of the tumors that were staged as "smaller" tumors, 43 were in situ, 38 ranged in size from 1.5 to 4 cm, and 92 were between 1 and 2 cm and were palpable. Therefore, only 43 (7%) could be considered minimal by either of the generally accepted criteria for minimal cancer that are currently in use. The remainder represent, by today's standards, large cancers.

Gautherie and coworkers state that it is acceptable to miss 24% of cancers smaller than 2 cm because some of the missed tumors were as small as 4 mm and probably had a slow growth rate. Perhaps that is so. It appears, however, that far more than 24% of cancers less than 2 cm in size were missed.

That 28% of 130 cancers larger than 1.5 cm in size were nonpalpable in their series is a remarkable observation. Given this perspective, it is easy to understand why 87% of these nonpalpable cases were thermographically positive. Sixty per cent of the few in situ carcinomas that they found were also regarded as positive. Given the low detection rate of these cancers by Gautherie and coworkers, it is safe to assume that for the most part they were reasonably large, probably multifocal, comedo carcinomas, many of which were probably palpable. In fact, in a blinded prospective study, Moskowitz and colleagues (1981) found some evidence to support this speculation.

Given the data by Threatt and coworkers (1980), Moskowitz and colleagues (1976a), Nyirjesy (1982), Feig and colleagues (1977), Haberman and coworkers (1980), Jones and colleagues (1975), Clark and associates (1978), and Stern and coworkers (1982) that expert thermographers do not find minimal breast cancers, and given the fact that most of the cancers in the series reported by Gautherie and colleagues developed within 18 months of an otherwise negative screen, it is far more likely that the apparent risk prediction of thermography is more an artifact of procedure than it is an indicator of risk.

In the author's hands, thermography does not appear to be a significant predictor of subsequent breast cancer risk. Although this alone does not indict thermography, the fact that so many authors cannot replicate the data found by Gautherie and associates or by Amalric and coworkers would indicate at least that this method is not ready for general use. From the data reviewed, the value of thermography in evaluation of the human breast has not been proved.

Thermography is an experimental tool for breast evaluation. Gautherie and coworkers' approach to standardizing interpretation represents at least a positive step. Circadian changes in breast heat in relation to breast conditions seem to be a promising area of research. Perhaps prospective trials adequately designed, asking appropriate questions,

and based on an adequately screened population can determine in an objective way, once and for all, what thermography can or cannot contribute to the diagnosis of diseases of the human breast.

Other Breast Imaging Modalities

Magnetic resonance imaging is still new on the scene. It appears to be quite specific for cysts, may be able to detect cancer in fatty breast, is limited in detection of cancer in dense breasts, and is not yet able to find cancer detected only by microcalcifications on mammography (Egan and Mosteller, 1977; Mansfield et al., 1980; Alcorn et al., 1985; and Wolfman et al., 1985). It may be helpful in planning surgery and in following patients (Heywang-Kobrunner, 1993; and Merchant, 1993). Magnetic imaging spectroscopy "is one of the most exciting new techniques under development . . . experimental work suggests possible future roles for P31 magnetic imaging spectroscopy as a tool for early detection and for prediction of response to treatment" (Gohagan and Shterm, 1992). At this time, however, it is still an immature technology. With the development of newer approaches and newer technology, and perhaps less emphasis on imaging and more on biology, magnetic resonance imaging can prove useful in clarifying the natural history of precancerous lesions and cancer (El Yousef et al., 1984, 1985; McSweeney et al., 1984a; and Orel and Troupin, 1993).

Computed tomography of the breast seems to require intravenous contrast media (Chang et al, 1980; and Kopans et al., 1984a). This requirement, the method's cost, and small number of patients examinable per hour sorely limit the use of computed tomography as a screening tool. In certain highly selected cases, it may prove useful as a diagnostic test or, occasionally, to localize in three-dimensional space a lesion that can be seen only on one mammographic view.

Digital mammography is on the horizon (McSweeney et al., 1984b; and Kopans, personal communication). Early work (Ackerman et al., 1985; and Watt et al., 1985) suggests that it may have an adjunctive diagnostic role when used with contrast media. It has the added potential advantages of (1) image enhancement; (2) expert system development; (3) perhaps automated prescreening; and (4) extremely low dose. Owing to its high initial costs, digital mammography "must be proven to offer substantial advantages over conventional systems in terms of improved detection [and diagnosis]* as well as in imaging archiving and technology (Gohagan et al., 1992)." Its ultimate role at this time is still conjectural.

SUMMARY

Breast imaging seems finally to have come of age. If it is used appropriately, fewer and fewer deaths from breast cancer should occur. Less bickering among the professionals (Baum, 1985; and Skrabanek, 1985) and a greater co-

---

*Added by the author.

operative effort are needed if the full benefit of the scientific advances in this area are to be realized.

References

Ackerman, L. V., Watt, A. C., Shetty, P., et al.: Breast lesions examined by digital angiography. Work in progress. Radiology, *155*:65, 1985.

Alberti, G. P., and Troiso, A.: Secreting breast: The role of galactography. Eur. J. Gynaecol. Oncol, *3*:96, 1982.

Alcorn, F. S., Turner, D. A., Clark, J. W., et al.: Magnetic resonance imaging in the study of the breast. Radiographics, *5*:631, 1985.

Almaric, C., Geraud, D., Thomassin, L., et al.: The persistently abnormal isolated infrared thermogram: The highest known risk for breast cancer. Acta Thermograph., *7*:91, 1983.

Anastassiades, O. T., Bouropoulou, V., Kontogeorgos, G., et al.: Microcalcifications in benign breast disease. A histological and histochemical study. Pathol. Res. Pract., *178*:237, 1984.

Andersson, I.: Mammographic screening for breast carcinoma: A cross sectional, randomized study of 45–69 year old women. University of Lund, Malmö General Hospital, S-214 01 Malmö, Sweden, 1980.

Andersson, I., Andren, L., Hildell, J., et al.: Breast cancer screening with mammography: A population based, randomized trial with mammography as the only screening mode. Radiology, *132*:273, 1979.

Angquist, K. A., Holmlund, D., and Liliequist, B.: Diaphanoscopy and diaphanography for breast cancer detection in clinical practice. Acta Chir. Scand., *147*:231, 1981.

Ashikari, R., Huvos, A. G., Snyder, R. E., et al.: A clinico-pathologic study of atypical lesions of the breast. Cancer, *33*:310, 1974.

Axtell, L., Asire, A., and Myers, M. (Eds.): Cancer patient survival. Report No. 5. Washington, D. C., U. S. Department of Health, Education and Welfare, Publ. No. (NIH) 77–992, 1976.

Baker, L. H.: Breast Cancer Detection Demonstration Project: Five year summary report. CA Cancer J. Clin., *42*:194, 1982.

Baines, C., McFarlane, D. V., and Miller, A. B.: The role of the reference radiologist: Estimates of interobserver agreement and potential delay in cancer detection in the National Breast Screening Study. Invest. Radiol., *25*:971–976, 1990*b*.

Baines, C. J., Miller, A. B., Kopans, D. B., et al.: Canadian National Breast Screening Study: Assessment of technical quality external review. Am. J. Roentgenol., *155*:743–747, 1990*a*.

Baral, E., Larsson, L. E., and Mattson, B.: Breast cancer following irradiation of the breast. Cancer, *40*:2905, 1977.

Bartrum, R. J., and Crow, H. C.: Transillumination light scanning to diagnose breast cancer: A feasibility study. Am. J. Roentgenol., *142*:409, 1984.

Baum, M.: Breast cancer controversies (letter to the editor). Lancet *ii*:564, 1985.

Black, M. M., Barclay, T. H. C., Cutler, S. J., et al.: Association of atypical characteristics of benign breast lesions with subsequent risk of breast cancer. Cancer *29*:338, 1972.

Blommers, T. J.: Transplant and dialysis: The cost/benefit question. Iowa Med., *74*:15, 1984.

Boice, J., Harvey, E. B., Blettner, M., et al.: Cancer in the contralateral breast after radiotherapy for breast cancer. N. Engl. J. Med., *326*:781–785, 1992.

Boisselier, P., Durand, J. C., Veith, F., et al.: Prognosis of breast epithelioma detected by microcalcifications in the absence of a palpable tumor. Presse Med., *12*:1411, 1983.

Boon, M. E., and deGraaf Guilloud, J. C.: Cost effectiveness of population screening and rescreening for cervical cancer in the Netherlands. Acta Cytol., *25*:539, 1981.

Boyd, N. F., O'Sullivan, B., Fishell, E., et al.: Mammographic patterns and breast cancer risk: Methodologic standards and contradictory results. J. Natl. Cancer Inst., *72*:1253, 1984.

Brisson, J., Morrison, A. S., Kopans, D. B., et al.: Height and weight, mammographic features of breast tissue, and breast cancer risk. Am. J. Epidemiol., *119*:371, 1984.

Broberg, A., Glas, U., Gustafsson, S. A., et al.: Relationship between mammographic pattern and estrogen receptor content in breast cancer. Breast Cancer Res. Treat., *3*:201, 1983.

Brooks, P. G., Gart, S., Heldfond, A. J., et al.: Breast screening in the

primary care office: A plea for early detection. J. Reprod. Med., *27*:685, 1983.

Campbell, I. D., Royle, G. T., Coddington, R., et al.: Technique and results of localization biopsy in a breast screening programme. Br. J. Surg., *78*:1113–1115, 1991.

Carlile, T., Kopecky, K. J., Thompson, D. J., et al.: Breast cancer prediction and the Wolfe classification of mammograms. J.A.M.A., *254*:1050, 1985.

Chang, C. H. J., Sibala, J. L., Fritz, S. L., et al.: Computed tomography in detection and diagnosis of breast cancer. Cancer, *46*:939, 1980.

Chaudary, M. A., Gravelle, I. H., Bulstrode, J. C., et al.: Breast parenchymal patterns in women with bilateral primary breast cancer. Br. J. Radiol., *56*:703, 1983.

Chu, K. C., and Connor, R. J.: Analysis of the temporal pattern of benefits in the Health Insurance Plan of Greater New York Trial by stage and age. Am. J. Epidemiol., *133*:1039–1049, 1991.

Clark, R. M., Rideout, D. F., and Chart, P. L.: Thermography of the breast: Experiences in diagnosis and follow up in a cancer treatment centre. Acta Thermograph., *3*:155, 1978.

Cole-Beauglet, C., Schwartz, G., Kurtz, A. B., et al.: Ultrasound mammography for the augmented breast. Radiology, *146*:737, 1983.

Committee on the Biological Effect of Ionizing Radiation: The effects on populations of exposure to low levels of ionizing radiation. Washington, D. C., National Academy of Sciences, National Research Council, 1980.

Coopmans de Yoldi, G. F., Andreoli, C., Costa, A., et al.: Lack of efficacy of xeroradiography to preoperatively detect axillary lymph node metastases in breast cancer. Breast Cancer Res. Treat. *3*:373, 1983.

Council on Scientific Affairs: Early detection of breast cancer. J.A.M.A., *252*:3008, 1984.

Danes, J.: Wolfe's risk groups and the incidence of breast carcinoma. Sb. Lek., *85*:24, 1983.

Dempsey, P. J., and Moskowitz, M.: Is there a role for breast sonography? *In* McGraham, J. P. (Ed.): Clinics in Diagnostic Ultrasound, Vol. 20. New York, Churchill Livingstone, 1987, pp. 17–36.

Dempsey, P. J., and Wilson, P. C.: The use of automated sonography in total clinical breast evaluation. Clin Diagn. Ultrasound, *12*:57, 1984.

de Haller, E. B., and Depeursinge, C.: Simulation of time-resolved breast transillumination. Med. Biol. Eng. Comput., *31*:165–170, 1993.

deWaard, F., Collette, H. J. A., Rombach, J. J., et al.: The DOM Project for the early detection of breast cancer, Utrecht, The Netherlands. J. Chron. Dis., *37*:1, 1984.

Devitt, J. E.: Mammography: A surgeon's experience. Can. Med. Assoc. J., *120*:1370, 1979.

DiPietro, S., Coopmans de Yoldi, G., Bergonzi, S., et al.: Nipple discharge as a sign of preneoplastic lesions and occult carcinoma of the breast: Clinical and galactographic study in 103 consecutive patients. Tumori, *65*:317, 1979.

Dodd, G. D.: Mammography. State of the art. Cancer, *53*(Suppl. 3):652, 1984.

Dowlatshahi, K., Yaremko, M. L., Kluskens, L. F., et al.: Nonpalpable breast lesions: Findings of stereotaxic needle-core biopsy and fine-needle aspiration cytology. Radiology, *181*:745–750, 1991.

Drexler, B., Davis, J. L., and Schofield, G.: Diaphanography in the diagnosis of breast cancer. Radiology, *157*:41, 1985.

Dupont, W. D., and Page, D. L.: Risk factors for breast cancer in women with proliferative breast disease. N. Engl. J. Med., *312*:146, 1985.

Eddy, D. M.: Screening for breast cancer. Proceedings of the Nineteenth Annual National Conference on the Diagnosis, Detection and Treatment of Breast Cancer, San Diego, CA, March 1981.

Eddy, D. M.: Finding cancer in asymptomatic people. Estimating the benefits, costs and risks. Cancer, *51*(Suppl. 12):2440, 1983.

Editorial: Lancet, *i*:851, 1985.

Egan, R. L., and Egan, K. L.: Detection of breast carcinoma: Comparison of automated water-path whole-breast sonography, mammography, and physical examination. Am. J. Roentgenol., *143*:493, 1984.

Egan, R. L., and Mosteller, R. C.: Breast cancer mammography patterns. Cancer, *40*:2087, 1977.

Egan, R. L., McSweeney, M. B., and Murphy, F. B.: Breast sonography and the detection of cancer. Recent Results Cancer Res., *90*:90, 1984.

El Yousef, S. J., Duchesneau, R. H., and Alfidi, R.: Nuclear magnetic resonance imaging of the human breast. Radiographics, *4*:113, 1984.

El Yousef, S. J., O'Connell, D. M., Duchesneau, R. H., et al.: Benign and malignant breast disease: Magnetic resonance and radiofrequency pulse sequences. Am. J. Roentgenol., *145*:1, 1985.

Evans, J.: Radiologic seminar CCXXXVIII: Mammography—benefit and risk. J. Miss. State Med. Assoc., *25*:151, 1984.

Fandos-Morera, A., Prats-Esteve, M., Tura-Soteras, J. M., and Traveria-Cros, A.: Breast tumors: Composition of microcalcifications. Radiology, *169*:325–327, 1988.

Feig, S. A.: Hypothetical breast cancer risk from mammography. Recent Results Cancer Res., *90*:1, 1984*a*.

Feig, S.: Radiation risk from mammography: Is it clinically significant? Am. J. Roentgenol., *143*:469, 1984*b*.

Feig, S.: Assessment of the hypothetical risk from mammography and evaluation of the potential benefit. Radiol. Clin. North Am., *21*:173, 1983.

Feig, S. A., Shaber G. S., Schwartz, G. F., et al.: Thermography, mammography and clinical examination in breast cancer screening: Review of 16,000 studies. Radiology, *122*:123, 1977.

Fleischer, A. C., Muhletaler, C. A., Reynolds, V. A., et al.: Palpable breast masses: Evaluation by high frequency, hand-held real-time sonography and xeromammography. Radiology, *148*:813, 1983.

Fox, S., Baum, J. K., Klos, D. S., et al.: Breast cancer screening: The underuse of mammography. Radiology, *156*:607, 1985.

Fox, S. H., Moskowitz, M., Saenger, E. L., et al.: Benefit/risk analysis of aggressive mammographic screening. Radiology, *128*:350, 1978.

Friedlander, M. L., and Tattersall, M. H.: Counting the costs of cancer therapy. Eur. J. Cancer Clin. Oncol., *18*:1237, 1982.

Gad, A., Thomas, D. A., and Moskowitz, M.: Screening for breast cancer in Europe: Achievements, problems, and future. Recent Results Cancer Res., *90*:179, 1984.

Galkin, B. M., Feig, S. A., Patchefsky, A. S., et al.: Ultrastructure and microanalysis of ''benign'' and ''malignant'' breast calcifications. Radiology, *124*:245, 1977.

Gautherie, M.: Improved system for the objective evaluation of breast thermograms. Prog. Clin. Biol. Res., *107*:897, 1982*a*.

Gautherie, M.: Temperature and blood flow patterns in breast cancer during natural evolution and following radiotherapy. Biomed. Thermol., *107*:21, 1982*b*.

Gautherie, M.: Thermobiological assessment of benign and malignant breast diseases. Chicago Gynecological Society, Holmes Lecture, April 1983.

Gautherie, M., and Gros, C. M.: Breast thermography and cancer risk prediction. Cancer, *45*:51, 1980.

Gautherie, M., Haehnel, P., Walter, J. P., et al.: Long term assessment of breast cancer risk by liquid crystal thermal imaging. Prog. Clin. Biol. Res., *107*:279, 1982.

Gautherie, M., Haehnel, P., and Walter, J. P.: Thermovascular disorders in in situ and minimal breast cancer. *In* Evaluation du Risque de Cancer Mammaire, Chimothérapie Première. Proceedings of the International Symposium of Senology, Liege, Belgium, November 1985.

Gautherie, M., Kotewicz, A., and Gueblez, P.: Accurate and objective evaluation of breast thermograms: Basic principles and new advances with special reference to an improved computer assisted scoring system. International Conference on Thermal Assessment of Breast Health, Washington, D. C., July 1983.

Geslien, G. E., Fisher, J. R., and Delaney, C.: Transillumination in breast cancer detection: Screening failures and potential. Am. J. Roentgenol., *144*:619, 1985.

Gohagan, J. K., Rodes, N. D., Blackwell, S. W., et al.: Individual and combined effectiveness of palpation, thermography, and mammography in breast cancer screening. Prev. Med. 9:713, 1980.

Gohagan, J., and Shterm, F.: Breast Imaging Workshop: State of the Art and Newer Technologies. September 1991: Summary Report. Bethesda, MD, Division of Cancer Prevention and Control, Early Detection Branch, National Institutes of Health, 1992.

Haberman, J. D.: Mass screening for breast cancer by electronic infrared pattern recognition. Final report, phase II (October 1976–June 1979). Oklahoma City, University of Oklahoma Health Sciences Center, Department of Radiological Sciences, 1979.

Haberman, J. D., Love, T. J., and Fracis, J. E.: Screening a rural population for breast cancer using thermography and physical examination techniques: Methods and results—a preliminary report. Ann. N.Y. Acad. Sci., *335*:492, 1980.

Haiart, D. C., and Henderson, J.: A comparison of interpretation of screening mammograms by a radiographer, a doctor, and a radiologist: Results and implications. Br. J. Clin. Pract., *45*:43–45, 1991.

Hajek, P., Binder, W., Kumpan, W., et al.: Lokalisationsgerät zur Feinnadelpunktion nicht papabler Veränderungen in der Mamma. Röntgenalatter, *36*:285, 1983.

Harper, A. P., and Kelly-Fry, E.: Ultrasound visualization of the breast in symptomatic patients. Radiology, *137*:465, 1980.

Harper, A. P., Kelly-Fry, E., Noe, J. S., et al.: Ultrasound in the evaluation of solid breast masses. Radiology, *146*:731, 1983.

Hebert, G., Carrier, R., McFarlane, D. V., et al.: Guidelines for detection of breast cancer: An update on investigative methods. A report to the Ad Hoc Committee on Mammography of The Canadian Association of Radiologists. J. Can. Assoc. Radiol., *35*:6, 1984.

Heywang-Kobrunner, S. H., Schlegel, A., Beck, R., Wendt, T., et al.: Contrast-enhanced MRI of the breast after limited surgery and radiation therapy. J. Comput. Assist. Tomogr., *17*:891–900, 1993.

Hinton, C. P., Roebuck, E. J., Williams, M. R., et al.: Mammographic parenchymal patterns: Value as a predictor of hormone dependency and survival in breast cancer. Am. J. Roentgenol., *144*:1103, 1985.

Hobbins, W.: INITIAL (quarterly newsletter for Thermal Image Analysis), *4*:1, 1983. Produced by Wisconsin Breast Cancer Detection Foundation, Madison.

Homer, M. J.: Nonpalpable breast lesion localization using a curved-end retractable wire. Radiology, *157*:259, 1985.

Horwitz, R. I., Lamas, A. M., and Peck, D.: Mammographic parenchymal patterns and risk of breast cancer in postmenopausal women. Am. J. Med., *77*:621, 1984.

Howe, G. R., Miller, A. B., and Sherman, G. J.: Breast cancer mortality following fluoroscopic irradiation in a cohort of tuberculosis patients. Cancer Detect. Prev., *5*:175, 1982.

Huppe, J. R., and Schneider, H. J.: Comparative film mammography and xeromammography (German). ROFO, *126*:361, 1977.

Jarlman, O., Andersson, I., Balldin, G., and Larsson, S. A.: Diagnostic accuracy of lightscanning and mammography in women with dense breasts. Acta Radiol., *33*:69–71, 1992.

Jarlman, O., Balldin, G., Andersson, I., et al.: Relation between lightscanning and the histologic and mammographic appearance of malignant breast tumors. Acta Radiol., *33*:63–68, 1992.

Jarlman, O., Berg, R., and Svanberg, S.: Time-resolved transillumination of the breast. Acta Radiol., *33*:277–279, 1992.

Jellins, J., Kossoff, G., and Reeve, T. S.: Detection and classification of liquid-filled masses in the breast by gray-scale echography. Radiology, *125*:205, 1977.

Jensen, S. R., and Mackey, J. K.: Xeromammography after augmentation mammoplasty. Am. J. Roentgenol., *144*:629, 1985.

Jones, C. H., Greening, W. P., Davey, J. B., et al.: Thermography of the female breast: A five year study in relation to the detection and prognosis of cancer. Br. J. Radiol., *48*:532, 1975.

Kalisher, L., Chu, A. M., and Peyster, R. G.: Clinico-pathological correlations of xeroradiography in determining involvement of metastatic axillary nodes in female breast cancer. Radiology, *121*:333, 1976.

Kambouris, T., Kotoulas, K., and Pontifex, G.: The diagnostic value of xeromammography in clinically occult breast cancer. Radiologe, *24*:L230, 1984.

Kasumi, F., Fukami, A., Kuno, K., et al.: Characteristic echographic features of circumscribed cancer. Ultrasound Med. Biol., *8*:369, 1982.

Kays, H. W.: Cost effective cancer screening. J. Indiana State Med. Assoc., *76*:324, 1983.

Kelly, M. E., Taylor, G. J., Moses, H. W., et al.: Comparative cost of myocardial revascularization: Percutaneous transluminal angioplasty and coronary artery bypass surgery. J. Am. Coll. Cardiol., *5*:16, 1985.

Key, H., Davies, E. R., Jackson, P. C., and Wells, P. N.: Optical attenuation characteristics of breast tissues at visible and near-infrared wavelengths. Phys. Med. Biol., *36*:579–590, 1991.

Key, H., Davies, E. R., Jackson, P. C., and Wells, P. N.: Monte Carlo modelling of light propagation in breast tissue. Phys. Med. Biol., *36*:591–602, 1991.

Kindermann, G., Paterok, E., Weishaar, J., et al.: Early detection of ductal breast cancer: The diagnostic procedure for pathological discharge from the nipple. Tumori, *65*:555, 1979.

Kobayashi, T.: Gray-scale echography for breast cancer. Radiology, *122*:207, 1977.

Kobayashi, T.: Diagnostic ultrasound in breast cancer: Analysis of retrotumorous echo patterns correlated with sonic attunuation by cancerous connective tissue. JCU J. Clin. Ultrasound, *7*:471, 1979.

Kojima, O., Majima, T., Uehara, Y., et al.: Radiographic parenchymal patterns in Japanese females as a risk factor for breast carcinoma. World J. Surg., *8*:414, 1984.

Kopans, D. B.: ''Early'' breast cancer detection using techniques other than mammography. Am. J. Roentgenol., *143*:465, 1984.

Kopans, D. B., Meyer, J. E., and Sadowsky, N.: Breast imaging. N. Engl. J. Med., *310*:960, 1984*a*.

Kopans, D. B., Meyer, J. E., Lindfors, K. K., et al.: Breast sonography to guide cyst aspiration and wire localization of occult solid lesions. Am. J. Roentgenol., *143*:489, 1984*b.*

Kopans, D. B., Meyer, J. E., and Lindfors, K. K.: Whole breast US imaging: Four year follow up. Radiology, *157*:505, 1985*a.*

Kopans, D. B., Lindfors, K. K., McCarthy, K. A., et al.: Spring hookwire breast lesion localizer: Use with rigid-compression mammographic systems. Radiology, *157*:537, 1985*b.*

Kopans, D. B., Meyer, J. E., and Steimbock, R. T.: Breast cancer: The appearance as delineated by whole breast water-path ultrasound scanning. J. Clin. Ultrasound, *10*:313, 1982.

Lansky, S. B., Black, J. L., and Cairns, N. U.: Childhood cancer. Medical costs. Cancer, *52*:762, 1983.

Layfield, L. J., Parkinson, B., Wong, J., et al.: Mammographically guided fine-needle aspiration biopsy of nonpalpable breast lesions: Can it replace open biopsy? Cancer, *68*:2007–2011, 1991.

LeGal, M., Chavanne, G., and Pellier, D.: Diagnostic value of clustered microcalcifications discovered by mammography (apropos of 227 cases with histological verification and without a palpable breast tumor). Bull. Cancer (Paris), *71*:57, 1984.

Lesnick, G. J.: Detection of breast cancer in young women. J.A.M.A., *237*:967, 1977.

Long, S. H., Gibbs, J. O., Crozier, J. P., et al.: Medical expenditures of terminal cancer patients during the last year of life. Inquiry, *21*:315, 1984.

Lundgren, B.: Population screening for breast cancer by single view mammography in a geographic region in Sweden. J. Natl. Cancer Inst., *62*:1373, 1379, 1979*a.*

Lundgren, B.: Positioning for oblique projection in mammography (letter to the editor). Am. J. Roentgenol., *132*:858, 1979*b.*

Lundgren, B., and Helleberg, A.: Single oblique view mammography for periodic screening for breast cancer in women. J. Natl. Cancer Inst., *68*:351, 1982.

Lundgren, B., and Jakobsson, S.: Repeat screening by single oblique view mammography. Breast Cancer Res. Treat., *1*:273, 1981.

Mahoney, L., and Csima, A.: Use and abuse of mammography in the early diagnosis of breast cancer. Can. J. Surg., *26*:262, 1983.

Mahoney, L. J., Bird, B. L., and Cooke, G. M.: Annual clinical examination. The best available screening test for breast cancer. N. Engl. J. Med., *301*:315, 1979.

Malberger, E., Edoute, Y., Toledano, O., et al.: Fine-needle aspiration and cytologic findings of surgical scar lesions in women with breast cancer. Cancer, *69*:148–152, 1992.

Mansfield, P., Moris, P. G., Ordidge, R. J., et al.: Human whole body imaging and detection of breast tumors by NMR. Phil. Trans. R. Soc. Lond. (Biol.), *289*:503, 1980.

Marshall, V., Williams, D. C., and Smith, K. D.: Diaphanography as a means of detecting breast cancer. Radiology, *150*:339, 1984.

Martin, J., Moskowitz, M., and Milbrath, J. R.: Breast cancer missed by mammography. Am. J. Roentgenol., *132*:737, 1979.

McSweeney, M. B., Small, W. C., Cerney, V., et al.: Magnetic resonance imaging in the diagnosis of breast disease: Use of transverse relaxation times. Radiology, *153*:741, 1984*a.*

McSweeney, M. B., Sprawls, P., and Egan, R. L.: Enhanced-image mammography. Recent Results Cancer Res., *90*:79, 1984*b.*

Mendell, L., Rosenbloom, M., and Maimark, A.: Are breast patterns a risk index for breast cancer? A reappraisal. Am. J. Roentgenol., *128*:547, 1977.

Merchant, T. E., Obertop, H., de Graaf, P. W.: Advantages of magnetic resonance imaging in breast surgery treatment planning. Breast Cancer Res. Treat., *25*:257–264, 1993.

Merritt, C. R., and Dempsey, P.: Presentation refresher course. Radiological Society of North America meeting, Chicago, IL, November 1985.

Merritt, C. R., Sullivan, M. A., Segaloff, A., et al.: Real time transillumination: Light scanning of the breast. Radiographics 4:989, 1984.

Meyer, J. E., Kopans, D. B., Stomper, P. C., et al.: Occult breast abnormalities: Percutaneous preoperative needle localization. Radiology, *150*:335 1984.

Miller, A. B.: Presentation at World Health Organization Committee meeting, Moscow, USSR, October 1985.

Mitnick, J. S., Vazquez, M. F., and Roses, D. F.: Recurrent breast cancer: Stereotactic localization for fine-needle aspiration biopsy. Radiology, *182*:103–106, 1992.

Monostori, Z., Herman, P. G., Carmody, D. P., et al.: Limitations in distinguishing malignant from benign lesions of the breast by systematic review of mammograms. Surg. Gynecol. Obstet., *173*:438–442, 1991.

Mooney, G. H.: Radiology and risk: An economist's perspective. Br. J. Radiol., *54*:861, 1981.

Mooney, G.: Breast cancer screening: A study in cost effectiveness analysis. Soc. Sci. Med., *16*:1277, 1982.

Morrone, D., Ambrogetti, D., Bravetti, P., et al.: Diagnostic errors in mammography: I. False-negative results. Radiol. Med. (Torino), *82*:212–217, 1991.

Moskowitz, M.: Guidelines for screening for breast cancer: Is a revision in order? Radiol. Clin. North Am., *30*:221–233, 1992.

Moskowitz, M.: Screening is not diagnosis. Radiology, *133*:265, 1979.

Moskowitz, M.: Mammographic parenchymal patterns: More controversy. J.A.M.A., *247*:210, 1982.

Moskowitz, M.: Minimal breast cancer redux. Radiol. Clin. North Am., *21*:93, 1983*a.*

Moskowitz, M.: Screening for breast cancer: How effective are our tests? CA Cancer J. Clin., *33*:26, 1983*b.*

Moskowitz, M.: The predictive value of certain mammographic signs in screening for breast cancer. Cancer, *51*:1007, 1983*c.*

Moskowitz, M.: Mammography to screen asymptomatic women for breast cancer. Am. J. Roentgenol., *413*:457, 1984.

Moskowitz, M., and Fox, S. H.: Cost analysis of aggressive breast cancer screening. Radiology, *130*:254, 1979.

Moskowitz, M., Fox, S. H., Brun del Re, R., et al.: The potential of liquid crystal thermography in detecting significant mastopathy. Radiology, *140*:659, 1981.

Moskowitz, M., Gartside, P., Gardella, L., et al.: The breast cancer screening controversy: A perspective. Am. J. Roentgenol., *129*:537, 1977.

Moskowitz, M., Gartside, P., and McLaughlin, C.: Mammographic patterns as markers for high risk benign breast disease and incident cancers. Radiology, *134*:293, 1980*a.*

Moskowitz, M., Gartside, P., Wirman, J. A., et al.: Proliferative disorders of the breast as risk factors for breast cancer in a self selected population: Pathologic markers. Radiology, *134*:289, 1980*b.*

Moskowitz, M., and Libshitz, H. I.: Mammographic screening for breast cancer by lateral view only: Is it practical? J. Can. Assoc. Radiol., *28*:259–261, 1977.

Moskowitz, M., Milbrath, J., Gartside, P., et al.: Lack of efficacy of thermography as a screening tool for minimal and stage 1 breast cancer. N. Engl. J. Med., *295*:249, 1976*a.*

Moskowitz, M., Saenger, E. L., Gartside, P. S., et al.: Benefit versus risk in mammographic screening: One approach. Proceedings of the Eighth Annual National Conference of Radiation Control, Springfield, IL, May 1976*b.*

Moskowitz, M., Russel, P., Fidler, J., et al.: Breast cancer screening: Preliminary report of 207 biopsies performed in 4128 volunteer screenees. Cancer, *36*:2245, 1975.

Muirhead, A., and Seright, W.: Clinical experience with the diaphanograph machine. Ann. R. Coll. Surg. Engl., *66*:123, 1984.

Myers, L. E., McLelland, R., Stricker, C. S., et al.: Reproducibility of mammographic classifications. Am. J. Roentgenol., *141*:445, 1983.

Myrden, J. A., and Hiltz, J. E.: Breast cancer following multiple fluoroscopies during artificial pneumothorax treatment of pulmonary tuberculosis. Can. Med. Assoc. J., *100*:1032, 1969.

Nielsen, N. S. M., and Poulsen, H. S.: Relation between mammographic findings and hormone receptor content in breast cancer. Am. J. Roentgenol., *145*:501, 1985.

Norton, L. W., Seligman, B. E., and Pearlman, N. W.: Accuracy and cost of needle localization breast biopsy. Arch. Surg., *123*:947–950, 1988.

Nyirjesy, I.: Breast thermography. Clin. Obstet. Gynecol., *25*:401, 1982.

O'Connor, G. T., Schneider-Jones, G. M., Leshen, M., et al.: The potential effects of mammographic screening as recommended by the American Cancer Society: A modeling study. Meeting abstract. Society of Medical Decision Making, 1985.

Orel, S. G., and Troupin, R. H.: Nonmammographic imaging of the breast: Current issues and future prospects. Semin. Roentgenol., *28*:231–241, 1993.

Pagani, J. J., Bassett, L. W., Gold, R. H., et al.: Efficacy of combined film screen/xeromammography. Am. J. Roentgenol., *135*:141, 1980.

Page, D. L., Vander Zwaag, R., Rogers, L. W., et al.: Relation between component parts of fibrocystic disease complex and breast cancer. J. Natl. Cancer Inst., *61*:1055, 1978.

Parker, S. H., Lovin, J. D., Jobe, W. E., et al.: Stereotactic biopsy with a biopsy gun. Radiology, *176*:741–747, 1990.

Parker, S. H., Lovin, J. D., Jobe, W. E., et al.: Nonpalpable breast lesions: Stereotactic automated large core biopsies. Radiology, *180*:403–407, 1991.

Paterok, E. M., Egger, H., and Willgeroth, F.: More than 1500 radiologically indicated breast biopsies: Microcalcifications and the pathologic galactogram, 1964–1982. Geburtshilfe. Fraunheilkd., *43*:721, 1983.

Paulus, D. D.: Conservative treatment of breast cancer: Mammography in patient selection and follow up. Am. J. Roentgenol., *143*:483, 1984.

Pelikan, S., Moskowitz, M.: Effects of lead time, length bias and false-negative assurance on screening for breast cancer. Cancer, *71*:1998–2005, 1993.

Peyster, R. G., Kalisher, L., and Cole, R.: Mammographic parenchymal patterns and the prevalence of breast cancer. Radiology, *125*:387, 1977.

Peyster, R. G., and Kalisher, L.: Galactography. Rev. Interam. Radiol., *4*:57, 1979.

Pollei, S. R., Mettler, F. A., Bartow, S., et al.: Occult breast cancer: Prevalence and radiographic detectability. Radiology, *163*:459, 1987.

Price, J.: Personal communication, 1985.

Prorok, J. J., Trostle, D. R., Scarlato, M., et al.: Excisional breast biopsy and roentgenographic examination for mammographically detected microcalcification. Am. J. Surg., *145*:684, 1983.

Rasanen, O., Auranen, A., and Gronross, M.: Screening for breast cancer in Finland. Presented at Third Meeting of the European Group for Breast Cancer Screening, Düsseldorf, Germany, August 1984.

Rasmussen, O. S., and Serrup, A.: Preoperative radiographically guided wire marking of nonpalpable breast lesions. Acta Radiol. Diagn., *25*:13, 1984.

Revesz, G.: Breast cancer screening: Predictive values and strategies. Acta Thermograph., *3*:150, 1978.

Rideout, D. F., and Poor, P. Y.: Patterns of breast parenchyma on mammography. J. Can. Assoc. Radiol., *28*:257, 1977.

Rodes, N. D., Farrell, C., and Blackwell, C. W.: Missouri's role in breast cancer detection. Missouri Med., *74*:689, 1977.

Romanini, A., and Bock E.: Mammography and xero-mammography. Min. Ginecol., *34*:851, 1982.

Rombach, J. J.: Breast cancer screening: Results and implications for diagnostic decision making. Brussels, Alphen Aan Den Rijn, Stafleu's Scientific Publishing Co., 1980.

Rosselli del Turco, M., Santoni, R., Ciatto, S., et al.: The role of infrared thermography, mammography, and physical examination in the diagnosis of breast cancer. Acta Thermograph., *8*:86, 1983.

Rossi, S., Cinini, C., Di Pietro, C., et al.: Diagnostic delay in breast cancer: Correlation with disease stage and prognosis. Tumori, *76*:559–562, 1990.

Rubin, E., Miller, V. E., Berland, L. L., et al.: Hand held real-time breast sonography. Am. J. Roentgenol., *144*:623, 1985.

Sandison, A. T.: An autopsy study of the adult human breast. National Cancer Institute Monograph. Washington, D. C., U. S. Department of Health, Education and Welfare, No. 8, June 1962.

Schalldach, U., and Schumann, E.: The significance of mammography in follow up care of mammary carcinoma patients for detection of bilateral carcinoma. Zentralbl. Chir., *107*:462, 1982.

Schroeder, S. A., Showstack, J. A., and Schwartz, J.: Survival of adult high-cost patients: Report of a follow up study from 9 acute care hospitals. J.A.M.A., *245*:1446, 1981.

Seidman, H.: Screening for breast cancer in younger women: Life expectancy gains and losses. An analysis according to risk indicator groups. Cancer, *27*:66, 1977.

Seltzer, S. E., McNeil, B. J., D'Orsi, C. J., et al.: Combining evidence from multiple imaging modalities: A feature-analysis method. Comput. Med. Imaging Graph., *16*:373–380, 1992.

Shapiro, S., Goldberg, J. D., and Hutchison, G. B.: Lead time in breast cancer detection and implications for periodicity of screening. Am. J. Epidemiol., *100*:357, 1974.

Shapiro S., Strax, P., Venet, L., et al.: Changes in 5 year breast cancer mortality in a breast cancer screening program: Seventh National Cancer Conference Proceedings. Philadelphia, J. B. Lippincott, 1973.

Shapiro, S., Venet, W., Strax, P., et al.: Ten to fourteen year effects of breast cancer screening on mortality. J. Natl. Cancer Inst., *69*:349, 1982.

Sickles, E. A.: Breast cancer detection with transillumination and mammography. Am. J. Roentgenol., *142*:841, 1984*a*.

Sickles, E. A.: Mammographic features of "early" breast cancer. Am. J. Roentgenol., *143*:461, 1984*b*.

Sickles, E. A., Filly, R. A., and Callen, P. W.: Breast cancer detection with sonomammography and mammography: Comparison using state-of-the-art equipment. Am. J. Roentgenol., *140*:843, 1983.

Sickles, E. A., Filly, R. A., and Callen, P. W.: Benign breast lesions: Ultrasound detection and diagnosis. Radiology, *151*:467, 1984.

Siu, O., Ghent, W. R., Colwell, B. T., et al.: Thermogram aided clinical examination of the breast—an alternative to mammography for women 50 or younger. Can. J. Publ. Health, *73*:232, 1982.

Skrabanek, P.: Screening for disease: False premises and false promises of breast cancer screening. Lancet, *ii*:316, 1985.

Snyder, R. E.: Specimen radiography and preoperative localization of nonpalpable breast cancer. Cancer, *46*:950, 1980.

Snyder, R. E., Watson, R. C., and Crux, N.: Graphic stress telethermography (GST): A possible supplement to physical examination in screening for abnormalities of the female breast. Am. J. Diagn. Gynecol. Obstet., *1*:197, 1979.

Spratt, J. S., Alagia, D. P., Greenberg, R. A., et al.: Association of chronic cystic mastopathy, xeromammographic patterns, and cancer. Cancer, *55*:1372, 1985.

Stamp, G. W., Whitehouse, G. H., McDicken, I. W., et al.: Mammographic and pathological correlations in a breast screening programme. Clin. Radiol., *34*:529, 1983.

Stark, A. M.: The significance of an abnormal breast thermogram. Acta Thermograph., *1*:33, 1976.

Stark, A. M., and Way, S.: The use of thermovision in the detection of early breast cancer. Cancer, *33*:1664, 1974.

Stern, E. E., Curtis, A. C., Miller, S., et al.: Thermography in breast diagnosis. Cancer, *50*:323, 1982.

Stomper, P. C., and Gelman, R. S.: Mammography in symptomatic and asymptomatic patients. Hematol. Oncol. Clin. North Am., *3*:611–640, 1989.

Strax, P.: Mass screening for control of breast cancer. Cancer, *53*(Suppl. 3): 665, 1984.

Swets, J. A., Getty, D. J., Pickett, R. M., et al.: Enhancing and evaluating diagnostic accuracy. *In* Swets, J. A., Getty, D. J., Pickett, R. M., et al. (Eds.): Medical Decision Making. Philadelphia, Hanley & Belfus, pp. 9–18, 1991.

Tabar, L., and Dean, P. B.: Mammographic parenchymal patterns: Risk indicators for breast cancer. J.A.M.A., *247*:185, 1982.

Tabar, L., Dean, P. B., and Pentek, Z.: Galactography: The diagnostic procedure of choice for nipple discharge. Radiology, *149*:31, 1983.

Tabar, L., and Gad, A.: Screening for breast cancer: The Swedish trial. Radiology, *138*:219, 1981*a*.

Tabar, L., Pentek, Z., and Dean, P. B.: The diagnostic and therapeutic value of breast cyst puncture and pneumocystography. Radiology, *141*:659, 1981*b*.

Tabar, L., Fagerberg, C. J. G., Gad, A., et al.: Reduction in mortality from breast cancer after mass screening with mammography. Lancet, *i*:829, 1985.

Texidor, H. S., and Kazam, E.: Combined mammographic-sonographic evaluation of breast masses. Am. J. Roentgenol., *128*:409, 1977.

Third National Cancer Survey: Incidence Data. National Cancer Institute Monograph No. 41, March 1975. Washington, D. C., U. S. Department of Health, Education, and Welfare, Publication No. (NIH) 75–787.

Thomas, B. A.: Breast transillumination using the sinus diaphanograph. Br. Med. J., *283*:1057, 1981.

Threatt, B., Norbeck, J. M., and Ullman, N. S.: Thermography and breast cancer: An analysis of a blind reading. Ann. N.Y. Acad. Sci., *335*:501, 1980.

Turnbull, A. D., Carlon, G., Baron, R., et al.: The inverse relationship between cost and survival in the critically ill cancer patient. Crit. Care Med., *7*:20, 1979.

Verbeek, A. L. M.: Population screening for breast cancer in Nijmegen: An evaluation of the period 1975–1982. Nijmegen, Netherlands: Katholieke Universiteit Nijmegen, 1985.

Verbeek, A. L. M., Henriks, J. H. C. L., Peeters, P. H. M., et al.: Mammographic breast pattern and the risk of breast cancer. Lancet, *i*:591, 1984.

Wagai, T.: Results of screening trials in Japan. *In* Jellins, J., and Kobayashi, T. (Eds.): Ultrasonic Examination of the Breast. New York, Wiley, 1983, p. 275.

Walker, Q. J., Gebski, V., and Langlands, A. O.: The misuse of mammography in the management of breast cancer revisited. Med. J. Aust., *151*:509–512, 1989.

Wallberg, H.: Diaphanography: A clinical and experimental study of benign and malignant mammary diseases. Huddinge, Sweden: Doctoral thesis, Department of Surgery, Karolinska Institute, 1984.

Ward, S. M.: Wall Street Journal, New York, NY, July 30, 1985.

Watanabe, H.: Current issues and future prospects of mass screening for breast cancer. Jpn. J. Cancer Res., *30*(Suppl. 6):598, 1984.

Watt, A. C., Ackerman, L. V., Shetty, P. C., et al.: Differentiation between benign and malignant disease of the breast using digital subtraction angiography of the breast. Cancer, *56*:1287, 1985.

Wellings, S. R., and Wolf, J. N.: Correlative studies of the histological and radiographic appearance of the breast parenchyma. Radiology, *129*:299, 1978.

Wenth, J., and Stein, M. A.: Efficacy of breast cancer screening by thermography. Acta Thermograph., *8*:76, 1983.

Whitehead, J., Carlile, T., Kopecky, K. J., et al.: Wolfe mammographic parenchymal patterns: A study of the masking hypothesis of Egan and Mosteller. Cancer, *56*:1280, 1985.

Wilkinson, E., Clapton, C., Gordonson, J., et al.: Mammographic parenchymal patterns and the risk of breast cancer. J. Natl. Cancer Inst., *59*:1397, 1977.

Witt, I., Hansen, S., and Brunner, S.: Risk of developing breast cancer in relation to the mammographic findings. Ugeskr. Laeger., *145*:237, 1983.

Witt, I., Hansen, H. S., and Brunner, S.: The risk of developing breast cancer in relation to mammography findings. Eur. J. Radiol., *4*:65, 1984.

Wolfe, J. N.: Breast patterns as an index of risk for developing breast cancer. Am. J. Roentgenol., *126*:1130, 1976*a*.

Wolfe, J. N.: Risk for cancer development determined by mammographic parenchymal pattern. Cancer, *37*:2486, 1976*b*.

Wolfe, J. N., Saftlas, A. F., and Salane, M.: Association of radiographic dysplasia and breast carcinoma: A case control study. *In* Evaluation du Risque de Cancer Mammaire, Chimothérapie Première. Proceedings of the International Symposium of Senology, Liege, Belgium, November 1985.

Wolfman, N. T., Moran, R., Moran, P. R., et al.: Simultaneous MR imaging of both breasts using a dedicated receiver coil. Radiology, *155*:241, 1985.

12 Gross and Microscopic Pathology

Carlos M. Perez-Mesa

New biologic concepts and contemporary technology have not diminished the importance of gross and microscopic characteristics of carcinoma of the breast. They remain an important source of information for treatment and prognostication (Fisher et al., 1977; Rilke et al., 1978; Monaghan and Roberts, 1985; and Page, 1991). It is the purpose of this chapter to highlight the most salient and clinically relevant of these features without attempting to cover, in scope or in depth, the information available in monographs or textbooks on breast disease (Azzopardi, 1979; Page, 1991; Rosen and Oberman, 1992; and Tavassoli, 1992).

CLASSIFICATION

Classification systems for breast cancer are all imperfect and incomplete. The continuous changes reflect both the complexity and the incomplete understanding of its pathobiology. Classifications have to take into account the heterogeneity of breast carcinoma and the variables that, singly or in combination, influence its behavior. New discoveries of diagnostic and prognostic importance will provide the basis for better approaches to classifications (Van Bogaert and Maldague, 1978; Azzopardi et al., 1982; McDivitt et al., 1986; and Page and Anderson, 1987).

Carcinoma of the breast originates from the epithelium of mammary ducts and acini; however, the studies by Wellings and colleagues (1974) have shown that a large percentage of breast carcinomas, both ductal and lobular, take origin in the terminal duct lobular unit rather than from larger ducts. Gross and microscopic morphology, together with the most likely topographic origin, permit the characterization of various types. In 1946, Foote and Stewart devised a classification that subsequent studies have corroborated; with minor modifications their schema is shown in Table 12–1.

INVASIVE DUCTAL CARCINOMA

Invasive ductal carcinoma is the most common type of invasive carcinoma, representing between 47% and 80% of all invasive types (Fisher et al., 1975; Azzopardi et al., 1982; Page and Anderson, 1987; and Rosen and Oberman, 1992). The diagnosis is based more on concept than on morphologic criteria, since it includes all carcinomas that cannot be assigned to another identifiable type. They are also referred to as *infiltrating duct carcinoma, infiltrating carcinoma of no special type* (NST) or *infiltrating carcinoma, not otherwise specified* (NOS).

On gross inspection this type of tumor appears predominantly as a poorly marginated mass whose consistency varies according to its fibrous content. When fibrous tissue is abundant it imparts a characteristic hardness (scirrhous; Fig. 12–1). The cut surface is retracted, grayish yellow, with radiating streaks running centrifugally; these streaks, which occur frequently though not exclusively in this type of tumor, represent condensation of elastic tissue along mammary ducts (elastosis). Necrosis, which is manifested as white chalky areas of softer consistency, is not uncommon.

Tumors vary widely in size. Those that are only a few millimeters in diameter can escape detection except with special imaging techniques or careful and experienced gross inspection. They can be so large as to occupy the entire mammary gland, including the skin and the subjacent musculature (Fig. 12–2). Several dominant masses can coexist in the breast, though this is not a frequent finding. The frequency increases in proportion to the size of the index tumor (Ingleby et al., 1960) (Fig. 12–3). The margins of the tumor can be circumscribed, indicating an expansile, pushing type of growth, but more frequently it is infiltrating

Table 12–1. CLASSIFICATION OF BREAST CARCINOMA

Invasive carcinoma
   Invasive ductal carcinoma not otherwise specified (NOS)
   Medullary carcinoma
   Mucinous (colloid) carcinoma
   Papillary carcinoma
   Invasive lobular carcinoma
   Tubular (orderly) carcinoma
Noninvasive carcinoma
   Intraductal carcinoma (ductal carcinoma in situ)
   Lobular carcinoma in situ (lobular neoplasia)
Rarer types of invasive carcinoma
   Adenocystic carcinoma
   Squamous cell carcinoma
   Metaplastic carcinoma
   Secretory carcinoma
   Signet ring cell carcinoma
   Lipid-rich carcinoma
   Sudoriferous (apocrine) carcinoma
   Carcinoma with neuroendocrine features
   Glycogen-rich clear cell carcinoma
Special manifestations of breast carcinoma
   Paget's disease of the nipple
   Inflammatory carcinoma

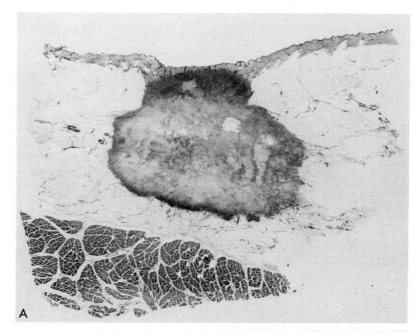

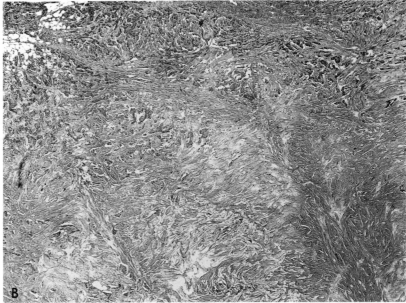

Figure 12–1. *A*, Whole section of the breast depicting invasive ductal carcinoma NOS with pronounced fibrosis in most of the tumor. Darker area, mostly toward the periphery, represents the epithelial component of tumor. *B*, Center of tumor, with intense fibrosis.

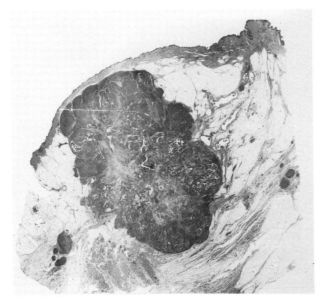

Figure 12-2. Whole mount of breast showing extensive tumor involvement, including fascia, muscle, and epidermis. The margins of the tumor are circumscribed. Notice the presence of other smaller tumors. The nipple is not retracted.

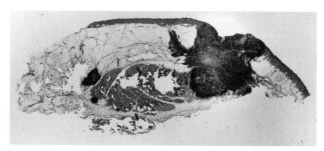

Figure 12-3. Notice large index tumor and the presence of other tumors in the whole mount of the breast. The skin is invaded by the tumor, as is the subjacent musculature.

This tumor also has been designated *infiltrating ductal carcinoma with productive fibrosis.* The frequency of this tumor makes it more available than any other type for study of parameters that have prognostic significance, particularly grade or differentiation. Among all types of ductal carcinoma, invasive ductal carcinoma, NOS, is associated with the largest risk of treatment failure.

MEDULLARY CARCINOMA

Medullary carcinoma has been also designated *encephaloid carcinoma, bulky carcinoma, circumscribed and solid carcinoma,* and *medullary carcinoma with lymphoid stroma.* It was described by Geschickter for the first time in 1945. Moore and Foote (1949) further defined their clinicopathologic characteristics. Ridolfi and coworkers (1977), however, are credited with establishing strict histopathologic

and serrated, with a stellate contour. Margins may be a combination of both types. Dentril-like extensions frequently are observed in tumors with infiltrating margins, making exact measurement of the tumor diameter difficult (Fig. 12–4). The microscopic appearance varies with the degree of cellularity and differentiation and the quantity and quality of stroma, necrosis, and inflammatory infiltrate.

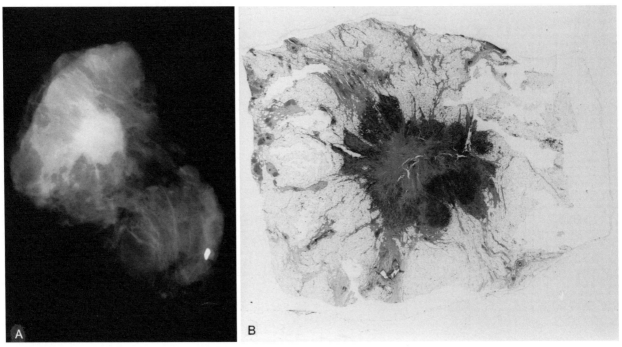

Figure 12-4. Montage of specimen radiograph, *A,* and whole mount of tumor, *B.* Notice in the latter the infiltrative margins and the extensions like dentrils into the neighboring adipose tissue. The actual measurement of the tumor can be imprecise and inexact.

criteria that permit this tumor to be distinguished from others with similar microscopic features but a different clinical outcome. Medullary carcinoma represents some 5% to 7% of all invasive carcinomas. The distinguishing gross characteristics consist of a globoid, homogeneous, soft, pinkish gray mass, with well-defined margins. When hemorrhage or necrosis has occurred, dark red or yellow areas may be observed. On gross inspection it can be confused with a fibroadenoma or with an intramammary lymph node. An expansile type of growth typifies these tumors (Fig. 12–5). The microscopic characteristics consist of anastomosing solid cords and sheets of medium to large anaplastic cells with syncytial growth, ill-defined borders, high-grade nuclei with marked pleomorphism, and frequent mitoses. The syncytial type of growth should represent 75% or more of the tumor. A pronounced lymphoplasmacytic stroma is one of the main characteristics of this tumor; intratumoral fibrosis should be negligible or absent, as should any glandular arrangement or intraductal component.

Atypical medullary carcinomas (Fisher et al., 1975; and Ridolfi et al., 1977) are a group of tumors with focally infiltrative margins composed of anaplastic cells with a syncytial type of growth occupying less than 75% of its volume. They are different from typical medullary carcinomas in showing milder lymphoplasmacytic stroma, intratumoral fibrosis, and areas of ductal carcinoma NOS.

Typical medullary carcinoma is associated with a good prognosis. The tumors have a lower frequency of lymph node metastases than patients with atypical medullary carcinoma or infiltrating ductal carcinoma of no special type. In one study by Rapin and coworkers (1988) patients with this tumor had a disease-free survival rate of 92%, in contrast with one of 51% for patients with nonmedullary types. Tumors smaller than 3 cm in diameter have a better prognosis than that of nonmedullary carcinomas of equal size; however, this difference disappears when they are larger than 3 cm in diameter with metastases to four or more

axillary lymph nodes. The biologic behavior of medullary carcinoma is so different from that of atypical medullary carcinoma that their distinction is critical; the most strict histopathologic criteria should be used for their diagnosis. In National Surgical Adjuvant Breast Project (NSABP) studies (Fisher et al., 1993), atypical medullary carcinoma had one of the highest rates of treatment failure and mortality. Hsu and colleagues (1981) found a qualitative difference in the type of plasma cells associated with medullary carcinoma and those associated with ductal carcinoma. The former were predominantly immunoglobulin A (IgA) plasma cells, and the tumor cells contained both IgA and secretory component (SC); plasma cells associated with ductal carcinoma were of IgG type. These differences express the degree of functional differentiation and may be related to the favorable prognosis of typical medullary carcinoma.

MUCINOUS CARCINOMA

This tumor, also designated *colloid, gelatinous, myxomatous,* and *mucoid,* was recognized in the early 19th century by its distinct appearance and biologic attributes (Saphir, 1941). It accounts for between 1% and 6% of all breast carcinomas. It occurs more frequently in older women, and its growth is slower than that of the usual invasive ductal carcinoma. In 1915, Halsted described its clinical signs as protrusion of the nipple and a sensation of ''swish'' on palpation; however, these signs are rarely observed (Fig. 12–6). The gross appearance of this tumor when pure is characterized by a nonencapsulated, well-circumscribed, soft, gray-yellow mass with a syrupy or gelatinous appearance (Fig. 12–7). The size varies from less than 1.0 cm to a mass that occupies the thickness of the entire breast. Microscopically, this carcinoma is composed of mucin pools divided into incomplete compartments by slender

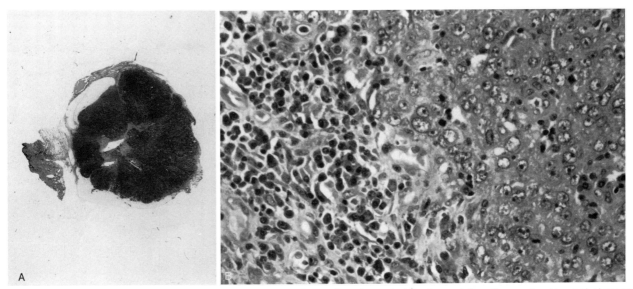

Figure 12–5. *A,* Whole mount of a medullary carcinoma exhibiting the characteristic sharp delineation and paler central areas representing necrosis. *B,* Microscopic features, including the syncytial pattern, nuclear high grade, and the plasmacytic interstitial component.

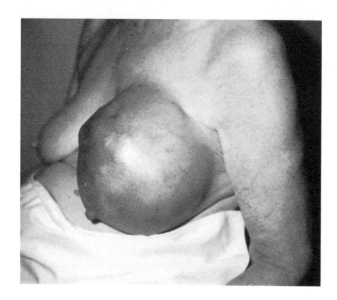

Figure 12–6. Clinical photograph of a pure mucinous carcinoma. A prominent nipple can be observed.

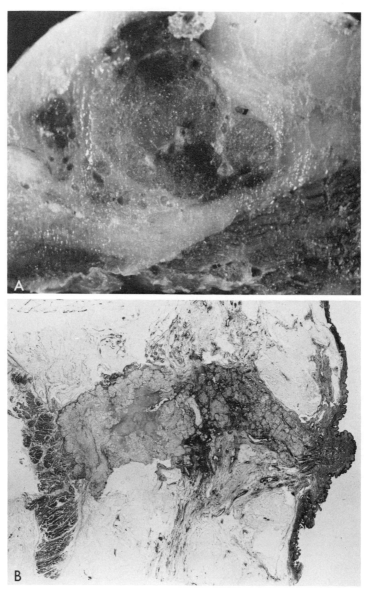

Figure 12–7. *A,* Close view of the cut surface, with the characteristic gelatinous appearance. *B,* Whole section of a breast depicting mucinous carcinoma infiltrating the skin and subjacent musculature. Darker areas toward center represent hemorrhage. Note the prominent nipple.

bands of fibrovascular tissue where small cells form nests, solid sheets, tubules, papillae, or sievelike patterns. The tumor cells are uniform, with a well-delineated membrane and are hyperchromatic, with regular nuclei but rare nucleoli. The cytoplasm is abundant and may contain mucin. The interface between tumor and neighboring tissue is characteristically sharp, without an inflammatory response; however, in the surrounding tissue an in situ component may be present. When infiltrating ductal carcinomas NOS coexist with mucinous carcinoma, the tumor is designated as *mixed.* The behavior of pure and mixed types is different; axillary metastases are associated with 3.1% to 15% of the pure type and with 33% to 46% of the mixed type (Rasmussen, et al., 1985, 1987; Haagensen, 1986; and Komaki et al., 1988). The clinical course of the mixed type is similar

to that of infiltrating ductal carcinoma NOS. The diagnostic criteria for pure mucinous carcinoma range from *pure mucinous carcinoma in which no infiltrating ductal carcinoma is present* (Melamed et al., 1961) to *carcinomas containing large amounts of extracellular epithelial mucus, sufficient to be visible grossly and recognizable microscopically around and within tumor cells* (World Health Organization, 1981). When reporting mucinous carcinoma, pathologists are obliged to state the proportion of pure and mixed types because of the different behavior of the two. In pure mucinous carcinoma the deoxyribonucleic acid (DNA) was diploid in 25 of 26 tumors in one report (Rosen and Wang, 1980), while more than 50% (11 of 19 cases) of the mixed variety were aneuploid, similar to infiltrating ductal carcinoma.

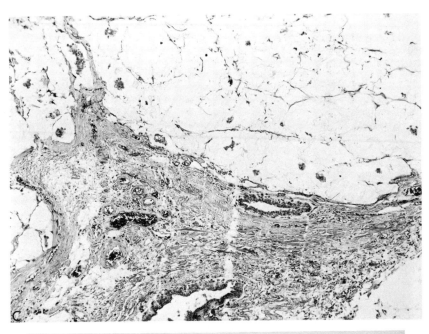

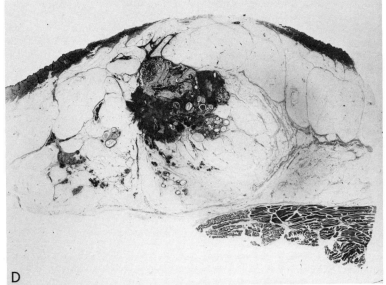

Figure 12–7 *Continued C,* Tumor margin is sharp and characteristically without inflammatory reaction. *D,* Whole mount of breast showing ``mixed'' mucinous carcinoma (lighter area).

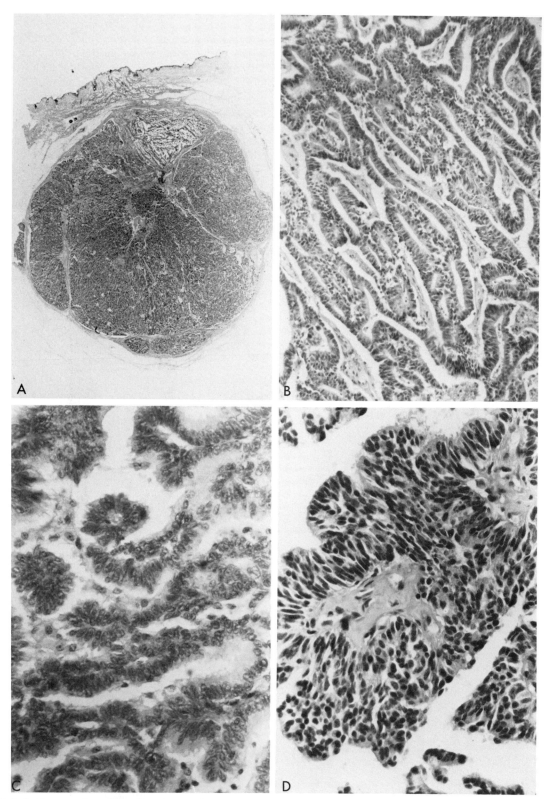

Figure 12–8. *A,* Cross section of papillary tumor, circumscribed with foci of invasion. Recognizable filiform structure is present. *B–D,* Various patterns (adenomatoid, papilliform). Note recognizable fibrous core and anaplasia in *D.*

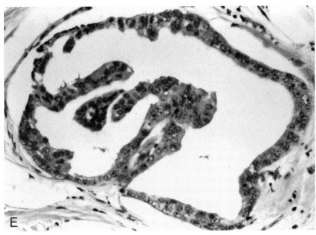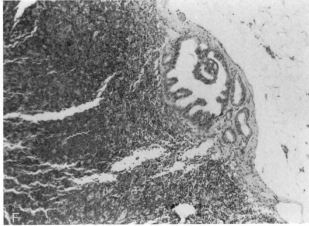

Figure 12-8 *Continued E,* Papillary carcinoma of the breast showing papilli lined by cells with prominent nucleoli. *F,* Axillary lymph node shows subcapsular metastatic deposit exhibiting a papillary pattern.

Pure mucinous carcinomas have an excellent short-term prognosis (Fisher et al., 1993), and more than 10 years' follow-up is necessary to appreciate the lethality of this tumor. In a group of 41 patients with pure mucinous carcinoma, nearly half died of tumor spread 12 years or more after the diagnosis (Rosen and Wang, 1980). In the author's files are six patients of a group of 15 who died of metastases from pure mucinous carcinoma 10 to 20 years after mastectomy.

Argyrophilic granules have been found in mucinous tumors, and attempts have been made to classify this tumor into subtypes (Capella et al., 1980) based on their presence. Type A has no argyrophilic granules, is hypocellular, and has minimal intracellular mucin. Type B is argyrophilic, more cellular, and has intracytoplasmic mucin. Nevertheless, no demonstrable differences, either clinical or morphologic, were found in a study of 202 tumors (Rasmussen et al., 1985).

INVASIVE PAPILLARY CARCINOMA

Invasive papillary carcinoma represents between 0.3% and 3% of all breast carcinomas (Fisher et al., 1980; and Azzopardi, 1983). There is a dearth of published studies on this tumor type, and, as others have commented, its distinction from other benign papillary lesions is controversial and difficult. It is not always possible to distinguish it from its noninvasive counterpart. The number of cases available to study is small, and the tumor is associated with a clinical behavior so favorable that correlation between morphology and clinical behavior is difficult. This tumor is more frequently found in postmenopausal, nonwhite women and is associated with nipple discharge, which in 25% of cases is blood tinged. The pattern of growth is expansile. Tumors are generally centrally located, most of the time are palpable, and depending on their size, they can protrude and affect the overlying skin, with dimpling and nipple retraction. The size varies: in one study it ranged from microscopic to 4.5 cm in diameter (Murad et al., 1981). In the author's cases, the mean size was 2.5 cm. Tumors are well-

demarcated and have been described as gray or tan, friable, and hemorrhagic. Occasionally their filiform structure can be recognized grossly (Fig. 12–8*A–D*). A papillary arrangement is the microscopic sine qua non. The proliferating cells form different patterns: *papilliform*, characterized by long or short blunt stalks, *adenomatoid*, in which the papilli fuse with the formation of glands, and *microcystic*, in which the lesion involves small ducts and the papilli are short. Combinations of patterns occur. The proliferating cells are of a single type, distributed in one or several rows. They exhibit good nuclear grade, generally without the features commonly observed in malignant processes. The existence of a single cell type, regardless of the number of layers, is of paramount importance to establish the diagnosis (Kraus and Neubecker, 1962). Important also is the absence of a myoepithelial cell layer, which in the opinion of some authors is the "quintessential morphologic feature of papillary carcinomas" (Tavassoli, 1992). The use of immunohistochemical stains for actin and S-100 to demonstrate the presence or absence of myoepithelial cells helps to distinguish benign from malignant papillary lesions of the breast. Coexistent areas of unequivocal invasion can show a papillary ductal NOS, or any other type of pattern. Although uncommon, axillary lymph node metastases can maintain a similar papillary pattern (Fig. 12–8*E, F*). The prognosis of this tumor is excellent; only three of 35 patients from a NSABP study had treatment failure, and only one patient died of tumor spread after 5 years (Fisher et al., 1993).

A variant of papillary carcinoma termed *intracystic papillary carcinoma* has been described (Gatchell et al., 1958; Squires and Betsill, 1981; Carter et al., 1983; Harris and Lessells, 1986; and McKittrick et al., 1969), which, despite its infrequency, has generated a larger number of publications than its more common congener. It is difficult in some of the publications to identify the malignant potential of this variant, as it is not clear whether the authors are describing an invasive or noninvasive carcinoma. The diagnosis should be restricted to tumors associated with a grossly visible cyst (Fig. 12–9). Carter and associates (1983) reviewed 41 cases of intracystic papillary carcinomas and found a favorable prognosis. The average age of

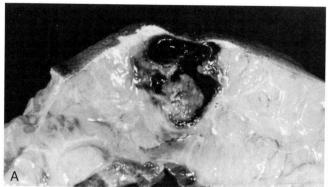
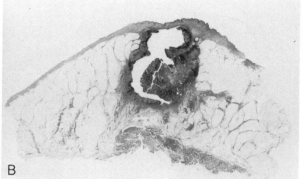

Figure 12–9. *A,* Gross photograph of intracystic papillary carcinoma showing tumor projecting as polypoid mass into cavity containing blood. *B,* Whole breast, exhibiting tumor and relation with cyst.

the patients was 63 years, and in 85% the presenting sign was a mass. Twenty-two per cent had nipple discharge and 15% pain. Eleven axillary dissections revealed no metastases. This tumor can be associated with ductal carcinoma in situ (DCIS); in three patients where this association occurred local resection was followed by local recurrence. Six of the seven cases reported by Hunter and Sawyer (1980), were treated with modified or radical mastectomy and one with simple mastectomy and postoperative radiotherapy. Only one patient had recurrence, and she died 2 years postoperatively with osseous metastases. Other authors (Czernobilsky, 1967; and McKittrick et al., 1969) report a 25% and a 36% rate of nodal metastasis.

INVASIVE LOBULAR CARCINOMA

The frequency of this tumor differs in various studies from 0.7% to 14% (Donegan and Perez-Mesa, 1972; Martinez and Azzopardi, 1979; and Dixon et al., 1983) of all breast cancers. Rather than ethnic or geographic differences, this reflects diagnostic criteria, and to some extent the inclusion of morphologic variants not initially or universally appreciated. In some studies it occurs less frequently in women under 35 years of age (2%) than in women older than 75 years (11%) (Rosen et al., 1977).

The clinical and gross features are variable; at one end, it can be manifested by a palpable mass large enough to occupy a great portion of the breast, appearing hard and gray and sharing some of the features of the so-called scirrhous carcinoma. At the other end of the spectrum, tumors are not detectable by visual inspection and are manifested only as diffuse induration without a dominant mass or as fine nodularity on palpation. Tumors not detected by mammography often belong to this category because calcifications frequently are not present and the pattern of invasion is diffuse, without margination (LeGal et al., 1992).

Microscopically, the tumor cell is characteristically small with round to oval nuclei. The cytoplasm is scanty although well-delineated, and occasionally it exhibits intracytoplasmic lumens. It infiltrates the breast parenchyma diffusely, sometimes rather inconspicuously. The tumor cells are dis-

tributed in a linear fashion (Indian files) or concentrically (bullseye pattern) around and between lobular units and ducts (Fig. 12–10A, B). All of the above represent the classic pattern, which is present in more than 90% of lobular carcinomas. Additional variants have been described including a *solid* (Fechner, 1975) pattern characterized by aggregates of tumor cells with similar characteristics but without intervening stroma and separated by delicate vascular channels (Fig. 12–10C). An alveolar pattern features solid nests of 30 or more cells separated by a delicate thin stroma (Martinez and Azzopardi, 1979) (Fig. 12–10D). A mixed variant shows a combination of the other patterns in various proportions. Fisher and associates (1977) described a variant of invasive lobular carcinoma that featured tubule formation *(tubulolobular)* (Fig. 12–10E). The distribution of the various types, classic, solid, alveolar, and mixed types are 30%, 22%, 19%, and 29%, respectively. An additional pattern has been recently described as *anaplastic.* To explain the morphologic variants it has been postulated that lobular carcinoma arises from the terminal secretory unit composed of the lobules and the terminal ducts. Infiltrating lobular carcinoma can occur in association with other types of breast carcinoma. An interesting feature of infiltrating lobular carcinoma is that the pattern of metastatic spread is different from that of infiltrating ductal carcinoma, showing preferential involvement of viscera (Figs. 12–11 and 12–12).

Estrogen receptor positivity has been noted in as many as 92% of infiltrating lobular carcinomas, including the classic type and the variants. Progesterone receptors are also positive in a large percentage.

Treatment should be patterned along the lines of other types of infiltrating ductal carcinomas, though multicentricity is common in this type of tumor and should be taken into consideration. The prognosis, according to various studies, is not different from that for infiltrating ductal carcinoma of no specific type when tumors of similar stage are compared. Claims have been made of prognostic differences according to the different microscopic patterns (variants worse than classic) (Dixon et al., 1983; and Di-Constanzo, 1990), but this needs to be confirmed with larger numbers of patients.

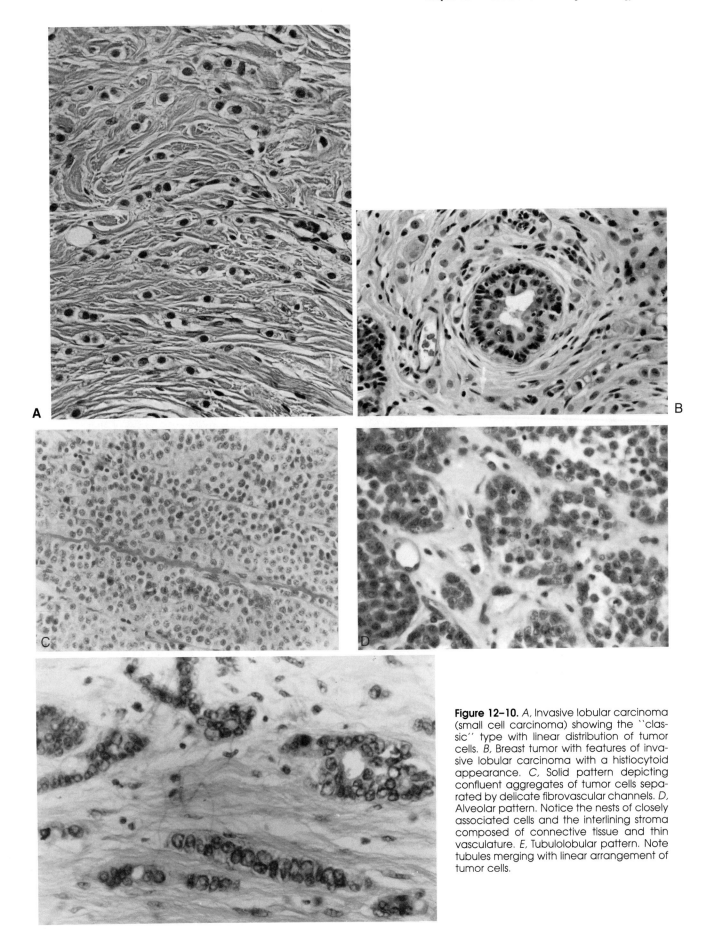

Figure 12–10. *A*, Invasive lobular carcinoma (small cell carcinoma) showing the ''classic'' type with linear distribution of tumor cells. *B*, Breast tumor with features of invasive lobular carcinoma with a histiocytoid appearance. *C*, Solid pattern depicting confluent aggregates of tumor cells separated by delicate fibrovascular channels. *D*, Alveolar pattern. Notice the nests of closely associated cells and the interlining stroma composed of connective tissue and thin vasculature. *E*, Tubulolobular pattern. Note tubules merging with linear arrangement of tumor cells.

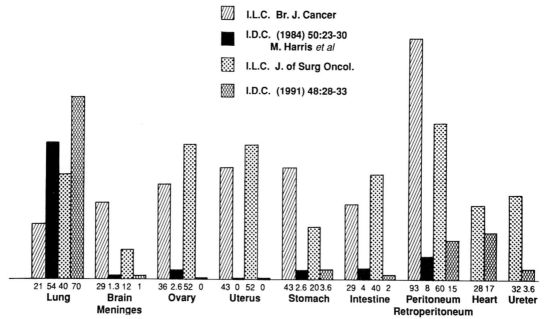

Pattern of Distribution of Metastasis of Infiltrating Lobular Carcinoma and Infiltrating Ductal Carcinoma N.O.S. Including 39 I.L.C.. and 271 I.D.C.

I.L.C. Br. J. Cancer
I.D.C. (1984) 50:23-30
        M. Harris *et al*
I.L.C. J. of Surg Oncol.
I.D.C. (1991) 48:28-33

| 21 54 40 70 | 29 1.3 12 1 | 36 2.6 52 0 | 43 0 52 0 | 43 2.6 20 3.6 | 29 4 40 2 | 93 8 60 15 | 28 17 | 32 3.6 |
| Lung | Brain Meninges | Ovary | Uterus | Stomach | Intestine | Peritoneum Retroperitoneum | Heart | Ureter |

Figure 12–11. Metastatic distribution of infiltrative ductal carcinoma NOS and invasive lobular carcinoma.

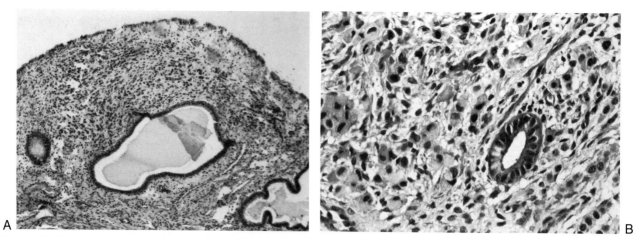

Figure 12–12. *A,* Endometrial polyp infiltrated by metastases from the breast tumor depicted in Figure 12–10*A. B,* Higher magnification of *A.* Notice linear distribution of tumor cells. (Courtesy of Dr. Marilyn Intengan.)

TUBULAR CARCINOMA

The distinctive characteristic of tubular carcinoma is well-delineated tubules or glands separated by a fibrous stroma. Because of its bland appearance it has been termed *well-differentiated carcinoma* or *orderly carcinoma,* and has been confused with other benign lesions of the breast such as sclerosing adenosis and radial scars. It was identified by Cornil and Ranvier in 1869. In symptomatic patients it is rare, comprising between 0.4% and 1% of breast cancers; however, the widespread use of mammography has resulted in increased detection of these tumors—to as high as 9% in asymptomatic patients subjected to mass screening (Patchetsky et al., 1977). The incidence is increased further when tubular carcinomas associated with other types of carcinoma are included (mixed variety) in reports. A 5% incidence of pure tubular carcinoma was recorded in the Breast Cancer Detection Demonstration Project (BCDDP) in Columbia, Missouri, whereas an 8% incidence was found nationwide (Beahrs et al., 1979). In another study (Rosen et al., 1985), tubular carcinoma accounted for 9% of carcinomas 1 cm or less in diameter.

On gross inspection this tumor is a poorly circumscribed grayish tan, hard or firm mass with retracted cut surface and with infiltrative margins. It cannot be distinguished on gross inspection from ductal carcinoma NOS with productive fibrosis.

The prognosis of tubular carcinoma is excellent. Metastases to the axillary lymph nodes occur in no more than 18.6% of cases, depending on the composition of the tumor (pure and mixed) and on its size. No axillary metastases occur when tubular carcinoma represents more than 75% of the tumor, and rarely when tumors are less than 1 cm in diameter. The dimensions of tubular carcinomas vary; they can be as small as 0.2 cm in diameter, or as large as 12 cm if the mixed variety is included. Haagensen reported that the average size of pure (100%) tubular carcinomas was less than 2 cm and that of the mixed variety was more than 2 cm (Haagensen, 1986). This observation has been confirmed (McDivitt et al., 1982) in more recent studies, where 80% and 52%, respectively, of pure and mixed tubular carcinomas were 1 cm or less in diameter (Tobon and Salazar, 1977; and Carsten et al., 1985).

The microscopic appearance is characteristically an irregular distribution of tubular structures, often with angulated contours, lined by a single row of monomorphous cells with good nuclear grade and rare mitoses (Fig. 12–13). Frequently, apocrine snouts project into the lumens of the tubules. Calcifications are observed in about 50% of cases. The intervening stroma is abundant, predominantly fibroblastic, and cellular. In situ carcinomas (lobular or ductal) are frequently associated with this type of tumor. Differentiating this lesion from sclerosing adenosis can be difficult; however, the lack of basal membrane and a myoepithelial layer, in addition to the features previously described, can help make the distinction. A rounded, lobular contour is always present in sclerosing adenosis. Tubular carcinoma should be distinguished from well-differentiated invasive ductal carcinomas NOS (Taylor and Norris, 1970). The criteria for defining pure tubular carcinoma are not univer-

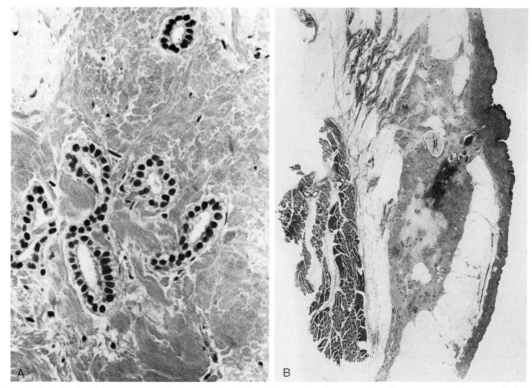

Figure 12–13. *A,* Tubular carcinoma; well-formed glands lined by a single row of cells, monomorphous, with bland nuclei. Apocrine snouts are visible. *B,* Whole breast section shows tubular carcinoma in the darkest area. In other segments of the specimen, lobular carcinoma in situ is also present.

sally accepted. Carsten and associates (1985) diagnose "pure" tubular carcinoma when 100% of the neoplasm is composed of tubules and the mixed tubular type when the lesion is at least 75% tubular. The size of tubular carcinomas appears to increase in proportion to the nontubular component, suggesting that some invasive ductal carcinomas are initially tubular carcinomas, that becoming larger, become less differentiated (Oberman and Fidler, 1979).

DUCTAL CARCINOMA IN SITU (INTRADUCTAL CARCINOMA)

The current diagnostic criteria for ductal carcinoma in situ (DCIS) include a heterogenous group. The common microscopic hallmark is the transformation or replacement of the ductal epithelial lining by a carcinomatous growth confined to the boundaries of pre-existing mammary ducts without invasion of the stroma. The diagnosis can only be established by careful microscopic examination of appropriate tissue samples. This type of carcinoma has been recognized for more than a century (Fechner, 1993); however, its natural history still remains largely uncertain. Before the mammographic era its frequency was 1% to 5.6% of all breast cancers (Rosner et al., 1980). The increasing use of mammography resulted in a rise to 15% to 33% in screened populations (Baker, 1982; and Schwartz et al., 1992). It can be manifested by a palpable mass, nipple discharge, or Paget's disease, but more frequently it is discovered as an incidental finding in biopsy material obtained for another lesion or as a mammographic abnormality. The manner of clinical detection is the basis used by some (Gump et al., 1987) for dividing intraductal carcinomas into a "gross group" (including symptomatic patients) and a "microscopic group" (those detected incidentally or by mammography). The gross features of intraductal carcinoma are best appreciated in the comedo type, which produces characteristic cylinders of necrotic material that is extruded when the tumor tissue is compressed.

Microscopically, several variants of DCIS can be identified: *comedo, micropapillary, papillary, cribriform, solid,* and *combinations* of patterns (Fig. 12–14). Comedocarcinomas consist of large pleomorphic cells with abundant cytoplasm, bizarre nuclei, and frequent mitoses. Focal central necrosis is the hallmark of this variant. Periductal fibrosis is a frequent component. This variant is the largest in size, most frequently palpable, and easiest to detect mammographically. It also has the greatest malignant potential. Cribriform DCIS is typically a monomorphic population of smaller cells with round nuclei exhibiting rare mitosis and showing a sievelike pattern. Necrosis is not common. The micropapillary type consists of monomorphic, proliferating cells, forming filiform fronds without central fibrovascular cores that project into the lumen of the duct. Necrosis and cellular atypia are not frequently present. The combination of cribriform and micropapillary patterns is so frequent that some authors consider them together. The papillary type of DCIS shows filiform excrescences composed of a fibrovascular core covered by atypical cells that project into the ductal lumen. The degree of atypia should be sufficient to qualify as carcinoma. The solid subtype consists of a solid growth pattern of pleomorphic cells with well-defined margins, atypical nuclei with prominent nucleoli, and abnormal mitoses. Combinations of subtypes are frequent. The most common single type is the comedo, representing about two-thirds of all DCIS, followed in decreasing order by cribriform or micropapillary, solid, and papillary. The morphologic criteria for classification are not standardized.

There is a spectrum in the biologic capability and the corresponding clinical behavior of the various types of intraductal carcinoma. The comedo type has the highest nuclear grade (irregular nuclei with coarse chromatin and prominent nucleoli) and the cribriform or micropapillary type at the other end of the scale exhibits the lowest nuclear grade. The micropapillary and cribiform variants are most frequently multicentric. The rate of growth of comedocarcinoma is rapid, with a high S-phase fraction on flow cytometry and a high thymidine-labeling index (TLI) (Meyer, 1986). Estrogen receptors have been reported in fewer than 20% of the comedo type and in more than 50% of the cribriform/micropapillary type (Giri et al., 1989). The comedo variant shows strong membrane staining for C-erb-B-2, whereas staining is weak or negative in the other variants (Tuluson et al., 1985). Similar differences are evident in the dimensions of nuclei, which are large (>20 μm) in the comedo type but smaller in the cribriform/micropapillary type (<10 μm) (Mayr et al., 1991). In the majority of studies the comedo variant is more prone to recurrence and to evolving into an invasive carcinoma. In a group of patients with DCIS treated with breast conservation (Sagebiel, 1969) 16% of 31 patients with the comedo type had recurrences, whereas 33 patients with cribriform or pleomorphic types had no recurrences. The available evidence is persuasive for the existence of a strong relationship between comedocarcinoma and invasive carcinoma. There is increasing evidence that the histologic patterns displayed by intraductal carcinoma correspond to variations in their biologic properties (Ottesen et al., 1992; Bellamy et al., 1993; and Solin et al., 1993). Careful assessment of histologic type and nuclear grade can provide information relevant to the type of treatment, the extent of the disease in the breast, and the risk of developing an invasive recurrence.

LOBULAR CARCINOMA IN SITU

Lobular carcinoma in situ (LCIS, lobular neoplasia) is a symptomless lesion of the breast that lacks distinguishing gross characteristics. The diagnosis is established by microscopic examination. Most of the time it is an incidental finding on a breast biopsy specimen that was removed because of a coexisting benign or malignant lesion. Although more than 50 years has elapsed since the initial description in 1941 (Foote and Stewart, 1941; and Muir, 1941), and despite recognition by others since early in the century as "acinar carcinoma" (Cornil and Ranviere, 1869), its clinical significance is elusive and its management, still controversial. Investigators agree, however, that it is multicentric in about 80% of cases and bilateral in some 15% to 40% (Lattes, 1980; and Rosner et al., 1980). This lesion gener-

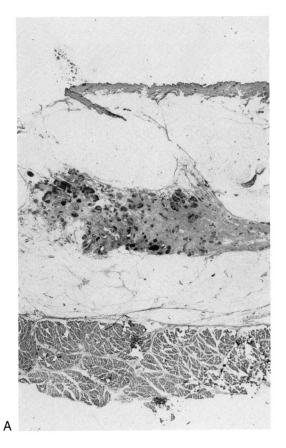

A

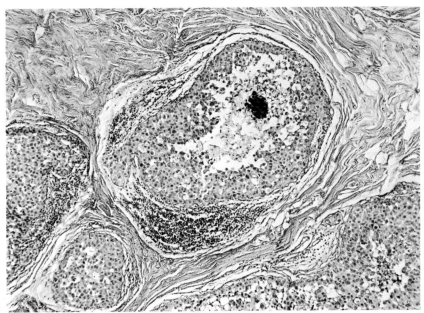

B

Figure 12–14. *A,* Whole breast mount, showing foci of intraductal carcinoma, comedo type. Tumor is represented by circular darker areas. *B,* Comedo pattern with central necrosis and calcification.

Illustration continued on following page

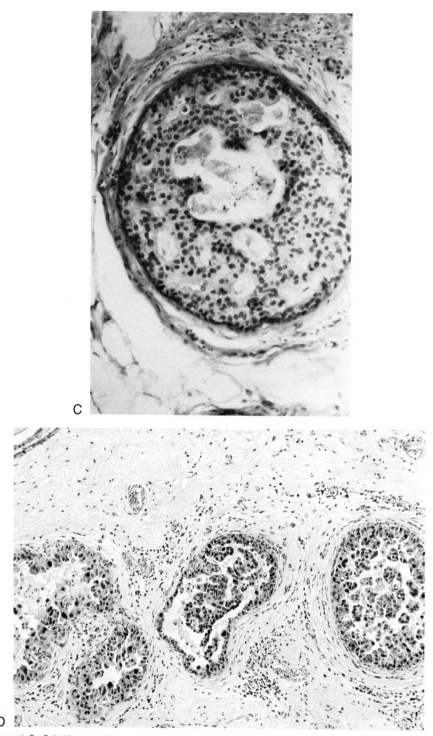

C

D

Figure 12–14 *Continued C,* Cribriform pattern with punched out round spaces. *D,* Papillary pattern with central necrosis and calcification.

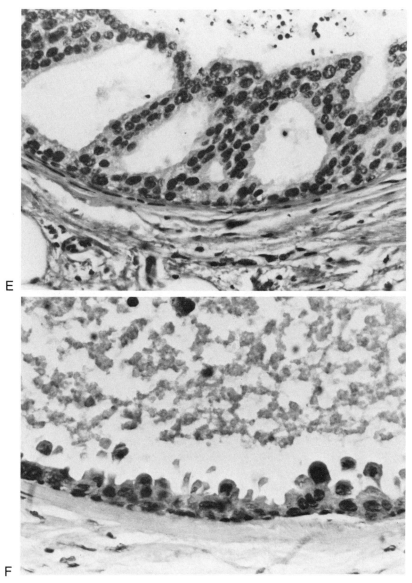

Figure 12-14 *Continued E,* Roman bridge pattern. *F,* "Clinging" type of DCIS.

ally is found in premenopausal women; 80% to 89% of patients are younger than 55 years. The average age of women with LCIS is 10 and 15 years younger, respectively, than that of patients with infiltrating ductal and infiltrating lobular carcinoma. Before mammography was widely used, 3% or less of breast biopsy specimens contained LCIS; now it is found in about 10% of specimens. Mammographic visualization is generally not diagnostic. Foci of calcification in adjacent mammary lobules may be the only abnormality detected on a mammogram.

The microscopic criteria consist of proliferation of small, round monomorphic cells, larger than the cells lining the normal ducts. The cells are loosely cohesive and obliterate the acini and distend the lobule. Extension may occur to the terminal duct and produce a pagetoid appearance (Fig. 12–15). The proliferating cells exhibit variable amounts of cytoplasm; they can be vacuolated and contain mucin, and they have uniform, bland-looking nuclei. Mitoses are rare

and necrosis even rarer. The differential diagnosis of LCIS includes ductal and lobular hyperplasia with various degrees of atypia. Their morphologic distinction from lobular neoplasia can be difficult, if not occasionally impossible. It is important to realize that both originate in the terminal duct lobular unit.

The phenomenon of coexistent LCIS and intraductal carcinoma has been reported to be as frequent as 22% in a study including 88 lesions (Ottesen et al., 1993); and they sometimes merge within a single lobular duct unit (Rosen, 1980). To some this association is not simply coincidental, since they also share other characteristics such as multicentricity and bilaterality, indicating "the carcinomatous character of the lobular as well as the ductal component" (Ottesen et al., 1993; and Rosen, 1980).

When patients with LCIS are treated by biopsy only, follow-up shows that their risk of developing invasive ductal or lobular carcinoma is 7 to 11 times that expected,

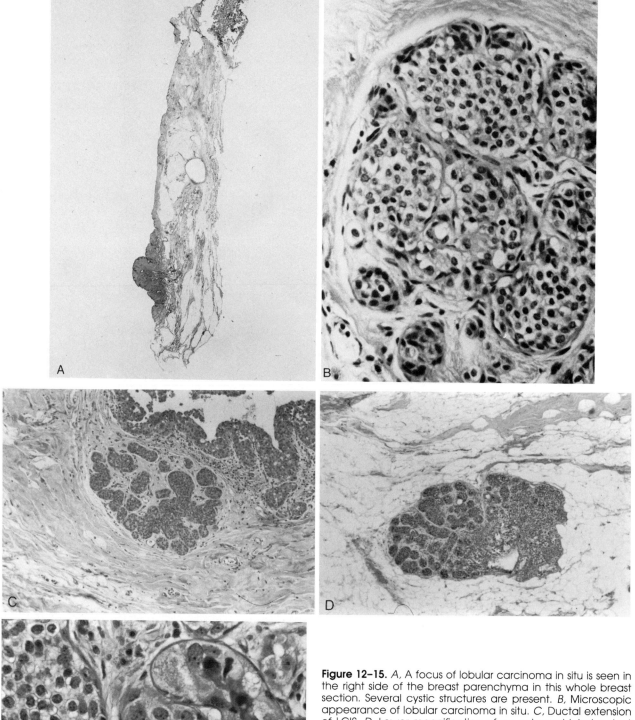

Figure 12–15. *A,* A focus of lobular carcinoma in situ is seen in the right side of the breast parenchyma in this whole breast section. Several cystic structures are present. *B,* Microscopic appearance of lobular carcinoma in situ. *C,* Ductal extension of LCIS. *D,* Lower magnification of an enlarged lobular duct unit containing both lobular carcinoma in situ and ductal carcinoma in situ. *E,* Notice toward left small monomorphic cells characteristic of LCIS, while toward the right the presence of larger-cell, higher–nuclear grade characteristic of intraductal carcinoma.

corresponding to 15% to 30% of the patients; approximately 50% of the invasive carcinomas arise in the contralateral breast. The interval between the diagnostic biopsy and the discovery of an invasive carcinoma varies. The prevalent view about management of patients with pure LCIS favors careful and periodic follow-up of both breasts; however, there is no consensus about what schedule is optimal.

RARE TYPES OF INVASIVE CARCINOMA

Adenocystic Carcinoma

Adenocystic carcinoma is an uncommon tumor that accounts for fewer than 0.2% of breast adenocarcinomas. The morphologic features are similar to those of other tumors known by the same name and more commonly observed in major and minor salivary glands, the tracheobronchial tree, lachrymal glands, tongue, nasopharynx, external ear canal, prostate, Bartholin's glands, and uterine cervix.

It is perplexing that despite similarities (light microscopic

and ultrastructural) with the salivary gland counterpart, their biologic behavior is vastly different. In a review of 106 cases of adenocystic carcinoma, distant metastases occurred in only seven instances, characteristically without involvement of the nodes of the axilla (Peters and Wolff, 1982). An authenticated case with metastases to the axillary lymph nodes has been reported (Wells et al., 1986).

Tumors are generally small (median 2.2 cm) and commonly appear as a small mass near the nipple. They are circumscribed, not encapsulated, of firm consistency, gray to yellow and without necrosis. They grow slowly. Microscopically (Fig. 12–16) the tumor is composed of two cell types. The first, a small basophilic cell with scanty cytoplasm, hyperchromatic monomorphic nuclei, and infrequent mitoses, and a second type that is smaller with bright eosinophilic cytoplasm. They are arranged in different patterns (cribriform, duct-forming, solid), pure or in combination. The stroma is an integral part of the tumor. It can be myxoid, hyaline, or a combination, forming "cylinders" around and within the nests of tumor cells and justifying the name *cylindroma* sometimes used to designate the tumor when it is found in other sites.

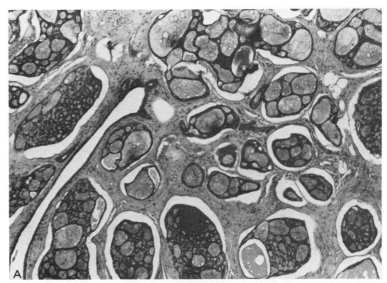

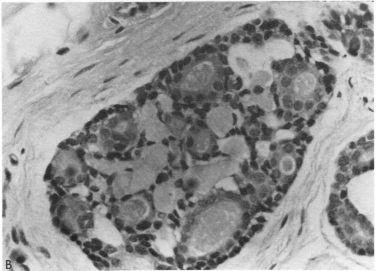

Figure 12–16. Low-, *A,* and high-, *B,* power views of adenocystic carcinoma. Notice the cribriform pattern and the stroma forming cylinders around and within the tumor.

The prognosis is excellent, but since recurrences and metastases have been described many years after treatment, long-term follow-up is mandatory. The practice of dividing the tumors into high- and low-grade ones has predictive value for the salivary congener but for the breast has been unproductive in short-term follow-up (Rosen, 1989).

Squamous Cell Carcinoma

While squamous metaplasia is perhaps the commonest metaplastic alteration of human breast carcinomas, pure squamous cell carcinoma is one of the rarest tumors (Fig. 12–17). Fisher and coworkers (1983) reported squamous metaplasia in 3.7% of 1665 invasive breast carcinomas; however, they did not observe a single case of pure squamous cell carcinoma, nor did Haagensen (1986) between 1919 and 1973. The main criteria for the diagnosis of squamous cell carcinoma of the breast are lack of connection with the overlying epidermis and the absence of any other type of coexisting breast cancer. The possibilities of origin from an old abscess and of being a metastasis should also be ruled out. About 55 cases have been reported in the English literature, representing fewer than 1% of all breast carcinomas. These tumors are up to 10 cm in diameter. Central necrosis and cyst formation can be observed in tumors larger than 2 cm. Microscopically, the conventional features of squamous cell carcinoma are observed—stratification, intercellular bridges, keratin production, and areas of acantholysis. Spindle cell metaplasia may be the dominant feature, requiring immunohistochemical stains to determine its epithelial nature.

It is difficult to predict the behavior, as few cases are reported. Only three pure primary squamous cell carcinomas were found among 4000 breast cancers by Toikanen (1981); all patients died of dissemination after radical mastectomy. Similar behavior was observed in three cases reported by Eusebi and colleagues (1986a) in which the tumors were an acantholytic variant of squamous cell carcinoma. In the three cases reported by Lafreniere and colleagues (1986) there was only one instance of metastasis to the axillary nodes. Most patients are treated with mastectomy, occasionally followed by chemotherapy or irradiation. The prognosis is comparable to that for invasive ductal carcinoma.

Metaplastic Carcinomas

Metaplastic carcinomas of the breast represent a heterogenous group of tumors that microscopically are composed of an admixture of epithelial and mesenchymal cells with varying degrees of differentiation. The epithelial component can be adenocarcinoma or squamous cell carcinoma, or both, or mixed adenosquamous carcinoma in combination with spindle cells. The mesenchymal component can show osseous or chondroid metaplastic changes (Figs. 12–18, 12–19). The morphologic appearance of all possible combinations is bewildering and confusing. The classification of these tumors proposed by Tavassoli (Table 12–2)

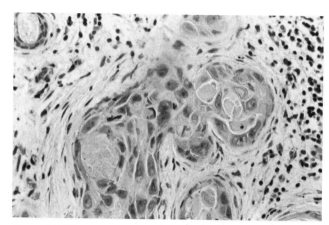

Figure 12–17. Moderately differentiated squamous cell carcinoma; notice abnormal mitotic figures.

serves as a practical guide for their study and understanding. The metaplastic nature of the mesenchymal component can be verified only by the use of immunohistochemistry to demonstrate an epithelial antigen. Ultrastructural studies are necessary in cases not clearly recognizable by their phenotypic character. Obviously, when the mesenchymal elements show no epithelial phenotype, those cases should be considered carcinosarcomas.

Secretory Carcinoma

Secretory carcinoma has distinct microscopic characteristics. It was described in 1966 by McDivitt and Stewart. It was designated in their publication as *juvenile carcinoma*, as it occurred in a group of seven patients ranging in age from 3 to 15 years; however, in subsequent publications about a third of the cases occurred in women older than 30 years. Consequently, the initial designation was replaced by the descriptive term *secretory carcinoma* (Tavassoli and Norris, 1980). Tumors of this sort also have been described in males (Akhtar et al., 1983). The usual presentation is as an indolent mass. On gross examination the tumor is a well-circumscribed, firm, grayish white mass with sharply delineated margins that can be confused with a fibroadenoma. The size ranges from 1 to 12 cm in diameter. The microscopic appearance is characterized by acinar structures containing secretory material within the lumens and in the cytoplasm (Fig. 12–20). The secretory material generally stains positive for mucopolysaccharides and for various milk proteins. The prognosis appears to be related to the

Table 12–2. CLASSIFICATION OF METAPLASTIC CARCINOMA

Squamous carcinoma (keratinizing, nonkeratinizing, spindle cell metaplasia)
Adenosquamous (high-grade and low-grade)
Adenocarcinoma with spindle cell metaplasia
Carcinoma with chondroid or osseous differentiation

(Modified from Tavassoli, F. A.: Pathology of the Breast. New York, Elsevier, 1992.)

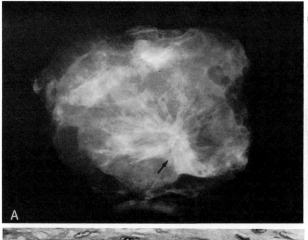

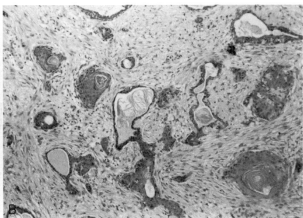

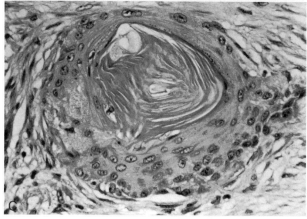

Figure 12-18. Squamous metaplasia of the breast. *A,* Specimen mammogram showing lesion with a stellate configuration *(arrow). B,* Foci of squamous metaplasia in numerous mammary ducts. *C,* Showing well-oriented squamous epithelium with keratin production. Patient remains free of abnormalities 6 years after simple excision.

patient's age and the tumor's size, according to the small number of cases reported. In children, tumors smaller than 2 cm are associated with a good prognosis and can be treated adequately with wide local excision. In older patients, because of the higher frequency of node involvement, more aggressive treatment should be considered, including mastectomy (Krausz et al., 1989).

Signet Ring–Cell Carcinoma

Signet ring–cell carcinoma was first described by Saphir in 1941 as a variety of mucinous carcinoma. Controversy exists about its histogenesis. Some authors (Steinbrecher and Silverberg, 1976), believe it represents part of the spectrum of invasive lobular carcinoma because of similarities in the pattern of growth such as the linear arrangement of the tumor cells, the coexistence of lobular carcinoma in situ, and the metastatic pattern in the lymph nodes (sinus catarrh). Other investigators (Harris et al., 1978) consider it a well-defined pathologic entity. The World Health Organization (1981) has not recognized it as a distinct tumor type. Its frequency, therefore, is difficult to determine. The clinical manifestations and gross appearance are not different from those of infiltrating ductal carcinomas NOS. The microscopic hallmark (Fig. 12–21) is signet ring cells. Pure tumors are rare; only two such examples were identified at Edinburgh (Page, 1991) during a review of 1050 breast

carcinomas. The criterion was that more than 90% of the tumor cells must exhibit the characteristic intracytoplasmatic vacuole that contained mucin and that compressed and indented the nuclei. The mucin stains with mucicarmine and with periodic acid–Schiff (PAS) and is diastase resistant. This tumor is associated with infiltrating ductal or lobular carcinomas (or their in situ forms) as well as with extracellular mucinous carcinoma. In its pure form it is more aggressive than the mucinous, ductal, and lobular invasive types. Bilaterality is a risk when these tumors are associated with lobular carcinoma. They have a poor prognosis; 60% of 24 patients studied by Merino and LiVolsi (1981) died of their cancers within 7 years.

Lipid-Rich Carcinoma

Lipid-rich carcinoma was first described by Aboumrad and coworkers in 1963. It is an aggressive tumor. Many patients already have metastases in axillary nodes when their cancer is discovered, and more than half die within 2 years after the diagnosis is established. The presenting clinical manifestation is a mass in the breast. The gross appearance is deceptive, lacking the conventional features of ductal carcinoma and sometimes mimicking a benign process. Microscopically, the tumor consists of large cells with small, round, oval nuclei and clear, vacuolated, foamy cytoplasm that contains material that stains positive for neutral lipids.

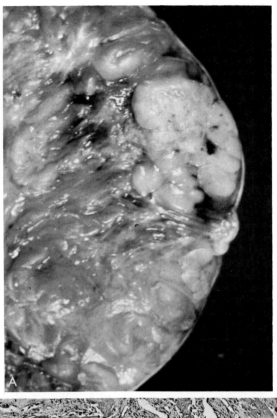

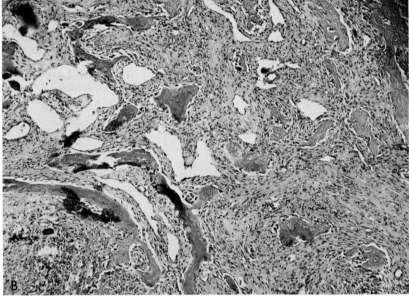

Figure 12–19. Metaplastic carcinoma with osseous differentiation. This carcinoma of the breast in a 67-year-old woman displayed considerable osseous formation and produced extensive metastases to the gastrointestinal tract. *A,* The primary tumor appeared circumscribed. *B,* Many bony spicules are present in the tissues.

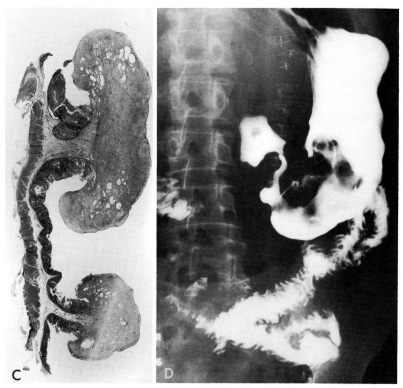

Figure 12–19 *Continued C,* Photomicrograph of the polypoid gastric metastases. *D,* Multiple polypoid metastases in the stomach demonstrated with a barium swallow. The patient developed dissemination 1 year after a radical mastectomy and died 2 years later.

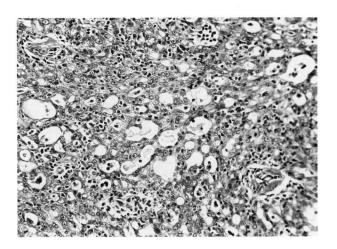

Figure 12–20. Low-power histologic section of secretory carcinoma. A 15-year-old girl had a 1.8 cm nodule removed from the left breast on 6-16-82 that was diagnosed as secretory carcinoma. After confirmation by the AFIP the biopsy site was widely re-excised 6-23-82 with tumor-free margins, and the patient has remained free of recurrence as of July 1989. ER was measured as 15.6 fmol/mg protein. (Courtesy of Paul Fox, M.D.)

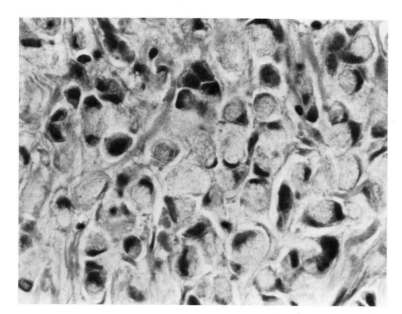

Figure 12–21. Intracellular mucinous carcinoma: Compact aggregate of signet ring cells with peripheral nuclei and foamy cytoplasm, positive for mucus.

Whether the latter represents a cell product or a degenerative product is an issue still unsettled. In the series reported by Ramos and Taylor (1974) areas of intraductal and lobular carcinoma in situ were found in some tumors (Fig. 12–22).

Sudoriferous Carcinoma

Sudoriferous carcinoma is a rare tumor also known as *apocrine carcinoma, sweat gland carcinoma, oncocytic carcinoma, carcinoma with apocrine metaplasia*, and *carcinoma with pink cells* (Archer and Omar, 1969; and Azzopardi, 1979). The gross characteristics do not distinguish it from the ordinary infiltrating ductal carcinoma. The microscopic appearance is characterized by cells with abundant opaque eosinophilic cytoplasm resembling the cells of apocrine glands of the skin (Fig. 12–23). Generally it is a well-differentiated tumor; when a glandular arrangement exists, apical snouts can be observed. Focal apocrine features have been observed in mucinous, lobular, medullary, and tubular carcinomas. The derivation and character of the apocrine type of tumor is still controversial. Some authors believe these tumors represent embryonal inclusion of sweat gland structures within the breast, focal degenerative changes, or metaplasia. There is disagreement about the ultrastructural features of these tumors in the limited number of studies that have been conducted (Eusebi et al., 1986*b*). Many others believe it represents a rare form of infiltrating ductal carcinoma with a characteristic light microscopic appearance and distinctive ultrastructural features. The prognosis of apocrine carcinoma, invasive or intraductal, is determined by prognostic factors not different from those pertaining to ductal carcinomas—for example, grade, size, and axillary lymph node status. Of interest is the apparent sensitivity of these tumors to androgen therapy, perhaps an important feature for making therapeutic decisions (Miller et al., 1985).

Carcinoma with Neuroendocrine Features

In 1963, Feyter and Hartman described for the first time two patients with mucinous carcinoma of the breast that exhibited carcinoid features (cited by Page and Anderson, 1987). The tumor cells showed cytoplasmic argyrophilic granules and both patients displayed clinical manifestations of endocrine activity. Serotonin was found in the tumors. In 1977, Cubilla and Woodruff reported eight patients whose breast tumors showed morphologic features of carcinoid tumors similar to those in other organs, with argyrophilic granules and dense-cored granules of neurosecretory type ultrastructurally. None of those patients displayed endocrine-related symptoms. This has been referred to as *biochemical* or *endocrine metaplasia*. During subsequent years, similar findings were reported in a variety of tumors without the morphology of carcinoid tumors, including ductal carcinomas without specific type and papillary and lob-

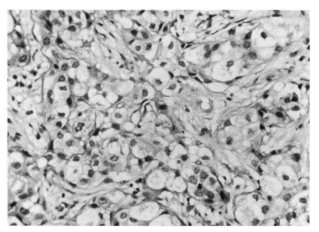

Figure 12–22. Lipid-rich carcinoma.

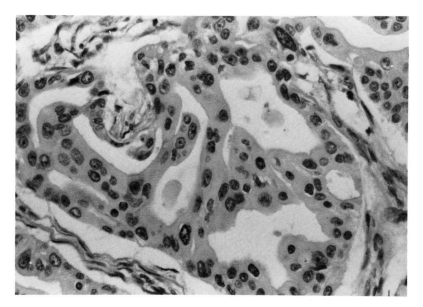

Figure 12–23. Sudoriferous carcinoma is a rare lesion that mimics sweat glands in its appearance. Tumor cells are large and possess eosinophilic cytoplasm.

ular carcinomas (both in situ and invasive), intraductal carcinoma, and mucinous carcinomas. Conversely there are breast carcinomas whose morphology is that of carcinoid tumors but that lack those immunohistochemical or ultrastructural characteristics. Their histogenesis remains uncertain. The designation for this tumor was suggested by the morphologic similarity to carcinoid tumors. No relationship has been established between the presence of cytoplasmic argyrophilia and the clinical behavior of the tumor.

Glycogen-Rich Carcinoma

Glycogen-rich carcinoma is a tumor characterized by cells with optically clear cytoplasm that contains glycogen but no mucin or lipids. The tumor cells are arranged predominantly in solid or papillary patterns. Similarities were noted to the breast bud epithelium of the 13-week embryo and to clear cell tumors of the salivary glands, lungs, and female genital tract. The clinical presentation and gross characteristics are not distinctive. Their frequency in two series (Fisher et al., 1981; and Toikanen and Joensuu, 1991) was reported between 1.4% and 3%, indicating a variation in diagnostic criteria. This tumor is more aggressive than invasive ductal carcinoma. Axillary metastases are more frequent. In one study the corrected 5-year survival rate of patients was 33%, while it was 56% for patients with other types of invasive carcinoma of the breast.

SPECIAL MANIFESTATIONS OF BREAST CARCINOMA

Paget's Disease of the Breast

Paget's disease occurs in some 1% to 5% of all breast carcinomas. The clinical description of James Paget's in 1874 remains unsurpassed. It is manifested clinically by an eczematoid and erosive lesion of the nipple and areola and

microscopically by the presence in the dermis of large pale cells with abundant cytoplasm, a large nucleus, and prominent nucleoli (Fig. 12–24). These are the histopathologic hallmarks of Paget cells, which are, in fact, cancer cells. It is of interest that, though James Paget described the clinical features of the lesion, the characteristic Paget's cells were not described until 1889 by Darier.

In almost all cases, Paget's disease is associated with an additional cancer within the breast. In half the cases a mass can be palpated in the subjacent mammary tissue. The underlying carcinomas vary in their clinical and pathologic features, but in most instances the lesion is an invasive ductal carcinoma of no specific type. It can be a favorable type such as medullary or papillary carcinoma or a DCIS still within the boundaries of the mammary ducts or limited to the nipple. It may occur with tumors associated with a dismal prognosis such as *inflammatory carcinoma*. Paget's disease is a manifestation of mammary duct carcinoma rather than an independent neoplastic entity (Ashikari et al., 1974).

Numerous views have been expressed concerning the histogenesis of Paget's cells (Muir, 1935; and Nadji et al., 1982). Some consider them an altered melanocyte, though results of immunostaining indicate otherwise (a positive reaction to cytokeratin and polyclonal carcinoembryonic antigen). An intraepidermal or in situ origin is supported by the occasional discontinuity between the tumor and the nipple epithelium, absence of an underlying tumor in some cases despite careful search, Paget's disease in ectopic nipples, the existence of heterotopies in the nipple epithelium, and desmosomal junctions between Paget's cells and keratinocytes. The prevalent view is that it represents an epidermotropic upward migration to the nipple of adenocarcinoma cells originating in the underlying tumor. The treatment and prognosis depend on the intercurrent tumor (Ridenhour et al., 1969; and Ashikari et al., 1974). When no tumor is palpable the 5- and 10-year survival rates are 92% and 87%, respectively; when a palpable mass exists they are 45% and 38%. Consequently, treatment is tailored

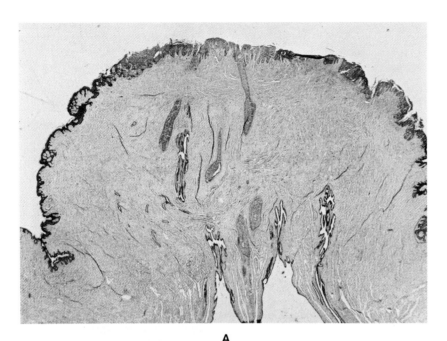

A

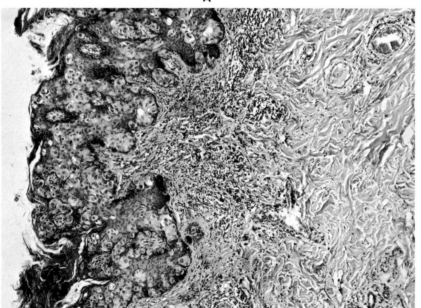

Figure 12–24. *A,* A low-power photomicrograph of the nipple shows lactiferous ducts engorged with ductal carcinoma and extensive changes characteristic of Paget's disease in the epidermis. *B,* High-power magnification of the epidermis of the nipple demonstrates extensive infiltration by the large cells with clear cytoplasm characteristic of Paget's disease.

to circumstances. Local excision of the nipple and areola, limited mastectomy with or without lymphadenectomy, and simple, total, and radical mastectomy have been the numerous therapeutic modes employed. Radiotherapy has been reported to be effective in cases when there were no palpable tumor and no mammographic alterations.

Inflammatory Carcinoma

Inflammatory carcinoma represents 1% to 4% of breast carcinomas and it occurs slightly more frequently in postmenopausal women. It is characterized clinically by erythema of the skin, *peau d'orange edema*, increased local temperature, pain and tenderness, and enlargement and induration of the affected breast (Taylor and Meltzer, 1938). Although the diagnosis is suspected on clinical grounds, a biopsy is necessary to exclude benign inflammatory conditions (Ellis and Teitelbaum, 1974). Conversely, the clinical manifestations can be so subtle that they go undetected (occult inflammatory carcinoma) (Saltzstein, 1974).

The identification of inflammatory carcinoma is based on a typical clinical appearance or on the demonstration of tumor invasion in dermal lymphatics, but inflammatory carcinoma represents a whole spectrum of clinical manifestations, and not all signs appear simultaneously or with the same intensity (Haagensen, 1986).

Its clinical appearance can lead to treatment for infection or for abscess; in a previous study, 20% of patients with inflammatory carcinoma were treated with antibiotics (Lucas and Perez-Mesa, 1978). Mammography shows thickening of the skin, which is almost always present.

The gross characteristics are variable. Frequently no dominant mass is present, only diffuse induration of the parenchyma and thickening of the skin (Fig. 12–25A–C). Microscopically, the presence of nests of tumor cells plugging the dermal and intramammary lymphatics constitutes the histopathologic hallmark. In the dermis a cellular inflammatory infiltrate may be present to variable degree or absent. Invasive ductal carcinomas, poorly differentiated or undifferentiated NOS, are mostly responsible. At the time of diagnosis tumor has frequently spread into the axillary lymph nodes.

Fewer than 5% of patients survive more than 5 years after surgery alone. Since the utilization of chemotherapy and radiotherapy, with or without surgery, the 5-year survival rate has been as high as 30% (McBride and Hortobagyi, 1985). Treatment induces characteristic morphologic changes in the tumor (Fig. 12–25D,E) (Kennedy et al., 1990).

Rarely, local "inflammatory" manifestations of carcinoma can occur in the skin of the breast from metastases. This has been designated *carcinoma erysipelatoides* (Hazelrigg and Rudolph, 1977). These inflammatory characteristics are also the result of plugging of lymphatics by the metastatic tumor.

CLINICOPATHOLOGIC CORRELATIONS

The morphologic characteristics of tumors can be of considerable prognostic importance if the data are recorded and collected uniformly and with consistency. The use of a protocol facilitates this (Rilke et al., 1978; and Royal College of Pathologists Working Group, 1991). A printed form on which to record data on the gross and microscopic details of breast specimens should be available in the cutting and the readout room of the laboratory. The basic information includes pertinent clinical details and what procedure was used to obtain the specimen, according to the surgeon. The need to maintain close communication between surgeons, radiologists, and pathologists has been underscored by the increasing number of nonpalpable lesions from asymptomatic patients and the growing frequency of lumpectomy as the sole ablative therapy. Obtaining and processing specimens accurately requires cooperation between the specialists involved. A brief description of the various specimens that are received in the laboratory of pathology follows:

Fine needle aspiration cytology (FNAC) in many instances is the initial diagnostic procedure for palpable and nonpalpable breast masses. In experienced hands fine needle aspiration can determine if the lesion under scrutiny is cystic or solid, benign or malignant. In addition, the cytologic material can be utilized for the determination of hormone receptors and for flow cytometric and morphometric analysis (Fig. 12–26). The accuracy of the method depends on the experience of the pathologist.

Core needle biopsy provides tissue that is suitable for histologic preparation; it permits assessment not only of cytologic details but of the architectural structure of tumors. In addition, in most instances it allows the pathologist to distinguish between in situ and invasive ductal carcinomas, something that is not possible with cytologic preparations alone. Incisional biopsies are obtained from palpable lesions and generally provide clear histologic evidence of the nature of the lesion.

Excisional biopsy is prompted by a palpable mass or an alteration in a mammogram, or both. It may be the only surgical procedure if breast-conserving therapy is selected; consequently, the assessment of the margins of excision becomes critical. When nothing palpable is detected a radiograph of the specimen, made by either the radiologist or the pathologist is obligatory to compare with the prebiopsy mammogram and determine if the mammographic alteration has been removed. The specimen should be received intact with the markings necessary for orientation in case further surgery is necessary. In the author's institution (Roswell Park Cancer Institute) the various surfaces of the specimen are painted with different colors, which helps locate the specific margin at which the tumor is transected.

There is no consensus on the ideal method of determining the adequacy of surgical margins. In most circumstances gross inspection of the lumpectomy specimen by an experienced observer can determine with considerable accuracy if the margins of excision are adequate and free of tumor. This assessment must be confirmed by microscopic examination. The main objective is to arrive at an accurate diagnosis, and this takes priority over all other considerations (Association of Directors of Anatomic and Surgical Pathology, 1993). The decision to perform a frozen section examination requires careful judgment. If the suspicious lesion is larger than 1 cm in diameter a frozen section

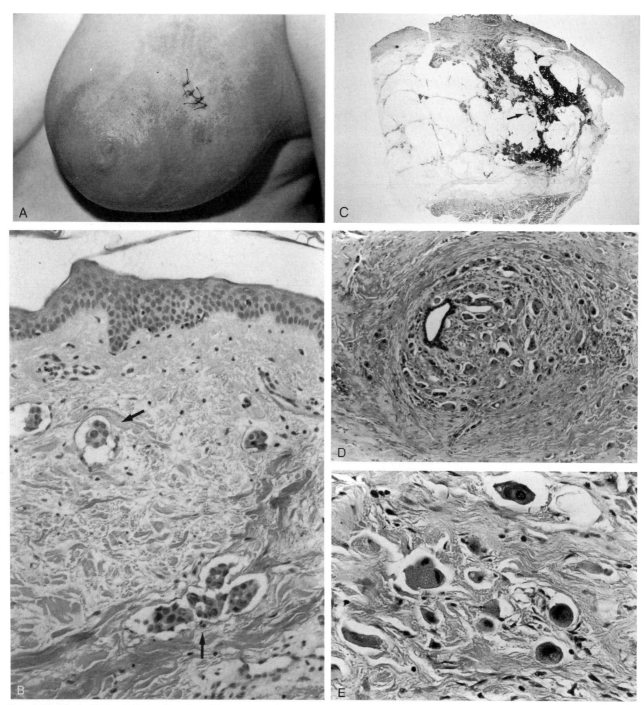

Figure 12–25. *A,* Clinical photo, showing enlargement of the breast, peau d'orange edema, and nipple retraction in a 28-year-old woman; *B,* Skin biopsy shows plugging of the dermal lymphatics by tumor *(arrows); C,* Whole mount of same breast exhibits extensive tumor infiltration. *D,* Effects of chemotherapy on inflammatory carcinoma of the breast. Notice degenerating tumor cells distributed in a concentric manner around a duct. *E,* Higher magnification shows extensive vacuolization of the cytoplasm.

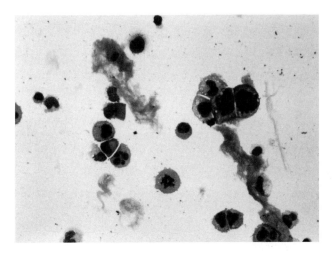

Figure 12-26. Fine needle aspiration of the breast shows clumps of hyperchromatic cells, exhibiting malignant features.

should be performed. A frozen section can be done if the lesion is large enough to permit a fresh tumor tissue sample for hormone receptor assay, flow cytometry, or other special procedures. No frozen section is done on lesions smaller than 1 cm in diameter. If the permanent sections show invasive carcinoma, hormone receptors can be determined from the fixed tissue with immunocytochemical methods. The artifact introduced by freezing tissue makes it difficult or impossible to evaluate the nature of the lesion on permanent section. Changes created by surgical cautery can also make margins difficult to evaluate.

The lumpectomy specimen should be handled with care, avoiding unnecessary pressure while drying its surface before applying the ink (Fig. 12–27). Undue pressure could result in artificial reduction of the thickness of the fat surrounding the tumor or seepage of the ink through a torn surface, creating a spurious surgical margin.

There is no uniform method of sectioning the specimen to evaluate the margins of excision. Different methods are used by various institutions. One I favor is the one recommended by the NSABP (Fisher et al., 1986), which provides a minimum of five lines of resection for histologic review, though variations can be introduced depending on the size of the specimen. I usually obtain radiographs of slices from the specimen, which also provide information on the margins of excision and an opportunity to correlate radiographic abnormalities with their gross and microscopic features (Fig. 12–28).

The size of a tumor should be determined as precisely as possible, including at least the greatest dimension. A mastectomy specimen should be carefully described, including what type of procedure was performed according to the surgeon, what structures were received, the dimensions of the specimen, and its skin and nipple characteristics. The existence of a recent or healed surgical scar should be recorded, including its length and location. The specimen should be sectioned from the deep margin to the skin in slices about 2.0 to 3.0 cm thick to facilitate fixation. The resulting slices can remain attached or separated depending

on preference or circumstances. If radiography equipment is available, selected slices should be radiographed to permit sampling of all suspicious alterations. The walls of any cavity from a previous biopsy should be examined carefully and representative samples obtained. Any other abnormalities should be noted and recorded. If a tumor is present its dimension should be determined precisely. It is recommended that the size be reassessed when microscopic sections are available. The tumor's relationship to and closest approach to margins of excision should be reported.

Lymph node levels should be identified by marks placed by the surgeon. Lymph nodes should be dissected carefully, since their status is the most important prognostic variable. The most productive approach to lymph node retrieval is dissolving the fat in special solutions, but this is a lengthy, expensive, and impractical procedure. An alternative method consists of washing the axillary tissues in running water for about 15 minutes (longer washing produces artifacts) and dissecting out the nodes over a translucent surface (plastic or glass) with a light source beneath. The nodes will stand out as dark structures on a yellow background. This procedure can be done rapidly since the nodes are readily identifiable.

Lymph Node Status

The most reliable index of aggressiveness of breast carcinoma is the presence of metastases in the axillary lymph nodes. Tumor recurrence, treatment failure, and patient survival are related to the status of the axillary lymph nodes. The number of positive lymph nodes appears to be more important than their level in the axilla or than the total number of lymph nodes found in the dissection. The 10-year survival rate for patients without axillary metastases is about 75%; it is reduced to 50% and then to 33%, respectively, when one to three and four or more lymph nodes contain metastases (Fisher et al., 1978). There are some qualifications. When metastasis occurs to a single node the survival rate is only slightly lower than when no axillary metastases are present, though when the involved node is larger than 2 cm in diameter (macrometastasis) the prognosis is equal to that for patients with two or more involved nodes (Huvos et al., 1971). The age of the patient plays a role. A decrease in survival is observed in postmenopausal women who have one or more nodal metastases, whereas for premenopausal women survival is affected unfavorably when two or more lymph nodes are involved. If the nodal deposit shows extracapsular extension into the perinodal fat, the prognosis is more dismal than when the tumor is confined within the boundaries of the node (Fig. 12–29) (Fisher et al., 1976). This finding, however, has been challenged (Mambo and Gallagher, 1977; and Donegan et al., 1993). The discovery of occult metastases in lymph nodes of patients considered negative on routine single section varies from 9% to 33% when the same nodes are examined with multiple sections. However, in many of the studies this did not alter prognosis significantly (Pickren, 1961). The International (Ludwig) Breast Cancer Study group found that patients with micrometastases in "negative"

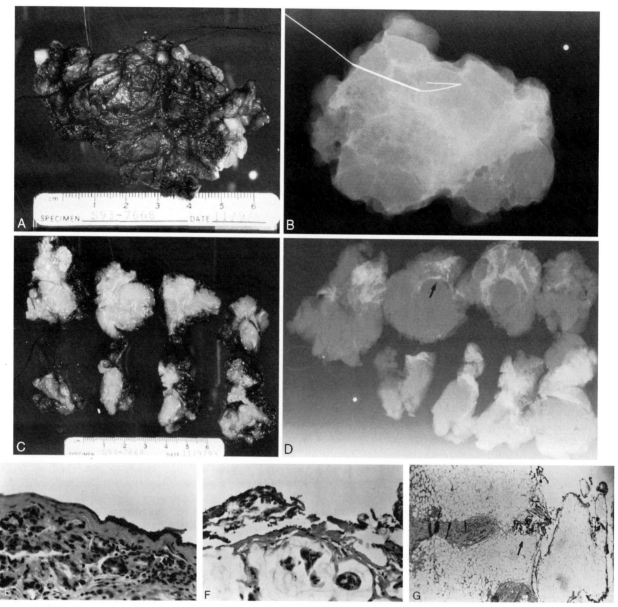

Figure 12–27. Lumpectomy specimen. *A,* India ink has been applied on surface. *B,* Specimen radiograph shows nidus of calcification near wire. *C,* Resulting segments after slicing of specimen. *D,* Radiograph of slices shows location of calcium in slices *(insets). E,* Tumor is separated from margin of excision by a fibrous band of nontumorous tissue. *F,* Tumor extends to the surgical margin. *G,* Ink seeping through fatty tissue due to torn surface.

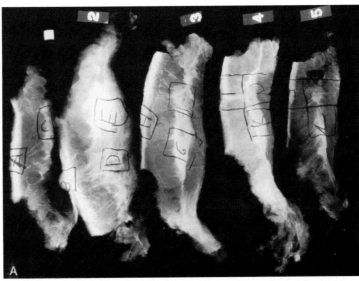

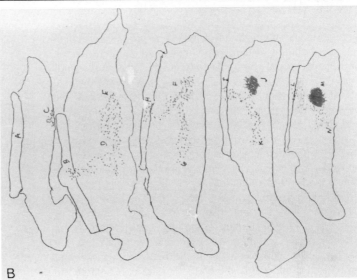

Figure 12–28. *A,* Roentgenograms of mastectomy specimen. *B,* Mapping of pathologic findings.

lymph nodes discovered by serial sectioning had a poorer disease-free survival rate at 6 years' median follow-up (75%) than the "nonconverted" group (86%) (Bettleheim et al., 1990). The impracticality of routine serial sectioning

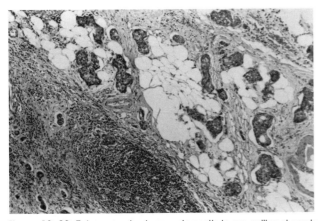

Figure 12–29. Extracapsular tumor deposits in an axillary lymph node. The capsule of the node is in the left lower area.

of lymph nodes remains a serious obstacle to more precise prognostication. Occult metastases are more frequent in patients younger than 50 years and in those with large tumors showing peritumoral vascular invasion (Bettleheim et al., 1984). Micrometastases overlooked by the routine hematoxylin and eosin–stained single-slice technique have also been detected utilizing immunochemical stains (Bussolati et al., 1986), and the recurrence and survival rates for such patients are similarly adverse.

Histologic Tumor Type

A gradient of aggressiveness is seen with carcinomas of various histologic types. "Special" histopathologic tumor types are prevalent in long-term survivors. Infiltrating ductal carcinomas predominate (Page and Anderson, 1987; Ellis et al., 1992; and Fisher et al., 1993). The special histologic types are easily identified by the pathologist as those that possess recognizable gross and microscopic features. Rosai (1981) classified carcinomas of the breast into four categories by their morphologic characteristics and their prognostic implications (Table 12–3).

The relative proportions of each tumor type have been estimated in various studies: ductal carcinoma NOS, 52% to 67%; medullary carcinoma, 3% to 6.2%; lobular carcinoma in situ, 3% to 8.5%; mucinous carcinoma 2% to 2.4%; papillary carcinoma, 0.3% to 3%; tubular carcinoma 1.2% to 1.5%; Paget's disease, 0.5% to 2.2%. These tumors exist in combination with ductal carcinomas NOS; co-existence has been estimated to occur in some 17% to 30% of cases. Carcinomas combined with ductal carcinomas most frequently were invasive lobular, 6%; tubular, 4.5%; papillary, 2%; or colloid, 0.5%. Fisher and colleagues noted that in "pure" ductal carcinomas NOS lymphatic invasion, palpable lymph nodes, and greater histologic differentiation occurred more frequently than in combined forms.

Tumor Size

Tumor size is one of the most important prognostic indicators of carcinoma of the female breast. Only axillary lymph node status surpasses it. Parenthetically, the interdependence of both factors is well-known (Say and Donegan, 1974). When tumors are less than 1 cm in diameter the prevalence of axillary metastases is between 5% and 25%, and about 90% of patients survive longer than 5 years. The 5-year survival rate is reduced to 65% when tumors are 2 to 2.5 cm in diameter. Further increments in tumor size produce further increases in metastases to the axillary lymph nodes and reductions in survival of patients. The importance of tumor size as a predictor of nodal metastases is evident in both symptomatic (Fig. 12–30) and asymptomatic (Fig. 12–31) patients. In the latter group tumors were detected during screening, whereas the former were referred because of a palpable mass in the breast. An increasing proportion of patients had metastases as tumors enlarged in both groups. Despite the importance of tumor size, the methods in use at present for this determination are approximate and crude.

Tumor Grade

For more than a century physicians have known there is a correlation between the microscopic differentiation of tumors and their clinical behavior. This was first formulated by Hansemann in 1890 (Fisher et al., 1975). In 1891 Dennis (Ashikari et al., 1974) applied it to breast tumors. He stated, "The more typical the structure the better the prognosis . . . the more embryonal the structure of the tumor the greater the possibility of recurrence." However, Greenough in 1925 (Azzopardi, 1979) was the first to use differentiation in a systematic manner, correlating the histologic features of 73 carcinomas of the breast with the patients' clinical outcome. The histologic criteria consisted of tubule formation and variations in size, shape, tinctorial affinity, and the mitotic rate of the tumor cells. He demonstrated the relationship between cancer "cures" and well-differentiated tumors. In subsequent years several studies using a similar or slightly modified schema found a comparable

Table 12–3. PROGNOSTIC CATEGORIES ACCORDING TO HISTOLOGIC TYPE

Type I (noninvasive)
   Intraductal carcinoma (with or without Paget's disease)
   LCIS (lobular neoplasia)
Type II (invasive, circumscribed margins, infrequent
   metastasis)
   Pure mucinous carcinoma
   Tubular carcinoma
   Invasive papillary carcinoma
   Medullary carcinoma
Type III (invasive, moderately metastasizing)
   Invasive ductal carcinoma NOS
   Intraductal carcinoma with invasion
   Invasive lobular carcinoma
Type IV (invasive, undifferentiated carcinoma)
   Tumors indisputably invading blood vessels, regardless of
   type

relationship between patient survival and histologic tumor grade. Scarff and Handley reported in 1938 that 31% of patients with Grade I breast carcinomas were alive 10 years after mastectomy, as compared with 13% of patients with Grade III tumors. In 1950, Bloom utilized a simplified version of Greenough's method with only three histologic factors: pattern of tubular arrangement, nuclear pleomorphism and hyperchromasia, and mitotic ratio. Each of these variables was assessed independently to produce three separate categories of grading: low (Grade I), intermediate (Grade II), and high (Grade III). In a study of 470 patients, 5-year survival rates of 79% and 25% were associated, respectively, with Grade I and Grade III tumors. The 10-year survival rates were 45% and 13%, respectively. Fur-

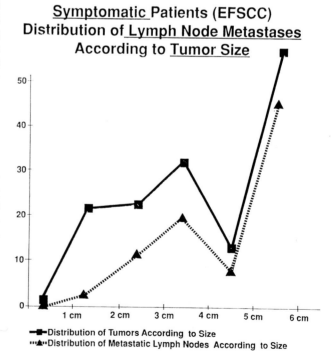

Symptomatic Patients (EFSCC) Distribution of Lymph Node Metastases According to Tumor Size

■—Distribution of Tumors According to Size
▲—Distribution of Metastatic Lymph Nodes According to Size

Figure 12–30. Symptomatic patients. Tumor size distribution is represented by solid line; metastasis according to tumor size is represented by *dotted line*. The ordinate represents numbers of cases. Abbreviation: EFSCC = Ellis Fischel State Cancer Hospital.

Asymptomatic Patients (BCDDP)
Distribution of Lymph Node Metastasis According to Tumor Size

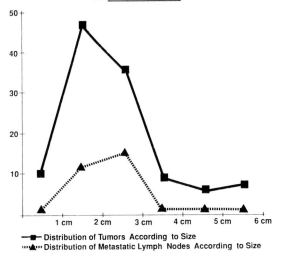

—■— Distribution of Tumors According to Size
····▲···· Distribution of Metastatic Lymph Nodes According to Size

Figure 12–31. Asymptomatic patients. *Solid line* represents distribution according to tumor size. Metastasis to lymph node is represented by *dotted line.* The ordinate represents numbers of cases.

ther prognostic refinement was achieved when Bloom combined the histologic grade with the axillary lymph node status (Bloom and Richardson, 1957). The 5-year survival rates for patients with Grade I and Grade III tumors were 95% and 55% when the axilla was free of tumor involvement; when metastases were present those rates were reduced to 65% and 16%. Further refinements resulted in the adoption of a scoring system, which provides more flexibility. Each of the three grades has a value from 1 to 3, for a total score of 9: Grade I, 3 to 5 points; Grade II, 6 to 7 points; and Grade III, 8 to 9 points. Numerous studies using this approach prove its ability to separate tumors according to prognostic potential. Other investigators give more im-

portance to characteristics of the nuclei of the tumor cells. Nuclear grade (Fig. 12–32), first used by Black and colleagues, assessed the variations in size, mitotic ratio, and chromatin pattern of the nucleus and the presence or absence of nucleoli. Grades were determined on a scale from 0 (the most undifferentiated) to 4 (the most differentiated). Their correlation with prognosis in 1409 cases showed survival rates two or three times greater for patients with low-grade tumors than for patients with poorly differentiated tumors. The prognostic influence of the axillary status was emphasized when the 5-year survival rate for patients with well-differentiated tumors and negative lymph nodes was 86% while it was 19% for patients with high-grade tumors and axillary lymph node involvement. Fisher and colleagues (1975, 1980) reversed the order of the nuclear grading to a more conventional schema and reduced the number of grades to three, Grade III being the least-differentiated. Tubule formation was also evaluated on a scale of 1 to 3. Although the results in 1984 showed a good correlation between grade and tumor behavior, case stratification was not adequate since two-thirds were classified as poorly differentiated. In a more recent publication both ''good'' nuclear and ''good'' histological grades showed a good correlation with outcome. Because of the small number of Grade I tumors, this group was merged with nuclear Grade II.

Thus, the histologic and nuclear grades of breast cancers are valuable and independent prognostic factors. Bloom showed that, coupled with axillary lymph node status, their value was improved. A prognostic index resulted from the Nottingham-Tenovous study (Elston and Ellis, 1991) that uses the following formula: PI = 0.2 X tumor size plus lymph node stage (1 to 3) plus histologic grade (1 to 3). The prognosis of the tumor is determined by the numerical value, which worsens with increase of the index. A separation into good, moderate, and poor-prognosis groups results from setting cutoff points of 3.4 and 5.4. Annual mortality rates of 3%, 7%, and 30%, respectively, were obtained for the groups.

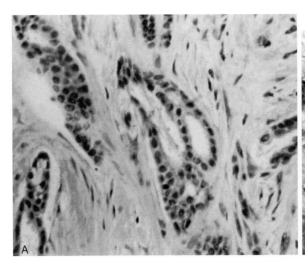
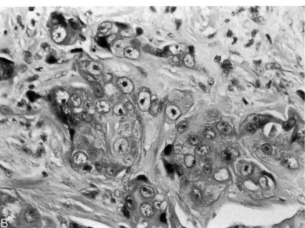

Figure 12–32. *A,* Well-differentiated ductal carcinoma NOS, exhibiting well-developed glandular structures and ''good'' grade nuclei. *B,* Poorly differentiated ductal carcinoma. Notice lack of glandular pattern and irregular nuclei with prominent nucleoli.

Tumor Margins

Invasive breast carcinomas with irregular, serrated margins have been noted to be more aggressive than tumors with well-circumscribed, knobby margins. This observation was made in several studies based both on histopathologic methods and mammographic images (Ingleby and Gershon-Cohen, 1960; and Gold et al., 1972). Tumors that exhibit well-delineated (Fig. 12–33), sharply defined contours with an expansile type of growth were less frequently associated with axillary lymph node metastasis than tumors whose margins were serrated and infiltrative (see Fig. 12–4). The 10-year survival rate for patients with circumscribed tumor margins was 80%, in contrast with only 38% for patients with irregular tumor contours. No direct relationship was found between lymph node metastasis, survival, and tumor size when the tumor had regular expansile borders. Patients whose tumor was smaller than 2.5 cm with irregular borders had a 10-year survival rate of 52%. For those with larger tumors and irregular borders survival was reduced to 25%. Lane and coworkers (1961) also found a direct relationship between tumor profile and axillary lymph node metastases. Fisher and colleagues (1975) found tumor circumscription, both gross and microscopic, to be associated with negative lymph nodes. Kouchoukos and associates (1967) found a significant difference in the incidence of metastasis to the axillary lymph nodes for tumors with pushing borders and those with infiltrative ones; however, no difference was found favoring survival of patients with circumscribed tumors, despite less axillary involvement. Subsequently, Carter and associates (1978) studied 330 patients with invasive tumors and found significant differences in axillary lymph node metastases and 10-year survival associated with circumscribed and infiltrative margins, but no differences when the characteristics of the tumor border were used as the sole discriminant. When tumor necrosis was included in the equation, tumors with necrosis and infiltrative margins behaved more aggressively than tumors with no necrosis and expansile borders. It appears that, although the quality of the margins of a tumor is a reflection of its pattern of growth, it is not the dominant force in tumor behavior. When considered in association with other variables it can provide useful prognostic information.

Inflammatory Infiltrate

In 1922 MacCarty suggested that cellular inflammatory infiltrate with breast tumors represented a sign of host reac-

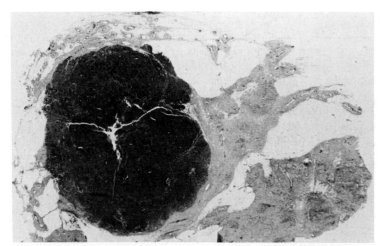

A

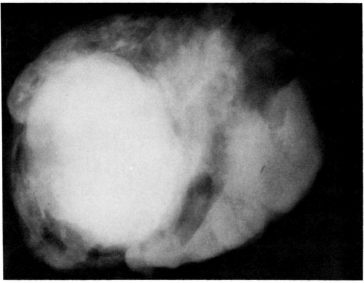

B

Figure 12–33. This photomicrograph *(A)* and specimen radiograph *(B)* illustrate a carcinoma (medullary) with a circumscribed margin.

tion analogous to the one he had observed in slow-growing stomach cancers. It represented host resistance against invasiveness, growth, and metastases. Subsequently, numerous studies attempted to assess the impact of inflammatory infiltrates on prognosis, with diverse results and conclusions. In an analysis of 348 patients, Black and coworkers (1975) concluded that an inflammatory cellular infiltrate was prognostically favorable. Berg (1971) found a relationship between plasma cell infiltration and survival. Hamlin (1968) considered various parameters from 222 tumors, including size, location, type, differentiation, patients' age, and clinical status and demonstrated a relationship between cellular response, prognosis, and tumor differentiation. Elston and coworkers (1982) and others were unable to prove such a relationship except in patients with poorly differentiated tumors. Shimokawara and colleagues (1982) utilized immunoperoxidase techniques on tissue sections and noticed that T-cell infiltration was frequent in patients without metastases in the axillary lymph nodes. Similar results were obtained by Bilik and associates in 1989. Fisher and collaborators of the NSABP concluded that absence of a cellular reaction was correlated with lack of nodal metastasis. Rosen and associates, in a study of 644 patients in 1989, also found that an intense lymphoplasmacytic reaction around the tumor was an unfavorable feature. In 1991 Rilke and colleagues studied 1210 patients to compare the prognostic significance of c-*erb*-B-2 *neu* with other prognostic factors and concluded that an inflammatory infiltrate is associated with a good prognosis.

Blood Vessel Invasion

There is no consensus on how frequently tumor cells invade blood vessels; it varies from 4% to 51%. This reflects the broad spectrum of diagnostic criteria utilized to make this determination (Fig. 12–34) (Fisher et al., 1975; Rosen et al., 1981; Roses et al., 1982; and Weigand et al., 1982). In some studies no distinction was made between small blood vessels and lymphatic channels. Early recurrence occurs in 70% of patients when both blood vessels and nodes are

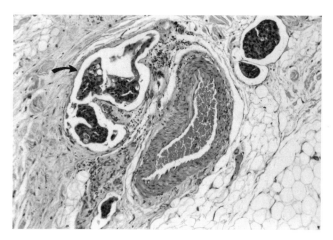

Figure 12–35. Perivascular lymphatics *(arrow)* containing tumor emboli.

involved by tumor. In one study only 12% of patients survived 5 years when both were present (Weigand et al., 1982), but Fisher and associates (1975) could not confirm this.

Lymphatic Invasion

Lymphatic invasion by tumor emboli is associated with local recurrence, lymph node metastases, and treatment failure (Fig. 12–35). In seven studies including 1602 patients with breast carcinomas staged T1 N0 M0, lymphatic tumor invasion failed to show prognostic value in only one (Table 12–4) (Azzopardi, 1983).

According to Fisher and associates, tumor extension to lymphatics is more closely associated with lymph node status than with treatment failure, as 33% of patients who survive 10 years exhibited such extension. In another study 63% of patients who survived 25 years after mastectomy had tumors that showed lymphatic invasion.

A consensus on what constitutes lymphatic invasion is paramount, and as Gilchrist and associates (1982) were unable to find unanimity among experienced pathologists. Artifacts due to poor fixation, including retraction of the stroma around tumors, can cause confusion. Strict morphologic criteria require spaces with an endothelial lining, a thin nonmuscular wall, and no erythrocytes in the lumen. Orbo and colleagues (1990) used these criteria and obtained 91% interobserver reproducibility. They concluded that lymphatic vessel invasion is a more powerful predictor of lymph node status than tumor size, margin contours, histologic grade, or tumor type. Immunohistochemical methods can be useful in identifying lymphatics; however, hematoxylin and eosin stain is still reliable for identifying lymphatic vessels if used with strict criteria.

Receptor Proteins

Determination of estrogen and progesterone receptors (ER and PR) on tumor tissue is presently part of the standard of practice for selection of treatment and a prognostic guide

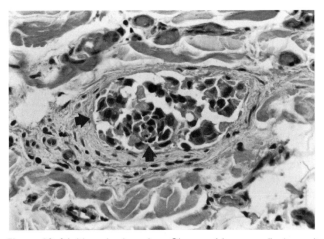

Figure 12–34. Vascular invasion. Clump of tumor cells *(arrow)* within the lumen of a vessel with muscular walls.

Table 12–4. HISTOPATHOLOGIC RISK FACTORS WITH PROGNOSTIC VALUE IN 1602 PATIENTS WITH T1N0M0 BREAST CANCER*

Author	Number of Patients	Tumor Grade	Histologic Type	Tumor Margin	Tumor Lymphoid Infiltrate	Tumor Lymphatic Invasion	Tumor Vascular Invasion	Other
Thomas, et al. Ann. Surg., *190*:129, 1979.	203	+		+		+	+	
Fracchia, et al. Surg. Gynecol. Obstet., *151*:375, 1980.	520	0		⊕		+		Tumor size +
Nealon, et al. Ann. Surg., *89*:279, 1981.	228	+		+		+	+	
Roses, et al. Am. J. Clin. Pathol., *78*:817, 1982.	122	0	+	0	0	+	0	Necrosis, cellularity, fibrous response, neural invasion
Ketterhagen, et al. Surg. Gynecol. Obstet., *188*:120, 1984.	69	+		+		+	+	
Rosen, et al. Ann. Surg., *193*:15, 1981.	382	+	+		0	+	+	
Bilik, et al. Am. J. Surg., *151*:460, 1986.	78	+			+		+	

+ Effect   0 No Effect   ⊕ Inconclusive

*Histopathologic parameters analyzed in seven separate studies encompassing 1602 patients.

for patients with invasive ductal carcinoma of the breast. Their value for tumors of special types, including mucinous, medullary, tubular, and intraductal, has not been established. The presence of receptor proteins indicates retention of the regulatory controls of the mammary epithelium. Tumors that are better differentiated are predominantly ER-positive and PR-positive and are associated with better prognosis. Some studies have shown that about 60% of women with ER-positive tumors respond to hormone manipulation, in contrast with 5% to 10% of women with ER-negative tumors. Progesterone receptors are equally valuable; the presence or absence of PR may even be a better predictor for endocrine therapy. Tumors with high labeling indices with rapid rates of cellular replication are less frequently positive for estrogen receptors. Still, there is controversy concerning its prognostic value as an independent variable. It requires evaluation in combination with age and tumor differentiation. In Stage I disease, ER and tumor size are useful for identifying a group at high risk for early recurrence and poor chances of survival. For Stage II the number of involved nodes and the PR are more important (McGuire, 1986).

MULTICENTRIC AND MULTIFOCAL CARCINOMA

The designations *multicentric* and *multifocal*, when applied to malignant tumors of the breast, commonly are used interchangeably, but biologic and therapeutic differences are implied in the semantic distinction. Multicentric carcinomas, according to Fisher and colleagues (1989), "are foci of cancer remote from the dominant mass," whereas mul-

tifocal carcinoma is "cancer in the vicinity of it or within the same quadrant" (Fig. 12–36). This definition has been quantified by considering invasive or in situ lesions as multifocal when more than a single focus occur within a distance of not more than 5 cm with respect to another. It is considered multicentric when a single focus of carcinoma, invasive or noninvasive, is located 5 cm or farther from the border of the index tumor. Because of the lack of uniformity in concept, definition, sampling, and methods, the frequency of multicentricity varies from 9% to 75%. The increasing use of breast-conserving surgery makes the notion of multicentricity relevant. In some studies it is not clear if the residual carcinoma was in the same quadrant of the excision or in a distant quadrant. In a group of patients treated by partial mastectomy for tumors 2 cm in diameter or smaller and followed for a minimum of 5 years, Crile and coworkers (1980) reported that 12% of patients developed local recurrence and 3% developed cancer in another site in the treated breast. In a study encompassing 286 total mastectomies Lagios and coworkers (1981) defined multicentricity as two independent carcinomas, invasive or noninvasive, separated by at least 5 cm. They found multicentricity in 28% of the cases. It is of interest that, when the same definition was applied to intraductal carcinomas, the rate of multicentricity was 17% when the tumor was less than 2.5 cm and 47% when it was larger. In a careful study of multicentricity Holland and coworkers (1985) correlated the expected rate of tumor recurrence with the amount of tissue removed around the tumor. No difference was found in the occurrence of multicentricity, whether the diameter of the index tumor was less than 2 cm or 2 to 4 cm. The therapeutic and clinical importance of these studies are obvious. It appears that coexisting carcinoma influences the success or failure of breast-conserving procedures.

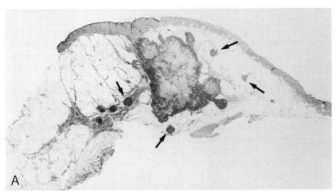
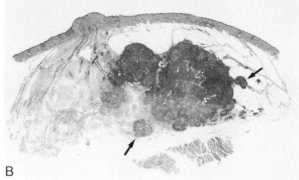

Figure 12–36. Whole mount of breasts showing large index tumors and other smaller ones located at varying distances. The distinction between multicentric *(A)* additional cancers in quadrants of the breast other than that of the dominant cancer *(arrows)* and multifocal *(B)* additional cancers in the same quadrant *(arrows)* is not always easily determined.

EVOLVING MARKERS OF PROGNOSIS

The last decades have witnessed an increasing need to develop new pathologic parameters that are capable of predicting prognosis and guiding treatment. Presently there are a number that are tested and validated. These include axillary lymph node status, tumor size, tumor grade (histologic and nuclear), mitotic rate, hormone receptors, S-phase fraction, and ploidy. The data are reproducible, amenable to quality control, and clinically relevant.

Additional markers are under study. The c-*erb*-B-2 protein, an oncogene of the *erb* B family similar in structure to, but different from, epidermal growth factor receptor (EGFR) has potential value (Perren, 1991). Its presence can be demonstrated by immunohistochemical or immunoblotting techniques: Slamon and colleagues utilized 86 lymph node–positive patients in 1986 and 345 lymph node–positive patients in 1989 to show that the overexpression of this oncogene was associated with a high rate of recurrence and a small chance of survival (Slamon et al., 1989). In a multivariate analysis c-*erb*-B-2 expression was second only to the number of positive lymph nodes as a predictor of both disease-free survival and survival overall. Overexpression is associated with poorly differentiated tumors, metastases to lymph nodes, large tumor size, and negative hormone receptors. No association with ploidy has been identified. Although its expression is more common in patients with advanced-stage tumors, it may prove a useful addition to the list of prognostic markers for groups considered to have a good prognosis according to conventional measures. Amplification of other oncogenes correlates with dismal prognosis, including c-*myc*, INT-2 and HST-1/INT.

Animal experiments suggest that after tumors reach a critical dimension their continued growth requires the formation of new vessels. These vessels increase the opportunity for tumor cells to enter the circulation. The relationship between intensity of angiogenesis and metastasis was reported for malignant melanomas of the skin. Similar observations have been made about breast carcinomas. Weidner and coworkers (1991) studied 49 patients with breast carcinoma, including 27 with and without metastases, and showed that microvessel count and density correlated with metastatic disease. It is a possible method for selecting patients with negative nodes for aggressive treatment.

The role of extracellular matrix, particularly basement membrane, in the process of tumor invasion and metastases has been the source of several studies (Monteagudo et al., 1990). Loss of the basement membrane is a common feature of invasion. Type IV collagen is one of the most important components of the basement membrane. Its enzymatic degradation is specifically initiated by a Type IV collagenase that is present in tumor and in normal cells. In a study of breast cancer samples from 55 patients, immunohistochemical stains showed a large percentage of positive cells, supporting the origin of the enzyme from the tumor cells and suggesting a role in tumor invasion and metastasis.

Expression of an estrogen-regulated protein known as the *27000-d heat shock protein* or *stress-response protein (srp-27)* was assessed in human breast cancer and established breast cancer cell lines. A correlation was noted between overexpression of srp-27 and tumor aggressiveness in the form of nodal metastases, lymphatic and vascular invasion, advanced stage, and short-lived disease-free survival (Thor et al., 1991).

Epidermal growth factor receptor is a polypeptide that participates in normal cell growth. In a study of 135 primary breast carcinomas, tumors that were EGFR positive were associated with shorter disease-free interval and overall survival than EGFR-negative tumors (Sainsbury et al., 1987). The effect was evident in patients with negative estrogen receptors and with negative and positive lymph nodes.

The loss of genetic heterozygosity in tumors has been used as a marker of tumor suppressor genes. The loss of this function, in combination with the activation of proto-oncogenes, has been proposed in colon carcinogenesis. Allelic imbalance of the chromosome 17 locus of the tumor suppressor gene p53 is observed in 60% of breast tumors. Overexpression of the p53 oncoprotein has been demonstrated in malignant tumors, including invasive carcinomas of the breast. In one study (Friedrichs et al., 1993) of tumor tissue from 156 patients with invasive carcinomas of the breast, overexpression of p53 nuclear protein was significantly related to poor differentiation and absence of steroid hormone receptors. Disease recurrence and survival were influenced regardless of axillary lymph node status. It appears to be an independent predictor for recurrence and diminished survival.

Cathepsin D, an estrogen-induced lysosomal protease, has growth-promoting activity and extracellular proteolytic activity (Tandon et al., 1990). Levels of this enzyme are elevated in proliferation of both benign and malignant cells. Overexpression of cathepsin D is associated with shorter disease-free and overall survival in patients with negative axillary nodes. It may represent an independent predictor of treatment failure and death in this group of patients.

References

Aboumrad, M. H., Horn, R. C., and Fine, G.: Lipid-secreting mammary carcinoma: Report of a case of associated with Paget's disease of the nipple. Cancer, *16*:521, 1963.

Akhtar, M. A., Robinson, C., Ali, M. A., et al.: Secretory carcinoma of the breast in adults. Light and electron microscopic study of three cases with review of the literature. Cancer, *51*:2245, 1983.

Archer, F., and Omar, M.: Pink cell (oncocytic) metaplasia in a fibroadenoma of the human breast: Electron microscopic observation. J. Pathol., *99*:99, 1969.

Ashikari, R., Park, K., Huvos, A. G., et al.: Paget's disease of the breast. Cancer, *26*:680, 1974.

Association of Directors of Anatomic and Surgical Pathology: Recommendation of the Association of Directors of Anatomic and Surgical Pathology. Part 1: Immediate management of mammographically detected breast lesions. Hum. Pathol., *24*:689, 1993.

Azzopardi, J. G.: Problems in Breast Pathology. Philadelphia, W. B. Saunders, 1979.

Azzopardi, J. G.: Benign and malignant proliferative lesions of the breast, a review. J. Cancer Clin. Oncol., *19*:1717, 1983.

Azzopardi, J. G., Chepick, O. F., Hartman, W. H., et al.: Histologic typing of breast tumors. Am. J. Clin. Pathol., *78*:806, 1982.

Baker, L. H.: Breast cancer detection demonstration project: 5-year summary report. CA, *32*:194, 1982.

Beahrs, O., Shapiro, S., and Smart, C.: Report of the working group to review the National Cancer Institute—American Cancer Society Breast Cancer Detection Demonstration Projects. J. Natl. Cancer Inst., *62*:640, 1979.

Bellamy, C. O. C., McDonal, C., Salter, D. M., et al.: Noninvasive ductal carcinoma of the breast: The relevance of histological characterization. Hum. Pathol., *24*:16, 1993.

Berg, J. W.: Morphological evidence for immune response to breast cancer. An historical review. Cancer, *28*:1453, 1971.

Bettelheim, R., Penman, H. G., Thornton-Jones, N. A. M., et al.: Prognostic significance of peritumoral vascular invasion in breast cancer. Br. J. Cancer, *50*:771, 1984.

Bettelheim, R., Price, K. W., Gelber, R. O., et al.: International (Ludwig) Breast Cancer Study Group. Prognostic importance of occult axillary lymph node micrometastases from breast cancers. Lancet, *335*:1565, 1990.

Bilik, R., Mor, C., and Moroz, C.: Characterization of T-lymphocyte subpopulations infiltrating primary breast cancer. Cancer Immunol. Immunother., *28*:143, 1989.

Black, M. M., Barclay, T. H. C., and Hankey, B. F.: Prognosis in breast cancer utilizing histologic characteristics of the primary tumor. Cancer, *36*:2048, 1975.

Black, M. M., Opler, S. R., and Speer, F. D.: Survival in breast cancer cases in relation to the structure of the primary tumor and regional lymph nodes. Surg. Gynecol. Obstet., *100*:543, 1955.

Black, M. M., and Speer, F. D.: Nuclear structure in cancer tissues. Surg. Gynecol. Obstet., *105*:97, 1957.

Bloom, H. J. G.: Prognosis in cancer of the breast. Br. J. Cancer, *4*:259, 1950.

Bloom, H. J. G.: Further studies on prognosis of breast carcinoma. Br. J. Cancer, *4*:347, 1950.

Bloom, H. J. G., and Richardson, W. W.: Histologic grading and prognosis in breast cancer: A study of 1709 cases of which 359 have been followed for 15 years. Br. J. Cancer, *2*:353, 1957.

Bussolati, G., Gugliotta, P., Morra, I., et al.: The immunohistochemical detection of lymph node metastases in breast cancer. Br. J. Cancer, *54*:631, 1986.

Capella, C., Eusebi, V., Mann, B., et al.: Endocrine differentiation in mucoid carcinoma of the breast. Histopathology, *4*:1613, 1980.

Carsten, P. H. B., Greenberg, R. A., Francis, D., et al.: Tubular carcinoma of the breast. A long-term follow-up. Histopathology, *9*:271, 1985.

Carter, D., Orr, S. L., and Merino, M. D.: Intracystic papillary carcinoma of the breast after mastectomy, radiotherapy or excisional biopsy alone. Cancer, *52*:14–19, 1983.

Carter, D., Pipkin, R. D., Shephard, R. H., et al.: Relationship of necrosis and tumor border to lymph node metastasis and 10-year survival in carcinoma of the breast. Am. J. Surg. Pathol., *2*:39, 1978.

Cornil, A. V., and Ranviere, L.: Manuel d'Histologie Pathlogique. Paris, Germer-Baillier, 1869, pp. 1167–1170.

Crile, G., Jr., Cooperman, A., and Esselstyn, C. B., et al.: Results of partial mastectomy in 173 patients followed for from five to ten years. Surg. Gynecol. Obstet., *150*:563–566, 1980.

Cubilla, A. C., and Woodruff, J. M.: Primary carcinoid tumor of the breast: A report of eight patients. Am. J. Surg. Pathol., *1*:283, 1977.

Czernobilsky, B.: Intracystic carcinoma of the female breast. Surg. Gynecol. Obstet., *124*:93, 1967.

DiConstanzo, D., Rosen, P. P., Gareen, I., et al.: Prognosis in infiltrating lobular carcinoma. An analysis of "classical" and variant tumors. Am. J. Surg. Pathol., *14*:12, 1990.

Dixon, J. M., Anderson, T. J., Page, D. L., et al.: Infiltrating lobular carcinoma of the breast. An evaluation of the incidence and consequences of bilateral disease. Br. J. Surg., *70*:513, 1983.

Donegan, W. L., and Perez-Mesa, C. M.: Lobular carcinoma: An indicator for elective biopsy of the second breast. Ann. Surg., *177*:178–187, 1972.

Donegan, W. L., Stine, S. R., and Santer, T. G.: Implications of extracapsular nodal metastases for treatment and prognosis of breast cancer. Cancer, *72*:778, 1993.

Ellis, I. O., Galea, M., Broughton, N., et al.: Prognostic factors in breast cancer. II. Histological type. Relationship with survival in a large study with long-term follow-up. Histopathology, *20*:479, 1992.

Ellis, D., and Teitelbaum, S. L.: Inflammatory carcinoma of the breast. A pathologic definition. Cancer, *33*:1045, 1974.

Elston, C. W., and Ellis, I. O.: Pathologic prognostic factors in breast cancer. I. The value of histological grade in breast cancer: Experience from a large study with long-term follow-up. Histopathology, *19*:403, 1991.

Elston, C. W., Gresham, C. A., Rao, G. S., et al.: The cancer research campaign (King's-Cambridge) trial for early breast cancer: Clinicopathological aspects. Br. J. Cancer, *45*:655, 1982.

Eusebi, V., Lamovec, J., Cattani, M. G., et al.: Acantholytic variant of squamous cell carcinoma of the breast. Am. J. Surg. Pathol., *10*:855, 1986a.

Eusebi, V., Mills, R. R., Cattani, M. G., et al.: Apocrine carcinoma of the breast. A morphologic and immunohistochemical study. Am. J. Pathol., *123*:532, 1986b.

Fechner, R. E.: Histologic variants of infiltrating lobular carcinoma of the breast. Hum. Pathol. *6*:373, 1975.

Fechner, R. E.: One century of mammary carcinoma in situ. What have we learned? Am. J. Clin. Pathol., *100*:654, 1993.

Fisher, E. R., Anderson, S., Redmond, C., et al.: Pathologic findings from the National Surgical Adjuvant Breast Project Protocol-B-06. 10-year pathologic and clinical prognostic discriminants. Cancer, *76*:2507, 1993.

Fisher, E. R., Gregorio, R. M., Fisher B., et al.: The pathology of invasive breast cancer: A syllabus derived from findings of the National Surgical Adjuvant Breast Project (Protocol No. 4). Cancer, *36*:1, 1975.

Fisher, E. R., Gregorio, R. M., Redmond, C., et al.: Pathologic findings from the national surgical adjuvant breast project (Protocol 4) III The significant of extranodal extension of axillary metastases. Am. J. Clin. Pathol., *65*:439, 1976.

Fisher, E. R., Gregorio, R. M., Redmond, C., et al.: Tubulolobular invasive breast cancer: A variant of lobular invasive cancer. Hum. Pathol., *8*:679, 1977.

Fisher, E. R., Plekar, A., Rockette, H., et al.: Pathologic findings from the National Surgical Adjuvant Breast Project (Protocol No. 4) vs significance of axillary nodal micro- and macrometastases. Cancer, *42*:2032, 1978.

Fisher, E. R., Palekar, A. S., Redmond, E., et al.: Pathologic findings from the national surgical adjuvant breast project protocol (No. 4) VI Invasive Papillary Carcinoma. Am. J. Clin. Pathol., *73*:313, 1980.

Fisher, E. R., Palekar, A. S., Gregorio, R. M., et al.: Mucoepidermoid and squamous cell carcinoma of breast with reference to squamous metaplasia and giant cells. Am. J. Surg. Pathol., 7:15, 1983.

Fisher, E. R., Redmond, C., and Fisher, B.: Histological grading of breast cancer. *In* Summers, J. G., and Rosen, P. P. (Eds.): Pathology Annual, Part I. New York, Appleton-Century-Crofts, 1980, p. 239.

Fisher, E. R., Sass, R., Fisher, K. B., et al.: Pathologic findings from National Surgical Adjuvant Project for Breast Cancers (Protocol No. 6). Intraductal carcinoma (DCIS). Cancer, 57:197, 1986.

Fisher, E. R., Sass, R., Fisher, B., et al.: Pathologic findings from the National Surgical Adjuvant Project (Protocol #6) 11. Relation of local breast recurrence to multicentricity. Cancer, 57:1717, 1989.

Fisher, E. R., Tavares, J., Bulatao, I. S., et al.: Glycogen-rich clear cell carcinoma of the breast. A light and electron microscopic study. Cancer, 78:2003, 1981.

Foote, F. W. Jr., and Stewart, F. W.: Lobular carcinoma in situ: A rare form of mammary cancer. Am. J. Pathol., 17:491, 1941.

Foote, F. W., and Stewart, F. W.: A histologic classification of carcinoma of the breast. Surgery, 19:74, 1946.

Friedrichs, K., Gluba, S., Eidtmann, H., et al.: Overexpression of p53 and prognosis in breast cancer. Cancer, 72:3641, 1993.

Gatchell, F. G., Dockerty, M. B., and Clagett, O. T.: Intracystic carcinoma of the breast. Surg. Gynecol. Obstet., 106:347, 1958.

Geschickter, C. F.: Diseases of the Breast: Diagnosis, Pathology and Treatment. 2nd ed. Philadelphia, J. B. Lippincott, 1945, p. 565.

Gilchrist, K. W., Gold, V. E., Hirsh, L. S., et al.: Intraobserver variation in the identification of breast carcinoma and intramammary lymphatics. Hum. Pathol., 13:170, 1982.

Giri, D. D., Dundas, S. A. C., Nottingham, J. F., et al.: Oestrogen receptors in benign epithelial lesions and intraduct carcinoma of the breast: An immunohistochemical study. Histopathology, 15:575, 1989.

Gold, R. H., Main, G., Zippin, C., et al.: Infiltration of mammary carcinoma as an indicator of axillary metastasis: A preliminary report. Cancer, 29:35, 1972.

Gump, F. E., Dicha, D. L., and Ozzello, L.: Ductal carcinoma in situ (DCIS): A revised concept. Surgery, 164:285, 1987.

Haagensen, C. D.: Diseases of the Breast. 3rd ed. Philadelphia, W. B. Saunders, 1986.

Halsted, W. S.: A diagnostic sign of gelatinous carcinoma of the breast. J.A.M.A., 64:1653, 1915.

Hamlin, I. M. E.: Possible host resistance in carcinoma of the breast. A histological study. Br. J. Cancer, 22:383, 1968.

Harris, M., and Lessells, A. M.: The ultrastructure of medullary, atypical medullary, and non-medullary carcinoma of the breast. Histopathology, 10:405, 1986.

Harris, M., Wells, S., and Vasudev, K. S.: Primary ring-cell carcinoma of the breast. Histopathology, 2:171, 1978.

Hazelrigg, D. E., and Rudolph, A. H.: Inflammatory metastatic carcinoma, carcinoma erysipelatoides. Arch. Dermatol., 11:69, 1977.

Holland, R., Veling, S. H. J., Mra-Vunac, M., et al.: Histologic multifocality of Tis, T1–2 breast carcinoma implications for clinical trials of breast conserving surgery cancer. 56:979, 1985.

Hsu, S. M., Raine, L., and Nayak, R. N.: Medullary carcinoma of breast: An immunohistochemical study of its lymphoid stroma. Cancer, 48:1368, 1981.

Hunter, C. E., Jr., and Sawyers, J. L.: Intracystic papillary carcinoma of the breast. South. Med. J., 73:1484, 1980.

Huvos, A. G., Hutter, R. V. P., and Berg, J. W.: Significance of axillary macrometastases and micrometastases in mammary cancer. Ann. Surg., 173:44, 1971.

Ingleby, H., and Gershon-Cohen, J.: Comparative Anatomy, Pathology and Roentgenology of the Breast. Philadelphia, University of Pennsylvania Press, 1960, p. 359.

Kennedy, S., Merino, M. F., Swain, S., et al.: The effects of hormonal and chemotherapy on tumoral and non-neoplastic breast tissue. Hum. Pathol., 21:192, 1990.

Komaki, K., Sakamoto, K. G., Sugano, H., et al.: Mucinous carcinoma of the breast in Japan. A prognostic analysis based on morphological features. Cancer, 61:989, 1988.

Kouchoukos, N. T., Ackerman, L. V., and Butcher, H. R. Jr.: Prediction of axillary lymph nodal metastases from the morphology of primary mammary carcinomas: Guide to operative therapy. Cancer, 20:978, 1967.

Kraus, F. T., and Neubecker, R. V.: The differential diagnosis of papillary tumors of the breast. Cancer, 15:444, 1962.

Krausz, T., Jenkins, D., Growtoft, O., et al.: Secretory carcinoma of the breast in adults. Emphasis on late recurrence and metastasis. Histopathology, 14:25, 1989.

LaFreniere, R., Moskowitz, L. B., and Ketcham, A. S.: Pure squamous cell carcinoma of the breast. J. Surg. Oncol., 31:113, 1986.

Lagios, M. D., Wesdhal, P. R., and Rose, M. R.: The concept and implications of multicentricity in breast carcinoma. Pathol. Annu., 16:83, 1981.

Lane, N., Goksel, H., Salerno, R. A., et al.: Clinical pathologic analysis of surgical curability of breast cancers: A minimum ten-year study of a personal series. Ann. Surg., 153:483, 1961.

Lattes, R.: Lobular neoplasia (lobular carcinoma in situ) of the breast: A histological entity of controversial clinical significance (Review article). Pathol. Res. Prat., 166:415, 1980.

LeGal, M., Ollivier L., Asselain, B., et al.: Mammographic features of 455 invasive lobular carcinomas. Radiology, 185:705, 1992.

Lucas, F. V., and Perez-Mesa, C.: Inflammatory carcinoma of the breast. Cancer, 41:1595, 1978.

MacCarty, W. C.: Factors which influence prognosis in cancer. Ann. Surg., 76:9, 1922.

Mambo, N. C., and Gallager, H. S.: Carcinoma of the breast: The prognostic significance of extranodal extension of axillary disease. Cancer, 39:2280, 1977.

Martinez, V., and Azzopardi, G.: Invasive lobular carcinoma of the breast: Incidence and variants. Histopathology, 3:467, 1979.

Mayr, N. A., Staples, J. J., Robinson, R. A., et al.: Morphometric studies in intraductal breast carcinoma using computerized image analysis. Cancer, 67:2805, 1991.

McBride, C. M., and Hortobagyi, G. N.: Primary inflammatory carcinoma of the female breast: Staging and treatment possibilities. Surgery, 98:792, 1985.

McDivitt, R. W., Boyce, W., and Gersell, D.: Tubular carcinoma of the breast: Clinical and pathological observations concerning 135 cases. Am. J. Surg. Pathol., 6:401, 1982.

McDivitt, R. W., and Stewart, F. W.: Breast carcinoma in children. J.A.M.A., 195:388, 1966.

McDivitt, R. W., Stone, K. R., Craig, R. B., et al.: A proposed classification of breast cancer based on kinetic information. Cancer, 57:209, 1986.

McGuire, W. L.: Prognostic factors in primary breast cancer. Cancer Surveys, 5:528, 1986.

McKittrick, J. E., Doane, W. A., and Failing, R. M.: Intracystic papillary carcinoma of the breast. Am. Surg., 35:195–202, 1969.

Melamed, M. R., Robbins, G. F., and Foote, F. W.: Prognostic significance of gelatinous mammary carcinoma. Cancer, 14:699, 1961.

Merino, M., and LiVolsi, V.: Signet-ring carcinoma of the female breast: A clinicopathologic analysis of twenty-four cases. Cancer, 48:1830, 1981.

Meyer, J. G.: Cell kinetics of histological variants of in situ breast carcinoma. Breast Cancer Res. Treat., 7:171, 1986.

Miller, W. R., Telford, J., Dixon, J. M., et al.: Androgen metabolism and apocrine differentiation in human breast cancer. Breast Cancer Res. Treat., 5:67, 1985.

Monaghan, P., and Roberts, J. D. B.: Immunohistochemical evidence for neuroendocrine differentiation in human breast carcinomas. J. Pathol., 147:281, 1985.

Monteagudo, C., Merino, M., San Juan, J., et al.: Immunohistochemical distribution of type IV collagenase in normal, benign and malignant breast tissue. Am. J. Pathol., 136:585, 1990.

Moore, O. S. Jr., Foote, F. W. Jr.: The relatively favorable prognosis of medullary carcinoma of the breast. Cancer, 2:635, 1949.

Muir, R.: The pathogenesis of Paget's disease of the nipple and associated lesions. Br. J. Surg., 22:728, 1935.

Muir, R.: The evolution of carcinoma in the mamma. J. Pathol. Bacteriol., 52:155, 1941.

Murad, T. M., Contesso, G., and Mourisse, H.: Papillary tumors of large lactiferous ducts. Cancer, 78:122, 1981.

Nadji, M., Morales, A. R., Girtanner, R. E., et al.: Paget's disease of the skin. A unifying concept. Cancer, 50:2203, 1982.

Oberman, H. A., and Fidler, W. J.: Tubular carcinoma of the breast. Am. J. Surg. Pathol., 3:387, 1979.

Orbo, A., Stalsberg, H., and Kunde, D.: Topographic criteria in the diagnosis of tumor emboli in intramammary lymphatics. Cancer, 66:972, 1990.

Ottesen, G. L., Graversen, H. P., Blichert-Toft, M., et al.: Ductal carcinoma in situ of the female breast. Short-term results of a prospective nationwide study. Am. J. Surg. Pathol., 16:1183, 1992.

Ottesen, G. L., Graversen, H. P., Blichert-Toft, M., et al.: Lobular carcinoma in situ of the female breast. Short-term results of a prospective nationwide study. Am. J. Surg. Pathol., 17:14–21, 1993.

Page, D. L.: Prognosis and breast cancer. Recognition of lethal and favorable prognostic types. Am. J. Surg. Pathol., *15*:334, 1991.

Page, D. L., and Anderson, T. J.: Diagnostic Histopathology of the Breast. New York, Churchill Livingston, 1987, pp. 198–205.

Paget, J.: On diseases of the mammary areola preceding carcinoma of mammary gland. St. Bart. Hosp. Rep., *10*:87, 1874.

Patchefsky, R. A., Shaber, G. S., Schwartz, G. J., et al.: The pathology of breast cancer detected by mass population screening. Cancer, *40*:1659, 1977.

Perren, T. J.: C-ERB2 oncogene as a prognostic marker in breast cancer (Editorial). Br. J. Cancer, *63*:328, 1991.

Peters, J. W., and Wolff, M.: Adenoid cystic carcinoma of the breast. A report of eleven new cases: A review of the literature. A discussion of biologic behavior. Cancer, *52*:680, 1982.

Pickren, J. N.: Significance of occult metastases. A study of breast cancer. Cancer, *14*:1266, 1961.

Ramos, C. V., and Taylor, H. B.: Lipid-rich carcinoma of the breast: A clinicopathological analysis of thirteen examples. Cancer, *33*:12, 1974.

Rapin, V., Contesso, G., Mouriesse, H., et al.: Medullary breast carcinoma, a reevaluation of 95 cases of breast cancer with inflammatory stroma. Cancer, *61*:2503, 1988.

Rasmussen, B. B.: Human mucinous carcinomas and their lymph node metastases. A histologic review of 247 cases. Pathol. Res. Pract., *180*:377, 1985.

Rasmussen, B. B., Rose, C., and Christensen, I.: Prognostic factors in primary mucinous carcinoma of the breast. Am. J. Clin. Pathol., 87:155, 1987.

Rasmussen, B. B., Rose, C., Thorpe, S. M., et al.: Argyrophilic cells in 202 human mucinous breast carcinomas. Relation to histopathologic and clinical factors. Am. J. Clin. Pathol., *84*:737, 1985.

Recommendations of the Association of Directors of Anatomic and Surgical Pathology—Part I: Immediate management of mammographically detected breast lesions. Hum. Pathol., *24*:689, 1993.

Ridenhour, C. E., Perez-Mesa, C. M., and Hori, J. M.: Paget's disease of the nipple. Cancer Bull., *21*:15, 1969.

Ridolfi, R. L., Rosen, P. P., Port, A., et al.: Medullary carcinoma of the breast: A clinicopathological study with 10 year follow-up. Cancer, *40*:1365, 1977.

Rilke, F., Andreola, S., Carbone, A., et al.: The importance of pathology in prognosis and management of breast cancer. Semin. Oncol., *5*:360, 1978.

Rilke, F., Colnaghi, M. I., Cascinelli, N., et al.: Prognostic significance of HER-2/neu expression in breast cancer and its relationship to other prognostic factors. Int. J. Cancer, *49*:44, 1991.

Rosai, J.: Ackerman's Surgical Pathology. 6th ed. St. Louis, C. V. Mosby, 1981.

Rosen, P. P.: Co-existent lobular carcinoma in situ and intraductal carcinoma in a single lobular duct unit. Am. J. Surg. Pathol., *4*:241, 1980.

Rosen, P. P.: Adenoid cystic carcinoma of the breast. A morphologically heterogeneous neoplasm. Pathol. Annu., *24*:237, 1989.

Rosen, P. P., Ashikari, R., Thaler, H., et al.: A comparative study of some pathologic features of mammary carcinoma in Tokyo, Japan and New York, USA. Cancer, *39*:429, 1977.

Rosen, P. P., Groshen, S., Saigo, P. E., et al.: Pathological prognostic factors in Stage I (T1N0M0) and Stage II (T1N1M0) Breast carcinoma: A study of 644 patients with median follow-up of 18 years. J. Clin. Oncol., *7*:1239, 1989.

Rosen, P. P., Lesser, M. L., and Kinne, D. W.: Breast carcinoma at the extremes of age: A comparison of patients younger than 35 years and older than 75 years. J. Surg. Oncol., *38*:90, 1985.

Rosen, P. P., and Oberman, H. A.: Atlas of Tumor Pathology. Tumors of the Mammary Gland. Washington, D.C., Armed Forces Institute of Pathology, 1992.

Rosen, P. P., Saigo, P. E., Braun, D. W. Jr., et al.: Predictors of recurrence in Stage I (T1N0M0) breast carcinoma. Ann. Surg., *193*:15, 1981.

Rosen, P. P., and Wang, T. Y.: Colloid carcinoma of the breast: Analysis of 64 patients with long-term follow-up (Abstract). Am. J. Clin. Pathol., *73*:304, 1980.

Roses, D. F., Bell, D. A., Flotte, T. J., et al.: Pathologic predictors of recurrence in Stage I (T1N0M0) breast cancer. Am. J. Clin. Pathol., *78*:817, 1982.

Rosner, D., Bedwani, R. N., Vana, J., et al.: Noninvasive breast carcinoma. Results of a national survey by the American College of Surgeons. Ann. Surg., *192*:139, 1980.

Royal College of Pathologists Working Group: Pathologic reporting in breast cancer screening. J. Clin. Pathol., *44*:710, 1991.

Sagebiel, R. W.: Ultrastructural observations on epidermal cells in Paget's disease of the breast. Am. J. Pathol., *57*:49, 1969.

Sainsbury, J. R. C., Farndon, J. R., Needham, G. K., et al.: Epidermal growth factor receptor status as predictor of early recurrence of and death from breast cancer. Lancet, *i*:1398, 1987.

Saltzstein, S. L.: Clinically occult inflammatory carcinoma of the breast. Cancer, *34*:382, 1974.

Saphir, D.: Mucinous carcinoma of the breast. Surg. Gynecol. Obstet., *72*:908, 1941.

Say, C., and Donegan, W. L.: Invasive carcinoma of the breast. Prognostic significance of tumor size and involved axillary lymph nodes. Cancer, *34*:468, 1974.

Scarff, R. W., and Handley, R. S.: Prognosis in carcinoma of the breast. Lancet, *ii*:582, 1938.

Schwartz, G. F., Finkel, G. C., Garcia, J. C., et al.: Subclinical ductal carcinoma in situ of the breast. Cancer, *70*:2468, 1992.

Shimokawara, I., Imamura, M., Yamanaka, N., et al.: Identification of lymphocyte subpopulations in human breast cancer and its significance: An immunoperoxidase study with anti–human T- and B-cell sera. Cancer, *49*:1456, 1982.

Slamon, D. J., Godolphin, W., Jones, L. A., et al.: Studies of the HER-2/neu proto-oncogene in human breast and ovarian cancer. Science, *244*:707–712, 1989.

Solin, L. S., Yeh, I-T, Kurtz, J., Fourquet, A., et al.: Ductal carcinoma in situ (intraductal carcinoma) of the breast treated with breast-conserving surgery and definitive irradiation. Cancer, *71*:2532, 1993.

Squires, J. E., and Betsill, W. L. Jr.: Intracystic carcinoma of the breast, a correlation of cytomorphology, gross pathology and clinical data. Acta Cytol., *25*:267, 1981.

Steinbrecher, J. S., and Silverberg, S. G.: Signet-ring cell carcinoma of the breast: The mucinous variant of infiltrating lobular carcinoma? Cancer, *37*:828, 1976.

Tandon, A. T., Clark, K. G. M., Chamness, G. C., et al.: Cathepsin D and prognosis in breast cancer. N. Engl. J. Med., *322*:297, 1990.

Tavassoli, F. A.: Pathology of the Breast. New York, Elsevier, 1992.

Tavassoli, F. A., and Norris, H. J.: Secretory carcinoma of the breast: A clinicopathologic study with ultrastructural findings. Cancer, *45*:2423, 1980.

Taylor, G., and Meltzer, A.: Inflammatory carcinoma of the breast. Am. J. Cancer, *33*:33, 1938.

Taylor, H. B., and Norris, H. J.: Well-differentiated carcinoma of the breast. Cancer, *25*:687, 1970.

Thor, A., Benz, C., Moore, D. II, et al.: Stress response protein (SRP-27) determination in primary human breast carcinomas: Clinical histologic and prognostic correlations. J. Natl. Cancer Inst., *83*:170, 1991.

Tobon, H., and Salazar, H.: Tubular carcinoma of the breast: Clinical, histological and ultrastructural observations. Arch. Pathol. Lab. Med., *101*:310, 1977.

Toikanen, S.: Primary squamous cell carcinoma of the breast. Cancer, *48*:1629, 1981.

Toikanen, S., and Joensuu, H.: Glycogen-rich clear cell carcinoma of the breast. A clinicopathologic and flow cytometric study. Hum. Pathol., *22*:81, 1991.

Tuluson, A. H., Ronay, G., Egger, H., et al.: A contribution to the natural history of breast cancer. V. Bilateral primary breast cancer. Incidence, risks and diagnosis of simultaneous primary cancer in the opposite breast. Arch. Gynecol., *237*:85, 1985.

Van Bogaert, L. J., and Maldague, P.: Histological classification of pure primary epithelial breast cancer. Hum. Pathol., *9*:175, 1978.

Weidner, N., Semple, J. P., Welch, W. R., et al.: Tumor angiogenesis and metastasis—correlation in invasive breast carcinoma. N. Engl. J. Med., *324*:1, 1991.

Weigand, R. A., Isenberg, W. M., Russo, J., et al.: Blood vessel invasion and axillary lymph node involvement as prognostic indicators for human breast cancer. Cancer, *50*:962, 1982.

Wellings, S. R., Jensen, H. M., and Marcum, R. G.: Atlas of subgross pathology of the human breast with special reference to possible precancerous lesions. J. Natl. Cancer Inst., *55*:231, 1974.

Wells, C. A., Nicoll, S., and Ferguson, D. J. P.: Adenoid cystic carcinoma of the breast: A case with axillary lymph node metastasis. Histopathology, *10*:415, 1986.

World Health Organization: Histological Typing of Breast Tumors. 2nd ed. International Histological Classification of Tumors No. 2. Geneva, World Health Organization, 1981.

13

Cell Kinetics of Breast and Breast Tumors

John S. Meyer

This chapter consists of three parts. The first part, *Overview of Cell Kinetics,* is intended for readers who are not conversant with the terminology and theory of cell kinetics and flow cytometry and for those who desire a review of these topics. The second section, *Cell Kinetics of Normal Breast and Benign Epithelial Hyperplasias,* provides a background against which the altered kinetics of cancers can be appreciated. The third section, *Cell Kinetic and DNA Flow Cytometric Measurements in Breast Carcinoma,* is a review of kinetic and deoxyribonucleic acid (DNA) flow cytometric data with a discussion of their clinical applicability.

OVERVIEW OF CELL KINETICS

Mitotic Counts

Initially, the counting of mitotic cells was the only approach to cell kinetic analysis. Mitotic counts are well established for prognosis of mesenchymal tumors (Stout, 1948; and Russell et al., 1977), including cytosarcomas of the breast (Norris and Taylor, 1967). Occasional earlier reports have associated high mitotic indices (MIs) with poor survival in breast carcinomas (Bloom and Richardson, 1957; Wallgren et al., 1976; and Parl and Dupont, 1982), but mitotic counts have not achieved widespread use in epithelial tumors of the breast.

Precise measurement of the MI is difficult in many breast carcinomas because mitoses are scarce. In some carcinomas, more than 10,000 cells must be counted to find five or more mitotic figures. Mitoses must be distinguished from pyknosis and karyorrhexis of dead or dying cells, a problem that becomes more troublesome as mitoses become increasingly infrequent. Mitotic index is a function of the proportion of cells in a population that are in the proliferative compartment (cycling cells), the duration of the cell cycle (time between mitoses), and length of time required to complete mitosis. The latter is brief compared with other segments of the cell cycle, but it can vary as much as fourfold or fivefold in carcinomas (Sisken et al., 1985). Prolonged duration of mitosis produces higher MIs, independent of the actual rate of cell proliferation. McDivitt and coworkers (1986) noted significant correlations between tritiated thymidine-labeling index (TLI) and S-phase fraction (SPF) by flow cytometry of DNA, on the one hand, and mitotic index per 10 high-power fields (HPF) on the other ($r = 0.43$, $r = 0.30$, respectively, $P = .0001$) in 168 primary breast carcinomas. The magnitude of these correlations indicates only partial correspondence of the three measurements.

Recently, success with more complex measurements of proliferation has led to renewed interest in the MI of breast carcinoma, and MI has proved to be a strong stage-independent prognostic indicator. Clayton (1991) counted mitoses per 50 HPF and found that variable was able to define a group of 30% of node-negative patients with poor prognosis; those with fewer than 4.5 mitoses per 10 HPF 0.412 mm in diameter in highly cellular areas (70% of patients) showed a 92% 5-year survival rate, whereas patients with more than that number had a 62% 5-year survival rate. These authors avoided areas of necrosis but did not compensate for relative volumes of stroma and carcinoma. Laroye and Minkin (1991) compared counting mitoses per HPF, per square millimeter of tumor section, and per calculated 10,000 cells. The number of cells was estimated as the product of the number per HPF and the number of HPF counted. Each method predicted survival to some extent in a group of 92 patients at various stages observed 10 years, but the per-square-millimeter method predicted best, though results were still short of statistical significance ($P = .07$). Baak and associates (Baak et al., 1985; and van Diest and Baak, 1991) developed a morphometric prognostic index for breast carcinoma of which the MI from the 10 HPF of the most mitosis-rich area was an important variable. The MI predicted cancer-specific survival at a significance level comparable to the number of axillary metastases and more strongly than tumor size, histologic grade, nuclear area, or standard deviation of nuclear area, all of which reached statistical significance as univariate predictors. Figure 13–1 shows the predictive power of MI for *cancer-specific* survival. (The reader should note that cancer-specific survival plots may exaggerate apparent prognostic effects because intercurrent deaths are censored. Therefore this plot should not be compared with those of Figs. 13–22 through 13–25, in which intercurrent deaths were considered treatment failures.)

In summary, mitotic counts are predictive of the course of breast carcinoma. This method of assessing proliferation has the advantages of not requiring special procedures and of being available in any laboratory and applicable for retrospective studies. It is less sensitive as a measure of proliferation than DNA precursor labeling (tritiated thymidine [^{3}H-TdR], 2′-deoxy-5-bromouridine [BrdUrd]), but whether it is less effective is not known. It has not been

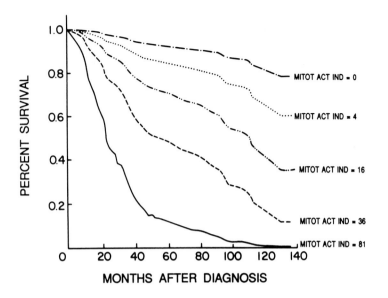

Figure 13-1. Effect of MI on tumor-specific survival of breast carcinoma patients. (After Baak, J. P. A., Van Dop, H., Kurver, P. H. J., et al.: The value of morphometry to classic prognosticators in breast cancer. Cancer, *56*:374–382, 1985, with permission.)

compared directly with the latter methods for predictive power.

Precursor of DNA and the Cell Cycle

The advent of radioactive labeling of DNA provided a practical means for assessing cellular proliferation that is particularly useful in epithelial tumors (Figs. 13–2 and 13–3). The first attempts to label cells during DNA synthesis (S-phase) employed radioactive phosphorus (Howard and Pelc, 1951) or carbon 14–labeled formate (Lajtha, 1957). Both of these labels were nonspecific but were preferentially incorporated into the DNA of S-phase cells (Lajtha, 1957). Thymidine labeled with tritium on the methyl group, introduced by Taylor and coworkers (1957), is a specific label for DNA because thymidine is incorporated only into DNA, and the methyl group evidently is not transferred to other pyrimidine bases. It soon was evident that all replicating cells engage in DNA synthesis during a discrete period

of the interval between mitoses. The S-phase is separated from mitosis by two intervals, G_1 and G_2. G_1 is relatively long and follows immediately after mitosis and ends at the beginning of the S-phase. G_2 is relatively short (usually 2 to 4 hours) and separates the S-phase from mitosis (M). (These two intervals in apparent activity were seen as gaps, thus the abbreviations G_1 and G_2.) The entire period between mitoses is termed the "cell cycle."

Bromodeoxyuridine and Iododeoxyuridine as Substitutes for Radiolabel

The thymidine analogue BrdUrd is chemically closely related to thymidine, the difference being replacement of the methyl group at the 5 position of the pyrimidine ring by a bromine atom. Steric properties of the bromine resemble those of the methyl group, and BrdUrd is handled by certain

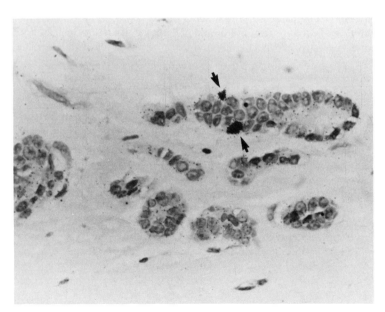

Figure 13-2. Autoradiograph of well-differentiated breast carcinoma with low TLI. S-phase nuclei appear black because of overlying silver grains activated by tritiated thymidine taken up during incubation. The only two labeled nuclei, marked by *arrows*, are in the tangentially sectioned tubule on the upper right. (Kodak NTB2 emulsion, hematoxylin and eosin stain, × 520.)

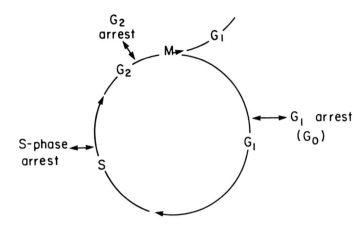

Figure 13–3. Cell cycle diagram. After mitosis (M), the daughter cells enter G_1, where they may become arrested (G_0). When conditions for growth improve, G_0 cells can re-enter the mitotic cycle. G_1 cells progress to DNA synthesis (S), but, if conditions deteriorate, may become arrested in the S-phase. On completion of DNA synthesis, a cell is in G_2 until the onset of the next mitosis.

enzymes, including thymidine kinase and DNA polymerases, as though it were thymidine. Thymidine kinase performs a phosphorylation step necessary for transport of BrdUrd into the cell, and DNA polymerase incorporates the triphosphate into DNA. The first monoclonal antibody to BrdUrd was developed by Gratzner (1982), and antibodies from a number of other clones have become available since. Affinities vary (Vanderlaan et al., 1986). Most antibodies bind only to single-stranded DNA labeled with BrdUrd or iododeoxyuridine (IdUrd), requiring denaturation of DNA, but one antibody has been found to bind without denaturation (Witzig et al., 1989). Not all antibodies react with both types of halogenated DNA. BR-3 reacts only with DNA labeled with BrdUrd. Used in conjunction with a cross-reacting antibody, for example IU-4, cells can be labeled sequentially and those labeled with either one or both precursors can be distinguished. This permits calculation of S-phase duration (Shibui et al., 1989) (see below). BrdUrd and IdUrd can be given parenterally for S-phase labeling in vivo (Wilson et al., 1985; and Hoshino et al., 1989). Results of S-phase labeling in vitro versus in vivo or by tritiated thymidine versus BrdUrd are equivalent for determination

of the proportion of cells in S-phase (labeling index [LI]) (Wilson et al., 1985; Meyer and Nauert, 1989; and Waldman et al., 1991).

BrdUrd labeling with direct microscopic assessment currently is the method of choice for determination of S-phase measurements in breast carcinoma, and it is the standard against which other methods should be compared. Labeling in vitro is effective, and the time required to carry out the entire procedure is not prohibitive. The microscope count takes approximately 25 minutes, and when specimens are batched for staining the total labor time per specimen is 1 hour or less. Preparations can be archived for future review. Figures 13–4 to 13–7 illustrate several types of breast carcinomas with S-phase cells labeled by BrdUrd.

Measurement of Duration of Cell Cycle and Its Segments

Several methods for measuring cell cycle segment transit times (durations for G_1, S, G_2, and M) have been developed and are thoroughly reviewed by Steel (1977). In general, these methods are not practical for routine clinical application because they require administering radioactive DNA

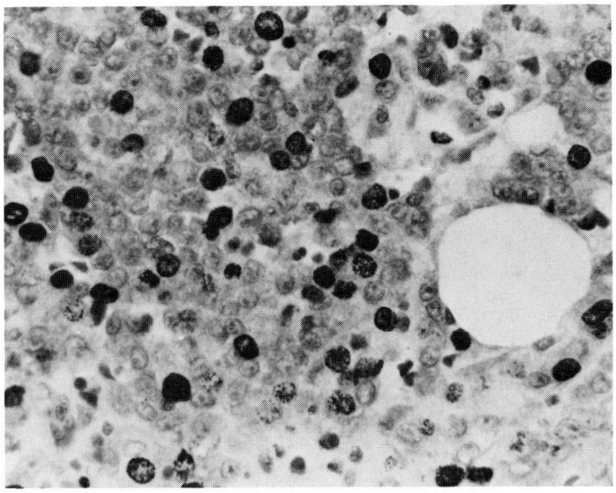

Figure 13–4. High-grade breast carcinoma labeled in vitro with BrdUrd. Note the high resolution of many S-phase nuclei that are marked black. BrdUrd incubation of slices, Carnoy fixation, hydrochloric acid DNA-denaturation, monoclonal anti-BrdUrd, immunogold-silver enhancement, nuclear-fast red, and light green counterstain. (× 520.)

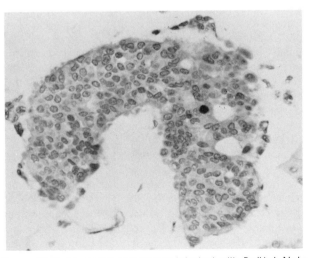

Figure 13–5. Mucinous carcinoma labeled with BrdUrd. Note the few labeled nuclei. This specimen was processed in the same manner as that in Figure 13–2. (× 520.)

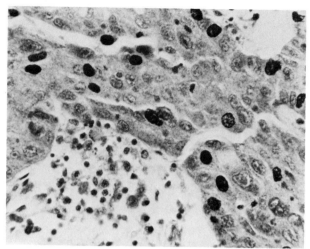

Figure 13–6. Medullary carcinoma labeled with BrdUrd. Many nuclei are labeled. This specimen was processed in the same manner as that in Figure 13–2. (× 520.)

precursors or mitosis-arresting agents (colchicine, vinca alkaloids) to patients and performing serial biopsies. Quastler and Sherman (1959) developed the classic fraction of labeled mitoses (FLM) method. A single injection of tritiated thymidine is administered and biopsies are taken at regular intervals for several days to plot the percentage of labeled mitoses (Fig. 13–8). From these data the duration of the cell cycle and its segments can be deduced (Mendelsohn and Takahashi, 1971; and Steel, 1977).

Introduction of halogenated pyrimidine DNA precursors BrdUrd and IdUrd has provided a new perspective for measurement of the duration of S-phase (T_s). By administering both precursors sequentially in vivo, preferably with an interval of 1 or 2 hours between infusions, cells in transit through S are doubly labeled. Cells that enter S after completion of the first infusion and before completion of the second infusion are labeled only with the second agent, and cells in S during the first infusion that progress beyond S before the second infusion are labeled only with the first agent. Chromogens of different colors are used to mark the BrdUrd and IdUrd labels distinctively during the immunohistochemical reactions (Miller et al., 1991; and Raza et al., 1991a). Knowing the durations of the infusions, which ordinarily are approximately 30 minutes to an hour, and the interval between them, the duration of S can be computed from the proportions of cells labeled with either agent or with both (Shibui et al., 1989; and Raza et al., 1991b). This method has the advantage of clear microscopic visualization of the neoplastic cells, which prevents inclusion of extraneous cells in the measurements.

Another technique utilizes flow cytometry of tissue labeled in vivo with BrdUrd a few hours prior to excision. The principle is that of movement of the labeled cells against the backdrop of the flow cytometric DNA histogram (Begg et al., 1985). Dual-parameter flow cytometry is employed after preparation of a cell or nuclear suspension, labeling of BrdUrd-positive nuclei with fluorescein immunohistochemically, and labeling of DNA stoichiometrically with propidium iodide. The red fluorescence of propidium

iodide and green fluorescence of fluorescein are discriminated by use of filters. As cells move through S after pulse labeling with BrdUrd, the amount of DNA in each labeled cell increases, causing the labeled cells to move from G_0–G_1 toward the G_2–M position. When the cells divide, they appear with halved prior green fluorescence in the G_0–G_1 position. Motion of the mean red fluorescence of BrdUrd-labeled cells to the right may remain linear as long as 8 hours (Fogt et al., 1991). Relative movement (RM) is calculated from the following equation:

$$RM = \frac{F_L - F_{G_1}}{F_{GM} - F_{G_1}} \quad (1)$$

where FL is the mean red fluorescence of labeled cells, F_{G_1} is the mean red fluorescence of the G_0–G_1 cells, and F_{GM} is the mean red fluorescence of the G_2–M cells (Begg et al., 1985; and Fogt et al., 1991). T_s can be calculated as follows:

$$T_s = \frac{0.5}{RM - 0.5} \times t \quad (2)$$

where t is the time between labeling and sampling. The numerator of the fraction is 0.5 because that is the value of RM when t is zero (Begg et al., 1985).

White and associates (1990) have presented an extensive analysis of the RM concept, and they have defined a function that relates T_s to cell cycle time when sufficient time has elapsed to permit BrdUrd-labeled cells to have divided. For an exponentially growing population with stable age distribution, fractions of labeled divided and undivided cells determine a variable, which, if T_s is known, permits calculation of potential doubling time. Provided that the great majority of S-phase cells in a specimen belong to the population of interest (i.e., tumor cells) as would be the case in most solid tumors, non-neoplastic cells dissociated from tumor specimens would not present consequential interference. Whether this method can work with fresh slices of

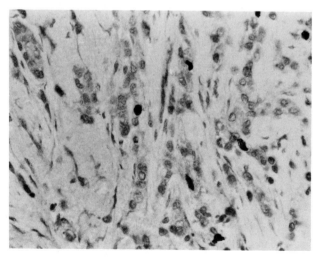

Figure 13–7. Infiltrating lobular carcinoma labeled with BrdUrd. The LI is low. This specimen was processed in the same manner as that in Figure 13–2. (× 520.)

Figure 13-8. Idealized and representative FLM curves for breast carcinoma. If the population of neoplastic cells all had the same invariable cell cycle transit times with total cycle time (T_c) of 43 h, G_1 of 20 h, T_s (DNA synthesis time) of 18 h, G_2 of 4 h, and mitosis of 1 h, the result would be a series of parallelograms. After a single injection of tritiated thymidine (^{3}H-TdR), at time zero, the first labeled mitotic figures would appear at 4 h, and the percentage of labeled mitoses would rise to 100% as the last unlabeled mitoses reached completion 1 h later. After 17 h, unlabeled mitoses, representing cells in late G_1 at the time of injection of ^{3}H-TdR, would appear, and within 1 h the last of the labeled cells would have completed mitosis. All of the mitoses would then be unlabeled. As the daughter cells from the first mitosis enter mitosis again, the second wave of the FLM curve develops.

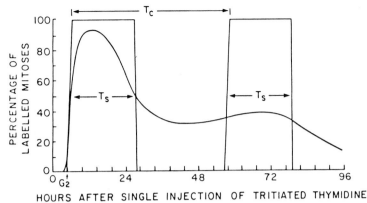

HOURS AFTER SINGLE INJECTION OF TRITIATED THYMIDINE

Because tumors have wide dispersions of durations of cell cycle phases, the actual FLM curve varies markedly from the ideal, and synchrony of the labeled cohort is lost so quickly that a clear second wave may not be seen. Variation in the length of G_2 may prevent the FLM from reaching 100% even in the first wave. Estimates for the cell cycle are derived from the FLM curve as follows: T_c from the distance between peaks, T_s from the width of the first peak as half height, G_2 from the time of first appearance of labeled mitoses, and G_1 by subtraction.

tumor incubated in vitro, thereby avoiding the need to administer BrdUrd to patients, is not yet known.

Little information is available from BrdUrd-IdUrd double labeling or BrdUrd relative motion flow cytometry concerning T_s of breast carcinomas, but a preliminary study with double labeling suggests that T_s may vary over a range of 18 to 33 hours (Raza et al., 1992). Work with leukemia has shown measurement of T_s to be useful in prognosis (Raza et al., 1991*a*), and the practicality of the method has been demonstrated in colorectal carcinoma (Yousuf et al., 1991).

Kinetic and Microenvironmental Heterogeneity

Populations of neoplastic cells invariably show a good deal of heterogeneity with regard to cell cycle transit times. Prolongation of cell cycle segments for nutritional and respiratory reasons is now firmly established for both in vitro and in vivo conditions. Trowell (1952) calculated that the theoretical limiting radius of a cluster of nonvascularized cells with ordinary rates of oxygen consumption would be 0.32 mm (weight, 0.14 mg). Tissue culture conditions can be adjusted to produce cell death, noncycling cells, or cells that move through the cycle at much reduced rates (Dell'Orco, 1974). Similar conditions occur in vivo as a result of imbalance between growth of neoplastic cells and nutrient blood vessels. In this context of heterogeneity, the FLM method is strongly influenced by rapidly cycling cohorts, which rise above the background of more slowly cycling cells in the FLM curve.

For this reason, as Hamilton and Dobbin (1983) have shown, the FLM method may grossly underestimate the mean cell cycle time. Sufficient heterogeneity is usually present among even the rapidly cycling cells in human tumors so that a second FLM peak seldom is seen (Mendelsohn and Takahashi, 1971; and Steel, 1977). Thus, the values for lengths of cell cycles and their segments derived from FLM curves are more representative of the healthier, more active cells than of the less well nourished cells.

Methods that compute cell cycle duration from measurement of T_s can also be influenced by microenvironmental heterogeneity, to the extent that T_s is prolonged by deprivation of oxygen and nutrients. Prolongation of T_s, even to the point of arrest under unfavorable environmental conditions, has been demonstrated in various cell lines. Shrieve and Begg (1985) showed that a period of hypoxia will stop DNA synthesis, and that after reoxygenation synthesis can be reinitiated but with markedly reduced rate of progression. Given the possibility of perfusional instability within tumors, it is clear that results are more reliable if multiple samples are taken from different areas.

Arrest of Progression in the Cell Cycle

Cells grown in culture as spheroidal aggregates show slowing of progression through the replicative cycle with increasing distance from the surface, finally progressing to complete arrest in one segment or another and still more centrally becoming necrotic. Wibe and coworkers (1981) found that the thickness of viable cells in tumors grown as spheroids is about 80 μm. Progressing inward from the surface, the relative number of cells in G_1 increased and the relative number in S decreased. Landry and coworkers (1982) and Allison and associates (1983) presented evidence for arrest also in the S and G_2 phases. Similar changes have been observed in thymidine labeling studies of experimental tumors with extensive necrosis and perivascular growth. In these so-called corded tumors (Tannock, 1968; and Jones and Camplejohn, 1983) found that the mean distance between zones of necrosis and blood vessels was 80 μm, similar to that of the zone of viability at the surface of spheroids. The mean number of layers of cells per cord was 10.3. Numbers of noncycling cells increased progressively with distance from blood vessels, and nonproliferative fractions were estimated as 64% in the inner zones and 94% in the outer zones. Cells with patterns of radioresistance typical of noncycling hypoxic cells exist in mouse mammary carcinomas as small as 1 mm in diameter (Suit and Shalek, 1963; and Rockwell et al., 1972). Therefore, they should be expected to occur in micrometastases as well as in clinically evident tumors.

The G_0 Concept and Growth Fraction

The concept of a facultatively nonproliferative compartment in tumors was elaborated by Mendelsohn (1960, 1962) as a means of explaining the differential sensitivities of oxygenated and hypoxic cells to radiation therapy. Evidence that hypoxic cells are nonproliferative or have prolonged cell cycle durations and can survive higher doses of potentially lethal radiation than well-oxygenated cells is well accepted among radiation biologists (Kennedy et al., 1980; Rockwell, 1983; and Moulder and Rockwell, 1984). It has led to a number of clinical studies using either high oxygen tensions (to decrease numbers of hypoxic cells), low oxygen tensions (to protect host tissues by rendering them hypoxic also), or drugs such as misonidazole that sensitize hypoxic cells to radiation (Chapman, 1979). Mendelsohn defined G_0 cells as cells that do not traverse the replicative cell cycle but are capable of doing so at some time when conditions become more favorable. A neuron would not be considered a G_0 cell because it is not capable of reentering the cycle; however, a liver cell can be considered as G_0 (although not for reason of hypoxia). Given the proper stimulus (partial hepatectomy, for example), the hepatocyte is capable of DNA replication and division. Initially, the G_0 compartment was considered to communicate with G_1. More recently, cells arrested in G_2 have been observed in both normal tissues (Sauerboern et al., 1978) and tumors (Coninx et al., 1983). S-phase–arrested cells have also been identified in tumors (Darzynkiewicz et al., 1980; and Allison et al., 1985). Whether these cells, arrested in cell cycle segments other than G_1, are capable of progression in the cell cycle and are therefore truly G_0 is not yet clear. Abundant evidence shows that hypoxic cells in experimental tumors under both in vivo and in vitro conditions are capable of growth when conditions become favorable and can reestablish tumors when transplanted into new hosts (Kennedy et al., 1980).

Recent studies by Amellem and Pettersen (1991) have clarified the status of cells arrested in S by hypoxia. They reported that cells in early and middle S-phase were killed by high-grade hypoxia but that cells in late G_1, late S, G_2, and M were able to survive 24 hours of hypoxia. Cells that were not in early or middle S when arrested by hypoxia were able to resume progression of the cell cycle when reoxygenated. Therefore, arrest prior to entry into S can protect cells from even severe hypoxia that would kill them if they progressed into S.

Duration of Cell Cycle and Its Segments

Summarized results from studies of human tumors both in vivo and in vitro show the following approximate dura-

tions: G_1, 58 hours; S, 19 hours; and G_2, 6 hours or less; total cell cycle, 85 hours (Meyer, 1981). These figures appear to apply to breast carcinoma, in addition to a spectrum of other tumors, but they are only generalizations and approximations, and they probably are representative of only the better-nourished cells.

From FLM studies of breast carcinomas, Post and coworkers (1977) reported a DNA synthesis time of 24 hours, Terz and coworkers (1977) reported 12.5 hours, and Straus and Moran (1977), 18 hours. Two studies in vitro by the double-labeling technique yielded results between 18 and 22 hours (Sklarew et al., 1977; and Schiffer et al., 1979). The FLM studies indicate a G_2 duration of approximately 4 or 5 hours (Post et al., 1977; and Terz et al., 1977).

Results with the more modern technique of BrdUrd DNA flow cytometry, using the relative motion of BrdUrd to define T_s, agree with the older data: T_s ranges from 10 to 31 hours for a variety of tumors, the mean being close to 18 hours. Melanomas were an exception: T_s was about 9 hours. (Wilson et al., 1988). Data from breast carcinomas are not yet available. A tendency for higher nuclear DNA contents to be associated with longer S-phase durations has been observed (Sklarew, 1984).

Time-lapse cinematographic studies of cell lines derived from human tumors show that the duration of mitoses (excluding prophase) is usually less than 30 minutes, the greater portion of this time being taken up by metaphase (Sisken et al., 1985). In three breast carcinoma lines, metaphases averaged 23, 40, and 60 minutes, anaphases lasted 4, 4, and 5 minutes, and cytokinesis lasted 3, 3, and 3 minutes, respectively. Total durations of histologically recognizable mitosis were 30, 47, and 68 minutes in the three cell lines (Sisken et al., 1985). As most measurements of the duration of the S-phase for breast carcinoma are near 19 hours, the number of S-phase cells is clearly approximately 20 times the number of M-phase cells at any given time. S-phase counts therefore have a great statistical advantage over M-phase counts.

The S-Phase Labeling Index (LI): In Vivo and in Vitro Labeling

The earliest TLIs were achieved by injection of ^{3}H-TdR into the patient shortly before biopsy or excision of the tumor (Baserga et al., 1962; Clarkson et al., 1965; Hoffman and Post, 1967; and Shirakawa et al., 1970). Straus and coworkers (Straus and Moran, 1980; and Straus et al., 1982) have published the only extensive studies of in vivo TLIs of breast carcinoma. They observed mean TLIs of 5.2% in 13 patients with T1–3 carcinomas, 9.0% in 10 patients with T4 carcinomas (local extension without distant spread), and 13.2% in nine patients with metastatic breast carcinoma (Straus and Moran, 1980). They also noted decreased survival rates in all stages, including metastatic disease, with TLIs in excess of 8%. Their frequency distribution of TLIs after in vivo labeling resembles the author's distribution from in vitro labeling (Meyer et al., 1986). These results have been confirmed by in vivo BrdUrd labeling studies by Waldman and coworkers

(1991). Convincing evidence that in vitro and in vivo TLIs are essentially the same is also furnished by several comparative studies with tumors in laboratory animals (Rajewsky, 1965; Steel and Bensted, 1965; Fabrikant et al., 1969; Meyer and Bauer, 1975; and Meyer and Connor, 1977).

Labeling indices with BrdUrd administered by intravenous infusion have also been shown to be equivalent to indices after in vitro incubation with BrdUrd (Waldman et al., 1991). Thus, the various combinations of in vivo versus in vitro and BrdUrd versus ³H-Tdr give equivalent labeling indices.

Effects of Oxygenation and Intracellular Precursor Pools on DNA Thymidine Labeling

DNA synthesis in mammalian cells requires oxygenation. Incubation of small blocks or slices with ³H-TdR at atmospheric oxygen tension may result in labeling only to a depth of 5 to 10 cells beneath the surface. Labeling tends to be deeper in poorly cellular tumors or in those with low TLIs than in tumors that are highly cellular and have high TLIs. When labeling is only superficial, the TLI is difficult to determine and may easily be underestimated. Fabrikant and coworkers (1969) demonstrated that the depth of labeling is increased by increasing the oxygen tension. Near maximum effects were achieved with 3 to 4 atmospheres (atm) of oxygen. Under these circumstances, well-labeled cells were found as far as 0.5 mm beneath the surface, but at atmospheric oxygen tension, labeling did not occur more than 0.1 mm beneath the surface. However, the author has observed in many highly cellular, high-TLI breast carcinomas that even with hyperbaric oxygenation the depth of labeling is relatively poor. This, presumably, is because of rapid degradation of ³H-TdR as it diffuses between the malignant cells (Rubini et al., 1966; and Maurer, 1981).

Large intracellular pools of thymidine phosphates dilute any ³H-TdR or BrdUrd transported into cells, and intensity of labeling of DNA is decreased thereby. Furthermore, high levels of thymidine triphosphate may inhibit thymidine kinase, the enzyme responsible for phosphorylation of exogenous ³H-TdR or BrdUrd and its transport across the cell membrane (Fig. 13–9). A second factor that may influence the success of labeling is intracellular synthesis of thymidylate. The principal precursor of thymidine phosphate is deoxyuridine phosphate (Heidelberger, 1982). Synthesis of thymidine phosphate is effected by the enzyme thymidylate synthetase from deoxyuridine phosphate in the presence of the coenzyme tetrahydrofolate reductase. One practical way to decrease intracellular thymidine phosphate pools is to block thymidylate synthetase with 5-fluorouracil (5-FU) or its derivative, 5-fluoro-2′-deoxyuridine (FUdR), thereby preventing synthesis of thymidylate (Heidelberger, 1982). Several studies have demonstrated that blockade of cellular thymidylate synthesis increases the incorporation of exogenously supplied thymidine or thymidine analogues (Dörmer et al., 1975; Meyer and Facher, 1977; Chavaudra and Malaise, 1979; Hamilton et al., 1984; and Ellward and Dörmer, 1985).

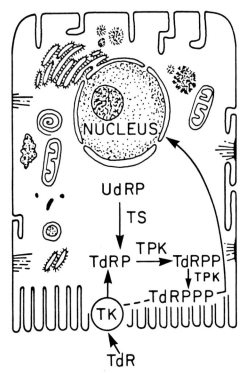

Figure 13–9. Simplified diagram of a cell showing paths for uptake and phosphorylation of thymidine (TdR) to thymidine monophosphate (TdRP) by the enzyme thymidine kinase (TK) located in the cell membrane. TdRP can also be produced within the cell through methylation of deoxyuridine monophosphate (UdRP) by the enzyme thymidylate synthetase (TS). TdRP is phosphorylated by thymidine phosphokinase to the diphosphate TdRPP (TPK) and again to the triphosphate TdRPPP, which serves as a substrate for DNA polymerase. TdRPPP in high concentrations inhibits thymidine kinase, a mechanism through which the cell avoids accumulation of excess levels of thymidine phosphates.

The data in Table 13–1 show that thymidylate synthetase blockade may enhance the detection of S-phase cells by thymidine labeling. Intracellular thymidylate synthesis may be particularly important in occasional tumors, as reported by Hamilton and Dobbin (1982). These murine mammary carcinomas were labeled very well with titrated deoxyuridine through the thymidylate synthetase pathway. When ³H-TdR was supplied, labeling was poor but was made equivalent to that achieved with tritiated deoxyuridine when thymidylate synthetase was blocked with FUdR (Hamilton et al., 1984). The author and colleagues have observed higher TLIs after in vitro labeling with use of hyperbaric oxygen and thymidylate synthetase inhibition than others have observed without these measures. Without blockade of thymidylate synthetase, DNA labeling with ³H-TdR or BUdR could give misleading results in certain carcinomas.

DNA Measurements by Static Cytometry

Static cytometry measures DNA content in single cells or nuclei on glass slides by spectrometry. The technique can be either microdensitometric, wherein the optical density of the nucleus at a given wavelength is proportional to DNA

Table 13-1. LABELING INDICES OF PRIMARY INVASIVE BREAST CARCINOMA

Investigator, Year	Method*	Number	TLI		
			Median	*Mean*	*Range*
Straus and Moran, 1980	1	13		5.2	
Gentili et al., 1981	2	541	2.8	4.8	0.09–40.7
Meyer and Hixon, 1979	3	128	2.1	3.7	0.05–18.6
Meyer et al., 1986	4	757	5.2	7.1	0.05–35.6
Hery et al., 1987	2	76	2.1	2.7	0.1–9.4
Goodson et al., 1991	5	66	5.6	7.7	0.1–23.9

*1, In vivo; 2, in vitro, atmospheric oxygen; 3, in vitro, hyperbaric oxygen; 4, in vitro, hyperbaric oxygen and thymidylate synthetase inhibition; 5, in vivo BrdUrd.

content, or microfluorimetric. In the latter case, DNA is stained stoichiometrically by a fluorescent dye and emission is measured at appropriate wavelength. Static cytometry permits visual selection of cells of interest, so that, to the degree that they can be distinguished in dissociated state, cancer cells can be included and inflammatory and stromal cells excluded. It is labor intensive because of the need to locate each cell by microscopy prior to measurement, but it has the advantage of selectivity and produces an archivable specimen—cells from which the measurements were made on a glass slide. Feulgen staining of DNA of breast carcinoma smears has been used most often (Auer et al., 1980a). Nuclei retrieved by digestion of paraffin-embedded tissue are also suitable (Hatschek et al., 1989). Figure 13–10 shows four types of DNA histograms obtained in breast carcinomas by Feulgen static photometry.

DNA Measurements by Flow Cytometry

The principle of DNA flow cytometry is analogous to that of the familiar Coulter counter of the hematology labora-tory, but fluorescence emission, rather than electrical con-ductance, is measured. As cells flow through the instrument rapidly and in single file, they intercept a beam of light. After staining with a fluorescent dye that is stoichiometric for DNA, the cells emit a pulse of light proportional to their DNA content. The light is allowed to pass through a filter toward a photoelectric detector and amplifier. The resultant electrical pulse is transmitted to a computer, and a histo-gram is generated by plotting the number of cells with different DNA contents (Figs. 13–11 to 13–15). For com-prehensive information, the reader is referred to reviews by Laerum and Farsund (1981), Braylan (1983), and Muirhead and colleagues (1985) and the detailed treatises of Shapiro (1988) and Melamed et al. (1990).

Flow cytometry offers the advantages of speed and au-tomation but has the disadvantage of nonselectivity. The instrument records data from all cells, both the malignant cells of interest and associated benign cells. Development of markers selective for breast carcinoma cells eventually may permit exclusion of contaminating cells, but at present the DNA histogram represents a mixture of neoplastic cells and the associated benign cells (lymphocytes, histiocytes, granulocytes, fibroblasts, endothelial cells, and others) that contaminate all breast carcinomas.

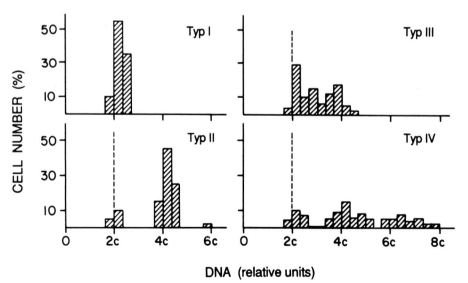

Figure 13-10. Four types of DNA histograms obtained in breast car-cinoma by static photometry fol-lowing staining of DNA by the Feulgen method. Types I and II are associated with good prognosis, and Types III and IV with poor prognosis. (From Fallenius, A. G., Auer, G. U., and Carstensen, J. M.: Prognostic significance of DNA measurements in 409 consecutive breast cancer patients. Cancer, 62:331–341, 1988a, with permission.)

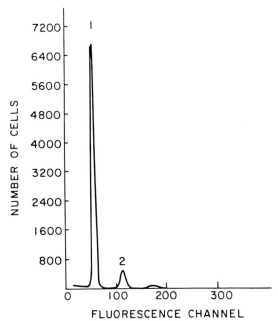

Figure 13–11. DNA histogram of breast carcinoma with diploid DNA content and a low percentage of S-phase cells (%S). Peak 1 represents G_1 and G_0 cells, and peak 2 G_2 and M cells. Because few S-phase cells are present, the curve between the two peaks approaches the baseline. The low peak to the right of peak 2 represents doublets or triplets. As computed from the histogram, SPF = 3%; TLI = 3%. This histogram and those in Figures 13–12 and 13–13 were obtained on cell suspensions stained with 4′, 6-diamidino-2-phenylindole (DAPI) and run on a Partec PAS II flow cytometer.

Ploidy Analysis of Flow Cytometric DNA Histograms

Flow cytometry resolves distinct peaks in the DNA histograms that correspond to G_1 and G_2 populations. Cell pop-

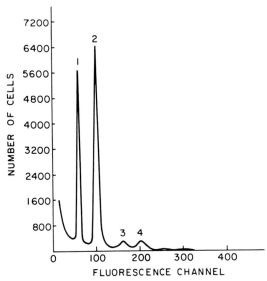

Figure 13–13. Breast carcinoma with an aneuploid (hyperdiploid) peak (peak 2). The diploid G_1-G_0 cells are to the right (peak 1). Peak 3 represents the G_2-M diploid cells and falls in the S region of the hyperdiploid portion of the histogram. Peak 4 represents the G_2-M hyperdiploid cells. SPF = 13%; TLI = 6.7%; DNA index = 1.69.

ulations fall into two classes, diploid and aneuploid. *Diploid,* as used in the context of flow cytometry, means DNA content indistinguishable from that of normal cells but does not imply a completely normal chromosomal pattern. Most of the aneuploid populations, which because of their tight DNA distributions are thought to be clonally derived, fall between G_1 diploid and G_2 diploid peaks or in the tetraploid (diploid G_2) position.

Roughly 20% to 40% of breast carcinomas have no detectable aneuploid cells ("diploid carcinomas"), and 60% have aneuploid cells detected ("aneuploid carcinomas").

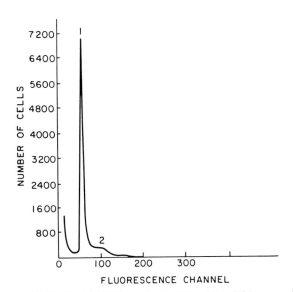

Figure 13–12. Diploid DNA content with a high %S in an adenocarcinoma of the lung. Such high S-phase fractions are unusual in diploid breast carcinomas. Peaks are identified as in Figure 13–11. Debris is seen to the left of peak. SPF = 23%; TLI = 24%.

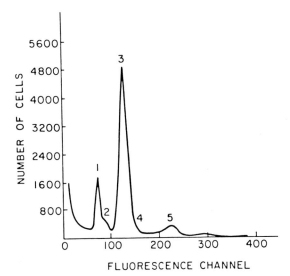

Figure 13–14. Breast carcinoma with two hyperdiploid populations. One (peak 3) has a DNA index of 1.74. The second is a small population with a DNA index of approximately 1.1 that appears as a shoulder on the G_1-G_0 diploid peak (peak 1). SPF = 13% for the major hyperdiploid population; TLI = 13%.

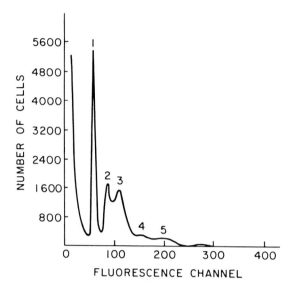

Figure 13–15. Breast carcinoma with two hyperdiploid peaks with DNA indices of 1.49 and 1.89 (peaks 2 and 3). The shoulder on peak 3 represents G_2-M diploid cells (peak 4), and peak 5 represents G_2-M cells of the hyperdiploid populations. SPF = 35%; TLI = 22%.

Of the aneuploid carcinomas, only about 1% are hypodiploid (less than normal DNA content), approximately 80% are hyperdiploid or tetraploid, and 20% are hypertetraploid (more than twice the normal DNA content). The rate of multiple aneuploidy (more than one distinct aneuploid population) is near 3% (Kute et al., 1981; Olszewski et al., 1981b; Raber et al., 1982; McDivitt et al., 1985; and Wenger et al., 1993).

Kinetic Information from Flow Cytometric DNA Histograms

The S-phase cells have a DNA content intermediate between those of G_1 and G_2 cells. In DNA histograms, they are distributed between the beginning of the G_1–G_0 peak and the G_2–M peak. Because of the relatively slow pace of DNA synthesis early and late in the S-phase, relatively more S-phase cells fall under the G_1–G_0 and G_2–M peaks than might be expected (Fig. 13–16) (Culpin and Morris, 1985). To account for the appearance of an S-phase cell in the extreme range of either peak, consider the multiple factors that can influence the size of the electronic pulse generated by a single fluorescent cell. These factors include the speed of flow through the light beam, variability in exciting beam intensity, course through the beam, orientation of the fluorescent nucleus and quenching within the cell and in its immediate environment, and output of the photomultiplier tube. Thus, a single G_1 cell that is repeatedly run through the instrument would produce a histogram with a normal distribution resembling the peaks generated by multiple cells. A very early S-phase cell with only a slight excess above the G_1 DNA content would produce a similar peak.

Various mathematical models have been proposed for analysis of DNA histograms, but for the most part they yield similar results (Baisch et al., 1982). Dean and associates (1982) observed inherent errors of 5% to 10% (coefficient of variation) for measurements of G_1–G_0, S, and G_2–M on replicate runs. A single measurement could produce an error as large as 40% for G_2–M and 15% to 20% for G_1–G_0 and S (Dean et al., 1982). With a low S-phase fraction (SPF), the relative error of measurement could be still greater.

In exponentially growing cell cultures, the percentage of S determined by flow cytometry is closely similar to the TLI, and cells in the S region of the DNA histogram have been shown to be uniformly labeled after exposure to ^{3}H-TdR (Sheck et al., 1980). When conditions for growth are not ideal, as in many neoplasms where zones of vascular insufficiency occur, cells may become arrested in the S-phase, as discussed earlier. This may result in an excess of the percentage of S from flow cytometry over the TLI. Although in some studies of breast carcinomas the mean SPF has been as low as 3.7% to 7.5% (Haag et al., 1984, 1987; and McDivitt et al., 1984), which is close to the mean TLI in the author's laboratory, in other studies the mean SPF has been reported as 9% to 14% (Kute et al., 1981; Olszewski et al., 1981b; Raber et al., 1982; Taylor et al., 1983; and Meyer et al., 1984a). The lowest results reflect methods of computation of percentage of S from DNA histograms that attempt to correct for presence of debris and other artifacts. When debris is subtracted, the distributions of SPF and TLI become closely similar (Haag et al., 1987). Whether these corrections are appropriate is controversial. It appears unlikely that cells in early or late S, when the pace of DNA synthesis is slow, are being missed by

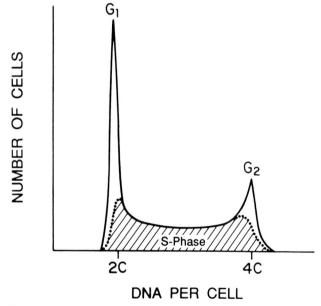

Figure 13–16. DNA histogram showing the U-shaped distribution of S-phase cells caused by the slow pace of DNA synthesis near the beginning and end of the S-phase. This results in a disproportionate fraction of S-phase cells being near the extremes of S rather than in the middle. The presence of many S-phase cells under the G_1 and G_2 peaks complicates the estimation of SPF from DNA histograms.

thymidine-labeling techniques that produce high grain counts over S-phase cells. Bose and coworkers combined computerized microfluorimetry for DNA analysis with autoradiography and showed that all mid-S cells of mouse bone marrow were labeled after 2 days' autoradiographic exposure and that all cells in early and late S were labeled after 8 days' exposure. Therefore debris subtraction, which reduces the median SPF to the level of the median TLI, appears to be necessary for accurate evaluation of breast carcinomas by flow cytometry.

Debris subtraction has been practiced frequently in breast carcinoma S-phase fraction calculations from DNA histograms in recent years (Dressler et al., 1988; Feichter et al., 1988*a;* and Clark et al, 1989). Nonetheless, the shape of the debris curve where it underlies the S-phase region is always uncertain, and recent sorting of particles in the debris regions has revealed that, in at least some tumors, the majority of these particles consist of cells with less than diploid DNA content (Heiden et al., 1991). If most of the so-called debris actually consists of subdiploid microcells, artificial construction of debris curves for subtraction from the S-region makes sense only to the extent that the microcells are counterbalanced by hyperdiploid macrocells in the S-region. That is to say, if faulty mitosis produces a hypodiploid microcell, the second daughter cell should be a hyperdiploid macrocell that would fall in the S-region of the histogram. The extent to which this phenomenon produces pseudo–S-phase cells is not known. SPF measurements by DNA flow cytometry of breast carcinomas correlate only moderately with TLIs, but nonetheless the two measurements have approximately equal value in prognosis of relapse (Meyer and Coplin, 1988; and Clark et al., 1989). Possibly, the flow cytometric measurement makes up what it lacks as a measure of proliferation by reflecting cytogenetic instability, which is also a factor in prognosis. Seen in these terms, the surprisingly strong prognostic power of flow cytometric SPF in comparison to TLI, which is a more direct measurement of DNA synthesis, may result from its relationship to genetic instability and mitotic errors, which play a role in evolution of heterogeneous and increasingly aggressive tumors.

CELL KINETICS OF NORMAL BREAST AND BENIGN EPITHELIAL HYPERPLASIAS

Breast epithelium has long been known to be responsive to ovarian hormones. Only recently has the proliferative activity been studied quantitatively. DNA synthesis takes place in epithelium of the lobule and the postlobular ducts ("breast ducts") at all stages of the menstrual cycle, but it is most intense during the progestational phase of the cycle (Masters et al., 1977; Meyer, 1977; Going et al., 1988; and Christov et al., 1991). In young women, the rate of cell production construed from the TLI is sufficient to renew all cells in the lobule in as little time as 1 month (Meyer, 1977). It is possible, however, that only a portion of the epithelium is renewed, in which case its turnover time would be even shorter. The rate of cell renewal decreases toward menopause and is markedly diminished after menopause. This helps explain the well-known atrophy of the

lobule that occurs at this time. The results of mitotic counting in the lobule are conflicting. Anderson and coworkers (1982) observed a peak in the MI during the progestational phase, a finding that fits with thymidine-labeling data. Vogel and coworkers' (1981) anomalous finding of a peak in MI late in the estrogenic phase has remained unexplained and unconfirmed and presumably is a result of difficulties in discriminating mitotic figures from artifacts.

The postlobular ducts show slower rates of cell renewal (lower TLIs) in premenopausal women than do the lobules (Table 13–2), but the TLIs of the postlobular ducts do not decrease appreciably after menopause. Meyer and Connor (1985) observed a mean TLI for all phases of the menstrual cycle of 1.0% of 59 premenopausal women, with a median of 0.44% and a range of 0.00 to 8.8%. Corresponding values for 16 postmenopausal women for the TLI of the lobular epithelium were a mean of 0.26%, median of 0.18%, and range 0.00% to 1.01%. In 50 premenopausal women, the postlobular ducts had a mean TLI of 0.75%, median of 0.29%, and range of 0.00% to 6.0%. In 16 postmenopausal women, the mean ductal TLI was 0.41%, the median was 0.34%, and the range was 0.00% to 0.93% (Meyer and Connor, 1985). These findings suggest that the postlobular ducts are less responsive to ovarian hormones than is the epithelium of the lobule.

Christov and colleagues (1991) administered bromodeoxyuridine preoperatively to 26 women in order to study normal breast epithelium after mastectomy for breast carcinoma. They confirmed a decline in LI of the lobular epithelium and in addition noted a decline of ductal epithelial LI after menopause. Both studies showed striking variability in LIs from one lobule or duct to another in certain specimens, but the mean indices of the in vitro and the in vivo studies are very similar. Proliferation increases in the breast lobule during pregnancy and is highest during the first 20 weeks, when the mean lobular TLI is approximately 6%, decreasing to approximately half that level for the remainder of pregnancy. With delivery and onset of lactation, levels drop dramatically, to approximately 0.2% (Battersby and Anderson, 1988).

Benign epithelial proliferations of the breast generally have TLIs that resemble those of normal breast epithelium. The TLIs of breast carcinomas, as will be shown later, may be as low as those of the normal breast epithelium and its benign proliferations, but some breast carcinomas have much higher TLIs than have been observed in the benign epithelium.

CELL KINETIC AND DNA FLOW CYTOMETRIC MEASUREMENTS IN BREAST CARCINOMA

Classic Cell Kinetics of Breast Carcinoma

The three fundamental kinetic characteristics to be considered in this section are cell cycle phase durations, growth fraction, and cell loss. Available information about these variables comes from a few FLM studies in vivo and in vitro studies using double-labeling techniques (Wimber and

Table 13–2. THYMIDINE-LABELING INDEX OF NORMAL AND BENIGN PROLIFERATIVE EPITHELIUM

Type of Epithelium	Number	TLI		
		Mean ± SE*	Median	Range
Normal lobule	101	0.09 ± 0.13	0.41	0.00–8.9
Normal postlobular duct	87	0.71 ± 0.12	0.36	0.00–7.2
Lobular hyperplasia	19	0.82 ± 0.22	0.60	0.00–3.1
Intraductal hyperplasia, nonpapillary	27	0.79 ± 0.16	0.33	0.00–2.5
Intraductal hyperplasia, papillary	15	1.02 ± 0.36	0.38	0.00–4.8
Blunt duct adenosis	7	0.68 ± 0.28	0.60	0.00–2.2
Sclerosing adenosis	6	0.47 ± 0.12	0.53	0.10–0.75
Cyst	34	0.56 ± 0.33	0.20	0.00–5.8
Intraductal papilloma	14	1.22 ± 0.33	0.71	0.00–5.9

*SE, Standard error of mean.

Quastler, 1963: Raza et al., 1992). Difficulties with giving radioactive precursors to patients and uncertainties about the reliability of in vitro results limit the scope and reliability of our knowledge (Table 13–3).

The duration of the S-phase is of potential clinical importance because a number of cytotoxic drugs (for example, arabinosyl cytosine and 6-thioguanine, and to a large extent 5-FU, its derivative FUdR, and methotrexate) specifically kill S-phase cells (Heidelberger, 1982). The proportion of S-phase cells in an exponentially growing population is related to the S-phase duration, as described by Steel (1977) in the following:

$$t_c = 0.75 \, (t_s/\text{TLI}) \qquad (3)$$

where t_c is the duration of the cell cycle, t_s is the duration of the S-phase, the TLI is a measure of the proportion of S-phase cells, and 0.75 is a constant related to the position of the S-phase in the cell cycle. This equation ignores the possibility of a G_0 population. Should such be present, the equation would overestimate the t_c for the cycling population.

The long duration of S-phase relative to M gives S-phase measurements a great advantage in speed and accuracy over M-phase measurements. Mitotic cells can be confused with relatively common pyknotic and fragmenting nuclei, and mitoses are so scarce in many breast carcinomas that many hours of work is required to measure MIs.

Growth Fraction

The growth fraction is theoretically important because noncycling cells are relatively insensitive to radiation therapy (Rockwell, 1983; and Moulder and Rockwell, 1984) or cycle-active cytotoxic agents (Laster et al., 1969; Schabel,

Table 13–3. ESTIMATES OF CYCLE PHASE TRANSIT TIMES OF BREAST CARCINOMA CELLS

Phase	Transit Time
Complete cycle	One to many days
G_1	One to many days
S	Approximately 18 hr
G_2	Approximately 5 hr
M, metaphase + anaphase	15 min to 1 hr
M, complete	30 min to 1.5 hr

1975; and Skipper and Schabel, 1982). Measurements of growth fraction of breast carcinoma from different laboratories have yielded values of 0.01 to 0.65. Mean and median values lie between 10% and 25% (Meyer, 1981; Lelle et al., 1987; McGurrin et al., 1987; Stumpp et al., 1992; and Kreipe et al., 1993).

Cell Loss

Cell loss is as important in determining the growth rate of a neoplasm as is cell production. Cells may be lost by death or migration. Necrosis and apoptosis (death of single cells) are prominent features of approximately one-third of infiltrating breast carcinomas (Meyer et al., 1986), but cell death may be inconspicuous and difficult to estimate by microscopic inspection. The only method whereby cell loss can be estimated in breast carcinoma at present is by comparing the proliferative rate of the neoplastic cells with the measured growth rate of the tumor (Steel, 1977). Steel (1967) wrote the following equation for calculation of cell loss (φ):

$$\phi = 1 - (t_c/t_d) \qquad (4)$$

where φ is the fractional rate of cell loss, t_c is the cell cycle time, and t_d is the measured doubling time. If no loss of cells occurred, a breast carcinoma with extremely high proliferative activity would double in volume in 36 hours. Because no clinically evident tumor even approaches this rate of growth, cell loss must be high in rapidly proliferating carcinomas. Mean volume-doubling times for breast carcinomas have ranged from 109 to 327 days, and measurements of cell cycle time range from less than 1 to 4 days. Even allowing for a large G_0 fraction, the mean rate of cell loss must be well over 50%. Measurements of cell loss in various human cancers have ranged from 15% to 85% (Meyer, 1981). The degree of histologically detectable cell loss (necrosis, apoptosis) increases in proportion to the TLI of breast carcinoma.

Frequency Distribution of the DNA-Labeling Index in Breast Carcinoma

Infiltrative and in situ breast carcinomas have a broad range of TLIs, which extend from 0.1% or less to 35% (Meyer et

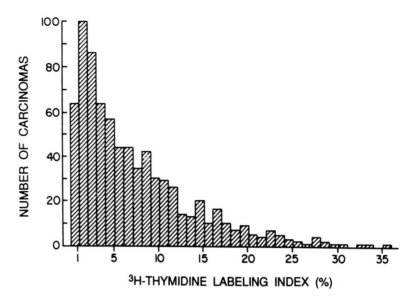

Figure 13–17. Frequency distribution of TLI in 757 primary, infiltrating breast carcinomas. (From Meyer, J.S., Prey, M.U., Babcock, D.S., et al.: Breast carcinoma cell kinetics, morphology, stage, and host characteristics: A thymidine labeling study. Lab. Invest., *54*:41, 1986. Reprinted with permission. Copyright 1986 by the U.S. and Canadian Academy of Pathology, Inc.)

al., 1986) (Fig. 13–17). Repeated studies have shown that the frequency distribution of the TLI of infiltrating breast carcinoma is highly positively skewed (Tubiana et al., 1975; Sklarew et al., 1977; Meyer and Hixon, 1979; Schiffer et al., 1979; Silvestrini et al., 1979; and Meyer et al., 1986). The author and colleagues have found the same to be true for in situ carcinoma, although their highest TLIs are lower than those for invasive carcinomas. Furthermore, the TLIs of in situ carcinomas have been found to be proportional to those of associated invasive carcinomas (Meyer, 1986). An in vivo BrdUrd-LI frequency distribution from invasive carcinomas recently reported (Goodson et al., 1991) (Fig. 13–18) resembles frequency distributions from in vitro ³H-TdR labeling (Fig. 13–19). LI values (mean 7.7%, median 5.6%) in this group of 66 patients were similar to those obtained in vitro by thymidine labeling (Meyer et al., 1986).

Special Histologic Types of Breast Carcinomas Have Characteristic Proliferative Indices

Table 13–4 describes the strong relationship between histologic type of carcinoma and the TLI. Certain carcinomas of established low-grade malignancy have low TLIs (Meyer et al., 1978, 1986). These include adenocystic, mucinous, papillary, and tubular carcinomas. Medullary carcinomas and tumors with some features of medullary carcinomas (atypical medullary carcinoma) consistently have high LIs (see Figs. 9–2 and 9–4 to 9–7). That medullary carcinomas have a relatively good prognosis despite rapid proliferative rates at first seems odd, but the good prognosis is explained by their low rates of metastasis, not by slow progression once metastases have occurred. Several authors have ob-

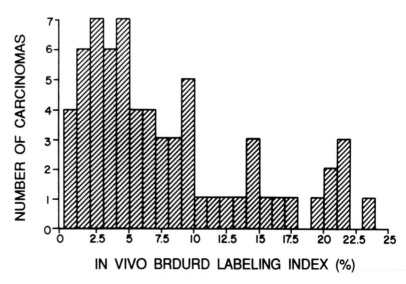

Figure 13–18. In vivo BrdUrd labeling index frequency distribution for 55 primary breast carcinomas. (From Goodson, W.H., Ljung, B.M., Waldman, F.M., et al.: In vivo measurement of breast cancer growth rate. Arch. Surg., *126*:1220–1223, 1991, with permission. Copyright 1991, American Medical Association.)

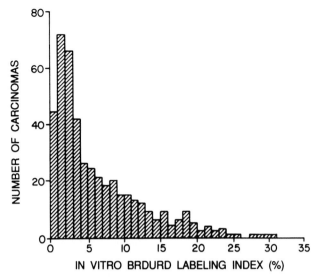

Figure 13-19. In vitro BrdUrd labeling index frequency distribution for 317 primary breast carcinomas. (Courtesy of St. Luke's Hospital, St. Louis, MO, 1988–1990.)

served that death from medullary carcinoma is restricted almost entirely to the first 5 years after diagnosis (Berg and Robbins, 1966; Hartviet, 1974; and Ridolfi et al., 1977). The author and coworkers have observed that circumscription of the tumor border is an important determinant of probability of relapse in carcinomas with high LI (Meyer et al., 1983).

Infiltrating lobular carcinomas have low TLIs but nonetheless do not have a particularly good prognosis, no doubt because of their highly infiltrative patterns and propensity to metastasize. However, their slow proliferative rates are reflected in long clinical courses. Ashikari and coworkers (1973) noted that in various clinical stages of infiltrating lobular carcinoma, nearly as many deaths occurred between 5 and 10 years after primary treatment as in the first 5 years. Lobular carcinomas with moderately anaplastic nuclei (Grade II) have higher LIs than those with minimal anaplasia (Grade I) (Meyer et al., 1986). Ladekarl and Sørensen (1993) found that high MI and large nuclear volume were prognostically unfavorable.

Only approximately 20% of breast carcinomas belong to any of the well-defined special histologic types. The proliferative indices of the residual group, best designated "not otherwise specified" (NOS) (Fisher and coworkers, (1975), reflect a broad range of LIs that extends from approximately 0.1% to 35%. Their behavior is as diverse as the spectrum of TLIs would suggest.

Proliferative Indices of Carcinoma in Situ

Carcinoma in situ within lobular ductules or postlobular ducts is associated with approximately two-thirds of invasive breast carcinomas. Three common histologic variants are recognized: comedo (large nuclei and necrosis), cribriform-papillary (small nuclei, glandular and papillary structures), and lobular (small nuclei, solid growth within lobular ductules). A fourth variant, solid, is less well-defined but differs from the others in its solid growth pattern within postlobular ducts and its relatively small nuclei. Like invasive carcinomas, different histologic types of breast carcinoma in situ have characteristic proliferative indices (see Table 13–5) (Meyer, 1986). Comedo intraductal carcinomas clearly have higher LIs than other variants, and in addition they are usually DNA aneuploid and overexpress the c-erb B_2 oncogene (*HEr-2/neu*) (Barnes et al., 1991). The comedo type, with its large nuclei, necrosis, high proliferative rate, lack of estrogen and progesterone receptors, c-erb B_2 overexpression and capability to evolve into highly proliferative invasive carcinoma, is the most aggressive and dangerous of the carcinomas in situ. Not all highly proliferative carcinomas arise from the comedo in situ variant, nor do they all overexpress c-erb B_2. Barnes and colleagues (1992) commented on an initially anomalous deficit of c-erb B_2 positive invasive carcinomas, noting that 60% of intraductal carcinomas are positive for the oncogene product but only 25% of invasive carcinomas are positive. Comedo intraductal carcinomas and their associated invasive carcinomas are routinely c-erb B_2 positive and rapidly proliferative, whereas other intraductal carcinomas and their associated invasive lesions are routinely c-erb B_2 negative and slowly proliferative. They accounted for the deficit in c-erb B_2 invasive carcinomas by defining a third group of invasive carcinomas with variable rates of proliferation that

Table 13–4. THYMIDINE-LABELING INDEX OF SPECIAL TYPES OF INVASIVE BREAST CARCINOMA

| Type | Number | TLI | | |
		Mean	Median	Standard Deviation
Adenocystic	3	1.7	0.6	1.9
Linear large cell*	4	9.9	11.2	6.3
Lobular	54	2.3	1.7	2.2
Medullary	24	16.6	16.2	5.6
Medullary, atypical	21	16.9	14.7	7.3
Metaplastic	2	10.1	10.1	2.1
Mucinous	20	2.0	1.5	1.4
Papillary	5	1.4	0.8	1.0
Tubular	10	1.3	1.0	1.0
Not otherwise specified (NOS)	581	7.1	5.5	5.9

*Resembles infiltrating lobular carcinoma but with large nuclei.

Table 13–5. LABELING INDEX OF BREAST CARCINOMA IN SITU*

Type	Number	Mean	Median	Range	DNA-aneuploidy† (%)
Comedo	41	7.2	6.0	0.5–22.8	92
Solid	18	3.3	2.4	0.1–9.8	
Cribriform-papillary	33	1.6	1.4	0.1–9.8	25
Lobular	11	1.6	1.4	0.2–5.5	

*By ^{3}H-TdR or BrdUrd labeling; the two are equivalent.

†Based on carcinomas in situ only; 25 comedo, 8 cribriform-papillary. Few flow cytometric data were available for pure lobular carcinoma in situ or solid intraductal carcinoma.

are c-*erb* B_2 negative and are not associated with intraductal carcinoma. Because of the latter group, C-*erb* B_2 expression is not a very useful prognostic marker (O'Reilly et al., 1991).

Ki-67 Antigen

A popular method, generally thought to measure growth fraction or an approximation of it, is Ki-67 monoclonal antibody. This reagent was developed by Gerdes and co-workers (1983) as a byproduct of studies of lymphocyte antigens and was found to react with cells in any of the four phases of the cell cycle, but not with nonproliferative cells. The antigen detected by this reagent has not been identified. It is evidently a large molecule (356–395 kd) that is distinct from cyclin, DNA topoisomerases, p53, c-*myc* gene product, and other known oncogene products related to cell proliferation (Gerdes et al., 1991). The antigen is found in the nuclear matrix, where it may play a role in structural organization (van Dierendonck et al., 1989). It is destroyed by formalin fixation and paraffin embedding. Recently it has been suggested that a rate-limiting enzyme for DNA synthesis, M_1 subunit of ribonucleotide reductase, is a better marker for cycling cells (Tay et al., 1991). Tay and associates reported that by use of a monoclonal M_1-ribosomal reductase antibody, more than 80% of breast carcinoma cells were marked as G_1 and fewer than 20% as G_0. In contrast, Ki-67 positivity ranges from less than 1% to 45% (80% in one study) in breast carcinoma cells (Lelle, 1989; Isola et al., 1990; Viehl et al., 1990; Sahin et al., 1991; and Wintzer et al., 1991). Although Ki-67 LIs relate strongly to other measures of proliferation in breast carcinoma and a variety of other human tumors, not all proliferating cells necessarily are marked by the antibody. Van Bockstaele and colleagues (1991) reported anomalously low Ki-67 indices in normal human bone marrow in which the Ki-67 index averaged 3.7% by microscopy, 4.8% by flow cytometry, in comparison with bromodeoxyuridine index of 11.6% by flow cytometry. This indicates that Ki-67 antigen may not be expressed by at least some differentiated, cycling cells. Further doubts of Ki-67's specificity for cycling cells have been raised. Van Dierendonck and associates (1989) showed that the antigen was undetectable at onset of S-phase in the MCF-7 breast carcinoma cell line and that it persisted in MCF-7 cells after arrest of proliferation. The sum of these opposing errors was an overestimation of the growth fraction by Ki-67 antibody staining.

Bruno and Darzynkiewicz (1992) were unable to detect Ki-67 antigen in a promyelocytic leukemic cell line at onset of S, and showed that in this cell line Ki-67 was synthesized predominantly during S-phase.

Despite evidence that Ki-67 measurements do not correspond to a true growth fraction, close correlations have been noted with other measures of proliferation in breast carcinoma, which include mitotic index (McGurrin et al., 1987; Isola et al., 1990; Verhoeven et al., 1990; Viehl et al., 1990; Di Stefano et al., 1991; and Sahin et al., 1991) and TLI (Kamel et al., 1989). Ki-67 indices have correlated less well with SPF by DNA flow cytometry (Lelle, 1989; Isola et al., 1990; and Viehl et al., 1990), although DNA-aneuploid carcinomas tended to have high Ki-67 indices (Isola, 1990; and Sahin et al., 1991). Inverse correlations of Ki-67 index and content of ERs and PgRs have been noted in some studies, in keeping with other proliferation markers (McGurrin et al., 1987; Lelle, 1989; Viehl et al., 1990; and Di Stefano et al., 1991). A weak positive relationship to tumor size was noted (Lelle, 1989). Relationship to number of positive axillary lymph nodes was suggestively positive but weak (Lelle, 1989; Lelle et al., 1987; and Viehl et al., 1990). Infiltrating lobular carcinomas were found to have lower Ki-67 indices than so-called ductal carcinomas (Lelle, 1989; Isola et al., 1990; and Sahin et al., 1991). Too few other special types of breast carcinoma were studied to enable us to draw conclusions about their characteristic Ki-67 indices. A tendency for the Ki-67 index to decline after menopause or with increasing age of the patient has been noted (Lelle, 1989). Ki-67 indices rose progressively with decreasing differentiation of tumors (Lelle, 1989) or increasing nuclear grade (McGurrin et al., 1987; Viehl et al., 1990; and Sahin et al., 1991). In all respects, the relationships between Ki-67 and other variables are similar to those noted with the TLI (Meyer, 1986; and Silvestrini et al., 1986).

Several studies have found Ki-67 indices to be prognostic for breast carcinoma (McGurrin et al., 1987; Lelle, 1989; Wintzer et al., 1991; and Sahin et al., 1991). The study by Sahin and associates concerned node-negative carcinoma. These results suggest that the Ki-67 index is slightly less effective or as effective as the TLI for prognosis of breast carcinoma, but the two have not been compared directly.

A present assessment of Ki-67 as a marker for breast carcinoma proliferation demonstrates that it is a practical measure of relative proliferative rates that can be applied clinically with relative ease when fresh frozen tissue is available. It probably overestimates but gives results proportional to those of growth fraction in unperturbed carcinomas, though it could provide misleading results if used as a measure of response to therapy because of retention of the antigen after arrest in the cell cycle.

PCNA/Cyclin

PCNA/cyclin is a phylogenetically highly conserved proliferation-related intranuclear protein. It can be demonstrated by monoclonal antibodies, which could provide a means for a simple assay performable in the histopathology laboratory on fixed tissue. PCNA was originally described as an antinuclear antigen in proliferating cells demonstrable by a circulating antibody present in a small minority of lupus erythematosus patients (Miyachi et al., 1978). Cyclin was independently identified as a proliferation-specific polypeptide (Bravo et al., 1981). PCNA and cyclin were shown to be identical by Matthews and coworkers (1984). Cyclin is thought to complex with DNA polymerase delta at entry into S-phase (Nakane et al., 1989). It is necessary for progression in G_1 and consists of two classes, A and B, the former apparently being involved in regulation of intracellular protein kinase activity by specific binding to transcription-regulating proteins (Ewen et al., 1992; and Faha et al., 1992). Galand and Degraef (1989) showed that a tightly bound cyclin entity, retained after methanol fixation, is essentially confined to S-phase cells, whereas some non–S-phase cells contain a second intranuclear cyclin component retained after formalin fixation. Landberg and Roos (1991) similarly noted two forms of cyclin and showed that with use of a lysing buffer prior to methanol fixation cyclin immunoreactivity corresponded closely to S-phase, but by other means of fixation the number of positive cells was increased and appeared to correspond to the growth fraction. Kamel and colleagues (1991) found that in human malignant lymphomas freshly fixed in formalin, proportions of Ki-67–positive and cyclin-positive cells were similar, and they concluded that immunocytochemical demonstration of cyclin positivity defined growth fraction. Dawson and coworkers (1990) used a monoclonal antibody to cyclin and observed mean cyclin-positive index of 10.2% in 54 breast carcinomas, which compared to SPF by flow cytometry of 7.9% and Ki-67 index of 21.6%. They reported modestly high correlation coefficients of 0.61 for cyclin versus Ki-67, 0.48 for cyclin versus SPF, and 0.48 for cyclin Ki-67 versus SPF. Evidence at present indicates that demonstration of cyclin by specific antibody binding in formalin-fixed tissues does not define an S-phase population, but it may define a growth fraction. Its practical importance in evaluation of breast carcinomas is not yet established, but two reports described high relapse rates associated with high PCNA index (Aaltomaa et al., 1993; and Tahan et al., 1993).

Relationships Between the Proliferative Index and Tumor Grade

Just as the histologic type of breast carcinoma relates to the LI, the grade of differentiation (histologic grade) and de-

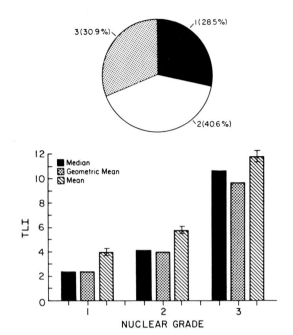

Figure 13–20. Relationship between the TLI of infiltrating breast carcinoma and the nuclear grade. The pie graph shows the relative proportions of patients with minimal (Grade 1), intermediate (Grade 2), and marked nuclear enlargement (Grade 3). The bar graph demonstrates that enlargement of nuclei is associated with high TLI. (From Meyer, J. S., Prey, M.U., Babcock, D.S., et al.: Breast carcinoma cell kinetics, morphology, stage, and host characteristics: A thymidine labeling study. Lab. Invest., *54*:41, 1986. Reprinted with permission. Copyright by the U.S. and Canadian Academy of Pathology, Inc.)

gree of nuclear anaplasia (nuclear grade) relate to LI. The small group of NOS carcinomas with predominant gland and tubule formation have low LIs, and the mean LI increases with decreasing participation of cells in formation of lumens. However, some histologic Grade III carcinomas (lobular carcinomas and also carcinomas with solid growth patterns) have low LIs. The mean LI increases impressively with progression of the nuclear grade from 1 to 3 (Meyer et al., 1986) (Fig. 13–20).

Relationship Between Age of the Patient and the DNA-Labeling Index

The LI shows an impressive inverse relationship to age (Silvestrini et al., 1979; Meyer and Lee, 1980; and Meyer et al., 1986) (Fig. 13–21). Young, premenopausal patients are likely to have high LIs, and older, postmenopausal patients are likely to have low LIs. Exceptions to this rule, however, are not rare.

Relationships Between the DNA-Labeling Index and Steroidal Receptor Content of Breast Carcinoma

An inverse relationship between the LI and content of either estrogen receptor (ER) or progesterone receptor (PgR) is

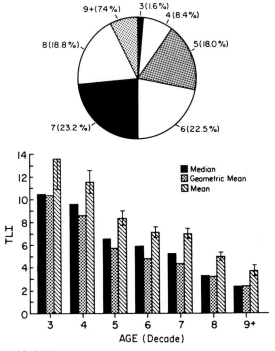

Figure 13–21. Relationship between TLI of infiltrating breast carcinoma and patient age at time of diagnosis. The pie graph shows the relative proportions of patients in each decade of age. The bar graph shows a steady decline in the median, geometric mean, and mean TLI with increasing age. (From Meyer, J. S., Prey, M.U., Babcock, D.S., et al.: Breast carcinoma cell kinetics, morphology, stage, and host characteristics: A thymidine labeling study. Lab. Invest., 54:41, 1986. Reprinted with permission. Copyright by the U.S. and Canadian Academy of Pathology, Inc.)

but not certain to be receptor negative, and carcinomas with low TLIs sometimes are not receptor positive. The relationship between PgR and TLI is not appreciably stronger than that between ER and TLI. Similar inverse relationships between ER content and percentage of S by flow cytometry of DNA (Kute et al., 1981; Olszewski et al., 1981*a;* Raber et al., 1982; and McDivitt et al., 1985), and by flow cytometric measurement of precursor uptake into DNA (Remvikos et al., 1991), have been observed.

DNA-Labeling Index and Stage of Disease

Tubiana and coworkers were the first to observe that locally aggressive breast carcinomas have high proliferative indices (Tubiana et al., 1975). This observation has been confirmed (Table 13–6). Nonetheless, only a weak relationship exists between the proliferative rate and number of axillary lymph node metastases (Tubiana et al., 1975; Schiffer et al., 1979; Bertuzzi et al., 1981; Raber et al., 1982; and Meyer et al., 1986), showing that the metastatic potential in breast carcinoma is not closely tied to proliferative rate. This fact accounts for the broad clinical spectrum of behavior. The author's data suggest, however, that metastasis to the brain is associated with high TLI (Meyer et al., 1984*b*).

We have found a positive relationship between tumor size and TLI (Meyer et al., 1986), subsequently confirmed in a second TLI series and a study of 450 tumors with BrdUrd labeling (Meyer et al., 1993). Although correlation coefficients were relatively low (r = 0.17, 0.28, and 0.29 in three studies, total of 1400 patients), they were highly significant (P < .0001). This relationship suggests that large breast carcinomas may result from rapid growth rather than neglect. Having observed a significant positive relationship between LI and number of metastatic axillary lymph nodes in our recent series of 559 patients (r = 0.23, P < .001), we are tempted to speculate that the striking relationship observed by Koscielny and coworkers (1984) between size of breast carcinoma and distant metastasis is explicable in part by association of large size with biologic characteristics indicative of aggressiveness. One of these characteristics certainly is proliferative rate.

well established (Meyer et al., 1977; Cooke et al., 1979; Silvestrini et al., 1979; and Meyer et al., 1986). The relationship is true for both premenopausal and postmenopausal patients (Silvestrini et al., 1986). The correlation coefficients that the author's group has observed between ER and TLI or PgR and TLI, although significant, are not particularly high (r = 0.2 to 0.4), which reflects a good deal of variability in receptor assay results for all proliferative classes. Thus, a breast carcinoma with a high TLI is likely

Table 13–6. RELATIONSHIP OF THYMIDINE-LABELING INDEX TO STAGE

| Investigator, Year | Method* | Number | Stage† | TLI | |
				Median	*Mean*
Straus and Moran, 1980	1	13	T1–3		5.2
	1	10	T4		9.0
	1	9	Metastasis		13.2
Meyer et al., 1986	3	325	A	4.5	6.7
	3	86	B	5.2	7.0
	3	22	C	8.5	8.0
	3	13	DL	12.2	12.7
	3	17	Metastasis	6.0	7.5

*1, In vivo; 3, in vitro, hyperbaric oxygen.
†Straus and Moran used the TMR system; T4 means local extension without distant spread. Meyer et al. used the Columbia Clinical Staging system; DL means local extension without distant spread.

DNA-Labeling Index of Breast Carcinoma as a Prognostic Feature

Since the first report by Tubiana and associates (1975), evidence has accumulated to establish the TLI as a powerful stage-independent indicator for the early course of breast carcinoma after primary treatment (Tubiana et al., 1975; Meyer and Lee, 1980; Straus and Moran, 1980; Gentili et al., 1981; Raber et al., 1982; and Tubiana et al., 1989). Most reports have dealt with patients observed for only a few years; a report by Silvestrini and coworkers establishes that the TLI remains prognostic over a 6-year period (Silvestrini et al., 1985), and Tubiana and associates (1984) have demonstrated a relationship between TLI and relapse-free survival continuing over 10 years' observation. The predictive power of the TLI appears to be most striking for low-stage patients (Fig. 13–22).

Limited association between the TLI and the stage of disease (Tubiana et al., 1975; Meyer and Hixon, 1979; Meyer and Lee, 1980; and Silvestrini et al., 1986) indicates that proliferative indices will not be useful in predicting the status of the axillary lymph nodes. However, patients are less likely to relapse when their TLIs are low and are more likely to relapse when their TLIs are high, regardless of the nodal status. Any relationship between the TLI and the clinical stage of the disease is expressed primarily locally. Locally advanced carcinomas, and inflammatory carcinomas in particular, have high TLIs (Meyer et al., 1986).

The TLI predicts relapse-free survival independently of ER and PgR, but ER supplements TLI for prediction of survival (Hery et al., 1987; Meyer and Province, 1988; Courdi et al., 1989; and Silvestrini et al., 1989) (Fig. 13–23). A probable explanation for retention of ER as a predictor for survival, whereas it drops out as a predictor of recurrence when TLI is included in multivariate analysis, is longer duration of life for patients with ER-positive tumors who are treated by hormone therapy. Therefore, LI, rather than ER or PgR, should be used for assessing probability of relapse of breast carcinoma. ER and PgR are most useful for assessing probability of responsiveness to hormone therapy and quite limited in utility for predicting relapse. Some evidence exists that LI may be useful as an adjunct to predicting probability of hormone response. Paradiso and coworkers (1988) observed significantly higher response rates in tumors with low TLI than with high TLI.

DNA Measurements in Breast Carcinoma

By microdensitometry of DNA in smears, breast carcinomas can be divided into four groups (Atkin, 1972; and Auer et al., 1980*a*) (Table 13–7). Survival is distinctly higher for patients with predominantly diploid-tetraploid DNA contents in their breast carcinoma cells than for those with clearly aneuploid DNA content (Atkin, 1972; Auer et al., 1980*a;* and Harvey et al., 1987). In addition, aneuploid carcinomas (Types II and IV) are poor in ER, whereas diploid-tetraploid carcinomas (Types I and II) are often ER rich (Auer et al., 1980*b*).

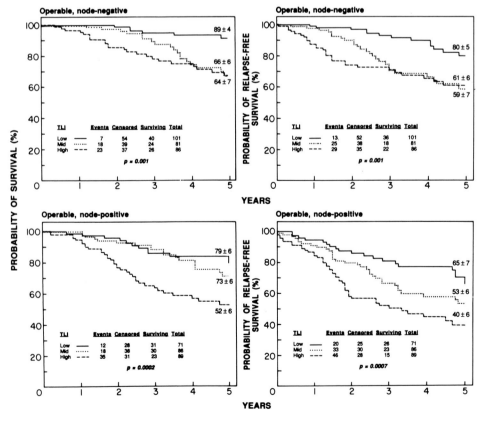

Figure 13–22. Probability of survival and relapse-free survival in patients with operable breast carcinoma with negative or positive axillary lymph nodes in relationship to the TLI of carcinoma. A TLI of 3% or less *(solid line)* compared with from 3.1% to 8% *(dotted line)* and with >8% *(broken line).* (After Meyer, J. S., and Province, M.: Proliferative index of breast carcinoma by thymidine labeling: Prognostic power independent of stage, estrogen and progesterone receptors. Breast Cancer Res. Treat., *12:*191–204, 1988, with permission.)

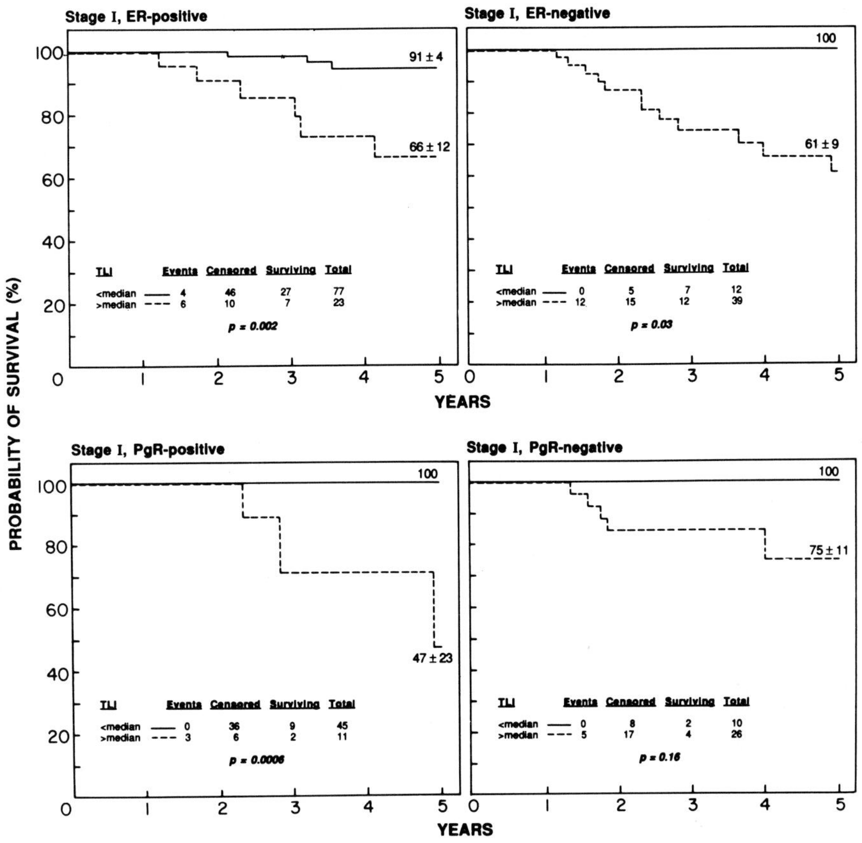

Figure 13–23. Probability of survival dependent on TLI in Stage I carcinomas that are positive or negative for estrogen and progesterone receptors. A TLI of 3% or less *(solid line)* compared with from 3.1% to 8% *(dotted line)* and with >8% *(broken line).* (After Meyer, J. S., and Province, M.: Proliferative index of breast carcinoma by thymidine labeling: Prognostic power independent of stage, estrogen and progesterone receptors. Breast Cancer Res. Treat., *12*:191–204, 1988, with permission.)

Subsequent studies by Auer's group (Erhardt et al., 1986; Harvey et al., 1987; Opfermann et al., 1987; and Feichter et al., 1988*b*) have confirmed these findings. Scattering of cells outside major peaks in DNA histograms, a finding that suggests genomic instability, was prominent in DNA-aneuploid tumors, and supplements major stemline position as a prognostic variable (Fallenius et al., 1988*a*). DNA-aneuploid tumors were noted to have a higher rate of axillary metastases than DNA-diploid tumors (Erhardt et al., 1986; and Berryman et al., 1987). These studies also observed increased rates of DNA aneuploidy in large and steroid receptor–negative tumors and in young women, relationships similar to those noted by flow cytometry (see below). A strong relationship was found between nuclear grade and DNA ploidy, but that between histologic grade and ploidy was weak (Fallenius et al., 1988*b*). Recent studies have shown that results comparable to those on smears may be obtained by analysis of nuclei released from formalin-fixed, paraffin-embedded tissue, and that results from image analysis agree reasonably well with those by flow cytometry (Fallenius et al., 1987; Roos et al., 1988; Dawson et al., 1990; and Lee et al., 1991). Static image analysis after Feulgen staining of DNA appears to be less effective than flow cytometry for resolving cell lines with minor degrees of DNA aneuploidy, but the former has the advantage of identifying the cell population of interest (Fallenius et al., 1987). Hatschek and colleagues (1989) used microfluorimetry to measure SPF in primary breast carcinomas and showed that SPF was predictive of survival after relapse.

The DNA flow cytometric patterns of breast carcinomas express the presence or absence of aneuploid stem lines and the number of S-phase cells. Figures 13–10 to 13–14 illustrate different types of flow cytometric histograms.

In various studies 44% to 92% of breast carcinomas have contained aneuploid cell populations (Kute et al., 1981; Olszewski et al., 1981*b;* Bichel et al., 1982; Fossa et al.,

Table 13–7. MICRODENSITOMETRIC CLASSIFICATION OF DNA CONTENT OF BREAST CARCINOMA CELLS*

DNA Type	Description	Frequency (%)	Estrogen Receptor	Long-Term Survival (%)
I	Single diploid modal DNA value	30%	Usually positive	50%
II	Both diploid and tetraploid DNA values	35%	Usually positive	50%
III	Modal DNA value between diploid and tetraploid	20%	Usually negative	25%
IV	Modal DNA value beyond tetraploid	15%	Usually negative	25%

*Based on data from Auer et al. (1980*a,b*); Atkin (1972); and Fossa et al. (1982).

1982; Raber et al., 1982; Barlogie et al., 1983; Taylor et al., 1983; Cornelisse et al., 1984; Coulson et al., 1984; Meyer et al., 1984a; and McDivitt et al., 1986). The variability from one series to another may be caused by differences in stage distribution, adequacy of sampling, and flow cytometric resolution. The aneuploidy rate averaged from nine different laboratories in early studies was 70%. A survey of 15 recent studies shows a mean of 63% aneuploid (Table 13–8). Ewers and coworkers (1984) have demonstrated increasing rates of aneuploidy with increasing stage from T1 to T4. Various methods of preparation of the cell suspensions have yielded similar proportions of aneuploid carcinomas (Chassevent et al., 1984; and Meyer et al., 1984a).

Nevertheless, other studies show that results are in part dependent on the method of preparing the single cell suspension. Mechanical dissociation by mincing tissue is more likely to kill cells than enzymatic dissociation and harvests proportionally more DNA-aneuploid cells in relationship to DNA-diploid cells. Enzymatic dissociation at physiologic pH harvests proportionally more DNA-diploid cells with high viability. Viability is also high in fine-needle aspirates (Ljung et al., 1989). The method of dissociation may affect rate of DNA aneuploidy and measurement of SPF. The latter is subject to variation based on proportion of DNA-aneuploid cells present because the S-phase proportions are approximately twice as high in DNA-aneuploid tumors as in DNA-diploid tumors, whether they are measured by DNA precursor incorporation as labeling index (Meyer et al., 1984a) or by DNA flow cytometry (Dressler, 1988). Witzig and coworkers (1991) detected a relatively large proportion of DNA-aneuploid carcinomas by gating on large nuclei, but Visscher's group (1990b) did not appear to increase detection of DNA aneuploidy by gating on cytokeratin-positive cells. SPF results also depend on the method of analysis of DNA histograms: lower results, comparable to ^{3}H-TdR or BrdUrd LI are obtained when debris

subtraction is used (Haag et al., 1987). Standardization of methods has not been achieved, and currently each laboratory must determine mean or other cutoffs for SPF analysis. Cytogenetic analysis has shown chromosomal abnormalities in diploid breast carcinomas (Barlogie et al., 1983; and Tribukait, 1984). These chromosomal abnormalities are too minor to result in change in DNA content of a magnitude detectable by flow cytometry.

Aneuploidy and high percentage of S by flow cytometry are consistently associated with ER negativity, although the relationship has not been statistically significant in all studies (Kute et al., 1981; Olszewski et al., 1981a,b; Raber et al., 1982; Taylor et al., 1983; Cornelisse et al., 1984; Coulson et al., 1984; Cornelisse et al., 1987; Visscher et al., 1990a; and Frierson, 1991). PgR and percentage of S are also negatively correlated, but to no greater degree than ER and percentage of S (Meyer et al., 1984b; and McDivitt et al., 1986). Breast carcinomas with diploid DNA indices are more likely to be ER positive and PgR positive than are those with aneuploid DNA indices. Aneuploidy is also associated with a high percentage of S (Kute et al., 1981; Olszewski et al., 1981a; and Moran et al., 1984) and high TLI (Meyer et al., 1984a; and McDivitt et al., 1985). Moran and coworkers (1984) have shown that the percentage of S, although consistently higher than the TLI, has the same relationships as the TLI to the age of the patient, histopathologic type of carcinoma, and nuclear grade.

A retrospective study in which nuclei were prepared from paraffin-embedded blocks demonstrated significantly increased relapse rates in patients with aneuploid tumors in comparison to diploid tumors (Hedley et al., 1984). Coulson and associates (1984) and Ewers and coworkers (1984) found the DNA index to be prognostic for short-term survival in prospective studies. Their findings paralleled the microdensitometric observations of Auer and coworkers (1980a) and Atkin (1972) in that the higher the DNA index, the greater was the risk of early relapse. These studies

Table 13–8. PROPORTION OF BREAST CARCINOMAS DETERMINED TO BE DNA ANEUPLOID BY FLOW CYTOMETRY

Investigator, Year	Material	Cases	Aneuploidy (%)
McDivitt, 1986	Fresh	168	55%*
Cornelisse, 1987	Frozen or paraffin	565	71%****
Hedley, 1987	Paraffin (node-positive)	490	65%***
Dressler, 1988	Frozen	1331	57%*
Feichter, 1988	Ethanol fixed	300	62%*
Kallioniemi, 1988	Paraffin	308	64%*
Roos, 1988	Paraffin T3, T4	72	58%*
Christov, 1989	Fresh	180	65%*
Joensuu, 1990	Paraffin	222	74%***
K.-Rofagha, 1990	Paraffin	165	57%**
Kute, 1990	Paraffin	197	52%**
O'Reilly, 1990	Paraffin	140	68%**
Visscher, 1990	Fresh	165	62%*
Eliason, 1991	Fine-needle aspiration	174	56%*
Fisher, 1991	Paraffin	398	57%**
Olsson, 1991	Premenopausal, frozen	175	58%*
Sharma, 1991	Paraffin	104	77%****
Witzig, 1991	Paraffin	167	71%[1]*

[1]Gated on large nuclei by light scatter. Ungated, 61% were aneuploid.
Key: Relationship of ploidy to clinical course: * = not reported; ** = not significant; *** = significant; **** = significant; independent of stage.

indicate that the probabilities of relapse and death within 3 to 5 years of primary treatment are increased twofold or more if the carcinoma is aneuploid rather than diploid.

A study with minimum follow-up of 22 years that utilized archived paraffin-embedded blocks found a 49% survival rate for 45 patients with diploid carcinomas and a 26% rate for 165 patients with nondiploid carcinomas (Toikkanen et al., 1989; and Joensuu et al., 1990). While the great majority of studies have shown DNA aneuploidy to be associated with relapse of carcinoma, the relationship often has not been statistically significant, and only about half have demonstrated that it is prognostic, independently of tumor size and axillary lymph nodal status (Joensuu, 1990). Frierson (1991) thoroughly reviewed publications on the topic and noted that only four of eight reports observed significantly reduced survival associated with DNA aneuploidy. In only three reports was ploidy an independent prognostic factor in multivariate analysis. DNA ploidy loses power in multivariate analysis because of the association between DNA aneuploidy and advanced stage. A positive relationship between DNA aneuploidy and size of tumor was noted in six studies (Frierson, 1991). Large carcinomas usually are DNA aneuploid, whereas small carcinomas usually have diploid DNA content. Fallenius and coworkers (1984) noted DNA aneuploidy in only 10% of 50 nonpalpable breast carcinomas sampled by stereotaxic needle aspiration biopsy. A tendency has been noted, statistically significant in some studies (Berryman et al., 1987), for lymph node metastases and inoperability to be associated with DNA aneuploidy. These associations help explain weakness of DNA ploidy as a stage-independent indicator.

Several studies recently have compared DNA ploidy and SPF by flow cytometry for prognosis of breast carcinoma (Table 13–9), but these reports are relatively few because of difficulties in measurement of SPF in archived specimens (Hedley et al., 1987; and Gonchoroff et al., 1990). Klintenberg and associates (1986) showed that after minimum follow-up of 60 months SPF contributed prognostic information independent of stage but DNA ploidy did not. Kallioniemi and coworkers (1988) found that DNA ploidy

was a strong predictor but that SPF contributed further information for both DNA-diploid and DNA-aneuploid carcinomas (Fig. 13–24 *A and B*). Tubiana and Courdi (1989) and Visscher and coworkers (1990*a*) reviewed reports of breast carcinoma proliferative measurements and noted that proliferation measurements were consistently stage-independent prognostic indicators whereas DNA ploidy was a weaker indicator. In five studies of node-negative patients, SPF was a significant prognostic variable in multivariate analysis (Frierson, 1991). Clark and coworkers (1992) (Fig. 13–25) showed in untreated controls of an intergroup cooperative study that flow cytometric SPF is effective for prognosis of small, node-negative, estrogen receptor–positive carcinomas, although DNA ploidy was not predictive. Their finding is consistent with those of earlier studies that showed that proliferation is prognostic independent of nodal status and ER (Meyer and Province, 1988; and Silvestrini et al., 1989). The predictive power of DNA ploidy appears to derive largely from its association with high proliferative rate, and proliferative rate emerges as the most important predictive variable. DNA aneuploidy is more strongly associated with advanced stage than is SPF (Hedley et al., 1987; and Visscher et al., 1990*a*). It is difficult to disprove some independent contribution of DNA ploidy, but scant evidence supports that it is independently important. In a recent review, O'Reilly and Richards (1992) were able to find studies by only two groups that showed a contribution of DNA ploidy to prognosis in multivariate analysis. In a more recent report, DNA ploidy failed as a univariate predictor but was a significant predictor for distant metastasis and relapse-free survival in multivariate analysis (Gnant et al., 1992). In this context the occurrence of DNA aneuploidy in benign tumors should be noted. Joensuu and Klemi (1988) demonstrated aneuploidy in 29% of pituitary adenomas, 25% of thyroid adenomas, 35% of parathyroid adenomas, and 53% of adrenal adenomas, findings that have been confirmed by others (Bronner et al., 1988; Cibas et al., 1990; and Obara et al., 1990). No evidence exists that DNA aneuploidy in these benign tumors has any prognostic meaning. Knowing this, it is not surpris-

Table 13–9. DNA PLOIDY AND S-PHASE FRACTION IN PROGNOSIS OF BREAST CARCINOMA

Principal Investigator, Year	Material	Cases (No.)	SPF Success Rate (%)	Prediction	
				Ploidy	*SPF*
Klintenberg, 1986	Frozen	191		Weak	Yes[1]
Hedley, 1987	Paraffin	490	58	Weak	Yes[2]
Kallioniemi, 1988	Paraffin	323	95	Yes	Yes[1]
Clark, 1989	Frozen	395	64	Yes	Yes[1, 3]
Hatschek, 1989	Paraffin	82	100[4]	No	Yes[4]
Joensuu, 1990	Paraffin	222	60	Weak	Yes
Kute, 1990	Paraffin	197	82	No	No[5]
O'Reilly, 1990	Paraffin	140	96	Weak	Yes[2]
Fisher, 1991	Paraffin	398	95	No	Yes[1]
Witzig, 1991	Paraffin	167	73	Yes[6]	Weak

1. Stage-independent predictor.
2. Independent of stage, not of tumor grade.
3. SPF independently predictive only in DNA-diploid carcinomas.
4. Measurements on breast carcinoma after relapse by static microfluorimetry. Other studies in this table were by flow cytometry.
5. All patients received adjuvant cytotoxic therapy.
6. By dual light scatter fluorescence. Ungated fluorescence did not predict. All patients received cytotoxic chemotherapy.

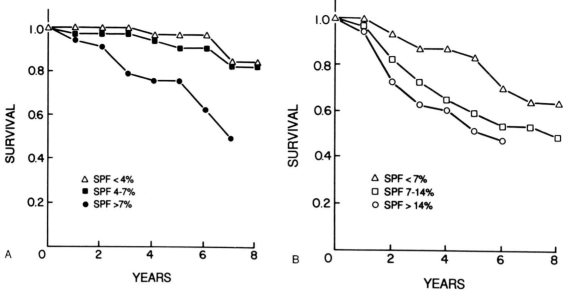

Figure 13-24. Survival of breast carcinoma patients with diploid *(A)* or aneuploid *(B)* DNA content depends on SPF. (After Kallioniemi, O. P., Blanco, G., Alavaikko, M., et al.: Improving the prognostic value of DNA flow cytometry in breast cancer by combining DNA index and S-phase fraction. Cancer, *62*:2183–2190, 1988, with permission.)

ing to find a preponderance of evidence that DNA ploidy, per se, apart from its associations with advanced stage and high proliferative rates, is not a strong prognostic indicator.

DNA ploidy and SPF correlate with histologic type of breast carcinoma. Review of 56 publications showed important differences in DNA aneuploidy rates for various histologic types. The aneuploidy rate was 64% for carcinoma of no special type (N = 1861), 18% for mucinous (N = 67), 33% for tubular (N = 24), 29% for papillary (N = 14), 35% for lobular (N = 100), and 92% for medullary (N = 40) carcinomas (Frierson, 1991). Infiltrating lobular, mucinous, papillary, and tubular carcinomas usually had low SPF, and medullary carcinomas had high SPF. These observations parallel those with ³H-TdR labeling (see above). Flow cytometric findings can be predicted with a good deal of assurance for special histologic types of breast

carcinoma, and evidence that flow cytometry helps in prognosis within the special histologic types is lacking.

Most breast carcinomas belong to no special type. In this group, frequency of DNA aneuploidy increases with decreasing histologic differentiation ([reviewed by] Visscher et al., 1990a; and O'Reilly and Richards, 1992). When tested against morphometrically determined histologic features, particularly MI and nuclear size, DNA ploidy proved to add little information for prognosis of breast carcinoma (Uyterlinde et al., 1988), although it might contribute in the case of small node-negative tumors (van der Linden et al., 1989). Hedley and colleagues (1987) observed that although SPF by DNA flow cytometry was a strong predictor in node-positive breast carcinoma, it lost its effect when the tumor grade was included in multivariate analysis, an observation that was confirmed by O'Reilly and colleagues

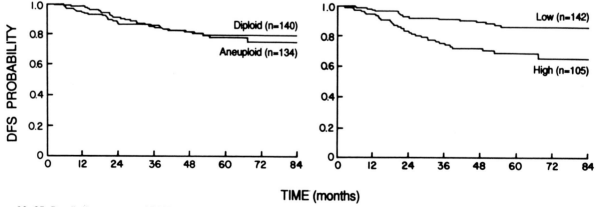

Figure 13-25. Predictive power of DNA ploidy and SPF (cutoff is 4.4% for diploid and 7.0% for aneuploid carcinomas) for disease-free survival in node-negative patients with a maximum tumor diameter of 3 cm who have undergone excisional therapy only. (After Clark, G. M., Mathieu, M. C., Owens, M. A., et al.: Prognostic significance of S-phase fraction of good-risk, node-negative breast cancer patients. J. Clin. Oncol., *10*:428–432, 1992, with permission.)

(1990*a*). Toikkanen (1989), Feichter et al. (1988*b*), and Visscher et al. (1990*a*) and their respective coworkers also noted strong correlation between high SPF and unfavorable histologic features. O'Reilly and Richards (1992) cited nine reports that associated high histologic grade and high SPF. The former observed that histologic grade was more important than SPF in prognosis of breast carcinoma on long-term (median = 27 years) follow-up, though SPF had some independent prognostic power by multivariate analysis. Our own experience indicated that a simple measurement of nuclear size was roughly coequal with TLI in effectiveness for breast carcinoma prognosis (Meyer and Province, 1992).

A few studies have addressed the question of prediction of chemotherapy response by DNA flow cytometry. Evidence that tumors with higher proliferative rates are more sensitive to chemotherapy is not firm, though such an effect is presumed from data on tumors in laboratory animals and has been reported for metastatic breast carcinoma (Sulkes et al., 1979; and Remvikos et al., 1989). In a group of patients who all received adjuvant cytotoxic therapy, Kute and associates (1990) reported that both DNA ploidy and SPF by flow cytometry were ineffective for prognosis. Fisher and colleagues (1983) noted a tendency for high–nuclear grade carcinomas, known to have relatively high proliferative rates, to respond well to chemotherapy. Hedley and coworkers (1987) observed no effects of ploidy or SPF on relapse-free survival within treatment arms for patients treated as part of Ludwig Breast Cancer Studies I through IV of adjuvant chemotherapy and endocrine therapy for node-positive carcinoma. On the other hand, Briffod and colleagues (1989) observed tumor regression in response to neoadjuvant chemotherapy more often in DNA-aneuploid than in DNA-diploid tumors. O'Reilly's group (1990) found that both low-SPF and high-SPF breast carcinomas benefited from adjuvant cytotoxic chemotherapy, although the magnitude of chemotherapeutic effect was greater among high-SPF tumors in premenopausal patients.

Both premenopausal and postmenopausal breast carcinomas show a spectrum of aggressiveness manifested by proliferative index. In southern Sweden, Olsson and colleagues (1991) found significant associations of DNA aneuploidy and high SPF with early use of contraceptive steroids. These results suggest an effect of the steroids at time of malignant transformation of breast duct cells that imprints them with a high proliferative rate. Use of contraceptive steroids does not increase the proliferative rate in breast ducts (Meyer, 1977; and Going et al., 1988), so the mechanism that results in a high rate of proliferation is not understood, and confirmation is required.

In summary, review of data on flow cytometric DNA measurements of breast carcinoma show complex relationships among DNA ploidy, SPF, tumor stage, and histologic features. DNA ploidy alone is not useful for prognosis of breast carcinoma. SPF is more useful, but it is not always obtainable for technical reasons and may not contribute if histologic evaluations are taken into account. The role of ploidy and SPF in predicting chemotherapeutic responsiveness is still unclear. A single study suggests that carcinomas originating during intake of exogenous sex steroid may be imprinted with a high proliferative rate.

Heterogeneity of Cell Kinetics and DNA Measurements In Breast Carcinoma

The proliferative index of various breast carcinomas is varied, though initially it was reported to be minimal from one sample to another or from primary to metastatic lesions (Auer et al., 1984; and Raber et al., 1982). A study of multiple samples of 59 breast carcinomas showed statistically significant differences of TLI between samples in 61%, but the differences were seldom great (Meyer and Wittliff, 1991). Regional differences in perfusion or presence of different stemlines could account for the differences. When primary tumors were compared with axillary metastases, similarity of TLIs was the rule in one study (Meyer and McDivitt, 1986); in another, considerable variation in both directions was noted (Diadone et al., 1990). Beerman and colleagues (1991) studied multiple archived paraffin-embedded samples, and in some cases frozen samples, from 44 primary breast carcinomas and found that all samples were DNA diploid for only 5 tumors. In two instances diploid tumors gave rise to aneuploid metastases. With a mean of 4.9 samples per tumor, 61% were judged heterogeneous for DNA index. Meyer and Wittliff (1991) noted heterogeneity for DNA index in 24% of 61 carcinomas. In these studies and that of Askensten and coworkers (1989), most of the heterogeneity involved multiple DNA-aneuploid stemlines. Finding of heterogeneity across the diploid-nondiploid boundary was unusual. Christov and coworkers (1989) noted disparity in ploidy between primary tumor and axillary nodal metastasis in 38% of 34 patients. Fuhr and associates (1991) reported that one or more samples from 18% of 74 DNA-aneuploid carcinomas showed diploid DNA content. Askensten and associates noted one example of apparent heterogeneity by DNA flow cytometry that could not be confirmed by static photometry. This underscores the problem of excessive numbers of benign inflammatory and stromal cells that may obscure a relatively minor population of DNA-aneuploid tumor cells in a given sample.

One can conclude from the various studies that the majority of breast carcinomas maintain stability of DNA ploidy over a fairly long time. A minority of them have stemlines that exhibit differences in DNA ploidy from one region to another. Thus, differences in DNA ploidy do not necessarily mean that the tumors from which the samples came have different origins. Small to moderate variability of proliferative rate is common, but large variations are unusual in a given tumor and its metastases.

Phyllodes Tumors

Phyllodes tumor, also known as cytosarcoma phyllodes, has the appearance of fibroadenoma with malignant-looking stromal change. Actually the majority of these tumors have only local malignant potential, and only a small minority have metastasized. Several authors have noted that the stromal mitotic index is predictive of the tumor's behavior (Norris and Taylor, 1967; Hart et al., 1978; and Pietruszka

Table 13–10. THYMIDINE-LABELING INDEX OF FIBROADENOMA AND PHYLLODES TUMOR

Tissue	Number	TLI Mean	Median	Range
Fibroadenoma, epithelium	13	1.7	0.95	0.05–4.2
Fibroadenoma, stroma	13	0.53	0.42	0.00–1.30
Primary phyllodes tumor, epithelium	5	2.0	2.7	0.35–3.15
Primary phyllodes tumor, stroma	5	3.7	1.3	0.10–13.11
Metastatic or recurrent phyllodes tumor, stroma	3	8.4	5.0	3.00–15.63

and Barnes, 1978). The TLI of the stroma of fibroadenomas is uniformly low, but most phyllodes tumors have higher stromal TLIs and also may have relatively high epithelial TLIs (Table 13–10). The author and colleagues have observed the highest proliferative indices in those cytosarcomas that exhibited malignant behavior.

Palko and coworkers (1990), in a flow cytometric study of archived paraffin-embedded tissue, further established the value of proliferative measurements in predicting the behavior of phyllodes tumor. In their study, none of nine tumors with SPF of 5% or less recurred or metastasized, but all six tumors with higher SPF either recurred locally or metastasized. El-Naggar and colleagues (1990) observed a significant relationship between DNA aneuploidy and malignant behavior, but Layfield and colleagues (1989) did not find DNA ploidy useful for prognosis.

COST EFFECTIVENESS IN BREAST CARCINOMA PROGNOSIS: LABELING INDEX VERSUS DNA STATIC OR FLOW CYTOMETRY VERSUS MORPHOLOGY AND MORPHOMETRY

The current status of surgical adjuvant therapy of breast carcinoma indicates the need to select patients who have little chance of relapse. Estimates indicate that approximately 25% or 30% of "operable patients" with lymph nodal metastases benefit from adjuvant cytotoxic therapy (Cuzick et al., 1988). Approximately the same number may benefit from adjuvant hormone therapy if ER or PgR are present, but the lesser side effects of modern hormone therapy make selection criteria less critical. Below some level, perhaps a 10% probability of relapse within 5 years, cytotoxic therapy might do more damage than good. The size of the carcinoma is a strong predictor for dissemination (Fig. 13–26), and the cutoff point for 10% probability of dissemination appears to be 10 mm diameter (Koscielny et al., 1984; and Kieback et al., 1990). Cell kinetic and DNA examinations have not been tested as predictors for smaller tumors, and with current knowledge, exclusion of invasive tumors smaller than 10 mm in diameter from adjuvant therapy would appear to be reasonable. Exclusion of patients with tubular carcinomas would be in accord with their excellent prognosis, even in the presence of axillary metastases showing tubular histology (McDivitt et al., 1982). Small medullary carcinomas could also reasonably be excluded (Ridolfi et al., 1977). After exclusion of these spe-

cial cases, kinetic measurements have strong prognostic value and currently have a place in decision making about adjuvant therapy for node-negative breast carcinomas.

DNA static and flow cytometry, in vitro DNA LI, and Ki-67 index all have repeatedly been demonstrated to be prognostic. The relative efficacy of these methods is unknown because of lack of direct comparisons. Flow cytometry has a serious disadvantage, in that DNA histograms adequate for interpretation of SPF are not obtainable in a considerable proportion, whereas in vitro thymidine or BrdUrd LI are nearly always successful. Flow cytometric ploidy, by itself, is of little value. Another disadvantage of flow techniques is interference by nonmalignant cells in analytic preparations unless secondary markers are used to exclude them. Static cytometry, LI, and Ki-67 index have the advantages of direct visualization of cells being measured and permanence of record, a glass slide that can be stored for re-examination. On the other hand, the requirement for viable tissue does not permit ready shipment of specimens for LI measurement. Frozen tissue can be used for Ki-67 studies. Static cytophotometry can use smears or archived, paraffin-embedded tissue. The LI is attractive because it measures a variable of direct biologic significance, fraction of cells in S-phase; the same is not true for either SPF by flow or static cytometry or Ki-67 index, at least not

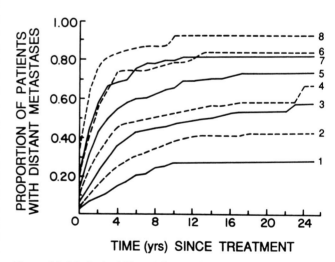

Figure 13–26. Probability of the metastatic dissemination of breast carcinoma in relationship to the size of the primary carcinoma (centimeters in diameter). (After Koscielny, S., Tubiana, M., Le, M. G., et al.: Breast cancer: Relationship between the size of the primary tumour and the probability of metastatic dissemination. Br. J. Cancer, *49*:709–715, 1984, with permission.)

until the nature and function of the Ki-67 antigen are known. Time required for analysis and interpretation of the various assays is a factor to be considered. Static photometry probably is the most labor intensive. We have found in our laboratory where BrdUrd LI and flow cytometry are both routinely performed on breast carcinomas that the latter is, at best, slightly less time consuming than the former.

A question of great importance—not yet answered—concerns the efficiency and efficacy of morphometric nuclear measurements versus cell kinetics. Comparative studies are lacking and need to be undertaken.

SUMMARY AND CONCLUSIONS

Much data has accumulated on relationships between (1) cell kinetic measurements and DNA measurements by flow cytometry and static cytometry and (2) course of breast carcinoma. At present, the following conclusions appear to be secure:

- Proliferation and DNA aneuploidy are strongly related to histologic features. Proliferative rate is a determinant of growth pattern and degree of necrosis.
- DNA ploidy is weakly related to breast carcinoma stage (tumor size, nodal status, and local extent), and proliferation even more weakly.
- DNA ploidy is a weak prognostic indicator and in most studies not stage independent. Measures of proliferation are superior to DNA ploidy for prognosis. The prognostic power of DNA ploidy comes largely from the association of DNA aneuploidy with high rates of proliferation.
- TLI and SPF by flow cytometry are equally strong prognostic indicators and are independent of stage, working well in both node-negative and node-positive patients. This is true despite the fact that the two measurements are only modestly correlated ($r = 0.6$). Because proliferation and metastatic potential are little correlated, proliferation is predictive of relapse and survival probabilities and pace of progression in various stages of disease.
- Since BrdUrd LI gives results equivalent to those of TLI, it can replace TLI.
- Either LI by measurement in vitro or in vivo or SPF by flow cytometry can be used to select patients as high risk in the node-negative group for treatment with surgical adjuvant therapy. These measurements of proliferation may be more effective for prognosis than assays of estrogen or progesterone receptors.
- LI and SPF by flow cytometry have not been evaluated sufficiently against morphometric nuclear measurements in breast carcinoma to determine whether one has an advantage over the other for breast carcinoma prognosis.
- SPF by flow cytometry is not purely a measurement of proliferation or S-phase fraction of breast carcinoma, but it should be looked on as an empiric result from mathematical analysis of DNA histograms.

References

Aaltomaa, S., Lipponen, P., Papinaho, S., et al.: Proliferating-cell nuclear antigen (PC10) immunolabelling and other proliferation indices as prognostic factors in breast cancer. J. Cancer Res. Clin. Oncol., *119*:288–294, 1993.

Allison, D. C., Yuhas, J. M., Ridolpho, P. F., et al.: Cytophotometric measurement of the cellular DNA content of ^{3}H thymidine-labeled spheroids. Cell Tissue Kinet., *16*:237, 1983.

Allison, D. C., Ridolpho, P. F., Anderson, S., et al.: Variations in the (^{3}H) thymidine labeling of S-phase cells in solid mouse tumors. Cancer Res., *45*:6010, 1985.

Amellem, O., and Pettersen, E. O.: Cell inactivation and cell cycle inhibition as induced by extreme hypoxia: The possible role of cell cycle arrest as a protection against hypoxia-induced lethal damage. Cell Prolif., *24*:127–141, 1991.

Anderson, T. J., Ferguson, D. J. P., and Raab, G. M.: Cell turnover in the "resting" human breast: Influence of parity, contraceptive pill, age and laterality. Br. J. Cancer, *46*:376, 1982.

Ashikari, R., Huvos, A. G., Urban, J. A., et al.: Infiltrating lobular carcinoma of the breast. Cancer, *31*:110, 1973.

Askensten, U. G., von Rosen, A. K., Nilsson, R. S., et al.: Intratumoral variations in DNA distribution patterns in mammary adenocarcinomas. Cytometry, *10*:326–333, 1989.

Atkin, N. B.: Modal deoxyribonucleic acid value and survival in carcinoma of the breast. Br. Med. J., *1*:271, 1972.

Auer, G. U., Caspersson, T. O., and Wallgren, A. S.: DNA content and survival in mammary carcinoma. Anal. Quant. Cytol., *2*:161, 1980*a*.

Auer, G. U., Caspersson, T. O., Gustafsson, S. A., et al.: Relationship between nuclear DNA distribution and estrogen receptors in human mammary carcinomas. Anal. Quant. Cytol., *2*:280, 1980*b*.

Auer, G. U., Fallenius, A. G., Erhardt, K. Y., et al.: Progression of mammary adenocarcinomas as reflected by nuclear DNA content. Cytometry, *5*:420–425, 1984.

Baak, J. P. A., Van Dop, H., Kurver, P. H. J., et al.: The value of morphometry to classic prognosticators in breast cancer. Cancer, *56*:374–382, 1985.

Baisch, H., Beck, H. P., Christensen, I. J., et al.: A comparison of mathematical methods for the analysis of DNA histograms obtained by flow cytometry. Cell Tissue Kinet., *15*:235, 1982.

Barlogie, B., Raber, M. N., Schumann, J., et al.: Flow cytometry in clinical cancer research. Cancer Res., *43*:3982, 1983.

Barnes, D. M., Meyer, J. S., Gonzalez, J. G., et al.: Relationship between c-*erb*B-2 immunoreactivity and thymidine labelling index in breast carcinoma in situ. Breast Cancer Res. Treat., *18*:11–17, 1991.

Barnes, D. M., Bartkova, J., Camplejohn, R., et al.: Overexpression of the c-*erb*B-2 oncoprotein: Why does this occur more frequently in ductal carcinoma in situ than in invasive mammary carcinoma and is this of prognostic significance? Eur. J. Cancer, *28*:644–648, 1992.

Baserga, R., Hennegar, G. C., and Kisieleski, W. E.: Uptake of tritiated thymidine by human tumors in vivo. Lab. Invest., *11*:360, 1962.

Battersby, S., and Anderson, T. J.: Proliferative and secretory activity in the pregnant and lactating human breast. Virchows Arch. A: Pathol. Anat., *413*:189–196, 1988.

Beerman, H., Bonsing, B. A., van de Vijver, J. M., et al.: DNA ploidy of primary breast cancer and local recurrence after breast-conserving therapy. Br. J. Cancer, *64*:139–143, 1991.

Begg, A. C., McNally, N. J., Shrieve, D. C., et al.: A method to measure the duration of DNA synthesis and the potential doubling time from a single sample. Cytometry, *6*:620–626, 1985.

Berg, J. W., and Robbins, G. F.: Factors influencing long and short term survival of breast cancer patients. Surg. Gynecol. Obstet., *122*:1311, 1966.

Berryman, I. L., Harvey, J. M., Sterrett, G. F., et al.: The nuclear DNA content of human breast carcinoma. Associations with clinical stage, axillary lymph node status, estrogen receptor status and outcome. Anal. Quant. Cytol. Histol., *9*:429–434, 1987.

Bertuzzi, A., Diadone, M. G., Di Fronzo, G., et al.: Relationship among estrogen receptors, proliferative activity and menopausal status in breast cancer. Breast Cancer Res. Treat., *1*:253, 1981.

Bichel, P., Poulsen, H. S., and Andersen, J.: Estrogen receptor content and ploidy of human mammary carcinoma. Cancer, *50*:1771, 1982.

Bloom, H. J. G., and Richardson, W. W.: Histologic grading and prognosis in breast cancer. Br. J. Cancer, *11*:359, 1957.

Bonadonna, G., Valagussa, P., Tancini, G., et al.: Current status of Milan adjuvant chemotherapy trials for node-positive and node-negative breast cancer. Natl. Cancer Inst. Monogr., *1*:45–50, 1986.

Bose, A. D., Ridolpho, P., and Meyne, J.: Lightly [^{3}H] TdR-labeled bone marrow cells are in G_1-G_2 (Abstract). Cell Tissue Kinet., *17*:669, 1984.

Bravo, R., Fey, S. J., Bellatin, J., et al.: Identification of a nuclear and of a cotyplasmic polypeptide whose relative proportions are sensitive to changes in the rate of cell proliferation. Exp. Cell Res., *136*:311–319, 1981.

Braylan, R. D.: Flow cytometry. Arch. Pathol. Lab. Med., *107*:1, 1983.

Briffod, M., Spyratos, F., Tubiana-Hulin, M., et al.: Sequential cytopunctures during preoperative chemotherapy for primary breast carcinoma. Cytomorphic changes, initial tumor ploidy and tumor regression. Cancer, *63*:631–637, 1989.

Bronner, M. P., Clevenger, C. V., Edmonds, P. R., et al.: Flow cytometric analysis of DNA content of Hurthle cell adenomas and carcinomas of the thyroid. Am. J. Clin. Pathol., *89*:764–769, 1988.

Bruno, S., and Darzynkiewicz, Z.: Cell cycle dependent expression and stability of the nuclear protein detected by Ki-s67 antibody in HL-60 cells. Cell Prolif., *24*:31–40, 1992.

Chapman, J. D.: Hypoxic sensitizers. Implications for radiation therapy. N. Engl. J. Med., *301*:1429, 1979.

Chassevent, A., Daver, A., Bertrand, G., et al.: Comparative flow DNA analysis of different cell suspensions in breast carcinoma. Cytometry, *5*:263, 1984.

Chavaudra, N., and Malaise, E. P.: In vitro incorporation of [³H]TdR in human and murine solid tumors. Influence of 5-fluorouracil and/or hyperbaric oxygen on special distribution of labelling. Cell Tissue Kinet., *12*:597, 1979.

Christov, K., Milev, A., and Todorov, V.: DNA aneuploidy and cell proliferation in breast tumors. Cancer, *64*:673–679, 1989.

Christov, K., Chew, K. L., Ljung, B. M., et al.: Proliferation of normal breast epithelial cells as shown by in vitro labeling with bromodeoxyuridine. Am. J. Pathol., *138*:1371–1377, 1991.

Cibas, E. S., Medeiros, L. J., Weinberg, D. S., et al.: Cellular DNA profiles of benign and malignant adrenocortical tumors. Am. J. Surg. Pathol., *14*:940–955, 1990.

Clark, G. M., Dressler, L. G., Owens, M. A., et al.: Prediction of relapse or survival in patients with node-negative breast cancer by DNA flow cytometry. N. Engl. J. Med., *320*:627–633, 1989.

Clark, G. M., Mathieu, M. C., Owens, M. A., et al.: Prognostic significance of S-phase fraction in good-risk, node-negative breast cancer patients. J. Clin. Oncol., *10*:428–432, 1992.

Clarkson, B., Ota, K., Ohkita, T., et al.: Kinetics of proliferation of cancer cells in neoplastic effusions in man. Cancer, *18*:1189, 1965.

Clayton, F.: Pathologic correlates of survival in 378 lymph node–negative infiltrating ductal breast carcinomas. Cancer, *68*:1309–1317, 1991.

Coninx, P., Liataud-Roger, F., Bousseau, A., et al.: Accumulation of noncycling cells with a G₂-DNA content in ageing solid tumors. Cell Tissue Kinet., *16*:505, 1983.

Cooke, T., George, D., Maynard, P., et al.: Hormone receptors and cell kinetics in breast cancer (Abstract). Cancer Treat. Rep., *63*:1190, 1979.

Cornelisse, C. J., de Koning, C. T., Moolenaar, A. J., et al.: Image and flow cytometric analysis of DNA content in breast cancer. Relation to estrogen receptor content and lymph node involvement. Anal. Quant. Cytol., *6*:9, 1984.

Cornelisse, C. J., van de Velde, C. J. H., Caspers, R. J. C., et al.: DNA ploidy and survival in breast cancer patients. Cytometry, *8*:225–234, 1987.

Coulson, P. B., Thornthwaite, J. T., Wooley, T. W., et al.: Prognostic indicators including DNA histogram type, receptor content and staging related to human breast cancer patient survival. Cancer Res., *44*:4187, 1984.

Courdi, A., Hery, M., and Dahan, E.: Factors affecting relapse in node-negative breast cancer: A multivariate analysis including the labeling index. Eur. J. Cancer Clin. Oncol., *25*:351–356, 1989.

Culpin, D., and Morris, V. B.: Pattern of DNA synthesis and its effect on the classification of cells by flow cytometry. Cell Tissue Kinet., *18*:1, 1985.

Cuzick, J., Stewart, H. J., Peto, R., et al.: Overview of randomized trials of postoperative adjuvant radiotherapy in breast cancer. Recent Results Cancer Res., *111*:108–129, 1988.

Darzynkiewicz, Z., Traganos, F., and Melamed, M. R.: New cell cycle compartments identified by multiparameter flow cytometry. Cytometry, *1*:98, 1980.

Dawson, A. E., Norton, J. A., and Weinberg, D. S.: Comparative assessment of proliferation and DNA content in breast carcinoma by image analysis and flow cytometry. Am. J. Pathol., *136*:1115–1129, 1990.

Dean, P. N., Gray, J. W., and Dolbeare, F. A.: The interpretation and misinterpretation of DNA distributions measured by flow cytometry. Cytometry, *3*:188, 1982.

Dell'Orco, R. T.: Maintenance of human diploid fibroblasts as arrested populations. Fed. Proc., *33*:1969, 1974.

Denekamp, J., and Kallman, R. F.: In vitro and in vivo labeling of animal tumours with tritiated thymidine. Cell Tissue Kinet., *6*:217, 1973.

Diadone, M. G., Silvestrini, R., Valentinis, B., et al.: Proliferative activity of primary breast cancer and of synchronous lymph node metastases evaluated by [³H]-thymidine labelling index. Cell Tissue Kinet., *23*:401–408, 1990.

Di Stefano, D., Mingazzini, P. L., Scucchi, L., et al.: A comparative study of histopathology, hormone receptors, peanut lectin binding, Ki-67 immunostaining, and nucleolar organizer region–associated proteins in human breast cancer. Cancer, *67*:463–471, 1991.

Dörmer, P., Brinkmann, W., Born, R., et al.: Rate and time of DNA synthesis of individual Chinese hamster cells. Cell Tissue Kinet., *8*:399, 1975.

Dressler, L. G., Seamer, L. C., Owens, M. A., et al.: DNA flow cytometry and prognostic factors in 1331 frozen breast cancer specimens. Cancer, *61*:420–427, 1988.

Eliasen, C. A., Opitz, L. M., Vamvakas, C., et al.: Flow cytometric analysis of DNA ploidy and S-phase fraction in breast cancer using cells obtained by *ex vivo* fine-needle aspiration: An optimal method for sample collection. Modern Pathol., *4*:196–200, 1991.

Ellward, J., and Dörmer, P.: Effect of 5-fluoro-2′-deoxyuridine (FdUrd) on 5-bromo-2′-deoxyuridine (BrdUrd) incorporation into DNA measured with a monoclonal BrdUrd antibody and by the BrdUrd/Hoechst quenching effect. Cytometry, *6*:513, 1985*a*.

El-Naggar, A. K., Mackay, B., Sneige, N., et al.: Stromal neoplasms of the breast: A comparative flow cytometric study. J. Surg. Oncol., *44*:151–156, 1990.

Erhardt, K., Auer, G., Folin, A., et al.: Comparison between histologic type, estrogen receptor, and nuclear DNA content in mammary carcinoma. Am. J. Clin. Oncol., *9*:83–89, 1986.

Ewen, M. E., Faha, B., Harlow, E., et al.: Interaction of p107 with cyclin A independent of complex formation with viral oncoproteins. Science, *255*:85–87, 1992.

Ewers, S.-B., Langstrom, E., Baldetorp, B., et al.: Flow-cytometric DNA analysis in primary breast carcinomas and clinicopathological correlations. Cytometry, *5*:408, 1984.

Fabrikant, J. I., Wisseman, C. L., III, and Vitak, M. J.: The kinetics of cellular proliferation in normal and malignant tissues. II. An in vitro method for incorporation of tritiated thymidine in human tissues. Radiology, *92*:1309, 1969.

Faha, B., Ewen, M. E., Tsai, L. H., et al.: Interaction between human cyclin A and adenovirus E1A–associated p107 protein. Science, *255*:85–87, 1992.

Fallenius, A. G., Skoog, L. K., Svane, G. E., et al.: Cytophotometrical and biochemical characterization of nonpalpable mammographically detected mammary adenocarcinomas. Cytometry, *5*:426–429, 1984.

Fallenius, A. G., Askensten, U. G., Skoog, L. K., et al.: The reliability of microspectrophotometric and flow cytometric nuclear DNA measurements in adenocarcinomas of the breast. Cytometry, *8*:260–266, 1987.

Fallenius, A. G., Auer, G. U., and Carstensen, J. M.: Prognostic significance of DNA measurements in 409 consecutive breast cancer patients. Cancer, *62*:331–341, 1988*a*.

Fallenius, A. G., Franzen, S. A., and Auer, G. U.: Predictive value of nuclear DNA content in breast cancer in relation to clinical and morphologic factors. A retrospective study of 227 consecutive cases. Cancer, *62*:521–530, 1988*b*.

Feichter, G., Czech, W., Haag, D., et al.: Comparison of S-phase fractions measured by flow cytometry and autoradiography in human transplant tumors. Cytometry, *9*:605–611, 1988*a*.

Feichter, G. E., Mueller, A., Kaufmann, M., et al.: Correlation of DNA flow cytometric results and other prognostic factors in primary breast cancer. Int. J. Cancer, *41*:823–828, 1988*b*.

Fisher, E. R., Gregorio, R. M., and Fisher, B.: The pathology of invasive breast cancer: A syllabus derived from the findings of the National Surgical Adjuvant Breast Project (Protocol No. 4). Cancer, *36*:1, 1975.

Fisher, E. R., Redmond, C., and Fisher, B.: Pathologic findings from the National Surgical Adjuvant Breast Project, VIII. Relationship of chemotherapeutic responsiveness to tumor differentiation. Cancer, *51*:181–191, 1983.

Fisher, B., Gunduz, N., Constantino, J., et al.: DNA flow cytometric analysis of primary operable breast cancer. Relation of ploidy and S-phase fraction to outcome of patients in NSABP B-04. Cancer, *68*:1465–1475, 1991.

Fogt, F., Wan, J., O'Hara, C., et al.: Flow cytometric measurement of cell cycle kinetics in rat Walker-256 carcinoma following in vivo pulse labelling with bromodeoxyuridine. Cytometry, *12*:33–41, 1991.

Fossa, S. D., Marton, P. F., Knudsen, O. S., et al.: Nuclear Feulgen DNA-content and nuclear size in human breast carcinoma. Hum. Pathol., *13*:626, 1982.

Frierson, H. F. Jr.: Ploidy analysis and S-phase fraction determination by flow cytometry of invasive adenocarcinomas of the breast. Am. J. Surg. Pathol., *15*:358–367, 1991.

Fuhr, J. E., Frye, A., Kattine, A. A., et al.: Flow cytometric determination of breast tumor heterogeneity. Cancer, *67*:1401–1405, 1991.

Galand, P., and Degraef, C.: Cyclin/PCNA immunostaining as an alternative to tritiated thymidine pulse labelling for marking S phase cells in paraffin sections from animal and human tissues. Cell Tissue Kinet., *22*:383–392, 1989.

Gentili, C., Sanfilippo, O., and Silvestrini, R.: Cell proliferation in relation to clinical features and relapse in breast cancers. Cancer, *48*:974, 1981.

Gerdes, J., Schwab, U., Lemke, H., et al.: Production of a mouse monoclonal antibody reactive with a human nuclear antigen associated with cell proliferation. Int. J. Cancer, *31*:13–20, 1983.

Gerdes, J., Li, L., Schlueter, C., et al: Immunobiochemical and molecular biologic characterization of the cell proliferation–associated nuclear antigen that is defined by monoclonal antibody Ki-67. Am. J. Pathol., *138*:867–873, 1991.

Gnant, M. F. X., Blijham, G., Reiner, A., et al.: DNA ploidy and other results of DNA flow cytometry as prognostic factors in operable breast cancer: 10 year results of a randomised study. Eur. J. Cancer, *28*:711–716, 1992.

Going, J. J., Anderson, T. J., Battersby, S., et al.: Proliferative and secretory activity in human breast during natural and artificial menstrual cycles. Am. J. Pathol., *130*:193–204, 1988.

Gonchoroff, N. J., Ryan, J. J., Kimlinger, T. K., et al.: Effect of sonication on paraffin-embedded tissue preparation for DNA flow cytometry. Cytometry, *11*:642–646, 1990.

Goodson, W. H., Ljung, B. M., Waldman, F. M., et al.: In vivo measurement of breast cancer growth rate. Arch. Surg., *126*:1220–1223, 1991.

Gratzner, H. G.: Monoclonal antibody to 5-bromo- and 5-iododeoxyuridine: A new reagent for detection of DNA replication. Science, *218*:474–475, 1982.

Haag, D., Goerttler, K., and Tschahargane, C.: The proliferative index (PI) of human breast cancer as obtained by flow cytometry. Pathol. Res. Pract., *178*:315, 1984.

Haag, D., Feichter, G., Goerttler, K., et al.: Influence of systematic errors on the evaluation of the S phase portions from DNA distributions of solid tumors as shown for 328 breast carcinomas. Cytometry, *8*:377, 1987.

Hamilton, E., and Dobbin, J.: [³H] thymidine labels less than half of the DNA-synthesizing cells in the mouse tumor, carcinoma NT. Cell Tissue Kinet., *15*:405, 1982.

Hamilton, E., and Dobbin, J.: The percentage labelled mitoses technique shows the mean cell cycle time to be half its true value in carcinoma NT. I. [³H]thymidine and vincristine studies. Cell Tissue Kinet., *16*:473, 1983.

Hamilton, E., Dobbin, J., and Kummermehr, J.: The relationship between the flash labelling index and the per cent S-phase cells in mouse tumors (Abstract). Cell Tissue Kinet., *17*:298, 1984.

Hart, W. R., Bauer, R. C., and Oberman, H. A.: Cystosarcoma phyllodes. A clinicopathologic study of twenty-six hypercellular periductal stromal tumors of the breast. Am. J. Clin. Pathol., *70*:211, 1978.

Hartviet, F.: Medullary carcinoma of the breast. Type I and type III tumors. Acta Pathol. Microbiol. Scand. A., *82*:319, 1974.

Harvey, J., de Klerk, N., Berryman, I., et al.: Nuclear DNA content and prognosis in human breast cancer: A static cytophotometric study. Breast Cancer Res. Treat., *9*:101–109, 1987.

Hatschek, T., Carstensen, J., Fagerberg, G. F., et al.: Influence of S-phase fraction on metastatic pattern and post-recurrence survival of a randomized mammography screening trial. Breast Cancer Res. Treat., *14*:321–327, 1989.

Hedley, D. W., Rugg, C. A., Alun, B. P., et al.: Influence of cellular DNA content on disease-free survival of stage II breast cancer patients. Cancer Res., *44*:5395, 1984.

Hedley, D. W., Rugg, C. A., and Gelber, R. D.: Association of DNA index and S-phase fraction with prognosis of nodes positive early breast cancer. Cancer Res., *47*:4729–4735, 1987.

Heidelberger, C.: Pyrimidine and pyrimidine nucleoside antimetabolites. In Holland, J. F., and Frei, E., III (Eds.): Cancer Medicine. 2nd ed. Philadelphia, Lea & Febiger, 1982, p 801.

Heiden, T., Schumann, J., and Goehde, W.: Flow sorting of tumor cells for morphometric analysis, particularly of rare cells. Virchows Arch. Cell Pathol., *61*:29–38, 1991.

Hery, M., Gioanni, J., Lalanne, C.M., et al.: The DNA labeling index: A prognostic factor in node-negative breast cancer. Breast Cancer Res. Treat., *9*:207–211, 1987.

Hoffman, J., and Post, J.: In vivo studies of DNA synthesis in human normal and tumor cells. Cancer Res., *27*:898, 1967.

Hoshino, T., Prados, M., Wilson, C. B., et al.: Prognostic implications of the bromodeoxyuridine labeling index of human gliomas. J. Neurosurg., *71*:335–341, 1989.

Howard, A., and Pelc, S. R.: Nuclear incorporation of ^{32}P as demonstrated by autoradiographs. Exp. Cell Res., *2*:178, 1951.

Isola, J. J., Helin, H. J., Helle, M. J., et al.: Evaluation of cell proliferation in breast carcinoma. Comparison of Ki-67 immunohistochemical study, DNA flow cytometric analysis, and mitotic count. Cancer, *65*:1180–1184, 1990.

Joensuu, H., Klemi, P. J.: DNA aneuploidy in adenomas of endocrine organs. Am. J. Pathol., *132*:145–151, 1988.

Joensuu, H., Toikkanen, S., and Klemi, P.J.: DNA index and S-phase fraction and their combination as prognostic factors in operable ductal breast carcinoma. Cancer, *66*:331–340, 1990.

Jones, B., and Camplejohn, R. S.: Stathmokinetic measurement of tumor cell proliferation in relation to vascular proximity. Cell Tissue Kinet., *16*:351, 1983.

Kallioniemi, OP., Blanco, G., Alavaikko, M., et al.: Improving the prognostic value of DNA flow cytometry in breast cancer by combining DNA index and S-phase fraction. Cancer, *62*:2183–2190, 1988.

Kamel, O. W., Franklin, W. A., Ringus, J. C., et al.: Thymidine labeling index and Ki-67 growth fraction in lesions of the breast. Am. J. Pathol., *134*:107–113, 1989.

Kamel, O. W., LeBrun, D. P., Davis, R. E., et al.: Growth fraction estimation of malignant lymphomas in formalin-fixed paraffin-embedded tissue using anti-PCNA/Cyclin 19A2: Correlation with Ki-67 labeling. Am. J. Pathol., *138*:1471–1477, 1991.

Kempson, R. L., and Bari, W.: Uterine sarcomas. Classification, diagnosis and prognosis. Hum. Pathol., *1*:331, 1970.

Kennedy, K. A., Teicher, B. A., Rockwell, S., et al.: The hypoxic tumor cell: A target for selective cancer chemotherapy. Biochem. Pharmacol., *29*:1, 1980.

Keyhani-Rofagha, S., O'Toole, R. V., Farrar, W. B., et al.: Is DNA ploidy an independent prognostic indicator in infiltrative node-negative breast adenocarcinoma? Cancer, *65*:1577–1582, 1990.

Kieback, D. G., Beller, F. K., Nitsch, C. D., et al.: [Therapy and prognosis of small breast carcinomas. Comparison of subcutaneous and standard mastectomy.] Geburtshilfe-Frauenheilkd., *50*:754–770, 1990.

Klintenberg, C., Stal, O., Nordenskjoold, B., et al.: Proliferative index, cytosol estrogen receptor and axillary node status as prognostic predictors in human mammary carcinomas. Breast Cancer Res. Treat., *7*(Suppl.):99–106, 1986.

Koscielny, S., Tubiana, M., Le, M. G., et al.: Breast cancer: Relationship between the size of the primary tumour and the probability of metastatic dissemination. Br. J. Cancer, *49*:709–715, 1984.

Kreipe, H., Alm, P., Olsson, H., et al.: Prognostic significance of a formalin-resistant nuclear proliferation antigen in mammary carcinomas as determined by the monoclonal antibody Ki-S1. Am. J. Pathol., *142*:651–657, 1993.

Kute, T. E., Muss, H. B., Anderson, D., et al.: Relationship of steroid receptor, cell kinetics and clinical status in patients with breast cancer. Cancer Res., *41*:3524, 1981.

Kute, T. E., Muss, H. B., Cooper, M. R., et al.: The use of flow cytometry for the prognosis of stage II adjuvant treated breast cancer patients. Cancer, *66*:2810–2816, 1990.

Ladekarl, M., Sørensen, F. B.: Prognostic, quantitative histopathologic variables in lobular carcinoma of the breast. Cancer, *72*:2602–2611, 1993.

Laerum, O. D., and Farsund, T.: Clinical application of flow cytometry: A review. Cytometry, *2*:1, 1981.

Lajtha, L. G.: Bone marrow cell metabolism. Physiol. Rev., *37*:50, 1957.

Landberg, G., and Roos, G.: Antibodies to proliferating cell nuclear antigen as S-phase probes in flow cytometric cell cycle analysis. Cancer Res., *51*:4570–4574, 1991.

Landry, J., Freyer, J. K. P., and Sutherland, R. M.: A model for the growth of multicellular spheroids. Cell Tissue Kinet., *15*:585, 1982.

Laroye, G. J., and Minkin, S.: The impact of mitotic index on predicting outcome in breast carcinoma: A comparison of different counting methods in patients with different lymph node status. Modern Pathol., *4*:456–460, 1991.

Laster, W. R., Jr., Mayo, J. G., Simpson-Herren, L., et al.: Success and failure in the treatment of solid tumors. II. Kinetic parameters and "cell cure" of moderately advanced carcinoma 755. Cancer Chemother. Rep., *53*:169, 1969.

Layfield, L. J., Hart, J., Neuwirth, H., et al.: Relation between DNA ploidy and the clinical behavior of phyllodes tumors. Cancer, *64*:1485–1489, 1989.

Lee, A. K. C., Dugan, J., Hamilton, W. M., et al.: Quantitative DNA analysis in breast carcinomas: A comparison between image analysis and flow cytometry. Modern Pathol., *4*:176–182, 1991.

Lelle, R. J., Heidenreich, W., Stauch, G., et al.: The correlation of growth fractions with histologic grading and lymph node status in human mammary carcinoma. Cancer, *59*:83, 1987.

Lelle, R. J.: Zellkinetische Befunde beim Mammakarzinom. Bestimmung der Wachstumsfraktion mit Hilfe des monoklonalen Antikorpers Ki-67. New York, Georg Thieme Verlag, 1989.

Ljung, B. M., Mayall, B., Lottich, C., et al.: Variations in tumor-cell viability and DNA ploidy cell dissociation techniques in human breast cancer. Breast Cancer Res. Treat., *13*:153–159, 1989.

Masters, J. R. W., Drive, J. O., and Scarisbrick, J. J.: Cyclical variations in DNA synthesis in human breast epithelium. J. Natl. Cancer Inst., *58*:1263, 1977.

Matthews, M. B., Bernstein, R. M., Franza, B. R., et al.: Identity of the proliferating cell nuclear antigen and cyclin. Nature, *309*:374–376, 1984.

Maurer, H. R.: Potential pitfalls of [³H] thymidine techniques to measure cell proliferation. Cell Tissue Kinet., *14*:111, 1981.

McDivitt, R. W., Boyce, W., and Gersell, D.: Tubular carcinoma of the breast. Clinical and pathological observations concerning 135 cases. Am. J. Surg. Pathol., *6*:401–411, 1982.

McDivitt, R. W., Stone, K. R., Craig, B., et al.: A proposed classification of breast cancer based on kinetic information. Cancer, *57*:269–276, 1986.

McDivitt, R. W., Stone, K. R., Craig, R. B., et al.: A comparison of human breast cancer cell kinetics measured by flow cytometry and thymidine labeling. Lab. Invest., *52*:287, 1985.

McDivitt, R. W., Stone, K. R., and Meyer, J. S.: A method for dissociation of viable human breast cancer cells that produces flow cytometric kinetic information similar to that obtained by thymidine labeling. Cancer Res., *44*:2628, 1984.

McGurrin, J. F., Doria, M. I. Jr., Dawson, P. J., et al.: Assessment of tumor cell kinetics by immunohistochemistry in carcinoma of breast. Cancer, *57*:1744–1750, 1987.

Melamed, M. R., Lindmo, T., Mendelsohn, M. L. (Eds): Flow Cytometry and Sorting. 2nd ed. New York, Wiley-Liss, 1990.

Mendelsohn, M. L.: The growth fraction: A new concept applied to tumors. Science, *132*:1496, 1960.

Mendelsohn, M. L.: Autoradiographic analysis of cell proliferation in spontaneous breast cancer of C3H mouse. III. The growth fraction. J. Natl. Cancer Inst., *28*:1015, 1962.

Mendelsohn, M. L., and Takahashi, M.: A critical evaluation of the fraction of labeled mitoses method as applied to the analysis of tumor and other cell cycles. *In* Baserga, R. (Ed.): The Cell Cycle and Cancer. New York, Dekker, 1971, p. 58.

Meyer, J. S.: Cell proliferation in normal human breast ducts, fibroadenomas, and other ductal hyperplasia measured by nuclear labeling with tritiated thymidine. Hum. Pathol., *8*:67, 1977.

Meyer, J. S.: Growth and cell kinetic measurements in human tumors. Pathol. Annu., *16*(Part 2):53, 1981.

Meyer, J. S.: Potential value of cell kinetics in management of cancers of unknown origin. Semin. Oncol., *9*:513, 1982.

Meyer, J. S.: Cell kinetics of histologic variants of in situ breast carcinoma. Breast Cancer Res. Treat., *7*:171, 1986.

Meyer, J. S., and Bauer, W. C.: In vitro determination of tritiated thymidine labeling index (LI). Cancer, *36*:1374, 1975.

Meyer, J. S., Bauer, W. C., and Rao, B. R.: Subpopulations of breast carcinoma defined by S-phase fraction, morphology, and estrogen receptor content. Lab. Invest., *39*:225, 1978.

Meyer, J. S., and Connor, R. E.: In vitro labeling of solid tissues with tritiated thymidine for autoradiographic detection of S-phase nuclei. Stain Technol., *52*:185, 1977.

Meyer, J. S., and Connor, R. E.: Cell proliferation in fibrocystic disease and postmenopausal breast ducts measured by thymidine labeling. Cancer, *50*:746, 1985.

Meyer, J. S., and Coplin, M. D.: Thymidine labeling index, flow cytometric S-phase measurement, and DNA index in human tumors. Am. J. Clin. Pathol., *89*:586–595, 1988.

Meyer, J. S., and Facher, R.: Thymidine labeling index of human breast carcinoma. Enhancement of in vitro labeling by 5-fluorouracil and 5-fluoro-2'-deoxyuridine. Cancer, *39*:2524, 1977.

Meyer, J. S., and Hixon, B.: Advanced stage and early relapse of breast carcinomas associated with high thymidine labeling indices. Cancer Res., *39*:4042, 1979.

Meyer, J. S., Friedman, E., McCrate, M. M., et al.: Prediction of early course of breast carcinoma by thymidine labeling. Cancer, *51*:1879, 1983.

Meyer, J. S., Koehm, S. L., Hughes, J. M., et al.: Bromodeoxyuridine labeling for S-phase measurement in breast carcinoma. Cancer, *71*:3531–3540, 1993.

Meyer, J. S., and Lee, J. V.: S-phase fraction of breast carcinoma in relapse: Relationships of remission duration, estrogen receptor content, therapeutic responsiveness, and duration of survival. Cancer Res., *40*:1890, 1980.

Meyer, J. S., and McDivitt, R. W.: Reliability and stability of the thymidine labeling index of breast carcinoma. Lab. Invest., *54*:160–164, 1986.

Meyer, J. S., McDivitt, R. W., Stone, K. R., et al.: Practical breast carcinoma cell kinetics: Review and update. Breast Cancer Res. Treat., *4*:79, 1984b.

Meyer, J. S., Micko, S., Craver, J. L., et al.: DNA flow cytometry of breast carcinoma after acetic-acid fixation. Cell Tissue Kinet., *17*:185, 1984a.

Meyer, J. S., and Nauert, J.: Cell kinetics of human tumors by in vitro bromodeoxyuridine labeling. J. Histochem. Cytochem., *37*:1449–1454, 1989.

Meyer, J. S., Prey, M. U., Babcock, D. S., et al.: Breast carcinoma cell kinetics, morphology, stage and host characteristics: A thymidine labeling study. Lab. Invest., *54*:41, 1986.

Meyer, J. S., and Province, M.: Proliferative index of breast carcinoma by thymidine labeling: Prognostic power independent of stage, estrogen and progesterone receptors. Breast Cancer Res. Treat., *12*:191–204, 1988.

Meyer, J. S., and Province, M.: Nuclear size (NS), thymidine labeling index (LI), estrogen and progesterone receptors (ER, PgR), tumor size (TS) and lymph node status (N) in long-term prognosis of breast carcinoma (Abstract). Breast Cancer Res. Treat., *23*:154, 1992.

Meyer, J. S., Rao, B. R., Stevens, S. C., et al.: Low incidence of estrogen receptor in breast carcinomas with rapid rates of cellular replication. Cancer, *40*:2290, 1977.

Meyer, J. S., and Wittliff, J. L.: Regional heterogeneity in breast carcinoma: Thymidine labelling index, steroid hormone receptors, DNA ploidy. Int. J. Cancer, *47*:213–220, 1991.

Miller, M. A., Mazewski, C. M., Yousuf, N., et al.: Simultaneous immunohistochemical detection of IUdR and BrdU infused intravenously to cancer patients. J. Histochem. Cytochem., *39*:407–412, 1991.

Miyachi, K., Fritzler, M. J., and Tan, E. M.: Autoantibody to a nuclear antigen in proliferating cells. J. Immunol., *121*:2228–2234, 1978.

Moulder, J. E., and Rockwell, S.: Hypoxic fractions of solid tumors: Experimental techniques, methods of analysis, and a survey of existing data. Int. J. Radiat. Oncol. Biol. Phys., *10*:695, 1984.

Muirhead, K. A., Horan, P. K., and Poste, G.: Flow cytometry: Present and future. Bio/Technology, *3*:337, 1985.

Moran, R., Black, M., Alpert, L., et al.: Correlation of cell-cycle kinetics, hormone receptors, histopathology and nodal status in human breast cancer. Cancer, *54*:1586, 1984.

Nakane, P. K., Moriuchi, T., Koji, T., et al.: Proliferating cell nuclear antigen (PCNA/cyclin): Review and some new findings. Acta Histochem. Cytochem., *22*:105–116, 1989.

Norris, H. J., and Taylor, H. B.: Relationship of histological features to behavior of cystosarcoma phyllodes: Analysis of ninety-four cases. Cancer, *20*:2090, 1967.

Obara, T., Fujimoto, Y., Kanaji, Y., et al.: Flow cytometric DNA analysis of parathyroid tumors. Implication of aneuploidy for pathologic and biologic classification. Cancer, *66*:1555–1562, 1990.

Olsson, H., Ranstam, J., Baldetorp, B., et al.: Proliferation and DNA ploidy in malignant breast tumors in relation to early oral contraceptive use and early abortions. Cancer, *67*:1285–1290, 1991.

Olszewski, W., Darzynkiewicz, Z., Rosen, P. P., et al.: Flow cytometry of breast carcinoma. II. Relation of tumor cell cycle distribution in histology and estrogen receptor. Cancer, *48*:985, 1981*a*.

Olszewski, W., Darzynkiewicz, Z., Rosen, P. P., et al.: Flow cytometry of breast carcinoma. I. Relation of DNA ploidy level to histology and estrogen receptor. Cancer, *48*:980, 1981*b*.

Opfermann, M., Brugal, G., and Vassilakos, P.: Cytometry of breast carcinoma: Significance of ploidy balance and proliferation index. Cytometry, *8*:217–224, 1987.

O'Reilly, S. M., Camplejohn, R. S., Barnes, D. M., et al.: DNA index, S-phase fraction, histological grade and prognosis in breast cancer. Br. J. Cancer, *61*:671–674, 1990*a*.

O'Reilly, S. M., Camplejohn, R. S., Millis, R. R., et al.: Proliferative activity, histological grade and benefit from adjuvant chemotherapy in node-positive breast cancer. Eur. J. Cancer, *26*:1035–1038, 1990*b*.

O'Reilly, S. M., Barnes, D. M., Camplejohn, R. S., et al.: The relationship between c-erbB-2 expression, S-phase fraction and prognosis in breast cancer. Br. J. Cancer, *63*:444–446, 1991.

O'Reilly, S. M., and Richards, M. A.: Is DNA flow cytometry a useful investigation in breast cancer? Eur. J. Cancer, *28*:504–507, 1992.

Palko, M. J., Wang, S. E., Shackney, S. E., et al.: Flow cytometric S fraction as a predictor of clinical outcome in cystosarcoma phyllodes. Arch. Pathol. Lab. Med., *114*:949–952, 1990.

Paradiso, A., Lorusso, V., Tommasi, S., et al.: Relevance of cell kinetics to hormonal response of receptor-positive advanced breast cancer. Breast Cancer Res. Treat., *11*:31–36, 1988.

Parl, F. F., and Dupont, W. D.: A retrospective cohort study of histologic risk factors in breast cancer patients. Cancer, *50*:2410, 1982.

Pietruszka, M., and Barnes, L.: Cytosarcoma phyllodes. A clinicopathologic analysis of 42 cases. Cancer, *41*:1974, 1978.

Post, J., Sklarew, R. H., and Hoffman, J.: The proliferative patterns of human breast cancer cells in vivo. Cancer, *39*:1500, 1977.

Quastler, H., and Sherman, F. G.: Cell population kinetics in the intestinal epithelium of the mouse. Exp. Cell Res., *17*:420, 1959.

Raber, M. N., Barlogie, B., Latreille, J., et al.: Ploidy, proliferative activity and estrogen receptor content in human breast cancer. Cytometry, *3*:36, 1982.

Rajewsky, M. F.: In vitro studies of cell proliferation in tumors. II. Characteristics of a standardized in vitro system for measurement of ³H-thymidine incorporation into tissue explants. Eur. J. Cancer, *1*:281, 1965.

Raza, A., Ucar, K., and Preisler, H. D.: Double labeling and in vitro versus in vivo incorporation of bromodeoxyuridine in patients with acute non-lymphocytic leukemia. Cytometry, *6*:633–640, 1985.

Raza, A., Miller, A., Mazewski, C., et al.: Observations regarding DNA replication sites in human cells *in vivo* following infusions of iododeoxyuridine and bromodeoxyuridine. Cell Prolif., *24*:113–126, 1991*a*.

Raza, A., Preisler, H., Lampkin, B., et al.: Biological significance of cell cycle kinetics in 128 standard risk newly diagnosed patients with acute myelocytic leukemia. Br. J. Hematol., *79*:33–39, 1991*b*.

Raza, A., Yousuf, N., Bokhari, A. J., et al.: Contribution of *in vivo* proliferation/differentiation studies toward the development of a combined functional and morphologic system of classification of neoplastic diseases. Cancer, *69*:1557–1566, 1992.

Remvikos, Y., Beuzeboc, P., Zajdela, A., et al.: Correlation of pretreatment proliferative activity of breast cancer with the response to cytotoxic chemotherapy. J. Natl. Cancer Inst., *81*:1383–1387, 1989.

Remvikos, Y., Vielh, P., Padoy, E., et al.: Breast cancer proliferation measured on cytological samples: A study by flow cytometry of S-phase fractions and BrdkU incorporation. Br. J. Cancer, *64*:501–507, 1991.

Ridolfi, R. L., Rosen, P. P., Port, A., et al: Medullary carcinoma of the breast. A clinicopathologic study with 10 year follow-up. Cancer, *40*:1365, 1977.

Rockwell, S.: Hypoxic cells as targets for cancer chemotherapy. *In* Cheng, Y.-C., Goz, B., and Minkoff, M. (Eds.): Development of Target-Oriented Anticancer Drugs. New York, Raven Press, 1983, p. 157.

Rockwell, S., Kallman, R. F., and Fajardo, L. F.: Characteristics of a

serially transplanted mouse mammary tumor and its tissue culture-adapted derivative. J. Natl. Cancer Inst., *49*:735, 1972.

Roos, G., Arnerlov, C., and Emdin, S.: Retrospective DNA analysis of T3/T4 breast carcinoma using cytophotometry and flow cytometry. A comparative study with prognostic evaluation. Anal. Quant. Cytol. Histol., *10*:189–194, 1988.

Rubens, R. D., and Richards, M. A.: DNA index, S-phase fraction, histological grade and prognosis in breast cancer. Br. J. Cancer, *61*:671–674, 1990.

Rubini, J. R., Wescott, E., and Keller, S.: In vitro DNA labeling of bone marrow and leukemic blood leukocytes with tritiated thymidine. II. H³ thymidine biochemistry in vitro. J. Lab. Clin. Med., *68*:566, 1966.

Russell, W. O., Cohen, J., Enzinger, F., et al.: A clinical and pathological staging system for soft tissue sarcomas. Cancer, *40*:1562, 1977.

Sahin, A. A., Ro, J., Ro, J. Y., et al: Ki-67 immunostaining in node-negative stage I/II breast carcinoma. Significant correlation with prognosis. Cancer, *68*:549–557, 1991.

Sauerboern, R., Balmain, A., Goerttler, K., et al: On the existence of "arrested G_2 cells" in mouse epidermis. Cell Tissue Kinet., *11*:291, 1978.

Schabel, F. M., Jr.: Concepts for systemic treatment of micrometastases. Cancer, *35*:15, 1975.

Schiffer, L. M., Braunschweiger, P. G., Stragand, J. J., et al.: The cell kinetics of human mammary cancers. Cancer, *43*:1707, 1979.

Shapiro, H.: Practical Flow Cytometry. 2nd ed. New York, Alan R. Liss, 1988.

Sharma, S., Mishra, M. C., Kapur, B. M. L., et al.: The prognostic significance of ploidy analysis in operable breast cancer. Cancer, *68*:2612–2616, 1991.

Sheck, L. E., Muirhead, K. A., and Horan, P.: Evaluation of the S-phase distribution of flow cytometric DNA histograms by autoradiography and computer algorithms. Cytometry, *1*:109, 1980.

Shibui, S., Hoshino, T., Vanderlaan, M., et al.: Double labeling with iodo- and bromodeoxyuridine for cell kinetics studies. J. Histochem. Cytochem., *37*:1007–1011, 1989.

Shirakawa, S., Luce, J. I., Tannock, I., et al.: Cell proliferation in human melanoma. J. Clin. Invest., *49*:1188, 1970.

Shrieve, D. C., and Begg, A. C.: Cell cycle kinetics of aerated, hypoxic and re-aerated cells *in vitro*. Cell Tissue Kinet., *18*:641–651, 1985.

Silvestrini, R., Diadone, M. G., and Di Fronzo, G.: Relationship between proliferative activity and estrogen receptors in breast cancer. Cancer, *44*:665, 1979.

Silvestrini, R., Daidone, M. G., and Gasparini, G.: Cell kinetics as a prognostic marker in node-negative breast cancer. Cancer, *56*:1982, 1985.

Silvestrini, R., Daidone, M. G., Di Fronzo, G., et al.: Prognostic implication of labeling index versus estrogen receptors and tumor size in node-negative breast cancer. Breast Cancer Res. Treat., *7*:161, 1986.

Silvestrini, R., Diadone, M. G., Valagussa, P., et al.: Cell kinetics as a prognostic indicator in node-negative breast cancer. Eur. J. Cancer Clin. Oncol., *25*:1165–1171, 1989.

Sisken, J. E., Bonner, S. V., Grasch, B. D., et al.: Alterations in metaphase durations in cells derived from human tumours. Cell Tissue Kinet., *18*:137, 1985.

Skipper, H. E., and Schabel, F. M., Jr.: Quantitative and cytokinetic studies in experimental tumor systems. *In* Holland, J. F., and Frei, E., III (Eds.): Cancer Medicine. Philadelphia, Lea & Febiger, 1982.

Sklarew, R. J.: Cytokinetics of subpopulations in mixed polyploid tumors by television imaging. I. Deconvolution of the S-phase DNA ploidy composition. II. Analysis of the S-emptying profile of ploidy subpopulations. J. Histochem. Cytochem., *32*:413–420, 1984.

Sklarew, R. J., Hoffman, J., and Post, J.: A rapid in vitro method for measuring cell proliferation in human breast cancer. Cancer, *40*:2299, 1977.

Steel, G. G.: Cell loss as a factor in the growth of human tumours. Eur. J. Cancer, *3*:381, 1967.

Steel, G. G.: Growth Kinetics of Tumours. Oxford, England, Clarendon Press, 1977.

Steel, G. G., and Bensted, J. P. M.: In vitro studies of proliferation in tumors. I. Critical appraisal of methods and theoretical considerations. Eur. J. Cancer, *1*:275, 1965.

Stout, A. P.: Fibrosarcoma. The malignant tumor of fibroblasts. Cancer, *1*:30, 1948.

Stumpp, J., Dietl, J., Simon, W., et al.: Growth fraction in breast carcinoma determined by Ki-67 immunostaining: correlation with pathological and clinical variables. Gynecol. Obstet. Invest., *33*:47–50, 1992.

Straus, M. J., and Moran, R. E.: Cell cycle parameters in human solid tumors. Cancer, *40*:1453, 1977.

Straus, M. J., and Moran, R. E.: The cell cycle kinetics of human breast cancer. Cancer, *46*:2634, 1980.

Straus, M. J., Moran, R., Muller, R. E., et al.: Estrogen receptor heterogeneity and the relationship between estrogen receptor and the tritiated thymidine labeling index in human breast cancer. Oncology, *39*:197, 1982.

Suit, H. D., and Shalek, R. J.: Response of anoxic C3H mouse mammary carcinoma isotransplants (1–35 mm^3) to X irradiation. J. Natl. Cancer Inst., *31*:479, 1963.

Sulkes, A., Livingstone, R.B., and Murphy, W.K.: J. Natl. Cancer Inst., *62*:513–515, 1979.

Tahan, S. R., Neuberg, D. S., Dieffenbach, A., et al.: Prediction of early relapse and shortened survival in patients with breast cancer by proliferating cell nuclear antigen score. Cancer, *71*:3442–3559, 1993.

Tannock, I. F.: The relation between cell proliferation and the vascular system in a transplanted mouse mammary tumor. Br. J. Cancer, *22*:258, 1968.

Tay, D.L.M., Bhathal, P.S., and Fox, R.M.: Quantitation of G_0 and G_1 cells in primary carcinomas. Antibody to M_1 subunit of ribonucleotide reductase shows G_1 phase restriction point block. J. Clin. Invest., *87*:519–527, 1991.

Taylor, I. W., Musgroove, E. A., Friedlander, M. L., et al.: The influence of age on the DNA ploidy levels of breast tumors. Eur. J. Cancer Clin. Oncol., *19*:623, 1983.

Taylor, J. H., Woods, P. S., and Hughes, W. L.: The organization and duplication of chromosomes using tritium-labeled thymidine. Proc. Natl. Acad. Sci. USA, *43*:122, 1957.

Terz, J. J., Curutchet, H. P., and Lawrence, W., Jr.: Analysis of the cycling and noncycling cell population of human solid tumors. Cancer, *40*:1462, 1977.

Toikkanen, S., Joensuu, H., and Klemi, P.: The prognostic significance of nuclear DNA content in invasive breast cancer—a study with long-term follow-up. Br. J. Cancer, *60*:693–700, 1989.

Tribukait, B.: Clinical DNA flow cytometry. Med. Oncol. Tumor Pharmacother., *1*:211, 1984.

Trowell, D. A.: The culture of lymph nodes in vitro. Exp. Cell Res., *3*:79, 1952.

Tubiana, M., and Courdi, A.: Cell proliferation kinetics in human solid tumors: Relation to probability of metastatic dissemination and long-term survival. Radiother. Oncol. *15*:1–18, 1989.

Tubiana, M., Chauvel, P., Ranaud, A., et al.: Vitesse de croissance et histoire naturelle du cancer du sein. Bull. Cancer, *62*:341, 1975.

Tubiana, M., Pejovic, M.H., Koscielny, S., et al.: Growth rate, kinetics of tumor cell proliferation and long-term outcome in human breast cancer. Int. J. Cancer, *44*:17–22, 1989.

Uyterlinde, A.M., Schipper, N.W., Baak, J.P.A., et al.: Limited prognostic value of cellular DNA content to classical and morphometrical parameters in invasive ductal breast cancer. Am. J. Clin. Pathol., *89*:301–307, 1988.

Van Boekstaehle, D.R., Lan, J., Snoeck, H.W., et al.: Aberrant Ki-67 expression in normal bone marrow revealed by multiparameter flow cytometric analysis. Cytometry, *12*:50–63, 1991.

Vanderlaan, M., and Thomas, C.B.: Characterization of monoclonal antibodies to bromodeoxyuridine. Cytometry, *6*:501–505, 1985.

Vanderlaan, M., Watkins, B., Thomas, C., et al.: Improved high-affinity monoclonal antibody to iododeoxyuridine. Cytometry, *7*:499–507, 1986.

van der Linden, J.C., Lindeman, J., Baak, J.P.A., et al.: The multivariate prognostic index and nuclear DNA content are independent prognostic factors in primary breast cancer patients. Cytometry, *10*:56–61, 1989.

van Dierendonck, J.H., Keijzer, R., van de Velde, C.G., et al.: Nuclear distribution of the Ki-67 antigen during the cell cycle: Comparison with growth fraction in human breast cancer cells. Cancer Res., *49*:2999–3006, 1989.

van Diest, P.J., and Baak, J.P.A.: The morphometric prognostic index is the strongest prognosticator in premenopausal lymph node–negative breast cancer patients. Hum. Pathol., *22*:326–330, 1991.

Verhoeven, D., Bourgeois, N., Derde, M.P., et al.: Comparison of cell growth in different parts of breast cancers. Histopathology, *17*:505–509, 1990.

Viehl, P., Chevillard, S., Mosseri, V., et al.: Ki-67 index and S-phase fraction in human breast carcinomas. Comparison and correlations with prognostic factors. Am. J. Clin. Pathol., *94*:681–686, 1990.

Visscher, D.W., Zarbo, R.J., Greenawald, K.A., et al.: Prognostic significance of morphologic parameters and flow cytometric DNA analysis in carcinoma of the breast. Pathol. Annu., *25*(Part 1):171–209, 1990a.

Visscher, D.W., Zarbo, R.J., Jacobsen, G., et al.: Multiparametric deoxyribonucleic acid cell cycle analysis of breast carcinomas by flow cytometry. Clinicopathologic correlations. Lab. Invest., *62*:370–378, 1990b.

Vogel, P. M., Georgiade, N. G., Fetter, B. F., et al.: The correlation of histologic changes in the human breast with the menstrual cycle. Am. J. Pathol., *104*:23, 1981.

Waldman, F.M., Chew, K., Ljung, B.M., et al.: A comparison between bromodeoxyuridine and ^{3}H thymidine labeling in human breast tumors. Modern Pathol., *4*:718–722, 1991.

Wallgren, A., Silfversward, C., and Eklund, G.: Prognostic factors in breast cancer. Acta Radiol. (Ther.), *15*:1, 1976.

Wenger, C. R., Beardslee, S., Owens, M. A., et al.: DNA ploidy, S-phase, and steroid receptors in more than 127,000 breast cancer patients. Breast Cancer Res. Treat., *28*:9–10, 1993.

White, R.A., Terry, N.H.A., Meistrich, M.L., et al.: Improved method for computing potential doubling time from flow cytometric data. Cytometry, *11*:314–317, 1990.

White, R.A., Terry, N.H.A., Baggerly, K.A., et al.: Measuring cell proliferation by relative movement. I. Introduction and in vitro studies. Cell Prolif., *24*:257–270, 1991.

Wibe, E., Lindmo, T., and Kaalhus, O.: Cell kinetic characteristics in different parts of multicellular spheroids of human origin. Cell Tissue Kinet., *14*:639, 1981.

Wilson, G.D., McNally, N.J., Dunphy, E., et al.: The labelling index of human and mouse tumours assessed by bromodeoxyuridine staining in vitro and in vivo and flow cytometry. Cytometry, *6*:641–647, 1985.

Wilson, G.D., McNally, N.J., Dische, S., et al.: Measurement of cell kinetics in human tumours in vivo using bromodeoxyuridine incorporation and flow cytometry. Br. J. Cancer, *58*:423–431, 1988.

Wintzer, H.O., Zipfel, I., Schulte-Monting, J., et al.: Ki-67 immunostaining in human breast tumors and its relationship to prognosis. Cancer, *67*:421–428, 1991.

Witzig, T.E., Gonchoroff, N.J., Greipp, P.R., et al.: Rapid S-phase determination of non-Hodgkin's lymphomas with the use of an immunofluorescence bromodeoxyuridine labeling index procedure. Am. J. Clin. Pathol., *91*:298–301, 1989.

Witzig, T. E., Gonchoroff, N. J., Therneau, T., et al.: DNA content flow cytometry as a prognostic factor for node-positive breast cancer. The role of multiparameter ploidy analysis and specimen sonication. Cancer, *68*:1781–1788, 1991.

Wimber, D. E., and Quastler, H.: A ^{14}C- and ^{3}H-thymidine double labelling technique in the study of cell proliferation in *Tradescantia* root tips. Exp. Cell Res., *30*:8, 1963.

Yousuf, N., Khan, S., Sheikh, Y., et al.: Cell cycle parameters and DNA ploidy in colorectal carcinomas. J. Surg. Res., *51*:457–462, 1991.

14

The Genetic Basis for the Emergence and Progression of Breast Cancer

George P. Studzinski
Janusz J. Godyn

Knowledge of the genetic controls of cell growth is important not only to the understanding of the evolution of a tumor but also to its precise diagnosis, treatment, and monitoring. In view of the enormous challenge of breast cancer as one of the diseases where, in many cases, the physician is often little more than a silent witness of human suffering, the genetic basis of mammary carcinoma is an area of intense current interest and investigation at both fundamental and clinical levels.

FAMILIAL OCCURRENCE

Development of a clinically recognizable tumor requires multiple genetic changes, or mutations. If one or more, but usually only one, such mutation is transmitted in the germ cell, the affected person has an increased chance of developing a malignancy, tends to develop this disease earlier in life than is usual, and may develop multiple primary tumors. Furthermore, if the mutated gene was present in one of the parents, rather than resulting from an accident of meiosis in germ cell formation, other members of the immediate family are also likely to be affected by some form of malignant disease.

Familial occurrence of breast carcinoma has been recognized for more than a hundred years (Broca, 1866). It is generally accepted that the risk of developing breast cancer is more than doubled for a woman whose mother, sister, or daughter had breast cancer, and the risk becomes 10-fold if that relative had bilateral cancer, or if more than one first-degree relative was affected (Anderson, 1972; 1974). This suggests that an abnormality in a gene, or more likely a set of genes, predisposes a woman to this disease. The search for the responsible genes has been long, but the genes have proved elusive, and only recently have several suspected culprits been rounded up.

The search for the genes whose mutations contribute to the development of breast cancer has been aided by the identification of families whose members are affected by cancer in numbers that much exceed the norm (Lynch et al., 1978; Li, 1988). In addition, the association of breast cancer with other diseases has provided important clues to the nature of the genetic basis for the disease. These include

Cowden's disease, characterized by keratoses on hands and feet, facial tricholemmomas, and oral papillomas or fibromas. Almost half of females so affected develop breast carcinoma, and prophylactic mastectomy has been suggested. Carcinoma of the breast is also frequent in association with ataxia-telangiectasia, estimated at 6.8 relative risk for heterozygous women. Since women homozygous for ataxia-telangiectasia have a short life span, breast cancer is not common in the homozygotes. It is also important to be aware that there is an association between the incidence of breast carcinoma and meningioma, and therefore symptoms of intracranial malignancy in a patient with breast cancer do not necessarily indicate the metastatic spread of the breast cancer to the brain. These associations are discussed at greater length in a detailed review by Wolman and Dawson (1991).

GENES INVOLVED IN BREAST CANCER

A very clear link between malfunctioning genes and breast carcinoma was provided by the description of predisposition to several types of cancer in families studied by Li and Fraumeni (1969). The original four families studied had nine cases of childhood sarcoma and 10 cases of breast cancer, several of which arose bilaterally at an early age. Additional families were later identified in which predisposition to cancer was transmitted in an autosomal dominant pattern. The syndrome was called SBLA (Lynch et al., 1978), a reference to the prominence of sarcomas of diverse soft tissue origin, breast cancer, leukemia, and adrenocortical carcinoma in various members of those families. Osteosarcomas and brain tumors were also seen with excessive frequency, and possible additional components include melanocarcinoma, gonadal germ cell tumors, and carcinomas of the lung, pancreas, and prostate. Components of the syndrome, more frequently referred to as the Li-Fraumeni syndrome, can occur as multiple primary cancers in one patient, or they can affect different members of the family, often at an unusually early age. For instance, for affected females the risk of developing breast cancer before age 45 years is 18 times greater than for the general population (Garber et al., 1991). Recently, inherited mutations in gene p53 have been found in patients with this syndrome (Malkin et al., 1990). The importance of this finding lies in the fact that the p53 gene is a known tumor suppressor gene and is the most commonly mutated gene identified so far in human cancer (Hollstein et al., 1991). Mutations in the p53 gene are also found in sporadic (i.e., nonfamilial) cases of breast cancer, but these mutations are somatic, being present in tumor cells but not in the normal tissues of the patient (Sidransky et al., 1992). Thus, it seems fairly certain that p53 is one of the key genes involved in the pathogenesis of breast carcinoma, though it is equally certain that it is not the only gene with that role.

The discoveries that have produced most recent excitement concern the two genes *BRCA1* and *BRCA2,* which are responsible for most of the 5% to 10% of breast carcinomas with familial background. *BRCA1* is present on the long arm of chromosome 17 (Miki et al., 1994), whereas *BRCA2* resides on the long arm of chromosome 13 (Wooster et al., 1994). Both of these genes have been cloned, but the function of the encoded proteins is still unknown. Affected family members, and a few of those who escape the disease, have a mutation in one of these genes. Abnormal *BRCA1* gene, unlike the *BRCA2* gene, also predisposes to ovarian carcinoma, but only *BRCA2* is linked to male breast cancer. Disappointingly to those clinicians who hoped for a broad advance in the knowledge of the molecular basis for the emergence of breast cancer, neither *BRCA1* nor *BRCA2* appears to be involved in the pathogenesis of nonfamilial (by far the most common) forms of this disease. Thus, proto-oncogenes, and "anti-oncogenes" also known as tumor suppressor genes, are being investigated for a possible role in the causation of nonfamilial breast cancer.

Rather remarkably, in view of the explosive acquisition of knowledge of oncogenes, antioncogenes, and other growth-related genes (e.g., Studzinski, 1989; Studzinski et al., 1990), their precise involvement in the formation of breast tumors is a matter of controversy or conjecture. The nuances of these arguments are meaningful only when the underlying principles of tumor clonality and progression, genetic instability, and the broad groups of genes involved in cancer are clearly understood.

CLONALITY AND TUMOR PROGRESSION

Maintenance of an epithelial structure, such as the lining of the ducts of the mammary gland, depends on the proliferative activity of cells in the basal layer, which have the ability to proliferate in such a way that some of the progeny retain the proliferative activity while other cells mature into terminally differentiated forms. The former, by definition, are stem cells. The proliferative activity of normal stem cells is subject to environmental control; nutrients and growth factors are permissive for replication, whereas hormones regulate their proliferation in a cyclical, temporal pattern. The fate of stem cells, determined by these controls, is essentially threefold (Fig. 14–1): (1) they can remain quiescent and serve as a reserve for future needs; (2) they can divide into two daughter cells, one of which remains a stem cell while the other travels along the differentiation pathway; or (3) they can form two daughter cells

with little ability to differentiate but with high proliferative activity. The last alternative is normally exceedingly rare, but the chance of its occurrence is increased by damage to the DNA or to a chromosome of the cell. Such damage may occur as an accident to the chromosomes during mitosis or as a result of exposure to environmental carcinogens (in humans principally noxious chemicals and radiation). Viral carcinogenesis, important in animal models of breast carcinoma, has not been completely excluded. Once the genome is altered by one or more of these factors, there is a progressively increasing chance of further alterations (e.g., Studzinski, 1977).

Such alterations are known as tumor progression, and it is important to realize that this term includes much more than the growth of the tumor in size, or its spread. The critical part of tumor progression is the acquisition of new properties that favor tumor growth, and new cell subclones may appear during this progression (Fig. 14–2). The new properties include more complex chromosome abnormalities leading to progressively hyperploid karyotypes with multiple marker chromosomes, decreasing dependence on growth factors, the ability to grow in new environments, which allows some cells to form micrometastases by gaining a foothold in distant tissues, and the secretion of proteins that affect the host's metabolism, such as calcium-mobilizing hormones. Importantly, progression occurs independently in different primary tumors, so with multiple primaries or with bilateral disease, examination of only one biopsy specimen may be misleading as to the extent of tumor progression in the other primaries.

One of the tenets of tumor progression is that new characteristics of malignant cells are acquired independently of one another. These characteristics pertain also to the cell's interaction with its environment. For instance, the ability to grow in one tissue (e.g., in the lymph node) is independent of its ability to establish a colony in another tissue (e.g., bone); therefore, the absence of regional metastases in the lymph nodes by no means precludes distant systemic metastases.

GENETIC INSTABILITY

Genetic instability is the force that drives tumor progression (Nowell, 1976). The first prerequisite for the development of clonal populations with genetic damage is proliferation. For reasons that are not at all clear, one genetic defect greatly increases the probability that other events will occur that result in further genetic damage. Perhaps this is the price the cell pays when it activates metabolic pathways that compensate for the original gene damage. Abnormalities in karyotype, such as extra or unpaired chromosomes, increase the difficulty of achieving an orderly distribution of the chromosomes to the daughter cells during mitosis, so superimposed mitotic errors lead to even more gross abnormalities of the karyotype. Many of these errors are not compatible with cell survival, but some endow the cell with an increased ability to outgrow its neighbors, and thus produce subclones that may replace the original neoplastic clone. This is illustrated in Figure 14–2. The genetic abnormalities that promote cell proliferation are those that lead

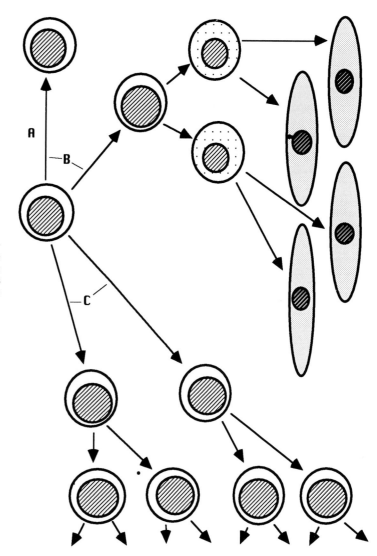

Figure 14-1. Possible fates of a stem cell. It can remain quiescent and serve as a reserve for future needs (A). It can undergo an asymmetric division into another stem cell and a cell that differentiates (B). It can divide into two stem cells (C). This has the potential to increase the population size.

to the activation of proto-oncogenes, to the loss of tumor suppressor genes, and to alterations in genes that regulate programmed cell death.

ACTIVATION OF PROTO-ONCOGENES

Several dozen cellular genes receive and propagate signals for cell proliferation and differentiation (Studzinski, 1989). They are also prone to malfunction and are thought to be responsible for the abnormal growth of neoplastic cells. When functioning normally, these genes are known as proto-oncogenes, but when the genes are "activated" to malfunction, they are referred to as oncogenes, or cancer-causing genes. Proto-oncogenes can be activated in several ways: (1) by somatic mutation, which is a change in the sequence of the bases in DNA—an exchange of one base for another, or loss/gain of a base or several bases; (2) by the formation of multiple copies of a gene in a process known as amplification, whereby expression of the gene is increased; and (3) by the activation of a gene by placement, nearby, of a strong promoter of gene transcription, which

can be provided by an invading virus but in human tumors is more commonly a result of a reciprocal chromosome translocation.

The known activations of proto-oncogenes in breast cancer are currently limited to somatic mutations of *ras* genes, and to the amplification of *erb* B$_2$, also known as *HER-2* or *neu* gene (Callahan & Campbell, 1989). Amplifications of c-*myc* and *int*-2 genes are also considered by some to be responsible for the neoplastic mode of growth of breast cancer cells (Table 14–1).

The oncogenes are known by a three-letter code, which usually relates to the means by which they were identified; the proto-oncogenes have the prefix *c*-, for cellular, to distinguish them from the activated oncogenes. The prefix "v-" signifies oncogenes originally identified as viruses. The pathway that transmits growth signals from the environment to the transcriptional machinery in the nucleus consists principally of proteins encoded by proto-oncogenes. For instance, proto-oncogene c-*sis* encodes a protein related to the beta subunit of the platelet-derived growth factor, *erb* B$_2$ is related to the gene that encodes a cell surface receptor for the epidermal growth factor, *ras* proteins transmit sig-

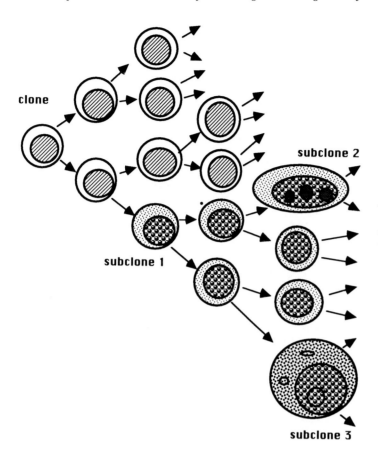

Figure 14–2. Appearance of clones with new phenotypes and properties during stem cell proliferation. The relative proportion of cells of any given clone depends on the growth advantage obtained as the result of the genetic change that caused the clone to arise.

nals from surface receptors toward the nucleus, and c-*myc* encodes a nuclear protein that binds to DNA and is involved in the reactions necessary for DNA replication. A fuller representation of the role of proto-oncogene products in growth signal transduction is shown in Figure 14–3.

Table 14–1. CHROMOSOME ABNORMALITIES IN BREAST CANCER CELLS

Aberration (Chromosome)	Chromosome Locus	Approximate Prevalence (%)
Deletion		
1p	1p36	40
1p	1p33–35	15
1p (L-*myc*)	1p32	35
1q	1q21	30
1q	1q23–32	25
1q	1q42–43	23
3p	3p21–25	30
11p	11p14	21–27
13q	13q14	7–20
17p	17p13.3	60
18q	?	?
Amplification		
c-*myc*	8q24	4–40
int-2	11q13	4–20
c-erb-2	17q21	10–40
Mutation		
Ha-*ras*	11p15.5	?
Ki-*ras*	12p12.1	3
BRCA2	13q12-13	<5
p53	17p13.1	?
"Prohibitin"	17p21	20
BRCA1	17q12-21	<5

DELETIONS OR FUNCTIONAL LOSS OF TUMOR SUPPRESSOR GENES

Deletions of portions of chromosomes or loss of entire chromosomes is frequent in cancer cells in general, and this is equally true in breast carcinoma cells (e.g., McGuire & Naylor, 1989) (see Table 14–1). An important consequence of these deletions is the loss of genes that are negative regulators of cell growth, since their protein products impede the passage of cells through the cell cycle, particularly the G_1–S-phase transition (Fig. 14–4). The tumor suppressor genes known to be important in breast cancer are the Rb-1 gene, responsible for the susceptibility to retinoblastoma in the hereditary forms of the disease (Hansen & Cavenee, 1987) and the previously discussed p53, *BRCA1*, and *BRCA2* genes. Unlike proto-oncogenes, only one of which needs to be activated or provide the uncontrolled growth signal, both copies (alleles) of most tumor suppressor genes need to be lost or inactivated by mutations to provoke abnormal growth. Thus, when an abnormal *BRCA1* gene is inherited, there is no disease, but a second "hit" that damages the DNA of the other allele of the *BRCA1* gene produces early-onset breast cancer, and it has been suggested that damage to the Rb-1 gene may be the cause of some cases of breast cancer (Lundberg et al., 1987; Varley et al., 1989). The evidence for such a role in breast neoplasms is also strong for the p53 gene (Malkin et al., 1990). This is an unusual tumor suppressor gene, since mutations in only one p53 allele are often sufficient to produce neoplastic growth. This can happen when the mutated p53 protein can neutralize the growth-restricting func-

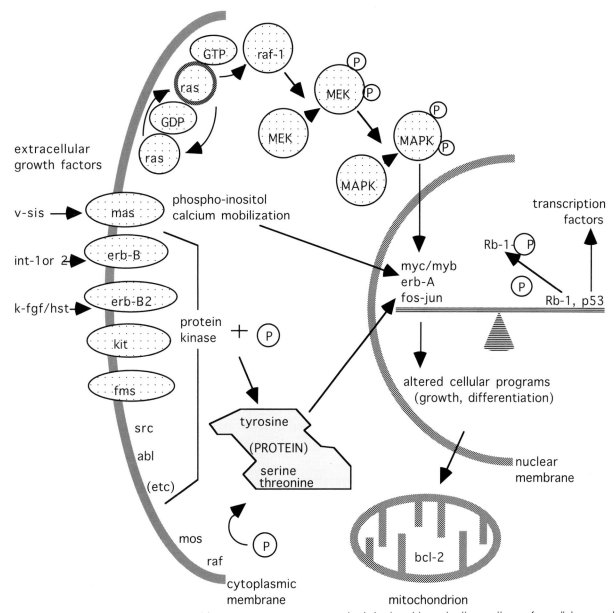

Figure 14–3. Role of proto-oncogene and tumor suppressor gene products in signal transduction pathway for cellular growth. Only representative gene products are shown from over 100 such genes. Nuclear-acting gene products are depicted over a fulcrum, with *myc/myb*, *erb* A, and *fos-jun* on one side, and tumor suppressing Rb-1 and p53 on the other side, opposing their actions.

tion of the normal ("wild-type") protein produced by the other allele. Interestingly, the mutated p53 protein is usually much more stable than the short-lived wild-type protein, so it can be more easily detected in the cell by immunocyto-chemical means (Thor et al., 1992). Its classification as a "dominant-negative" regulator of cell growth is derived from the fact that one mutation is sufficient to produce the malignant phenotype. On the other hand, the Rb-1–damaged gene is "recessive" because both alleles have to be lost or inactivated to produce malignant growth, and proto-oncogenes are "dominant" but positive in their action on growth regulation.

Recent studies have uncovered the mechanisms of the growth-inhibitory activity of Rb-1 and p53 proteins. It seems that these proteins have the ability to form complexes with, and thus sequester, transcription factors such as the E2F factor, which are necessary for the synthesis of proteins required for DNA replication, for example, thymidine kinase, thymidylate, and c-*myc* protein (Nevins, 1992). Normal progression from the G_1 phase to the S-phase involves activation of cellular enzymes that phosphorylate the sequestering complexes and therefore liberate the E2F transcription factor. These phosphorylating enzymes consist of catalytic subunits that belong to the cdc-2 protein kinase family of proteins, and to activating subunits known as cyclins C, D_1, D_2, D_3, E, and A. Loss of Rb-1 or p53 proteins removes this hurdle to the cell's progress to the S-phase and results in uncontrolled proliferation. Thus, we

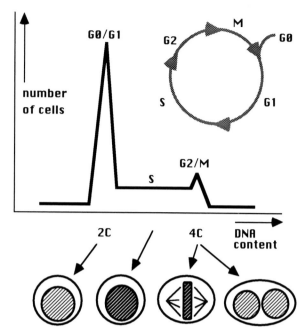

Figure 14–4. A schematized outline of the cell cycle, and an illustration of DNA content in each cell cycle phase as determined by flow cytometry.

see the propensity toward early-onset, bilateral breast cancer in women with Li-Fraumeni syndrome.

ACTIVATION OF GENES THAT CONTROL CELL DIFFERENTIATION AND CELL DEATH

Tumor growth results from an imbalance of cell proliferation and cell attrition by terminal differentiation and by cell death (Fig. 14–5). Little is known about genes that control either of these processes in breast cancer cells, but they appear to be promising targets for future investigation. Significant progress in this area has already been made for other malignancies. Induction of differentiation by retinoic acid is important in the control of promyelocytic leukemia and several types of skin carcinoma (Bloch et al., 1990; Clarkson, 1991). The genes involved in regulation of differentiation by retinoic acid belong to families of proteins known as RAR and RXR, which are related to steroid receptors and act as ligand (i.e., retinoic acid)–activated transcription factors (Mangelsdorf et al., 1990). Human myeloid leukemia cells have been shown to differentiate in response to vitamin D derivatives (Miyaura et al., 1981; Studzinski et al., 1985), and some studies indicate that breast cancer cells have receptors for vitamin D and that their growth may be subject to control by this compound (Frampton et al., 1983).

Another area of expanding knowledge is the control of cell death by the cell's own genes. In some instances it can be shown that cell death is regulated by gene expression and is considered to be a physiologic process required for normal development and tissue turnover (Kerr et al., 1972). The protein encoded by the proto-oncogene bcl-2 has been

shown to counteract this form of cell death, known as apoptosis. The overexpression of the bcl-2 gene leads to abnormal proliferation of some cell types, such as lymphocytes (Hockenberry et al., 1990). Impaired apoptosis is known to be involved in the involution of the lactating breast in mice and rats (Walker et al., 1989), and its role in human breast cancer is suggested by induction of apoptosis in mammary adenocarcinoma by the tumor necrosis factor (Bellomo et al., 1992).

SUMMARY

It is now possible to present a scenario for the genetic basis of the emergence of a breast carcinoma. The hormone-sensitive cells in the terminal duct–lobular unit (Wellings et al., 1975; Russo et al., 1982)—the interface between the mammary gland duct system and the origin of the lobules—contain the stem cells that generate the lactating lobules. These cells are responsive to estrogen and progesterone, which provide abortive signals for growth during the menstrual cycle and elicit overt growth and proliferation during pregnancy. Should the individual inherit, through a germ cell, a defective p53, *BRCA1*, or *BRCA2* gene, the stem cells in the terminal ductal–lobular unit are predisposed to malignancy, but since these cells are quiescent in prepubertal life, no tumor can form. When these cells are subjected to hormone stimulation during puberty, their DNA is replicated to permit cell proliferation; however, the control of DNA replication is defective, because the mutated p53 protein not only fails in its "guard dog" role in DNA replication, but usually also prevents the protein produced by the undamaged allele from discharging this function. As the abnormal cells proliferate, genetic instability in some cells may result in the activation of proto-oncogenes by somatic mutation (the *ras* genes) or by gene amplification (*erb* B$_2$, c-*myc*, *int*-2 genes). Now, the cells *appear* to receive a growth signal, although there is none; deceived by the activated oncogene, they increase their already uncontrolled rate of proliferation. Most of the genetic damage that occurs secondarily to the p53 mutation is not compatible with cell survival, and those cells perish; other cells, however, acquire growth advantage over their neighbors and thrive. This explains the multiple primaries and bilateral disease in women who inherit a mutated p53 gene. In nonfamilial breast cancer, the p53 gene can mutate in the abortively proliferating cells of the terminal ductal–lobular unit, but this event is rare, and therefore sporadic breast cancer usually takes the form of a single tumor that is manifested later in life, as years of exposure to the environmental carcinogens and endogenous hormones take their toll on the population of susceptible cells.

Breast carcinomas increase in size slowly. They can take as long as 10 years to reach 1 cm in diameter, and, as they grow larger, they acquire properties that allow the cells not only to proliferate inexorably but also to spread. These phenomena arise owing to alterations in proto-oncogenes and tumor suppressor genes that may be inherited, or arise de novo, and are exacerbated by a vicious circle of ever-increasing chromosome abnormalities.

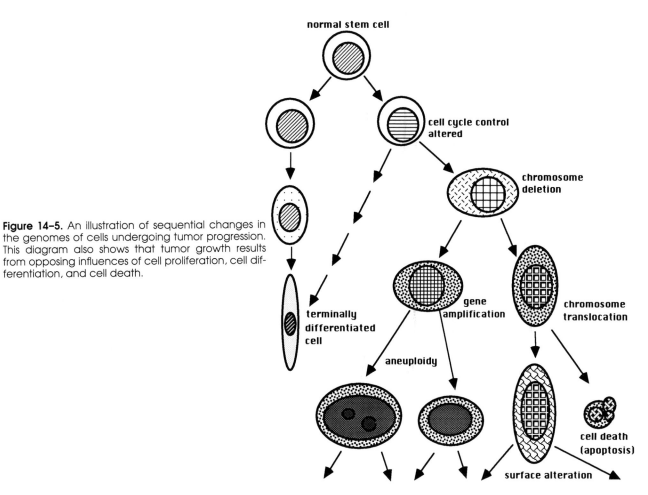

Figure 14-5. An illustration of sequential changes in the genomes of cells undergoing tumor progression. This diagram also shows that tumor growth results from opposing influences of cell proliferation, cell differentiation, and cell death.

Acknowledgments

We are grateful to Drs. Sandra Wolman and Peter Dawson for a copy of their manuscript prior to its publication, and to our colleagues for their helpful comments on this manuscript: Drs. R. Athwal, K. M. Klein, M. Lyons, G. M. Mulcahy, and H. Ozer. Experimental work of the first author was supported by grant RO1-CA-44722 from the National Cancer Institute.

References

Anderson, D. E.: A genetic study of human breast cancer. J. Natl. Cancer Inst., 48:1029–1034, 1972.

Anderson, D. E.: Genetic study of breast cancer. Identification of a high risk group. Cancer, 34:1090–1097, 1974.

Bellomo, G., Perotti, M., Taddei, F., et al.: Tumor necrosis factor-α induces apoptosis in mammary adenocarcinoma cells by an increase in intranuclear free Ca²⁺ concentration and DNA fragmentation. Cancer Res., 52:1342–1346, 1992.

Bloch, A., Koeffler, H. P., Pierce, G. B., et al.: Ninth Annual Sapporo Cancer Seminar. Cell differentiation and cancer control. Cancer Res., 50:1346–1350, 1990.

Broca, P. P.: Traité des Tumeurs. Vols. 1 and 2. Paris: Asselin, 1866.

Callahan, R., and Campbell, G.: Mutations in human breast cancer: An overview. J. Natl. Cancer Inst., 81:1780–1786, 1989.

Clarkson, B.: Retinoic acid in acute promyelocytic leukemia: The promise and the paradox. Cancer Cells, 3:211–220, 1991.

Frampton, R. J., Omond, S. A., and Eisman, J. A.: Inhibition of human cancer cell growth by 1,25-dihydroxyvitamin D₃ metabolites. Cancer Res., 43:4443–4447, 1983.

Garber, J. E., Goldstein, A. M., Kantor, A. F., et al.: Follow-up study of twenty-four families with Li-Fraumeni syndrome. Cancer Res., 51:6094–6097, 1991.

Hansen, M. F., and Cavenee, W. K.: Genetics of cancer predisposition. Cancer Res., 47:5518–5527, 1987.

Hockenberry, D., Nunez, G., Milliman, C., et al.: Bcl-2 is an inner mitochondrial membrane protein that blocks programmed cell death. Nature, 348:334–336, 1990.

Hollstein, M., Sidransky, D., Vogelstein, B., et al.: p53 Mutation in human cancers. Science, 253:49–53, 1991.

Kerr, J. F. R., Wylie, A. H., and Currie, A. R.: Apoptosis: A basic biological phenomenon with wide ranging implications in tissue kinetics. Br. J. Cancer, 26:239–257, 1972.

Li, F. P.: Cancer families: Human models of susceptibility to neoplasia—The Richard and Hinda Rosenthal Foundation Award Lecture. Cancer Res., 48:5381–5386, 1988.

Li, F. P., and Fraumeni, J. F., Jr.: Rhabdomyosarcoma in children: Epidemiologic study and identification of a familial cancer syndrome. J. Natl. Cancer Inst., 43:1365–1373, 1969.

Lundberg, C., Skoog, L., Cavenee, W. K., et al.: Loss of heterozygosity in human ductal breast tumors indicates a recessive mutation on chromosome 13. Proc. Natl. Acad. Sci. U.S.A., 84:2372–2376, 1987.

Lynch, H. T., Mulcahy, G. M., Harris, R. F., et. al.: Genetic and pathologic findings in a kindred with hereditary sarcoma, breast cancer, brain tumors, leukemia, lung, laryngeal, and adrenal cortical carcinoma. Cancer, 41:2055–2064, 1978.

Malkin, D., Li, F. P., Strong, L. C., et al.: Germ line p53 mutations in a familial syndrome of breast cancer, sarcomas, and other neoplasms. Science, 250:1233–1238, 1990.

Mangelsdorf, D. J., Ong, E. S., Dyck, J. A., et al.: Nuclear receptor that identifies a novel retinoic acid response pathway. Nature, 345:224–229, 1990.

McGuire, W. L., and Naylor, S. L.: Loss of heterozygosity in breast cancer: Cause or effect? J. Natl. Cancer Inst., 81:1764–1765, 1989.

Miki, Y., Swensen, J., Shattuck-Eidens, D., Futreal, et al.: A strong candidate for the breast and ovarian cancer susceptibility gene BRCA1. Science, *266*:66–71, 1994.

Miyaura, C., Abe E., Kuribayashi, T., et al.: 1α,25-Dihydroxyvitamin D_3 induces differentiation of human myeloid leukemia cells. Biochem. Biophys. Res. Commun., *102*:937–943, 1981.

Nevins, J. R.: E2F: A link between the Rb tumor suppressor protein and viral oncoproteins. Science, *258*:424–429, 1992.

Nowell, P. C.: The clonal evolution of tumor cell populations. Science, *194*:23–28, 1976.

Russo, J., Tay, L. K., and Russo, I. H.: Differentiation of the mammary gland and susceptibility to carcinogenesis. Breast Cancer Res. Treat., 2:5–73, 1982.

Sidransky, D., Tokino, T., Helzlsouer, K., et al.: Inherited p53 gene mutations in breast cancer. Cancer Res., *52*:2984–2986, 1992.

Studzinski G. P.: Viral transformation. *In* Cristofalo, V. J., and Rothblat, G. (Eds.): Growth, Nutrition, and Metabolism of Cells in Culture. Vol. III. New York, Academic Press, 1977.

Studzinski, G. P.: Invited review. Oncogenes, growth, and the cell cycle: An overview. Cell Tissue Kinet., *22*:405–424, 1989.

Studzinski, G. P., Bhandal, A. K., and Brelvi, Z. S.: A system for monocytic differentiation of leukemic cells HL 60 by a short exposure to 1,25-dihydroxycholecalciferol. Proc. Soc. Exper. Biol. Med., *179*:288–295, 1985.

Studzinski, G. P., Moore, D. C., and Carter, D. L.: Suppressor genes: Restraint of growth or of tumor progressions (Editorial). Lab. Invest., *63*:279–282, 1990.

Thor, A. D., Moore, D. H. II, Edgerton, S. M., et al.: Accumulation of p53 tumor suppressor gene protein: An independent marker of prognosis in breast cancers. J. Natl. Cancer Inst., *84*:845–855, 1992.

Varley, J. M., Armour, J., Swallow, J. E., et al.: The retinoblastoma gene is frequently altered leading to loss of expression in primary breast tumors. Oncogene, *4*:725–729, 1989.

Walker, N. I., Bennett, R. E., and Kerr, J. F. R.: Cell death by apoptosis during involution of the lactating breast in mice and rats. Am. J. Anat., *185*:19–32, 1989.

Wellings, S. R., Jensen, H. M., and Marcum, R. G.: An atlas of subgross pathology of the human breast with special reference to possible precancerous lesions. J. Natl. Cancer Inst., *55*:231–243, 1975.

Wolman, S. M., and Dawson, P. J.: Genetic events in breast cancer and their clinical correlates. Crit. Rev. Oncogenesis, 2:277–291, 1991.

Wooster, R., Neuhausen, S. L., Mangion, J., et al.: Localization of a breast cancer susceptibility gene, BRCA2, to chromosome 13q12-13. Science, *265*:2088–2090, 1994.

15

Growth Rates

John S. Spratt
John A. Spratt

Growth is a characteristic of all true cancers, and the rate of growth is a fundamental determinant of the time required by any cancer to reach a threshold size sufficiently large for it to be detected, to produce symptoms, or to expand to lethal proportions. Cancers are thought to originate from a single cell (Gould et al., 1978). Cancer development is at least a two-step process. First, the normal cell is "immortalized" and is capable of dividing indefinitely without ever becoming fully differentiated or mature. This conversion of the normal cell to a cancer cell occurs through induction by chemical or physical carcinogens or by certain oncogenes. Second, growth in the immortalized cell that results in the disorganized structure of cancer is promoted. True cancer has the capacity to induce angiogenesis, and cancer cells have reduced contact inhibition. Differentiation of immortalized cells is an intensely researched subject, and the findings of its study have significant implications for prevention and treatment of cancer patients. Currently, work in this area has only limited clinical application. Clinicians are encountering only the end results of the molecular processes.

Appreciating the geometry of cancer growth requires an appreciation for the magnitude of change that occurs in size when a geometric or exponential variable changes. The double helix of deoxyribonucleic acid (DNA) would fit into a box that is about 10^{-18} m^2, the nucleus of a cell into a box 10^{-16} m^2, and a red blood cell into a box 10^{-15} m^2. In comparison, a person could easily fit in a box that is 10^0 m^2 and the human hand into a box that is 10^{-1} m^2.

An adult human is composed of approximately 10^{13} cells. A cancer that is 1 cm^3 in size contains approximately 10^9 cells. Death from cancer can usually be expected in a patient with a tumor burden of 10^{12} cells (equivalent to 2^{40} cells, or 40 net generations). Occasionally, a cancer exceeds this size; however, a certain proportion of cancer cells to host cells always exists, and if this proportion is exceeded, death of the individual will result. The upper limit of this lethal proportion is on the order of 10^{12} to 10^{13} cells, or approximately one-tenth of the body's cell composition. This would be less than 10% of body weight when extracellular mass is considered. Anatomically critical locations and variable endocrine output allow for some variance in the lethal mass.

In many scientific discussions, powers of 2 rather than powers of 10 are used. The following relationship permits conversion between the two powers:

$$10^x = 2^y, \tag{1}$$

$$x \ln 10 = y \ln 2, \tag{2}$$

$$y = \frac{x\ln10}{\ln2}, \quad x = \frac{y\ln2}{\ln10} \tag{3}$$

Most human cancer cells undergo binary division and grow to a certain size or a certain age and repeat the process. In a variety of circumstances, subsets of cells may become nonproliferating. Growth is a multiplicative or geometric increase in proliferating cells; random errors in such a system are to be expected. Cell death is a prominent phenomenon in growing cancers. In the clinical arena, net accumulations of cells are observed.

The cell cycle can be divided into four phases: the presynthetic (G_1) phase, the DNA synthesis (S) phase, the postsynthetic (G_2) phase, and the mitotic (M) phase. M-phase time, the shortest segment of the cycle, may be regarded as the fourth phase of a cell's reproductive cycle or as the brief interval in the cycle during which two daughter cells appear. The time a cell spends in each phase is subject to biologic variation, which leads to a frequency distribution of cycle times that Steel (1967 and 1972) considered normal, lognormal, gamma, or other.

The relationship between the mitotic index (MI) and tissue growth measurement was considered by Hoffman (1949). MI is defined as the ratio of the number of cells containing mitotic figures (m) to the total number of cells counted (N). The index m/N is proportional to the ratio of the time in mitosis (T) and the cell doubling time (DT), or cell cycle time (t_c). The duration of intermitotic interval can be highly variable, affecting the value of t_c proportionately. T is also susceptible to considerable variation. These changes in relationships limit the ability of the MI to quantify growth rates accurately. However, correlations between the MI and the aggressiveness of breast cancer have been shown. Parl and Dupont (1982) concluded that a high MI was the "single most important factor indicating high risk for death from cancer." Patients whose breast cancers had a high MI had a standardized mortality ratio (SMR) that was 2.7 times the mortality ratio of the base population studied. Absence of tubule formation and nuclear anaplasia were associated with SMRs of 2.0 and 1.9 times the base rate, respectively. A combination of a high MI and an absence of tubule formation was associated with an SMR of 2.9, whereas a high MI and nuclear anaplasia had an

SMR of 2.5. Well-defined tubules were associated with an SMR of 0.2; when combined with a low MI, the SMR was only 0.17. Thus, although the MI is only a crude parameter for measuring growth rates, it has great prognostic significance when considered alone or in conjunction with other histopathologic variables.

Meyer and Bauer (1976) reported correlations among in vitro thymidine labeling indices (TLIs) and the S-phase fraction (SPF) of cells and patient age, various staging and histopathologic characteristics, estrogen and progesterone receptor assay levels, and survivorship (Chapter 13). The TLI frequency distributions were consistently lognormal. Cancers associated with high TLIs are larger, exhibit more inflammatory cell reactions, consist of more undifferentiated histologic patterns, show greater nuclear anaplasia, and contain more necrosis at time of diagnosis than cancers with low TLIs. The higher TLIs were also associated with cancers that tended to be well circumscribed. The TLIs did not correlate significantly with race, axillary lymph node status, or the invasion of lymphatics and blood capillaries. TLIs were higher in younger women than in older women and tended to be reciprocally related to estrogen and progesterone receptor values.

The TLI was found to be directly related to the intensity of the inflammatory cell response around a cancer and to cell death. For Meyer and Bauer (1976), this suggested that inflammatory cell response was a secondary phenomenon, possibly relating to cell death. They concluded that the TLI values were an important, possibly causative determinant of morphologic patterns. The TLI is definitely associated with the modulation of the disease's progress but is a weak determinant of metastasis.

Post and associates (1977) studied the proliferative patterns of human breast cancer cells in vivo and used intravenous tritiated thymidine (^{3}H-TdR) delivered as a pulse and continuously. Tumor cells engaged in DNA synthesis ranged from 4% to 11%. The periods from G_2 + (½M) and for DNA synthesis were estimated at 4 hours each. They also observed a wide range of intermitotic intervals.

The three main parameters that determine the net rates of growth of cancer are the cell cycle time, the proportion of proliferating cells, and the extent of cell loss. Cell loss results from exfoliation, metastasis, or cell death (Spratt and Ackerman, 1961; and Pearlman, 1976). The shedding of cells into the circulation and the development of metastases are stochastic processes that can be defined by mathematical models (McGuire et al., 1974). A very small percentage of all cancer cells that are shed actually survive.

Recent data reaffirm the process of metastasis from human breast cancer. A longitudinal evaluation of the association of tumor volume, status of the axillary lymph nodes, and remote metastases has been analyzed for 2663 women with breast cancer (Atkinson et al., 1986). The sample was drawn from 4609 women with mammographically measurable tumors at initial diagnosis who had no evidence of lymph node metastasis (76% of the total population). Distant metastases were defined as any cancer outside the breast and its regional lymph nodes (axillary, internal mammary, and supraclavicular). Tumor volume was calculated from the measurements of length and width obtained from the mammograms. The data accessed were recorded be-

tween 1955 and 1979. Certain categories of breast cancer in a total population of breast cancers have probably been excluded: those surfacing in intervals between mammographic examinations and those not visible on mammograms; the authors' own data suggest that these are the more virulent cancers. The second critical omission is descriptions of the histopathologic characteristics of small cancers.

The study by Atkinson and coworkers (1986) shows the extremes of kinetic and metastatic behavior. There was an "extraordinarily large contribution to metastasis of very small tumors." The metastatic potential per cancer cell actually *decreased* with increasing tumor size. These investigators concluded that very small primary cancers exhibit a propensity for rapid diversity, with cloning of cell lines with high metastatic potential, as do tumors that are subject to strong selection pressure (Fidler and Hart, 1982). At the opposite extreme, over 20% of the very largest cancers had not produced diagnosable metastases within 300 months of follow-up. "Large" is defined as a chordal dimension of 7.5 to 8 cm and a volume of 200 mL. The volume effect differed according to nodal status.

The simple relationship of a small, predetectable cancer to its source of nutrition has an unequivocal but incompletely measured impact on the rates of growth and rapid deceleration in growth. When tumors grow as cords of cells, the cords generally appear around capillaries. However, necrosis of the cord cells occurs whenever the distance of the cells from the capillaries exceeds 200 μm. Tissue oxygen approaches zero at this distance (Tannock and Steel, 1969). Whenever V_2 carcinoma is implanted into the avascular vitreous, a neoplastic node evolves; this node develops a necrotic center when it reaches a diameter of 0.5 mm (Brem et al., 1976).

The mean distance of cells from their nearest blood vessel is greater for large tumors. Cells in mitosis are closer to blood vessels, but even with higher vascular density, necrosis is common. Intact blood vessels are often seen in areas of necrosis. When red blood cells are labeled with chromium-51, few of them appear in the blood vessels in necrotic regions, suggesting that necrosis and intravascular stasis are commonly associated. A cell's average distance from its nearest capillary is 100 μm for large tumors.

The diffusion length for any nutrient is the distance from an isolated blood vessel to the point where the nutrient's concentration falls to zero (Breur et al., 1966a). Gullino (personal communication, 1985) estimated that a spherical conglomerate of cells with a diameter of 300 to 400 μm would have trouble maintaining uniform cell survivorship if it were totally dependent on diffusion of oxygen and nutrients. Angiogenesis, therefore, becomes essential for the sustained growth of a cancer. With angiogenesis comes the avenue for metastasis.

Thus, cell loss accelerates as the tumor enlarges. The loss seems predetermined by the distance oxygen and other nutrients can diffuse through tissues. If the rate of diffusion cannot keep up with the demands of cell metabolism, central cell death occurs, and a decelerating influence on the net growth rate of the neoplasm is effected (Gullino et al., 1967).

MICROVASCULAR ANATOMY AND GROWTH RATES

The relationship between microvascular anatomy and breast cancer growth rates has been studied by a number of investigators. There are many complex intratumoral forces at work in determining growth (Peterson, 1991). The geometric relationship of replicating cancer cells to the vascular morphology of a cancer is an important determinant of both anatomy and growth. The vascular space constitutes from 1.0% to 12.4% of a tumor's mass and varies with tumor type. For murine mammary tumors, the proportion of vascular volume to viable tumor volume remains at a stable 17%. The volume of necrotic tumor increases progressively with increasing tumor mass. The average vessel diameter increases with tumor growth, while the length and surface area of vasculature per mm^3 of tumor decreases with growth. The interstitial water space varies from 30%–60% of the total tumor water. Interstitial fluid pressure in tumors tends to be greater than in normal tissue. The arterial pressure approximates that of normal tissue, but the venous pressure is low. These pressure gradients considered in combination with data from diffusion studies indicate a high vascular permeability within tumors. An intratumoral lymphatic system does not exist. The intratumoral blood vessels are all newly formed, and the growing tumor often destroys existing blood vessels. Frequent intercellular fenestrations in tumor capillaries have been observed. The heterogeneity of tumor vasculature is associated with variable intratumor oxygen tension. The growth of all tumors is angiogenesis-dependent. Viable tumor cells must remain close to these new vessels if they are to be sustained by diffused nutrients and oxygen. The vessels also serve as conduits for the dissemination of cancer cells through the vascular system.

The vascularity of a breast cancer correlates with both the growth rate and the propensity to metastasize. Weidner and colleagues (1991) concluded that the number of microvessels in invasive breast cancer fields correlate with the propensity to metastasize.

In a model using implantation of human breast cancer in nude mice, Kallinowski and coworkers (1989) observed a 10-fold variation in tumor perfusion, supporting the existence of a large variation in the degree of angiogenesis in small cancers. Furthermore, a ninefold variation in oxygen and a fourfold variation in glucose consumption were observed in the implants. However, blood flow was the major modulator of the consumption of oxygen and glucose. The authors concluded that high metabolic rates and high flow rates were associated with rapid growth rates.

The microvascular anatomy of breast carcinomas has features that are different from normal microvascular architecture. The differences in various parts of the same tumor are sufficiently great to affect the concentrations of delivered drugs and, thus, to influence the efficacy of treatment (Less et al., 1991).

HYPOXIC COMPARTMENT WITH INTRADUCTAL CARCINOMA AND RESISTANCE TO RADIATION

Seeking an explanation for the resistance of intraductal carcinoma to radiation, Mayr and associates (1991) con-ducted a morphometric study of intraductal carcinoma using computerized image analysis. Necrosis was found in 56% of the ducts that contained intraductal carcinoma. This necrosis was surrounded by a rim of viable tumor cells. Their observations support the hypothesis that a zone of hypoxic tumor cells exists adjacent to the zone of necrosis. Hypoxic cancer cells are more resistant to radiotherapy. If their conclusions are correct, then radiotherapy should be less effective for intraductal carcinomas that have central necrosis than for those that do not.

GEOMETRIC RELATIONSHIPS

The geometric relationships that occur as a cancer grows are defined by the following equation:

$$N = 2^n \qquad (4)$$

where N equals the number of cells, and n equals the number of net generations of cancer cells.

If the specific volume of a primary locus of cancer is known, the number of cells in the locus may be estimated crudely by dividing its volume by the approximate volume of a cell (10^{-6} mm^3). More concise estimates of N have been obtained in the laboratory.

Meyskens and colleagues (1984) provided an estimate of the number of cells that grew in tissue culture. The colonies grew into shapes, such as oblate spheroids. The relationship of cells to colony size fitted the following linear regression equation with a correlation coefficient of 0.92:

$$\ln \text{(number of cells per colony)} = \qquad (5)$$
$$0.87 - 2.80 \ln \text{(colony cells' axis)} +$$
$$2.38 \ln \text{(colony axis)}$$

This provided an accurate prediction of the total number of cells counted. Estimations of the total number of cells based on a spherical shape resulted in an overestimation of the number of cells.

Estimating the number of cells in a colony growing in vivo in humans cannot approach this accuracy. With the data available, we can only estimate orders of magnitude and use Equation 4. The method of Meyskens and colleagues lends itself to clonogenic assays of cells in tissue culture, but it can be applied only to cancer that is relatively free of noncancerous stroma.

Consistent with the foregoing observations, Heuser and coworkers (1979a,b) have shown that the xeromammographic dimensions of mammary cancer fit best those of a spheroid. In determining the tumor's volume, the geometric formula for calculating the volume of spheroids was used. For estimating the number of cells, the volume was divided by the volume of a single cell rounded off to 10^{-6} mm^3 (Heuser et al., 1979a).

For various colonies of cancer cells, the spread in the cell cycle time has been measured. The geometric mean of this spread is the value usually quoted as the actual spread. Cell cycle time, which is measured using tritiated thymidine to label DNA during its synthesis, gives a wealth of information about the cytokinetics of both normal and neoplastic tissues (Steel, 1972). Additional cytokinetic terms and their relations are as follows:

t_c = cell cycle time

t_s = duration of DNA synthesis of proliferating cells

LI or TLI = the labeling index. This is the ratio of the number of cancer cells that incorporated tritiated thymidine into DNA during the period of thymidine exposure to the total number of cancer cells. The ratio is expressed as the percentage of cells in the synthesis of DNA. LI = $\mu t_s/t_c$ for proliferating cells, when DT is more than 19 days and μ, the constant for the equation, is in the range of 0.7 to 0.8.)

DT_{pot} = potential DT, or the time required for the volume to double when cell loss is absent (i.e., when all dividing cells survive)

DT_{act} = actual DT, or the actual time required for a cancer to double its volume. (The DT_{act} represents the net effect of all cytokinetic parameters. Cell loss is a major and variable factor, and DT_{act} is of longer duration than DT_{pot}. DT_{act} frequently can be calculated from gross serial measurements of growing human cancer taken from radiographs or the direct measurement of tumor masses. A margin of error is always present in measuring growth rates, but if this margin stays relatively constant, its effect on calculated rates is minimal.)

If cell loss is the major variable, and if DT_{act} is of longer duration than DT_{pot}, then the relation between DT_{act} and DT_{pot} can be defined for a parameter of the rate of cell loss, ρ (rho). Cell loss is defined as a fraction of the rate at which cells enter mitosis. For a 100% loss of new cells, DT_{act} would be static. The relation is indicated by the following equation:

$$\rho = 1 - \frac{DT_{pot}}{DT_{act}} \tag{6}$$

If the approximate number of newly generated cancer cells per 1000 cells per day can be estimated from the tritiated thymidine labeling index, from the S-phase fraction from DNA analysis by flow cytometry, or from the mitotic index, DT_{pot} can be estimated. The above parameters have to be converted into the decimal form approximating the growth constant, b, a decimal representation of the number of dividing cells per thousand. This b can then be divided into the natural logarithm of 2 to estimate DT_{pot}. When this is done, the source of data for b should be specified. According to Hoffman (1949), at least 10 times as many cells are in the division cycle as exhibit mitotic figures requiring a decimal adjustment in b. With TLI and SPF verification of DNA synthesis, the number of cells in the synthesis phase may exceed Hoffman's estimate.

The inaccuracy of the approach lies in the variable capacity of flow cytometry to measure SPF. Heterogeneity in the cell population and the overlap of distributions in the populations confound the attainment of greater accuracy. The mathematical considerations for determining SPF have been well reviewed by Dean (1985). The utility of flow cytometric analysis should continue to improve in accuracy and clinical applicability.

Dressler (1992) addressed the importance of predicting the propensity of node-negative breast cancers to recur. Identifying those cancers that have a high probability of recurrence would permit selection of candidates for controlled clinical trials of adjuvant therapy. A great number of women would avoid adjuvant treatment with no potential benefit. Dressler considers the absence of national standards for DNA analysis by flow cytometry to be a limiting factor in the use of DNA flow cytometry to assay ploidy and proliferative capacity.

Much more accurate methods of estimating DT_{pot} exist but are not yet in clinical use. Shibamoto and Streffer (1991) reported on eight breast cancer cell lines and compared DT_{pot} calculations performed using flow cytometry after 5-bromodeoxyuridine and cytokinesis block macronucleus assay with actual tumor volume DTs for each line. The DT_{pot} yielded by the 5-bromodeoxyuridine method ranged from 0.8 ± 1 to 7.9 ± 3.3 days. With the cytokinesis block method, the range was from 0.9 ± 0.1 to 9.5 ± 1.9 days. Comparable actual tumor volume DTs ranged from 1.2 ± 0.1 days to 7.8 ± 1.2 days. These in vitro systems demonstrate just how short DT_{pot} can be.

Other methods for calculating DT_{pot} using Chinese hamster ovarian cells have been demonstrated by White and associates (1990). Their basic equation is as follows:

$$DT_{pot} = \ln 2 \frac{T_s}{V} \tag{7}$$

where T_s is the DNA synthesis time determined through the use of double labeling techniques using 5-bromodeoxyuridine and monoclonal antibodies against 5-bromodeoxyuridine. The letter V represents the fraction of labeled divided and labeled undivided cells. For Chinese hamster ovarian cells, White and associates reported a DT_{pot} ranging from 14.6 ± 2 hours to 20.2 ± 5.5 hours, depending on certain assumptions in their calculations.

SPF was observed to be an independent predictor of the duration of disease-free survival in cancers discovered in a mammographic screening trial. After first recurrence, the median survival was 31.3 months when the SPF was below 6%, and was 10.7 months when the SPF exceeded 10% (Hatschek et al., 1989).

The correlation of mammographically measured growth rates, the S-phase fraction, and histologic factors among breast cancers in a screened population has been reported by Arnerlov and colleagues (1992a). These authors calculated the DT_{act} of the tumor volume for 158 breast cancers detected by mammographic screening. The fastest growing cancer that they observed had a DT_{act} of 0.6 months, and 11 cancers showed no growth. The median DT_{act} was 9 months, and the mean was 10.9 months. For patients under the age of 50 years, the DT_{act} was shorter than the median in 70%; in older women, the DT_{act} was shorter in 48%. They observed a significant correlation between rapid growth rates and pathologic stage. They found no correlation between DT_{act} and the presence or absence of metastases in the axillary lymph nodes. Aneuploidy was increased in cancers with a short DT_{act}. However, all 11 cancers with extremely slow growth were aneuploid. Arnerlov and colleagues were able to determine the S-phase fraction for 122 of the cancers. They found a significant correlation between SPF and pathologic stage and tumor size. An SPF equal to or greater than 7.5% correlated weakly with the presence of axillary metastases and strongly with histologic grade and short DT_{act}. Seventy-four per cent of the cancers with an SPF greater than 7.5% were aneuploid, but only 23% of them with a lower SPF were aneuploid. Among cancers diagnosed by mammographic screening, a significantly greater representation of euploid cancers and a tendency toward long DT_{act} and low SPF were demonstrated when compared with interval and clinically detected cancers.

In a second study, Arnerlov and coworkers (1992*b*) reported the prognostic significance of the factors assayed in their previous study. They concluded that the S-phase fraction, stage, and lymph node status were prognostic for small and node-negative cancers. DNA ploidy and DT_{act} were less significant. They found no difference in survival when they compared women whose breast cancers were detected by screening with those whose cancers were discovered clinically. Cancers with a high SPF not only had faster growth rates but also possessed the potential to metastasize.

In a multivariate study of factors associated with prognosis, the presence of a DNA index of 2.1 and an SPF of less than 14% were associated with a more favorable prognosis (ρ = .0002) and were predictors independent of tumor size and the status of axillary lymph nodes (Joensuu et al., 1990).

Bosari and associates (1992) reported the prognostic significance of flow cytometric analysis of breast cancer for 158 women followed for a minimum of 9 years. They stratified their results into three groups according to prognosis. For small diploid ($\leq$ 2 cm with a low SPF) and small tetraploid tumors, the recurrence rate was only 12%. For aneuploid tumors with a low SPF, the recurrence rate was 21%. The highest recurrence rate (49%) was associated with cancers having a high SPF or with large tetraploid cancers.

Tabbane and colleagues (1989) observed that regardless of growth rate, the existence of inflammatory signs was associated with "frequent and precocious" metastases.

In a more general study, Tubiana and coworkers (1989) observed that through the 25th year of follow-up, the tumor growth and proliferation rates correlated with the probability of metastatic proliferation. Vollmer and associates (1989) reported an inverse relationship between the hormone receptor content of breast cancers and the growth fraction expressed as the percentage of breast cancer cells labeled with Ki − 67.

Williams and Daly (1990) provided the best available summary of this subject in the conclusions of a comprehensive review of the current literature. Aneuploid populations of cells have been observed in 52% to 92% of breast cancer specimens. Aneuploidy seems to be a predictor of shorter disease-free survival, and recurrence rates for aneuploid cancers are double those for cancers with no aneuploidy. In addition, aneuploid cancers tend to present with a greater number of positive lymph nodes than do those without aneuploidy.

The percentage of cancer cells in the SPF is of even greater predictive value. First, cancers with a high SPF are more likely to be aneuploid. Cancers with high steroid receptor values are more likely to be diploid and to have a lower SPF. The mean SPF for diploid tumors is 2.66%, whereas it is 6.12% for aneuploid cancers. Tritiated TLI and SPF tend to parallel one another, and a higher value for either is predictive of shorter disease-free survival. With increasing histologic grade, both the SPF and TLI tend to be increased. Diploid cancers are less likely to have metastases in the regional lymph nodes. The SPF value correlates less well with the presence or absence of lymph nodes positive for cancer. Estrogen receptor–negative cancers have significantly higher SPF values (mean 7.1%) than do estrogen receptor–positive tumors (mean = 3.8%). In comparing progesterone receptor–positive and progesterone receptor–negative cancers, there is no difference in SPF values. Obviously, these DNA flow cytometric characteristics, particularly the SPF, tend to correlate with the behaviors predicted for faster and slower growing cancers. The technology to use these cytokinetic parameters to assess the clinical behavior of individual breast cancers is now available.

The frequency distribution that best describes cytokinetic parameters, as well as other characteristics of cancers and their hosts, is the logarithm of the variate. Such a distribution occurs whenever the random errors of the variate are geometric or logarithmic rather than arithmetic or linear (i.e, a product rather than a sum of random events).

All standard statistical tests applicable to the more common arithmetic normal distribution can be applied (Spratt, 1969). The probability that a frequency distribution is, in fact, lognormal can be calculated by using the Kolmogovov-Smirnov test (Bradley, 1968). Various growth equations express the pattern of growth within a cancer. The pattern is determined by the complex and changing interactions of variables that affect the division and accumulation of cancer cells. Descriptions of the more commonly used growth equations follow.

Linear Growth Equation

A cancer that grows linearly has its dimensions increased by a specific daily linear increment regardless of its size. Examples include the Jensen's rat sarcoma (Mayneord, 1932) and some human lung cancers (Spratt and Spratt, 1976). This pattern occurs when all cellular proliferation is restricted to the periphery of the cancer. The equation is as follows:

$$R = \frac{d_1 - d_0}{t} \qquad (8)$$

where R = linear rate of change in the tumor's diameter, usually expressed as millimeters per day
d_0 = greatest chordal dimension; or, in the case of spherical tumors, the diameter at first observation
d_1 = greatest chordal dimension or diameter at second observation
t = time elapsing between the measurement of d_0 and of d_1

If the rate of a single growth vector or radius is desired, R must be divided by 2.

Exponential Growth Equation

A cancer that is growing exponentially or geometrically has a random, steady increase in volume. Any cell population whose number of cells increases owing to the random, steady, binary division of cells and that has negligible or at least steady-state cell loss would be described by the equations that follow:

$$V_1 = V_0 e^{bt} \text{ or } d_1^3 = d_0^3 e^{bt} \quad (9)$$

$$b = \frac{\ln V_1 - \ln V_0}{t} \text{ or } b = \frac{3(\ln d_1 - \ln d_0)}{t} \quad (10)$$

$$DT_{act} = \frac{\ln 2}{b} \quad (11)$$

where $\ln 2 = 0.69315$

V_0 = volume at first measurement, expressed in cubic millimeters (mm^3)

V_1 = volume at second measurement, expressed in cubic millimeters

d_0 = diameter at first measurement, expressed in millimeters

d_1 = diameter at second measurement, expressed in millimeters

t = time in days elapsing between the measurement of V_0 and V_1 or between the measurement of d_0 and d_1

b = exponential growth constant expressed in cubic millimeters per cubic millimeters per day (mm^3/mm^3 per day)

$\ln$ = a prefix indicating the natural logarithm of the variate

e = base of the natural logarithm, 2.71828.

By moving the decimal point of b three places to the right, the constant becomes a measure of the number of new cells per 1000 existing cells per day. When b is divided into the natural logarithm of 2 (0.69315), the DT_{act} is obtained in days. When more than two measurements exist, the growth equation is more accurately determined by the use of regression analysis.

Decelerating and Gompertz Growth Equations

Use of the Gompertz equation is one of many techniques for determining decelerating growth (Gompertz, 1825). Very few tissues can sustain exponential growth indefinitely, and deceleration of growth with increasing size becomes a necessity. Skehan (1984) concluded that decelerating growth must be a relatively universal phenomenon. The phenomenon expresses itself grossly by the gradual lengthening of tumor volume DT_{act} with increasing tumor size. Decelerating growth is the most frequent pattern exhibited by metazoa. All of the mechanisms that mediate or control such growth are not known; however, patterns of communication between cells are essential, even though they are incompletely understood. In addition to the Gompertz equation, decelerating growth in cancer systems has also been modeled by the inverse cube root (ratio of volume to surface area) and by logistic and simple power functions. The various growth models are given in Table 15–1.

The relationship between the specific growth rate (SGR) and DT_{act} can be determined in successive pairs of data points or size measurements, which are separated by an observation time, T_{obs}. Thus,

$$SGR = 100 \left[-1 + 2^{Tu(\ln[S2/S1])/(0.69315)T_{obs}} \right] \quad (12)$$

$$DT_{act} = 16.636/\ln(1 + 0.01 \, SGR) \quad (13)$$

where Tu is the unit of time (1 day). DT_{act} with this relationship is calculated in hours. Three growth phases are identified: accelerating (increasing SGR), exponential (constant SGR), and decelerating (decreasing SGR). Using data from the literature and Equations 12 and 13, Skehan ana-

Table 15–1. MATHEMATICAL MODELS OF CANCER GROWTH

Family of Equation	Value of Root (N)	Equations
1. Nth root	N = 1	$SGR = R(1 - S^N/K^N)$
2.	1/2	
3.	1/3	
4.	1/4	
5. Inverse Nth root	N = −1	$SGR = \theta(1 - K^{-N}S^N)$
6.	−1/2	
7.	−1/3	
8.	−1/4	
9. Nth power	N = 2	$SGR = R(1 - S^N/K^N)$
10.	3	
11.	4	
12. Inverse Nth power	N = −2	$SGR = \theta(1 - K^{-N}S^N)$
13.	−3	
14.	−4	
15. Gompertz		$SGR = G(\ln K - \ln S)$
16. Exponential decay		$SGR = Re^{-GS}$
17. Hyperbolic		$SGR^{1/2} = G(1 - (\ln S/\ln K))$
18. Simple power		$\ln SGR = \ln G - (1/b)\ln S$

(Adapted from Skehan, P.: *In* Skehan, P., and Friedman, S. J. (Eds.): Growth, Cancer, and the Cell Cycle. Clifton, NJ, Humana Press, 1984, p. 323.)

Abbreviations: SGR = Specific (to size) growth rate; R = SGR at infinitesimal size (single cell level); S = tumor size; θ = SGR at infinite size; K = final size attained by tumor; G,b = arbitrary rate coefficients.

lyzed 58 databases for normal tissue growth and 49 databases for neoplastic tissue growth. Table 15–2 gives a comparison of these analyses.

Cancer growth rates have significant chronologic implications for cancer behavior. Skehan's model (1984) considers the implications of growth rates for the growth rates of the tissue of origin and provides an explanation for the survival of mutant cells when cancers develop in metazoa. Also, Skehan (1984) observed that exponential growth is rarely observed in vivo. The pattern for normal tissue and for cancer is one of nonexponential kinetics in which growth decelerates continuously with time. This results in a progressive increase in the length of the DT_{act} with the passage of time and in an increase in tumor size. Growth-inhibiting negative feedback is predominantly responsible for this. Skehan used a variety of equations to describe the growth of normal and neoplastic tissue (see Table 15–2). He consistently observed that cancers do not grow faster than their tissues of origin and that organized tissue growth is required for the maintenance of phenotypic homogeneity in the cells of metazoa. When feedback controls and contact inhibition are lost, progressive phenotypic heterogeneity is tolerated and becomes a characteristic of a true cancer.

Furthermore, Skehan (1984) observed insignificant qualitative and quantitative differences between the growth of normal and neoplastic tissues (see Table 15–2). Meyer and Bauer (1976) provided evidence for the existence of nearly identical TLIs for both normal and cancerous breast tissue. Because the rates are basically the same, Skehan hypothesized that the error in cancer growth lies in the failure of the body to recognize and inhibit proliferation of cancer cells, not in the actual rates of proliferation. Replication rates of cells in cancerous and normal tissues are too similar for the nature of cancerous growth to be attributed to growth rates alone. Tumors behave like new types of tissue, with normal growth regulating parameters and control mechanisms, but, according to Skehan, they have an altered "recognitive determinant." Some cancers could even be a disorder of tissue neogenesis. Growth spurts come with the loss of decelerating feedback. Proponents of this theory consider that the contemporary use of antiproliferative drugs may be both valueless and counterproductive because of the similarity of growth rates of normal tissues and

cancers. These drugs generally fail to improve the prognosis of most solid neoplasms even though they are often effective for neoplasms of lymphatic and hematopoietic cell origin as well as for pediatric neoplasms, which have a larger percentage of cells undergoing division compared with populations of non-neoplastic cells of the same type.

By applying the various decelerating growth equations to various cancer growth data sets, Skehan found the best "fits" to occur with Equations 1, 2, and 13 in Table 15–1) (ρ = .560–.669). Equations 4 and 15 of Table 15–1 were second best in this regard. We selected Equation 15 of Table 15–1, the Gompertz equation, to evaluate the implications of decelerating growth for a breast cancer growth database. This equation is a specific decelerating growth rate formula. It is the exact solution to the following two differential equations:

$$\frac{dV}{dt} = \lambda V \tag{14}$$

$$\frac{d\lambda}{dt} = \alpha \lambda \tag{15}$$

Equation 14 states that tumor growth rate is the product of relative growth rate and volume. This is what is seen in exponential growth, where λ is constant. In the second equation, relative growth rate is time-dependent. The rate of decay of the relative growth rate (α) is a constant. Thus, the Gompertz growth equation is derived as follows:

$$V = V_0 e^{(1 - e^{act})\beta/\alpha} \tag{16}$$

The independent variables that describe a given curve are α and β. Comparative plots of Gompertz and exponential growth curves are shown in Figure 15–1. A cancer whose rate of growth is described by the Gompertz equation grows rapidly while small and more slowly as its size increases. The curve approaches a horizontal asymptote determined by a size ($V = V_{max}$ as $t \to \infty$) that it never exceeds. The curve shows a steady decrease in the tumor's actual growth rate as it approaches the asymptote. A nomogram showing the interrelationship of tumor volume and diameter, net number of cell generations, net or actual DT assuming a constant DT_{act}, and tumor duration is provided in Figure 15–2.

As the relative growth rate constantly decreases, the DT_{act} continuously increases. The DT equation can be solved as a function of time (Equation 17) or as a function of tumor size (Equation 18):

$$DT_{act} = \frac{-1}{\alpha}\left(1 - \frac{\alpha}{\beta}\ln 2e^{\alpha t}\right), \tag{17}$$

for $t < t_{1/2}$

$$DT_{act} = \frac{-1}{\alpha}\ln\left(1 - \frac{\ln 2}{\ln(V_{max}/V)}\right), \tag{18}$$

for $V < 1/2 V_{max}$.

DT_{act} has meaning only for a tumor that is smaller than one-half of its maximum size ($V < 1/2V_{max}$).

Table 15–2. COMPARISON OF THE GROWTH OF NORMAL AND NEOPLASTIC TISSUES

Characteristic	Tissue Growth	
	Normal	Neoplastic
Exclusively or predominantly decelerating	Yes	Yes
Deceleration related to mass inhibition	Yes	Yes
Most of growth inhibition or deceleration occurs while tissue of tumor mass still quite small	Yes	Yes
Inverse Nth root equations constitute the family of growth equations providing the best fit to observed data; Nth power equations provide the poorest fit	Yes	Yes

(Adapted from Skehan, P.: In Skehan, P., and Friedman, S. J. (Eds.): Growth, Cancer, and the Cell Cycle. Clifton, NJ, Humana Press, 1984, p. 323.)

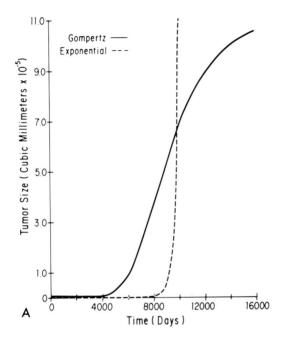

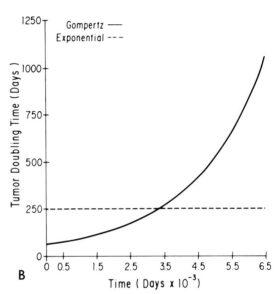

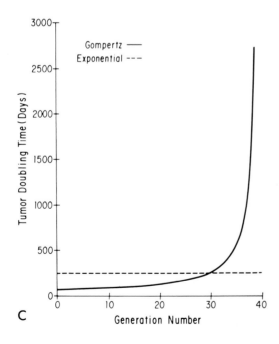

Figure 15–1. *A–C,* Graphic demonstration of the differences between exponential and Gompertzian growth with respect to tumor size and tumor duration *(A)*, actual tumor volume doubling time and tumor duration *(B)*, and actual tumor volume doubling time and the net number of tumor cell generation *(C)*. (From Spratt, J. A., von Fournier, D., Spratt, J. S., and Weber, E. E.: Decelerating growth and human breast cancer. Cancer, *71*:2013–2019, 1993*a.* Reprinted with permission.)

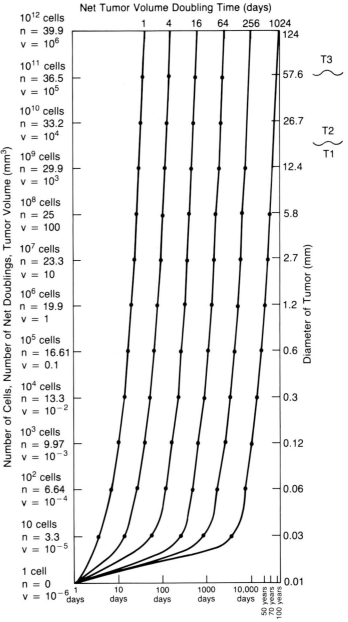

Net Tumor Volume Doubling Time (days)

Figure 5–2. A nomogram showing the interrelations of number of cancer cells, net number of generations of cancer cells, tumor volume, tumor diameter, time elapsing from the inception of a cancer, and the net actual tumor volume doubling time. (From Spratt, J. S., Greenberg, R. A., Heuser, L.: Geometry, growth rates, and duration of cancer and carcinoma in situ of the breast before detection by screening. Cancer Res., *46*:970, 1986. Reprinted by permission.)

Time Elapsing from Inception of One Cancer Cell (days)

The time necessary for a tumor to grow to one-half of its maximum size ($1/2V_{max}$) is calculated by using the following equation:

$$t_{1/2} = \frac{1}{\alpha} \ln\left(\frac{\beta}{\alpha \ln 2} \right) \qquad (19)$$

At the University of Heidelberg (Germany) and the University of Louisville (Kentucky), 448 patients underwent sequential mammography and demonstrated breast cancers on two or more mammograms, permitting the measurement of cancer sizes (Spratt et al., 1993a). A series of logistic equations that define decelerating growth was fitted to these data. The data used for the testing of "best fits" were known to be truncated for several reasons. In the study

population, no assessment of growth rates was possible in women with cancers that were observed only once, cancers that did not grow, cancers not visible on mammograms, and cancers appearing in the intervals between mammographic evaluations. Thus, the fits only apply to cancers that were observed to grow on successive mammograms. Great natural variability was observed. At least 10% of tumors grew to near lethal proportions within 1 year, whereas 11% of tumors had a less than 10% change in diameter by the end of the same period. Some cancers grew so slowly that they were considered to constitute no predictable threat to patient life (Tables 15–3 to 15–7). The maximum tumor size attainable (S_∞) was assumed to contain 2^{40} cells. The adult human body is composed of approximately $2^{40.8}$ cells.

DT_{act} as a function of tumor size can be expressed as follows:

Table 15–3. DOUBLING TIMES OF PRIMARY MAMMARY CANCERS OBSERVED BY MAMMOGRAPHY

Case Number	Observation Period (mo)	Diameter at Operation (cm)	Doubling Time (d)	Natural Log of Doubling Time
1	6	2.0	23	3.1355
2	6	3.0	36	3.5835
3	12	3.0	37	3.6109
4	12	2.5	49	3.8918
5	23	2.0	57	4.0431
6	16	1.2	63	4.1431
7	20	3.2	75	4.3175
8	12	1.0	90	4.4998
9	20	0.4	120	4.7875
10	6	1.0	120	4.7875
11	30	0.8	130	4.8675
12	12	1.8	144	4.9698
13	12	2.0	144	4.9698
14	21	0.8	160	5.0752
15	30	0.6	180	5.1930
16	18	1.0	180	5.1930
17	54	2.0	200	5.2983
18	16	1.0	205	5.3230
19	6	0.7	209	5.3423

(From Spratt, J. S., Kaltenbach, M. L., and Spratt, J. A.: Cytokinetic definition of acute and chronic breast cancer. Cancer Res., 37:226, 1977. Reprinted with permission.)

$$DT_{act} = -(1/bN)\{\ln[(S_\infty/2S)^n - 1] - \ln[(S_\infty/S)^n - 1]\}. \quad (20)$$

This curve has an inflection point at $S_\infty/(N+1)^{1/N}$. For decreasing positive values of N, the decelerating portion of a curve becomes more pronounced (see Fig. 15–1). Reciprocally, with increasing values of N, deceleration becomes less prominent. When N becomes very great, the exponential equation results. We let N range from 4 to 1/4. For N < 0, tumor growth is longer than the human lifespan. The resultant generalized logistic equation with the least standard error of the mean was as follows:

$$S = 1.1(10)^6 [1023e^{-1/4bt} + 1]^{-4} \quad (21)$$

The results of the least squares regression analysis for each growth model are provided in Table 15–8 and the resultant

growth curves calculated from the best-fitting model are shown in Figure 15–3 (Spratt et al., 1993a,b).

Irregular Growth

Irregular growth is not described by any specific rate formula. Different segments of the curve for a tumor with irregular growth may demonstrate varying growth patterns and growth rates. Such patterns and rates may occur with episodes of necrosis, slough, infection, spontaneous regression, regression under treatment, and unexplained accelerations and decelerations of growth. Random errors in measurement would contribute to some of the observed "irregularity."

Table 15–4. CHARACTERISTICS OF THE FREQUENCY DISTRIBUTION OF THE ACTUAL DOUBLING TIMES (DT$_{act}$) OF PRIMARY MAMMARY CANCERS, ASSUMING LOGNORMALITY AND LINEAR NORMALITY

Deviation	Logarithmic		Linear (d)
	Logarithm	*Days*	
+ 3σ	6.6011	736	304
+ 2σ	5.9276	375	242
+ 1σ	5.2541	191	179
μ	4.5806	98	117
− 1σ	3.9071	50	55
− 2σ	3.2336	25	
− 3σ	2.5601	13	

(From Spratt, J. S., Kaltenbach, M. L., and Spratt, J. A.: Cytokinetic definition of acute and chronic breast cancer. Cancer Res., 37:226, 1977. Reprinted with permission.)

Table 15–5. ACUTE AND CHRONIC SURVIVORSHIP IN DAYS AS CALCULATED FROM THE LOGNORMAL FREQUENCY DISTRIBUTION OF ACTUAL DOUBLING TIMES OF PRIMARY MAMMARY CANCERS

Probability of Surviving	Survivorship*
0.005 (+ 3σ)†	29,440
0.025 (+ 2σ)	15,000
0.158 (+ 1σ)	7640
0.500 (μ)	3920
0.842 (− 1σ)	2000
0.975 (− 2σ)	1000
0.995 (− 3σ)	520

(From Spratt, J. S., Kaltenbach, M. L., and Spratt, J. A.: Cytokinetic definition of acute and chronic breast cancer. Cancer Res., 37:226, 1977. Reprinted with permission.)

*These figures are calculated by multiplying the number of days in Table 15–4, column 3, by 40. Forty net doublings of a malignant clone of cells are estimated to produce a lethal mass of cancer cells. Thus, the time required to produce this lethal mass determines host survivorship.

†In parentheses μ = mean, σ = standard deviation about the mean.

Table 15–6. ACUTE AND CHRONIC SURVIVORSHIP IN DAYS AS CALCULATED FROM THE LINEAR NORMAL FREQUENCY DISTRIBUTION OF ACTUAL DOUBLING TIMES OF PRIMARY MAMMARY CANCERS

Probability of Surviving	Survivorship*
0.005 (+3σ)†	12,160
0.025 (+2σ)	9680
0.158 (+1σ)	7160
0.500 (μ)	4680
0.842 (−1σ)	2200
0.975 (−2σ)	
0.995 (−3σ)	

(From Spratt, J. S., Kaltenbach, M. L., and Spratt, J. A.: Cytokinetic definition of acute and chronic breast cancer. Cancer Res., *37*:226, 1977. Reprinted with permission.)

*These figures are calculated by multiplying the number of days in Table 15–4, column 4, by 40.

†In parentheses μ = mean, σ = standard deviation about the mean.

Data Sources

Basic data on the rates of growth of human mammary cancer have been obtained indirectly by radiography and from TLIs for human breast cancer in vivo or in vitro. Direct measurements of skin and lymph node metastases have been made with calipers. A collection of growth curves derived from the measurement of pulmonary metastases from mammary cancer is given in Figure 15–4 (Spratt and Spratt, 1964). These data were used to calculate the DT_{act} of the pulmonary metastases. The values for DT_{act} are plotted in Figure 15–5.

Data of this type generally form lognormal frequency distributions, but this cannot be shown unequivocally with the small sample sizes used in this instance. The data and the implications that they might have on host survivorship (assuming both normal and lognormal frequency distributions) are given in Tables 15–4 to 15–6 and Table 15–8. These estimates also assume constant exponential growth based on DTs determined after the cancers had become sufficiently large to be measured grossly. Since this approach does not allow for rapid early growth and deceleration with time and size, the estimates are considered high.

The thermal properties of growing neoplasms have also

Table 15–7. ESTIMATED NUMBER OF DAYS ELAPSING BETWEEN THE INCEPTION OF A CLONE OF MAMMARY CANCER CELLS AND THE SMALLEST SIZE DISCERNIBLE BY MAMMOGRAPHY (ABOUT 22 DOUBLINGS)

Doubling Times from Table 15–4, Column 3	Table 15–4, Column 3 × 22
736	16,192
375	8250
191	4202
98	2156
50	1100
25	550
13	286

(From Spratt, J. S., Kaltenbach, M. L., and Spratt, J. A.: Cytokinetic definition of acute and chronic breast cancer. Cancer Res., *37*:226, 1977. Reprinted with permission.)

Table 15–8. RESULTS OF LEAST SQUARES REGRESSION ANALYSIS FOR EACH TUMOR GROWTH MODEL

Order of Best Fit	Growth Model	Per Cent Increase in Total Mean Squared Error
1	GL (¼)*	—
2	GL (⅓)*	0.3
3	GL (½)*	2.7
4	GOM†	7.8
5	GL (1)†	10.8
6	GL (2)†	15.9
7	GL (3)†	16.4
8	GL (4)†	16.4
9	EXP†	16.5

(From Spratt, J. A., von Fournier, D., Spratt, J. S., and Weber, E. E.: Decelerating growth and human breast cancer. Cancer, *71*:2013–2019, 1993a.)

Abbreviations: GL (N) = generalized logistic equation for value N; GOM = Gompertz equation; EXP = exponential equation.

Models indicated by an asterisk (*) have significantly better fit than do those indicated by a dagger (†; P = .04). Differences in degree of fit within the two groups are not significant.

been used for measuring tumor growth indirectly (Chato, 1980; Eberhart et al., 1980; Gautherie, 1980; and Gullino, 1980). The theory of and observations made in the thermobiology of breast cancer as well as the differences between cancer tissue and normal tissue formed the basis for the promotion of thermography as a diagnostic tool. Methods also confirm that breast cancer cells have a greater sensitivity to heat than do normal tissue cells. The combination of the greater sensitivity of cancer cells to death from increased heat and the increase in temperature that occurs in a growing breast cancer provides one theoretical explanation for the high rate of cell death in growing cancer.

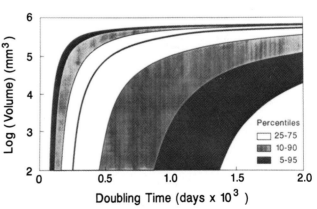

Figure 15–3. Tumor volume shown as a function of doubling time. The median value is represented by a *solid line*. Doubling time is seen to be relatively constant from 100 to 1000 mm³, after which it increases progressively. The shapes of the curves above 10⁴ mm³ were determined by extrapolation based on the model and the assumption of maximal tumor size. (From Spratt, J. A., von Fournier, D., Spratt, J. S., and Weber, E. E.: Mammographic assessment of human breast cancer growth and duration. Cancer, *71*:2020–2026, 1993b. Reprinted with permission.)

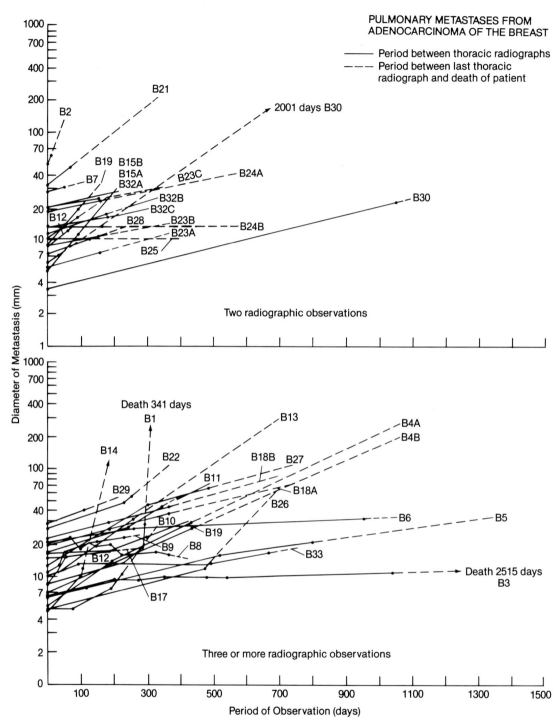

Figure 15–4. Each *dot* represents the measurement of the diameter of a specific pulmonary metastasis from a breast cancer. The *broken line* beyond the last dot records the time between the last chest radiograph and the death of the host. These curves are for the fastest growing pulmonary metastasis in 29 different hosts. The frequency distribution of the growth rates was lognormal. The log mean (or linear median) doubling time (actual) was 82 days with a 99% confidence range of 7 to 969 days. Equivalent exponential growth constant is 0.0085 with a 99% confidence range from 0.0007 to 0.099. Moving the decimal point of these constants three places to the right gives the number of new breast cancer cells surviving each day per 1000 existing breast cancer cells, as varying from less than one to as many as 99 new cancer cells per 1000 existing cells per day. (From Spratt, J. S., and Spratt, T. L.: Rates of growth of pulmonary metastases and host survival. Ann. Surg., *159*:161, 1964. Reprinted with permission.)

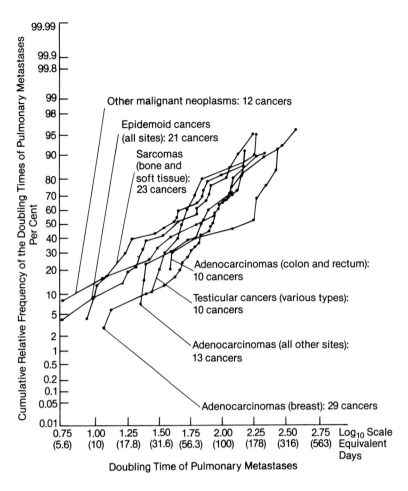

Figure 15–5. Accumulative relative frequency of the doubling times of pulmonary metastases from cancer of various sites, showing the comparative plot for metastatic adenocarcinoma of the breast. (From Spratt, J. S., and Spratt, T. L.: Rates of growth of pulmonary metastases and host survival. Ann. Surg., *159*:161, 1964. Reprinted with permission.)

Other malignant neoplasms: 12 cancers

Epidemoid cancers (all sites): 21 cancers

Sarcomas (bone and soft tissue): 23 cancers

Adenocarcinomas (colon and rectum): 10 cancers

Testicular cancers (various types): 10 cancers

Adenocarcinomas (all other sites): 13 cancers

Adenocarcinomas (breast): 29 cancers

Cumulative Relative Frequency of the Doubling Times of Pulmonary Metastases Per Cent

Doubling Time of Pulmonary Metastases

Log₁₀ Scale Equivalent Days

Observations of Actual Doubling Times

The first gross measurements of the rates of growth of primary human breast cancers were provided by Gershon-Cohen and coworkers (1963). They studied 18 patients who had not undergone biopsy until two or more mammographic procedures had been performed. Gross DTs were calculated. One case from the Cancer Research Center at Ellis Fischel State Cancer Hospital was added (see Tables 15–3 to 15–7). The median DT observed for 19 cases was 120 days; however, the range was from 23 to 209 days (Spratt et al., 1977). Von Fournier and associates (1980) studied DTs of 147 patients with primary breast cancers who were examined using serial mammography. Although unable to correlate the histologic characteristics of breast cancers with DTs as measured by serial mammography, they did note that thermographic changes were more likely to be abnormal in quickly growing breast cancers. Their measurements were based on multiple mammograms obtained from the examination of 163 women. The longest period of observation of a single neoplasm was 11 years; the cancer did not increase in size during this period. The accuracy of their measurements varied by ±0.6 mm. The smallest cancer was 2 mm in diameter. They observed considerable variation with respect to tumor size, growth deceleration, regression, and nongrowth.

By 1982, the database of von Fournier and associates contained measurements and the dates of measurement for tumor nucleus shadows observed on mammograms for each of 202 patients. Data on 32 patients from the Breast Cancer Detection and Demonstration Project–Louisville (BCDDP-L) were added. These data were evaluated assuming the existence of exponential, decelerating, and Gompertzian growth patterns.

Tumor size measurements were made in three dimensions. Volume was calculated as an ellipsoid. Exponential DTs were calculated by performing a linear regression analysis between ln V and the times between the various observations. The slope of this relationship is the relative growth rate.

DT_{act} is the natural logarithm of 2 divided by the relative growth rate and is constant with exponential growth. The distribution of the DTs was assessed with the Kolmogorov-Smirnov test (Bradley, 1968). The distribution was lognormal with a log mean of 5.53 ± 0.81 days (which corresponds to 252 days).

To plot the curves demonstrating decelerating growth and the special case of Gompertzian growth, it was assumed that (1) each cancer originated as one cell (2^0) (Gould et al., 1978) and that (2) the maximum size attainable was 2^{40} cells ($V_{max} = 2^{40}$). The usual lethal tumor mass is roughly 10^{12} cells or 40 net cellular generations (2^{40}). The total body cell composition of an adult is about 10^{13} cells, or $2^{40.8}$ cells. A lethal number of breast cancer cells would have a total body distribution equivalent to 10% of all of the cells in the host. Our measurements, unfortunately, are only of the tumor nucleus shadows seen on mammograms and, predictably, represent a decreasing smaller percentage of the total body mass composed of cancer cells. By specifying 2^{40} to equal V_{max}, it can be shown that

$$\alpha = \beta/(40 \ln 2) \qquad (22)$$

Hence, the Gompertz equation becomes

$$V = V_0 e^{(1 - e^{-\alpha t})40 \ln 2} \qquad (23)$$

The DT formula in Equations 16 and 17 can be simplified by substituting Equation 19. In addition, DT could then be expressed as a function of the net generation number:

$$DT_{act} = \frac{-1}{\alpha} \ln \left(1 - \frac{1}{40 - n} \right) \qquad (24)$$

where n is the net generation number.

The Gompertz equation can be converted into linear form by taking the logarithm of each side of Equation 16 twice. This resultant equation is as follows:

$$\ln \ln (V_{max}/V) = -\alpha t + \ln(\beta/\alpha) \qquad (25)$$

From our assumptions, β/α and V_{max} are known. Thus, the resultant equation is the relationship between tumor size and time where $-\alpha$ is the slope of the relationship. A standard regression analysis on $\ln[\ln (V_{max}/V)]$ versus time between observations was calculated for each patient studied.

Using the Kolmogorov-Smirnov test, the distribution of α's was examined. Although the distribution closely approximated a lognormal distribution, the test was significant because of kurtosis and a slight skew to the right. The mean was -7.813 ± 0.844 day^{-1}. The antilog of this number, the geometric mean of α, was $4.034 (10)^{-4}$ day^{-1}.

With Gompertzian growth, tumor DT_{act} is a function of tumor size. To compare sojourn time and DT_{act} when assuming Gompertzian or exponential growth, the parameters must be specified. For example, DT_{act} could be compared with the size of a tumor when the tumor is first detected. The mean diameter of the first mammographic tumor shadow detected in our study was 8.7 mm. This corresponds to a volume of 345 mm^3, which is the 28th net cellular generation of the tumor. It should be emphasized that most tumors in this study were first detected when they were of a larger size and that they were only verified to be present at the 345-mm^3 size retrospectively. A graph of the mean tumor growth for all patients, assuming both exponential and Gompertzian growth, is shown in Figure 15–1A. With Gompertzian growth, the cancer's growth rate progressively decreases as tumor size increases. The exponential growth curve shows tumor size to be very small until a sojourn time of approximately 8000 days is reached. The tumor then undergoes a rapid increase in size for the next 2000 days. DT_{act} is plotted as a function of sojourn time in Figure 15–1B. With exponential growth, mean DT

was constant at 252 days. Assuming Gompertzian growth, however, the mean DT_{act} for the first cellular division was 62 days. DT_{act} slowed to approximately 231 days at the time the tumors were discovered; it then slowed even more to a mean of over 1000 days by the 6500th day of growth.

This same effect is illustrated in Figure 15–1C, in which DT_{act} is plotted as a function of generation number. Exponential DT_{act} is constant, regardless of generation number. Gompertzian growth begins with a DT_{act} of 62 days for the first generation but approaches infinity at the 39th generation, the last generation for which DT_{act} has significance.

Tissue culture and thymidine labeling studies have shown that the initial DT_{pot} of mammary cancer cells ranges from 12 to 48 hours (Tseng, 1986). Tumors approximately 1 cm^3 in size double by a mean of 261 days. Many large tumors have no demonstrable growth, indicating a further prolongation of the DT_{act}. Although exponential growth curves can be fitted accurately to some data in the range of clinical observation, they cannot be used to describe the rapid growth rates of smaller tumors. Gompertzian or other decelerating growth curves may be fitted to available data to reflect more accurately a tumor's growth throughout its entire lifespan.

An important result of this type of analysis is estimating the sojourn time of a tumor from one cell through its clinically detectable size. Assuming Gompertzian growth, the mean sojourn time from one cancer cell to the development of a tumor mass 1 cm^3 in size was 3428 days (with 95% confidence intervals of 633 days to 18,569 days).

Other decelerating growth rate formulas suggested by Skehan (see Table 15–1) may allow more accurate mathematical modeling of breast cancer growth. Growth rates calculated from the measurements of tumor nucleus shadows on mammograms would be expected to be lower than the actual rates of increase in total body tumor burdens if cells are being shed rapidly from cancers to incite metastatic growth elsewhere.

Von Fournier and associates (1980) reported a mean DT_{act} of 311 days. Their data, which were composed of measurements of mammographically visible cancers, formed a *lognormal* frequency distribution of DT_{act} with a coefficient of correlation of 0.8899. The coefficient of correlation for a *linear* frequency distribution of these authors' data was 0.4763. Mammography was repeated annually for the patients whose tumor growth was measured. This bias results in a significant truncation of the growth rate measurements owing to the exclusion of very rapidly developing cancers; this can be assessed by considering the frequency with which cancers are diagnosed within the interval between annual mammographic examinations. A population-based study is required to quantify this bias by identifying all cancers that are diagnosed during the intervals between annual mammographic examinations.

INTERVAL CANCERS

Panoussopoulas and associates (1977) reported the interval cancer discovery rates of one of the BCDDPs. The percentage of cancers diagnosed *between* annual mammographic examinations was 29% of all cancers diagnosed (24 of 89).

Monitoring rates at which breast cancers were discovered between annual mammographic examinations were essential for evaluating the value of mammography and for estimating the potential truncation of the frequency distribution of mammographically measured growth rates by identifying the percentage of very rapidly appearing cancers (Spratt, J. S., in the discussion of Panoussopoulas et al., 1977). As an extension of this observation, data were later provided by Spratt and coworkers (1983) on "acute carcinoma of the breast." More acute cancers, or "fast"-growing carcinomas, were associated with a greater anaplastic nuclear grade, the absence of mammographically and microscopically identifiable calcifications in tumors, a patient age of less than 50 years, mammographically dysplastic breasts, the absence of a family history of breast cancer, and a poorer prognosis when they were compared with slowly growing cancers. Significantly, more slowly growing cancers were associated with a circumscribed tumor margin and a papillary growth pattern. In this same population, the absence of calcifications and the presence of lymphatic invasion around the periphery of the primary cancer were associated with the early development of metastases in the axillary lymph nodes (Heuser et al., 1984).

The potential truncation of the DT_{act} data, which originates from the exclusion of the rates of acute, rapidly growing interval cancers, can be estimated in several ways. Dividing 365 days by the lethal number of net doublings (about 40) yields a value of 9. Any breast cancer with a net DT_{act} of less than 9 days could arise de novo and kill the host during the interval between annual mammographic examinations. If this estimate is recalculated from the threshold of mammographic detection (i.e., a range of about 2 mm, or 20 to 22 doublings), 365 could be divided by 20 (40 minus 20), giving 18 days. Any breast cancer that could sustain a net DT_{act} of 18 days or less could grow from the threshold of mammographic detectability to cause death of its host in less than 365 days. If the majority of breast cancers were characterized by Gompertzian or decelerating growth in their predetectable period, the truncation problem would be even more serious. Not only can accurate reporting of breast cancer development rates *between* annual mammographic examinations help in the evaluation of the degree of truncation, but careful follow-up of interval cancer cases can also confirm whether faster growing cancers are more rapidly lethal as well. Eventually, it will be possible to determine to what degree mammographic screening produces a reduction in the lethality of mammary cancer or simply divides breast cancers into subsets of fast-growing and slow-growing carcinomas.

The BCDDP-L study provided an opportunity to define the entire frequency distribution of actual growth rates for primary mammary cancers. This distribution falls into three subsets. The first consists of cancers growing too rapidly to permit measurement by annual mammography; these include the interval surfacing cancers and at least some of the cancers observed only once. The second subset comprises cancers for which two or more annual mammographic observations permitted measurement of growth and calculation of growth rates. The third subset includes very slowly growing cancers for which no measurement of growth could be made on mammographic observations conducted at intervals of 1 year or greater in duration.

During the BCDDP-L study (Heuser et al., 1979*a,b*), 115 cancers were identified among 10,128 women who collectively received more than 30,000 mammograms over a 4-year period of annual screening. When the pathologic material was reviewed by a panel of national experts appointed for a quality control check on pathologic diagnoses, the University of Louisville had the lowest exception rate in the country (among the 27 centers), giving the pathologic diagnoses a high degree of reliability. Serial measurements were possible with xeromammography in 32 patients. DT_{act}s ranged from 109 to 944 days, with a median value of 324 days. The log mean DT_{act} was 327 days. The predominant geometric shape of small primary breast cancers was a spheroid, with the long axis following the direction of the ducts. The frequency distribution of the DT_{act}s of these spheroids was lognormal.

Of these tumors, 43% (49 of 115) were interval cancers. Nine of the 115 (7.8%) or 9 of the 32 cancers measured serially (28%) had cancers growing too slowly to permit measurement of growth. Incidence in interval cancers increased from 6.4% to 23.9% over the first 3 years of the project and dropped to 14.4% in the fourth year, when women who were younger than 50 years of age were excluded.

Galante (1986) summarized his continuing clinical characterization of breast cancers with different DT_{act}s (Tables 15–9 and 15–10). He established some clear associations among DT_{act}, histopathologic cancer characteristics, nodal metastases, anatomic foci of metastases, and multicentricity. His data show that cancers with the shortest DT_{act}s had more tumor necrosis, more frequent multicentricity, more

Table 15–9. CHARACTERISTICS OF THE DIFFERENT GROUPS OF GROWTH FOR CANCER OF THE BREAST— EXPERIENCE WITH 193 CASES

Fast (16%): DT_{act} 1 to 30 days	
Highest percentage of necrosis (48.4%)	NS
Highest percentage of multicentricity (50%)	$P = .02$
Lowest percentage of estrogen receptor positivity (44.4%)	$P = .007$
Highest percentage of second tumor (16%)	$P = .03$
Intermediate (42%): DT_{act} 30.1 to 90	
High rate of ductal carcinomas (46%)	$P = .009$
Highest percentage of PLI (48.9%)	NS
Highest percentage of positive nodes (70%)	$P = .01$
Highest percentage of LI values	Mean, 7.6
High percentage of metastases to soft tissues (62.5%)	NS
Slow (17.6%): DT_{act} 90.1 d to $< \infty$	
Low percentage of necrosis (38.2%)	NS
High percentage of estrogen receptor positivity (77.8%)	$P = .007$
Very Slow (24.4%): DT_{act} ∞	
High percentage of mixed forms (43.2%)	$P = .09$
Lowest percentage of necrosis (36.2%)	NS
Lowest percentage of PLI (25%)	NS
Lowest percentage of multicentricity (8.7%)	$P = .02$
Highest percentage of estrogen receptor positivity (95%)	$P = .007$
Lowest LI values	Mean 2.3
Lowest percentage of second tumor (2%)	$P = .03$

(Courtesy of E. Galante, Milan, Italy, 1986.)
Abbreviations: PLI = Peritumoral lymphatic infiltration; LI = labeling index; ∞ = infinity; NS = not significant.

Table 15–10. RELATIONSHIP BETWEEN HISTOLOGIC TYPE OF BREAST CANCER AND THE DOUBLING TIME

	Infiltrative Duct	Mixed Ductal	Lobular	Others	Mixed	Total
Fast	10	10	3	5	3	31
Intermediate	44	19	1	3	14	81
Slow	17	9	3	1	4	34
Very Slow	16	12	2	1	16	47
Total	87	50	9	10	37	193

(Courtesy of E. Galante, Milan, Italy, 1986.)
$P = .009$

frequent peritumoral lymphatic invasion, higher labeling indices, lower estrogen receptor assay values, more frequent nodal metastases, and more frequent soft tissue metastases than did cancers with longer DT_{act}s. The data generally parallel many of Meyer's conclusions, which are summarized in Chapter 13.

In summary, a very large percentage of all breast cancers are characterized by exceedingly rapid growth in their early or predetectable stages, and annual mammography has primarily subdivided breast cancers into subsets of quickly growing and slowly growing tumors. Quickly growing cancers are much more likely to metastasize. These observations have numerous implications on the natural history of early breast cancer and on the development of mathematical models for the detection of tumors and for the evaluation of treatment. The BCDDP-L data provide the first report of a full spectrum of growth rates in a defined population of women whose ages range from 35 to 70 years (Heuser et al., 1979a,b).

Intensified, effective training in breast self-examination (BSE) at monthly intervals may be the only cost-effective method for earlier detection of interval cancers. However, the cancers discovered by BSE are relatively large. After correcting for lead time bias, the question that needs to be answered by the results of a controlled trial is, "Will the earlier self-discovery of palpable cancers by BSE lead to a higher percentage of nondisseminated cancers that are curable by local-regional treatment?" Threshold size for discovery varies with the screening method and with the contrast between cancer-containing and non–cancer-containing breasts.

Thoracic Radiographs

Coincident with the report by Gershon-Cohen and coworkers (1963) on mammographically measured DT_{act} were studies done at the Ellis Fischel State Cancer Hospital (Spratt et al., 1962, 1963; Spratt and Spratt, 1964; and Spratt, 1969). The data from these studies consisted of two or more thoracic radiographs for each of 21 patients who had 22 primary lung cancers and for 176 patients who had various types of cancer metastatic to the lung. The sizes of the metastases were lognormally distributed, and the limits on observed size were determined by the threshold of radiographic resolution and by lethal size. Initially, no tumor was diagnosed by the radiologist if it was 3 mm in diameter or smaller. Generally, diagnosis was not established until tumors achieved a diameter of 6 mm. This is equivalent to

26.7 doublings of a 1000-μm^3 cell. A tumor 200 mm in diameter, equivalent to 40.8 doublings, was uniformly lethal. Thus, the segment of the growth curve amenable to gross measurement was determined by the terminal 14 doublings in the life of the cancers ($40.8 - 26.7 = 14.1$).

The growth of pulmonary metastases from breast cancer were studied in 29 patients (Spratt and Spratt, 1964). The distribution of growth rates was lognormal, with a geometric mean of 83 days and with 95% confidence limits of 16 to 426 days. The number of cells dividing each day was estimated to be small compared with the total number of cells in a tumor mass. Growth curves for these 29 different breast cancers are shown in Figure 15–4. Growth rates were compared for all types of tumors. In this study, sex, age, and tumor type did not affect the growth rate of primary pulmonary cancers or of metastases developing in the lungs. Exceptions were bone and soft tissue sarcomas, testicular and epidermoid carcinomas, and cancers in patients younger than 29 years of age. These tumors grew significantly more quickly than did cancers in other categories. A comparison of the frequency distribution of the DT_{act}s of pulmonary metastases from breast cancer with those of metastases from other sites is shown in Figure 15–5.

Breur (1966a,b) reported the DT_{act}s of six mammary cancers metastatic to the lung in patients who were between 52 and 71 years of age. DTs ranged from 23 to 745 days. With the administration of sublethal doses of radiation, regrowth started immediately after the last fractionated treatment. Breur used the rate of cancer regression that occurred with the fractionated treatments to estimate the dose needed to eradicate specific tumors. The same approach could be applied to estimate the tumoricidal dose of a chemotherapeutic agent that is needed to produce varying percentages of tumor cell destruction based on observed regression with fractional doses.

Cutaneous Metastases

Phillipe and Le Gal (1968) reported on the growth rates of cutaneous nodules of mammary cancer that recurred after mastectomy. They reported an order of magnitude of growth rates similar to that calculated from radiographic measurements of pulmonary metastases. For 78 nodules, the average gross DT was 40 days, varying from 3 to 211 days.

Pearlman (1976) calculated the DT of breast cancers recurrent in mastectomy scars for 82 patients (Figs. 15–6 and 15–7). The scar recurrences observed by Pearlman and

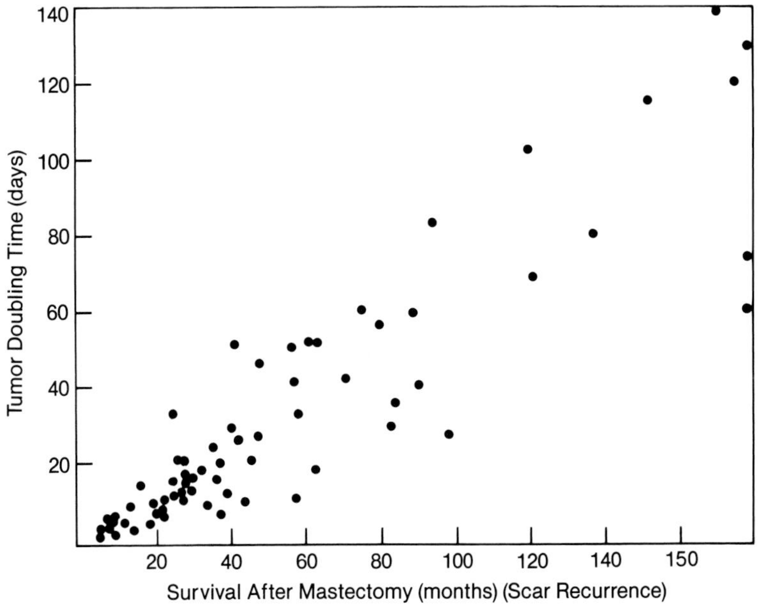

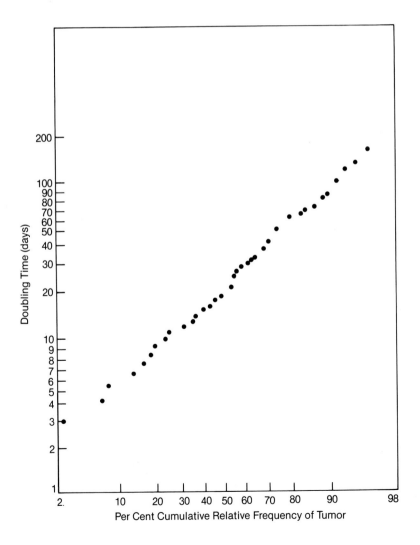

Figure 15–6. In this scattergram, survival in months after mastectomy has been correlated with the tumor growth rate in 67 patients with a mastectomy scar recurrence. An approximately linear relationship exists between doubling time and longevity. The distribution becomes scattered especially in the range of the longer doubling times. (From Pearlman, A. W.: Breast cancer—influence of growth rate on prognosis and treatment evaluation. Cancer, *38*:1826, 1976. Reprinted with permission.)

Figure 15–7. Cumulative relative frequency of the actual tumor volume doubling time for pulmonary metastases from breast cancers. (From Pearlman, A. W.: Breast cancer—influence of growth rate on prognosis and treatment evaluation. Cancer, *38*:1826, 1976. Reprinted with permission.)

by Phillipe and Le Gal had greater growth rates than did primary cancers observed on mammography. Pearlman concluded that the 5-year survival rate would not be a meaningful parameter for such extreme variances in tumor growth rates and in survivorship. The same can be said for any fixed-endpoint survival rates for cancer patients.

Peer and associates (1993) reviewed the literature on mammographically measured growth rates and reported that the geometric mean of the DT_{act} for women under 50 years of age was 80 days (95% confidence interval with a range from 44 to 147 days), for women between 50 and 70 years of age was 157 days (95% confidence interval with a range from 121 to 204 days) and for women older than 70 years of age was 188 days (95% confidence interval with a range from 120 to 295 days). Their data are truncated by the absence of growth rate data on cancers observed only once, on interval cancers, on nongrowing cancers, and on cancers not visible on mammograms. With faster DT_{act}s seen in young patients, they speculated on the possible value of more frequent mammographic examinations in the young. They did consider the value of the threshold size for breast cancers potentially diagnosable through the use of mammography. In a breast of low density, the threshold was 5 mm.

Multiple Sites

Kusama and colleagues (1972) compared the median actual DTs of metastatic breast cancers at various sites. They also considered the association between the DT_{act}s and various characteristics in the population from which the data were derived. In each group, the frequency distribution of DT_{act}s for a population of cancer patients was lognormal. The median DT_{act}, which was longest for primary cancers, was progressively shorter for pulmonary metastases, metastases in lymph nodes, and local metastases. The DT_{act}s were shorter for patients under the age of 30 years and longer for those over the age of 60 years. DT_{act}s were no different among married and single women, parous and nulliparous women, and whites and blacks. No relationship could be established between DT_{act} and the presence or absence of axillary metastases. With the exception that tumors with DT_{act}s greater than 8 months recurred infrequently, no relationship could be established between the probability of recurrence and DT_{act}. Cancers with 8-month DT_{act}s might take more than 15 years to produce a grossly visible neoplastic mass. Survival time was more favorable in patients with slowly growing cancers.

In a study of the Ellis Fischel State Cancer Hospital data, the gross growth rates of 171 soft tissue metastases have been reported (Lee, 1970, 1972; and Lee and Spratt, 1972). The frequency distribution of observed growth rates was lognormal. Sixty-six metastases were measured in patients who were not treated with systemic therapy; the DT_{act} was 17.1 days (geometric mean), with a 95% confidence range of 3.4 to 86.1 days. For cancers treated subsequently, the ratios of the tumor shrinkage rates after therapy to the growth rates before therapy had means of approximately 1 but varied from 0.2 to 4.2 (with 95% confidence).

Indirectly Measured Doubling Times

DTs estimated indirectly are related to DT_{act}s in an expected order of magnitude. Malaise and coworkers (1973) described the application of DNA labeling to human solid tumors, and reviewed data available from the literature. In most cases, cell division was measured by assessing the need for thymidine in DNA production and mindful of the fact that DNA is manufactured by the cell only during the active S-phase of cell division. By tagging thymidine with tritium, cell nuclei that incorporate thymidine during DNA synthesis can be recognized owing to the radioactive emission of the tritium. Thus, tritiated thymidine, which is either given to a patient with cancer or included in the nutrient media into which viable cancer tissue specimens are placed, permits the measurement of the percentage of cells in the DNA synthesis phase of the cell cycle, and hence the tritiated TLI. The distribution of TLIs for cancers with histologic characteristics in common tends to be lognormal or to follow other skewed frequency distributions. The labeling indices of groups of proliferative cells are proportional to the duration of DNA synthesis and to the cell cycle time. The TLI data can be used to estimate the *potential* DT of a tumor cell population as noted earlier in this chapter. Applying such considerations to laboratory data, Steel (1967) concluded that the duration of DNA synthesis in human tumors is not much greater than 15 hours and that the cell loss from many human cancers may exceed 50%.

Seventy-five breast cancers were found among the 121 patients with adenocarcinoma reported by Malaise and coworkers (1973). The DT_{act} was 83 days, but the DT_{pot}, based on labeling data, was about 23.8 days.

Meyer and Bauer (1976) reported the TLI obtained with in vitro pulse labeling. The TLI of terminal breast ducts without neoplasm was significantly greater during the second half of the menstrual cycle than during the first half, with a geometric mean of 1.5. This is equivalent to a 47% turnover of duct cells during a menstrual cycle. Fibroadenomas showed a similar menstrual variation of TLI. The TLI range for cancers was from 0.04 to 18.6. The arithmetic mean was 3.7, and the geometric mean was 2.1. TLIs tended to be greater in women younger than 50 years of age ($\rho > .05$) than in older women and also when two or more axillary lymph nodes contained metastases.

CLINICAL DATA, AND THE INDIRECT ASSESSMENT OF GROWTH RATES

The application of an indirect method for assessing breast cancer growth rates that relies on the clinical histories of patients was emphasized by Charlson and Feinstein (1984). These investigators reconstructed entire chronologies of patients' cancers, including data regarding the history, physical examination, initial treatment, tumor histology, nodal involvement, and follow-up events as well as data pertaining to additional treatments. The cancers were classified according to the tumor-node-metastasis (TNM) system. The index of cancer progression was developed for 219 women and validated for 465 additional women. By using the Cox proportional hazard model (Cox, 1972), they created prog-

Table 15–11. ASSOCIATION OF LYMPH NODE METASTASES WITH PRIMARY CANCERS 10 MM IN DIAMETER OR LESS AS CONFIRMED BY CLEARING STUDIES AND STEP SECTIONS

Greatest Chordal Dimension of Primary Cancer (mm)	Number of Cancers	Number with Metastasis
10	5	1
9	1	1
8	7	2†
7	1	0
5	2	0
4	1	0
0*	2	0
Total	19	4

(From Pickren, J. W.: Significance of occult metastases: A study of breast cancer. Cancer, *14*:1266, 1961. Reprinted with permission.)

*The cancers listed as "0" mm were microscopic in size and not recognized as gross nodules.

†The two cancers 8 mm in diameter with metastases had respectively 1 and 11 axillary nodes containing metastatic cancer.

nostic distinctions within staging groups by relying on anatomic size and extent of tumors and on the presence or absence of nodal metastases. Using a qualitative method for comparing rates of cancer progression before treatment, they showed that the indices had a prognostic validity "independent of anatomic stage, nodal status, type of treatment, and other variable." Boyd and coworkers (1981) confirmed the validity of their indices. They divided cancers into categories for "slow," "intermediate," and "rapid" growth. These divisions must be regarded as arbitrary, as extant data consistently exhibit a continual spectrum of growth rates that are distributed lognormally (Spratt, 1969). This spectral phenomenon results in an overlap of the characteristics of arbitrary subdivisions. However, even with overlap, the concepts are useful in appreciating the importance of growth rate with respect to prognosis. A cancer of long pretreatment duration may have a better prognosis than a cancer with a short pretreatment duration. Even in screening, this phenomenon occurs with the acute cancers that are self-detected by patients during the intervals between annual examinations (Spratt et al., 1983).

Indirectly, growth rates may be expressed as rate of progression in evaluating survival, as noted by Pearlman and Jochimsen (1979). These authors studied 464 patients with recurrent breast cancer and used a convention of the R_1-R_2 intervals to compare different subsets of cases. The *R_1-R_2 interval* is defined as the period of time elapsing between the diagnosis and treatment of the first recurrence (R_1) and the appearance of a second recurrence (R_2). For Pearlman and Jochimsen, the most important determinants were the anatomic site of the first recurrence and the tumor progression rate as quantified by the R_1-R_2 interval. Type of treatment had less influence on survival than these other factors. The median survival from R_1 was 22 to 26 months for bone or soft tissue recurrences; 10 to 12 months for involvement of the pleura or lung, or both; and 4 to 6 months for hepatic or intracranial metastases, or both. Patients with longer R_1-R_2 intervals had better survival times than did patients with shorter intervals for each anatomic site. Long R_1-R_2 inter-

vals were present in about 50% of patients with bony or soft tissue metastases. For patients with long R_1-R_2 intervals, survival was independent of the treatment method. Long R_1-R_2 intervals were present in only 16% to 20% of the patients with visceral metastases who had undergone only local-regional treatment and in 37% to 38% of those who received systemic therapy. Survivorship was similar for patients who received local treatment and for those who received systemic treatment. Of those with visceral metastases, systemic treatment yielded superior results. Pearlman and Jochimsen concluded that knowledge of the anatomic site of first recurrence combined with the R_1-R_2 interval provided a way of relating prognosis to the rate of metastatic tumor progression for metastases at different loci.

Potential Relation Between the Size and Duration of Primary Mammary Cancers and the Development of Metastases

Several approaches have been used to estimate how small a breast cancer is when it begins to metastasize. From clearing studies of axillary contents removed at mastectomy, Pickren (1961) identified all nodes in the axilla and step-sectioned each. Of the 200 patients in his series, 19 had a primary breast cancer that was 10 mm in size or smaller. The smallest cancer with axillary metastases was 8 mm in size. Of the 2 patients whose cancers were 8 mm in diameter and who had metastases, 1 had 11 lymph nodes positive for the disease (Table 15–11). The selection of these cases would introduce length-biased sampling as a result of truncation due to the exclusion of the most rapidly growing cancers that might metastasize at undetectably small sizes.

There is also a biologic variant of breast cancer that never seems to metastasize no matter how large the primary tumor. In reviewing the Ellis Fischel State Cancer Hospital data, Donegan identified a subset of women who had mammary cancers larger than 9 cm in greatest chordal dimension and no lymph node metastases; the 5-year survival of these women after radical mastectomy was 70% (Donegan, 1977).

Campbell and associates (1976) noted bone scans positive for cancer in 30% of women with Stage I breast cancer and in 35% of women whose cancers were less than 2 cm in greatest chordal dimension. In both the study of Pickren and that of Campbell and associates, the first metastasis must have occurred early, when the primary cancers were relatively small. From the Ellis Fischel State Cancer Hospital data, only seven patients who had radical mastectomies had primary cancers that were smaller than 1 cm in diameter. Distant dissemination developed in three of these seven patients during follow-up. Rosen and colleagues (1980) documented the early expression of adverse cellular characteristics for T1N0M0 cancers that recur and cause death. Tumor emboli in lymphatics was most strongly linked with recurrence. Other factors were poor differentiation, marked lymphoid reaction to the cancer, and menarche beginning either before age 12 years or after age 14 years. A very low risk of recurrence was observed for tumors 1.0

cm or smaller in size and for tubular, medullary, or colloid cancers up to 2.0 cm in size. The patients were diagnosed and treated with at least modified radical mastectomy. This selection pattern would be characterized by length-biased sampling because more indolent cancers would be extant longer at a detectable size of under 2.0 cm. A population-based assessment of all cancers under 2.0 cm in size might be expected to present a higher proportion of adverse characteristics.

Cell Shedding and Cell Death with Decelerating Growth Rate

In the cytokinetics of mammary cancer, the rate of cell shedding from the primary neoplasm into the circulation and its relation to growth rates are significant factors. A number of breast cancers disseminate before detection (Spratt et al., 1983). Breast cancer cells circulating in the blood have been reported on a number of occasions; however, in humans the rate of shedding is difficult to quantify. The work of Butler and Gullino (1975) has provided insight into cell death and shedding. These authors' model was an isolated hormone-dependent MTW9 rat mammary cancer from which all efferent blood could be collected. Regression could be induced by reduction of the mammotropin level in the rat. Tumor cells were identified in blood by immunofluorescence. The growing tumors shed at a rate of 3.2×10^6 cells per gram of cancer per 24 hours. The cell shedding rate from growing and regressing tumors was not significantly different. The number of cells in arterial blood was one-twelfth of that in efferent tumor blood. Butler and Gullino concluded that the shedding of cancer cells into the vascular system begins with the onset of angiogenesis. They observed that the largest cancer cell mass that can subsist on diffused nutrients alone without the ingrowth of new blood vessels comprises approximately 10^4 cells.

Butler and Gullino concluded that cell shedding via the bloodstream has only a minor role in the total cell loss from growing cancers, that the hormone-produced regression was not associated with increased cell shedding, that the shed tumor cells were rapidly cleared from circulating blood, and that a 2-g carcinoma shed a sufficient number of cells into the circulation to transplant itself every 24 hours. Cell loss during growth and regression was primarily attributable to cell death within the primary neoplasm rather than the rate of shedding. The estimated cell destruction and necrosis within the tumor were consistent with measured amino acid nitrogen loss during regression. This loss accounted for 60% to 90% of the tumor protein loss during regression. Furthermore, the rate of cell loss by shedding into the efferent venous blood remained constant whether tumor was growing or regressing. Although similar data do not exist for human mammary cancer, the same processes are at work and must start very early in the evolution of a breast cancer. Cancer cells are identified in the venous blood–draining human mammary cancer in 26% of the patients with Stage I and II disease (Golinger et al., 1977). With sampling errors and intermittent shedding taken into consideration, it can be assumed that the true cumulative presence of venous shedding from early human cancers is much greater than 26%.

Determining Growth Rates of Predetectable Cancers Using Composite BCDDP Data

The accumulation of program data in the BCDDPs provided an opportunity to assess the duration and biologic behavior of preclinical breast cancer. The National Cancer Institute contracted with 27 separate BCDDP groups for each to screen 5000 asymptomatic self-referred women during the first year of the Projects and 5000 more women during the second year. These women had no prior history of breast cancer and were between the ages of 35 and 70 years. The sample was not population-based and was non-randomly selected, and thus introduced sources of bias. As a demonstration project to determine the feasibility of mass screening, no controls were used. It was, therefore, not possible to test hypotheses as to the benefit of this program.

Screening consisted of a standard history and physical examination followed by mammographic and thermographic examinations of the breasts on admission into the Project. At the time of the first screening, women were taught the technique of BSE. The first screening resulted in the discovery of accumulated cancers. When the number of accumulated cancers was divided by the total number of women screened, the prevalence rate for the population was obtained at the very first screening examination. In each of the next 4 years of screening, additional cancers were discovered. These cancers fell in two subsets that were combined to obtain the total number of newly diagnosed cancers in a single year. These subsets included cancers that were self-discovered in the intervals between annual screens and cancers discovered at annual screens. When the number of cancers discovered yearly was divided by the number of women screened that year, the annual incidence of cancers was obtained. When these rates were divided into the prevalence rates measured at the entry year, an estimate of disease duration before discovery was obtained (Spratt et al. 1986). This period, defined as the *sojourn time from threshold* (ST_t), approximates the time elapsing between the time that the tumor reaches the threshold size and the time of its actual detection. Gould and coworkers (1978) reaffirmed that extant knowledge on breast cancer supported its origin from a single cell but that the time between origin from the single cell and the attainment of threshold size could not be estimated with these data.

Two separate sets of data were available for this study. The first set of data is from the BCDDP-L (Louisville) and is a subset of the second set of composite data from all BCDDP studies. The characteristics of the first subset have been reported (Heuser et al., 1979a,b; Spratt et al., 1983; and Heuser et al., 1984). This subset contained too few cases to allow stratification of many factors that might be associated with growth rates. The accumulated data for all 27 centers (Baker, 1984) gave meaningful stratification for patient age (Table 15–12). In all instances, time between the attainment of threshold size that might permit detection

Table 15–12. ESTIMATION OF THE DURATION OF BREAST CANCERS BEFORE DETECTION IN BCDDP PROGRAMS OBTAINED BY DIVIDING FIRST YEAR (PREVALENCE) RATES BY ANNUAL INCIDENCE RATES IN YEARS 2 TO 5 ACCORDING TO AGE RANGES

Age (y)	Year 1 Prevalent*	Year 2–5 Incident* (Range)	Prevalence Over Incidence (Year 1/Incidence in Years 2–5)	Previous Column Converted to Days and Inverted†
35–39	1.0	0.8–1.0	1.25–1.00	365–456
40–44	2.4	1.6–2.1	1.50–1.14	416–548
45–49	5.1	2.1–2.8	2.43–1.82	664–887
50–54	6.6	2.4–3.0	2.75–2.20	803–1004
55–59	7.9	3.2–3.6	2.47–2.00	750–902
60–64	9.4	3.6–3.8	2.61–2.47	902–953
65–69	9.6	3.7–4.1	2.59–2.34	854–945
70–74	12.9	3.4–5.0	3.79–2.58	942–1383

(Data from Baker (1982). From Spratt, J. S., Greenberg, R. A., and Heuser, L. S.: Geometry, growth rates, and duration of cancer and carcinoma *in situ* of the breast before detection by screening. Cancer Res., *46*:970, 1986. Reprinted with permission.)

*See definitions of "prevalent" and "incident" in the text.

†Ranges in this column provide an age-specific estimate of the sojourn time elapsing between mammographic threshold size and size at detection of breast cancers discovered in the BCDDP programs. For an unknown increment of this estimated duration, cancers would have been below the threshold size permitting detection. Considerable variation around these values would be expected. The entire duration of the cancer from inception as a single cell to detection cannot be estimated with these data.

and the time of actual detection (ST_t) was estimated by dividing the prevalence rate in the first year of screening by the annual incidence rates in the same population. This calculation was done under the assumption that the incidence rate remained constant. Incidence does increase with age and probably with other factors; however, in a short-term study, there was little reason to assume a major change in the incidence within the population.

A previous report on BCDDP-L data identified the significance of the association of younger age at mastectomy and the absence of microcalcifications with the more acute cancers that appeared in the interval between annual screening examinations (Spratt et al., 1983). Other factors associated with interval cancers were anaplastic nuclear grade, mammographically classified dysplastic breasts, and the absence of a family history of breast cancer. Survivorship was also poor for patients with quickly growing cancers (Heuser

et al., 1979a,b; Buchanan et al., 1983; Spratt et al., 1983; and Heuser et al., 1984). The threshold size below which mammary cancers were not diagnosed on mammography ranged from 2.1 to 1.6 mm (Heuser et al., 1979a).

In the BCDDP-L data, the prevalence of breast cancers discovered at first screen was 0.40% (41 cancers ÷ 10,128 women × 100). From the second through the fifth screens, the incident cancers (those discovered at annual screening in combination with those that were diagnosed in the 12 months preceding the annual screening) exhibited an incidence rate ranging from 0.18% to 0.37%. The data from the BCDDP-L are provided in Tables 15–13 through 15–24.

The times elapsing between the attainment of threshold size and detection (ST_t) from the BCDDP-L are provided in Tables 15–14 and 15–15. The authors separated invasive cancers (CA) and carcinoma in situ (CIS) to calculate the

Table 15–13. ACCUMULATIVE SCREENING EXPERIENCE FOR INVASIVE CANCER AND CIS IN THE BCDDP-L

Screen	Cancers at Screen	Cancers Surfacing in the 12 mo Preceding Screen	Total Cancers	CIS at Screen	CIS in the 12 mo Preceding Next Screen	Total CIS
1 prevalent (10,128)*	41	—	41	6		6
2 (9497)	15	6	21	6	1	7
3 (8878)	23	10	33	4	2	6
4 (8483)	10	7	17	2	2	4
5 (7725)	20	4	24	3	0	3
No sixth screen	—	6†	—	—	—	—
Totals	109	27	136‡	21‡	5	26

(From Spratt, J. S., Greenberg, R. A., and Heuser, L. S.: Geometry, growth rates, and duration of cancer and carcinoma *in situ* of the breast before detection by screening. Cancer Res., *46*:970, 1986. Reprinted with permission.)

Abbreviation: CIS = carcinoma in situ.

*Numbers in parentheses represent number screened.

†Cancers known to have occurred in the 12 mo following the fifth screen, but there was no sixth screen; thus, true incidence is indeterminable for this period.

‡In three cases with cancer and one case with CIS, bilateral simultaneous lesions were present. These cases are tabulated singly rather than as two separate cancers.

Table 15–14. ESTIMATION OF SOJOURN TIME OF CIS FROM THRESHOLD SIZE TO SIZE AT DETECTION IN BCDDP-L

Mathematical Step	Data from Table 15–12*	Prevalence Rate / Incidence Rate	ST_t	
			Years	Days
Prevalence rate at first screen	$\dfrac{6}{10{,}128}$			
Composite incidence rate in years 2–5	$\dfrac{20}{34{,}583}$	$\dfrac{0.0005924}{0.0005783}$	1.0243818	373
Annual incidence rate for next 4 y				
Year 1	$\dfrac{7}{9497}$	$\dfrac{0.0005924}{0.0007371}$	0.80363901	293
Year 2	$\dfrac{6}{8878}$	$\dfrac{0.0005924}{0.0006758}$	0.8765907	320
Year 3	$\dfrac{4}{8483}$	$\dfrac{0.0005924}{0.0004715}$	1.2564157	459
Year 4	$\dfrac{3}{7725}$	$\dfrac{0.0005924}{0.0003883}$	1.5256245	557

(From Spratt, J. S., Greenberg, R. A., and Heuser, L. S.: Geometry, growth rates, and duration of cancer and carcinoma *in situ* of the breast before detection by screening. Cancer Res., *46*:970, 1986. Reprinted with permission.)
*Number of cases with CIS divided by number of women screened.

prevalence and incidence rates for each separately and to estimate the ST_t of each category. The estimated time lapsing between CIS and invasive cancer (CA) was determined and designated $ST_{tCIS-CA}$. The estimated $ST_{tCIS-CA}$ for CA detected in the BCDDP-L is given in Table 15–16. The difference between the ST_t for CA and the ST_t for CIS estimates the span of time elapsing after CA transgresses the CIS stage but before the point of detection (see Table 15–15). This estimation is predicated on the assumption that CIS progresses to CA and that CAs go through a CIS phase. If a significant number of cancers bypass a detectable CIS period, the effect would simply negate the value of these estimates. The estimates in Table 15–12 are based on the accumulated data from all BCDDP studies. Previous

studies on cancer data were affected by tumor size at first observation. Growth rates of both CIS and CA form lognormal frequency distributions (Spratt, 1969). If this general tendency were applicable to the estimates of duration, the existence of a highly skewed distribution of ST_t and DT_{act} before detection could be assumed around the estimates in Table 15–12. The estimates approximate averages. The data in Table 15–12 provide the 95% confidence limits of a lognormal distribution. Age, the only stratification performed on the composite data from all of the contracted centers, does make a difference. The authors estimated that over 50% of the invasive CAs occurring in women under the age of 40 years (and probably under the age of 45 years) were present for less than 1 year before they were

Table 15–15. ESTIMATION OF THE SOJOURN TIME OF INVASIVE CA FROM THRESHOLD SIZE TO SIZE AT DETECTION IN BCDDP-L

Mathematical Step	Data from Table 15–12	Prevalence Rate / Incidence	ST_t*	
			Years	Days
Prevalence rate at first screen / Composite incidence	$\dfrac{41 \div 10{,}128}{95 \div 34{,}583}$	$\dfrac{0.0040482}{0.002747}$	1.473804	538
Prevalence rate at first screen / Annual incidence rate for next 4 y				
Year 1	$\dfrac{41 \div 10{,}128}{21 \div 9497}$	$\dfrac{0.0040482}{0.0022112}$	1.8307706	668
Year 2	$\dfrac{41 \div 10{,}128}{33 \div 8878}$	$\dfrac{0.0040482}{0.0037171}$	1.0890748	398
Year 3	$\dfrac{41 \div 10{,}128}{17 \div 9483}$	$\dfrac{0.0040482}{0.0017927}$	2.2581581	824
Year 4	$\dfrac{41 \div 10{,}228}{24 \div 7725}$	$\dfrac{0.0040482}{0.0031068}$	1.3030127	475

(From Spratt, J. S., Greenberg, R. A., and Heuser, L. S.: Geometry, growth rates, and duration of cancer and carcinoma *in situ* of the breast before detection by screening. Cancer Res., *46*:970, 1986. Reprinted with permission.)
Abbreviation: CA = invasive cancer.
*Sojourn time (ST_t) equals time elapsing between the moment the cancer reaches threshold size and the actual time of detection.

Table 15–16. ESTIMATION OF SOJOURN TIME (ST$_{CA-CIS}$) ELAPSING BETWEEN DETECTION OF CIS IN BCDDP-L AND INVASIVE CANCER (DAYS)

| Year of Screen | ST$_i$ in Days | | Difference (ST$_{CA-CIS}$ in days) |
	Invasive Cancer	CIS	
1	668	293	375
2	398	320	78
3	824	459	365
4	475	557	(Negative)
Composite	538	373	165

(From Spratt, J. S., Greenberg, R. A., and Heuser, L. S.: Geometry, growth rates, and duration of cancer and carcinoma *in situ* of the breast before detection by screening. Cancer Res., *46*:970, 1986. Reprinted with permission.)

detected. With much longer durations for breast cancers in women 45 years of age and older, we must assume that both length and lead time bias would be highly significant factors in the assessment of any reduced mortality attending screening in this age group. The longer duration might permit less frequent screening.

The next step was to use the volumes of cancers at the time of their discovery on screening mammography (Heuser et al., 1979*a*). The volume was calculated in cubic millimeters on the basis of radiographic dimensions and shape (Tables 15–17 to 15–19). The cancers assumed the shape of spheroids, and the volumes were calculated using the formula for a spheroid (Heuser et al., 1979*a*). The volume of a single cell was then assumed to be 10^{-6} mm^3. The number of cells was estimated by dividing 10^{-6} mm into the volume of the cancer. Tumor volume for the threshold size below which breast cancers were not detectable by mammography (2.1 mm) was calculated and is provided in Table 15–20. The number of significant figures for all data depends on the methods of measuring tumor size on mammograms. The dimensions of the tumor on the mammograms were measured in two dimensions to the nearest millimeter with a millimeter scale. The next step uses the formula fundamental to exponential growth (see Equation 4 [$N = 2^n$]), where n is the net number of doublings of the original cancer cell, and N is the estimated number of cells,

Table 15–17. RELATION OF VOLUME, NUMBER OF CANCER CELLS, AND NUMBER OF NET CELL GENERATIONS AT FIRST OBSERVATION FOR CIS OF THE BREAST DETECTED BY XEROMAMMOGRAPHY

Case Code	Volume (mm^3)	Number of Cells (N)*	Number of Cell Generations (n)†
6352 (1)	24	2.4×10^7	24.52
0050 (2)	28	2.8×10^7	24.74
5318 (3)	42	4.2×10^7	25.32
7014 (4)	113	1.13×10^8	26.75

(From Spratt, J. S., Greenberg, R. A., and Heuser, L. S.: Geometry, growth rates, and duration of cancer and carcinoma *in situ* of the breast before detection by screening. Cancer Res., *46*:970, 1986. Reprinted with permission.)
*Mean (1n) = 3.2571 ± 0.0298; 95% limits = 3.1735 to 3.3408.

Table 15–18. RELATION OF VOLUME, NUMBER OF CANCER CELLS, AND NUMBER OF NET CELL GENERATIONS AT FIRST OBSERVATION FOR CA WITH AXILLARY LYMPH NODE METASTASES (AX+) DETECTED BY XEROMAMMOGRAPHY

Case Code	Volume (mm^3)	Number of Cells (N)*	Number of Net Cell Generations (n)†
2147 (1)	335	3.35×10^8	28.32
8807 (2)	681	6.8×10^8	29.34
6129 (3)	824	8.24×10^8	29.62
6580 (4)	3535	3.54×10^9	31.72
2147 (5)	14,509	1.45×10^{10}	33.76
7069 (6)	179,646	1.80×10^{11}	37.39

(From Spratt, J. S., Greenberg, R. A., and Heuser, L. S: Geometry, growth rates, and duration of cancer and carcinoma *in situ* of the breast before detection by screening. Cancer Res., *46*:970, 1986. Reprinted with permission.)
*Mean (log) = 3.4514 ± 0.0426; 95% limit = 3.3413 to 3.5615.
†n̄ = 31.55 (28.26 to 35.22).

as calculated in the previous paragraph. To solve for n, conversion to the Naperian logarithmic form is performed as follows:

$$nln2 = \ln N \text{ or } n = \frac{\ln N}{\ln 2} \qquad (26)$$

The n value for breast cancers of threshold size, n$_t$ (22 from

Table 15–19. RELATION OF VOLUME, NUMBER OF CANCER CELLS, AND NUMBER OF NET CELL GENERATIONS AT FIRST OBSERVATION FOR CA WITHOUT AXILLARY LYMPH NODE METASTASES (AX—) DETECTED BY XEROMAMMOGRAPHY

Case Code	Volume (mm^3)	Number of Cells (N)*	Number of Net Cell Generations (n)†
9601 (1)	79	7.9×10^7	26.24
2074 (2)	79	7.9×6^7	26.24
5264 (3)	92	9.2×10^7	26.46
2684 (4)	151	1.51×10^8	27.17
7320 (5)	151	1.51×10^8	27.17
7059 (6)	189	1.89×10^8	27.49
4833 (7)	335	3.35×10^8	28.32
5607 (8)	448	4.48×10^8	28.74
1165 (9)	513	5.13×10^8	28.93
1818 (10)	760	7.6×10^8	29.50
3210 (11)	760	7.6×10^8	19.50
7324 (12)	943	9.43×10^8	29.81
4981 (13)	1,508	1.508×10^9	30.49
8748 (14)	1,593	1.59×10^9	30.57
0071 (15)	1,659	1.66×10^9	30.63
4489 (16)	1,767	1.77×10^9	30.72
2015 (17)	2,121	2.121×10^9	30.98
0266 (18)	3,394	3.39×10^9	31.66
3116 (19)	3,784	32.78×10^9	31.82
7673 (20)	6,285	6.29×10^9	32.55

(From Spratt, J. S., Greenberg, R. A., and Heuser L. S.: Geometry, growth rates, and duration of cancer and carcinoma *in situ* of the breast before detection by screening. Cancer Res., *46*:970, 1986. Reprinted with permission.)
*Mean (ln) = 3.3737 ± 0.0151; 95% limits = 3.3421 to 3.4053.
†n̄ = 29.19 (28.28 to 30.12).

Table 15–20. NUMBER OF NET GENERATIONS OF CANCER CELLS AT THRESHOLD SIZE (n$_t$)

Range of Diameters at Earliest Detection (mm)*	Tumor Volume (mm³)	N	n
2.1	4.85	4.85 × 10⁶	22

(From Spratt, J. S., Greenberg, R. A., and Heuser L. S.: Geometry, growth rates, and duration of cancer and carcinoma *in situ* of the breast before detection by screening. Cancer Res., 46:970, 1986. Reprinted with permission.)

*No breast cancer was diagnosed by mammographic exam at a size smaller than this in all categories (P <.005).

Table 15–20) can be subtracted from the n values at actual discovery, n$_d$, and the differences may be divided into the ST$_t$ to estimate the average DT$_{act}$ in this period (see Tables 15–21 to 15–23). These estimates are shorter by manyfold than those obtained from the direct mensuration of larger neoplasms reported previously and are consistent with the predictions of growth rates that decelerate as neoplasms enlarge.

As uniform quality control was exercised over mammography in the 27 BCDDPs, the assumption was made that estimates of n in the BCDDP-L would be approximately the same as n for the composite data for all BCDDP studies. The net difference for the n value at threshold size (n$_t$) and the n value of the detection size (n$_d$) (n$_d$ − n$_t$), can be divided into the ranges of ST$_t$ for the national data from all centers. Table 15–24 shows the potential variations in net DT$_{act}$ for the predetectable growth of breast cancers among women of different ages. Greater reliability exists for these composite data, as a greater number of cases were studied. The variations are an expression of the randomness of incidence rates.

That estimated values of DT$_{act}$ are shorter in the ST$_t$ period is expected. Many breast cancers develop so rapidly that they are diagnosed in the intervals between annual examinations. This observation provides additional justification for accepting that cancers follow decelerating growth, with growth undergoing time- and size-dependent retardation. The net effect is that growth becomes progressively slower as the cancers approach a maximum size. The growth rates achieved by cancers before they are large enough to be detected would be the fastest rates that these cancers attain. The rates would most likely be even faster in the period of growth preceding the achievement of mammographically detectable size and could possibly approach the mammalian cell replication rate.

In the BCDDP-L, the measurement of the DT$_{act}$ of breast cancers observed serially on mammography after they had become large and observable resulted in a mean DT$_{act}$ of 325 days (range = 109 to 944 days for 23 cases). For nine additional cancers, no measurable growth in mammographic tumor shadows was observed for as long as 4 years (Heuser et al., 1984). The actual rate of cell division at the time of onset of a cancer in the human breast is not known. According to Tseng (personal communication, 1986), human mammary cancer cells in tissue culture may exhibit

cell DTs of 24 to 36 hours with decelerating growth of the total cell mass. Present data support the thesis that after the cancer is large enough to be seen on a mammogram, the DT$_{act}$ is longer than in the predetectable period.

Limitations on Breast Self-Examination Imposed by Rapid Early Growth and Metastasis

More rapid growth in predetectable breast cancer has immediate relevance to the relationship between BSE practices and breast cancer survival (Foster and Constanza, 1975). At 5 years, the survivorship of monthly BSE performers was 75% (±3%) compared with 57% (±3%) for nonperformers. Death due to breast cancer was 14% at 5 years for women performing BSE in contrast to 26% for those not performing the test (ρ < .001). Women performing BSE discovered their cancers when they were at an average size of 2.1 cm; in contrast, those who did not perform BSE discovered their cancers when they were 3.2 cm in size. In adjusting survivorship for lead time bias, Foster and Constanza concluded that survivorship remained significantly better in women who performed BSE. However, these authors used a *uniform* cancer volume DT of 100 days to estimate lead time. This does not allow for the extreme variance in the DTs and the change in DT$_{act}$ with increasing tumor size. Their conclusions that BSE survivors had significantly better survivorship for lead times up to 3 years cannot be defended by their calculations.

Accumulating evidence supports the thesis that a significant number of new breast cancers grow rapidly and metastasize in the predetectable period. As a consequence, many cancers that appear in the intervals between annual screening examinations will already have metastasized. This problem is more significant for women younger than 45 years of age. The enormous variations in average DT$_{act}$ of grossly measurable cancers also complicate the defining of an optimum time interval between screening examinations. The clonogenic kinetic events that occur before a breast cancer is detectable undoubtedly have a major impact on prognosis, which may override the prognostic utility of anatomic staging. The prognostic differences with various anatomic stages may be an illusion that incompletely considers numerous sources of sampling bias and variations in kinetic and biologic behavior. Paralleling the early rapid increase in total cell mass is the tendency to metastasize

Table 15–21. DIFFERENCE BETWEEN NUMBER OF NET CELLULAR GENERATIONS (n$_d$) AT DETECTION AND AT THRESHOLD SIZE (n$_t$ = 22 or 23)

	n$_t$ = 22		n$_t$ = 23	
CIS	4.022	± 1.769808	3.022	± 1.769808
Ax(−)	7.2495	± 1.9596172	6.2495	± 1.9596172
Ax(+)	9.70033	± 3.4042704	8.70033	± 3.4042704

(From Spratt, J. S., Greenberg, R. A., and Heuser, L. S.: Geometry growth rates, and duration of cancer and carcinoma *in situ* of the breast before detection by screening. Cancer Res., 46:970, 1986. Reprinted with permission.)

Table 15–22. ESTIMATIONS BY XEROMAMMOGRAPHY OF THE DT$_{act}$ WITH 95% RANGE FOR A LOGNORMAL DISTRIBUTION FOR CANCERS GROWING FROM THRESHOLD SIZE TO DETECTABLE SIZE

Age (y)	ST$_t$ (d)*	CIS $n_d - n_t$†	CIS DT$_{act}$‡	Cancer Ax − $n_d - n_t$†	Cancer Ax − DT$_{act}$‡	Cancer Ax + $n_d - n_t$	Cancer Ax + DT$_{act}$
35–39	365–465	3.98	92–117	7.19	51–65	9.55	38–49
40–44	416–547	1.89–6.24	105–137	6.28–8.12	58–76	6.26	44–57
45–49	664–887	(95%)	167–223	(95%)	92–123	13.22	70–93
50–54	803–1004		201–252		112–140	(95%)	84–105
55–59	750–902		188–227		104–125		79–94
60–64	902–953		227–239		125–133		94–100
65–69	854–945		215–237		119–131		89–99
70–74	942–1383		237–347		131–192		99–145
Extremes (95%)			59–732		50–220		28–221

(From Spratt, J. S., Greenberg, R. A., and Heuser, L. S.: Geometry, growth rates, and duration of cancer and carcinoma *in situ* of the breast before detection by screening. Cancer Res., *46*:970, 1986. Reprinted with permission.)

*ST$_t$, Sojourn time, or time elapsing from the time a cancer reaches threshold size to time it is detected.

†n_d, Number of doublings or net cell generations required to attain the volume of a cancer at the threshold of detection by xeromammography; n_t, Number of doublings or net cell generations required to attain the volume of a cancer at the time actually detected by xeromammography.

‡DT$_{act}$, Mean time (d) for a cancer to double its volume.

that may be greater with faster growing cancers. It is possible that many breast cancers metastasize before the cancer reaches detectable size.

Using data from an older study (see Table 15–3), the shortest DT$_{act}$ measured for any primary breast cancer observed by mammography was 23 days; the longest was 209 days. Few persons survive after their tumor cells have undergone a net of 40 doublings; thus, 40 times this DT$_{act}$ was used to speculate about the extreme duration of human breast cancer from inception to death. In the series of Gershon-Cohen and coworkers (1963), the shortest survival time was 23 × 40 = 920 days and the longest was 209 × 40 = 8320 days (22.8 years). Decelerating growth rather than exponential growth would affect this variation in that the sojourn time from inception of the cancer would be much shorter than these estimates.

Applying the DT$_{act}$ of only 3 days reported by Phillipe and Le Gal (1968) for a cutaneous metastasis from breast cancer, breast cancers could be acutely lethal. Three days times 40 doublings could conceivably be associated with a mammary cancer growing from inception to lethal proportions in as little as 120 days. At the opposite extreme, Breur (1966a) reported a breast cancer with DT$_{act}$ of 745 days. This value times 40 equals 29,000 days, a period longer than the normal life span (27,375 days). A person with such a slowly growing cancer would be likely to die from other causes before the cancer reached lethal proportions. In fact, long survivals are seen clinically without relying on the

dormant cell theory to account for very long symptom-free intervals. These slower growing cancers would be the ones most likely discovered by screening. Thus, cancers discovered by annual screening would be a biased group not representative of the entire population of cancers. Cancers of the breast discovered at autopsy stand a higher probability of being slowly growing neoplasms.

Survival of patients at Ellis Fischel State Cancer Hospital from the time of first radiographic diagnosis of pulmonary metastases was also found to be lognormal with respect to time (Spratt and Spratt, 1964). Mean survival, corrected for measurement from a common point (a metastasis of 10 mm in diameter), was 310 days with 95% confidence limits and ranged from 20 to 4780 days without treatment. This extreme variance in survival of patients with mammary cancer must be considered before attributing benefit to newer therapeutic methods or combinations of such methods. As length of survival and rates of growth both show extreme natural variance, the rate of growth and the time required to produce a lethal neoplastic mass may be the two most important characteristics of mammary cancer (Spratt et al., 1977). Data on growth rates and survivorship are not yet of the quality and quantity necessary to describe the type of linear relation that probably exists between these two variables, but seeking this relationship is a useful area of research.

A simple relationship between DT$_{act}$ and survivorship from first radiographic observation of pulmonary metastasis

Table 15–23. ESTIMATION OF DT$_{act}$ FOR CANCERS GROWING BETWEEN THRESHOLD SIZE (n_t) AND SIZE OF DETECTION (n_d) IN BCDDP-L

	ln (mean) $n_d = e$	95% Limits	d.f.	n_t	$n_d - n_t$	$n_d - n_t$ (95%)	ST$_t$	DT$_{act}$	DT$_{act}$ (95%)
CIS	25.98	23.89–28.24	45	22	3.98	1.89–6.29	373	94	197–60
Ca AX (−)	29.19	28.28–30.12	19	22	7.19	6.28–8.12	538	75	86–66
Ca Ax (+)	31.55	28.26–35.22	5	22	9.55	6.26–13.22	538	56	86–41

(From Spratt, J. S., Greenberg, R. A., and Heuser, L. S.: Geometry, growth rates, and duration of cancer and carcinoma *in situ* of the breast before detection by screening. Cancer Res., *46*:970, 1986. Reprinted with permission.)

Table 15-24. ESTIMATIONS OF THE DT$_{act}$ FOR MAMMARY CANCERS DURING ST$_t$ ACCORDING TO THE AGE OF WOMEN, CIS, OR CANCER BY AXILLARY NODE STATUS

Age (y)	ST$_t$ (d)	CIS		Cancer Ax −		Cancer Ax +	
		$n_d - n_t$	DT$_{act}$ (d)	$n_d - n_t$	DT$_{act}$ (d)	$n_d - n_t$	DT$_{act}$ (d)
35–39	365–465	4.02	90–116	7.25	50–64	9.7	38–48
40–44	416–547	4.02	103–136		56–75		43–56
45–49	664–887	4.02	105–221		91–122		68–91
50–54	803–1004	4.02	200–250		110–138		83–104
55–59	750–902	4.02	167–224		103–124		77–93
60–64	902–953	4.02	224–237		124–131		93–98
65–69	854–945	4.02	212–235		118–130		88–97
70–74	942–1383		234–344		130–191		97–143

(From Spratt, J. S., Greenberg, R. A., and Heuser, L. S.: Geometry, growth rates, and duration of cancer and carcinoma *in situ* of the breast before detection by screening. Cancer Res., *46*:970, 1986. Reprinted with permission.)

was determined for a small series of patients at Ellis Fischel State Cancer Hospital. A DT$_{act}$ of 100 days was a critical point in the lethality of these cancers. With a DT$_{act}$ of less than 100 days, 10 of the 24 (41%) patients died within a year. With a DT$_{act}$ of over 100 days, 5 of 5 patients, or 100%, lived longer than 1 year.

Cytokinetics, Genetics, Heterogeneity, and Drug Resistance

Cytokinetics, genetics, cellular heterogeneity, and drug resistance are interrelated. Each cellular generation has a mutation rate that fosters greater phenotypic heterogeneity. The mutation rate, which seems related to cancer cell division, cannot be reduced. By the time a cancer has undergone 30 net generations (and consists of about 10^9 cells), there is a zero probability that it contains no cells resistant to chemotherapy (Goldie and Coldman, 1979; Goldie and Coldman, 1984; and Goldie and Coldman, 1985). By the time new cancers have reached a threshold of size that permits discovery, the number of existing cells is very great, and the cancer has progressed through thirty generations or more. Goldie and Coldman reviewed the importance of overall tumor growth kinetics to determine the response of a tumor to chemotherapeutic agents. The theoretical relationship to the chances of cure can be expressed as follows:

$$\text{function } C \text{ (cure)} = e^{-\alpha N} \tag{27}$$

where α is the mutation rate per cell generation
N is the number of cells in the cancer
e is the base of the natural logarithms.

Goldie and Coldman's model (1985) attempts to integrate the stem cell and somatic mutation hypotheses and thus provide an explanation for the emergence of drug resistance in cancer. The model recognizes the capacity of neoplasms to assume a great range of phenotypic diversity compared with normal cell systems. Skehan's (1984) arguments address the inherent reasons for this phenotypic diversity and for the survival of mutants. The achievement of

chemotherapeutic resistance by a cancer is similar to the development of antibiotic resistance by bacteria.

The probability that zero resistant cells are present is expressed by the following relationship:

$$P_0 = \exp[-\alpha(N - 1)], \tag{28}$$

where P_0 is the probability, α is the mutation rate per cell generation, and N is the size of the cell population.

The model assumes that no resistant cells are present at the onset of the neoplasm. If the original cell is not sensitive, drug resistance would be an initial phenotypic property of the neoplasm. The plot of this function provides a sigmoid-shaped curve in which the probability of cure from drugs falls very quickly. Any treatment strategy that does not control the neoplasm increases the likelihood of double or even multiple levels of mutation, which in turn increases the probability of incurability, assuming that the cancer was curable by drugs at the time of onset.

The stem cell model of tumor growth may be applicable to neoplasms that mimic the normal cell removal system, in which the end cell is differentiated, nonrenewing, or dead, as in the hematopoietic system. Random stem cell loss magnifies the risk of drug resistance. A patient with cancer characterized by a relatively high clonogenic cell mass, relatively low renewal probability, and high rates of mutation relative to resistance probably cannot be cured by current drug protocols.

The Goldie-Coldman model has been used to simulate many different treatment strategies. The disturbing constraint implied by this model is that it predicts a high probability of drug incurability by the time that the number of cell generations is greater than 30. This yields a neoplasm containing 10^9 (or 2^{30}) cells, for which the probability of zero drug resistance falls to zero. When all 10^9 cells are found together, this yields a neoplasm of less than 1 cm^3 in size. Actually, with angiogenesis and the early propensity for vascular seeding, 10^9 cells diffused throughout the breast and body could be associated with an exceedingly small primary neoplasm but still represent a body tumor burden well in excess of 10^9 cells. From the standpoint of detection and screening strategy, the number of cell generations elapsing between the attainment of threshold size visible on mammograms (2^{22} cells) and the development of a tumor consisting of 2^{30} cells is no greater than eight. The actual time lapsing between the attainment of threshold size and the discovery of cancer by screening varied from between 365 and 465 days for patients aged 35 to 40 years to between 942 and 2383 days for patients aged 70 to 74 years (Spratt et al., 1986). The authors suspect that this time period for patients under the age of 35 years is much shorter than that for older patients. Clearly, these cytokinetic factors near the threshold of detectability impose persistent limitations on the ability to control breast cancer by "early" detection (Spratt et al., 1986). As Goldie and Coldman (1984) observed, "the upper limit of curable size (by chemotherapy) of many solid tumors appears to be only at the lower range of *even microscopic tumor burden.*" Because of the complex issue identified theoretically and in laboratory models, there are "still many unresolved questions in the area of drug resistance, especially as applied to the behavior of human cancer *in vivo.*" In both the laboratory and clinical situation, drug resistance is a multifactorial problem.

Duration of Symptoms, Growth Rate, and Survival

The relationship between duration of symptoms before the treatment of breast cancer and survivorship also is related to growth rate. Dennis and coworkers (1975) reported no significant correlation ($\rho > .005$) between delay attributable to either physician or patient and survivorship after treatment when survivorship is measured from the onset of symptoms to correct for lead time. They also reviewed the contradictory literature that antedated their report. Fisher and colleagues (1977) noted that both tissue necrosis within the cancer and the prevalence of highly malignant histologic grade decreased when the duration of symptoms antedating treatment exceeded 9 months. Although the appearance of "ominous" prognostic findings increased with long delay, the average monthly treatment failure rate was not altered. A trend was even noted toward a decline in monthly treatment failure rates when the duration of symptoms antedated treatment by more than 9 months. Thus, there is a documented trend for the rapidly appearing cancers to be more virulent, and for the more chronic, more slowly growing cancers with longer duration of symptoms before treatment to progress more slowly after treatment.

Clinical Application of Growth Rates

Precise measurements of in vivo growth of most human breast cancers are at present insufficient to define an absolute relationship between gross rates of growth, tumor cell proliferation, cell loss, and survivorship in a specific host. Multiple events occur continuously in the life of a cancer and its host, and the net effect reflects the interaction of these variables. The slope of the growth curves mirrors the net effect of many variables; these curves also reflect the changing relationship among these variables with the growth of cancer. Attempts to extrapolate growth curves beyond the observed data are subject to serious error.

The extreme variation in the prelethal duration of a breast cancer casts further doubt on the value of fixed-endpoint survival rates (such as 5-year survival rates) as a parameter for assaying the value of treatment. This is particularly true when fixed-endpoint (5-year) survival rates are reported for specific anatomic stages (e.g., tumor-node-metastasis stages). Slower growing cancers are more likely to be discovered while they are small and are at an earlier stage. Similarly, when the fixed-endpoint survival rates of successive stages are compared, a highly variable lead time bias exists. Relative rates of dying describe and compare survivorship more accurately. In summary, the cytokinetic properties of cancer cells are significant determinants of cancer behavior and patient prognosis.

References

Arnerlov, C., Emdin, S. O., Lundgren, B., et al.: Breast carcinoma growth rate described by mammographic doubling time and S-phase fraction: Correlations to clinical and histopathologic factors in a screened population. Cancer, 70:1928–1934, 1992a.

Arnerlov, C., Emdin, S. O., Lundgren, B., et al.: Mammographic growth rate, DNA ploidy, and S-phase fraction analysis in breast cancer: A prognostic evaluation of a screened population. Cancer, 70:1935–1942, 1992b.

Atkinson, E. N., Brown, B. W., and Montague, E. O.: Tumor volume, nodal status, and metastasis in breast cancer in women. J. Natl. Cancer Inst., 76:171, 1986.

Baker, L. H.: Breast cancer detection demonstration project: Five year summary report. Cancer, 53:96, 1984.

Bosari, S., Lee, A. K. C., Tahan, S. R., et al.: DNA flow cytometric analysis and prognosis of axillary lymph-node negative breast carcinoma. Cancer, 70:1943–1950, 1992.

Boyd, N. F., Meakin, J. W., Hayward, J. L., et al.: Clinical estimation of the growth rate of breast cancer. Cancer, 48:1037, 1981.

Bradley, J. V.: Distribution Free Statistical Tests. Englewood Cliffs, NJ, Prentice-Hall, 1968, p. 296.

Brem, S., Brem, H., Folkman, J., et al.: Prolonged tumor dormancy by prevention of neovascularization in the vitreous. Cancer Res., 36:2807, 1976.

Breur, K.: Growth rate and radiosensitivity of human tumours: I. Growth rate of human tumours. Eur. J. Cancer, 2:157, 1966a.

Breur, K.: Growth rate and radiosensitivity of human tumours: II. Radiosensitivity of human tumours. Eur. J. Cancer, 2:173, 1966b.

Buchanan, J. B., Spratt, J. S., and Heuser, L. S.: Tumor growth, doubling times and the inability of the radiologists to diagnose certain cancers. Radiol. Clin. North Am., 21:115, 1983.

Butler, T. P., and Gullino, P. M.: Quantitation of cell shedding into efferent blood of mammary adenocarcinoma. Cancer Res., 35:312, 1975.

Campbell, D. J., Banks, A. J., and Oates, G. D.: The value of preliminary bone scanning in staging and assessing prognosis of breast cancer. Br. J. Surg., 63:811, 1976.

Charlson, M. E., and Feinstein, A. R.: Rate of disease progression in breast cancer: A clinical estimate of prognosis within nodal and anatomical stages. J. Natl. Cancer Inst., 72:225, 1984.

Chato, J. C.: Measurements of the thermal properties of growing neoplasms. Ann. N. Y. Acad. Sci., 335:67, 1980.

Cox, D. R.: Regression models and life tables. J. R. Stat. Soc., 34:187, 1972.

Dean, P. N.: Methods of data analysis in flow cytometry. *In* Van Dilla, M. A., Dean, P. N., Laerum, O. D., et al. (Eds.): Flow Cytometry: Instrument and Data Analysis. London, Academic Press, 1985, pp. 195–221.

Dennis, C. R., Gardner, B., and Lim, B.: Analysis of survival and recurrence vs. patient and doctor delay in treatment of breast cancer. Cancer, 35:714, 1975.

Donegan, W. L.: Personal communication, 1977.

Dressler, L. G.: Are DNA flow cytometry measurements providing useful information in the management of the node-negative breast cancer patient? Cancer Invest., 10:477–486, 1992.

Eberhart, R. C., Shitzer, A., and Hernandez, E. J.: Thermal dilution methods: Estimation of tissue blood flow and metabolism. Ann. N. Y. Acad. Sci., *335*:67, 1980.

Fidler, I. J., and Hart, I. R.: Biological diversity in metastatic neoplasms: Origins and implications. Science, *217*:998–1003, 1982.

Fisher, E. R., Redmond, C., and Fisher, B.: A perspective concerning the relation of duration of symptoms to the treatment failure in patients with breast cancer. Cancer, *4*:3160, 1977.

Foster, R. S., and Constanza, M. C.: Breast self-examination and breast cancer survival. Cancer, *53*:999, 1975.

Galante, M.: Personal communication, 1982.

Gautherie, M.: Thermopathology of breast cancer: Measurement and analysis of in vivo temperature and blood flow. Ann. N. Y. Acad. Sci., *335*:383, 1980.

Gershon-Cohen, J., Berger, S. M., and Klickstein, H. S.: Roentgenography of breast cancer moderating concepts of "biologic predeterminism." Cancer, *16*:961, 1963.

Goldie, J. H., and Coldman, A. J.: A mathematical model for relating the drug sensitivity of tumors to their spontaneous mutation rate. Cancer Treat. Res., *63*:1727, 1979.

Goldie, J. H., and Coldman, A. J.: The genetic origin of drug resistance in neoplasms: Implicatons for systemic therapy. Cancer Res., *44*:3643, 1984.

Goldie, J. H., and Coldman, A. J.: A model for tumor response to chemotherapy: An integration of the stem cell and somatic mutation hypotheses. Cancer Invest., *3*:553, 1985.

Golinger, R. C., Gregorio, R., and Fisher, E. R.: Tumor cell in venous blood draining mammary carcinoma. Arch. Surg., *223*:707, 1977.

Gompertz, B.: On the nature of the function expressive of the law of human mortality, and on a new mode of determining the value of life contingencies. Philos. Trans. R. Soc. Lond. Biol., *115*:513, 1825.

Gould, M. N., Jirtle, R., Crowley, J., et al.: Reevaluation of the number of cells involved in the neutron induction of mammary neoplasms. Cancer Res., *38*:189, 1978.

Gullino, P. M.: Influence of blood supply on thermal properties and metabolism of mammary carcinoma. Ann. N. Y. Acad. Sci., *335*:1, 1980.

Gullino, P. M., Grantham, F. H., and Courtney, A. H.: Utilization of oxygen by transplanted tumors in vivo. Cancer Res., *27*:1028, 1967.

Gullino, P. M.: Personal communication, 1985.

Hatschek, T., Carstensen, J., Fagerberg, G., et al.: Influence of S-phase fraction on metastatic pattern and post-recurrence survival in a randomized mammography screening trial. Breast Cancer Res. Treat., *14*:321–327, 1989.

Heuser, L. S., Spratt, J. S., Kuhns, J. G., et al.: The association of pathologic and mammographic characteristics of primary human breast cancers with "slow" and "fast" growth rates and with axillary lymph node metastases. Cancer, *53*:96, 1984.

Heuser, L. S., Spratt, J. S., and Polk, H. C., Jr.: Growth rates of primary breast cancers. Cancer, *43*:1888, 1979*a*.

Heuser, L. S., Spratt, J. S., Polk, H. C., Jr., et al.: Relation between mammary cancer growth kinetics and the intervals between screenings. Cancer, *43*:857, 1979*b*.

Hoffman, J. G.: Theory of mitotic index and its application to tissue growth measurement. Bull. Math. Biophys., *11*:139, 1949.

Joensuu, H., Toikkanen, S., and Klemi, P. J.: DNA index and S-phase fraction and their combination as prognostic factors in operable ductal breast cancer. Cancer, *66*:331–340, 1990.

Kallinowski, F., Schlenger, K. H., Rundel, S., et al.: Blood flow, metabolism, cellular microenvironment and growth rate of human tumor xenografts. Cancer Res., *49*:3759–3764, 1989.

Kusama, S., Spratt, J. S., Jr., Donegan, W. L., et al.: The gross rates of growth of human mammary carcinoma. Cancer, *30*:594, 1972.

Lee, Y. T.: The lognormal distribution of growth and shrinkage rates of soft tissue metastases of breast cancer. Trans. Mo. Acad. Sci., *4*:33, 1970.

Lee, Y. T.: The lognormal distribution of growth rates of soft tissue metastases of breast cancer. J. Surg. Oncol., *4*:81, 1972.

Lee, Y. T., and Spratt, J. S., Jr.: Rate of growth of soft tissue metastases of breast cancer. Cancer, *29*:344, 1972.

Less, J. R., Skalak, T. C., Sevick, M., and Jain, R. K.: Microvascular architecture in mammary carcinoma: Branching patterns and vessel dimensions. Cancer Res., *51*:265–273, 1991.

Malaise, E. P., Chavaudra, N., and Tubiana, M.: The relationship between growth rate, labelling index and histological type of human solid tumors. Eur. J. Cancer, *9*:305, 1973.

Mayr, N. A., Staples, J. J., Robinson, R. A., et al.: Morphometric studies in intraductal breast carcinoma using computerized image analysis. Cancer, *67*:2805–2812, 1991.

Mayneord, W. V.: On a law of growth of Jensen's rat sarcoma. Am. J. Cancer, *16*:841, 1932.

McGuire, W. L., Channess, G. C., Costlow, M. E., et al.: Hormone dependence in breast cancer. Metabolism, *23*:75, 1974.

McGuire, W. L., Carbone, P. P., and Vollmer, E. (Eds.): Estrogen Receptors in Human Breast Cancer. New York, Raven Press, 1975.

Meyer, J. S., and Bauer, W. C.: Tritiated thymidine labelling index of benign and malignant human breast epithelium. J. Surg. Oncol., *8*:165, 1976.

Meyskens, F. L., Jr., Thomson, S. P., and Moon, T. E.: Quantitation of the number of cells within tumor colonies in semisolid medium and their growth as oblate spheroids. Cancer Res., *44*:271, 1984.

Panoussopoulas, D., Chang, J., and Humphrey, L. J.: Screening for breast cancer. Ann. Surg., *186*:356, 1977.

Parl, F. P., and Dupont, W. D.: A retrospective cohort study of histologic risk factors in breast cancer patients. Cancer, *50*:2410, 1982.

Pearlman, A. W.: Breast cancer—influence of growth rate on prognosis and treatment evaluation: A study based on mastectomy scar recurrences. Cancer, *39*:1826, 1976.

Pearlman, N. W., and Jochimsen, P. R.: Recurrent breast cancer: Factors influencing survival, including treatment. J. Surg. Oncol., *11*:21, 1979.

Peer, P. G. M., van Dijck, J. A. A. M., Hendriks, J. H. C. L., et al.: Age-dependent grown rate of primary breast cancer. Cancer, *71*:3547–3551, 1993.

Phillipe, E., and Le Gal, Y.: Growth of seventy-eight recurrent mammary cancers: Quantitative study. Cancer, *21*:461, 1968.

Peterson, H.-I.: The microcirculation of tumors. *In* Orr, F. W., Buchanan, M. R., and Weiss, L. (Eds.): Microcirculation in cancer metastases. Boca Raton, CRC Press, 1991, pp. 278–298.

Pickren, J. W.: Significance of occult metastases: A study of breast cancer. Cancer, *14*:1266, 1961.

Post, J., Sklarew, R. J., and Hoffmann, J.: The proliferative patterns of human breast cancer cells in vivo. Cancer, *39*:1500, 1977.

Rosen, P. P., Saigo, P. E., Braun, D. W., et al.: Predictors of recurrence in Stage I (TIN0M0) breast carcinoma. Ann. Surg., *193*:15, 1980.

Shibamoto, Y., and Streffer, C.: Estimation of the dividing fraction and potential doubling time of tumors using cytochalasin B. Cancer Res., *51*:5134–5138, 1991.

Skehan, P.: Cell growth tissue neogenesis and neoplastic transformation. *In* Skehan, P., and Friedman, S. J. (Eds.): Growth, Cancer and the Cell Cycle. Clifton, NJ, Humana Press, 1984, p. 323.

Spratt, J. S., and Ackerman, L. V.: The growth of a colonic adenocarcinoma. Am. Surg., *17*:23, 1961.

Spratt, J. S.: The lognormal frequency distribution and human cancer. J. Surg. Res., *9*:151–157, 1969.

Spratt, J. S., and Spratt, J. A.: The prognostic value of measuring the gross linear radial growth of pulmonary metastases and primary pulmonary cancers. J. Thorac. Cardiovasc. Surg., *71*:274, 1976.

Spratt, J. S., and Spratt, T. L.: Rates of growth of pulmonary metastases and host survival. Ann. Surg., *159*:161, 1964.

Spratt, J. S., Chang A. F.-C., Heuser, L. S., et al.: Acute carcinoma of the breast. Surg. Gynecol. Obstet., *157*:220, 1983.

Spratt, J. S., Greenberg, R. A., and Heuser, L. S.: Geometry, growth rates and duration of cancer and carcinoma in situ of the breast before detection by screening. Cancer, *46*:970, 1986.

Spratt, J. S., Kaltenbach, M. L., and Spratt, J. A.: Cytokinetic definition of acute and chronic breast cancer. Cancer Res., *37*:226–230, 1977.

Spratt, J. S., Spjut, H. J., and Roper, C. L.: The frequency distribution of the growth and the estimated duration of primary pulmonary carcinomas. Cancer, *16*:687, 1963.

Spratt, J. S., Spjut, H. J., Ter-Pogossian, M., et al.: Correlation of primary pulmonary neoplastic growth curves with morphology, necrosis, survival and aetiology: Proceedings of the VIIIth International Cancer Congress, Moscow, 1962, p. 281.

Spratt, J. A., von Fournier, D., Spratt, J. S., and Weber, E. E.: Decelerating growth and human breast cancer. Cancer, *71*:2013–2019, 1993*a*.

Spratt, J. A., Von Fournier, D., Spratt, J. S., and Weber, E. E.: Mammographic assessment of human breast cancer growth and duration. Cancer, *71*:2020–2026, 1993*b*.

Steel, G. G.: Cell loss as a factor in the growth rate of human tumours. Eur. J. Cancer, *3*:381, 1967.

Steel, G. G.: The cell cycle in tumours: An examination of data gained by technique of labelled mitosis. Cell Tissue Kinet., *5*:87, 1972.

Tabbane, F., Bahi, J., Rahal, K., et al.: Inflammatory symptoms in breast cancer: Correlations with growth rates, clinicopathologic variables, and evolution. Cancer, *64*:2081–2089, 1989.

Tannock, I. F., and Steel, G. G.: Quanitative techniques for study of the anatomy and function of small blood vessels in tumors. J. Natl. Cancer Inst., *42*:771–782, 1969.

Tseng, M.: Personal communication, 1986.

Tubiana, M., Pejovic, M. H., Koscielny, S., et al.: Growth rate, kinetics of tumor cell proliferation and long-term outcome in breast cancer. Int. J. Cancer, *44*:17–22, 1989.

Vollmer, G., Gerdes, J., and Knuppen, R.: Relationship of cytosolic estrogen and progesterone receptor content and the growth fraction in human mammary carcinomas. Cancer Res., *49*:4011–4014, 1989.

von Fournier, D., Kubli, F., and Barth, V.: Growth rates of 147 mammary carcinomas. Cancer, *45*:2198, 1980.

von Fournier, D.: Personal communication, 1982.

Weidner, N., Semple, J. P., Welch, W. R., et al.: Tumor angiogenesis and metastasis: Correlation in invasive breast cancer. N. Engl. J. Med., *324*:2–8, 1991.

White, R. A., Terry, N. H. A., Meistrich, M. L., et al.: Improved method for computing potential doubling time for flow cytometric data. Cytometry, *11*:314–371, 1990.

Williams, N. N., and Daly, J. M.: Flow cytometry and prognostic implications in patients with solid tumors. Surg. Gynecol. Obstet., *171*:257–266, 1990.

16

Hormone and Growth Factor Receptors

James L. Wittliff

Since Beatson's original observations (1896), the hormonal milieu of a patient has been known to influence significantly the growth rates of certain breast cancers. Clinical observations by Huggins and Bergenstal (1952), Luft and Olivecrona (1955), and others (Dao, 1972; and Kennedy, 1974) since the turn of the century indicated that 25% to 40% of breast cancers respond to the surgical removal of hormone-producing glands, such as the ovaries in premenopausal women or the adrenals or anterior pituitary in postmenopausal patients. Pharmacologic doses of estrogens, androgens, and so-called antihormones such as tamoxifen (Nolvadex) and toremifene also brought about remissions (Hall, 1968; Fisher et al., 1983; and Santen et al., 1990). Endocrine ablative surgery has been replaced largely by administration of antihormones, owing to increased knowledge of steroid hormone action and its relationship to hormone response (Jensen et al., 1971; Wittliff et al., 1972, 1974; and McGuire et al., 1975, 1977).

Oncologists treating breast cancer must identify which patients are most likely to respond to endocrine manipulation (Polk, 1986). Endocrine treatment of breast cancer in women utilizes a variety of agents, such as the antiestrogens, progestins such as medroxy-progesterone acetate and Megestrol acetate (PAR), aromatase inhibitors such as aminoglutethimide, and gonadotropin-releasing hormones (LH-RH) analogs (cf. Santen, 1990). Emerging treatments utilizing endocrine activities include the antiprogestin RU486 (mifepristone, Horwitz, 1992), somatostatin analogs (Lamberts et al., 1991), and bromocriptine. Earlier, clinical factors such as previous response to hormone therapy, disease-free interval, age and menopausal status, and location of the dominant metastatic lesion were the principal criteria for selecting therapeutic regimens for women with breast cancer.

Investigations during the past 20 years have made significant progress toward elucidating the mechanism by which steroid hormones influence the differentiation and development of target organs (Buller and O'Malley, 1976; Clark and Pack, 1979; Wittliff et al., 1980; and Moudgil, 1985). A prerequisite for responsiveness appears to be a cellular protein termed the *steroid receptor* or *steroid-binding protein*. Receptor proteins are found in a variety of concentrations, ranging from 50 to 50,000 sites in target cells, but they are virtually absent in nontarget tissues. An important property is that the steroid hormones associate with their characteristic receptor proteins in a manner characterized by high affinity and ligand specificity.

Since the original report of Folca and coworkers (1961)

indicating a greater uptake of labeled hexoestrol by breast tumors of patients who showed a response to ablative therapy, numerous studies have shown that approximately half of all biopsy specimens of malignant breast tumors contained estrogen receptors (Jensen et al., 1971; Wittliff, 1974, 1984; and McGuire et al., 1975, 1977). Furthermore, 55% to 60% of the patients who exhibited estrogen receptors were responsive to either administrative or ablative hormone therapy. The oncologist's use of this single biochemical criterion (presence of estrogen receptors) has increased by twofold or threefold the accuracy of selecting the patients with advanced breast cancer who are most likely to respond objectively to endocrine manipulation. Addition of the results of progestin receptor determinations further defines the endocrine-responsive breast carcinomas (Proceedings of the NIH Consensus Development Conference, 1980; Clark et al., 1983; Fisher et al., 1983; and Wittliff, 1984).

At present, both estrogen and progestin receptors are used routinely in the clinical management of breast cancer as predictive indices of a patient's response to endocrine therapy and as prognostic indicators of a patient's clinical course. Clearly, this is a decade of enormous progress in the application of molecular endocrinology to clinical medicine. Soon, additional receptor tests will be added to the oncologist's armamentarium to combat breast cancer and other hormone-responsive neoplasms.

STEROID HORMONE–TARGET CELL INTERACTION

The normal breast is an organ in which both peptide and steroid hormones influence the molecular processes involved in proliferation, differentiation, and secretion (Wittliff, 1975). The major stages in the differentiation of the breast involve both parenchymatous and mesenchymal components. Although the specific role of each hormone is unknown, estrogens, progesterone, and glucocorticoids are known to influence these processes. Likewise, androgen is known to exert a negative control on the proliferation of breast epithelium during early development.

Several peptide hormones, such as insulin, prolactin, growth hormone, and certain growth factors, act in concert with the steroid hormones to bring about the orderly differentiation of the resting female breast cell to a structurally and functionally differentiated state. The functionally differentiated state is characterized histologically by an alveolar secretory appearance and by increased rates of synthesis of milk proteins, lipids, and lactose. Before the onset of lactation, the breast is composed predominantly of adipose cells surrounding a branched system of ducts of epithelial cells with connective tissue elements. As the gland differentiates during pregnancy and lactation, the tissue shifts its composition toward a higher concentration of lobuloalveolar cells, which are responsible for the synthesis of milk. At the culmination of lactation, the mammary epithelium undergoes involution. These events appear to be regulated by a host of factors, of which hormone receptors are central to organized differentiation and development.

The concept underlying endocrine therapy is that certain tumor cells have retained the molecular mechanisms (receptors) to respond to the same hormones as their normal progenitor cells. With specific hormone-binding data, it is possible to derive information about the natural history of the lesion, such as transformation (dedifferentiation), which may result in the loss of receptors; it is also possible to exploit their presence by employing hormone therapy.

Current understanding of the sequence of events that follows the interaction of a steroid hormone with a target cell (Fig. 16–1) evolved from the original "two-step mechanism" suggested independently by Gorski and coworkers (1968) at the University of Illinois and by Jensen and colleagues (1968) at the University of Chicago. Uterine tissue from rodents was used for these early studies. Investigations from many laboratories with rodents and human tissues suggest that a similar cascade of events exists in normal and neoplastic mammary cells. Steroid hormones are transported in the plasma compartment by several proteins, including albumin, testosterone-estradiol–binding globulin (TeBG, formerly sex steroid–binding globulin), and corticosteroid-binding globulin (CBG), each with a characteristic affinity and capacity. Albumin binds estradiol-17β (Fig. 16–2), the native female sex hormone, reversibly, with a dissociation constant (K_d) value of 10^{-5} to 10^{-6} M, whereas TeBG associates with the hormone exhibiting a (K_d) value of 10^{-7} to 10^{-8} M.

The unbound steroid enters the cell, apparently by passive diffusion, and combines with its specific receptor protein in a reaction termed *uptake* (see Fig. 16–1). This step is characterized by a high degree of ligand affinity with and specificity for the intracellular receptor. The exact location of the receptor in normal or neoplastic target cells is not clearly understood, although most data utilizing immunohistochemistry suggest a nuclear location (e.g., King and Greene, 1984; and Welshons et al., 1984). Prior to high-affinity association within the nuclear matrix, the steroid-receptor complex must be activated, which may involve phosphorylation of the receptor (Moudgil, 1985). The activated steroid hormone–receptor complex then associates with the chromatin at specific sites termed *hormone response elements* (Shepel and Gorski, 1988). This interaction stimulates RNA biosynthesis in a manner yet unknown, resulting in the formation of certain target cell proteins. Thus, the steroid receptor is a biologic prerequisite for responsiveness to hormonal perturbations; in its absence, alterations in macromolecular synthesis do not occur at physiologic hormone concentrations. Normal breast cells contain specific binding proteins for estrogen, progestin, glucocorticoids, and androgens in variable quantities, depending on the stage of mammary gland differentiation (Wittliff, 1975; and Moudgil, 1985, 1994). Representative examples of radiochemically labeled ligands for estrogen and progestin receptors are shown in Figure 16–2.

HORMONE RECEPTOR ANALYSIS

Tissue specimens should be transported from the operating suite and pathology laboratory to the clinical chemistry laboratory either frozen or chilled in a Petri dish or plastic bag placed in ice. If possible, the specimen should be frozen immediately upon excision at the time of frozen section diagnosis; however, specimens transported directly to the pathologist for permanent section should be processed quickly and chilled to retard receptor degradation. Recent studies indicate that the half-lives of estrogen and progestin receptors are highly variable in intact tumor specimens, ranging from as little as 30 minutes to no change in 6 hours at room temperature (Wittliff, 1987). Generally, the tissue should be frozen within 30 to 45 minutes after surgery and, preferably, maintained on ice or in a refrigerator in the interim. If a specimen is to be shipped to a distant laboratory for analysis, the snap-cap vials used by electron microscopists for grid storage are superb for freezing in liquid nitrogen or on dry ice. This treatment preserves receptor activity for ligand binding, *enzyme-linked immunoassay* (EIA), and immunohistochemistry (e.g., Wittliff, 1987).

The pathologist plays an important role in preserving the biologic integrity of the specimen until it arrives in the laboratory. The specimen sent for steroid receptor analyses should be representative of the tumor and large enough for receptor analysis. Usually 200 to 400 mg of tumor is required to determine both estrogen and progestin receptors by either ligand binding or EIA (Pasic et al., 1990). This size specimen allows sufficient cytosol for analyses of the protease cathepsin D and c-*erb* B-2 protein as well (Wittliff et al., 1991). Regional intratumor differences in steroid receptor status have been observed (Locher et al., 1984; and Meyer and Wittliff, 1991) emphasizing the need for submission of a representative sample. These results and others (Wittliff and Savlov, 1975; Meyer, 1986; and Meyer and Wittliff, 1977, 1983) suggest a clonal heterogeneity relative to receptor status.

Because human breast tumors are heterogeneous with regard to cell type, the author and colleagues examined the relationship between estrogen-binding capacity and the proportion of tumor epithelium in a breast biopsy specimen (Wittliff et al., 1976). No apparent correlation existed between the quantity of estrogen receptors in a biopsy specimen and the proportion of tumor epithelium. It was noted, first, that numerous specimens containing less than 25% tumor epithelium exhibited very great estrogen-binding capacity. Second, the results indicated that the specific estrogen-binding capacities of individual tumor specimens containing the same quantity of tumor epithelium were highly variable. The quantity of estrogen receptors in these tumors varied from undetectable levels to several hundred femtomoles (fmol = 10^{-15} moles) per milligram of cytosol pro-

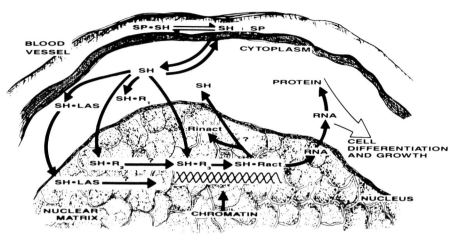

Figure 16–1. Proposed intracellular cascade of events following steroid hormone interaction with its receptor in a target cell. Steroid hormones (SH) normally circulate in the blood bound to albumin and certain specific serum proteins (SP) such as testosterone-estradiol–binding globulin (TeBG) and corticosteroid-binding globulin (CBG). Being lipids, steroids move across the cell membrane into the cytoplasm in a passive fashion and interact with their intracellular receptor proteins (R) in a reaction exhibiting high affinity and specificity. The exact location of the true receptor protein is unknown, but possibilities include sites associated with the nuclear membrane (R_1), nuclear matrix (R_2), and the chromatin (R_3). Following association with the steroid, activation takes place, which may involve phosphorylation. The activated steroid-receptor complex (Sh·Ract) associates with acceptor sites in chromatin and stimulates the synthesis of nucleic acids and subsequently proteins characteristic of the biologic response (differentiation and growth) to the specific steroid hormone. In addition, steroid hormones may associate with low-affinity sites (LAS), whose subsequent pathway is uncertain. The presence of a receptor protein in a cell appears to be a prerequisite for response to a steroid hormone stimulus.

tein. Although it may be expected that the estrogen-binding capacity of normal mammary gland increases with increasing cellularity, this is not true of breast cancers. Thus, the quantitative differences in estrogen-binding capacity are not due simply to the number of tumor cells in a biopsy specimen. Rather, this variation in activity reflects differences in the number of binding sites per breast tumor cell. Numerous

studies using immunohistochemistry now confirm this using monoclonal antibodies directed against the receptor proteins (cf. Symposium on estrogen receptor determination, 1986). This author has long recommended that, routinely, a small sample of the biopsy material sent for receptor analysis be fixed and stained to confirm the presence of tumor and its pathology (Wittliff et al., 1972, 1976).

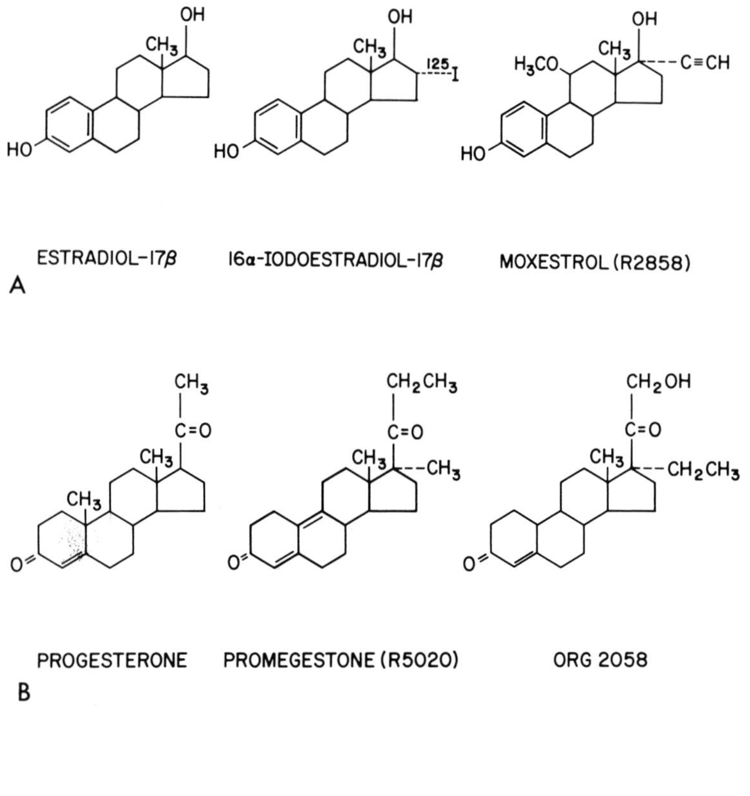

ESTRADIOL–17β   l6α–IODOESTRADIOL–17β   MOXESTROL (R2858)

A

Figure 16–2. Ligands used in the determination of estrogen receptors, *A*, and progestin receptors, *B*.

PROGESTERONE   PROMEGESTONE (R5020)   ORG 2058

B

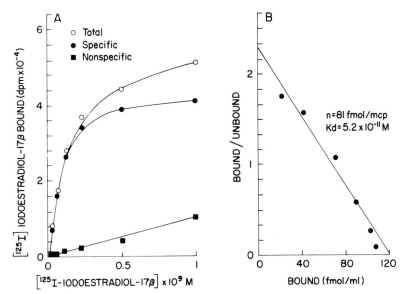

Figure 16–3. Titration analysis of estrogen receptors in human breast carcinoma. *A*, Aliquots (0.1 mL) of cytosol prepared from frozen human breast tumors were incubated in triplicate with 0.1 mL ^{125}I-iodoestradiol-17β solutions in homogenization buffer containing increasing amounts of radioactive ligand, in either the absence (○) or the presence (■) of a 200-fold excess of unlabeled diethylstilbestrol. Specific binding (●) was estimated as the difference between total binding (○) and binding in the presence of the competitor (■). *B*, The titration data from *A* were plotted according to the method of Scatchard. This dissociation constant (K_d) determined from the slope of the curve was 5.2 × 10^{-11} M for this preparation. The specific binding capacity (*n*) of the estrogen receptor complexes was estimated from the intercept on the *x* axis and gave a value of 81 fmol/mg of cytosol protein. (Reproduced by permission from Wittliff, J. L.: Steroid hormone receptors. *In* Pesce, A., and Kaplan, L. (Eds.): Clinical Chemistry Methods. St. Louis, C. V. Mosby, 1987.)

After the biopsy specimen arrives in the laboratory, an extract is made of the tumor cells by homogenization in buffer. The thermostability of steroid receptors in tumor specimens has been difficult to assess, owing partially to the heterogeneous nature of the tissue and the quantity of steroid receptors. It is clear, however, from studies in vitro that steroid receptors are labile proteins that undergo degradation or ligand dissociation in a temperature-dependent manner (Wittliff, 1975, 1987). Association of the ligand with the receptor clearly aids in stabilization, which suggests that the interval between cytosol preparation and introduction of the ligand should be as short as possible. Addition of sodium molybdate to the homogenized and buffered mixture also helps to stabilize receptors released during cellular extraction (Raam and Teixeira, 1985).

Other aspects of tissue selection include a comparison of receptor levels in tumors obtained from fresh mastectomy specimens and in biopsy specimens (Meyer et al., 1983). Apparently only a small reduction occurs in the proportion of estrogen receptor–positive tumors from mastectomy specimens compared with biopsy specimens, suggesting that either source is clinically useful if the specimen is maintained properly.

Ligand Titration Technique

The two accepted methods for quantitative determination of steroid receptors are ligand titration and the sucrose gradient analysis (DeSombre et al., 1979; and Wittliff, 1984, 1987). The titration procedure is the most commonly employed and uses labeled steroid (Fig. 16–2) with dextran-

coated charcoal to remove steroid that is not bound to intracellular receptors (Fig. 16–3).

The location of steroid receptors in a target cell continues to be debated, although increasing evidence suggests a nuclear association (King and Greene, 1984; and Welshons et al., 1984). Receptors are soluble proteins found in cytosolic extracts of target cells. Cytosol is accepted as an operational definition referring to the soluble portion of the cell, both nuclear and cytoplasmic. Most steroid receptors exist in the presence of other binding components, complicating measurements of their binding properties. Receptors associate with their particular steroid hormone in a reversible fashion and with high affinity and ligand specificity.

$$\text{Ligand + Receptor} \underset{k_{-1}}{\overset{k_1}{\rightleftharpoons}} \text{[Ligand-Receptor]}$$

$$\downarrow k_3 \qquad\qquad\qquad \downarrow k_2$$

$$\text{degradation} \qquad\qquad \text{degradation}$$

The rates of association and dissociation of steroid hormones with specific binding sites in cytosol from a target tissue depend on incubation time and temperature.

For example, the binding of ^{3}H-estradiol to its receptor is maximal after 4 hours at 0° to 3° C and remains virtually unchanged for 16 additional hours of incubation. At 25° C, apparent equilibrium is reached in 30 minutes and is maintained for 30 additional minutes before a gradual loss in binding activity is observed. Presumably, this loss is due to the degradation of the receptor protein itself, whether or not its binding sites are occupied by steroid, though it is possible that irreversible dissociation of the steroid receptor complexes also occurs in some tumors. As a result of the temperature sensitivity of the estrogen receptor and progestin receptor complexes, the majority of binding reactions are performed at 0° to 3° C.

To demonstrate the affinity and concentration of steroid receptors in a cytosol preparation, aliquots are incubated with increasing concentrations of various labeled steroids for 5 to 18 hours at 0° to 3° C (see Fig. 16–2). Routinely, 2,4,6,7-^{3}H-estradiol-17β and 17-methyl-^{3}H-promegestone (R5020) are used as labeled ligands to measure estrogen and progestin receptors, respectively (see Fig. 16–3). An iodine-125–labeled estrogen (see Fig. 16–2) has been synthesized, which is also a satisfactory ligand for estrogen receptor determinations (Hochberg, 1979). Binding observed in the presence of an excess of unlabeled inhibitor is related to nonreceptor or nonspecific (low-affinity, high-capacity) association of the ligand. Specific binding is estimated as the difference between total and nonspecific binding (see Fig. 16–3). The use of a double-label procedure also increases sensitivity (Grill et al., 1984; and Folk and Wittliff, 1992).

Using Scatchard analysis, the dissociation constant (K_d) or the association constant (K_a) may be determined from the slope of the plot according to the following equation:

$$\text{Slope} = 1/K_d, \text{ where } K_d = 1/K_a = k_{-1}/k_1$$

Here, k_1 represents the rate constant for the association reaction, while k_{-1} represents the rate constant for dissociation. The binding capacity is estimated from the intercept of the abscissa. By definition, the higher the affinity of the binding site, the lower the dissociation constant, which is a measure of the tendency of the steroid receptor complex to dissociate. The rate of this first-order process is highly dependent on both the type of ligand used in the assay and the kind of receptor being measured (Table 16–1). When K_d values of 10^{-10} to 10^{-11} M for the estrogen receptors and of 10^{-9} to 10^{-10} M for progestin receptors are found on a patient's chart, they indicate that the biopsy specimen contains high-affinity components.

Usually specific binding capacity is expressed in femtomoles of labeled steroid bound per milligram of cytosol protein. It is generally accepted that less than 3 fmol/mg

cytosol protein represents a quantity correlated with the lack of response of a breast cancer patient to endocrine therapy of either the ablative or additive type (NIH consensus development conference, 1980; Wittliff, 1984). Although there is a ''borderline'' range of values from 3 to 10 or 20 fmol/mg cytosol protein, estrogen-binding capacities of more than 10 fmol of estrogen appear to represent a clinically significant level (Fisher et al., 1981, 1983). The author's group has observed values of more than 5000 fmol/mg cytosol protein for the estrogen receptor and 6000 fmol/mg cytosol protein for progestin receptors in certain tumors (Table 16–2). The levels of estrogen receptors in breast tumor biopsy specimens from premenopausal patients appear considerably lower than those from postmenopausal women. In general, greater progestin-binding capacity was observed in tumor specimens from both premenopausal and postmenopausal women when the estrogen receptor was present in the tumor; however, a lower progestin receptor level was measured in the absence of estrogen receptors, supporting the suggestion that the formation of the progestin receptors is dependent on estrogen action (Horwitz et al., 1975).

Sucrose Gradient Technique

Sucrose gradient centrifugation separates the various isoforms of the steroid receptors (Fig. 16–4). This method, which is largely used for research currently, demonstrated that the sedimentation profiles of both estrogen and progestin receptors in human breast carcinomas fall into four categories (Wittliff, 1974): tumors that contain specific steroid-binding components that migrate at either 8 Svedberg units (S) only, at 4 S only, or at both 8 and 4 S (see Fig. 16–4), and those in which receptors are undetectable. The sedimentation coefficients of 8 and 4 S are only approximate and are used operationally. Most breast tumors containing estrogen receptors exhibit both the 8 and 4 S isoforms (see Fig. 16–4). Some 10% to 15% of biopsy specimens contain only the 4 S specimens using sucrose gradient centrifugation with conditions of low ionic strength (Wittliff et al., 1978). Since two kinds of steroid receptors exist, and each has four different types of profiles, there are at least 16 possible combinations.

Table 16–1. STEROID HORMONES AND ANALOGUES USED AS LIGANDS FOR STEROID HORMONE RECEPTORS

Estrogen Receptors	Progestin Receptors	Androgen Receptors	Glucocorticoid Receptors
^{3}H-estradiol-17β*	^{3}H-progesterone	^{3}H-testosterone	^{3}H-hydrocortisone
^{3}H-estrone	^{3}H-R5020 (promegestone)*	^{3}H-5α-dihydrotestosterone	^{3}H-corticosterone
^{3}H-estriol	^{3}H-R27987	^{3}H-R1881	^{3}H-dexamethasone*
^{125}I-iodoestradiol-17β*	^{3}H-Org 2058	(methyltrienolone)*	^{3}H-dexamethasone
^{3}H-R2858 (moxestrol)	^{3}H-medroxyprogesterone	^{3}H-cyproterone acetate	mesylate
^{3}H-tamoxifen	acetate	^{3}H-mibolerone*	^{3}H-triamcinolone
^{3}H-tamoxifen-40H			acetonide*
^{3}H-tamoxifen aziridine			

*Most often employed in clinical assays.

(Reproduced by permission from Wittliff, J. L.: Clinical analysis of steroid hormone receptors. *In* Pesce, A., and Kaplan L. (eds.): Clinical Chemistry—Methods. St. Louis, C. V. Mosby, 1987.)

Table 16-2. SPECIFIC BINDING CAPACITIES OF STEROID RECEPTORS IN BREAST TUMOR BIOPSY SPECIMENS ACCORDING TO PATIENT ENDOCRINE STATUS

Steroid-Binding Capacity	(fmol/mg Cytosol Protein)*	Endocrine Status of Patient	Receptor Status of Tumor
Estrogen	Progestin		
90 ± 9 (10–1335)	237 ± 22 (10–3038)	Premenopausal	ER+, PR+
83 ± 16 (10–568)	—	Premenopausal	ER+, PR−
—	84 ± 18 (10–1151)	Premenopausal	ER−, PR+
286 ± 18 (10–5693)	337 ± 28 (10–5922)	Postmenopausal	ER+, PR+
176 ± 29 (10–2807)	—	Postmenopausal	ER+, PR−
—	75 ± 26 (10–977)	Postmenopausal	ER−, PR+

*Measured by multipoint titration analyses using Scatchard plots. Mean ± standard error of the mean of number of determinations shown in Table 16-6. Range shown in parentheses. A level of > 10 frmol/mg cytosol protein was taken as an arbitrary cut-off point for the presence of receptors as utilized by the NSABP (Fisher et al., 1983).
(From Wittliff, J. L.: Steroid hormone receptors in breast cancer. Cancer, *53*:630, 1984. Reprinted with permission.)

Experimental Methods

Since experimental methods were reviewed in detail in several reports (Wittliff, 1985, 1986, 1987; and Wittliff and Wiehle, 1985), only brief mention will be made of them here. Table 16–3 outlines various methods of steroid receptor determination that may be used with the ligands listed in Table 16–1.

Steroid receptors are dynamic proteins whose properties of size, shape, surface charge, and hydrophobicity vary with conditions in their environment. Using various types of chromatography, these properties can be exploited so that the various species (isoforms) of the receptors can be separated. Early chromatographic methods used conventional gel filtration and ion-exchange chromatography (Wittliff, 1975); however, because of the extended time required for separation, many of the receptor species reported may have been products of reactions that occurred with the packing matrices or as a result of the long incubation times.

To circumvent the problem of prolonged manipulation in receptor preparations, high-performance liquid chromatography (HPLC) for size exclusion, ion exchange, chromatofocusing, and hydrophobic interaction modes were developed for rapid, effective separation of receptor isoforms, (Wittliff, 1985, 1986, 1987; and Wittliff and Wiehle, 1985).

HPLC separation has shown that receptors exhibit polymorphism. This indicates that their composition is far more complicated than was originally assumed. The author suggested the use of the term *fractionated receptors* to designate the pattern of the various steroid hormone–binding components (isoforms) displayed by a single receptor type (Wittliff, 1984). Sophisticated separation procedures, such as HPLC and Western blotting techniques, will be the new generation of methods for assay of steroid receptor isoforms and variants in a tumor specimen.

A representative profile of estrogen receptor isoforms separated on the basis of properties of size and shape using higher-performance size exclusion chromatography (HPSEC) is shown in Figure 16–5. Note the large variation in molecular weights of the receptor isoforms, similar to that seen with sucrose gradient centrifugation (see Fig. 16–4).

Polymorphism of steroid hormone receptors also may be demonstrated by separating isoforms on the basis of surface charge properties using either ion exchange chromatography (HPIEC) (Wittliff and Wiehle, 1985) or chromatofocusing (HPCF) (Wittliff, 1986). Representative profiles of receptor isoforms are shown in Figures 16–6 and 16–7, which illustrate the two separation modes. The molecular heterogeneity of receptors in a tumor extract are easily

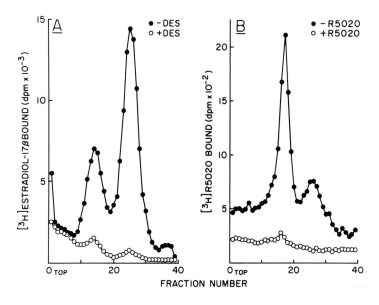

Figure 16–4. Sucrose density gradient separation of the isoforms of estrogen and progestin (R5020) receptors in human breast carcinoma. Tumor cytosol was reacted either with ³H-estradiol-17β, *A*, or with ³H-R5020, *B*, for 4 hours at 3° C in the presence (○) or absence (●) of a 200-fold excess of unlabeled competitor. Note the presence of both 8 S and 4 S forms of these steroid receptors in the single breast carcinoma analyzed. (Reprinted with permission from The Clinical Biochemistry of Cancer. Washington, D.C., American Association for Clinical Chemistry, Inc. 1979.)

Table 16–3. METHODS OF DETERMINING PRESENCE OF STEROID HORMONE RECEPTORS

Method	Principle	Usage	Comments
Titration	Sample incubated with increasing amounts of labeled steroid, with and without the presence of unlabeled inhibitor. Amount of specific binding plotted by Scatchard plot and the total number of binding sites and dissociation constant (K_d) are calculated.	Frequently used	Requires largest sample size Results dependent on ligand used
Sucrose density gradient	Molecular forms of receptors of different sizes are separated on sucrose gradient following centrifugation. Location and number of sites present are determined by labeled ligand binding (with and without inhibitor).	Infrequently used	Cannot calculate K_d by this method
High-performance liquid chromatography (HPLC) methods	Different receptor isoforms are separated by specific molecular property of receptors.	Research of molecular properties	Calculation of K_d values approximate by these methods
Size exclusion	Following binding with labeled ligand, receptors are separated on basis of molecular size and shape.		
Ion exchange	Following binding with labeled ligand, receptors are separated on basis of their surface charge properties.		
Chromatofocusing	Following binding with labeled ligand, receptors are separated on basis of their isoelectric points.		
Hydrophobic interaction	Following binding with labeled ligand, receptors are separated on basis of different surface hydrophobicity.		
Immunofluorescence	Fluorescein-labeled steroid is bound to tissue steroid receptors. Amount of bound steroid is visualized by fluorescence microscopy.	Rare, experimental	Used for qualitative identification on small tissue biopsy specimens
Immunohistochemistry	Monoclonal antibody, specific for a steroid receptor, binds to tissue steroid receptor. Second antibody, labeled with peroxidase, is used to localize first antibody binding. Visualization of receptor in tissue with substrates for peroxidase stain.	Most frequent alternative to titration method	Used for qualitative identification on small tissue samples
Enzyme-linked immunoassay	Sandwich assay with immobilized monoclonal antibody to receptor. Following binding of specific receptor, second monoclonal antibody labeled with horseradish peroxidase is bound. Quantitation using appropriate substrate is performed.	Frequently used	Cannot be used to calculate K_d

(Reproduced by permission from Wittliff, J. L.: Clinical analyses of steroid hormone receptors. *In* Presce, A., and Kaplan, L. (Eds.): Clinical Chemistry—Methods. St. Louis, C. V. Mosby, 1987.)

detected in hours, and a small tissue sample (100 mg) is satisfactory for a complete assay. Table 16–4 summarizes some of the molecular properties of estrogen receptors in breast cells.

The clinical significance of receptor isoform or variant profiles is currently the subject of considerable research in our group. Various physiologic conditions appear to alter the relative amounts and distribution of isoforms of both estrogen and progestin receptors. Some of these parameters

include the patient's age, endocrine status, and history of therapeutic manipulation. Application of "fractionated receptor" profiles to clinical management of breast cancer must await additional investigation.

Fluorescein-Linked Steroid Ligands

Often breast carcinomas that contain an insufficient amount of tissue for titration analysis of estrogen and progestin

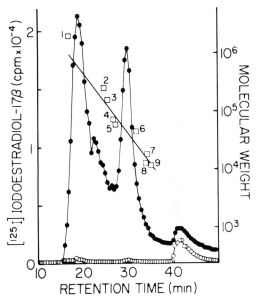

Figure 16–5. Identification and characterization of isoforms of the estrogen receptor from human breast cancer by high-performance size exclusion chromatography (HPSEC). Cytosol was prepared from a sample of human breast cancer and incubated with 3 to 4 nM of ^{125}I-iodoestradiol-17β in the presence (○) and absence (●) of excess diethylstilbestrol (DES). A 200-μL aliquot of incubate was cleared of free steroid with dextran-coated charcoal and applied to a TSK 3000 SW chromatography column. Hemoglobin was added to all samples before analysis or reanalysis as an internal marker. In addition, the HPSEC system was calibrated using a series of pure proteins: (1) thyroglobulin, (2) catalase, (3) aldolase, (4) bovine serum albumin, (5) hemoglobin, (6) ovalbumin, (7) lysozyme, (8) myoglobin, and (9) cytochrome C. (From Wittliff, J. L., and Wiehle, R. D.: Analytical methods for steroid hormone receptors and their quality assurance. *In* Hollander, V. P. (Ed.): Hormonally Responsive Tumors. New York, Academic Press, 1985, p. 383. Reprinted with permission.)

receptors are discovered. Another approach to estimating the level of receptors in small biopsy specimens has been the use of fluorescein-linked steroid hormones (Chamness et al., 1980). This provides a nonradiochemical means of detecting receptors in histologic preparations of breast and endometrial cancer. The method involves the incubation of tissue slices with a fluorescein-linked estrogen and the visualization of the ''receptor-bound'' steroid under a fluorescence microscope.

Although the use of a fluorescein-linked steroid as a ligand for steroid hormone receptors would be desirable, especially for tissue biopsy sections of tumors, this procedure has been employed with very little success (Lonsdorfer et al., 1983). Thus far, the use of these compounds has two major disadvantages: (1) formation of estradiol as a derivative in the 17β position reduces the affinity of the ligand for the specific binding sites on the receptor and (2) bonds between the fluorescent steroid ligand and the spacer are labile, so assessment of the affinity constant is made difficult because of the presence of contaminated free estradiol. The unequivocal determination of estrogen receptors in tissue preparations has not been possible because of these and other complicating factors such as tissue autofluorescence and low-affinity association (Berns et al., 1984).

Immunocytochemical Techniques

Most immunohistochemical techniques for localization of steroid hormone receptors use highly specific monoclonal antibodies directed against the partially purified receptor (Greene et al., 1980). Sections of freshly frozen tumor samples are prepared in a cryostat, and the slides are immersed immediately in 3.7% formaldehyde phosphate–buffered saline at 25° C for 10 minutes. The tissue sections are then transferred to 100% methanol for 4 minutes at −10° C, followed by a 1-minute soak at −10° C in acetone. A peroxidase-antiperoxidase method for immunocytochemical staining has been employed. Normal goat serum serves as the blocking antibody, and the primary antibody is a monoclonal antibody to human estrogen receptor (e.g., Greene et al., 1980, 1984; and King and Greene, 1984). The bridging antibody is goat antirat immunoglobulin; thus, the peroxi-

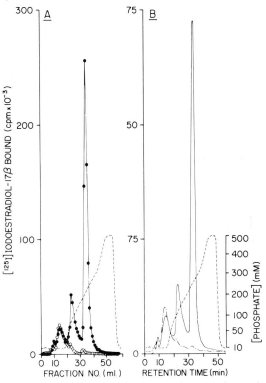

Figure 16–6. High-performance ion exchange chromatography (HPIEC) separation of ionic isoforms of estrogen receptors from human breast cancer. Cytosol was prepared and incubated with 5 nM ^{125}I-iodoestradiol-17β, as described earlier. Elution of the AX-1000 ion exchange column was performed on 200 μL of cytosol cleared of unbound ligand at 1.0 mL/min using a gradient of potassium phosphate at pH 7.4 *(dashed line).* A, Fractions of 1 mL were collected and radioactivity was measured manually with a gamma counter. B, Radioactivity was recorded continuously using the Beckman Model 170 radioisotope detector on line with a conductivity flow cell. Total binding is indicated by ● in *A* and by a solid line in *B,* and nonspecific binding is indicated by ○ in *A* and by -●-, in *B.* Recovery rate of radioactivity from the column was 97%. Specific binding was 167 fmol of receptor/mg cytosol protein determined by multipoint titration analysis. (From Boyle, D. M., et al.: Rapid, high-resolution procedure for assessment of estrogen receptor heterogeneity in clinical samples. J. Chromatogr., *327:*369, 1985. Reprinted with permission.)

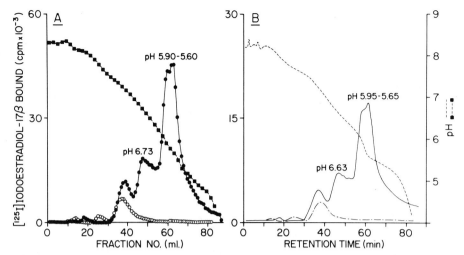

Figure 16–7. High-performance chromatofocusing (HPCF) separation of ionic isoforms of estrogen receptors from human breast cancer. The sample of breast tissue and conditions used in this experiment were the same as described in the legend to Figure 16–6. The curves of bound ^{125}I-iodoestradiol-17β shown are the results of receptors separated in the presence (● in *A;* -●-● in *B*) or absence (○ in *A;* — in *B*) of 200-fold excess of DES. Elution of the AX-500 column by a pH gradient was performed isocratically on 200 μL of cleared cytosol at 1.0 mL/min. The pH gradient is indicated as ■ in *A* and as — in *B*. *A,* Fractions of 1 mL were collected and radioactivity or pH was measured manually. *B,* Radioactivity and pH were recorded continuously using on-line Model 170 radioisotope detector with flow-through electrode. Recovery rate of radioactivity from the column was 97%. Specific binding was 167 fmol of receptor/mg cytosol protein, determined by multipoint titration analysis. (From Boyle, D. M., et al.: Rapid, high-resolution procedure for assessment of estrogen receptor heterogeneity in clinical samples. *J. Chromatogr., 327;369,* 1985. Reprinted with permission.)

dase-antiperoxidase complex must be of rat origin. Serial sections of breast tissue should be prepared as control slides by incubation with rat immunoglobulin. Peroxidase activity is detected by use of the substrate diaminobenzidine. Evaluation of the immunohistochemical analysis is largely qualitative, though some workers (McCarty et al., 1985) divide the percentage of positively stained epithelial cells into various intensity categories using a system of 0, 1+, 2+, and so on.

Although this represents a nonradiochemical means of detecting these receptors in histologic preparations of tumors, the method is largely qualitative. The procedure is being developed as a more quantitative test that requires calibration with conventional ligand-binding assays and enzyme immunoassay (King et al., 1985; and McCarty et al., 1985). It is unclear whether these commercially prepared monoclonal antibodies (Abbott Laboratories, North Chicago, IL) react with the various isoforms of the steroid

Table 16–4. COMPARISON OF PROPERTIES OF ESTROGEN RECEPTORS SEPARATED BY CONVENTIONAL METHODS AND VARIOUS MODES OF HPLC

Tissue	Sucrose Density Gradient Centrifugation	Sephacryl S-300	HPSEC (TSK 3000 SW Column)	DEAE-Celulose	HPIEC (AX-1000 Column)	HPCF (AX-500 Column)
Human breast carcinoma	4-5 S and 8-9 S*		>61 A and 29-32 A§	0.03 M KCl 0.09 M KCl 0.22 M KCl‖	52, 100, 190 mM phosphate**	pH 6.3, 5.3 4.8-3.5 shoulder††
MCF-7 cells	4-5 S and 8-9 S†	85 A and 65-70 A†	68 A†		55 and 180 mM phosphate†	pH 6.3 and 4.3†
Rat lactating mammary gland	4-5 S and 8-9 S‡	>85 A, 70-72 A, and 28-30 A	>61 A§	0.02-0.05 M MCl 0.18-0.20 M KCl¶	90 and 205 mM phosphate**	pH 6.8 and 6.5†‡

*Wittliff et al. (1972).
†Shahabi et al. (1984).
‡Wittliff (1975).
§Wiehle et al. (1984).
‖Kute et al. (1978).
¶Wittliff et al. (1978).
**Wiehle and Wittliff (1984).
††Boyle et al. (1985).
‡‡Hutchens et al. (1983).
   HPSEC, High performance size exclusion chromatography; DEAE, Diethylaminoethylcellulose; HPIEC, high performance ion exchange chromatography; HPCF, high performance chromatofocusing; S, Svedberg units; A, Angstrom; KCl, potassium chloride.

hormone receptors to the same extent (Sato et al., 1986). The immunohistochemical procedure may be used with specimens that are too small (e.g., 10 to 50 mg) for conventional quantitative receptor analysis. A technique (Hedley, 1987; and Helin, 1989) that permits flow cytometric and sex steroid–receptor analyses on paraffin-embedded tissue allows archival tissue to be evaluated.

Enzyme-Linked Immunochemical Assay

This procedure is based on a "sandwich" technique that involves two specific monoclonal antibodies generated against different epitopes of the sex hormone receptors (Greene et al., 1980, 1984). The first antibody is immobilized on a polystyrene bead. Cytosol is prepared in either Tris or phosphate buffer containing 5 to 10 mM sodium molybdate and incubated with the polystyrene bead for 18 hours at 3° C. After incubation and complexing of the receptor with the monoclonal antibody, the bead is washed and a second monoclonal antibody that has previously been labeled with horseradish peroxidase is incubated with the bead. The peroxidase enzyme linked to the second antibody serves as a marker for the presence of the receptor protein. The intensity of the color produced as a result of the enzymatic action of the horseradish peroxidase on the substrate indicates the quantity of the receptor present in the cytosol.

This procedure measures the mass of the receptor, in contrast to radioligand-binding techniques, which measure steroid-binding capacity and affinity. However, most workers relate the enzyme immunoassay results to specific steroid-binding capacity, expressed as femtomoles per milligram of cytosol protein. There appears to be considerable variation in the receptor levels measured by the multipoint titration assay as compared with that observed with EIA (Mirecki and Jordan, 1985; Nakao et al., 1985; Raam and Vrabel, 1986; and Pasic et al., 1990) with a greater receptor level by the EIA method. The molecular basis of this difference is unclear and requires further investigation.

Quality Control of Steroid Receptor Analyses

For years, the lack of uniformity in the methods of receptor analyses in the clinical laboratory and in the expression of specific steroid-binding data was a problem (Wittliff et al., 1980, 1981a; Sarfaty et al., 1981; and Leclercq et al., 1984). Some common sources of variability in steroid receptor analyses are these:

1. Type and range of steroid ligand concentrations
2. Concentration and type of competitive inhibitor
3. Incubation time and temperature
4. Concentration of cytosol protein and type of assay selected

Other parameters that may complicate steroid receptor analyses if not properly controlled are these:

1. Metabolism of the ligand
2. Contribution of nonspecific (low-affinity, high-capacity) binding
3. Ligand-receptor dissociation
4. Ligand association with specific serum proteins such as TeBG and CBG
5. Thermal lability both in the biopsy and cell-free preparations
6. Ion strength lability
7. Occupancy of binding sites by endogenous hormone
8. Receptor "inhibiting" substances
9. Proteolysis

To ensure accurate quantification of the number of steroid-binding sites in a biopsy specimen using a titration procedure and dextran-coated charcoal to remove unbound steroid, it is necessary to use a broad range of ligand concentrations. These must include a sufficient number of points below the saturation level so that an interpretable Scatchard plot is generated (see Fig. 16–3). If too many saturating concentrations of either ^{3}H-estradiol or ^{3}H-R5020 are employed, the points will be "grouped" near the abscissa of the Scatchard plot, making it difficult to estimate the dissociation constant. However, the number of specific binding sites will be estimated in a reasonable manner.

Other common sources of variation are the concentration and type of competitive inhibitor used to estimate the contribution of nonspecific (low-affinity, high-capacity) binding. It appears this is largely due to contamination of tumor biopsy specimens by necrotic material and blood, which may contain albumin and other proteins, such as TeBG and CBG, known to associate specifically with steroid hormones (Wittliff et al, 1979.) Diethylstilbestrol (DES) is a potent synthetic estrogen that does not bind to plasma proteins with high affinity. Thus, it is a useful inhibitor in estrogen receptor analyses (see Fig. 16–3), as it associates only with intracellular binding components. The dissociation constant (K_d) of the DES receptor complexes in cytosol from breast tumors is approximately 10^{-9} M, which is higher than that of estradiol receptor complexes (Wittliff et al., 1978, 1979). Routinely, the author uses a 200-fold excess of unlabeled DES in a titration assay.

A similar quantity (200-fold excess) of unlabeled R5020, a synthetic progestin, is utilized with ^{3}H-R5020 to estimate low-affinity, high-capacity binding. Since R5020 and certain glucocorticoids may associate with similar binding sites (McGuire et al., 1977), it is advisable to use low nanomolar (nM) concentrations of ^{3}H-R5020, to avoid also measuring glucocorticoid receptors (Horwitz and McGuire, 1975). The principal advantage of utilizing ^{3}H-R5020 as a ligand for the progestin receptor is that it does not associate to any great extent with CBG, known to bind progesterone, the natural progestin (Wittliff et al., 1981a). Furthermore, it does not dissociate readily from the progestin receptor of mammary gland, as has been observed for progesterone, nor is it metabolized under the conditions of most clinical assays (Wittliff et al., 1981*a*).

If the sucrose gradient procedure (see Fig. 16–4) is used to quantify steroid receptors, the investigator must be sure to use a saturating concentration of the labeled ligand, usually 3 to 5 nM for either estradiol-17β or R5020, as suggested from titration analyses (see Fig. 16–2). Furthermore, it is imperative to use a competitive inhibitor of ligand binding to estimate the receptor proteins clearly. Because albumin and other contaminating proteins sediment in the 4 to 5 S region of the sucrose gradient, where certain receptor species migrate as well (see Fig. 16–4), the receptor's specificity should be evaluated, using the newer techniques of HPLC for receptor isoform separation (Wittliff and Wiehle, 1985; and Wittliff, 1985, 1986). Unlabeled inhibitors are also employed to ensure specificity (see Figs. 16–5 to 16–7).

Quality Assurance Programs

Currently, estrogen and progestin receptors are analyzed annually in tens of thousands of breast tumor biopsy specimens in the United States. To examine the correlations of these data with responses to specific therapeutic techniques, certain clinical cooperative groups, particularly the National Surgical Adjuvant Breast and Bowel Project (NSABP) and the Southeastern Cancer Study Group (SECSG), in the late 1970s initiated experimental therapeutic protocols requiring analyses of estrogen and progestin receptors of breast tumors (Wittliff et al., 1980, 1981a). Thus, the establishment of assay uniformity and quality control was imperative to ensure meaningful correlations between laboratory results and clinical response.

Among the conclusions drawn from the 1979 NIH Consensus Development Conference on Steroid Receptors in Breast Cancer (DeSombre et al., 1979; NIH Consensus development conference on steroid receptors, 1980) was this: "There is a need for quality control of steroid receptor assays."

Regarding this point, in 1977 the author's laboratory (Wittliff et al., 1980, 1981a) developed a national reference program for establishing uniformity in steroid receptor analyses. A variety of tissue reference powders were prepared that were composed of various quantities of frozen, pulverized organs such as uterus, breast, muscle, and liver, as well as certain types of sera (e.g., of pregnancy), using tissue grinders and liquid nitrogen. Breast tumors also were added to certain powders. Each reference powder was formulated to contain different combinations of estrogen and progestin receptors (e.g., estrogen receptor positive, progestin receptor negative; estrogen receptor positive, progestin receptor positive, and so forth) at different test levels. The exact composition was based on the specific need of each clinical cooperative trial group. Thus far, this laboratory has cooperated with the NSABP, SECSG, Southwest Oncology Group (SWOG), Cancer and Leukemia Group B (CALGB), North Central Cancer Treatment Group (NCCTG), Eastern Cooperative Oncology Group (ECOG), and the College of American Pathologists to bring about greater uniformity in the analyses of steroid receptors and the expression of binding capacity data. Currently, more than 400 laboratories in North America have participated in this quality assurance program. The author's group has also cooperated with laboratories on virtually every continent to bring about standardized methods (Wittliff, 1987) and quality assessment of results for clinical management of breast cancer.

Briefly, a laboratory from an institution participating in a treatment trial of one of the cooperative groups was sent a set of two to four different tissue powders frozen in dry ice. Often, three vials of each powder were included to evaluate the intra-assay variability of each receptor measurement. A vial of unknown protein concentration was included to assess the influence of variation in this important determination. The laboratory analyzed these using "in-house" methods and returned the results to the headquarters of the cooperative group for comparison with data generated by other laboratories and by the reference laboratory. Criteria for evaluating agreement of the results were established by committees in each of the cooperative groups. Either the committee or the reference laboratory reported to each participating laboratory on its performance relative to that of the other laboratories participating in the clinical trial. A representative survey report is shown in Table 16–5. This information is available to physicians by contacting the author's reference laboratory. It is essential that receptor assays on breast tumor tissue be conducted by laboratories that meet the compliance criteria of one or more of the quality assurance programs. Currently our laboratory conducts a volunteer survey and a biennial survey for the College of American Pathologists.

FACTORS THAT INFLUENCE THE LEVEL OF STEROID RECEPTORS

Clinical and Physiologic Factors

Numerous clinical and physiologic factors must be considered when assessing the significance of a steroid receptor level: race, sex, age, menopausal status, day of cycle for premenopausal women, pregnancy and lactation, organ site, tumor cellularity and histologic differentiation, and history of drug therapy.

As discussed earlier (see Table 16–2), the concentration of estrogen receptors in biopsy specimens of infiltrating ductal carcinoma shows a broad spectrum of values, ranging from zero to almost 6000 fmol/mg cytosol protein. Thus far, no single histologic feature has been found to explain the variation in the levels of estrogen receptors in human breast cancers. Black and coworkers (1983) suggested that tumor cellularity and estrogen receptor levels were related to prognosis for operable breast cancer. The prognosis was actually better for patients with low cellularity.

Relative to histopathology, Chua and associates (1985) reported a strong correlation among estrogen receptor level, age, and histologic grade of breast tumors from women in Singapore. Silfversward and coworkers (1980) reported a positive correlation between estrogen receptor content and degree of differentiation of ductal carcinoma. Cancers associated with lymphoid infiltration generally showed low estrogen receptor levels. Other studies (Rosen et al., 1975; Wittliff et al., 1976; Meyer et al., 1977; Mills, 1980; Chabon et al., 1982; Howat et al., 1983; Ponsky et al., 1984; and Meyer and Wittliff, 1991) have investigated the relationship between pathologic features and receptor status. There is much variability in the reported results, and a well-controlled interlaboratory study is recommended for assessing the relationship of parameters such as histologic class,

Table 16–5. INTERNATIONAL ONCOLOGY GROUP, STEROID RECEPTOR REFERENCE LABORATORY, UNIVERSITY OF LOUISVILLE, SUMMARY RESULTS FROM DECEMBER 15, 1986, SHIPMENT OF TISSUE REFERENCE POWER

Laboratory	Specific Estrogen-Binding Capacity (fmol/mg Cytosol Protein)		Specific Progestin-Binding Capacity (fmol/mg Cytosol Protein)		Protein Unknown (mg/mL)
	Mean ± SD Ref. Powder I*	Mean ± SD Ref. Powder III†	Mean ± SD Ref. Powder I*	Mean ± SD Ref. Powder II†	
IN-AA	101 ± 6	0	145 ± 18	0	3.9
IN-AB	67 ± 24	4	137 ± 40	4	5.5
IN-AC	104 ± 32	18	46 ± 4	0	4.0
IN-AD	57 ± 6	0	220 ± 53	14	3.9
IN-AE	85 ± 29	0	133 ± 12	2	3.9
IN-AF	100 ± 4	0	72 ± 9	1	3.3
IN-AG	97 ± 4	2	121 ± 7	15	3.4
IN-AH	96 ± 6	2	162 ± 21	2	3.8
IN-AI	90 ± 17	0	147 ± 24	0	4.7
IN-AJ	44 ± 33	0	182 ± 31	0	6.2
U of L #1	95 ± 2	2	150 ± 8	2	3.1
Return shipment #2	104 ± 4	3	164 ± 2	3	3.0
Target values	98 ± 10	2	155 ± 5	2	3.6 ± 0.3
Kd values (× 10 − 10M)	1.9 ± 0.4		2.4 ± 0.7		(Bradford)
Participating labs	84 ± 28		137 ± 54		4.3 ± 0.9
range	44 − 104		46 − 220		3.3 − 6.2

*Reference Powder I designated as IN-225, IN-227, IN-228 (n = 3).   Reference Powder Assays n = 15
†Reference Powder II deisgnated as In-226, IN-229 (n = 2).   Reference Powder Assays n = 15
‡Sucrose density gradient centrifugation method.
Target and Kd values generated by multipoint titration analysis using dextran-coated charcoal.
Please note these were analyzed over a period of at least 10–12 weeks and may reflect some degradation.

Compliance Criteria					
Within	7 of 10	9 of 10	6 of 10	8 of 10	7 of 10
Above	0 of 10	1 of 10	1 of 10	2 of 10	3 of 10
Below	3 of 10		3 of 10		0 of 10

nuclear grade, DNA content, ploidy, and lymphocytic infiltration to receptor status. In general, it may be concluded that the presence of both estrogen and progesterone receptors implies retention of the regulatory mechanisms operating in normal breast epithelium. Thus, a loss of receptor may be taken with other neoplastic features as a means of identifying patients at increased risk of tumor recurrence or death (Parl et al., 1984).

In the author's experience, the proportion of tumor cells to surrounding connective tissue and adipose cells does not correlate with estrogen-binding capacity (Wittliff et al., 1976; and Meyer and Wittliff, 1991), although connective tissue appears to contribute to the quantity of progesterone receptors estimated in a specimen. This observation relates to the finding that fibroblasts may contain significant levels of specific progestin-binding components. For this reason, it is imperative to use a specimen that contains as much of the malignant lesion as is possible. It is known that the adipose cells of normal breast do not contain specific estrogen receptors (Wittliff, 1975), although these cells have the ability to take up a large amount of the steroid hormones, presumably because of their lipid solubility. The level of a steroid receptor in a tumor specimen can reflect either a heterogeneous cell population, in which a variable number of tumor cells exhibit hormone sensitivity, or a more homogeneous cell population in which individual cells contain variable numbers of estrogen receptor molecules. Analysis of this point is progressing through use of immunocyto-

chemical methods for detecting steroid receptors (King et al., 1985b; McCarty et al., 1985; and Symposium on estrogen receptor determinations, 1986).

Several studies have not found a correlation between steroid receptor status and either the size or location of the tumor in the breast, or the axillary node status, or the clinical stage of the disease. It was initially reported (McGuire et al., 1975) that larger tumors contained fewer estrogen receptors, presumably because of increased necrosis, but this was not supported in later, more thorough investigations (NIH Consensus Development Conference, 1980).

The endocrine status of the patient influences the endogenous concentration of estrogens in the plasma and in the tumor. Circulating estrogen and progesterone levels are known to influence the number of specific binding sites on receptor proteins occupied in vivo by the steroid hormones. Early studies by Maass and colleagues (Maass et al., 1972; and Trams and Maass, 1976) and Pollow and associates (1980) found that the estrogen-binding capacity in target organs varied during the menstrual cycle; it was low in midcycle and reduced further in the second phase. Trams and Maass and their colleagues (1976; Stegner et al., 1980) also demonstrated insignificant binding of ^{3}H-estradiol to receptors in breast tumors from patients with plasma estradiol-17β levels exceeding 300 mg/ml.

Most studies indicated that both the incidence and the concentration of steroid receptors in breast tumors were lower in premenopausal women than in postmenopausal ones (Table 16–6; see also Table 16–2). Clearly, patient age influences the level of receptors, higher concentrations being exhibited by tumors from elderly patients (Wittliff, 1974; McCarty et al., 1983; and Alghanem and Hussain, 1985). Apparently, this is partly due to the elevated levels of endogenous estrogen in plasma of premenopausal women, which may mask receptor-binding sites; however, since estrogen is known to stimulate the formation of its own receptor as well as the progesterone receptor (Horwitz and McGuire and Horowitz et al., 1975 a,b), the level of circulating estrogen may not be the only factor. Elevated circulating progesterone in premenopausal patients with breast cancer may reduce the formation of estrogen receptors in comparison with the level known to occur in postmenopausal women, whose progesterone levels are lower (NIH consensus development conference, 1980). Thus, it seems prudent to consider the menstrual status of the patient when evaluating the significance of the specific steroid-binding capacity of a tumor. EIA results of a breast specimen from a premenopausal patient appear to be particularly dependable.

In general, the levels of specific steroid receptors in specimens of metastatic breast carcinomas are similar to those observed in primary tumors (NIH consensus development conference, 1980; Wittliff and Dapunt, 1980; and Hull et al., 1983). There is general agreement that the numbers of estrogen and progestin receptors are somewhat elevated in tumor specimens from postmenopausal patients as compared with those from premenopausal women (see Table 16–6). This may be due to the fact that metastatic lesions are often less differentiated than primary breast tumors. During malignant transformation, there may have been a loss of steroid hormone receptors, reflecting a more endocrine-independent growth pattern. A few studies reported at the NIH Consensus Development Conference (1980) and later (Hull et al., 1983; Young et al., 1985) using multiple sequential biopsy specimens suggest that there may be a progressive loss of estrogen receptors in breast tumors as the disease progresses.

Hähnel and Twaddle (1985) provided an excellent review of the relationship between estrogen receptors in primary and secondary breast carcinomas and in sequential primary breast cancers. No major discordance in estrogen receptor

status was observed in 48 cases from their laboratory. In the majority (80%) of cases reviewed, estrogen receptor status of the asynchronous secondary tumor was the same as that of the primary tumor, even though variations in quantifiable receptor levels were observed in approximately half the tumors. There was no consistent influence of site or time interval between primary and secondary tumor appearance on the variation in estrogen receptors. This author agrees with Hähnel and Twaddle's recommendation that whenever feasible steroid receptors should be evaluated in the metastatic lesion.

Thus, most investigations support the view that the presence of steroid receptors in a primary tumor correlates well (75–85%) with the presence of receptors in metastatic lesions, even though the interval between the two events may be years. These data clearly indicate that every primary breast tumor should be analyzed for steroid receptors, even if the patient does not have metastatic disease. If, later, metastases appear, receptor levels from the primary tumor may prove useful if the metastatic lesions have disseminated to organs such as bone and brain, which are not easily accessible for biopsy.

The influence of interim therapies using cytotoxic drugs or antihormones must be considered (e.g., Green, 1990). Studies by Allegra and coworkers (1978) suggested that intervening hormone therapy selectively eliminates estrogen receptor–containing cells, but chemotherapy apparently has little or no effect on the specific estrogen-binding capacity of tumor biopsy specimens.

Wilking and colleagues (1984) observed that tamoxifen exhibited a small influence on estradiol-17β production in human breast tumors. Burke and coworkers (1978) reported that estrogen receptor levels were not altered by irradiation of human breast cancer cells and, further, that they reappeared after removal of antiestrogen inhibition. Because of the long half-life of tamoxifen receptor complexes in vivo, it is recommended that administration be discontinued at least 3 weeks before biopsy for steroid receptor analyses. Literature from studies on cells in culture (Allegra and Lippman, 1980) and in patients (Carlson et al., 1984; and Jordan et al., 1992) clearly indicates that tamoxifen may work as either an estrogen agonist or an estrogen antagonist, depending on its concentration. Furthermore, it may be used therapeutically to induce progestin receptors in human tumors (Mortel et al., 1981; and Carlson et al., 1984). The development and clinical use of new progesterone antagonists (e.g., RU486 [Horwitz, 1992]) will require assessment of their effect on receptor levels in cancer specimens.

Criteria used to select therapy for the breast cancer patient include sites of metastases. This author and others (NIH consensus development conference, 1980; and Wittliff, 1984) demonstrated the presence of estrogen and progestin receptors in breast carcinoma metastases from the adrenal gland, bone, colon, contralateral breast, kidney, liver, lung, lymph nodes, muscle, omentum, ovary, skin, stomach, and thyroid gland. The incidence and specific steroid-binding capacities of these metastatic lesions varied considerably; however, the ligand affinities and specificities of the sex hormone receptors were characteristic of those in normal tissues. At no time has a correlation been observed

Table 16–6. DISTRIBUTION OF STEROID RECEPTORS IN TUMOR BOPSIES ACCORDING TO PATIENT ENDOCRINE STATUS*

Receptors Status of Tumor Biopsy Specimen	Endocrine Status of Patient	
	Premenopausal	*Postmenopausal*
ER+, PR+	222 (45%)	520 (63%)
ER+, PR–	58 (12%)	128 (15%)
ER–, PR–	136 (28%)	137 (17%)
ER–, PR+	72 (15%)	41 (5%)
Total	488	826

*Fifty-five years of age was chosen as an age at which virtually every woman may be considered postmenopausal.

(From Wittliff, J. L.: Steroid hormone receptors in breast cancer. Cancer, 53:630, 1984. Reprinted with permission.)

between the presence of steroid receptors and the organ site of metastatic lesions in breast cancer patients.

The race of the patient seems to influence prognosis (Wynder et al., 1963; Morrison et al., 1973; Nemoto et al., 1980; and Walker et al., 1984) and steroid receptor status (Nomura et al., 1977, 1984; Savage et al., 1981; Mohla et al., 1982; Pegoraro et al., 1986*a, b*). At this time the relationship between receptor level and survival considering White, Black, and Asian patients is unclear.

Reference Ranges

As the ligand titration assay and the EIA described have been used in the author's laboratory for 25 years on tens of thousands of biopsy specimens from breast cancer patients, well-defined reference ranges have been developed. Specific binding capacity is expressed as femtomoles of labeled steroid bound per milligram of cytosol protein. Because menopausal status influences receptor level (see Table 16–2), the reference ranges should be considered in terms of this factor (Bland et al., 1981; and McCarty et al., 1983). Table 16–2 and Figure 16–8 provide examples of the range of steroid-binding capacity in breast tumors from premenopausal patients (range, 10 to 3038 fmol/mg cytosol protein) and postmenopausal patients (range, 10 to 5922 fmol/mg). It is generally accepted (McGuire et al., 1975, 1977; NIH consensus development conference, 1980; and Wittliff, 1984) that a level greater than 10 fmol/mg cytosol protein of receptor establishes the presence of these receptors

(Fisher et al., 1981, 1983). The sensitivity of the assay and the biologic data suggest that less than 3 fmol/mg cytosol protein is a clinically insignificant quantity in human breast cancers. K_d values of 1 to 9×10^{-10} M to 1 to 9×10^{-11} M are representative of the estrogen receptor, whereas 1 to 9×10^{-9} M to 1 to 9×10^{-10} M are indicative of the presence of high-affinity progestin-binding components.

Some tumors exhibit both estrogen and progestin receptors whereas others exhibit only one of them (NIH consensus development conference, 1980), as illustrated in Table 16–6. A fourth category exhibits neither steroid hormone receptor. This distribution of receptor types is important to note, particularly that of the progestin receptor, for which the level is high in tumors from premenopausal patients in the presence of the estrogen receptor but considerably lower and rarely observed in patients who do not exhibit the estrogen receptor (see Table 16–6). An example of the distribution of the two receptor types in premenopausal and postmenopausal patients with breast cancer is shown in Figure 16–8. In general, steroid hormone receptors are seen more often and in higher concentrations in breast tumors from postmenopausal patients than in those from premenopausal patients. In addition, the curious distribution in which the estrogen receptor is lacking and the progestin receptor is present is seen three times more often in biopsy specimens from premenopausal patients than in those from postmenopausal patients (Bland et al., 1981). This appears to be due in part to the presence of circulating estrogens in the plasma in premenopausal patients, which mask the steroid hormone receptors in a specimen (Maass et al., 1972;

Figure 16–8. Distribution of estrogen and progesterone receptors in human breast tumors determined by multipoint titration analyses using dextran-coated charcoal to remove unbound steroids. Specific steroid-binding capacities are expressed as fmol/mg cytosol protein. ³H-estradiol-17β and ³H-R5020 were used to measure estrogen and progestin receptors, respectively. (From Wittliff, J. L.: Steroid hormone receptors in breast cancer. Cancer, *53*:630, 1984. Reprinted with permission.)

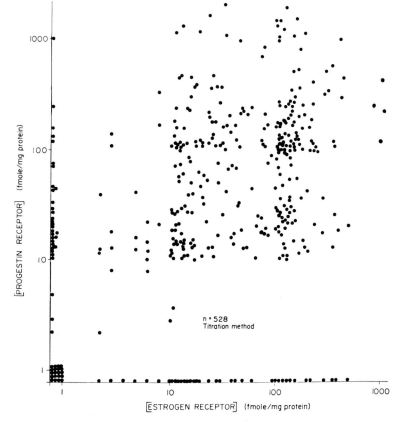

and McCarty et al., 1983). We suggest that the EIA procedure be used for these biopsies (e.g., Pasic et al., 1990).

In the presence of endogenous ligand or drugs such as tamoxifen or toremifene the steroid hormone receptor associates more tightly with nuclear components, and radioligand-binding procedures would be expected to underestimate the number of receptors, but EIA using monoclonal antibodies (Greene et al., 1984; and Raam and Vrabel, 1986) provides a sound means for estimating both ligand-associated and nonassociated forms of the receptor. Enzyme immunoassays, like ligand-binding procedures, require standardization (Wittliff, 1987).

The stage of differentiation of the normal mammary gland influences the level of receptor concentration in target tissue (Wiehle and Wittliff, 1983; and Wittliff et al., 1991). There are few data that define the influence of tumor differentiation on the level of estrogen and progestin receptors (NIH consensus development conference, 1980), but the relationship of tumor differentiation to patient age, menopausal status, day of cycle, and associated therapy complicates interpretations of the results. Therefore, it is essential that the relevant information be indicated on the assay request form prior to analysis.

Three early studies indicated that ethnic origin influenced steroid-binding capacity in tumors (Savage et al., 1981; Mohla et al., 1982; Pegoraro et al., 1986a,b). Another study (Crowe et al., 1986) reported a striking relationship between estrogen receptor status and race in predicting prognosis for Stage I breast cancers. These data suggested that reference ranges may vary in different areas of the world, depending on the population distribution; however, more studies will be needed to define these reference ranges.

This author highly recommends that an individual laboratory develop its own distribution profiles of steroid hormone receptors, such as those presented in Figure 16–8, including the levels found in the various types of tumors (see Tables 16–2, 16–6). These should be compared with published studies to ensure that a laboratory is generating comparable information. Results from other receptors, such as those for androgen and glucocorticoid, may help establish the degree of loss of hormone regulatory mechanisms in breast cancer cells (Wittliff, 1984, 1986). Allegra and colleagues (1979 a,b) evaluated relationships among all the steroid hormone receptors.

CLINICAL SIGNIFICANCE OF ESTROGEN RECEPTORS

It has been demonstrated conclusively that the presence of estrogen receptors provides a molecular basis for the distinction between human breast carcinomas that are responsive to hormone therapy or to endocrine organ ablation and those that are not. From studies of these steroid-binding proteins in hormonally responsive tumors of rodents, Jensen and coworkers (1971) originally suggested that the ability of a breast carcinoma to bind estrogen predicted a patient's response to endocrine therapy. This was supported by their findings in which the presence of estrogen receptors in tumor biopsy specimens from patients was correlated with a favorable response to adrenalectomy. Since the orig-

Table 16–7. RELATIONSHIP BETWEEN ESTROGEN RECEPTOR (ER) STATUS OF BREAST TUMOR AND PATIENT'S OBJECTIVE RESPONSE TO ENDOCRINE THERAPY

Estrogen Receptor Status	
Responses/ER+ Tumors	Responses/ER− Tumors
522/977 (53%)	36/567 (6%)

Based on the collective papers presented at the NIH Consensus Development Conference on Steroid Receptors in Breast Cancer (DeSombre et al., 1979; Proceedings of NIH Consensus Development Conference, 1980).

inal report of Folca and coworkers in 1961, numerous studies (NIH consensus development conference, 1980) have shown that approximately half of all malignant breast tumors contain estrogen receptors.

Analysis of approximately 8000 breast cancer specimens over a 10-year period indicates that 60% to 65% of primary lesions and 45% to 55% of metastatic breast cancers exhibit more than 10 fmol/mg cytosol protein binding of estrogen receptors. Furthermore, 53% of patients with breast tumors containing estrogen receptors were responsive to hormone therapies of the additive or ablative types (Wittliff et al., 1978). The data given in Table 16–7 are the collective results from investigators participating in the NIH Consensus Development Conference in 1979. They represent the level of response (50–60%) that may be expected of a breast cancer patient to hormone manipulation when only estrogen receptor status is considered. These results also agree with the data presented in 1974 at the first International Workshop on Estrogen Receptors in Human Breast Cancer (Table 16–8).

Numerous investigations support the thesis that the percentage of objective remissions in breast cancer patients given hormone therapy may be expected to increase with the specific estrogen-binding capacity of the tumor. When the collective results from the NIH Consensus Development Conference (1980) were summarized, there was a spectrum of responses, which ranged from less than 6% when estrogen receptor levels were below 10 fmol/mg cytosol protein to more than 80% objective remissions when tumors contained more than 200 fmol/mg. Results suggest that only

Table 16–8. RELATIONSHIP BETWEEN ESTROGEN-BINDING CAPACITY OF BREAST TUMOR BIOPSY SPECIMENS AND OBJECTIVE REMISSION AFTER AN ENDOCRINE MANIPULATION

Therapeutic Manipulation	Specific Estrogen-Binding Capacity	
	Positive	Negative
Additive hormone treatment	59/105 (56%)	12/109 (11%)
Ablative endocrine therapy	59/107 (55%)	8/94 (8%)
Total	118/212 (56%)	20/203 (10%)

Based on the collective papers presented at the National Cancer Institute Workshop on Estrogen Receptors in Human Breast Cancer (McGuire et al, 1975).

analyses providing quantification of the estrogen and progestin receptors should be used in the clinical laboratory. Likewise, the clinician should appreciate that the potential of the patient for hormone response depends on both the specific binding capacity and the K_d (or K_a) values of estrogen and progestin receptors.

The prognostic value of estrogen receptors in primary lesions evolved from the work of Knight and coworkers (1977). Patients with breast cancers containing estrogen receptors exhibited longer disease-free survival when compared with patients whose tumors did not contain estrogen receptors. The disease-free interval of Stage II patients appeared to be independent of the patient's menopausal status and of the presence of metastases in the axillary lymph nodes. These data, supported by several studies (Bishop et al., 1979; Hähnel et al., 1979; Blamey et al., 1980; Gapinski and Donegan, 1980; Palshof et al., 1980; and Stewart et al., 1983), indicate clearly that the estrogen receptor is useful as a predictive index of a patient's response to endocrine manipulation and as a prognostic index of the course of the disease. Thus, quantitative results from receptor analyses play a major role in the management of carcinoma of the breast (Fisher et al., 1981, 1983).

The relationship between estrogen receptor content of a tumor and either disease-free survival or overall survival is at present unclear. However, Fisher and coworkers (1987) showed the benefit of prolonging tamoxifen therapy for primary breast cancer in patients whose cancers contained more than 10 fmol/mg cytosol protein of the steroid hormone receptors. Women aged 50 years or older receiving a third year of tamoxifen had a better disease-free survival rate and overall survival rate through their fifth postoperative year. Other investigations suggest that these parameters also may be related to the stage of breast cancer and the race of the patient. Crowe and associates (1986) reported that estrogen receptor status and race interact to influence survival. They concluded that Black patients with estrogen receptor–negative tumors, particularly postmenopausal ones, were at high risk of recurrence and death.

The reader is referred to Chapter 22 for a more detailed treatment of the clinical significance of these receptors.

CLINICAL SIGNIFICANCE OF PROGESTIN RECEPTORS

Some women with breast tumors containing sex-hormone receptors do not respond to hormone therapy. One explanation is that there may be a defect in the intracellular cascade of events that normally controls biologic response to an endocrine stimulus. One approach taken to assess whether the estrogen response mechanism is intact has been the determination of progestin receptors. (Horwitz et al., 1975). The assumption is that progestin receptor formation is regulated by estrogen receptors in a fashion similar to the mechanism in rodent uterine tissues, as described by Rao and Meyer (1977). Thus, the simultaneous determination of the progestin receptor with the estrogen receptor (see Fig. 16–8) should increase the accuracy of selecting the patients who are most likely to respond to hormone therapy.

If the presence of a functional estrogen receptor is re-

Table 16–9. RELATIONSHIP BETWEEN STEROID RECEPTOR (ER, PR) STATUS OF BREAST TUMOR AND PATIENT'S OBJECTIVE RESPONSE TO ENDOCRINE THERAPY

Steroid Receptors Status*			
ER+, PR+	ER+, PR−	ER−, PR−	ER−, PR+
135/174 (78%)	55/164 (34%)	16/165 (10%)	5/11 (45%)

*Number of patients responding to treatment/number of women with receptor status designated.

Based on the collective papers presented at the NIH Consensus Development Conference on Steroid Receptors in Breast Cancer (Proceedings of the NIH Consensus Development Conference, 1980).

quired for the formation of a progestin receptor, there should be a direct relationship between these two receptors in responsive cells. Breast tumors containing both receptors would be assumed to retain hormone responsiveness (Degenshein et al., 1980).

A summary of results presented at the NIH Consensus Development Conference (1980) is shown in Table 16–9. Studies of the steroid receptor status of tumor specimens found that 78% of patients with breast tumors containing both receptors responded objectively to hormone therapy. If only the estrogen receptor was present, a 34% response rate was observed, whereas only 10% of patients responded to endocrine manipulation if neither receptor was present in the breast tumor. Use of quality assurance programs for receptor determination has improved this relationship whereby less than 3% of patients respond if neither receptor is present. Surprisingly, 5 of 11 (45%) patients responded objectively to hormone therapy when only the progestin receptor was present. This appears puzzling if there is a relationship between estrogen and progestin receptors in responsive tumors, but it may be related to the endocrine status of the patient (McCarty et al., 1983; and Alghanem and Hussain, 1985), as discussed earlier (see Table 16–2). The data suggest that presence of the progestin receptor may be particularly important in selecting premenopausal patients for endocrine manipulation (Bland et al., 1981).

An adjuvant trial that compared cytotoxic chemotherapy with and without tamoxifen also suggested that the progestin receptor may have particular significance (Fisher et al., 1983, 1987). Patients with increased levels of progestin receptors who received both cytotoxic chemotherapy and tamoxifen exhibited increased disease-free survival. Clark and associates (1983) and the review by Osborne (1991) also concluded that progestin receptor level was of equal or greater value than that of the estrogen receptor for predicting the disease-free survival of breast cancer patients.

STEROID RECEPTORS IN MALE BREAST CANCER

Breast cancer in men is often hormone dependent: approximately 65% of patients with advanced disease respond to orchiectomy or adrenalectomy. Because these tumors are encountered infrequently, relatively few analyses correlating endocrine manipulation with the presence of steroid hormone receptors have been reported. The collective study reported by Everson and colleagues (1980) found that estrogen receptors were present in tumor specimens from 29 of 34 cases (85%) of male breast cancers. There was a negative correlation between estrogen receptor concentration and patient age. Although the quantity of estrogen receptor appeared to be related to the level of progesterone receptor, the disease-free interval, and the duration of response, these were not statistically significant. Clinical results from this report and that of Pegoraro and coworkers (1982) are not sufficient justification for basing a therapeutic maneuver on the sex hormone receptor status of a biopsy specimen in a manner analogous to that used for breast cancer in women. More detailed analyses of both cytoplasmic and nuclear levels of these receptors may be useful, as suggested by Pegoraro and colleagues (1982).

Nine of 14 breast cancer specimens (64%) from male patients had significant levels of progesterone receptors, and several exhibited androgen and glucocorticoid receptors (Everson et al., 1980). Concentrations of estrogen receptors are elevated in both primary and metastatic tumors. It has been the author's experience and that of others that few gynecomastia specimens exhibit estrogen receptors, and usually these are limited to the 4 S species as detected by sucrose gradient centrifugation.

The presence of estrogen receptors in the breast cancers of men indicates that these patients are candidates for hormone or endocrine manipulation. Orchiectomy, adrenalectomy and inhibitors of estrogen binding such as tamoxifen or toremifene can prove useful (e.g., Jordan et al., 1990, 1992).

STEROID RECEPTORS IN BENIGN BREAST TISSUES

During the past decade, numerous workers have investigated the presence of steroid receptors in nonmalignant lesions of the breast, such as chronic cystic mastopathy (fibrocystic changes) or fibroadenoma (Spratt et al., 1985). From determinations in more than 200 biopsies using either the titration method or sucrose gradient centrifugation, the author has rarely detected more than 10 fmol/mg cytosol protein (Wittliff et al., 1972, 1976). The majority of studies from other workers agree with these findings (NIH consensus development conference, 1980). However, significant binding of labeled estradiol has been reported in a few specimens of benign breast disease when measured by the tissue slice procedure. In general, it may be concluded that benign breast disease peripheral to the malignant lesion will not contribute significantly to the estrogen-binding capacity. Thus, the possibility of a false-positive estrogen receptor assay is excluded. However, fibroblasts may contain a significant level of progestin receptors, complicating this measurement if excessive nontumorous tissue is present in the specimen (Wittliff, 1984, 1987).

Although normal breast tissue from women is known to concentrate ^{3}H-estradiol in vivo, the level of steroid retained is considerably lower than that found in tumor tissue. One explanation for this reduced binding is that normal breast tissue contains few epithelial cells except during pregnancy and lactation. Furthermore, it contains a predominance of adipose and connective tissue cells, as compared with most malignant breast tumors. To date, this author has detected specific estrogen receptors sedimenting at 8 S in normal breast tissue in only one patient. Results obtained in the author's laboratory suggest that lack of cellularity may not be the reason for the absence of estrogen receptors in normal breast tissue. Examination of the specific binding capacities of mammary glands from rats revealed that the levels of estrogen receptors were low in breast tissue from virgin and pregnant animals (Wiehle and Wittliff, 1983). These receptors increased throughout lactation, reaching a maximum just before weaning of the young, to levels comparable to that of infiltrating ductal carcinoma of the human breast. Normal breast tissue from pregnant or lactating women was not examined, however, for the obvious reason that it is rarely, if ever, available. The prediction is that these tissues would exhibit estrogen receptors that have properties similar to those found in breast tumors. Since virtually all breast tumors are removed from women who are not pregnant or lactating, the inclusion of normal breast tissue in the biopsy specimen does not pose a problem so long as the sample is representative of the malignant lesion. Using immunohistochemical determination of estrogen and progestin receptors, Khan and coworkers (1994) evaluated benign breast samples from 120 women. Receptor positivity was defined as the presence of nuclear immunoreaction with the monoclonal antibodies. This interesting study suggested that the presence of estrogen receptors in benign breast epithelium is a risk factor for breast malignancy.

ESTROGEN RECEPTORS AND RESPONSE TO CHEMOTHERAPY

The concept that the estrogen receptor may be useful for predicting a patient's response to chemotherapy is based on the assumption that the absence of one or more steroid hormone receptors reflects a loss of differentiated function (hormone control mechanisms), which might be correlated with a more rapid growth rate. Thus, these rapidly growing tumors may be more sensitive to chemotherapy than tumors that possess steroid hormone receptors. In support of this idea, Meyer and coworkers (1977, 1983) showed that breast tumors without estrogen receptors exhibited faster growth, as measured by thymidine labeling and mitotic indices.

Knight and colleagues (1977) reported that patients whose primary breast cancer contained estrogen receptors had a longer period of disease-free survival than women with receptor-negative tumors, independent of their menopausal status or the involvement of the axillary lymph nodes with metastases. These workers also postulated that the lower incidence of estrogen receptors in breast tumor specimens from premenopausal women may account for their increased survival with adjuvant therapy as opposed to that of postmenopausal patients. This implies that the higher incidence of estrogen receptor–negative tumors in premenopausal patients may be associated with greater sensitivity to cytotoxic chemotherapy. Several randomized trials of adjuvant chemotherapy conducted by the NSABP (Fisher et al., 1977) and by Bonadonna and coworkers

(1977) in Europe, showed that the major beneficiaries of this therapy were premenopausal patients. Although chemotherapy is known to cause ovarian suppression, this does not appear to be the reason for the increased survival of premenopausal women.

Allegra and coworkers (1978) were among the first to determine whether a correlation existed between lack of estrogen receptors in breast cancers and response to chemotherapy. Using a group of patients carefully matched with regard to age, menopausal status, Karnofsky performance index, disease-free interval, number of sites involved with metastases, and prior therapy, they found that premenopausal patients with tumors predominantly negative for estrogen receptor may be more sensitive to chemotherapy than postmenopausal women with estrogen receptor–positive tumors. The distribution of the treatments was similar for the two groups and consisted of doxorubicin hydrochloride (Adriamycin) and one or more additional chemotherapeutic agents. Thirty-four of 45 patients (75%) with estrogen receptor–negative tumors responded objectively, compared to only three of 25 women (12%) with breast tumors containing estrogen receptors. Regardless of visceral involvement, patients whose tumors lacked estrogen receptors had a higher response rate to chemotherapy. Furthermore, the presence of progestin receptors in a tumor does not appear to influence the response rate of patients given combination chemotherapy.

The relationship between specific estrogen-binding capacity of a tumor and a patient's response to cytotoxic chemotherapy remains controversial. Many investigators (cf. Osborne, 1991) have studied this question since the original suggestion by Allegra and coworkers (1978). Although a few groups reported results that agreed with this study during the 1979 NIH Consensus Development Conference (1980), others reached different conclusions. The studies of Kiang and Kennedy (1977) and others gave virtually opposite results; patients with breast tumors containing estrogen receptors more often responded to chemotherapy than did patients whose tumors lacked them. Other studies were unable to demonstrate any relationship between the estrogen receptor status of a breast tumor and a patient's response to cytotoxic chemotherapy, further complicating the picture. Differences in the mode of patient selection may have considerable bearing on the lack of consensus.

POLYMORPHISM OF ESTROGEN RECEPTORS AS A MOLECULAR BASIS OF ENDOCRINE RESPONSIVENESS

In 1969, the author and coworkers began a long-term study to examine the hypothesis posed by Jensen and colleagues (unpublished until 1971) that the presence of estrogen-binding components in breast carcinomas could predict a patient's response to endocrine therapy.

The distribution and levels of estrogen receptor isoforms in tumors were examined and correlated with a patient's response to endocrine therapy (Wittliff and Savlov, 1975; Wittliff et al., 1978; and Wittliff, 1984). No objective re-

missions were observed in patients with advanced breast carcinoma whose tumors were estrogen receptor negative, regardless of the type of hormone therapy administered. Approximately 75% of patients whose specimen revealed either 8 S species or both the 8 S and 4 S forms of the estrogen receptors exhibited objective remissions after receiving various types of hormone therapy. Of the 23 patients whose tumors contained exclusively or predominantly the 4 S species of estrogen receptors, only four responded objectively to hormone therapy. These data suggested that the molecular forms of estrogen receptors in human breast cancer have clinical significance. In 1981 (1981*b*) the author suggested the use of the term *isoform* to describe this variability in receptor species.

Steroid hormone receptors are proteins that show a great deal of heterogeneity in size, shape, and charge (see Table 16–4). To characterize further the estrogen-binding components in the cytosol of breast tumors, DEAE-cellulose chromatography (Kute et al., 1978; and Wittliff et al., 1981*b*) and more sophisticated procedures such as HPLC (Wittliff 1985, 1986) were employed to study the interrelationships of these elusive receptor proteins. The number of binding components, (i.e., isoforms) and their relative specific estrogen-binding capacities were highly variable from tumor to tumor (see Figs. 16–4 to 16–7). Whether these binding components represent distinct subunits or cleavage products owing to proteolytic digestion of the estrogen receptors is unknown (Sluyser and Wittliff, 1992). Similar molecular heterogeneity has been observed in progestin receptors (van der Walt and Wittliff, 1986). The findings using partially purified forms of estrogen receptors from human breast carcinoma suggest that the molecular composition of the 8 S species from hormonally responsive tumors is different from that of unresponsive neoplasms. Monoclonal antibodies to estrogen receptors helped determine the interrelationships of various receptor isoforms (Greene et al., 1980, 1984).

Numerous workers in the field, particularly those working with uterine tissue (Puca et al., 1972; and Notides et al., 1981), favor a model that contains a single type of subunit (Fig. 16–9). The dimer is the species most likely to occur at physiologic ion strength. Regardless of the ionic strength of the environment in vitro, it is assumed that no more than four types of components are possible. These include the meroreceptor (3.5 S), which is presumed to arise from proteolytic cleavage of higher–molecular weight species (Sherman et al., 1978).

Employing a monoclonal antibody that Greene and coworkers (1980, 1984) produced against estrogen receptors from the MCF-7 human breast cancer cell line, the author and associates demonstrated that immunopurified isoforms of the estrogen receptors from extracts of these cells were associated with both protein kinase (Fig. 16–10) and phospholipid kinase activities (Baldi et al., 1986, 1992). These enzyme activities were easily ascertained in vitro on femtomolar quantities of the receptors because the isoform–monoclonal antibody complexes were immobilized on a single polystyrene bead (Sato et al., 1986). A further novelty was that the receptor could be associated with ^{125}I-iodoestradiol-17β and could easily be measured in a gamma counter by placing the bead coated with labeled receptor

COMPOSITION OF ESTROGEN RECEPTORS

Assuming a single type of subunit:

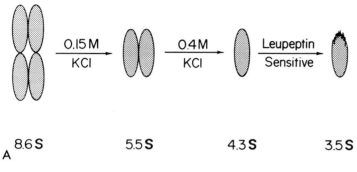

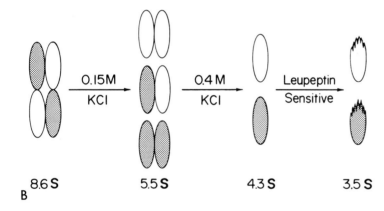

Figure 16-9. Proposals regarding the composition of the estrogen receptor in hormone target organs of eukaryotes. (From Wittliff, J. L., Feldhoff, P. A., Fuchs, A., et al.: Polymorphism of estrogen receptors in human breast cancer. *In* Soto, R., DeNicola, A. F., and Blaquier, J. A. (Eds.): Physiopathology of Endocrine Diseases and Mechanisms of Hormone Action. New York, Alan R. Liss, 1981*b*, p. 375. Reprinted with permission.)

COMPOSITION OF ESTROGEN RECEPTORS

Assuming two types of subunits:

into the counting well (Sato et al., 1986). The receptor directed a phosphorylation reaction requiring adenosine triphosphate (ATP) rather than guanosine triphosphate (GTP) as the phosphoryl donor (see Fig. 16–10) and was highly dependent on the presence of Mg^{2+}. As seen in Figure 16–10, three phosphopeptides were eluted by detergent from the monoclonal antibody–coated bead associated with the purified estrogen receptor. Only estrogen receptor–positive cell lines (MCF-7) exhibited the protein kinase activity; estrogen receptor–negative breast cancer cell lines, such as the MDA and the T-47D, showed little or no activity (Baldi et al., 1986, 1992).

Recent observations from several groups implicate steroid receptor phosphorylation as a possible regulatory mechanism that alters the binding capacity of these molecules (Auricchio et al., 1981). Furthermore, an increasing number of protein hormone receptors, growth factors, and oncogenic transforming products have been shown to have autophosphorylating activity and to exhibit the ability to phosphorylate exogenous substrates. The observation that two oncogenic products, p68[v-ras] (Macara et al., 1984) and pp60[v-src] (Sugimoto et al., 1984), contained phospholipid kinase activity, has brought new insight into the phosphate transfer reaction related to oncogenesis.

The evidence that the immunopurified estrogen receptor directs autophosphorylating activity and phosphorylates phosphoinositides (Baldi et al., 1986, 1992) leads us to postulate a mechanism by which steroid hormone receptors may share similar properties with oncogene products (Sluyser and Mester, 1985). It should be mentioned, however, that the kinase activity exhibited by estrogen receptor molecules from MCF-7 breast cancer cells is a serine-type kinase (Baldi et al., 1992), in contrast to the tyrosine kinase mode exhibited by most oncogenic transforming products (Hunter and Cooper, 1985). Of course, considerable work is needed to establish a relationship between steroid hormone receptors and the synthesis of oncogenic products; however, these results suggest that the steroid-binding site of the estrogen receptor represents only a portion of a more complex regulatory molecule.

The author's data from ion-exchange chromatography, isoelectric focusing, and, more recently, HPLC, are more consistent with the model shown in Figure 16–9B (Wittliff et al., 1981*b*), illustrating protein polymorphism. In this model, the molecular heterogeneity of the estrogen receptor arises as a result of the various possible combinations of two different subunits. It is unclear, at present, which are the so-called native forms and which are proteolytic frag-

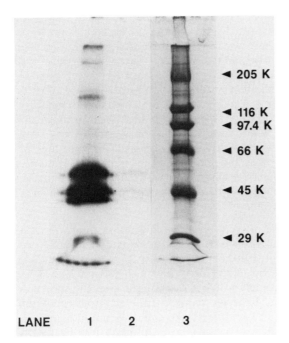

Figure 16-10. Nucleotide dependence of estrogen receptor (ER) autophosphorylation activity from MCF-7 cells. ER was purified from MCF-7 cytosol using immobilized monoclonal antibody. The immune complexes were washed extensively and incubated either with Y-^{32}P-ATP or Y-^{32}P-GTP. Reactions were terminated by removal of the reaction medium and the ^{32}P-labeled polypeptides were solubilized and separated by polyacrylamide-SDS gel electrophoresis. The slab gels used were dried and autoradiography was performed for 16 hours at 25° C. *Lane 1*, MCF-7 MAb-receptor complex incubated with Y-^{32}P-ATP as substrate, shows the presence of phosphorylated proteins with molecular weights of 57, 47, and 43 kd. *Lane 2*, Same as Lane 1, but Y-^{32}P-GTP was used as substrate. Note absence of phosphorylation activity. *Lane 3* shows the corresponding molecular weight standards. Numbers on the right indicate the position of molecular weight standards in kilodaltons. (From Baldi, A., Boyle, D. M., and Wittliff, J. L.: Estrogen receptor is associated with protein and phospholipid kinase activities. Biochem. Biophys. Res. Commun., *135*:597, 1986. Reprinted with permission.)

As many as 30% to 40% of human breast cancers are resistant to endocrine therapy, in spite of the fact that they contain steroid receptors (McGuire, et al., 1975). Earlier, we demonstrated that both ER and PR exhibit polymorphism (isoforms) and suggested that their distribution may be related to endocrine responsiveness (Wittliff, 1984). Using HPLC in various separation modes, we characterized the molecular heterogeneity of estrogen and progestin receptors and identified several variant forms (Wittliff et al., 1989, 1991). Studies using Northern blot analysis have shown that there are variant estrogen receptor mRNA molecules in certain human breast cancers (Murphy and Dotzlaw, 1989). Similar findings have been made for progesterone receptor mRNA species (i.e., that certain progestational agonists autoregulate the levels of their own receptor proteins by inhibiting the transcription of the PR gene) (Wei et al., 1988). Evidence from Gronemeyer and colleagues (1991) suggests that certain antihormones, such as RU-486, express their actions depending on association with specific receptor isoforms.

It is now possible to use a variety of biochemical and molecular biologic approaches to detect variant receptors with aberrant function in human breast cancers (McGuire, et al., 1992). The field is sufficiently equipped also to investigate the clinical significance of the receptor variants.

There is increasing interest in receptors for other members of the superfamily such as 1,25-dihydroxyvitamin D_3 in gynecologic neoplasms (Saunders et al., 1992). The Ah receptor, which appears to exhibit polymorphism, binds to halogenated aromatic hydrocarbons in a variety of species and produces tissue-specific toxic and biologic responses (Dennison, 1992). Androgen receptors have long been predictive indices for selecting endocrine therapy for patients with prostate cancer (Benson et al., 1987). As a result of cloning these genes, many of the protein products are candidates as predictive indicators of therapeutic response to their cognate ligands (e.g., thyroid antagonists and the triiodothyronine-thyroxine [T_3-T_4] receptor). Retinoic acid and its analogs, and their interrelationships with their receptors, also appear to be of interest in chemoprevention.

HORMONE RECEPTOR PROFILES

Analyses of sex hormone receptors are important for identifying which breast cancer patients are most likely to respond to additive or ablative endocrine manipulation. Steroid hormone receptors are used in conjunction with clinical factors such as previous response to hormone therapy, disease-free interval, age, menopausal status, and location of the dominant metastatic lesion to make therapeutic decisions.

The author suggested the use of the term *receptor fingerprint* or *isoform profile* to designate the pattern of specific steroid hormone–binding components (isoforms) displayed by a single receptor type when separated according to properties of size, shape, surface charge, and hydrophobicity (Wittliff et al., 1981*b*, 1989, 1991). For example, Figures 16–4 to 16–7 illustrate the isoform profiles of the estrogen receptors in several tissue specimens. The author predicts that methods that separate receptor isoforms and variants

ments retaining the ligand-binding domain in HPLC profiles of these receptors (Boyle et al., 1985). These differences in separation characteristics may be due to a variety of physiologic reasons, including phosphorylation, protein-protein interaction such as subunit association-dissociation, and possible protein–nucleic acid association. The authors have preliminary evidence that a high–molecular weight component (larger than 400 kd) exists in cytosol from studies with molybdate using ^{125}I-iodoestradiol-17β and HPLC. This binding protein may be a precursor of the functional estrogen receptor. The author's current research is directed toward understanding the interrelationships of receptor isoforms and variants and their role in target cell response. HPLC, ^{125}I-labeled ligands, receptor-specific monoclonal antibodies, and DNA band shift assays provide the means of exploring these receptor proteins at a molecular level that was not possible earlier. Using both bacterial and yeast expression systems, we have produced full-length biologically active human estrogen and progestin receptors with a gene fusion technology (Wittliff et al., 1990, 1994).

based on size and shape (PAGE-Western blotting, DNA band-shift assays, and high-performance size exclusion chromatography) or on surface ion charge (isoelectric focusing, IEC, and chromatofocusing) will play a greater role in the clinical laboratory in this decade. In contrast to a receptor fingerprint, the term *receptor profile* is suggested to indicate the presence of the different types of hormone receptors (e.g., those for estrogen, progestin, EGF, and LH-RH) in a single tumor specimen.

In general, when estrogen receptors were present in a specimen, greater progestin-binding capacity was observed in both premenopausal and postmenopausal women. In the absence of estrogen receptors, a lower progestin receptor level was measured, supporting the suggestion that the formation of estrogen receptor is dependent on estrogen action. Similar values have been reported for biopsies of endometrial cancers.

SUMMARY OF INFORMATION ON SEX HORMONE RECEPTORS

The following findings summarize current information on sex hormone receptors:

- Reliable methods of quantifying estrogen and progestin receptors are (1) multipoint titration analysis with radiolabeled ligand using dextran-coated charcoal and (2) enzyme immunoassay with monoclonal antibodies.
- Some 55% to 65% of primary breast cancers contain more than 10 fmol/mg cytosol protein of estrogen receptors.
- Some 45% to 55% of metastatic breast cancers contain more than 10 fmol/mg cytosol protein of estrogen receptors.
- Estrogen receptors are more often present in breast cancers of postmenopausal women than in those of premenopausal women.
- Benign breast lesions, such as fibrocystic changes and fibroadenomas, usually contain less than 10 fmol/mg cytosol protein of estrogen receptor.
- Ninety per cent of male breast carcinomas contain estrogen receptors and fewer than 50% contain progestin receptors.
- Approximately 55% of women with breast cancers containing estrogen receptors respond with measurable tumor regression to endocrine therapy, either additive or ablative.
- Fewer than 3% of women with breast cancers lacking estrogen receptors respond objectively to hormone therapy.
- Some 45% to 60% of primary or metastatic breast cancers contain progestin receptors.
- The presence of both estrogen and progestin receptors in a breast cancer indicates a 75% to 80% likelihood that the patient will respond to endocrine manipulation, either additive or ablative.
- Both estrogen and progestin receptors exhibit polymorphism (isoforms or variants) based upon separation and characterization using properties of size, shape, surface ion charge, and hydrophobicity. Molecular heterogeneity appears in part due to receptor modification, such as

phosphorylation, and to association with nonreceptor activities, such as heat-shock proteins.

- Immunocytochemical methods should be used as a confirmatory test of receptor status. If only small samples (less than 20 mg tissue) are available, such as those from needle biopsy specimens, fine-needle aspiration, or paraffin-embedded specimens, immunohistochemistry may be utilized for qualitative assessment using monoclonal antibodies specific for these receptors.
- There is a relationship between the quantities of both estrogen and progestin receptors in a breast tumor and a patient's response to endocrine therapy. The incidence of response to hormone therapy increases with increasing receptor levels.

It is recommended that both estrogen and progestin receptor analyses be performed on all tumor specimens from patients with confirmed or suspected breast carcinoma prior to therapeutic manipulation. Laboratories should be used that comply with criteria assigned by quality assurance programs. Receptor profiles (i.e., the presence of different types of hormone receptors) may be useful in the diagnosis of certain neoplasms. Receptor results may be used as (1) a *predictive* indicator of an endocrine-responsive tumor, and (2) a *prognostic* index of a patient's clinical course. Elevated levels of these receptors in a tumor specimen are associated with a greater probability of disease-free survival.

GROWTH FACTORS AND MACROMOLECULES

Epidermal Growth Factor Receptors

Several steroid and peptide hormones appear to be involved in the differentiation and proliferation of normal breast cells throughout their natural history. Pregnancy and lactation are dependent upon hormones such as estradiol-17β, progesterone, prolactin, and human chorionic gonadotropin for their initiation and maintenance. Some of these same signal-transducing molecules, as well as growth factors such as epidermal growth factor (EGF), now appear to be important in the normal physiologic response of human breast cells. The EGF receptor is the product of a proto-oncogene referred to by some authors as c-*erb* B-1 (Carpenter, 1987).

EGF is a single polypeptide chain containing 53 amino acids with M_r of 6000 that is highly heat stable, particularly because of three disulfide bridges. EGF is known to act as a mitogen for human breast cancer cells in culture (Davidson et al., 1987), and it interacts with a number of organs in the body, including reproductive tissues.

EGF receptor is a complicated molecule consisting of multiple domains, including a large extracellular portion responsible for the association with EGF (Carpenter and Cohen, 1979; and Carpenter, 1987). The conformation of this domain is maintained by a large number of disulfide bridges and glycosylated residues. The transmembrane portion secures the receptor in the cytoplasmic membrane. The internal domain contains an adenosine triphosphate (ATP)-binding site and exhibits tyrosine kinase activity. Interestingly, the receptor molecule autophosphorylates itself on tyrosine residues located near the carboxyl terminal as well as on tyrosine residues of certain intracellular proteins when EGF occupies the binding site. The glycoprotein has a molecular weight of approximately 170 kd (Cohen et al., 1982). Transforming growth factor-alpha (TGFα), which is produced by certain breast cancer cells growing in culture, binds to the EGF receptor, producing a similar response (Todaro et al., 1980).

Fitzpatrick and colleagues (1984) first demonstrated that membrane preparations from primary and metastatic breast cancers contain EGF receptors. These early studies were expanded to a large series of human breast, endometrial, and ovarian cancers, using a sensitive ligand-binding assay in a competition mode (Fekete et al., 1989; and Srkalovic, et al., 1990). Currently this assay serves as a standard by which other types of EGF receptor assays, such as those employing monoclonal antibodies, may be evaluated. At least two antibody-based assays are under development. One uses an EIA format developed by Ciba Corning Diagnostics while the other utilizes an enzyme-linked immunosorbent assay (ELISA) format developed by Oncogene Science.

Although the cutoff values for clinical significance have not been determined for the monoclonal-based assays, a study of the relationship between these results and those of the ligand-binding assay is progressing (Yang et al., 1992). Based on early clinical results and a ligand-binding assay, Harris and coworkers (1989) suggested a cutoff value of 10 fmol/mg. Using this value, patients with breast tumors containing elevated levels of EGF receptor had significantly shorter periods of relapse-free survival and overall survival (Sainsbury et al., 1985, 1987; Nicholson et al., 1988a,b, 1989, 1991; and Harris et al., 1989).

Many studies have reported the presence of epidermal growth factor receptors in human breast cancer biopsies (e.g., Perez et al., 1984; Macias et al., 1986; and Fekete et al., 1989) and cells in tissue culture since the original finding of Fitzpatrick and co-workers in 1984. A review of the investigations since 1984 (Klijn et al., 1992a,b, 1993) indicated that approximately half of human breast cancers expressed EGF receptors. The majority of these results suggested an inverse relationship between EGF receptors and estrogen receptor levels in biopsies of human breast cancers. In general, no significant relationship was observed between EGF receptor expression and patient age, menopausal status, tumor histologic subtypes, tumor size, grade, or DNA content, or lymph node involvement. Most reports reviewed by Klijn and investigators suggested the value of EGF receptors as a prognostic factor with respect to disease-free survival and overall survival. The greatest clinical significance appeared to be the association of EGF receptor expression and hormone resistance. Correlations of laboratory data with clinical response seeking to extend the promising findings of the British group (Sainsbury et al., 1985, 1987) were obtained with a variety of ligand-binding, monoclonal antibody–based, and immunohistochemical methods to detect EGF receptors (Klijn, 1992, 1993). Currently, it appears that standardization of the EGF procedure is possible, and the availability of commercially developed kits should complement these approaches. Evaluation of the

clinical utility of EGF receptors in cooperative clinical trials is necessary to determine its value as a routine prognostic factor.

The c-*erb* B-2 (HER-2/*neu*) Oncogene Product

Almost 100 proto-oncogenes have been described, and their protein products appear to play fundamental roles in the control of cell growth and differentiation (Bishop, 1987). Activation of certain cellular proto-oncogenes appears to be related to the induction or progression of certain human carcinomas. Genetic alterations contributing to malignant transformation and tumor progression include activation of oncogenes and loss or mutation of suppressor genes. Activation may occur by a number of different mechanisms, including mutations in the DNA itself resulting in a functionally altered protein product, a change in the manner of expression of the proto-oncogene, chromosome translocation, or gene amplification. The proto-oncogene and oncogene protein products regulating growth and differentiation may be divided into functional categories. Some protein products act as growth factors or as hormone receptor proteins themselves, whereas others are intracellular signal transduction proteins or nuclear transcriptional factors. Measurement of a proto-oncogene product may be useful as a prognostic factor in human breast cancer.

The *neu* oncogene, originally isolated from rat neuroblastomas that were chemically induced, encodes a 185-kd surface glycoprotein termed p185 *neu* (Schechter et al., 1984; and Maguire and Greene, 1989). The protein product exhibits tyrosine kinase activity with a structure similar to that of the EGF receptor (Coussens et al., 1985; Akiyama et al., 1986). When various molecular properties and chromosomal localization studies were conducted, it was revealed that the new protein was distinct from the EGF receptor (Schechter et al., 1984; Bargmann et al., 1986; and Yamamoto et al., 1986). The identity of the native ligand for p185 *neu* is the focus of research in many laboratories (Lupu et al., 1990, 1992). Various designations have been given to the oncogene expressing the protein product related to the EGF receptor; these include *neu*, HER-2, and c-*erb* B-2. Overexpression of c-*erb* B-2 protein was related to transformation and tumorigenesis of cells in culture (DiFiore et al., 1987; Hudziak et al., 1987).

Gene amplification is detected by Southern blotting DNA (Southern, 1975) extracted from breast cancer specimens, whereas mRNA overexpression may be assessed by Northern blotting. Both techniques require considerable care in tissue handling and technical skill. Both polyclonal and monoclonal antibodies have been prepared against the c-*erb* B-2 protein to evaluate its expression in human breast carcinomas. Two commercial kits are under development that employ these reagents—an ELISA procedure by Oncogene Science and an EIA method by Ciba Corning Diagnostics. Several workers have employed the antibodies in immunohistochemical procedures (Venter et al., 1987; Barnes et al., 1988; Paik et al., 1990; and Nicholson et al., 1991).

The human homolog of c-*neu* gene, c-*erb* B-2, is expressed in human breast cancer (Slamon et al., 1987). This gene, which is located on chromosome 17, appears to be amplified (increased number of copies) in certain breast carcinomas (King et al., 1985; Yokota et al., 1986; Varley et al., 1988; Berger et al., 1988; Slamon et al., 1987, 1989; and van de Vijver, 1988). However, c-*erb* B-2 was not overexpressed in benign breast tissue (Gusterson et al., 1988). The observation by Slamon et al. (1989) that c-*erb* B-2 gene amplification was correlated with decreased disease-free survival and lower overall survival appeared important to the management of breast cancer. Several studies did not confirm these results (e.g., Zhou et al., 1989; Heintz et al., 1990; and Parkes et al., 1990). Methods for assessing gene amplification have not been developed suitably for routine application in the clinical laboratory. Therefore, numerous investigators began to pursue a correlation between the expression of the protein product of the oncogene and the clinical course of breast cancer patients.

Overexpression of the HER-2/neu protein product was weakly correlated with amplification of the oncogene but was strongly related to decreased disease-free survival and diminished overall survival (Tandon et al., 1989). Other investigators confirmed these results (Slamon et al., 1989; Borg et al., 1990; Paik et al., 1990; and Nicholson et al., 1991), while a few did not (e.g., Barnes et al., 1988). Overall, elevated levels of the oncoprotein appear to be associated with poor prognosis of breast cancer patients.

Since the EGF receptor exhibits a structure related to that of the protein product of the c-*erb* B-2 gene, several workers have questioned the importance of measuring both of these putative markers. Our laboratory and that of Harris and coworkers (Nicholson et al., 1991) have shown that there is no relationship between the expression of the EGF receptor and the c-*erb* B-2 oncoprotein when measured simultaneously on the same breast cancer specimen. More important, Nicholson and coworkers (1991) provided evidence that patients who overexpressed both EGF receptors and c-*erb* B-2 protein had much diminished disease-free survival as compared with patients whose tumors overexpressed only one of the proto-oncogene products. These data strongly suggest that both of these proteins are prognostic factors. Elledge's group (1992) and Henderson (1991) suggest caution about the use of EGF receptors and c-*erb* B-2 gene amplification or protein overexpression in the management of breast cancer. While not classifiable as a prognostic factor, these proteins appear to help define the biology and natural history of breast carcinoma.

Cathepsin D

When a carcinoma invades its local environment, certain proteases play an important role (Liotta et al., 1980; Goldfarb, 1986). A few studies have suggested that proteases belonging to the cathepsin family are secreted in larger amounts by carcinoma cells than by their normal counterparts (Poole et al., 1978; and Matrisian et al., 1986). Cathepsin D is a member of this protease family (Rochefort et al., 1987, 1988). This enzyme belongs to a class of acidic lysosomal proteases that are found in all cells. The cathepsin D gene is located at the extremity of the short arm of

chromosome 11, near the Ha-*ras* oncogene (Rochefort, 1990). Faust and associates (1985) determined that the amino acid sequence of human kidney cathepsin D contained 87% homology with that of cathepsin D isolated from porcine spleen. Other workers (e.g., Augereau et al., 1988) showed that cDNA clones of pro–cathepsin D from MCF-7 human breast cancer cells share more than 99% sequence homology with human kidney cathepsin D. Apparently there is little species differences in the primary structure (Rochefort et al., 1990).

Henri Rochefort's laboratory is largely responsible for the identification of this enzyme as a potential prognostic factor in cancer (Rochefort et al., 1989). His group demonstrated that certain breast cancer cell lines secrete a-52 kd precursor of cathepsin D that was identified as the proenzyme (Capony et al., 1987a, 1989). The pro–cathepsin D is a phosphoglycoprotein that is cleaved to mature forms of the enzyme with molecular weights of 48, 34, and 14 kd. Rochefort and coworkers also demonstrated a relationship between the incubation of estrogen receptor–positive cell lines, such as MCF-7 and ZR75-1, and the induction of pro–cathepsin D (Capony et al., 1989; and Rochefort et al., 1987a, 1988). Another important observation was that certain cell lines (MDA-MB231 and BT20), which are known to grow in a steroid hormone–independent environment, produced elevated levels of pro–cathepsin D (Vignon et al., 1986).

The final data suggesting the prognostic significance of this protease came from their studies (Rochefort et al., 1987, 1988) showing that certain primary breast cancer cell preparations exhibited pro–cathepsin D as detected by specific monoclonal antibodies. Rochefort and his coworkers produced a series of monoclonal antibodies against the different forms (Rochefort et al., 1990) of cathepsin D, and these have been assimilated into an (IRMA) kit format by CIS bio International.

The digestive pattern of cathepsin D appears to be similar in breast cancer and in normal breast cells. Some other interesting properties of pro–cathepsin D include autocrine mitogenic activity in MCF-7 human breast carcinoma cells (e.g., Morriset et al., 1986; Vignon et al., 1986; Capony et al., 1989) and the ability to recognize the mannose 6-phosphate/insulin-like growth factor (IGF)-II receptor (Capony et al., 1989; Mathieu et al., 1991). Researchers propose that this novel receptor is saturated as a result of treatment with pharmacologic doses of estrogen. This suggests that the estrogen-induced secretion of pro–cathepsin D and other lysosomal proenzymes may be closely associated with the sorting efficiency of the transport system responsible for these macromolecules.

Since the development of a clinical kit for measuring cathepsin D and its related molecules using specific monoclonal antibodies, many laboratories have been assessing these proteases in primary and metastatic breast cancers (e.g., Maudelonde et al., 1988; Spyratos et al., 1989; Thorpe et al., 1989; Brouillet et al., 1990; Tandon et al., 1990; Namer et al., 1991; Duffy et al., 1991, 1992; and Kute et al., 1992). Though it is unclear what level of cathepsin D represents overexpression in human breast cancer, data from some laboratories (e.g., Thorpe et al., 1989) suggest that premenopausal patients who exhibit more than

78 pmol/mg cytosol protein and postmenopausal patients who exhibit more than 24 pmol/mg cytosol protein experience a shorter disease-free interval and shorter survival overall. Many laboratories have now reported results using a variety of cutoff values. Most employ the cytosol from human breast biopsies that is used for estrogen and progestin determinations (Wittliff et al., 1991). Because of the sensitivity of the monoclonal antibody–based assays, cathepsin D can easily be measured on 200 mg of tissue.

Review of the literature suggests that there is a good correlation between the overexpression of cathepsin D in node-negative breast cancer and decreased disease-free and overall survival (e.g., Maudelonde et al., 1988; Spyratos et al., 1989; Thorpe et al., 1989; Rochefort et al., 1990; Tandon et al., 1990; Duffy et al., 1991, 1992; Granata et al., 1991; and Kute et al., 1992). Cathepsin D detected by immunohistochemical means also seems to be an independent prognostic factor for node-negative cases of breast cancer (Elledge et al., 1992; Leto et al., 1992; and Isola et al., 1992). When cathepsin D was evaluated relative to the expression of other prognostic factors, no association was found with estrogen or with progestin receptor levels, EGF receptors and c-*erb* B-2 protein expression, tumor size, or with the age of the patient (Duffy et al., 1991; and Kute et al., 1992). Using multivariant analysis, Tandon and coworkers (1990) found by flow cytometry that expression of cathepsin D was associated with aneuploidy. The combination of these two prognostic factors should be incorporated into the laboratory studies used for the management of patients with breast cancer.

OTHER POSSIBLE MARKERS

Experimental and clinical studies suggest that analogs of luteinizing hormone–releasing hormone (LH-RH), such as Zoladex, buserelin, leuprolide and [D-Trp⁶]LH-RH and of somatostatins such as Sandostatin are useful for treatment of certain breast cancers (e.g., Klijn et al., 1985, 1992*a*; Vickery and Lunenfeld, 1989; Lamberts et al., 1991; Schally et al., 1991; and Höffken, 1992;). Microanalytic methods of measuring LH-RH and somatostatin receptors in these tumors (Fekete et al., 1989; and Srkalovic et al., 1990) now allow correlation of the levels of these regulatory proteins with clinical parameters to better identify endocrine-responsive carcinomas (Schally, 1988; Vickery and Lunenfeld, 1989; Lamberts et al., 1991; and Höffken, 1992). Klijn and coworkers, (1992*a*) indicated that treatment with LH-RH analogs produced an objective response in approximately 40% of 419 breast cancer patients. Patients exhibiting estrogen receptor–positive breast carcinomas had a greater than 50% objective response, the longest one lasting more than 5 years.

The finding that more than half of primary breast tumors exhibit specific LH-RH receptors suggests that LH-RH analogs may have a direct inhibitory effect on tumor growth (Fekete et al., 1989; and Srkalovic et al., 1990). Synthesis of new LH-RH analogs with antagonistic activity and longer durations of action than LH-RH agonists may improve their therapeutic effectiveness (Schally et al., 1991). Regardless, there is sufficient evidence that measurements of LH-RH and somatostatin receptors in human breast cancers may be valuable predictive indices for selecting patients for treatment with LH-RH and somatostatin analogs.

Clinical trials suggest treatment with Zoladex plus tamoxifen promotes longer disease-free survival than treatment with the LH-RH analog alone (Nicholson, et al., 1990; and Blamey et al., 1991). If a correlation is found between clinical response to an LH-RH analog and LH-RH receptor expression, certain breast cancer patients could be treated more efficiently after analysis of both sex hormone and LH-RH receptors.

SUMMARY

Investigations in the past decade have provided biochemical and clinical evidence that estrogen and progestin receptors, EGF receptors, the protein product of the c-*erb* B-2 oncogene, and cathepsin D represent a panel of biochemical markers that is useful for ascertaining the biologic status of a carcinoma. Thus, laboratory medicine continues to play an important role in the management of the patient with breast carcinoma.

Acknowledgments

I acknowledge the devoted assistance of Ms. Carole Hall and Ms. Madeleine Marcum in the preparation of this chapter's revision. I am especially grateful to my wife, Mitzie, who has been my right hand in the laboratory and at home.

This chapter is dedicated to Dr. Thomas C. Hall, my first clinical mentor, who shared his knowledge of and devotion to the application of basic science to problems of clinical medicine.

References

Akiyama, T., Sudo, C., Ogawara, H., et al.: The product of the human c-*erb* B-2 gene: A 185 kilodalton glycoprotein with tyrosine kinase activity. Science, *232*:1644, 1986.

Alghanem, A.A., and Hussain, S.: The effect of age on estrogen and progesterone receptors in primary breast cancer. J. Surg. Oncol., *30*:29, 1985.

Allegra, J.C., and Lippman, M.E.: The effects of 17β-estradiol to tamoxifen on the ZR-75-1 human breast cancer cell line in defined medium. Eur. J. Cancer, *16*:1007, 1980.

Allegra, J.C., Lippman, M.E., and Thompson, E.B.: An association between steroid hormone receptors and response rate to cytotoxic chemotherapy in metastatic breast cancer. Cancer Treat. Rep., *62*:1281, 1978.

Allegra, J.C., Lippman, M.E., Thompson, E.B., et al.: Distribution, frequency and quantitative analysis of estrogen, progesterone, androgen and glucocorticoid receptors in human breast cancer. Cancer Res., *39*:1447, 1979*a*.

Allegra, J.C., Lippman, M.E., Thompson, E.B., et al.: Relationship between the progesterone, androgen, and glucocorticoid receptor and response rate to endocrine therapy in metastatic breast cancer. Cancer Res., *39*:1973, 1979*b*.

Allred, D., Clark, G., Tandon, A., et al.: HER-2/neu expression identified a group of node-negative breast cancer patients at high risk for recurrence (Abstract). Proc. Am. Soc. Clin. Oncol., *9*:23, 1990.

Augereau, P., Garcia, M., Mattei, M.G., et al.: Cloning and sequencing of the 52K cathepsin D cDNA of MCF7 breast cancer cells and mapping on chromosome 11. Molec. Endocrinol., *2*:186, 1988.

Auricchio, F., Migliaccio, A., and Castoria, G.: Dephosphorylation of oestradiol nuclear receptor in vitro. Biochem. J., *198*:699, 1981.

Baldi, A., Boyle, D.M., and Wittliff, J.L.: Estrogen receptor is associated with protein and phospholipid kinase activities. Biochem. Biophys. Res. Commun., *135:*597, 1986.

Baldi, A., Boyle, D.M., Annibali, N.V., et al.: A novel protein kinase activity identified from human breast cancer cell lines. *In* Li, J.J., Nandi, S., and Li, S.A. (Eds.): Hormonal Carcinogenesis. New York, Springer-Verlag, 1992, p. 58.

Bargmann, C.I., Hung, M.-C., and Weinberg, R.A.: The new oncogene encodes an epidermal growth factor receptor–related protein. Nature, *319:*226, 1986.

Barnes, D.M., Lammie, G.A., Millis, R.R., et al.: An immunohistochemical evaluation of c-erb B-2 expression in human breast cancer. Br. J. Cancer, *58:*448, 1988.

Beatson, G.T.: On the treatment of inoperable cases of carcinoma of the mamma; suggestions for a new method of treatment with illustrative cases. Lancet, *2:*104, 1896.

Benson, R.C., Jr., Gorman, P.A., O'Brien, P.C., et al.: Relationship between androgen receptor binding activity in human prostate cancer and clinical response to endocrine therapy. Cancer, *59:*1599, 1987.

Berger, M.S., Locher, G.W., Sauer, S., et al.: Correlation of c-erb B-2 gene amplification and protein expression in human breast carcinoma with node status and nuclear grading. Cancer Res., *48:*1238, 1988.

Berns, E.M.J.J., Mulder, E., Rommerts, F.F.G., et al.: Fluorescent ligands, used in histocytochemistry, do not discriminate between estrogen receptor–positive and receptor-negative human tumor cell lines. Breast Cancer Res. Treat., *4:*195, 1984.

Bishop, H.M., Blamey, R.W., Elston, C.W., et al.: Relationship of oestrogen-receptor status to survival in breast cancer. Lancet, *2:*283, 1979.

Bishop, J.M.: The molecular genetics of cancer. Science, *235:*305, 1987.

Black, R., Prescott, R., Bers, K., et al.: Tumor cellularity, oestrogen receptors and prognosis in breast cancer. Clin. Oncol., *9:*311, 1983.

Blamey, R.W., Bishop, H.M., Blake, J.R.S., et al.: Relationship between primary breast tumor receptor status and patient survival. Cancer, *46:*2765, 1980.

Blamey, R.W., Forbes, J., Jonat, W., et al.: Randomized trial comparing Zoladex with Nolvadex plus Zoladex in premenopausal advanced breast cancer (Abstract 77). 5th EORTC Breast Cancer Working Conference, 1991.

Bland, K.I., Fuchs, A., and Wittliff, J.L.: Menopausal status as a factor in the distribution of estrogen and progestin receptors in breast cancer. Surg. Forum, *32:*410, 1981.

Bonadonna, G., Rossi, A., Valagossa, P., et al.: The CMF program for operable breast cancer with positive axillary nodes: Updated analysis on the disease-free interval, site of relapse and drug tolerance. Cancer, *39:*2904, 1977.

Borg, A., Tandon, A.K., Signurdsson, H., et al.: HER-2/neu amplification predicts poor survival in node-positive breast cancer. Cancer Res., *50:*4332, 1990.

Boyle, D.M., Wiehle, R.D., Shahabi, N.A., et al.: Rapid, high-resolution procedure for assessment of estrogen receptor heterogeneity in clinical samples. J. Chromatogr., *327:*369, 1985.

Brouillet, J.-P., Theillet, C., Maudelonde, T., et al.: Cathepsin D assay in primary breast cancer and lymph nodes: Relationship with c-myc, c-erb B-2, and int-2 oncogene amplification and node invasiveness. Eur. J. Cancer, *26:*437, 1990.

Buller, R.E., and O'Malley, B.W.: The biology and mechanism of steroid hormone receptor interaction with the eukaryotic nucleus. Biochem. Pharmacol., *25:*1, 1976.

Burke, R.E., Miva, J.G., Datta, R., et al.: Estrogen action following irradiation of human breast cancer cells. Cancer Res., *38:*2813, 1978.

Capony, F., Morisset, M., Barrett, A.J., et al.: Phosphorylation, glycosylation and proteolytic activity of the 52K estrogen-induced protein secreted by MCF7 cells. J. Cell Biol., *104:*253, 1987.

Capony, F., Rougeot, C., Moncourier, P., et al.: Increased secretion, altered processing and glysylation of pro–cathepsin D in human mammary cancer cells. Cancer Res., *49:*3904, 1989.

Carlson, J.A., Allegra, J.C., Day, T.G. Jr., et al.: Tamoxifen and endometrial carcinoma alterations in estrogen and progesterone receptors in untreated patients and combination hormonal therapy in advanced neoplasia. Am. J. Obstet. Gynecol., *149:*149, 1984.

Carpenter, G.: Receptors for epidermal growth factor and other polypeptide mitogens. Ann. Rev. Biochem., *56:*881, 1987.

Carpenter, G., and Cohen, S.: Epidermal growth factor. Annu. Rev. Biochem., *48:*193, 1979.

Chabon, A.B., Goldberg, J.D., and Venet, L.: Carcinoma of the breast:

Interrelationship among histopathologic features, estrogen receptor activity and age of the patient. Hum. Pathol., *14:*368, 1982.

Chamness, G.C., Mercer, W.D., and McGuire, W.L.: Are histochemical methods for estrogen receptor valid? J. Histochem. Cytochem., *28:*792, 1980.

Chua, D.Y.F., Pang, M.W.Y., Rauff, A., et al.: Correlation of steroid receptors with histologic differentiation in mammary carcinoma. Cancer, *56:*2228, 1985.

Clark, G.M., McGuire, W.L., Hubay, C.A., et al.: Progesterone receptors as a prognostic factor in stage II breast cancer. N. Engl. J. Med., *309:*1343, 1983.

Clark, J.H., and Peck, E.J. Jr.: Female Sex Steroids: Receptors and Functions. New York, Springer-Verlag, 1979.

Cohen, S., Ushiro, H., Stoscheck, C., et al.: A native 170,000 epidermal growth factor receptor–kinase complex from shed plasma membrane vesicles. J. Biol. Chem., *257:*1523, 1982.

Coussens, L., Yang-Feng, T.L., and Liao, Y.-C., et al.: Tyrosine kinase receptor with extensive homology to EGF receptor shares chromosomal location with neu oncogene. Science, *230:*1132, 1985.

Crowe, J.P. Jr., Gordon, N.H., Hubay, C.A., et al.: The interaction of estrogen receptor status and race in predicting prognosis for stage I breast cancer patients. Surgery, *100:*599, 1986.

Dao, T.L.: Ablation therapy for hormone-dependent tumors. Annu. Rev. Med., *23:*1, 1972.

Davidson, N.E., Gelmann, E.P., Lippman, M.E., et al.: Epidermal growth factor receptor gene expression in estrogen receptor–positive and negative human breast cancer cell lines. Molec. Endocrinol., *1:*216, 1987.

Degenshein, G.A., Bloom, N., and Tobin, E.: The value of progesterone receptor assays in the management of advanced breast cancer. Cancer, *46:*2789, 1980.

Denison, M.S.: Heterogeneity of rat hepatic Ah receptor: Identification of two receptor forms which differ in their biochemical properties. J. Biochem. Toxicol., *7:*249, 1992.

DeSombre, E.R., Carbone, P.P., Jensen, E.V., et al.: Steroid receptors in breast cancer. N. Engl. J. Med., *301:*1011, 1979.

DiFiore, P.P., Pierce, J.H., Kraus, M.H., et al.: erb-B2 is a potent oncogene when over-expressed in N1H/3T3 cells. Science, *237:*178, 1987.

Donegan, W.L., and Spratt, J.S. (Eds.): Cancer of the Breast. 3rd ed. Philadelphia, W.B. Saunders, 1988.

Duffy, M.J., Brouillet, J.-P., Reilly, D., et al.: Cathepsin D concentration in breast cancer cytosols: Correlation with biochemical, histological and clinical findings. Clin. Chem., *37:*101, 1991.

Duffy, M.J., Reilly, D., Brouillet, J.-P., et al.: Cathepsin D concentration in breast cancer cytosols: Correlation with disease-free interval and overall survival. Clin. Chem., *38:*2114, 1992.

Elledge, R.M., McGuire, W.L., and Osborne, C.K.: Prognostic factors in breast cancer. Semin. Oncol., *19:*244, 1992.

Everson, R.B., Lippman, M.E., Thompson, E.B., et al.: Clinical correlations of steroid receptors and male breast cancer. Cancer Res., *40:*991, 1980.

Faust, P.L., Kornfeld, S., and Chirgwin, J.M.: Cloning and sequence analysis of cDNA for human cathepsin D. Proc. Natl. Acad. Sci. USA, *82:*4910, 1985.

Fekete, M., Wittliff, J.L., and Schally, A.V.: Characteristics and distribution of receptors for [D-TRP^6] luteinizing hormone-releasing hormone, somatosatin, epidermal growth factor, and sex steroids in 500 biopsy samples of human breast cancer. J. Clin. Lab. Anal., *3:*137, 1989.

Fisher, B., Brown, A., Wolmark, N.A., et al.: Prolonging tamoxifen therapy for primary breast cancer. Ann. Intern. Med., *106:*649, 1987.

Fisher, B., Redmond, C., Brown, A., et al.: Treatment of primary breast cancer with chemotherapy and tamoxifen. N. Engl. J. Med., *305:*1, 1981.

Fisher, B., Redmond, C., Brown, A., et al.: Influence of tumor estrogen and progesterone receptor levels on the response to tamoxifen and chemotherapy in primary breast cancer. J. Clin. Oncol., *1:*227, 1983.

Fisher, B., Sherman, B., Rockette, H., et al.: L-Phenylalanine mustard (L-PAM) in the management of premenopausal patients with primary breast cancer: Lack of association of disease-free survival with depression of ovarian function. Cancer, *44:*847, 1977.

Fitzpatrick, S.L., Brightwell, J., Wittliff, J.L., et al.: Epidermal growth factor binding by breast tumor biopsies and relationship to oestrogen receptor and progestin receptor levels. Cancer Res., *44:*3448, 1984.

Folca, P.J., Glascock, R.F., and Irvine, W.T.: Studies with tritium-labeled hexoestrol in advanced breast cancer. Lancet, *2:*796, 1961.

Folk, P., Dong, J., and Wittliff, J.L.: Simultaneous identification of estrogen and progesterone receptors by HPLC using a double isotope assay. J. Steroid Biochem. Molec. Biol., *42:*141, 1992.

Gapinski, P.V., and Donegan, W.L.: Estrogen receptors and breast cancer: Prognostic and therapeutic implications. Surgery, *88:*386, 1980.

Goldfarb, R.H.: Proteolytic enzymes in tumor invasion and degradation of host extracellular matrices. *In* Honn, K.V., Powers, W.E., and SLoane, B.F. (Eds.): Mechanisms of Cancer Metastasis. Boston, Martinus Nijhoff, 1986, p. 341.

Gorski, J., Toft, D., Shyamala, G., et al.: Hormone receptors: Studies on the interaction of estrogen with the uterus. Recent Progr. Hormone Res., *24:*45, 1968.

Granata, G., Coradini, D., Cappelletti, V., et al.: Prognostic relevance of cathepsin D versus oestrogen receptors in node-negative breast cancers. Eur. J. Cancer, *27:*970, 1991.

Greene, G.L., Fitche, F.W., and Jensen, E.V.: Monoclonal antibodies to estrophilin: Probes for the study of estrogen receptors. Proc. Natl. Acad. Sci. USA, *77:*157, 1980.

Greene, G.L., Sobel, N.B., King, W.J., et al.: Immunochemical studies of estrogen receptors. J. Steroid Biochem., *20:*51, 1984.

Green, S.: Modulation of oestrogen receptor activity by oestrogens and anti-oestrogens. J. Steroid Biochem. Molec. Biol., *37:*747, 1990.

Grill, H., Manz, B., Belozsky, O., et al.: Criteria for establishment of the double labeling assay for simultaneous determination of estrogen and progesterone receptors. Oncology, *41:*25, 1984.

Gronemeyer, H., Meyer, M.-E., Boequel, M.-T., et al.: Progestin receptors: Isoforms and antihormone action. J. Steroid Biochem. Mol. Biol., *40:*271, 1991.

Gusterson, B.A., Machin, L.G., Gullick, W.J., et al.: c-*erb* B-2 expression in benign and malignant breast tissue. Br. J. Cancer, *58:*453, 1988.

Hähnel, R., and Twaddle, E.: The relationship between estrogen receptors in primary and secondary breast carcinomas and insequential primary breast carcinomas. Breast Cancer Res. Treat., *5:*155, 1985.

Hähnel, R., Woodings, T., and Vivian, A.B.: Prognostic value of estrogen receptors in primary breast cancer. Cancer, *44:*671, 1979.

Hall, T.C.: Chemotherapy of breast cancer. Clin. Obstet. Gynecol., *11:*401, 1968.

Harris, A.L., Nicholson, S., Sainsbury, J.R.C., et al.: Epidermal growth factor receptors in breast cancer: Association with early relapse and death, poor response to hormones and interactions with neu. J. Steroid Biochem., *34:*123, 1989.

Hedley, D., Rugg, C., and Gelber, R.: Association of DNA index and S-phase fraction with prognosis of nodes positive early breast cancer. Cancer Res., *47:*4729, 1987.

Heintz, N.H., Leslie, K.D., Roger, L.A., et al.: Amplification of the c-erb B-2 oncogene and prognosis in breast cancer. Arch. Pathol. Lab. Med., *114:*1603, 1990.

Helin, H., Helle, M., Kalliomieni, O., et al.: Immunohistochemical determination of estrogen and progesterone receptors in human breast carcinoma. Cancer, *63:*1761, 1989.

Henderson, I.C.: Prognostic factors. *In* Harris, J.R., Hellman, S., Henderson, I.C., and Kinne, D.W. (Eds.): Breast Diseases. 2nd ed. Philadelphia, J. B. Lippincott, 1991, p. 332.

Hochberg, R.B.: Iodine-124-labeled estradiol: A gamma-emitting analog of estradiol that binds to the estrogen receptor. Science, *205:*1138, 1979.

Höffken, K.: Peptides in Oncology: LH-RH Agonists and Antagonists. Heidelberg, Springer-Verlag, 1992.

Horwitz, K.B.: The molecular biology of RU486. Is there a role for antiprogestin in the treatment of breast cancer? Endocrine Rev., *13:*136, 1992.

Horwitz, K.B., and McGuire, W.L.: Specific progesterone receptors in human breast cancer. Steroids, *25:*497, 1975*a*.

Horwitz, K.B., McGuire, W.L., Pearson, O.H., et al.: Predicting response to endocrine therapy in human breast cancer: A hypothesis. Science, *189:*726, 1975*b*.

Howat, J.M.T., Barnes, D.M., Harris, M., et al.: The association of cytosol oestrogen and progesterone receptors with histological features of breast cancer and early detection of disease. Br. J. Cancer, *47:*629, 1983.

Hudziak, R., Schlessinger, J., and Ullrich, A.: Increased expression of the putative growth factor receptor p185 HER2 causes transformation and tumorigenesis of H1H/3T3 cells. Proc. Natl. Acad. Sci. USA, *84:*7159, 1987.

Huggins, C., and Bergenstal, D.M.: Inhibition of human mammary and prostatic cancer by adrenalectomy. Cancer Res., *12:*134, 1952.

Hull, D.F. III, Clark, G.M., Osborne, C.K., et al.: Multiple estrogen receptor assays in human breast cancer. Cancer Res., *43:*413, 1983.

Hunter, T., and Cooper, J.A.: Protein-tyrosine kinases. Annu. Rev. Biochem., *54:*897, 1985.

Hutchens, T.W., Wiehle, R.D., Shahabi, N.A., et al.: Rapid analysis of estrogen receptor heterogeneity by chromatofocusing with high performance liquid chromatography. J. Chromatogr., *266:*115–128, 1983.

Isola, J., Weitz, S., Visakorpi, T., et al.: Cathepsin D expression detected by immunohistochemistry has independent prognostic value in axillary node–negative breast cancer. J. Clin. Oncol., *11:*36, 1993.

Jensen, E.V., Block, G.E., Smith, S., et al.: Estrogen receptors and breast cancer response to adrenalectomy. Natl. Cancer Inst. Monogr., *34:*55, 1971.

Jensen, E.V., Suzuku, T., Kawashima, T., et al.: A two-step mechanism for the interaction of estradiol with rat uterus. Proc. Nat. Acad. Sci., *59:*32, 1968.

Jordan, V.C., and Murphy, C.S.: Endocrine pharmacology of antiestrogens as antitumor agents. Endocrine Rev., *11:*49, 1990.

Jordan, V.C., Jeng, M.-H., Jing, S.-Y., et al.: Hormonal strategies for breast cancer: A new focus on the estrogen receptor as a therapeutic target. Semin. Oncol., *19:*299, 1992.

Kennedy, B.J.: Hormonal therapies in breast cancer. Semin. Oncol., *1:*19, 1974.

Khan, S.A., Rogers, M.A.M., Obando, J.A., et al.: Estrogen receptor expression of benign breast epithelium and its association with breast cancer. Cancer Res., *54:*993, 1994.

Kiang, D.T., and Kennedy, B.J.: Factors affecting estrogen receptors in breast cancer. Cancer, *40:*1571, 1977.

King, C.R., Kraus, M.H., and Aaronson, S.A.: Amplification of a novel c-*erb* B-related gene in a human mammary carcinoma. Science, *229:*974, 1985*a*.

King, W.J., and Greene, G.L.: Monoclonal antibodies localize oestrogen receptor in the nuclei of target cells. Nature, *307:*745, 1984.

King, W.J., DeSombre, E.R., and Jensen, E.V.: Comparison of immuno-cytochemical and steroid-binding assays for estrogen receptor in human breast tumors. Cancer Res., *45:*293, 1985*b*.

Klijn, J.G.M., Berns, P.M.J.J., Bontenbal, M., et al.: Clinical breast cancer, new developments in selection and endocrine treatment of patients. J. Steroid Biochem. Molec. Biol., *43:*211, 1992*a*.

Klijn, J.G.M., Berns, P.M.J.J., Schmitz, P.I.M., et al.: The clinical significance of epidermal growth factor receptor (EGF-R) in human breast cancer: A review on 5,232 patients. Endocrine Rev., *13:*156, 1992*b*.

Klijn, J.G.M., Berns, P.M.J.J., Schmitz, P.I.M., et al.: Epidermal growth factor receptor (EGF-R) in clinical breast cancer: Update 1993. Endocrine Rev., *1:*171, 1993.

Klijn, J.G.M., De Jong, F.H., Lamberts, S.W.J., et al.: LH-RH agonist treatment in clinical and experimental human breast cancer. J. Steroid Biochem., *23:*867, 1985.

Knight, W.A., Livingston, R.B., and Gregory, E.J.: Estrogen receptor as an independent prognostic factor for early recurrence in breast cancer. Cancer Res., *37:*4669, 1977.

Kute, T.E., Heidemann, P., and Wittliff, J.L.: Molecular heterogeneity of cytosolic forms of estrogen receptors from human breast tumors. Cancer Res., *38:*4307, 1978.

Kute, T.E., Shao, Z.-M., Sugg, N.K., et al.: Cathepsin D as a prognostic indicator for node-negative breast cancer patients using both immunoassays and enzymatic assays. Cancer Res., *52:*5198, 1992.

Lamberts, S.W.J., Krenning, E.P., and Reubi, J.-C.: The role of somatostatin and its analogs in the diagnosis and treatment of tumors. Endocrine Rev., *12:*212, 1991.

Leclercq, G., Toma, S., Paridaens, R., et al. (Eds.): Clinical Interest of Steroid Hormone Receptors in Breast Cancer. New York, Springer-Verlag, 1984.

Leto, G., Gebbia, N., Rausa, L., et al.: Cathepsin D in the malignant progression of neoplastic diseases (Review). Anticancer Res., *12:*235, 1992.

Liotta, L.A., Tryggvason, K., Garbisa, S., et al.: Metastatic potential correlates with enzymatic degradation of basement membrane collagen. Nature (Lond.), *284:*67, 1980.

Locher, G.W., Davis, B., Zava, D.T., et al.: Intratumoral regional differences in hormone receptor status of breast cancer. Geburtshilfe Fraunheilkd., *44:*304, 1984.

Lonsdorfer, M., Clements, N.C. Jr., and Wittliff, J.L.: Use of high performance liquid chromatography in the elevation of the synthesis and binding of fluorescein-linked steroids to estrogen receptors. J. Chromatogr., *266:*129, 1983.

Luft, R., and Olivecrona, H.: Hypophysectomy in man; experiences in metastatic cancer of the breast. Cancer, *8:*261, 1955.

Lupu, R., Colomer, R., Zugmaier G., et al.: Direct interaction of a ligand for the erbB2 oncogene product with the EGF receptor and p185erbB2. Science, *249:*1552, 1990.

Lupu, R., Dickson, R.B., and Lippman, M.E.: The role of *erb* B-2 and its ligands in growth control of malignant breast epithelium. J. Steroid Biochem. Molec. Biol., *43:*229, 1992.

Maass, H., Engel, B., and Hohmeister, H.: Estrogen receptors in human breast tissue. Am. J. Obstet. Gynecol., *113:*377, 1972.

Macara, I.G., Marinetti, G.V., and Balduzzi, P.C.: Transforming protein of avian sarcoma virus UR2 is associated with phosphatidylenositol kinase activity: Possible role in tumorigenesis. Proc. Natl. Acad. Sci. USA, *81:*2728, 1984.

Macias, A., Azavedo E., Perez, R., et al.: Receptors for epidermal growth factor in human mammary carcinomas and their metastases. Anticancer Res., *6:*849, 1986.

Maguire, H.C., and Greene, M.I.: The *neu* (c-*erb* B-2) oncogene. Semin. Oncol., *16:*148, 1989.

Mathieu M., Vignon, F., Capony, F., et al.: Estradiol down-regulates the mannose-6-phosphate/insulin-like growth factor-II receptor gene and induces cathepsin D in breast cancer cell: A receptor saturation mechanism to increase the secretion of lysosomal proenzymes. Molec. Endocrinol., *5:*815, 1991.

Matrisian, L.Y., Bowden, G.T., Krieg, P., et al.: The mRNA coding for the secreted protease transin is expressed more abundantly in malignant than in benign tumors. Proc. Natl. Acad. Sci. USA, *83:*9413, 1986.

Maudelonde, T., Khalaf, S., Garcia, M., et al.: Immunoenzymatic assay of Mr 52,000 cathepsin D in 182 breast cancer cytosols. Low correlation with other prognostic parameters. Cancer Res., *48:*462, 1988.

Maudelonde, T., Martinez, P., Brouillet, J.P., et al.: Cathepsin D in human endometrium: Induction by progesterone and potential value as a tumor marker. J. Clin. Endocrinol. Metab., *70:*115, 1990.

McCarty, K.S. Jr., Silva, J.S., Cox, E.B., et al.: Relationship of age and menopausal status to estrogen receptor content in primary carcinoma of the breast. Ann. Surg., *197:*123, 1983.

McCarty, K.S. Jr., Miller, L.S., Cox, E.B., et al.: Estrogen receptor analyses: Correlation of biochemical and immunohistochemical methods using monoclonal antireceptor antibodies. Arch. Pathol. Lab. Med., *109:*716, 1985.

McGuire, W.L., Carbone, P.O., and Vollmer, E.P. (Eds.): Estrogen Receptors in Human Breast Cancer. New York, Raven Press, 1975.

McGuire, W.L., Chamness, G.C., and Fuqua, S.A.W.: Abnormal estrogen receptor in clinical breast cancer. J. Steroid Biochem. Molec. Biol., *43:*243, 1992.

McGuire, W.L., Raynaud, J.P., and Baulieu, E.-E. (Eds.): Progesterone Receptors in Normal and Neoplastic Tissues. New York, Raven Press, 1977.

Meyer, J.S.: Hormone receptors in human malignancy of unknown origin: Potential utility in clinical management. *In* Fer, M.F., Oldham, D., and Greco, A. (Eds.): Tumors of Unknown Origin and Poorly Differentiated Neoplasms. Orlando, FL, Grune & Stratton, 1986, p. 519.

Meyer, J.S., Rao, B.R., Stevens, S.C., et al.: Low incidence of estrogen receptor in breast carcinomas with rapid rates of cellular replication. Cancer, *40:*2290, 1977.

Meyer, J.S., Schechtman, K., and Valdes, R. Jr.: Estrogen and progesterone receptor assays on breast carcinoma from mastectomy specimens. Cancer, *52:*2139, 1983.

Meyer, J.S., and Wittliff, J.L.: Regional heterogeneity in breast carcinoma: Thymidine labelling index, steroid hormone receptors, DNA ploidy. Int. J. Cancer, *47:*213, 1991.

Mills, R.R.: Correlation of hormone receptors with pathological features in human breast cancer. Cancer, *46:*2869, 1980.

Mirecki, D.M., and Jordan, V.C.: Steroid hormone receptors and human breast cancer. Lab. Med., *16:*287, 1985.

Mohla, S., Sampson, C.C., Kahn, T., et al.: Estrogen and progesterone receptors in breast cancer in black Americans. Cancer (Phila.), *50:*552, 1982.

Morriset, M., Capony, F., and Rochefort, H.: Processing and estrogen regulation of the 52-kilodalton protein inside MCF-7 breast cancer cell. Endocrinology, *119:*2773, 1986.

Morrison, A.S., Black, M.M., Lowe, C.R., et al.: Some international differences in histology and survival in breast cancer. Int. J. Cancer, *11:*261, 1973.

Mortel, R., Levy, C., Wolff, J.-P., et al.: Female sex steroid receptors in postmenopausal endometrial carcinoma and biochemical response to an antiestrogen. Cancer Res., *41:*1140, 1981.

Moudgil, V.K. (Ed.): Molecular Mechanisms of Steroid Hormone Action (German). Berlin, Walter de Gruyter, 1985.

Moudgil, V.K. (Ed.): Steroid Hormone Receptors: Basic and Clinical Aspects. Boston, Birkhäuser, 1994.

Murphy, L.C., and Dotzlaw, H.: Variant estrogen receptor mRNA species detected in human breast cancer biopsy samples. Molec. Endocrinol., *3:*687, 1989.

Nakao, M., Sato, B., Koga, M., et al.: Identification of immunoassayable estrogen receptor lacing hormone-binding ability in tamoxifen-treated rat uterus. Biochem. Biophys. Res. Commun., *132:*336, 1985.

Namer, M., Ramaioli, A., Fontana, X., et al.: Prognostic value of total cathepsin D in breast tumors. Breast Cancer Res. Treat., *19:*85, 1991.

Nemoto, T., Vana, J., Bedwani, R.N., et al.: Management and survival of female breast cancer: Results of a national survey by the American College of Surgeons. Cancer, *45:*2917, 1980.

Nicholson, R.I., Walker, K.J., McClelland, R.A., et al.: Zoladex plus tamoxifen versus Zoladex alone in pre- and peri-menopausal metastatic breast cancer. J. Steroid Biochem. Molec. Biol., *37:*989, 1990.

Nicholson, S., Halcrow, P., Sainsbury, J.R.C., et al.: Epidermal growth factor receptor (EGFr) status associated with failure of primary endocrine therapy in elderly postmenopausal patients with breast cancer. Br. J. Cancer, *58:*810, 1988a.

Nicholson, S., Harris, A.L., and Farndon, J.R.: Role of receptors in the management of patients with breast cancer. Diagn. Oncol., *1:*43, 1991.

Nicholson, S., Sainsbury, J.R.C., Needham, G.K., et al.: Quantitative assays of epidermal growth factor receptor in human breast cancer: Cutoff points of clinical relevance. Int. J. Cancer, *42:*36, 1988b.

Nicholson, S., Sainsbury, J.R.C., Halcrow, P., et al.: Expression of epidermal growth factor receptors associated with lack of response to endocrine therapy in recurrent breast cancer. Lancet, *i:*182, 1989.

NIH consensus development conference on steroid receptors in breast cancer. Cancer, *46:*2759, 1980.

Nomura, Y., Kobayashi, S., Takatani, O., et al.: Estrogen receptor and endocrine responsiveness in Japanese versus American breast cancer patients. Cancer Res., *37:*106, 1977.

Nomura, Y., Tashiro, H., Hamada, Y., et al.: Relationship between estrogen receptors and risk factors in breast cancer in Japanese pre- and postmenopausal patients. Breast Cancer Res. Treat., *4:*37, 1984.

Notides, A.C., Lerner, N., and Hamilton, D.E.: Positive cooperativity of the estrogen receptor. Proc. Natl. Acad. Sci. USA, *78:*4926, 1981.

Osborne, C.K.: Receptors. *In* Harris, J.R., Hellman, S., Henderson, I.C., and Kinne, D.W. (Eds.): Breast Diseases. 2nd ed. Philadelphia, J.B. Lippincott, 1991.

Paik, S., Hazen, R., Fisher, E.R., et al.: Pathologic findings from the National Surgical Adjuvant Breast and Bowel Project: Prognostic significance of c-*erb* B-2 protein overexpression in primary breast cancer. J. Clin. Oncol., *8:*103, 1990.

Palshof, T., Mouridsen, H.T., and Daehnfeldt, J.L.: Adjuvant endocrine therapy of primary operable breast cancer. Report on the Copenhagen breast cancer trials. Eur. J. Cancer, *16* (Suppl. 1):183, 1980.

Parkes, H.C., Lillycrop, K., Howel, A., et al.: c-*erb* B-2 mRNA expression in human breast tumours: Comparison with c-*erb* B-2 DNA amplification and correlation with prognosis. Br. J. Cancer, *61:*39, 1990.

Parl, F.F., Schmidt, B.P., Dupont, W.D., et al.: Prognostic significance of estrogen receptor status in breast cancer in relation to tumor stage, axillary node metastasis, and histopathologic grading. Cancer, *54:*2237, 1984.

Pasic, R., Djulbegovic, B., and Wittliff, J.L.: Comparison of sex steroid receptor determinations in human breast cancer by enzyme immunoassay and radioligand binding. J. Clin. Lab. Anal., *4:*430, 1990.

Pegoraro, R.J., Karnan, V., Nirmul, D., et al.: Estrogen and progesterone receptors in breast cancer among women of different racial groups. Cancer Res., *46:*2117, 1986a.

Pegoraro, R.J., Nirmul, D., and Joubert, S.M.: Cytoplasmic and nuclear estrogen and progesterone receptors in male breast cancer. Cancer Res., *42:*4812, 1982.

Pegoraro, R.J., Nirmul, D., Reinach, S.G., et al.: Breast cancer prognosis in three different racial groups in relation to the steroid hormone receptor status. Breast Cancer Res. Treat., *7:*111, 1986b.

Perez, R., Pascual, M., Macias, A., et al.: Epidermal growth factor receptors in human breast cancer. Breast Cancer Res. Treat., *4:*189, 1984.

Polk, H.C. Jr.: Improved understanding of mammary cancer and exemplar for surgical oncology. Cancer, *57:*411, 1986.

Pollow, K., Schmidt-Gollwitzer, M., and Pollow, B.: Progesterone- and estradiol-binding proteins from normal human endometrium and endometrial carcinoma: A comparative study. *In* Wittliff, J.L. and Dapunt, O. (Eds.): Steroid Receptors and Hormone-Dependent Neoplasia. New York, Masson Publishing, 1980, p. 69.

Ponsky, J.L., Gliga, L., and Reynolds, S.: Medullary carcinoma of the breast: An association with negative hormonal receptors. J. Surg. Oncol., *25:*76, 1984.

Poole, A.R., Tiltman, K.J., Recklies, A.D., et al.: Differences in secretion of the proteinase cathepsin B at the edges of human breast carcinomas and fibroadenomas. Nature (Lond.), *273:*545, 1978.

Puca, G.A., Nola, E., Sica, V., et al.: Estrogen-binding proteins of calf uterus. Interrelationship between various forms and identification of a receptor-transforming factor. Biochemistry, *11:*4157, 1972.

Raam, S., and Teixeira, T.: Effect of sodium molybdate on protein measurements: Quality control aspects of steroid hormone receptor assays. Eur. J. Cancer Clin. Oncol., *21:*1219, 1985.

Raam, S., and Vrabel, D.M.: Evaluation of an enzyme immunoassay kit for estrogen receptor measurements. Clin. Chem., *32:*1496, 1986.

Rao, B.R., and Meyer, J.S.: Estrogen and progestin receptors in normal and cancer tissue. *In* McGuire, W.L., Raynaud, J.P., and Baulieu, E.E. (Eds.): Progesterone Receptors in Normal and Neoplastic Tissues. New York, Raven Press, 1977, p. 155.

Rochefort, H.: Cathepsin D in breast cancer. Breast Cancer Res. Treat., *16:*3, 1990.

Rochefort, H., Augereau, P., and Briozzo, R.: Structure, function, regulation and clinical significance of the 52 kd pro–cathepsin D secreted by breast cancer cells. Biochimie, *70:*943, 1988.

Rochefort, H., Capony, F., and Garcia, M., et al.: Estrogen-induced lysosomal proteases secreted by breast cancer cells: A role in carcinogenesis. J. Cell Biochem., *35:*17, 1987*a*.

Rochefort, H., Capony, F., and Garcia, M.: Cathepsin D in breast cancer: From molecular and cellular biology to clinical applications. Cancer Cells, *2:*383, 1990.

Rochefort, H., Cavailles, V., Freiss, G., et al.: Detection and assay of the 52K estrogen-regulated protease in mammary tumors. *In:* Ceriani, R.L., (Ed.): Immunological Approaches to the Diagnosis and Therapy of Breast Cancer. New York, Plenum Publishing Corp., 1987*b*, p. 85.

Rochefort H., Cavailles V., Augereau P., et al.: Overexpression and hormonal regulation of pro–cathepsin D in mammary and endometrial cancer. J. Steroid Biochem., *34:*177, 1989.

Rosen, P.P., Menendez-Botet, C., Nisselbaum, J.S., et al.: Pathological review of breast lesions analyzed for estrogen receptor protein. Cancer Res., *35:*3187, 1975.

Sainsbury, J.R.C., Farndon, J.R., Needham, G.K., et al.: Epidermal growth factor receptor status as predictor of early recurrence of and death from breast cancer. Lancet, *i:*1398, 1987.

Sainsbury, J.R.C., Malcolm, A.J., Appleton, D.R., et al.: Presence of epidermal growth factor receptor as an indicator of poor prognosis in patients with breast cancer. J. Clin. Pathol., *38:*1225, 1985.

Santen, R.J., Manni, A., Harvey, H., et al.: Endocrine treatment of breast cancer in women. Endocrine Rev., *11:*1, 1990.

Sarfaty, G.A., Nash, A.R., and Keightly, D.D. (Eds.): Estrogen Receptor Assays in Breast Cancer: Laboratory Discrepencies and Quality Assurance. New York, Masson Publishing, 1981.

Sato, N., Hyder, S.M., Chang, L., et al.: Interaction of estrogen receptor isoforms with immobilized monoclonal antibodies. J. Chromatogr., *359:*475, 1986.

Saunders, D.E., Christensen, C., Lawrence, W. D., et al.: Receptors for 1,25-dihydroxyvitamin D₃ in gynecologic neoplasms. Gynecol. Oncol., *44:*131, 1992.

Savage, N., Levin, J., De Moor, N.G., et al.: Cytosolic oestrogen receptor content of breast cancer tissue in blacks and whites. S. Afr. Med. J., *59:*623, 1981.

Schally, A.V.: Oncological applications of somatostatin analogs. Cancer Res., *48:*6977, 1988.

Schally, A.V., Comaru-Schally, A.M., Hollander, V.: Hypothalamic and other peptide hormones. *In* Holland, J.F., Frei, E. III, Bast, R.C., et al. (Eds.): Cancer Medicine. 3rd ed. Philadelphia, Lee & Febiger, 1991.

Schecter, A.L., Stern, D.F., Vaidyanathan, L., et al.: The *neu* oncogene: An *erb*-B–related gene encoding a 185,000-M$_r$ tumor antigen. Nature (Lond), *312:*513, 1984.

Shahabi, N.A., He, Y.J., Wiehle, R.D., et al.: Characteristics of estrogen receptors in MCF-7 breast cancer cells. Amsterdam, Excerpta Medica, 1984, p. 1469.

Shepel, L.A., and Gorski, J.: Steroid hormone receptors and oncogenes. BioFactors, *1:*71, 1988.

Sherman, M.S., Pickering, L.A., Rollwagen, F.M., et al.: Meroreceptors: Proteolytic fragments of receptors containing the steroid-binding site. Fed. Proc., *37:*167, 1978.

Silfversward, C., Gustafsson, J.-A., Gustafsson, S.A., et al.: Estrogen receptor concentrations in 269 cases of histologically classified human breast cancer. Cancer, *45:*2001, 1980.

Slamon, D.J., Clark, G.M., Wong, S.G., et al.: Human breast cancer: Correlation of relapse and survival with amplification of the Her-2/*neu* oncogene. Science, *235:*177, 1987.

Slamon, D.J., Godolphin W., Jones, L.A., et al.: Studies of the HER-2/*neu* proto-oncogene in human breast and ovarian cancer. Science, *244:*707, 1989.

Sloane, B.F., Sadler, J.G., Evens, C., et al.: Cathepsin-B–like cysteine proteinases and tumor metastasis. Cancer Bull., *36:*196, 1984.

Sluyser, M., and Mester, J.: Oncogenes homologous to steroid receptor (Letter to the editor)? Nature, *315:*546, 1985.

Sluyser, M., and Wittliff, J.L.: Influence of estrogen receptor variants in mammary carcinomas on the prognostic reliability of the receptor assay. Molec. Cell. Endocrinol., *85:*83, 1992.

Southern, E.M.: Detection of specific sequences among DNA fragments separated by gel electrophoresis. J. Molec. Biol., *98:*503, 1975.

Spratt, J.S., Damian, P.A., Greenberg, R.A., et al.: Association of chronic cystic mastopathy, xeromammographic patterns, and cancer. Cancer, *55:*1372, 1985.

Spyratos F., Brouillet, J.P., Defrenne A., et al.: Cathepsin D: An independent prognostic factor for metastasis of breast cancer. Lancet, *2:*1115, 1989.

Srkalovic, G., Wittliff, J.L., Schally, A.V.: Detection and partial characterization of receptors for [D-Trp⁶]-luteinizing hormone–releasing hormone and epidermal growth factor in human endometrial carcinoma. Cancer Res., *50:*1841, 1990.

Stegner, H.E., Maass, H., Trams, G., et al.: Estrogen receptors and ultrastructural pathology of mammary carcinoma. *In* Dallenback-Hellweg, G. (Ed.): Functional Morphological Changes in Female Sex Organs Induced by Exogenous Hormones. Berlin, Springer-Verlag, 1980.

Stewart, J.F., Rubens, R.D., Millis, R.R., et al.: Steroid receptors and prognosis in operable (Stage I and II) breast cancer. Eur. J. Cancer Clin. Oncol., *19:*1381, 1983.

Sugimoto, Y., Whitman, M., Cantly, L.C., et al.: Evidence that the Rous sarcoma virus transforming gene product phosphorylates phosphatidylinositol and diacylglycerol. Proc. Natl. Acad. Sci. USA, *81:*2117, 1984.

Symposium on estrogen receptor determination with monoclonal antibodies. Cancer Res., *46*(Suppl 1):4231, 1986.

Tandon, A.K., Clark, G.M., Chamness, G.C., et al.: HER-2/*neu* oncogene protein and prognosis in breast cancer. J. Clin. Oncol., *7:*1120, 1989.

Tandon, A.K., Clark, G.M., Chamness, G.C., et al.: Cathepsin D and prognosis in breast cancer. N. Engl. J. Med., *322:*297, 1990.

Thorpe, S.M., Rochefort, H., Garcia, M., et al.: Association between high concentrations of M 52,000 cathepsin D and poor prognosis in primary human breast cancer. Cancer Res., *49:*6008, 1989.

Todaro, G.J., Fryling C., and Delsarco, J.E.: Transforming growth factors produced by certain human tumour cells: Polypeptides that interact with epidermal growth factor receptors. Proc. Natl. Acad. Sci. USA, *77:*5258, 1980.

Trams, G., and Maass, H.: Specific binding of estradiol and dihydrotestosterone receptors in human mammary cancers. Cancer Res., *37:*258, 1976.

van de Vijver, M.J., Peterse, J.L., Mooi, W.J., et al.: *Neu*-protein overexpression in breast cancer. N. Engl. J. Med., *319:*1239, 1988.

van der Walt, L.A., and Wittliff, J.L.: Assessment of progestin receptor polymorphism by various synthetic ligands using HPLC. J. Steroid Biochem., *24:*377, 1986.

Varley, J.M., Swallow, J.E., Brammer, W.J., et al.: Alterations to either c-*erb* B-2 (*neu*) or c-*myc* proto-oncogenes in breast carcinomas correlate with poor short-term prognosis. Oncogene, *1:*432, 1988.

Venter, D.J., Tuzi, N.L., Kumar, S., et al.: Over-expression of the c-*erb* B-2 oncoprotein in human breast carcinomas: Immunohistologic assessment correlates with gene amplification. Lancet, *2:*69, 1987.

Vickery, B.H., and Lunenfeld, B.: GnRH Analogues in Cancer and Human Reproduction: Basic Aspects. Vol. 1. Dordrecht, Kluwer Academic Publishers, 1989.

Vignon F., Capony F., Chambon M., et al.: Autocrine growth stimulation by the MCF-7 breast cancer cells by the estrogen-regulated 52 K protein. Endocrinology, *118:*1537, 1986.

Walker, A.R.P., Walter, B.F., Tshyabalala, E.N., et al.: Low survival of

South African urban black women with breast cancer. Br. J. Cancer, *49:*241, 1984.

Wei, L.L., Krett, N.L., Francis, M.D., et al.: Multiple human progesterone receptor messenger ribonucleic acids and their autoregulation by progestin agonists and antagonists in breast cancer cells. Molec. Endocrinol., *2:*62, 1988.

Welshons, W.V., Lieberman, M.E., and Gorski, J.: Nuclear localization of unoccupied oestrogen receptors. Nature, *307:*747, 1984.

Wiehle, R.D., Hofmann, G.E., Fuchs, A., et al.: High performance size exclusion chromatography as a rapid method for the separation of steroid hormone receptors. J. Chromatogr., *307:*39, 1984.

Wiehle, R.D., and Wittliff, J.L.: Alterations in sex-steroid hormone receptors during mammary gland differentiation in the rat. Comp. Biochem. Physiol., *768:*409, 1983.

Wiehle, R.D., and Wittliff, J.L.: Isoforms of estrogen receptors by high-performance ion-exchange chromatography. J. Chromatogr., *297:*313, 1984.

Wilking, N., Carlström, H., Sköldefors, H., et al.: Estradiol formation and estrogen receptors in breast tumor tissue: Effect of tamoxifen on estrogen interconversions in breast tumor homogenate in vitro. Breast Cancer Res. Treat., *4:*149, 1984.

Wittliff, J.L.: Specific receptor of the steroid hormones in breast cancer. Semin. Oncol., *1:*109, 1974.

Wittliff, J.L.: Steroid-binding proteins in normal and neoplastic mammary cells. *In* Busch, H. (Ed.): Methods in Cancer Research. Vol. II. New York, Academic Press, 1975, p. 293.

Wittliff, J.L.: Steroid hormone receptors in breast cancer. Cancer, *53:*630, 1984.

Wittliff, J.L.: Separation and characterization of isoforms of steroid hormone receptors using high-performance liquid chromatography. *In* Moudgil, V.K. (Ed.): Molecular Mechanisms of Steroid Hormone Action. Berlin, Walter de Gruyter, 1985, p. 791.

Wittliff, J.L.: HPLC of steroid-hormone receptors. LC-GC Magazine Liquid Gas Chromatogr., *4:*1092, 1986.

Wittliff, J.L.: Steroid hormone receptors. *In* Pesce, A., and Kaplan, L. (Eds.): Methods in Clinical Chemistry. St. Louis, C.V. Mosby, 1987, p. 767.

Wittliff, J.L., and DaPunt, O. (Eds.): Steroid Receptors and Hormone-Dependent Neoplasia. New York, Masson, 1980.

Wittliff, J.L., and Savlov, E.D.: Estrogen-binding capacity of cytoplasmic forms of the estrogen receptor in human breast cancer. *In* McGuire, W.L., Carbone, P.O., and Vollmer, E.P. (Eds.): Estrogen Receptors in Human Breast Cancer. New York, Raven Press, 1975, p. 73.

Wittliff, J.L., and Wiehle, R.D.: Analytical methods for steroid hormone receptors and their quality assurance. *In* Hollander, V.P. (Ed.): Hormonally Responsive Tumors. New York, Academic Press, 1985, p. 383.

Wittliff, J.L., Beatty, B.W., Savlov, E.D., et al.: Estrogen receptors and hormone dependency in human breast cancer. Recent Results Cancer Res., *57:*59, 1976.

Wittliff, J.L., Durant, J.R., and Fisher, B.: Methods of steroid receptor analyses and their quality control in the clinical laboratory. *In* Soto, R., DeNicola, A.F., and Blaquier, J.A. (Eds.): Physiopathology of Endocrine Diseases and Mechanisms of Hormone Action. New York, Alan R. Liss, 1981*a*, p. 397.

Wittliff, J.L., Feldhoff, P.A., Fuchs, A., et al.: Polymorphism of estrogen receptors in human breast cancer. *In* Soto, R., DeNicola, A.F., and Blaquier, J.A. (Eds.): Physiopathology of Endocrine Diseases and Mechanisms of Hormone Action. New York, Alan R. Liss, 1981*b,* p. 375.

Wittliff, J.L., Fisher, B., and Durant, J.R.: Establishment of uniformity in steroid receptor analyses used in cooperative clinical trials of breast cancer treatment. Recent Results Cancer Res., *71:*198, 1980.

Wittliff, J.L., Folk, P., Dong, J., et al.: Characteristics of the human estrogen receptor protein produced in microbial expression systems. *In* Moudgil, V.K. (Ed.): Steroid Hormone Receptors: Basic and Clinical Aspects. Boston, Birkhäuser, 1994, p. 473.

Wittliff, J.L., Heidemann, P.H., and Lewko, W.M.: Molecular basis of endocrine responsiveness in normal and neoplastic breast tissues. *In* Fleisher, M.F. (Ed.): The Clinical Biochemistry of Cancer. Washington, DC: The American Association for Clinical Chemistry, 1979, p. 179.

Wittliff, J.L., Hilf, R., Brooks, W.F. Jr., et al.: Specific estrogen-binding capacity of the cytoplasmic receptor in normal and neoplastic tissues of humans. Cancer Res., *32:*1983, 1972.

Wittliff, J.L., Lewko, W.M., Park, D.C., et al.: Steroid binding proteins of mammary tissues and their clinical significance in breast cancer. *In* McGuire, W.L. (Ed.): Hormones, Receptors, and Breast Cancer. New York, Raven, 1978, p. 325.

Wittliff, J.L., Pasic, W., and Bland, K.I. Steroid and peptide hormone receptors identified in breast tissue: *In* Bland, K.I., and Copeland, E.M. III. (Eds.): The Breast: Comprehensive Management of Benign and Malignant Diseases. Philadelphia, W. B. Saunders, 1991, pp. 900–936.

Wittliff, J.L., Wenz, L.L., Dong, J., et al.: Expression and characterization of an active human estrogen receptor as a ubiquitin fusion protein from *Escherichia coli.* J. Biol. Chem., *265:*22016, 1990.

Wittliff, J.L., Wiehle, R.D., and Hyder, S.M.: HPLC as a means of characterizing the polymorphism of steroid hormone receptors. *In* Kerlavage, A.R., (Ed.): The Use of HPLC in Receptor Biochemistry. New York, Alan R. Liss, 1989, p. 155.

Wynder, E.L., Kajitani, T., Kuno, J., et al.: Comparison of survival rates between American and Japanese patients with breast cancer. Surg. Gynecol. Obstet., *117:*196, 1963.

Yamamoto, T., Ikawa, S., Akiyama, T., et al.: Similarity of protein encoded by the human c-*erb* B-2 gene to epidermal growth factor receptor. Nature, *319:*230, 1986.

Yang, A.-R., Wiehle, R.D., Lee, O.-H., et al.: Over-expression of EGF receptors and the protein product of the related c-*erb* B-2 oncogene in breast, endometrial and ovarian carcinomas (Abstract). 1992.

Yokota, J., Yamamoto, T., and Toyoshima, K.J., et al.: Amplification of c-*erb* B oncogene in human adenocarcinomas in vivo. Lancet *1:*765, 1986.

Young, S.C., Burkett, R.J., and Stewart C.: Discrepancy in ER levels of breast carcinoma in biopsy vs mastectomy specimens. J. Surg. Oncol., *29:*54, 1985.

Zhou, D.J., Ahuja, H., and Cline, M.J.: Proto-oncogene abnormalities in human breast cancer: c-*erb* B-2 amplification does not correlate with recurrence of disease. Oncogene, *4:*105, 1989.

17 Staging and Primary Treatment

William L. Donegan

Primary treatment of breast cancer pertains to the initial management of the breast and regional lymph nodes. A decision regarding primary treatment is reached on the basis of a secure histologic diagnosis of cancer and on the stage of the disease. This chapter addresses the treatment of carcinomas, which constitute 95% of all malignancies of the breast. Because the terms used to designate operations for cancer of the breast are varied and often confusing, Table 17–1 matches procedure names with the anatomic parts that are removed.

The objectives of primary treatment are control of the tumor in local and regional tissues and achievement of an optimal chance for cure. These are the criteria against which alternative treatments are evaluated. In the past, treatment of breast cancer routinely included removal of the breast. The possibility of losing a breast or breasts was so socially and emotionally disturbing to women that it may have contributed to delays in both diagnosis and treatment. The focus of recent investigations has been on techniques of breast conservation, and the results of these studies have made conservation techniques viable alternatives for many women with breast cancer. In the public's interest, lawmakers in most states have passed laws obligating physicians who manage breast cancer to fully inform patients about alternative treatments. Following are excerpts of some states' laws:

Massachusetts, 1979: Every patient ''suffering from any form of breast cancer'' has a right to ''complete information on all alternative treatments which are medically viable.''

California, 1980: ''Failure . . . to inform a patient by means of a standardized written summary . . . of alternative efficacious methods of treatment . . . when the patient is being treated for any form of breast cancer . . .'' is unprofessional conduct.

Michigan, 1986: ''A physician who is administering the primary treatment for breast cancer to a patient who has been diagnosed as having breast cancer shall inform the patient, orally and in writing, about alternative methods of treatment of the cancer, including surgical, radiological or chemotherapeutic treatments, or any other generally accepted medical treatment. The physician also shall inform the patient about the advantages, disadvantages and risks of each method of treatment.''

In addition to defining alternative treatments, the information provided to patients should include anticipated risks, benefits, and expected outcomes. Patients should be made aware that despite the best available treatment and the earliest of stage of cancer, in no case can cure be guaranteed. Public interest in the problem of breast cancer and the sources of public information are sufficiently great that patients seeking surgical consultation are often already well informed about the subject, aware of recent developments, and prepared to ask cogent questions. They are likely to have had a biopsy and an established diagnosis. A radiation therapist and a medical oncologist may already have been consulted. They may well seek more than one surgical opinion. When mammography and biopsies have been performed, it is essential to review the reports as well as the films and slides before making a final recommendation for any patient.

The reliability of information on treatment alternatives has greatly improved since the introduction of randomized prospective trials, and trials continue to provide important guidelines for making clinical decisions. The limitations of trials should also be appreciated. They usually pertain to a narrow spectrum of disease, the elderly are excluded from them, and concurrent illness, so prevalent in clinical practice, is often a basis for candidate ineligibility. It is not entirely from reluctance that only 1% or 2% of women with breast cancer are included in clinical trials. One must also be aware that statistically significant differences in outcome are not always clinically relevant and that information is forever incomplete and subject to revision or reinterpretation. In short, the exercise of sound clinical judgment remains indispensable.

STAGING

Staging refers to classification of breast cancer by anatomic extent. The premise that underlies staging is that breast cancer progresses anatomically in an orderly manner and that its progression is related to prognosis. In the course of events that lead to disease, normal ductal epithelium progresses to epithelial hyperplasia, then to atypical epithelial hyperplasia, and next to noninvasive carcinoma (Gallager and Martin, 1969). Noninvasive cancer then penetrates the basement membrane of the duct to become invasive cancer and gains access to lymphatics and blood vessels. Via these conduits, it reaches regional lymphatics and more distant parts of the body. With each step of the process, the prospects of survival and the probability of cure for a patient

Table 17–1. ANATOMIC STRUCTURES REMOVED IN VARIOUS OPERATIONS FOR CANCER OF THE BREAST

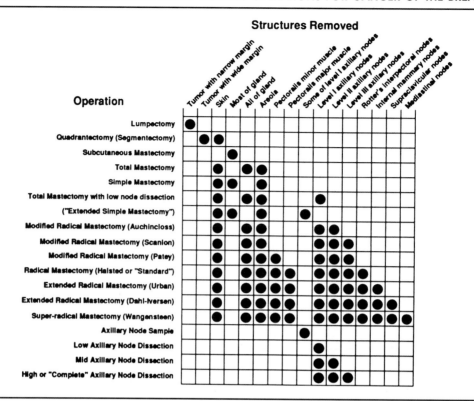

Operation	Tumor with narrow margin	Tumor with wide margin	Skin	Most of gland	All of gland	Areola	Pectoralis minor muscle	Pectoralis major muscle	Some of level I axillary nodes	Level I axillary nodes	Level II axillary nodes	Level III axillary nodes	Rotter's interpectoral nodes	Internal mammary nodes	Supraclavicular nodes	Mediastinal nodes
Lumpectomy	●															
Quadrantectomy (Segmentectomy)		●	●													
Subcutaneous Mastectomy				●												
Total Mastectomy			●		●	●										
Simple Mastectomy			●		●	●										
Total Mastectomy with low node dissection			●		●	●				●						
("Extended Simple Mastectomy")			●		●	●			●							
Modified Radical Mastectomy (Auchincloss)			●		●	●				●	●					
Modified Radical Mastectomy (Scanlon)			●		●	●				●	●	●				
Modified Radical Mastectomy (Patey)			●		●	●	●			●	●	●				
Radical Mastectomy (Halsted or "Standard")			●		●	●	●	●		●	●	●	●			
Extended Radical Mastectomy (Urban)			●		●	●	●	●		●	●	●	●	●		
Extended Radical Mastectomy (Dahl-Iversen)			●		●	●	●	●		●	●	●	●	●	●	
Super-radical Mastectomy (Wangensteen)			●		●	●	●	●		●	●	●	●	●	●	●
Axillary Node Sample									●							
Low Axillary Node Dissection										●						
Mid Axillary Node Dissection										●	●					
High or "Complete" Axillary Node Dissection										●	●	●				

diminish. The close link between stage and prognosis is apparently a function of increasing occult dissemination.

In addition to being a basis for estimating prognosis, staging serves to simplify communication, to provide a means for selecting a patient's treatment, and to permit comparison of treatment results in comparable cases. It provides a continuing stimulus for the investigation of cancer because effective staging requires careful examination of clinical and pathologic information and an accurate knowledge of end results (Beahrs, 1991). Clinical stage is determined solely on the results of clinical evaluation, which includes data from physical examinations and analysis of radiographs and scans. Determination of pathologic stage relies on additional information obtained from surgical resections. Surgical resection yields data that are more accurate and precise than those obtained from clinical evaluation, but the data from the latter are in some respects more useful than those of the former. *Clinical staging* can be determined prior to treatment and therefore makes possible the equitable comparison of diverse methods of treatment, both resective and nonresective. *Pathologic staging* is based on the detailed examination of resected tissues and provides a basis for comparison only among patients with resections of equal extent.

Staging has a number of important limitations. It is perhaps obvious that relegating a disease as complex as cancer of the breast to a few categories is artificial and simplistic. Each stage contains cases that progress to dissemination and death and other cases that do not. However, a strong association exists between increasing anatomic extent and the proportion of cases that prove lethal within a fixed period. Furthermore, not only does the prevalence of treatment failure increase with increases in stage, but also the rapidity with which failures occur (e.g., more patients with Stage II cancers die than do those with Stage I cancers, and they die faster). This accounts for the fact that the slopes of survival curves for each stage differ, and it suggests that a relationship exists between anatomic extent and growth rate (Mueller, 1988).

Although stages appear to represent the natural history of the disease, this is only implied; the orderly progression of patients' disease through all stages cannot be expected. For example, a tumor may disseminate without ever involving regional lymph nodes in the process. Again, it is assumed that each tumor develops as in situ carcinoma before it becomes invasive; however, this is not regularly demonstrable. It is also apparent that staging based exclusively on assessment of anatomic features omits biologic factors of prognostic importance such as hormone receptor status, histologic grade, and rapidity of tumor growth. These factors determine how quickly a tumor reaches a particular stage and how quickly it advances. Tumors with rapid rates of growth can prove lethal rapidly despite their having been discovered at a small, "favorable" size. Investigations continue to explore measures of growth and genetic alteration within cancers to obtain prognostic information that is independent of stage. Finally, staging is not static; it changes with new insights. It is not a substitute for recording accurate and factual information; rather, it is simply a means for organizing that information—that is, it is a useful abstraction.

Staging has a long history. As a practical matter, surgeons originally divided patients into two groups, "operable" or "inoperable," depending on whether they believed there was a chance of surgical cure or not. However, what was "operable" varied considerably in the perceptions of surgeons, encompassed a diverse mix of patients, and proved to be a poor basis on which to compare results. It was plain that, within this broad category, certain patients fared far better than others. Patients in whom the cancer was apparently confined to the breast were more likely to be cured than those who had axillary adenopathy. The latter in turn fared better than others with more widespread involvement. On the basis of these observations, Steinthal of Stuttgart (1905) suggested three groupings:

Steinthal's Groupings (author's translation)
Group 1 Slowly growing tumors not larger than a plum confined to glandular tissue and not involving skin. Axillary lymph nodes are not clinically evident and are generally found only during an operation.
Group 2 Obvious tumors adherent to the overlying skin. Enlarged axillary lymph nodes are clearly evident.
Group 3 Most of the breast is diseased, and the tumor has extended to the skin and deep tissues. Supraclavicular lymph nodes often are involved.

The majority of cases qualified for Group 2. Recurrences after resection were noted in 27.3% of Group 1, 76% of Group 2, and 100% of Group 3 cases, and because of the discouraging results in Group 3, Steinthal recommended operation at this stage only when required for palliation. This classification was widely adopted in Germany and Scandinavia, but as it became plain that clinical evaluation of the axilla was inaccurate, Stages 1 and 2 were redefined in Scandinavia to mean the histologic absence or presence of metastases in axillary lymph nodes, in effect changing a clinical to a pathologic classification.

Later, Lee and Stubenbord (1928) proposed a cumbersome classification called the *clinical index of malignancy,* which was based not only on the extent of the disease but also on the age of the patient and on the rate of tumor growth. This "biologic" system did not gain widespread acceptance.

In 1940, the Manchester classification was developed at the Christie Hospital and Holt Radium Institute in Manchester, England. The Manchester system adhered strictly to clinical criteria for defining four stages, and therefore provided a common denominator for comparing diverse methods of management (Windeyer, 1949). The introduction of this four-stage system served to define two prognostically favorable categories and two poor ones. Stage III was characterized by contiguous advancement of the primary tumor into adjacent tissues and Stage IV by unremovable disease, either because of obvious dissemination or technical unresectability. The Manchester classification enjoyed wide acceptance in the British literature.

The Manchester System
Stage I The growth is confined to the breast. Involvement of the skin directly over and in continuity with the tumor may be present provided the area is small in relation to the size of the breast.
Stage II The growth is confined to the breast, but palpable mobile lymph nodes are present in the axilla.
Stage III The growth extends beyond the mammary parenchyma, as shown by
　(a) skin invasion or fixation over an area large in relation to the size of the breast, or skin ulceration.
　(b) tumor fixation to the underlying muscle or fascia; axillary nodes, if present, are mobile.
Stage IV The growth extends beyond the breast area, as shown by fixation or matting of the axillary nodes, complete fixation of tumor to chest wall, deposits in supraclavicular nodes or in the opposite breast, satellite nodules, or distant metastases.

Three years later Portmann (1943) of the Cleveland Clinic introduced a four-stage system based on both clinical and pathologic features; the system took into consideration the extent of the primary tumor, skin involvement, and the extent of metastases. This mixed classification was symptomatic of continuing dissatisfaction with the inaccuracies of clinical staging.

Portmann Classification
Group or Stage I
Skin: Not involved
Tumor: Localized in breast and movable
Metastases: None in axillary lymph nodes or elsewhere
Group or Stage II
Skin: Not involved
Tumor: Localized in breast and movable
Metastases: Few axillary lymph nodes involved, no other metastases
Group or Stage III
Skin: Edematous; brawny red induration and inflammation not obviously due to infection; extensive ulceration; multiple secondary nodules
Tumor: Diffusely infiltrating breast; fixation of tumor or breast to chest wall; edema of breast; secondary tumors
Metastases: Many axillary lymph nodes involved or fixed; no clinical or radiographic evidence of distant metastases
Group or Stage IV
Skin: As in any other group or stage
Tumor: As in any other group or stage
Metastases: Axillary and supraclavicular lymph nodes extensively involved, and clinical or radiographic evidence of more distant metastases

Portmann found that 25% of cases were Group I, 25% were Group II, 30% were Group III, and 20% were Group IV, and survivals at 5 years after surgical treatment were 90%, 50%, 5%, and 5%, respectively. He recommended radical mastectomy alone for Group I, radical mastectomy and postoperative irradiation for Group II, and irradiation alone for Groups III and IV.

The Columbia Clinical Classification evolved from Haagensen and Stout's criteria for inoperability first published in 1943. These criteria were derived from careful study of 568 cases treated with radical mastectomy at Columbia–Presbyterian Medical Center in New York City from 1915 to 1935. At a time when radical mastectomy was being performed indiscriminately, this work served to define features of breast cancer that identified them as incurable with this operation. Breast cancer accompanied by pregnancy appeared on the original list but was removed subsequently, and the list reached final form as follows:

Haagensen and Stout's Criteria of Inoperability
1. Extensive edema of the skin over the breast (involving more than one-third of the skin of the breast)
2. Satellite nodules present in the skin
3. Carcinoma of the inflammatory type
4. Parasternal tumor nodules
5. Proven supraclavicular metastases
6. Edema of the arm
7. Distant metastases
8. Two or more of the following five grave signs of locally advanced carcinoma:
   a. Ulceration of the skin
   b. Edema of the skin of limited extent (less than one-third of the skin of the breast)
   c. Fixation of the axillary lymph nodes to the skin or to the deep structures of the axilla
   d. Axillary lymph nodes measuring 2.5 cm or more in transverse diameter
   e. Solid fixation of the tumor to the chest wall

To these strictly clinical criteria of inoperability were added biopsy proof of metastases in parasternal lymph nodes or lymph nodes at the apex of the axilla, with such biopsies becoming a part of some patients' pretreatment evaluation. Haagensen and Stout's ''triple biopsy'' (biopsy of the primary tumor, apical axillary nodes, and internal mammary nodes), however, was not widely adopted.

The continuation of this work and the statistical assistance of Cooley ultimately resulted in the four-stage Columbia Clinical Classification, in which the foregoing criteria of inoperability defined Stage D, and the five ''grave signs'' of advancement identified Stage C.

The Columbia Clinical Classification
Stage A No skin edema, ulceration, or solid fixation of tumor to chest wall; axillary lymph nodes not clinically involved
Stage B No skin edema, ulceration, or solid fixation of tumor to chest wall; clinically involved axillary lymph nodes, but smaller than 2.5 cm in transverse diameter and not fixed to overlying skin or deeper structure of axilla
Stage C Any one of the five grave signs of comparatively advanced carcinoma:
   1. Edema of skin of limited extent (less than one-third of the skin over the breast)
   2. Skin ulceration
   3. Solid fixation of tumor to chest wall
   4. Massive involvement of axillary lymph nodes (2.5 cm or greater in transverse diameter)

   5. Fixation of the axillary lymph nodes to overlying skin or deeper structures of the axilla
Stage D All other more advanced carcinomas, including the following:
   1. A combination of any two or more of the five grave signs listed in Stage C
   2. Extensive edema of skin (involving more than one-third of the skin over the breast)
   3. Satellite skin nodules
   4. The inflammatory type of carcinoma
   5. Supraclavicular metastases, clinically apparent
   6. Parasternal metastases, clinically apparent
   7. Edema of the ipsilateral arm
   8. Distant metastases

This classification was carefully conceived. It was widely accepted and in 1974 was used in an international cooperative study to compare results of various treatment methods in the United States and abroad (Haagensen et al., 1969). A long-term follow-up of personal experience with radical mastectomy and the Columbia Clinical Classification (CCC) was published by Haagensen and Bodian in 1984. Stage-specific 10-year survival rates were as follows: A, 80% (727 cases); B, 50% (208 cases); C, 28.2% (85 cases); and D, 25% (16 cases). Their ultimate assessment was that only cancers of Stages A and B were suitable for radical mastectomy; tumors of Stages C and D should be treated with irradiation. In this author's experience with the CCC, the four stages provide clear separation of survival with a continuum of deterioration from Stages A to D (Fig. 17–1). Cancers in the subcategories of Stage C treated surgically are prognostically homogeneous, and the same can be said of Stage D cancers (Fig. 17–2).

The CCC may be criticized for ignoring the prognostic importance of tumor size in early stages of the disease. The influence of this important variable is shown in Figure 17–3. The CCC likewise does not discriminate between objective findings in the axilla and the examiner's subjective

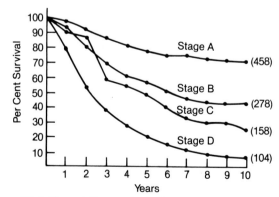

Figure 17–1. The relative survival of patients with invasive carcinoma at EFSCH, 1940–1965, treated with radical mastectomy according to the Columbia Clinical Classification (CCC). Relative survival deletes natural mortality; thus, when mortality from the disease ceases, the curve becomes flat. It is evident that this generally does not occur even after 10 years of observation. Stage D was composed of highly selected cases without obvious dissemination. The distinction between stages B and C is not as great as it is between others.

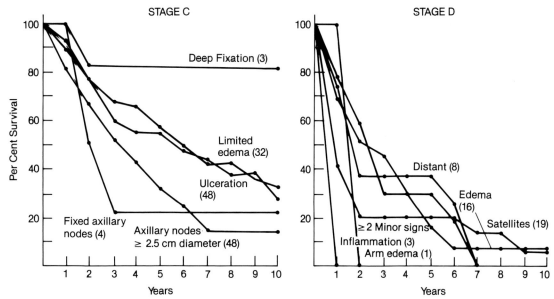

Figure 17-2. The relative survival of patients in subcategories of the CCC Stages C and D at EFSCH, 1940–1965, after radical mastectomy. Numbers in parentheses indicate number of cases. The patients are women with unilateral invasive carcinomas of the breast who have no previous mammary cancer, no pregnancies during symptoms or treatment, no simultaneous malignancies elsewhere, no previous therapy, and no adjuvant therapy with either irradiation or chemotherapy. Some overlap is evident (e.g., patients with large axillary nodes in Stage C have approximately the same survival as those with satellite nodules and edema in Stage D). Patients with limited edema of the breast or ulceration in Stage C, however, clearly have superior survival to all groups in Stage D. The few patients with either inflammatory carcinoma or edema of the arm in Stage D died rapidly, and none with distant metastases or two or more minor signs of local advancement survived for 10 years.

opinion regarding involvement of the axillary lymph nodes. Furthermore, it does not distinguish between invasive and noninvasive cancers, having evolved during a period when in situ carcinomas were rare. These shortcomings are addressed in the more complex TNM system.

THE TNM CLASSIFICATION

In 1954 the International Union Against Cancer (UICC) initiated an effort to perfect a staging classification that would have worldwide acceptability (UICC Committee on Clinical Stage Classification, 1961). At the instigation of Denoix of France, a system based on meticulous description of the primary tumor (T), the regional lymph nodes (N), and distant metastases (M) was adopted. The subcategories of T, N, and M were then grouped in various combinations to describe four stages. The TNM concept was adopted by the American Joint Committee for Cancer Staging and End Results Reporting (AJC), but published in a somewhat different form in 1962, a year after the UICC version appeared. Efforts to evaluate the two systems and to reconcile differences generated several revisions. Using data collected from the California Tumor Registry, Zippin (1966) demonstrated that the AJC version failed to give sufficient consideration to tumor size, a feature it simply dichotomized as 2.0 cm or smaller versus 2.0 cm or greater. A joint AJC-UICC TNM classification published in 1972 was encumbered by a large Stage III, which encompassed 50% of all cases and was composed of many subgroups that overlapped prognostically with Stages II and IV. A further revision endorsed by both organizations appeared in 1977.

Tumors with direct extension to the chest wall or skin were moved out of Stage III into Stage IV, as were those associated with edema of the arm and those with supraclavicular or infraclavicular adenopathy. Inflammatory carcinoma, requiring histologically proved dermal lymphatic invasion, remained in Stage IV.

The current version of the TNM system, which has been

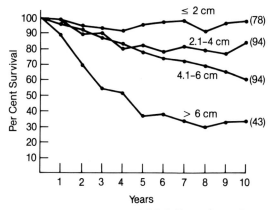

Figure 17-3. Relative survival of CCC Stage A carcinomas by tumor size after radical mastectomy for invasive carcinoma, EFSCH, 1940–1965. The prognosis of patients with Stage A carcinomas varies considerably, depending on the maximum diameter of the primary tumor, a feature not considered in the staging system. Patients with carcinomas 2 cm or less in diameter fare well, and those with carcinomas greater than 6 cm in diameter fare poorly. Tumors with diameters of greater than 2 cm but not more than 6 cm appear to be a relatively homogeneous group prognostically.

Table 17-2. TNM STAGING SYSTEM FOR BREAST CANCER—1992

I. Primary Tumor (T)
Definition: Classification of the primary tumor is the same for clinical and for pathologic classification.
TX Primary tumor cannot be assessed
T0 No evidence of primary tumor
Tis Carcinoma in situ: Intraductal carcinoma, lobular carcinoma in situ, or Paget's disease of the nipple with no tumor.
(Paget's disease with a tumor is classified according to the size of the tumor.)
T1 Tumor 2.0 cm or less in greatest dimension
  T1a 0.5 cm or less
  T1b >0.5 cm, but not >1.0 cm
  T1c >1.0 cm, but not >2.0 cm
T2 Tumor >2.0 cm, but not >5.0 cm in greatest dimension
T3 Tumor >5.0 cm in greatest dimension
T4 Tumor of any size with direct extension to chest wall or skin
  T4a Extension to chest wall
  T4b Edema (including peau d'orange) or ulceration of the skin of the breast or satellite skin nodules confined to the same breast
  T4c Both T4a and T4b
  T4d Inflammatory carcinoma (diffuse brawny induration of the skin of the breast with an erysipeloid edge, usually without an underlying palpable mass)

II. Regional Lymph Nodes (N)
NX Regional nodes cannot be assessed (e.g., previously removed or no information on them can be obtained)
N0 No metastases
N1 Metastases in movable ipsilateral axillary lymph node(s)
N2 Metastases in ipsilateral axillary lymph node(s) fixed to each other or to other structures
N3 Metastases to ipsilateral internal mammary lymph node(s)

III. Pathologic Classification of Regional Lymph Nodes (pN)
pNx Cannot be assessed (previously removed, or not removed)
pN0 No metastases
pN1 Metastases to mobile ipsilateral axillary node(s)
  pN1a Only micrometastasis (i.e., none >0.2 cm)
  pN1b Metastasis with any >0.2 cm
    pN1bi Metastases in 1–3 nodes (all <2.0 cm)
    pN1bii Metastases in 4 or more nodes (all <2.0 cm)
    pN1biii Metastases <2.0 cm with extension beyond the capsule of a lymph node
    pN1biv Metastases >2.0 cm in diameter
pN2 Metastasis to ipsilateral axillary nodes fixed to one another or to other structures
pN3 Metastasis to ipsilateral internal mammary lymph node(s)

IV. Distant Metastasis (M)
MX Cannot be assessed
M0 None
M1 Distant metastasis present (includes metastasis to ipsilateral supraclavicular lymph node(s))

Histopathologic Grade (G)

G X	Cannot be assessed
G 1	Well differentiated
G 2	Moderately differentiated
G 3	Poorly differentiated
G 4	Undifferentiated

accepted by the UICC and the American Joint Committee on Cancer (AJCC, previously the AJC), is shown in Tables 17–2 and 17–3 (American Joint Committee on Cancer, 1992). Microscopic confirmation of the diagnosis is mandatory; histologic type and grade are also recorded. In this system, pathologic staging requires removal of the entire gross tumor and removal of at least the low (Level I) axillary lymph nodes. *Pathologic stage* applies only to lymph nodes and is indicated by the prefix p. The complexity of this system is noteworthy as are some of its peculiarities. The measurement of tumor size applies only to invasive cancer. Hence, only the invasive component of a tumor is considered in measuring its diameter; any in situ component is ignored. Clinical tumor size may be based on results of either palpation or mammography, whichever is considered ''more accurate,'' but opinions on this point vary. The

Yorkshire Breast Cancer Group (1974) found that surgeons and pathologists agreed on the T category in only 54% of cases and that radiologists and pathologists concurred in only 59%. In the TNM system, only the largest primary tumor is considered for the staging of multiple primary tumors, and such cases are considered separately. Metastases present in fat adjacent to primary tumors qualify as nodal metastases, and metastases to supraclavicular nodes are considered distant metastases rather than regional metastases. It is also noteworthy that the subclassifications of the N1 category are neither mutually exclusive nor independently prognostic (Donegan et al., 1993). In some publications, it is not always clear whether the current version of the TNM system is used. Comparability of cases depends on clarity and consistency in this regard. A simplified representation of the TNM system is shown in Figure 17–4.

Table 17-3. TNM STAGE GROUPING—1992

Stage 0	Tis	N0	M0
Stage I	T1	N0	M0
Stage IIA	T0	N1	M0
	T1	N1	M0
	T2	N0	M0
Stage IIB	T2	N1	M0
	T3	N0	M0
Stage IIIA	T0	N2	M0
	T1	N2	M0
	T2	N2	M0
	T3	N1	M0
	T3	N2	M0
Stage IIIB	T4	N (any)	M0
	T (any)	N3	M0
Stage IV	T (any)	N (any)	M1

TNM Stages 1992

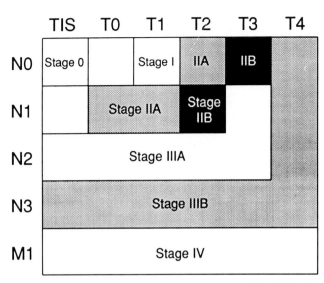

Figure 17-4. A diagrammatic representation of the TNM (*Tumor, Node, Metastasis*) staging system.

Survival of 50,834 cases registered with the Surveillance, Epidemiology and End Results (SEER) program of the National Cancer Institute (NCI) according to TNM stage is shown in Figure 17–5. Clinicians should consult the most recent publications of the AJCC so that their knowledge of the TNM system remains current.

An unofficial and imprecise but generally understood four-stage system is often used for convenience in discussing breast cancer. Noninvasive (in situ) tumors are specified as such and without further reference to stage. Stage I is understood to mean an invasive cancer confined to the breast without involvement of the skin or chest wall. Stage II indicates such a tumor with early spread to axillary nodes, and Stage IV indicates the presence of distant metastases. Stage III includes variations of local and regional advancement that are between Stages II and IV.

THE PROCESS OF CLINICAL STAGING

A complete physical examination is essential for clinical staging. It includes not only an examination of the breast and its regional lymphatics but also of likely sites of distant metastases. These sites include the bones, lungs and pleura, liver, and brain; thus, particular attention is given to exam-

BREAST CANCER
SURVIVAL ACCORDING TO AJCC STAGE

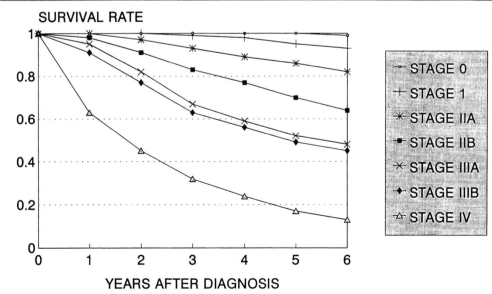

Figure 17-5. Survival by TNM stage of 50,834 cases of breast cancer from the SEER registry. (Reprinted with permission from American Joint Committee on Cancer: Manual for Staging of Cancer. 4th ed. J. B. Lippincott, 1992, pp. 149–154.)

ination of the lungs and liver as well as to any sites of new bone pain. Headaches or dizziness suggests the need for more complete neurologic examination. The physical examination is supplemented with chest radiography, serologic testing of liver function, and bilateral mammography. Mammography is necessary, despite the presence of an obvious cancer, to detect clinically occult lesions in the same or opposite breast (Young et al., 1986). Bone scanning is not performed in patients with in situ cancer. Most everyone would agree that bone scanning is needed if a tumor is large or regionally advanced or if symptoms suggest the possibility of bone metastases. This author obtains bone scans in all patients with invasive cancer to serve as a baseline. Although true-positive results are few, many patients have changes due to arthritis or other causes; if not documented, these changes may complicate the interpretation of bone scans obtained later. The studies required prior to a general anesthesia include a complete blood count and urinalysis, pregnancy testing for premenopausal women, electrolyte assessment, and electrocardiography (depending on a patient's age). Neurologic symptoms are an indication for performing computed tomography (CT) of the head, and suggestive changes on chest radiographs or in levels of hepatic enzymes are evaluated with CT of the chest and abdomen. Detection of distant metastases has a major influence on prognosis and on treatment planning. It changes the prognosis of the disease from potentially curable to incurable, and the objectives of treatment from cure to palliation.

Chest Radiography

Pulmonary and pleural metastases may be asymptomatic or betrayed by a cough (see Fig. 17–6). The most frequent signs are pleural effusions and parenchymal densities. Lymphangitic spread within the lung is suggested by dyspnea but may be evidenced by minimal radiographic signs. Diffuse streaking from the hilar areas is characteristic; blood gas determinations and pulmonary function studies demonstrate reduced pulmonary compliance and compromised ventilatory function. A solitary lesion of the lung in a woman with otherwise clinically localized cancer of the breast is more likely to be a primary carcinoma of the lung than a metastasis (Cahan and Castro, 1975). Among 42 women with breast cancer who had a solitary pulmonary nodule either initially or during follow-up, Casey and associates (1984) found that 52% had primary lung cancer, 5% had a benign lesion, and 43% had metastatic breast cancer. This fact is of considerable significance for staging and treatment. It can be attributed to the rising frequency of lung cancer among women in the United States and to the low frequency with which breast cancer produces a solitary pulmonary metastasis. Histologic diagnosis of a solitary pulmonary nodule is necessary (with thoracotomy if required). A considerable number of women with asymptomatic lung cancers can be successfully treated with resection, and the breast cancer can also be treated for cure. Abnormalities seen on a chest radiograph that are equivocal for metastases require clarification with special views, use of nipple markers, or CT of the chest, as appropriate.

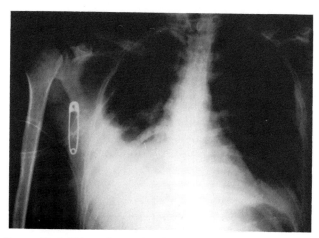

Figure 17–6. This radiograph of the chest shows the typical ellipse of a right pleural effusion resulting from metastasis.

Skeletal Radiography and Bone Scanning

A skeletal radiography series (ribs, skull, spine, pelvis, femora, and humeri) is unnecessary unless a patient has symptoms suggestive of osseous metastases. Thirty per cent to 50% of mineral loss is necessary before a metastasis is visible on a radiograph. Gibbons and coworkers (1961) examined 85 consecutive asymptomatic patients within 6 weeks after mastectomy and found that only 1 had a possible asymptomatic metastasis. The lesion had not progressed after 18 months. Radiographs are essential for evaluating bone abnormalities detected with bone scanning.

Radioisotopic bone scanning is highly sensitive but is not specific for metastases (Fig. 17–7). Metastases can be detected on bone scans before they are symptomatic and up to 12 months before they are detectable on radiographs, but any osteoblastic activity (e.g., fractures, trauma, arthritis, Paget's disease of bone, cartilagenous lesions, and primary or metastatic bone tumors) produces abnormalities. Thus, radiography of abnormalities is necessary for reliable interpretation, and sometimes CT or magnetic resonance imaging must be performed. Joints often show increased activity due to arthritis; thus, activity where no arthritis is expected (e.g., ribs, long bones, and skull) is suggestive of the presence of metastases, as is the combination of an abnormal bone scan and normal radiographs. Bone scans suggestive of metastases are associated with poor prognosis but not necessarily with initial recurrence in bones (Komaki et al., 1979). Because discovery of unsuspected metastases is infrequent in early stages of breast cancer, most investigators recommend selective use of bone scanning and confine its use to patients with axillary adenopathy, signs of local advancement, or symptoms suggestive of metastases (Lee, 1981; Khansur et al., 1987; and Bassett et al., 1989). Ciatto and coworkers (1988) reported that only 1 of 633 patients with T1 tumors and 2 of 189 patients with T2 tumors had asymptomatic bone metastases that were discovered on routine bone scanning. In their study, preoperative bone scans of 2450 asymptomatic patients provided 22 true-positive results and 125 false-positive results (see Fig. 17–7). Using

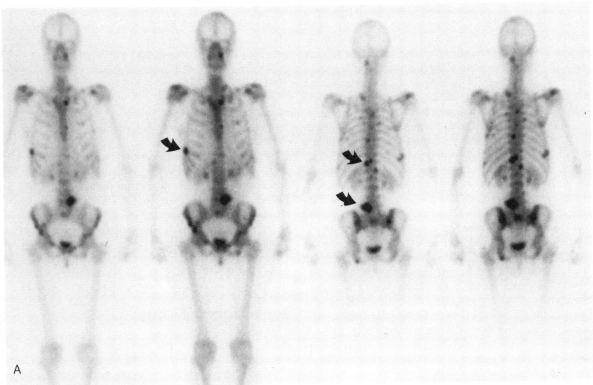

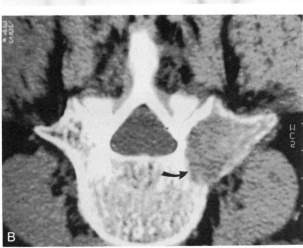

Figure 17-7. *A,* A bone scan performed for staging shows multiple sites of increased uptake in the ribs and vertebrae because of osseous metastases (*arrows*). Bone scans are sensitive but not specific, and radiography or CT is necessary for confirmation of metastases. *B,* A CT scan demonstrates a large lytic lesion in a vertebra (*arrow*).

routine bone scanning, Brar and associates (1993) studied 133 patients with operable breast cancers and found the scans to be abnormal in 23% of cases. Only four patients (3%) were found to have true-positive results. Two were in 67 otherwise Stage II cases (3%), and 2 were in 43 Stage III cases (5%). A focal abnormality detected in radiologically normal bone should not preclude potentially curative treatment in the absence of histologic proof that it represents a metastasis.

Hepatic Function and Liver Scanning

Thirty-five per cent to 65% of autopsied patients with breast cancer have hepatic metastases (Haagensen, 1971); however, few patients have such metastases at diagnosis. Abnormal results on serologic testing of hepatic function are not specific for hepatic metastases, and the utility of such testing for early detection is questionable; however, serologic testing is a quick and relatively inexpensive means of increasing the possibility of early detection. Normal function does not guarantee that metastases are not present, and the reliability of test results is diminished by the presence of concurrent disease and by the use of medications with hepatic effects. Clark and associates (1988) screened 220 patients with operable breast cancer using liver function tests and identified 1 patient (Stage III) who had hepatic metastases. Function test results were abnormal in 15% of the population (including the patient with metastases, who had an elevated lactate dehydrogenase level). Alkaline phosphatase level was not a sensitive indicator of bone or hepatic metastases in the study of Brar and associates (1993). It was elevated in 58% of operable patients and in 54% of those with normal bone scans, and it was normal in

30% of patients with abnormal bone scans. The positive predictive value of alkaline phosphatase levels for bone metastases was a low 27%, although levels tended to be high when bone scan results were abnormal. The solitary patient with hepatic metastases had a normal alkaline phosphatase level. Other serologic tests (e.g., for determining aspartate aminotransferase, lactate dehydrogenase, and gamma glutamyltransferase levels) were not useful.

CT of the liver has replaced radionuclide scanning because of its superior accuracy and definition (Fig. 17–8). Cysts can be distinguished from solid lesions, and when scans are enhanced with the use of intravenous contrast media, the size and number of metastases can be discerned with considerable accuracy. Hepatic metastases from various cancers are detected with an accuracy of up to 92% (Kemeny and Schneider, 1989). False-negative results are most often attributable to diffuse involvement and to small lesions located between the planes that are imaged.

Ultrasonography of the liver is capable of detecting hepatic metastases as small as 1 to 2 cm in diameter. It has the advantages of no radiation exposure and of being less expensive than CT. Routine sonography is not often productive, however, and its results can be misleading. Colizza and associates (1985) reported 2 positive results on sonography of the liver in 97 patients with operable breast cancer but considered them to be false-positive because the patients were alive and well 24 months later. Clark and associates (1988) screened a similar population of 220 patients with ultrasonography and found that the results of only 3 examinations (1.3%) were consistent with metastasis, and results on 2 of these were confirmed to be false-positive. In direct comparisons, CT of the liver proves to be superior to technetium-99 sulfur colloid scintigraphy, ultrasonography, and magnetic resonance imaging for the detection of hepatic metastases (Zeman et al., 1985).

CT is generally reserved for patients suspected to have metastases on the basis of hepatomegaly or abnormal results on serologic testing (Felix et al., 1976; and Wiener and Sachs, 1978). Focal defects suggestive of metastases, particularly when unaccompanied by clear evidence of dis-

turbed hepatic function, require histologic confirmation. Percutaneous needle biopsy can be used for this purpose. CT enhanced with the use of intravenous contrast media provides optimum sensitivity but still detects fewer than 50% of metastases discovered at laparotomy (Foley et al., 1983).

CT of the Brain

Intracranial metastases become manifest quickly and are rarely detected with present imaging techniques in the absence of symptoms. This is true for radionuclide scanning (Muss et al., 1976) and for CT of the head. Lewi and coworkers (1980) reviewed the CT scans of 61 asymptomatic patients and detected no occult metastases. Weisberg (1986) found that all but one of 17 patients with evidence of metastases to the brain on CT already had clinical symptoms (Fig. 17–9).

Bone Marrow Biopsy

Bones are the most frequent and often the first site of distant metastasis. This fact has stimulated several studies of bone marrow aspiration in patients with newly diagnosed breast cancers. Their results have indicated that sampling without some indication of bone involvement is unproductive. In a study of 532 cases by Ridell and Landys (1979), routine biopsy analysis of the posterior iliac crest demonstrated the presence of cancer cells in 28% of patients when skeletal radiographs were abnormal, but in only 1.6% of patients when results were normal. When results on both bone scanning and radiography are normal, routine bone biopsies reveal the presence of metastases in 2.8% to 4% of cases (Ingle et al., 1978; and DiStefano et al., 1979). Using a monoclonal antibody against the tumor-associated glycoprotein TAG12 to identify cancer cells, Diel and coworkers (1992) examined bone marrow aspirates and biopsy samples from 260 patients with breast cancer. Tumor cells were found in 44% of patients, and their presence correlated with tumor size, nodal status, and histologic grade. Their presence was also associated with the development of distant metastases, but not necessarily in bone. Whether such information allows more accurate prediction of prognosis than is otherwise possible is uncertain.

This Author's Personal Experience with Staging

The vagaries of clinical staging were evident in the author's review of 100 consecutive new cases of breast cancer. Despite many abnormal test results and more than a few secondary procedures, in only one case was an asymptomatic metastasis discovered. In 64% of the 76 patients in whom chest radiography, liver function tests, and bone scanning were performed, the results of at least 1 of the 3 tests were abnormal. Twelve (13%) of 94 chest radiographs were abnormal, and 3 of these suggested the presence of metastases. Pulmonary resection in one patient revealed a ham-

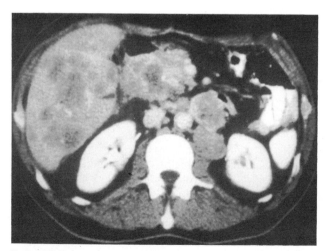

Figure 17–8. Hepatic metastases from carcinoma of the breast appear as multiple dark areas in the liver on a CT scan of the upper abdomen.

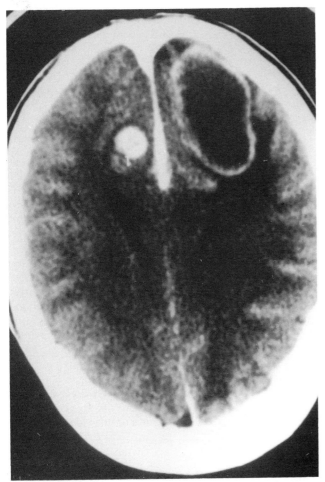

Figure 17–9. This CT scan of the head shows an enhancing lesion in the right frontal lobe and a large metastasis with dark central necrosis in the left frontal lobe. CT scans of the head rarely show metastases in the absence of neurologic symptoms.

artoma, and CT in the second demonstrated a bone island in a rib. In the third patient, mediastinal adenopathy was found; mediastinoscopy proved this to be metastatic adenocarcinoma. Liver function testing in 89 cases detected no metastases, but the results in 28 cases (32%) were abnor-

mal. An elevated lactate dehydrogenase level was the most frequent abnormality; an elevated alkaline phosphatase level was the second most frequent. Abnormal liver functions prompted four CT scans, all of which were normal; and in 36% of the cases, hepatic functions returned to normal within the next 14 months. One of 80 bone scans demonstrated metastases, but the patient for whom the scan was performed was symptomatic with bone pain. One-half (50%) of the 80 bone scans revealed an abnormality. Twenty-six of the 80 patients who underwent bone scanning (32%) were examined further with radiography, and the majority were found to have benign changes. In one patient, radiography demonstrated the presence of symptomatic metastases; and in two patients, it showed suspicious changes. One of the latter two patients underwent a rib biopsy that showed that no cancer was present, and the other patient had no sign of progression after 46 months. Although bone metastases are rarely detected in the absence of symptoms, many patients have symptoms related to the bones and joints that are the result of other problems. The problem most often found is arthritis; less often, Paget's disease of bone, cartilaginous lesions, and an assortment of other problems are seen. The ultimate distribution of clinical stages in the 100 cases reviewed by this author is shown in Table 17–4. The frequency of nodal metastases increased progressively with stage in those patients who were treated surgically. Five-year survival was 68% overall, and 65% of this was disease-free. Twenty-seven per cent of patients treated surgically for cure had recurrence within 5 years.

CLASSIFICATION OF DISSEMINATED BREAST CANCER

Considerable variation is observed in the survival of patients with disseminated and incurable cancer of the breast, that is, TNM stage IV. Differing prospects for morbidity and survival influence both the selection of treatment and its urgency. Proper classification in this regard also permits more meaningful evaluation of palliative treatments. The most important influences on prognosis are (1) the organs involved, (2) their number, and (3) the tumor growth rate. Patients with metastases in the liver, peritoneum, brain, or

Table 17–4. TNM CLINICAL STAGE OF 100 CONSECUTIVE CASES OF BREAST CARCINOMA—PERSONAL SERIES

Stage	No. and Per Cent of Cases	Axillary Nodes		
		No. with Positive Nodes/ No. that Had Nodes Removed	*Per Cent with Positive Nodes*	Median No. of Positive Nodes
0	16	0/13	0	0
I	35	6/33	18	2.5
IIA	31	11/28	39	2.0
IIB	9	7/9	78	3.0
IIIA	2	2/2	100	9
IIIB	5	2/2	100	4
IV	2*	?	?	?

*One case had supraclavicular metastases, and one case had painful bone metastases.

spinal cord have a rapid demise, generally having a median survival of no greater than 6 months. The survival of those with metastases to other sites is directly related to the number of organ systems involved. Cutler and colleagues (1974) placed patients with dissemination into three groups with declining prospects for survival:

Group I Metastases in only one organ system (median survival of 15 months)
Group II Metastases in two or more organ systems (median survival of 12 months)
Group III Metastases in the liver or central nervous system (median survival of 4 months)

A classification was also suggested for postoperative dissemination. This classification takes into consideration that a long disease-free interval (DFI) was associated with longer survival after recurrence.

Group I (Median survival of 14–40 months)
    DFI = 5 or more years, or
    DFI = 2 to 5 years, with one organ system involved
Group II (Median survival of 11–16 months)
    DFI = 2 to 5 years, with two or three organ systems involved, or
    DFI = 1 to 2 years, with one or two organ systems involved, or
    DFI = less than 1 year, with one organ system involved

Group III (Median survival of 5–7 months)
    DFI = 2 to 5 years, with four or more organ systems involved, or
    DFI = 1 to 2 years, with three or four organ systems involved, or
    DFI = less than 1 year, with two or more organ systems involved
Group IV (Median survival of 5–11 months)
    DFI of any duration, with the liver or central nervous system involved

The influence of specific organ involvement on survival after recurrence was also evident in a review by Tomin and Donegan (1987). The poorest survival was seen in cases with recurrence in the liver, peritoneum, or gastrointestinal tract. Median survival was 6 months, and no patient lived longer than 3 years. Patients with the most favorable outlook were those with local recurrence followed by those with recurrence in the lymph nodes. Outlook for patients with recurrence in bones was more favorable (median survival = 30 months) than that for patients with recurrence in the lung or pleura (median survival = 21 months) (Fig. 17–10). Osseous metastases generally have a more indolent course than do extraosseous metastases (Leone et al., 1988). As observed by others, the presence of tumor estrogen receptors indicated a more favorable prognosis. Understandably, the growth of tumor in vital organs is more serious than growth in ones that are not so vital, and the rapidity of such growth is also of considerable importance.

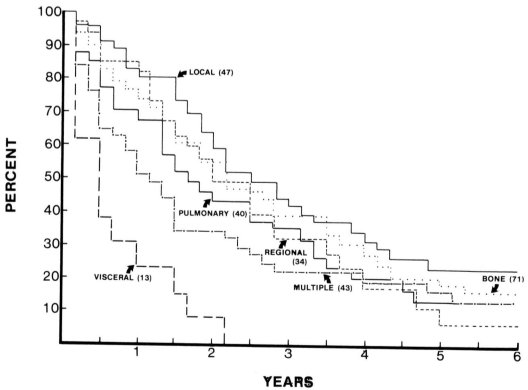

Figure 17–10. The survival of 248 patients with recurrent breast cancer at the Medical College of Wisconsin demonstrates that prognosis varies according to the site of initial recurrence. Recurrence in viscera (e.g., liver, brain, and intraperitoneal organs), has the most unfavorable prognosis; survival associated with recurrence at multiple sites is also poor. (Data from Tomin, R., and Donegan, W. L.: Screening for recurrent breast cancers—Its effectiveness and prognostic value. J. Clin. Oncol., 5:62–67, 1987.)

DFI, estrogen receptors, differentiation, and other measures of aggressive tumor kinetics, such as histologic grade, S-phase fraction, and thymidine labeling, correlate with prognosis after recurrence. DeLena and coworkers (1993) found aneuploid tumors to be associated with shorter survival than diploid tumors in patients with extraosseous metastases.

PATHOLOGIC STAGING

A critical judgment that a pathologist must make is whether a tumor is invasive. Noninvasive (in situ) cancers as a group are associated with highly favorable prognoses. They are identified with some reservation, however, because although invasion is readily recognized, its absence cannot be determined with equal confidence. Histologic examination of the entire tumor is not always feasible when specimens are large. Cases in which nodal metastases are found in conjunction with in situ cancer are assumed to be instances in which invasion was missed or not recognized. *Microinvasive* is a term applied to invasive cancers no larger than 5 mm in diameter or to in situ cancers with a focus of invasion that penetrates a distance no greater than 5 mm; however, these tumors are included along with other invasive cancers for the purpose of staging.

The appeal of pathologic staging is the histologic certainty that it provides about tumor size and node status. One might assume that a pathologist provides results of the greatest accuracy; however, tumors can be ill-defined, and measurements can be compromised by previous incisional biopsies and by eccentric section. In some cases, the mammographically or clinically determined size may more accurately reflect a tumor's true dimensions. The presence of cancer in the axillary and the internal mammary nodes is prognostically important, but more attention has been given to pathologic staging of cancer in the former because they are readily accessible to the surgeon. In a review of 641 cases, Fisher and associates (1981) found an overall discrepancy of 33.5% between the results of clinical and pathologic staging of the axilla. Metastases were present on histologic examination in 38.6% of cases judged clinically negative for cancer and were absent in 27.3% of cases in which metastases were clinically suspected. In almost one-fifth (17.2%) of clinically negative cases, more than three nodes were found to be involved. An error of similar magnitude was confirmed in Sugarbaker's cases (Fig. 17–11). A judgment that the axilla is clinically negative for cancer becomes more accurate when tumors are small and the likelihood of metastasis is small (Sariego et al., 1993). The internal mammary nodes often contain metastases, but since they lie deep to the bone thorax, they are hidden from clinical examination (the exception is in rare cases of gross involvement when they create subcutaneous mounds of tumor between the ribs along the sternal border). Factors that receive attention when metastases are present in the lymph nodes include the number of involved nodes, the size of the metastases, the axillary level of involved nodes, and the presence or absence of tumor growth through the capsule of the node.

Axillary Lymph Nodes

The presence of metastases in axillary lymph nodes is the single most important influence on prognosis (Joensuu et al., 1990). Fisher and coworkers (1992) considered 21 clinical and pathologic features of 620 Stage I and II invasive breast cancers and found only 3 had any independent prognostic value (i.e., the number of involved nodes, tumor size, and the presence or absence of nipple involvement). The number of nodal metastases was found to have the greatest influence. Recurrence within 10 years of radical mastectomy was seen in 76% of patients in another series (Fisher, 1976) when involvement was present compared with 24% when it was not. The risk of treatment failure rose with increases in the number of nodes that contained metastases. When the number was one to three, the 10-year failure rate was 65%, and when it was 4 or more, the 10-year failure rate was 86%. Although the count of involved nodes is aggregated in various ways (most recently, 1 to 3, 4 to 10, 11 +), a direct and continuous correlation exists between the absolute number of positive nodes and treatment failure (Nemoto et al., 1980; and Wilson et al., 1984) (Fig. 17–12). Data indicate that survival, local recurrence, and total treatment failure after mastectomy correlate precisely with the total number of involved nodes (Table 17–5). Even after preoperative chemotherapy, the strong correlation between the number of involved nodes and prognosis persists (McCready et al., 1989).

Patients with extensive involvement of regional nodes not only are more likely to have recurrence but are more likely to have it sooner than those who do not. Figure 17–13 plots the disease-free survival of this author's patients after radical mastectomy according to nodal status. Patients with 11 or more diseased nodes had rapid recurrence and a median disease-free survival of only 10 months. The median disease-free survival increased to 16 months in patients with from 5 to 10 positive nodes; to 22 months in those with from 1 to 4 involved nodes; and to 26 months in patients with no metastases in lymph nodes. The rapid recurrence in patients with abundant regional metastases suggests more rapid tumor growth or a greater residual tumor burden, or both.

Other features of nodal metastases have prognostic importance but are less important than their number. The presence of gross metastases is less favorable than that of micrometastases (i.e., metastases smaller than 2.0 mm in diameter) (Attiyeh et al., 1977; and Rosen et al., 1981), the growth of metastases through the capsules of lymph nodes is unfavorable (Fisher et al., 1976; and Mambo and Gallager, 1977), and metastasis at Level III of the axilla is less favorable than metastasis at lower levels (Table 17–6) (Haagensen, 1971; and Donegan, 1972). These findings are interrelated, however, and the influence on prognosis of any one is not independent of that of the others. For example, involvement of Level III occurs almost entirely in patients with many involved nodes. Micrometastases are found only in patients with three or fewer nodal metastases. Extracapsular metastases influence prognosis independently of number of metastases only in patients with few (from one to three) involved nodes (Donegan et al., 1993a). A single,

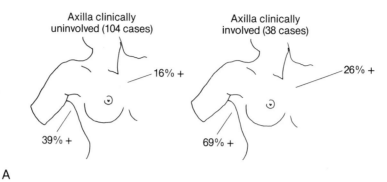

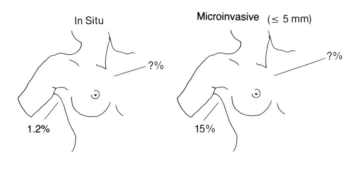

Figure 17–11. *A,* The frequency of metastatic cancer in axillary and internal mammary lymph nodes as determined from extended mastectomies performed by E. D. Sugarbaker. The axillary nodes contained metastases in 39% of cases when they were considered clinically negative, and were free of metastases in 31% of cases when they were believed clinically positive. The internal mammary nodes, which cannot be evaluated clinically, contain metastases in 16% of patients with clinically localized tumors and 26% of cases with axillary adenopathy.

B, The frequency of axillary nodal metastases is shown for 96 cancers in a review at the Medical College of Wisconsin. One of 83, or 1.2%, of apparently noninvasive ductal carcinomas produced axillary metastases, and 2 of 13 microinvasive carcinomas produced them (15%).

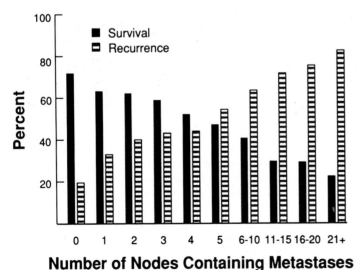

Five Year Recurrence and Survival Versus Number of Positive Axillary Nodes

Figure 17–12. The number of axillary nodes that contain metastases is directly related to recurrence and inversely related to survival and is the single most important indicator of prognosis. (Based on 20,547 cases reported by Nemoto, T., Vana, J., Bedwani, R. N., et al.: Management and survival of female breast cancer: Results of a national survey by the American College of Surgeons. Cancer, *45*:2917–2924, 1980.)

Table 17-5. RECURRENCE AND SURVIVAL AFTER RADICAL MASTECTOMY BASED UPON THE NUMBER OF AXILLARY LYMPH NODES WITH METASTASES (EFSCH 1940 TO 1965)*

No. of Axillary Metastases	No. of Cases	Survival		Relative Survival		Local Recurrence (%)	Overall Recurrence (%)
		5 y	10 y	5 y	10 y		
None	332	70	52	82	74	11	27
Any	456	41	22	47	30	36	67
1–2	171	52	34	60	46	21	52
3–4	71	51	27	58	38	38	66
5–6	49	41	22	47	30	49	74
7–8	38	24	11	28	14	47	87
9–10	32	38	21	42	26	47	66
11–12	20	26	0	31	0	40	85
13–15	23	30	4	34	6	52	83
15–20	23	22	8	24	9	39	87
21 +	29	7	0	8	0	59	90

Note: The presence of metastases in axillary lymph nodes and the number of involved nodes are the most important and sensitive pathologic indicators of prognosis following surgical treatment of mammary carcinoma. It is clear that prognosis progressively deteriorates as the number of involved nodes increases.
*After 5 to 24 years of observation.

gross metastasis leads to a less favorable prognosis than does a single micrometastasis, but the influence of the latter varies with the size of the tumor that produced it (Rosen et al., 1981).

Rotter's (Interpectoral) Lymph Nodes

Interpectoral lymph nodes lying along the thoracoacromial vessels between the pectoralis major and pectoralis minor muscles can be found in 65% of radical mastectomy specimens. However, these nodes are so seldom involved when the axillary nodes are not that their independent influence

SPEED OF RECURRENCE ASSOCIATED WITH NUMBER OF INVOLVED AXILLARY LYMPH NODES, EFSCH, 1940-1965

Number of Positive Nodes	Number of cases	Median Disease-Free Survival (Months)
0	66	26
1–4	124	22
5–10	85	16
≥ 11	81	10

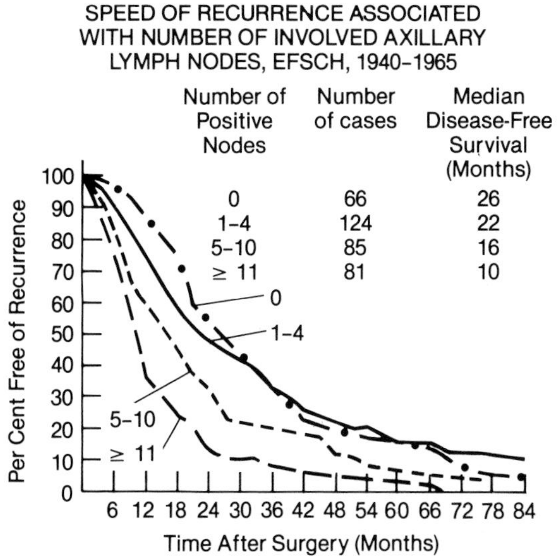

Figure 17–13. The disease-free survivals of patients with recurrence after radical mastectomy indicate that recurrences are more rapid in patients with large numbers of involved lymph nodes. These curves can be interpreted to mean that patients with the fewest nodes involved have the least residual tumor burden after radical mastectomy, or that cancers with the greatest metastatic ability have the most rapid growth rates. Both may be true.

on prognosis is difficult to demonstrate (Kay, 1965). Cody and associates (1984) found metastases in Rotter's nodes in 0.5% of patients whose axillary nodes were free of metastases and considered their removal inconsequential to surgical therapy. Rotter's nodes are removed in the course of a radical mastectomy. They are not routinely removed in a modified radical mastectomy, although they can be.

Extent of Axillary Dissection Necessary for Staging

The extent of axillary dissection necessary for accurate pathologic staging is a matter of importance because unnecessary dissection of the axillae risks lymphedema of the upper extremities. In patients with in situ carcinomas, axillary metastases are not expected and, in fact, are found in only 2% or 3% of axillary dissections. For this reason, surgeons are increasingly reluctant to dissect the axilla in patients with ductal carcinoma in situ (DCIS) unless microinvasion is suspected, the tumor is large, or the axillary nodes are clinically suspicious. Otherwise, a dissection is omitted or confined to Level I. An abbreviated Level I dissection that is confined to tissues inferior to the intercostobrachial nerve has been described (Kinne, 1993).

For patients with invasive carcinomas, prognosis is closely related to the absolute number of nodes that contain metastases but neither to the total number of nodes recovered nor to the per cent of total nodes that contain metastases (Fisher and Slack, 1970) (Fig. 17–14). The lack of correlation of prognosis with the total number of nodes recovered seems to minimize the importance of extensive axillary dissection; however, the patients providing this data all had radical mastectomies, and differences in node count resulted from variations in specimen examination, anatomic differences among patients, and perhaps other factors, but not from variations in the extent of dissection.

The extent of dissection that is necessary for staging depends on whether the objective is simply to determine whether metastases are present or to determine the total

Table 17–6. RECURRENCE AND SURVIVAL AFTER RADICAL MASTECTOMY ACCORDING TO THE HIGHEST LEVEL OF AXILLARY LYMPH NODES WITH METASTASES (EFSCH, 1940 TO 1965)

Axillary Level*	No. of Cases	10-y Survival (%)	10-y Relative Survival (%)	Local Recurrence (%)	Overall Recurrence (%)
I (Low)	93	29	42	28	50
II (Mid)	129	32	43	33	64
III (High)	177	10	13	45	80

Note: The highest level of involved axillary nodes divided according to the convention of Berg (1955) is of prognostic importance. At least 80% of patients with metastases in the high axillary lymph nodes experienced treatment failure. Little difference prognostically, however, can be appreciated between involvement of low nodes only and that of midaxillary nodes.

*Axillary levels: Lateral and inferior to the pectoralis minor muscle (low, or Level I), behind the pectoralis minor (mid, or Level II) and medial and superior to the pectoralis minor muscle (high, or Level III).

number of metastases. If metastases progress in a stepwise manner up the axillary node chain, a Level I dissection should be sufficient to detect nodal involvement; however, the evidence does not entirely support this conjecture; skip metastases do occur. The problem has been addressed with tagged axillary dissections, in which the findings at each level are compared with the results of the completed (Level III) dissection. As most of the studies addressing this included patients who underwent modified radical mastectomies, which do not remove Rotter's interpectoral nodes, a small 1% or 2% false-negative error is introduced at the outset. The investigations indicate that "sampling," an ill-defined procedure equivalent to the removal of some Level I nodes, fails to detect nodal metastases in up to 42% of patients in whom they exist (Davies et al., 1980) and that dissection of Level I nodes alone fails to detect metastases in as many as 29%. Dissection of Levels I and II nodes

RECURRENCE WITHIN 5 YEARS
OF RADICAL MASTECTOMY
VERSUS
TOTAL NUMBER OF AXILLARY
LYMPH NODES REMOVED

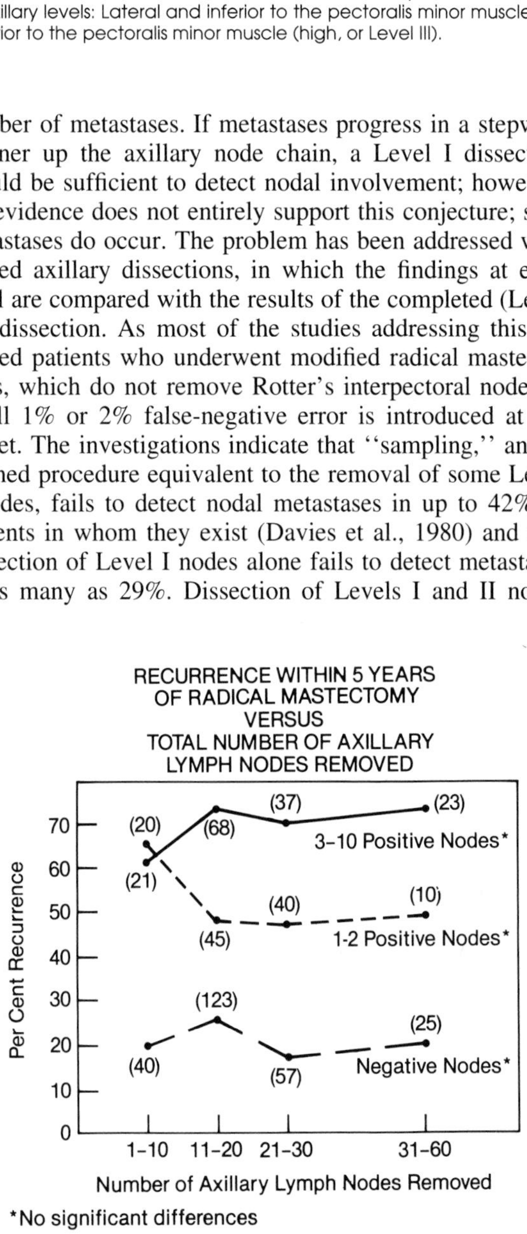

Figure 17–14. Cases of invasive carcinoma of the breast treated with radical mastectomy at Ellis Fischel State Cancer Hospital demonstrating that the prognosis of patients based on the number of axillary nodes that contain metastases is constant despite the total number of lymph nodes examined. The graph also shows that if metastases were present, the distinction in number of involved nodes became more accurate when more than 10 nodes were examined. Parentheses indicate number of cases.

fails to detect metastases in only 2% or 3% of patients, according to most researchers (Table 17–7). For this reason, removal of nodes from Levels I and II is considered the minimum acceptable procedure for detection of axillary metastases.

With respect to the determination of the number of nodes that contain metastases, leaving involved nodes at any level can be expected to produce an inaccurately low count of metastasis-containing nodes. Fisher and associates (1981) reported that as increasing numbers of nodes were examined, the likelihood of finding four or more positive nodes increased. In a study of 539 cases, Veronesi and colleagues (1987) determined that if nodes were positive for cancer at Level I, then higher levels were involved in 41% of patients. If Levels I and II were involved, nodes positive for cancer could be expected at Level III as well. The risk of leaving nodal metastases with an incomplete dissection increased with increases in tumor size and in the number of metastases at Level I. It is clear that in the presence of clinical adenopathy or intraoperative findings that suggest the presence of axillary metastases, a dissection of all three levels of the axilla must be performed if an accurate count is to be obtained. A complete dissection in this circumstance is also desirable because it can achieve tumor control in the axilla. Unremoved nodal metastases can be expected to undergo progressive growth and to invite regional recurrence in the axilla in a substantial number of patients. If the

Table 17–7. SENSITIVITY OF VARYING LEVELS OF AXILLARY LYMPH NODE DISSECTION IN IDENTIFYING METASTASES WHEN THEY ARE PRESENT

Reference	No. of Cases	Level I (%)	Level II (%)
Senofsky et al., 1991	92		95
Danforth et al., 1986	65	71	97
Smith et al., 1977	304	73	90
Pigott et al., 1984	72	75	99
Schwartz et al., 1986	127	87	98
Boova et al., 1982	80	91	99
Rosen et al., 1983	281	98	100
Veronesi et al., 1987	539	99	100

Note: Consensus is lacking on the sensitivity of a Level I (low) dissection in detecting metastases: estimates of false-negative results range from 1% to 29%. Better accord is seen with a Level II dissection. Overall accuracy of axillary dissection depends on the proportion of cases with metastases.

axilla is left untreated when it is clinically negative for cancer, the axilla is the first site of treatment failure in 18% of patients (about 50% of those expected to have occult nodal involvement) (Fisher et al., 1981). Abbreviated axillary dissections compromise detection of nodal metastases, yield inaccurate information on the number of nodal metastases, and provide inadequate tumor control. Comparison of treatment results by pathologic stage among patients who have undergone different levels of axillary dissection is at best imperfect and at worst misleading.

A source of inaccuracy in pathologic staging of interest to pathologists is sampling error. In a few cases, metastases identified in routine histologic sections of nodes are simply missed by the original observer; moreover, several reviews of cases with tumor-negative nodes demonstrate that with multiple rather than the usual single section of each node, metastases can be found in from 17% to 33% of cases (Wilkinson et al., 1982). Despite the increased accuracy multiple-section examinations provide for pathologic staging, they are not routinely employed because they are time consuming and expensive and because the prognosis of cases with metastases so identified is not substantially different from that of cases considered node-negative on routine examination.

Internal Mammary Nodes

Information from survey biopsies and therapeutic excisions firmly establish the prognostic importance of metastases in the internal mammary lymph nodes (IMNs). These nodes were involved in 19.1% of 1119 extended radical mastectomies reviewed by Veronesi and associates (1985) and in 22.4% of 7070 cases collected from the literature by Morrow and Foster (1981). The probability of metastasis is increased by the presence of primary tumors located in the medial side of the breast and of large tumors; by youth; and by the presence of metastases in axillary lymph nodes. Morrow and Foster found that the IMNs were the only site of nodal involvement identified in 4.9% of 7070 patients who had extended mastectomy or IMN biopsy and that they contained metastases in 9.9% of 3512 patients with axillary nodes negative for cancer. This means that as a staging procedure, complete axillary dissection carries the possibility of substantial error; indeed, about 10% of patients with tumors identified pathologically as node-negative based on axillary dissection do in fact have regional metastases (Table 17–8). This accounts for the poor survival of some ''node-negative'' patients and leads some to recommend IMN biopsy in selected cases to identify patients who are part of this poor prognostic group.

The prognosis associated with IMN metastases is approximately that of axillary node involvement; however, when both sites contain metastases, the prognosis is materially worse. Fifty-six per cent of Cacere's (1959) patients with only IMN metastases and 52% of those with only axillary metastases survived 5 years after extended mastectomies; in contrast, only 24% with involvement at both sites survived for this length of time. Only 10% of the latter survived 10 years. The involvement of both sites likely reflects more extensive regional advancement. If the number of

Table 17–8. FREQUENCY OF INTERNAL MAMMARY NODE (IM) BUT NO AXILLARY NODE (AX) METASTASES BY LOCATION OF PRIMARY TUMOR

Source	Medial Primary		Lateral Primary	
	No.	IM + (%)	No.	IM + (%)
Handley and Thackray (1949)	17	17.6	33	3.0
Andreassen et al. (1954)	37	10.8	63	0.0
Wyatt et al. (1955)	27	25.9	33	0.0
Handley et al. (1956)	55	20.0	2	0.0
Caceres (1959)	89	4.5	118	1.7
Pavrovsky et al. (1969)	70	8.6	0	0.0
Urban and Marjani (1971)	267	13.1	34	2.9
Bucalossi et al. (1971)	570	5.8	621*	2.7
Livingston and Arlen (1974)	97	10.3	296	2.7
International Cooperative Study (Lacour et al., 1976)	630	5.2	796	3.4
Valagussa et al. (1978)	110*	6.4	197	4.1
Total	1969	7.6	2193	2.9

(From Morrow, M., and Foster, R. S. Jr.: Staging of breast cancer. A new rationale for internal mammary node biopsy. Arch. Surg., *116*:748, 1981. Reprinted with permission.)
*Includes central lesions.

IMN metastases were added to the number of involved axillary nodes, the total count may well be a more sensitive indicator of prognosis than merely the fact that dual involvement is present. In a multivariate analysis of multiple prognostic factors, including ploidy, c-*erb* B$_2$ oncogene expression, and tumor size, Noguchi and coworkers (1993) found the presence of IMN metastases to be second only to the presence of axillary nodal metastases as an independent predictor of survival. Evaluation of the IMNs with lymphoscintigraphy has received some attention; however, the technique has not found a place in routine clinical practice (Bassett et al., 1989).

Supraclavicular Nodes

Ordinarily, tumor metastasis to supraclavicular nodes occurs only after extensive involvement of axillary nodes or IMNs, and the presence of metastases at this site strongly implies that wider dissemination has occurred. In the current TNM staging system, these nodes are given an M1 designation, equating them with distant dissemination. Papaioannou and Urban (1964) reported that none of 28 patients with positive biopsies of prescalene lymph nodes lived longer than 1 year without progressive disease. In the experience of Fentiman and coworkers (1986), the 5- and 10-year survival of 35 patients with ipsilateral supraclavicular metastases was 30% and 23%, respectively. However, the presence of such metastases does not preclude prolonged survival of some patients. One of this author's most recent five patients with isolated supraclavicular recurrence after mastectomy (20%) lived for more than 10 years afterward (139 mo), and two survived for longer than 5 years. One was still alive at 54 months and a third may prove to live at least 5 years. Interestingly, in three of these patients, no axillary metastases were found at the time of mastectomy.

Tumor Size

Whether measured clinically by palpation or mammographically, or on cut section by a pathologist, the gross size (diameter) of invasive primary carcinomas is a sensitive indicator of prognosis. It is second only to the presence of nodal metastasis in importance and is a prominent anatomic feature in staging (Joensuu et al., 1990). The prognostic influence of tumor size likely reflects both the dynamics of neoplastic growth and the biases of detection. Tumors may not only become more aggressive as they enlarge, but they may be found large because they are more aggressive. Conversely, slowly growing, indolent tumors are likely to be found at a small size and to have a favorable prognosis. (Spratt, 1994). When tumor size is considered as a single variable, increasing diameter is associated with a progressive deterioration in disease-free survival after treatment (Fig. 17–15). The explanation for this lies largely in the direct relationship between tumor size and the presence of regional metastasis. Published series indicate that the frequency of metastasis in axillary nodes rises from 3% to 27% for tumors less than 0.5 cm in diameter to 78% for those greater than 10 cm in diameter (Fig. 17–16). Associated with the increasing risk of nodal involvement is a gradual increase in the mean number of positive nodes at each progressively greater tumor size, a further indication of increasing aggressiveness as disseminating tumors enlarge (Fig. 17–17).

Although tumor size is closely related to nodal metastasis, its influence on prognosis is expressed whether or not nodal metastases are present (Carter et al., 1989). This apparently reflects a relationship between tumor size and occult blood vascular dissemination, which is measurable only in eventual outcome. In patients with pathologically

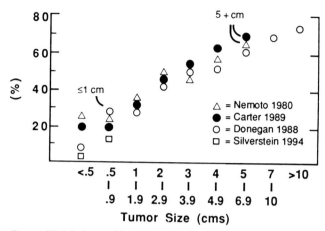

Figure 17–16. A graphic representation of the results from four published series shows a direct relationship between tumor diameter and histologically confirmed metastases in axillary lymph nodes. The relationship is independent of the method of detection (physical examination or mammography alone). There is less agreement about the frequency of metastasis from tumors smaller than 5 mm in diameter than from larger ones. (Modified from Donegan, W. L.: Prognostic factors: Stage and receptor status in breast cancer. Cancer, 70:1755–1764, 1992.

negative axillary nodes, tumor size remains the single most important prognosticator for survival (Joensuu et al., 1990). Figure 17–18 shows the relationship between tumor size and survival in node-negative and node-positive cases registered with the NCI's SEER tumor registry.

INFLUENCES ON PROGNOSIS OTHER THAN STAGE

Histologic and biologic features of breast cancer also influence prognosis. One of the most important is *histopathologic grade*. The majority of breast cancers are ductal carcinomas of no special type and are distinguished only by varying degrees of histologic differentiation: well-differentiated, or grade one (G1), moderately differentiated, or grade two (G2), poorly differentiated, or grade three (G3), or undifferentiated, or grade four (G4). Using SEER data, Henson and colleagues (1991) were able to correlate increasing grade with both increasing tumor size and stage and with decreasing survival. Ten-year survival for patients with G1 tumors was 90% compared to 53% for patients with G3 and G4 tumors. In addition, patients with Stage I and G1 tumors had a 10-year survival of 95%. Since G3 and G4 differ little with regard to prognostic significance, a three grade system was preferred. A similar relationship is seen with the classification of nuclear grade, in which Grades I, II, and III are used to indicate declining differentiation and prognosis. Fisher and associates (1975a) graded breast carcinomas based on their nuclear features and on tubule formation and found that 70% were poorly differen-

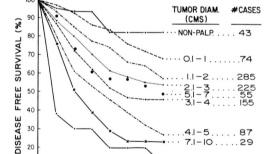

Figure 17–15. Survival after primary treatment is directly related to the maximum diameter of the primary tumor (cases treated at the Medical College of Wisconsin (MCW)). Only the small 5 to 7 cm category, shown with unconnected dots, is out of sequence. This simple relationship provides a strong impetus for diagnosis of tumors at their smallest size.

RELATIONSHIP BETWEEN TUMOR SIZE, AXILLARY
NODE INVOLVEMENT, AND MEAN NUMBER OF
POSITIVE NODES

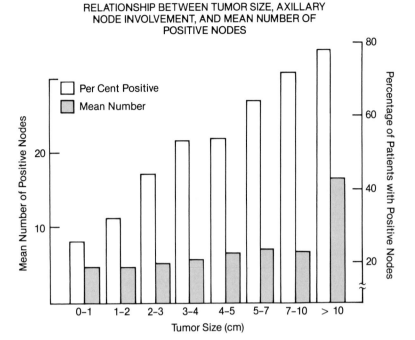

Figure 17–17. As tumor size increases, so does the frequency of histologically confirmed metastases in axillary nodes. In patients with axillary metastases, the mean number of involved nodes also increases with increases in tumor size, suggesting that tumor size reflects total-body tumor burden. (Case data in this analysis are the same as those represented in Figure 17–15.)

tiated (Grade III) and that only 2.5% were well differentiated (Grade I). Poor nuclear grade was associated with early treatment failure. The 1992 version of the TNM staging system categorizes information on the histopathologic type and grade of mammary carcinomas (Tables 17–2 and 17–9).

A few special histologic types of breast cancer are considered to be associated with a relatively favorable prognosis (McDivitt et al., 1968; and Adair et al., 1974). These include mucinous, tubular, and papillary carcinomas. Typical medullary carcinoma is also a favorable type, but the more frequent "atypical" medullary carcinoma is not (Rubens et al., 1990). Unfortunately, special types consti-

tute fewer than 15% of all breast cancers. The less aggressive behavior of these tumors is attributable to their reduced metastatic potential rather than to their small size.

Similarly, biologic characteristics of mammary carcinoma are important prognostically (McGuire et al., 1990; Osborne, 1990; and Robert, 1990). The absence of estrogen receptors is less favorable than their presence (Donegan, 1992). Rapid tumor growth is associated with a less favorable course than is slow growth. Rapid growth is reflected by a short net tumor doubling time (Kusama, 1972; and Pearlman, 1976), a high mitotic index (number of mitoses per 10,000 cells or per 10 high-power fields) (Laroye and Minkin, 1991), a high thymidine labeling index (Meyer and

Survival vs Tumor Size and Node Category

Figure 17–18. Survival is influenced by tumor size independent of the number of involved axillary lymph nodes. Survival decreases as tumor diameter increases in each nodal category. (Based on 24,730 cases from the SEER registry.) (From Carter, C. L., Allen, C., and Hensen, D. E.: Relation of tumor size, lymph node status, and survival in 24,730 breast cancer cases. Cancer, 63:181–187, 1989.)

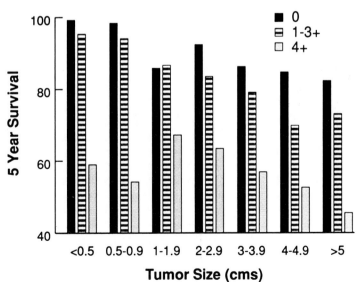

Table 17-9. HISTOLOGIC TYPES OF BREAST CANCER

Carcinoma, NOS (not otherwise specified)
Ductal
    Intraductal (in situ)
    Invasive with predominant intraductal component
    Invasive, NOS
    Comedo
    Inflammatory
    Medullary with lymphocytic infiltrate
    Mucinous (colloid)
    Papillary
    Scirrhous
    Tubular
    Other

Lobular
    In situ
    Invasive with predominant in situ component
    Invasive

Nipple
    Paget's disease, NOS
    Paget's disease with intraductal carcinoma
    Paget's disease with invasive ductal carcinoma
    Other
    Undifferentiated carcinoma

(From American Joint Committee on Cancer: Manual for Staging of Cancer. 4th ed. Philadelphia, J. B. Lippincott, 1992, p. 152.)

Province, 1988), and a high S-phase fraction (Clark et al., 1992; and Johnson et al., 1992). Other characteristics associated with poor prognosis include abnormal amounts of deoxyribonucleic acid (DNA) (aneuploidy), a high DNA index (ratio of tumor DNA to normal DNA), and abnormal oncogene expression (e.g., *HER-2/neu,* epidermal growth factor receptor, and p53) (Bosari et al., 1992; Gasparioni et al., 1992; and Toikkanen et al., 1992). Neovascularization provides avenues for dissemination of tumors, and the extent of angiogenesis within primary breast cancers (i.e., the number and concentration of microvessels) correlates directly with the presence of metastasis in nodes and at distant sites (Weidner et al., 1991). In node-negative cases, the presence of tumor in lymphatic channels and blood vessels around the primary tumor is associated with a substantially increased frequency of recurrence and death. Serum levels of the tumor-associated antigen CA 15-3 correlate with clinical and pathologic stage but lack independent prognostic value (Gion et al., 1991). The presence of carcinoembryonic antigen also reflects tumor burden. The frequency of elevation of this antigen increases with clinical and pathologic stage, and such elevation is associated with recurrence and a high death rate (Myers et al., 1978). Controversy exists regarding the reliability of biologic factors and how they should be used for making therapeutic decisions. Some have prognostic value only for node-negative cases. In a single individual, they are not always in accord in signaling a good or bad prognosis, and the influence of a particular combination of values on prognosis is uncertain. Their most important potential application is as a means of accurately identifying patients who will or will not have recurrence. To date, these factors have not proved sufficiently reliable compared with the accuracy of tumor size and node status to replace the latter. They do provide sup-

plementary information (Fig. 17–19) (McGuire and Clark, 1992).

The precise location of a primary tumor within the breast—specifically, whether it is located laterally or medially—has no consistent influence on prognosis. The experience with radical mastectomy at Ellis Fischel State Cancer Hospital (EFSCH) suggests that a slightly less favorable survival exists for patients with medial lesions, but this factor has not been controlled for other variables (Table 17–10). The series of Sugarbaker and of Handley, when reviewed by the author, revealed no poorer prognosis for patients with medial tumors (Donegan, 1970). In large studies, neither Fisher and coworkers (1985b) nor Veronesi and Valagussa (1981) were able to find a significant difference in prognosis related to the position of a tumor either medially or laterally.

Age and body habitus influence prognosis. Competing causes of death are substantial among the elderly. This creates the impression that breast cancer is less lethal than in younger patients. However, the elderly are not spared from excess deaths due to breast cancer, and it has not been established whether breast cancer follows a more benign course in the elderly. At EFSCH, advanced age was associated with improved survival (when correction for natural mortality was considered) and with decreasing frequency of axillary metastases (Table 17–11). Host and Lund (1986) found poorer survival both among patients younger than 35 years of age and among those older than 75 years of age. They speculated that the older patients had received less aggressive treatment. In Milwaukee, this author confirmed that elderly patients were treated with less complete operations than young patients and received adjuvant therapy less frequently than young patients (Donegan, 1983). Goodwin and associates (1986) documented the same findings in a review of cases in New Mexico. What is still uncertain is how often optimal treatment is prevented by infirmity and associated illness.

Women who are overweight not only have a greater risk of developing cancer of the breast but also a greater risk of recurrence and death (deWaard, 1975; and Donegan et al., 1978). The influence of obesity is independent of pathologic nodal status and is expressed most strongly in node-negative patients. The adverse effect of obesity is poten-

Table 17-10. RESULTS OF RADICAL MASTECTOMY ACCORDING TO LOCATION OF PRIMARY CARCINOMA

Quadrant	No.	Relative Survival (%)		Local Recurrence (%)
		5 y	10 y	
Upper outer	369	64	50	25
Lower outer	86	63	45	28
Upper inner	114	58	44	32
Lower inner	42	50	40	21
Central	129	62	59	18
Diffuse	37	41	19	65

Note: The prognosis of patients with diffuse carcinomas at EFSCH was less favorable than that of other patients. No patients were treated with postoperative radiation.

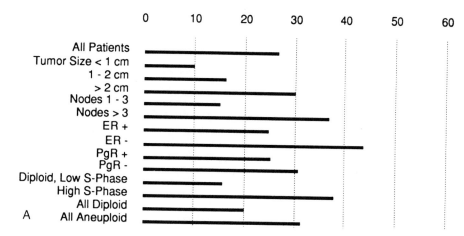

Node Positive Breast Cancer
% Probability of Recurrence (3 yr) in Variously Treated Patients

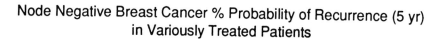

Figure 17-19. Five-year recurrence rates related to various prognostic factors in patients with (A) and without (B) axillary metastases. (From Owens, M. A., Beardslee, S., Wenger, C. R., et al.: A prognostic index for patients with node-positive breast cancer. Breast Cancer Research and Treatment, *16*:193, 1990, and McGuire, W. L., and Clark, G. M.: Prognostic factors and treatment decisions in axillary node-negative breast cancer. N. Engl. J. Med., *326*:1756–1761, 1992. Reprinted by permission of *The New England Journal of Medicine*.)

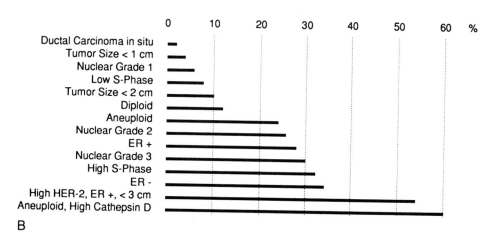

Node Negative Breast Cancer % Probability of Recurrence (5 yr) in Variously Treated Patients

Table 17-11. AGE VERSUS SURVIVAL AFTER RADICAL MASTECTOMY FOR MAMMARY CARCINOMA (EFSCH, 1940 TO 1958)*

| Age | Total | With Positive Axillary Lymph Nodes (%) | 5-y Survivors | | Per Cent of General Population Expected to Survive 5 y† | Corrected Survival‡ (%) |
			No.	Per Cent of Total		
20–29	3	100.0	0	0.0	100.0	0.0
30–39	38	84.2	16	42.1	99.4	42.4
40–49	106	63.5	59	55.7	98.0	56.8
50–59	143	60.0	79	55.2	95.2	58.0
60–69	211	47.9	124	58.8	90.4	65.0
70–79	179	53.1	92	51.4	73.1	70.3
80–89	24	50.0	8	33.3	48.8	66.9

Note: The survival of elderly patients after surgical treatment of mammary carcinoma is lowered by deaths due to intercurrent disease. If survivals are corrected for age, the prognosis of younger patients is less favorable than that of the elderly.

*Age-specific survival after radical mastectomy corrected for natural mortality is directly correlated with age but falls short of statistical significance.

†Calculated for the average in each age category from the Missouri Life Tables: 1949–1951. United States Department of Health, Education and Welfare.

‡Corrected for natural mortality by method derived from Abbott's formula. Finney, D. J.: Probit Analysis. 2nd ed. New York, Cambridge Press, 1962, p. 88.

tiated by high serum cholesterol levels and, by implication, a diet high in fat (Tarter et al., 1981).

UNTREATED CANCER OF THE BREAST

The clinical course of mammary cancer when the disease is untreated (that is, the natural history), provides a baseline against which the value of therapy can be assessed. At present, almost all patients are treated in some fashion; hence, most information on this point stems from the 19th and early 20th centuries. Patients with cancers too advanced for treatment when surgical removal was the only recourse (oophorectomy was not used until 1896, and irradiation was not generally available before 1916), those who refused treatment, and those who were institutionalized in terminal stages of disease have provided information. At least seven authors have published works on this subject since 1926 (Greenwood, 1926; Daland, 1927; Forber, 1931; Nathanson and Welch, 1936; Wade, 1946; Phillips 1959; and Bloom et al., 1962). Bloom and coworkers estimated that in slightly more than 5% of cases in England seen between 1950 and 1962, the patients were untreated, and an additional 60% were treated only with endocrine therapy or chemotherapy.

Bloom (1968) reviewed earlier reports as well as 250 cases from the cancer charity ward of the Middlesex Hospital, which operated between 1792 and 1933, and from the Royal Marsden Hospital of London. The 1728 collected cases had a mean survival of 39.9 months and a median survival of 2.5 years. Absolute survivals reported from the different sources varied from 12% to 22% at 5 years, from 3.6% to 6.6% at 10 years, and from 0.8% to 3.8% at 15 years.

None of Bloom's own series of 250 patients had surgery or irradiation during their lives, and all were autopsied to prove the presence of cancer. Some lived many years without specific treatment; the 5-, 10-, and 15-year absolute survival rates were 18%, 3.6%, and 0.8%, respectively. The median survival was 2.7 years, and not until 19 years after the onset of disease had the last patient died. Survivorship was inversely correlated with age and appeared definitely related to the histologic grade of the tumors, with median survivals of 47.3 months for patients with Grade I cancers, 39.2 months for those with Grade II cancers, and 22 months for those with Grade III cancers. A spontaneous regression was not recorded in any of the cases, and 95% of the patients died as a direct result of their cancer (only 5% died as a result of intercurrent disease). It is worthy to note that 73% of the patients had marked ulceration of the breast prior to death; in 21%, it was so extensive that it sometimes destroyed the breast and chest wall and exposed the pleura.

In seeking to assess the impact of radical surgery on the natural history of untreated breast cancer, it can be observed that radical mastectomy results in a 55% to 65% 5-year survival rate overall, whereas for untreated cases the rate is only about 20%. This favorable comparison must be viewed in light of the biases that promote it. It is likely that the data pertaining to untreated patients are weighted with rapidly progressive cancers. Many women with slowly growing cancers may have escaped documentation by dying of other causes before seeking consultation. Second, selection operates in favor of mastectomy, as women with rapidly progressing tumors that quickly become inoperable are not chosen for mastectomy. Finally, untreated cases were collected from a time when expected survival was considerably less than it is today. To address this problem, Henderson and Cannelos (1980) compared cases treated with radical mastectomy at Johns Hopkins Hospital between 1889 and 1931 with Bloom's untreated cases seen between 1805 and 1933 and found no more than a modest 12% improvement in survival with surgery. A personal review of the records of Halsted's first 50 cases treated with radical mastectomy between 1889 and 1894 that calculated actuarial survival from first symptom (as in the untreated cases) revealed that the 5- and 10-year survivals of Halsted's patients were 40.4% and 32.3%, respectively (Fig. 17–20). This suggests that Halsted doubled 5-year survival and increased 10-year survival 10-fold, a substantial improvement.

Sixty-four per cent of 2618 patients reviewed at EFSCH were treated with radical surgery. Based on computed survival for all cases from the first symptom, patients treated with radical surgery fared better than those treated with all other palliative measures by about 25% at 5 years (Fig. 17–21). If it is assumed that the opportunity for surgical intervention was present at some point in all cases, it is possible to conclude that surgical intervention had a favorable influence.

The 945 patients who had unsuccessful radical surgery fared no more poorly than those who had none, suggesting that although surgery may fail to cure, when it is unsuccessful it has no detrimental influence on the patient's course. In fact, the patients with treatment failures fared somewhat better in their early years than did patients who were not surgical candidates, although at 10 years the survival was comparable.

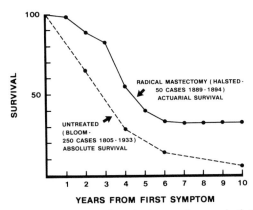

Figure 17-20. This comparison between the survival of Halsted's first 50 cases treated with radical mastectomy and Bloom's untreated cases of breast cancer, plotted from first symptom in both series, suggests that radical mastectomy was associated with an improved prognosis. The long follow-up of Bloom's cases permitted computation of absolute survival as opposed to actuarial survival in those treated surgically. The untreated cases span a broad period that encompassed the introduction of radical surgery.

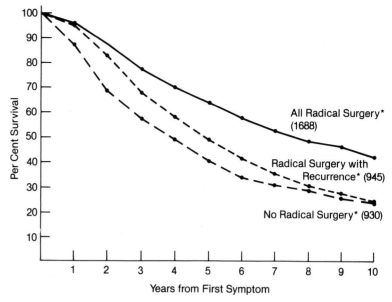

Figure 17-21. The actuarial survival of 2618 patients (EFSCH, 1940–1965) from the time of their first symptom illustrates that patients with treatment failures after radical surgery fared somewhat better than those who were never candidates for radical surgery. All radical operations are included. An operation that failed to cure the patient had no deleterious influence on the clinical course.

*Radical Surgery: Standard, Extended, or Modified Radical Mastectomy

When surgery fails to cure, it can still permanently eliminate cancer from the chest wall. In no more than 43% of patients who were radical mastectomy failures at EFSCH was cancer present in the surgical area at the time of death.

NONINVASIVE (IN SITU) CARCINOMA (TNM STAGE 0)

Noninvasive in situ carcinoma is the earliest recognizable form of carcinoma: its preinvasive phase. The period of transition from noninvasive carcinoma to invasive disease may be protracted or very brief. The difference in mean age between patients with in situ carcinoma and those with invasive breast cancer and the time to appearance of invasive carcinoma after local excision of noninvasive carcinoma suggest that this period averages 6 years in duration. Two forms of noninvasive carcinoma are recognized: ductal carcinoma in situ (DCIS) and lobular carcinoma in situ (LCIS). The forms are histologically distinct, have a dissimilar age distribution, and have different natural histories (Fig. 17–22). The distinguishing clinical features of these two forms are summarized in Table 17–12. Diagnosis of in situ carcinoma using frozen section is fraught with difficulty. Rosen and coworkers (1979) reviewed 129 diagnoses of in situ carcinoma based on the study of frozen sections or permanent sections and found that of 46 cases diagnosed using frozen section, 7 (15%) were later found to be invasive on analysis of paraffin sections. The remaining 83 cases (64%) had been diagnosed as atypical or benign lesions on frozen section analysis. DCIS was more often recognized on frozen section analysis than was LCIS.

Lobular Carcinoma in Situ

LCIS arises from ducts in the lobules of the breast and is the precursor of invasive lobular carcinoma (Fig. 17–23).

LCIS produces few if any clinical signs and is usually an incidental finding in breast tissues. In this author's cases, most LCISs were found in the study of biopsy specimens for microcalcifications; however, in 36% of cases biopsy was conducted for diagnosis of a palpable mass or of thickening due to fibrocystic changes. LCIS is highly multifocal and almost always present in both breasts. Lambird and Shelley (1969) found LCIS to be most often located in the superior periareolar region. In 4% to 6% of patients with a biopsy-confirmed diagnosis of LCIS, unsuspected invasive carcinoma is found in the breast if a mastectomy is performed. Axillary metastases from LCIS are rare.

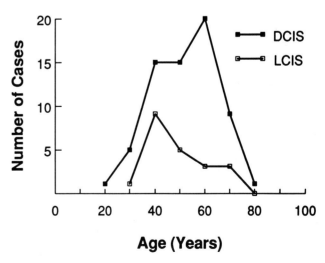

Figure 17-22. The age distribution of patients with DCIS and LCIS examined at the MCW indicate that LCIS occurs in a younger population. Average ages of patients with DCIS and LCIS are 57 years and 51 years, respectively.

Table 17-12. COMPARISON OF DUCTAL CARCINOMA IN SITU AND LOBULAR CARCINOMA IN SITU OF THE BREAST

	LCIS	DCIS
Per cent of in situ cases	20%	80%
Physical signs	Incidental	Varied
Younger than 54 years of age	80%	50%
Multicentricity	Almost always	Often
Bilaterality	Usually	Often
Estrogen receptor–positive	90%	50%
Occult invasion	0–13%	2–28%
Axillary metastasis	Rare	1–3%

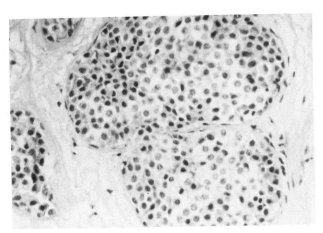

Figure 17-23. LCIS. The typical histologic features of LCIS are distinctly different from those of DCIS. Crowded, uniformly round cells fill the lobule, expand it, and eliminate the lumens.

Attitudes about LCIS have changed since its discovery early in this century. In 1919, James Ewing described it as the "atypical proliferation of acinar cells" without further definition (Haagensen, 1986). It received little attention until 1941, when both Muir in Scotland and Foote and Stewart in New York defined it as a form of preinvasive carcinoma. The studies of McDivitt and coworkers (1967) and Hutter and Foote (1969) then documented that women with LCIS were highly likely to develop invasive breast cancer. This seemed to confirm LCIS's role as a preinvasive malignancy and initiated a period of aggressive treatment of the disease. On the basis of further observations, Haagensen (1983) encouraged use of the term "lobular neoplasia" instead of LCIS to emphasize the unique features of this lesion. In his view, LCIS was not cancer but rather a histologic marker of high risk for future cancer. The current concept is that LCIS is both a marker for high risk and the precursor for some future cancers.

The natural history of LCIS is reflected in the courses of women treated with local excision. In a study of 285 patients observed for an average of 16.3 years, Haagensen (1986) found that 18.6% of them developed breast cancers, and that both the right and left breasts were affected equally. One-half of the cancers were invasive lobular carcinomas, and the others were ductal carcinomas (the latter being equally divided between in situ and invasive ductal forms). Nearly 4% of patients (3.9) died of breast cancer, and an additional 0.7% were living with tumor dissemination. The fact that only 41% of subsequent cancers were invasive lobular carcinomas supported the concept that

LCIS is a marker for carcinoma rather than its precursor. These observations and those of others confirm that the risk for development of subsequent invasive cancer and the number of deaths from it are increased—in some instances, the death rate is up to 11-fold that expected (Table 17–13). Among women with a diagnosis of LCIS, breast cancer can be expected to appear in approximately 1% per year. Furthermore, this risk continues indefinitely. A particularly relevant observation is that risk for future carcinoma is not concentrated in the breast that yielded the diagnosis but is shared almost equally between the two breasts; this no doubt reflects the diffuse distribution of LCIS. No good indicators exist to identify those patients destined to develop future cancers; however, breast cancer in a close relative of a woman with LCIS doubles that woman's risk of developing invasive breast cancer (Haagensen et al., 1978).

It is clear that treatment with local excision alone entails a continuing risk for the development of carcinoma and some risk of dying from it. Thorough removal of both breasts eliminates this risk and is regularly curative (Table 17–14). Less-than-complete removal of all breast tissue, however, carries a continuing risk for the development of cancer, and the development of invasive lobular carcinoma in residual breast tissue after "simple" mastectomy has been reported (Giordano and Klopp, 1973). Bilateral sub-

Table 17-13. RISK OF INVASIVE CANCER SUBSEQUENT TO LOBULAR CARCINOMA IN SITU

Reference	Average Follow-up (y)	Ipsilateral		Contralateral		Overall Risk of Invasive Breast Cancer (X expected)
		Total No.	*Per Cent*	*Total No.*	*Per Cent*	
Rosen et al. (1978)	24	99	18%	96	14%	9×
Andersen (1977)	16	44	20%	44	9%	11.9×
Haagensen et al. (1978)	14	192	10%	204	9%	7.2×
Wheeler et al. (1974)	18	25	4%	32	9%	3.7×

The risk of developing invasive breast cancer subsequent to a biopsy diagnosis of lobular carcinoma in situ is high, reaching 25% to 35%, and the risk is shared almost equally between the two breasts.

Table 17–14. TREATMENT OF LOBULAR CARCINOMA IN SITU WITH UNILATERAL AND WITH BILATERAL MASTECTOMY

	No. of Cases	Local Recurrence	Deaths	Follow-up
I. Unilateral Mastectomy				
Giordano et al., 1973	105	1	1	?
Carter and Smith, 1977	27	0	0	?
Davis et al., 1979	5	0	0	?
Rosen et al., 1981	84	0	2	15 y
Sunshine et al., 1985	15	0	0	>10 y
Total	236	1	3 (1.3%)	
II. Bilateral Mastectomy				
Carter and Smith, 1977	22	0	0	?
Rosen et al., 1981	24	0	0	14 y
Sunshine et al., 1985	21	0	0	>10 y
Total	67	0	0	

Note: Treatment with bilateral total mastectomy generally cures LCIS. Unilateral mastectomy risks the development of cancer in the second breast and a low probability of death from it. Twenty per cent of the cases reviewed by Rosen, Braun, and Lyngholm (1981) developed cancer in the remaining breast.

cutaneous mastectomy with the implantation of prostheses (Blevins, 1981) yields good cosmetic results but does not remove all breast tissue; thus, the risk of developing cancer continues, possibly undiminished (Klamar et al., 1983; and Eldar et al., 1984). Unilateral mastectomy, which has often been used in the past, addresses the occult invasive cancers found in some of the breasts. However, this procedure treats only half the problem, as the remaining breast has an equal potential to be the source of future cancers that could lead to death. In five series that studied a total of 236 cases of unilateral mastectomy, at least three women (1.3%) died of cancers that developed in the remaining breast (see Table 17–14). Supplementing unilateral mastectomy with elective (''blind,'' ''mirror image,'' ''random'') biopsy of the remaining breast to detect and treat possible bilateral involvement has been largely unsuccessful. At Memorial Sloan-Kettering Cancer Center in New York City, as many women developed cancer in the second breast after negative contralateral biopsies (17.2%) as did when no biopsy was performed (17.6%) (Rosen et al., 1981). Irradiation of the breasts has no role in the treatment of LCIS.

Treatment of LCIS is based on its diffuse distribution and bilaterality. The premise is that the treatment for one breast is equally appropriate for the other. The only choice for women who wish to avoid the risk of future breast cancer is bilateral total mastectomy. An axillary dissection is not necessary, and breast reconstruction is available for those who desire it. For other women, observation alone is favored (Swain et al., 1989). All other treatment options have the disadvantage of entailing morbidity without either eliminating risk or possibly even reducing it compared with no treatment at all. Frykberg and colleagues (1987) summarized the case for observation alone in the management of LCIS as follows:

1. Patients are young and have a long life expectancy.
2. Despite the increased risk, only a minority of patients will develop breast cancer in the future.
3. The occurrence of future cancers is delayed: 50% of them develop only after 15 years of follow-up.

4. The risk of death is small: only 5% of patients die of breast cancer within 10 years after diagnosis of LCIS.
5. Bilateral mastectomy seems an excessive preventive measure.
6. The prognosis for cure of future cancers is good with close follow-up.

It is worth emphasizing that a patient's commitment to observation must be lifelong and involves a program of conscientious monthly breast self-examinations, periodic physical examinations, and regular mammography. The intervals recommended in the literature for physical examination vary from 3 to 6 months, and those for mammography range from 6 to 12 months (Hutter, 1984). This author favors physical examination every 6 months and annual mammography. Seven patients on this regimen have been followed by this author for a median of 37 months. Two of them developed further LCIS, and after excision, follow-up was continued. The experience of all has not been rewarding. Six of eight cancers in women being followed for LCIS in one outpatient department were staged as T2 or greater at the time of discovery (Davis and Baird, 1984). A final option for patients with LCIS in the future may be chemoprevention with antiestrogens. These patients are included with other women at high risk in the international Breast Cancer Prevention Trial with tamoxifen being conducted by the National Surgical Adjuvant Breast and Bowel Project. As LCIS is often estrogen receptor–positive, it may be particularly susceptible to suppression.

Ductal Carcinoma In Situ

DCIS arises in the extralobular ducts. It can extend into the lobules secondarily in a process termed ''cancerization of the lobules''; however, it is easily distinguished from LCIS. Several histologic types of DCIS are recognized (Table 17–15). The *comedo* variety is noteworthy as being the most sinister (Fig. 17–24). It is poorly differentiated, lacks estrogen receptors, and is likely to harbor occult invasion (Bur et al., 1992). Noncomedo types constitute about 75% of

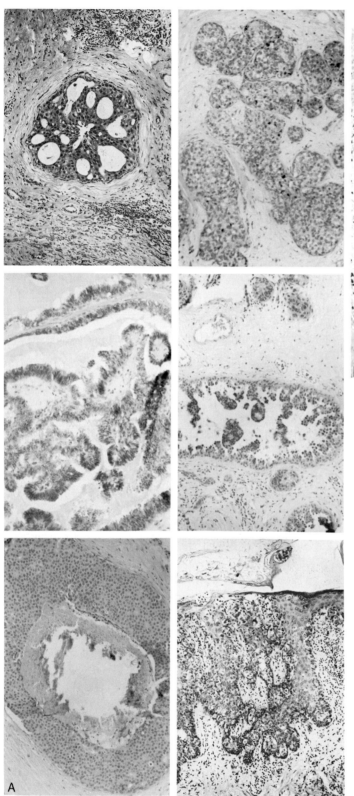

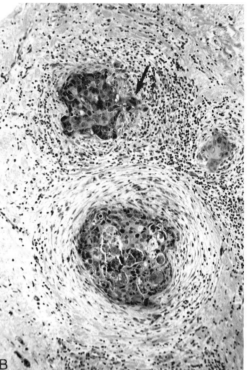

Figure 17-24. *A,* Various histologic types of ductal carcinoma in situ. Cribriform *(upper left),* solid *(upper right),* papillary *(middle left),* micropapillary *(middle right),* comedo *(lower left),* and Paget's disease *(lower right).* Combinations are present in most cases. Clinically, it is important to distinguish between comedo and noncomedo types. (Courtesy of Dr. Henry Ravello and Dr. Thomas G. Peters.) *B,* Ductal carcinoma in situ of the solid type with possible microinvasion *(arrow).*

Table 17-15. HISTOLOGIC TYPES OF DUCTAL CARCINOMA IN SITU

Solid
Comedo
Clinging
Papillary
Cribriform
Intracystic
Micropapillary
Paget's disease without invasion

Note: Two or more histologic types are often seen in combination. The comedo type is poorly differentiated and most likely to be characterized by occult invasion.

DCIS cases, and these types often occur in combination. Cribriform and micropapillary types are associated most frequently (Lennington et al., 1993).

Occult invasion, multicentricity, and occasional metastasis to axillary nodes (1–2% of cases) serve to make management of DCIS more complicated than at first might appear to be the case. Minimal invasion is easily overlooked but is often found in a diligent microscopic search. Lagios (1989) found microinvasion to be associated with large tumor size (i.e., larger than 5.5 cm in diameter). In a review of 50 cases, Schwartz and coworkers (1989) identified microinvasion in 26% of the cases and found it most likely to occur in the comedo type of DCIS (53%) and far more so than in the solid or micropapillary types (14%). The micropapillary, comedo, and papillary types of DCIS were most likely to be multicentric, having frequencies of 86%, 42%, and 33%, respectively. In addition to multicentricity in 18% of cases and obvious but unsuspected invasive carcinoma in 2% of cases, Schuh and associates (1986) found Paget's disease in 8% of cases of DCIS, and LCIS in 13%. These frequencies were somewhat higher in patients with microinvasion. Lagios and coworkers (1982) reported Paget's disease of the nipple in 20% of patients with DCIS. Paget's disease of the nipple is a special form of DCIS. In fewer than 5% of cases, it is isolated to the nipple. Almost always, more extensive in situ or invasive carcinoma is found within the breast. After studying 82 cases of DCIS

with serial section analysis, Holland and associates (1990) concluded that what appeared to be multicentricity was actually growth through ducts in continuity and could be extensive: two or more quadrants were involved in 23% of patients. The extent of involvement confirmed histologically exceeded that estimated by mammography in almost one-half of cases (46%) and exceeded clinical estimates in 38% of cases. More than one-half the tumors were greater than 5.0 cm in diameter, and the center of the breast was involved in 11% of cases. These observations are highly relevant to treatment of DCIS with breast-conserving techniques.

Extensive screening with mammography has increased the proportion of breast cancers detected as DCIS. If detected only as Paget's disease, nipple discharge, or a palpable lump, DCIS accounts for about 5% of breast cancers; however, in populations screened with mammography, the frequency of DCIS triples. Almost a third of cancers discovered with mammography are DCIS, and DCIS accounts for 20% to 77% of cancers discovered on mammography as microcalcifications. This author's own review at three Milwaukee hospitals in 1985 indicated that 9 of every 10 cases of DCIS were discovered with mammography. The tumor can present either as microcalcifications or as a mammographic mass (Fig. 17–25). Patients with DCIS on average are several years older than those with LCIS, and a larger proportion are postmenopausal. Unlike with LCIS, recurrences after local excision of DCIS remain ductal in type and regularly reappear in the same breast, predominantly at the site of excision. Approximately one-half of recurrences are invasive. Whether the second breast is at exceptional risk for the development of new primary tumors is controversial (Webber et al., 1981). This author's personal review of 112 cases of DCIS at the Medical College of Wisconsin suggested an increased risk; the actuarial occurrence of cancer in the second breast reached 20% after 10 years of follow-up (Fig. 17–26).

DCIS is almost completely curable with mastectomy. In four published series, 294 patients with DCIS were treated with total mastectomy with or without axillary node dissection. After a long follow-up, only one patient (0.3%) had local recurrence and six (2%) died of metastatic breast

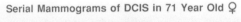
Serial Mammograms of DCIS in 71 Year Old ♀

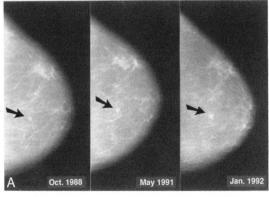

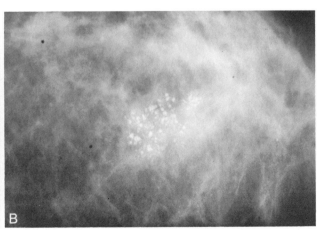

Figure 17–25. *A,* Mammograms showing how DCIS as a mass enlarged during the course of 4 years. *B,* DCIS detected on mammography as a cluster of microcalcifications.

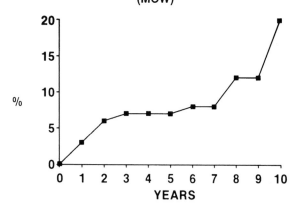

CONTRALATERAL BREAST CA* AFTER TREATMENT OF 112 CASES OF DCIS (MCW)

Figure 17–26. The cumulative incidence of carcinoma in the second breast of patients with an initial diagnosis of DCIS at MCW suggests a higher-than-usual risk for involvement.

cancer (Table 17–16). In the author's experience, the occasional local recurrence after mastectomy usually proves to be persistence or progression in unremoved breast tissue after a less-than-thorough operation; this is preventable. Because nodal metastases are infrequent and axillary dissection risks lymphedema, recommendations are varied (Table 17–17). Some authors feel that axillary dissection is not necessary. Others confine dissections to patients with extensive tumors and those with suspected microinvasion. Surgeons who do perform dissection generally limit it to Level I, which minimizes the risk of lymphedema. A Level I dissection limited to the nodes inferior to the intercostobrachial nerve has been suggested (Kinne, 1993). If no dissection is performed initially, an occasional patient will develop adenopathy that requires axillary dissection. Overlooked or occult sites of invasion apparently account for nodal metastases and the few patients who develop dissemination.

Breast conservation is considered an option for some women with DCIS, largely owing to the favorable results that have been obtained with its use for the treatment of early invasive carcinomas. No randomized prospective trial has compared it with mastectomy, but retrospective and uncontrolled data seem to justify its use. Table 17–18 shows data from reports of local tumor removal with and without irradiation. Case selection, technique, and duration of follow-up varied; however, when breast irradiation was not used, recurrence in the breast was as high as 43%, and

survival in some series was inferior to that expected after mastectomy. Irradiation of the breast after tumor excision reduced breast recurrences (allowing more breasts to be preserved), and survival approximated that expected with mastectomy. It must be noted that a potential staging bias attends reports that compare mastectomy with local excision. Mastectomy offers the opportunity to examine the entire breast and to eliminate the cases of unsuspected invasive carcinoma; this is not true when treatment is with local excision.

Whether irradiation is necessary in all cases of DCIS treated with local excision is uncertain. In a series of 79 carefully selected cases confined to small tumors that were treated with local excision only, Lagios (1990) reported breast recurrences in only 12.6% of cases after a median follow-up of 68 months as well as no deaths. High nuclear grade and comedo type were associated with a high (25%) risk of breast recurrence. Six recurrences were noninvasive, and five of these were treated with local re-excision. One of the four invasive recurrences had metastasized to an axillary node (Lagios et al., 1989). Lagios and coworkers recommended the following criteria be satisfied if treatment with excision alone is to be performed:

1. Occult DCIS detected as microcalcifications on mammography.
2. Histologic tumor size of 2.5 cm or smaller.
3. Complete excision with histologically uninvolved surgical margins.
4. No residual microcalcifications on postoperative mammography.
5. A breast favorable for follow-up with physical examination and mammography.
6. A patient fully aware of the status of this treatment approach and willing to accept its risks.

Others also have proposed local excision alone for nonpalpable or incidentally discovered DCIS. Schwartz and colleagues (1992) treated 70 patients with tumors smaller than 2.5 cm in diameter with local excision alone and observed a 15.3% breast recurrence rate after a median follow-up period of 47 months. All but 1 of 11 breast recurrences were due to the presence of a comedo-type tumor. Recurrences were treated variously with mastectomy, local excision, or breast irradiation.

In the only study of DCIS comparing breast conservation with mastectomy that resembles a randomized prospective trial, Fisher and associates (1991a) confirmed the higher local recurrence associated with breast conservation and the role of irradiation in reducing it. The cases were gleaned

Table 17–16. MASTECTOMY ± AXILLARY DISSECTION FOR DUCTAL CARCINOMA IN SITU

	No. of Cases	Follow-up (mo)	Local Recurrence	No. of Deaths (%)
Sunshine et al., 1985	68	>120	0	3 (4.4)
Kinne et al., 1989	101	138	0	1 (0.9)
Silverstein et al., 1990	97	45	1	1 (1.0)
Fisher et al., 1991	28	85	0	1 (3.6)
Total	294		1 (0.3%)	6 (2.0)

Table 17-17. RECOMMENDATIONS FOR AXILLARY DISSECTION FOR DUCTAL CARCINOMA IN SITU

Schnitt et al., 1988	Not indicated for limited DCIS treated with lumpectomy; reserve for invasive breast recurrence
Lagios et al., 1989	Indicated for extensive DCIS
Temple et al., 1989	Not indicated
Schwartz et al., 1989	Indicated for comedo histologic type
Kinne et al., 1989	Indicated for gross DCIS or microinvasion.
Silverstein et al., 1990	Indicated for microinvasion

Table 17-19. LUMPECTOMY VERSUS LUMPECTOMY COMBINED WITH BREAST IRRADIATION FOR DUCTAL CARCINOMA IN SITU* (NSABP TRIAL [PROTOCOL B-17], 43 MONTHS AVERAGE FOLLOW-UP†)

	Lumpectomy	Lumpectomy Combined with Irradiation
Total No. of cases	391	399
Breast recurrences	64	28
DCIS	32	20
Invasive ductal carcinoma	32	8
5-y cumulative breast recurrence	20.7%	10.4%
Axillary recurrence	1	2
Distant metastases	2	1
Carcinoma of the second breast	8	10
Deaths from breast carcinoma	1	2

*Axillary dissection optional.
†Data from Fisher, B., Constantino, J., Redmond, C., et al.: Lumpectomy compared with lumpectomy and radiation therapy for the treatment of intraductal breast cancer. N. Engl. J. Med., *328*:1581–1586, 1993.

from National Surgical Adjuvant Breast Project (NSABP) Protocol B-06, which was conducted for invasive carcinoma. On pathologic review, 78 patients' tumors were reclassified as noninvasive but had been treated randomly, according to protocol, with modified radical mastectomy, lumpectomy with breast irradiation, or lumpectomy without breast irradiation. All tumors were removed with normal margins, and all patients underwent a Level II or III axillary lymph node dissection. After 85 months of observation, no local recurrences were found after treatment with modified radical mastectomy. Breast recurrences did follow lumpectomy and were sixfold more frequent in those treated with lumpectomy alone (43%) compared with those with breast irradiation added (7%). Six of the 11 patients with breast recurrences (55%) had invasive rather than in situ cancers, and 2 of these 6 patients subsequently died of dissemination. One death from dissemination occurred in the mastectomy group. No differences in overall survival with individual treatments were evident. Comedo-type carcinomas produced a high rate of local recurrence; this finding is in accord with the experience of other researchers. Baird and associates (1990) and Silverstein and colleagues (1991) reported breast recurrence rates that ranged from 11% to 25%, even with the use of irradiation.

The breast-conserving value of irradiation was also evident in the prospective randomized trial of lumpectomy with or without breast irradiation for DCIS (Protocol B-17) conducted in the NSABP (Fisher et al., 1993). Tumor-free

surgical margins were required, but axillary node dissection was optional. The breast was treated postoperatively with 50 Gy of irradiation with or without a boost to the site of excision. Eighty per cent of the tumors were discovered on mammography alone, and 74% were 1 cm or less in diameter. After a mean follow-up of 43 months, irradiation had prevented approximately 50% of breast recurrences (Table 17–19). However, it was more effective in preventing invasive recurrences than in situ recurrences (75% of invasive recurrences were prevented compared with only 37.5% of in situ recurrences). Death rates for breast cancer were similar in the two groups, but the 5-year, "event"-free survival of irradiated patients ("events" being deaths, local or distant recurrences, and cancers of the second breast) was superior owing to a reduction in breast recurrences (Fig. 17–27A). Three patients without axillary dissections had axillary recurrences. Since many DCISs cannot be

Table 17-18. RESULTS OF BREAST CONSERVATION FOR DUCTAL CARCINOMA IN SITU

Series	No. of Cases	Follow-up (mo)	No. (%) of Local Recurrences	No. (%) of Deaths
Lumpectomy				
Gallagher et al., 1989	13	100	5 (38)	3 (23)
Lagios et al., 1990	79	68	10 (13)	0
	20	124	4 (20)	0
Fisher E. R. et al., 1991	21	85	9 (43)	2 (10)
Lumpectomy plus radiation				
Montague, 1984	54	>36	0	—
Zafrani et al. 1985	54	55	4 (7)	1 (2)
Silverstein et al., 1990	104	51	7 (7)	0
Bornstein et al., 1991	38	81	8 (21)	—
Fisher et al., 1991	27	85	2 (7)	0
Solin et al., 1991	259	78	28 (16)*	— (3)*

*Ten-year actuarial rates.
(Modified from Donegan, W. L.: Symposium—Recent Trends in the Management of Breast Cancer: 1. Carcinoma In Situ of the Breast. Can. J. Surg. *35*:361–365, 1993*b*.)

completely removed with satisfactory cosmetic results, the subsequent NSABP Protocol (B-24) did not require complete tumor removal. Lumpectomy and irradiation were used in all patients, who were then randomized to receive tamoxifen or a placebo. No results are available.

In considering treatment alternatives for DCIS, it is clear that total mastectomy with axillary dissection of some extent avoids the need for irradiation, can be applied to all patients, offers almost complete protection from local-regional recurrence, and results in excellent prospects for cure, even when microinvasion is present (Wong et al., 1990; and Rosner et al., 1991). Loss of the breast is the major disadvantage of the procedure, but one which can be partially alleviated with breast reconstruction. At the least, low axillary dissection is considered for those likely to have microinvasion either on the basis of tumor size or the presence of comedo type as demonstrated histologically.

Breast-conserving therapy using the same principles as for treatment of invasive carcinoma is an option for some women who are motivated to avoid mastectomy and offers prospects for survival not obviously different from those expected from mastectomy. Local resection that includes the nipple necessarily sacrifices most of the cosmetic advantage of breast conservation, and therefore patients with Paget's disease are not ideal candidates for such a procedure. A high per cent of patients have residual disease in the breast after local excision, and recurrence in the breast remains a problem. An occasional recurrence in the axilla can also be expected if axillary dissection is not performed. Irradiation of the breast is necessary if breast tumor recurrence is to be minimized; however, it does not eliminate it. Breast tumor recurrence remains a concern not only because it represents failure to conserve the breast but also because one-half of all recurrences are invasive cancers, which pose a greater threat to a patient's continued well-being than the original tumor. Solin and coworkers (1991)

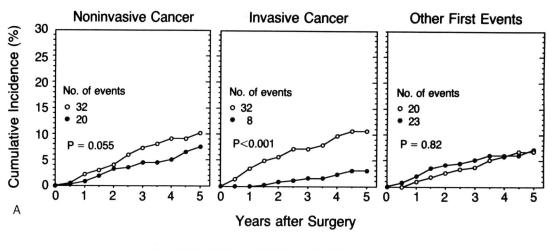

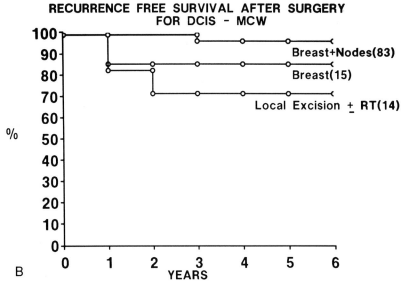

Figure 17-27. *A,* Cumulative breast recurrence after lumpectomy with (•) and without (○) breast irradiation for DCIS in NSABP Protocol B-17. Irradiation reduced the overall frequency of tumor recurrence in the breast; however, it was more successful in preventing invasive than in situ recurrences. (From Fisher, B., Constantino, J., Redmond, C., et al.: Lumpectomy compared with lumpectomy and radiation therapy for the treatment of intraductal breast cancer. N. Engl. J. Med., *328*:1581–1586, 1993. Reprinted with permission from *The New England Journal of Medicine*.) *B,* Owing to tumor recurrence in the breast, disease-free survival of patients with DCIS treated at the MCW with breast conserving operations is shorter than that of patients receiving mastectomy. No relationship was found between survival and the type of operation.

reported on the management of 28 breast tumor recurrences after irradiation for DCIS, one-half of which were invasive. Twenty-six of the patients were treated with mastectomy, and 2 with further local excision. After 29 months median follow-up, three patients (11%) had chest wall recurrences, and four (14%) had distant metastases. The full implications of breast tumor recurrence have yet to be clarified.

The potential morbidity of irradiation remains a concern with breast-conserving techniques, and whether irradiation can be omitted for some patients without excessive subsequent recurrence is of interest. Patients whose tumors are small, isolated, and unlikely to be multifocal or microinvasive may be candidates for lumpectomy alone; however, experience in this area is limited, and guidelines for patient selection are tentative. If further experience proves that breast tumor recurrence does not jeopardize survival, then the penalty for not irradiating may simply be the need to perform more salvage procedures and the preservation of fewer breasts. Re-excision with irradiation might be reserved for those tumors that recur after lumpectomy alone. Lumpectomy alone with tumor-free margins serves reasonably well for patients whose general condition does not permit mastectomy or irradiation. It offers cure for some patients and useful periods of disease-free survival for others.

EARLY INVASIVE CARCINOMA (TNM STAGES I AND II)

TNM Stages I and II are the earliest stages of invasive carcinoma—the so-called "operable" stages. Together, they constitute 75% to 80% of all cases of breast cancer. In contrast to other stages, the large number of patients with Stage I and II disease has permitted many large-scale randomized trials to address critical issues of surgical treatment. The following sections discuss the operations used for these stages, both in the past and at present, their rationale, and their indications.

Radical Mastectomy

The radical mastectomy of Halsted has been largely abandoned for treatment of early breast cancer (Wilson et al., 1984). It is still used to treat some locally advanced cancers, notably those with direct involvement of the pectoralis major muscle or extensive axillary lymph node involvement. In 1990, only 0.4% of all operations for breast cancer in the United States were radical mastectomies (Osteen et al., 1994), but the operation is of interest historically and as a point of departure for more recent operations.

Halsted's "complete" mastectomy was first mentioned in the surgical literature in 1891 within the text of an article in the Johns Hopkins Hospital Report entitled "The treatment of wounds with especial reference to the value of the blood clot in the management of dead spaces." Halsted had performed 13 such operations and had narrowed the large skin defect by means of a pursestring suture, allowing the remaining wound to granulate through an overlying blood

clot. Between 1889 and 1894, Halsted performed 50 such mastectomies and reported his experience in the same year (1894) that Meyer of New York reported a similar operation developed independently in 1891.

These operations removed the entire breast with the overlying skin, the pectoralis major muscle, and the axillary contents in one piece (Fig. 17–28). They differed in that Halsted dissected the breast and muscles from the chest wall first, leaving the axilla until last, whereas Meyer proceeded in the reverse order. In addition, Halsted (1912) removed a large quantity of skin, ultimately using skin grafts to close the wound, and simply divided the pectoralis minor muscle. In contrast, Meyer closed the wound primarily by removing less skin with the specimen, and he also removed the pectoralis minor muscle. Each subsequently modified his skin incision, and Halsted adopted Meyer's practice of removing the pectoralis minor muscle. Later, surgeons developed a variety of incisions, and Raffl (1952) introduced suction catheters for skin flap decompression.

The "radical" mastectomy, as this operation came to be known, was adopted enthusiastically in the United States and abroad. The operation resulted in an immediate and dramatic reduction in chest wall recurrences, which were at this time as high as 82% after lesser operations. Little evidence can be found, however, that it provided better survival than lesser operations. On the contrary, a number of surgeons subsequently reviewed their experience to find that survival rates after Halsted's "complete" operation were, in fact, inferior to those after less extensive operations (Matas, 1898; and Greenough et al., 1907). These disappointing results stemmed from an initial tendency to reserve

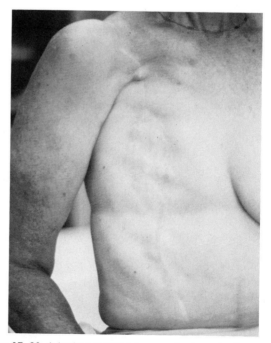

Figure 17–28. A typical Halsted-type radical mastectomy with vertical incision reaching to the shoulder, removal of the pectoral muscles, and removal of a large amount of skin with the breast, necessitating closure with a split thickness skin graft. This results in obvious deformity that is difficult to correct with a prosthesis or surgical reconstruction of the breast.

Halsted's operation for relatively advanced cases and its ambitious application to cases that might formerly have been considered inoperable. Accurate comparisons with earlier operations were hampered by the absence of staging and of randomized trials.

In ensuing decades, two notable trends served to improve results: (1) diagnosis of breast cancer at increasingly earlier stages; and (2) selective use of the operation. The scholarly work of Haagensen helped to confine radical surgery only to those patients for whom it promised cure. This selectivity, however, created the paradox of constant improvement in the results of treatment but with undiminished overall death rates. McWhirter (Page, 1948) and Smithers and associates (1952) commented on this illusion, which is now recognized as "stage shift"; to wit, as surgery is confined to increasingly favorable cases with better results, more favorable ones are perforce referred for irradiation or nonsurgical therapy, with the result that both surgical and nonsurgical therapies appear to yield improved results without any overall increase in cures. For example, assume that cases of cancer are divided into three stages and that Stages I and II are customarily treated with surgery, with observed survival rates of 75% (three of four) and 50% (two of four), and Stage III is treated with irradiation, with a survival rate of 25% (one of four). The surgical "cures" are, therefore, five of eight (63%) and irradiation cures are one of four (25%). Cures overall are 6 of 12, or 50%. If surgery is then restricted only to Stage I cases, the surgical cure rate becomes 75% and irradiation cures become 3 of 8, or 37.5%. The apparent progress on both fronts is achieved without improving the overall cure rate of 50%. Feinstein and co-workers (1985) designated this finding the "Will Rogers phenomenon" after the popular commentator's remark, "When the Okies left Oklahoma and moved to California, they raised the average intelligence level in both states."

After 1903, the radical mastectomy was often supplemented with postoperative irradiation, particularly if axillary lymph nodes contained metastases or if primary tumors were situated in the medial hemisphere of the breast, where they were likely to have produced metastases to the internal mammary nodes. Later, other surgical adjuvants were introduced, so that the operation constituted the sole treatment only in particularly favorable cases.

Modern experience with radical mastectomy has been reported from many centers. Fisher and associates (1975*b*) reported the 5- and 10-year results with 370 cases collected from 23 medical centers in the United States after 1958. All patients were treated with radical mastectomy alone and represented a spectrum of practice throughout the country. Recurrence was observed in 49.5% of the patients during the 10-year period. Radical mastectomy failed to cure 76.1% of patients with axillary metastases and almost regularly failed (86.2%) if more than three nodes contained metastases. These disappointing long-term results illustrate the limitations of local therapy even of this extent and the high likelihood of treatment failure when cancer is found in regional lymph nodes.

Schottenfeld and associates (1976) reported 5- and 10-year survival rates after radical mastectomy combined with selective postoperative irradiation according to the 1972 TNM clinical classification. These rates were, respectively: Stage I, 95.6% and 90.9%; Stage II, 71.8% and 57.1%; and Stage III, 53% and 33.9%.

Much experience with radical mastectomy was accumulated at EFSCH between 1940 and 1970, when it was the principal method of treating operable cases of breast cancer. By 1965, 2621 cases of breast cancer had been seen, of which 1291 were treated with Halsted's operation. The operations were performed by numerous surgeons and surgical residents and included many improvements in anesthesia, surgical technique, and postoperative care. Overall, an average of 3 hours 48 minutes was required to perform the operation, during which 1.3 units of whole blood (average) were transfused. Hospital deaths were recorded in 1.2% of cases, most often from pulmonary emboli, myocardial infarctions, and cerebrovascular accidents.

The indications for the operation fluctuated considerably during these years. It was at times performed in the presence of locally advanced cancer with the intention of giving the benefit of a doubtful chance for cure, and on occasion it was used for palliation. Rarely was it supplemented with postoperative irradiation or adjuvant systemic therapy.

Recurrence, relative survival, and local treatment failure rates are shown in Figures 17–29 to 17–31 as a function of several features of the disease. Because the population was elderly (average age: 63.8 years) survival rates were age-corrected and reported as relative survivals, that is, observed survival ÷ expected survival of Missourians of similar sex and age × 100. From these data, it is evident that a large number of variables pertaining to both the tumor and the patient can be correlated with end results. It is likewise evident that success is not ensured in any stage, and in no situation is freedom from local recurrence a certainty.

In 1984, Haagensen and Bodian reported their personal experience with the Halsted radical mastectomy, which involved 1036 patients with a follow-up of 47 years. All of the patients with carcinoma of the central and inner portions of the breast had prophylactic radiotherapy to the internal mammary region following this operation if the axillary nodes revealed metastases. The study began in 1935 and when, after 20 years, it was found that only 28.2% of 85 patients with CCC Stage C carcinomas remained alive for 10 years, further operations were limited to CCC Stages A and B, and the study continued to 1975. The 10-year survival of 727 patients with clinical Stage A was 80% and of 208 with clinical Stage B was 50%. Ten-year local recurrence was 4.3% in Stage A and 13.4% in Stage B. The axillary dissection was meticulous in these cases, and none of the patients in CCC Stage A developed axillary recurrence during follow-up. Despite the fact that 72% of 208 Stage B patients had axillary metastases, only one patient developed axillary recurrence, a tribute to the therapeutic value of a meticulous axillary dissection. Local recurrence on the chest wall was correlated with the number of histologically involved axillary lymph nodes, rising to 21.9% in patients with eight or more involved nodes in Stage A and to 42.2% in patients with eight or more involved nodes in Stage B. The extent of nodal involvement also influenced 10-year survival in both clinical stages. Haagensen reported

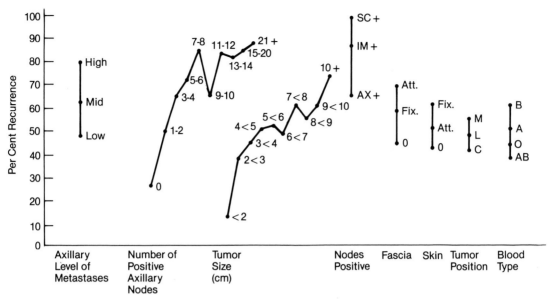

Figure 17–29. Treatment failure after radical mastectomy (i.e., recurrence after 5–24 years of observation), is correlated with the presence, number, and level of axillary metastases, the size of the primary tumor, the sites of regional node involvement, fixation of the primary tumor to fascia and skin, the position in the breast, and the patient's blood type. Recurrence occurred in more than 90% of cases when 21 or more axillary lymph nodes contained metastases and was virtually certain if supraclavicular metastases were present.

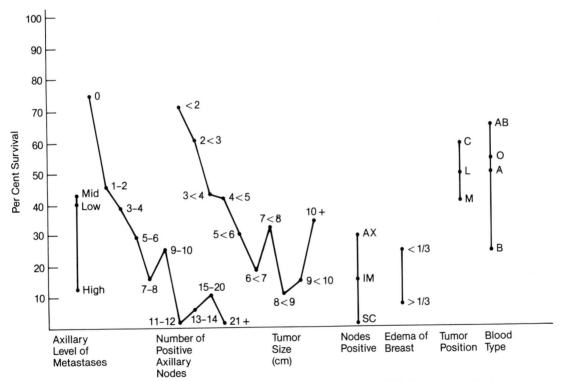

Figure 17–30. Ten-year relative survival of 801 patients after radical mastectomy at EFSCH was most highly correlated with the number of axillary nodes that contained metastases and with the size of the primary tumor. Unfavorable characteristics were metastases in high axillary nodes, supraclavicular metastases, edema of more than one-third of the breast, primary tumors located in the medial portion of the breast, and blood type B. Little prognostic differential was observed in patients with metastases in the middle portions of the axilla compared with those with metastases in the lower portions of the axilla.

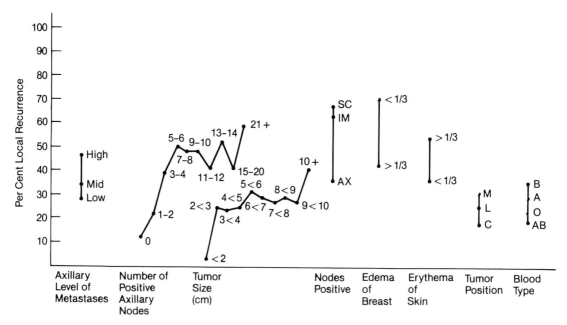

Figure 17–31. Local recurrence after 5 to 24 years of observation is illustrated according to a number of selected variables. Metastases in high axillary nodes, many axillary metastases, metastases in supraclavicular nodes, edema of more than one-third of the breast, erythema of the skin of the breast, medial position of the tumor in the breast, and blood type B were most highly correlated with local recurrence. Tumor position M stands for medial hemisphere, L for lateral hemisphere, and C for central.

edema of the arm in only 5% of the patients when the operation was "well done" and wound healing was uncomplicated.

After being the standard of treatment for eight decades, radical mastectomy was compared in prospective trials with most therapeutic alternatives and found to offer no advantage in early stages of the disease. The most prominent of these trials are discussed in the sections that follow.

EXTENDED RADICAL MASTECTOMY

The internal mammary lymph node chain constitutes one of the primary routes of lymphatic drainage from the breast and frequently is the seat of metastatic disease. This anatomic fact and its possible contribution to treatment failure and local recurrence formerly induced many surgeons to include resection of the internal mammary nodes. Other surgeons ambitiously pursued metastatic disease to secondary nodal areas, the supraclavicular and mediastinal groups. These versions of the radical mastectomy became known as "extended radical mastectomies." They now are rarely used (Osteen et al., 1994).

Halsted was aware of the anatomic shortcomings of his original operation, and for a period he extended its scope, as did Meyer (1905), who frequently dissected the supraclavicular nodes. Halsted reported in 1898 to the American Surgical Association, "Our present method of operating for the cure of breast cancer is even more radical than it was at the time of the writer's first publication on this subject. The supraclavicular area is almost invariably cleaned out. I fail to see why the neck involvement in itself is more serious than the axillary. The neck can be cleaned out just as

thoroughly as the axilla." At this time, Halsted had performed 53 primary supraclavicular dissections and 14 secondary dissections after supraclavicular nodes had become involved clinically. The mediastinum had also been dissected. "Dr. Bloodgood, Instructor in Surgery, has on the necks of two patients done as many as three operations on each for glandular involvement and apparently saved his patients. In one of the cases he entered the mediastinum from above to remove a cancerous gland and had to excise a piece of the innominate vein. Dr. H. W. Cushing, my House Surgeon, has in three instances cleaned out the anterior mediastinum on one side for recurrent cancer. It is likely, I think, that we shall in the near future remove the mediastinal content at some of our primary operations." Halsted subsequently ceased to pursue supraclavicular dissections.

In 1918, interest was renewed in extra-axillary routes of lymphatic drainage from the breast. In this year, W. S. Handley in London reported diagnostic biopsies of internal mammary nodes during 5 mastectomies and subsequently implanted intercostal radium tubes at the time of mastectomy, reporting 77 cases in 1927 (Handley, 1927).

In 1933, Prudente (1949) in Brazil added interscapulothoracic amputation and supraclavicular dissection to mastectomy for patients with mammary cancer with fixed axillary and mobile supraclavicular adenopathy. Two of 12 patients (17%) were cured for prolonged periods, but neither had supraclavicular metastases.

R. S. Handley and Thackray called attention to the less obvious internal mammary nodes with their report in 1949 of internal mammary lymph node biopsies in 50 unselected cases of mammary carcinoma. Metastases were found in 38% of the cases, ostensibly making them incurable with radical mastectomy. More than one-half (51.6%) of inner quadrant lesions associated with positive axillary nodes had metastases to the internal mammary nodes. This information spurred efforts to treat these nodes effectively, either with surgical removal or with postoperative irradiation.

Margottini and Bucalossi of Rome are credited with first practicing internal mammary node dissection as a routine part of radical mastectomy, which they began performing in 1948 (Margottini and Bucalossi, 1949). In 1950, Dahl-Iversen and colleagues in Denmark, who had already appended supraclavicular dissections to their radical mastectomies, added internal mammary dissection and culminated their efforts in 1952 with dissection of both internal mammary and supraclavicular nodes (Dahl-Iversen, 1963). After 1951, Urban, Sugarbaker, and others in the United States began removing the internal mammary chain and an overlying portion of the chest wall en bloc with the radical mastectomy specimen. This became the most widely practiced version of the extended operation. The most ambitious practitioner of the early period was Wangensteen (1949, 1950, 1956; and Wangensteen et al., 1957), who began performing a two-stage "super-radical" mastectomy, removing the specimen in four parts: (1) breast and axillary contents, (2) internal mammary artery and vein with accompanying lymph node chain, (3) upper mediastinal lymph nodes, and (4) low supraclavicular lymph nodes. The procedure was subsequently reduced to one stage with a decrease in mortality from 12.5% to 3.6% and then abandoned.

It is plain that medial (or central) location of the primary tumor in the breast and the presence of metastases in axillary lymph nodes are the two most important determinants of internal mammary lymph node metastases. Eight surgeons' published data relative to these two variables on a total of 2742 cases are summarized in Figure 17–32. Primary tumors located in the central (subareolar) area of the breast and medial quadrants metastasized to the internal mammary nodes in 28% of patients, and lateral primary tumors did so in 18%. When axillary metastases were present, the frequency of internal mammary metastases from centromedial lesions reached 50%, compared with 25% for lateral lesions. In the absence of axillary lymph node metastases, the frequency of involvement from medial and lateral primary tumors was 13% and 4%, respectively. Handley's and E. D. Sugarbaker's data suggest that metastases to these nodes also can be correlated with clinical stage (9–16% in CCC Stage A, 19–26% in CCC Stage B, and 28–42% in CCC Stage C), and this author's data relate it with tumor size (20% if smaller than 2.0 cm and 33% if larger than 5.0 cm) (Donegan, 1972). On the basis of these observations, some surgeons thought that resection of internal mammary nodes was indicated with all mastectomies. Other surgeons confined dissections to lesions with the highest frequency of parasternal metastases, those located centromedially in the breast (Urban and Marjani, 1971) (Fig. 17–33).

This operation did not increase the small mortality rate associated with the standard radical mastectomy. Sugarbaker had one death in 262 cases (0.4%).

Extended mastectomies varied in scope and technique. The principal issues were whether removal of the parasternal lymph nodes (1) improved disease control on the chest

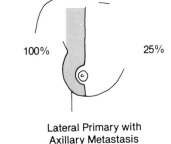

100%   25%

**Lateral Primary with
Axillary Metastasis**

100%   50%

**Central or Medial Primary
with Axillary Metastasis**

Figure 17–32. Frequency of internal mammary metastasis related to location of primary tumor and axillary metastasis. Derived from 2742 reported cases of extended radical mastectomy.

0%   4%

**Lateral Primary Without
Axillary Metastasis**

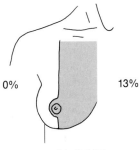

0%   13%

**Central or Medial Primary
Without Axillary Metastasis**

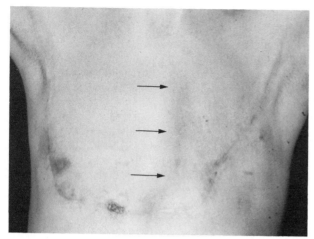

Figure 17–33. Postoperative appearance of a patient with a radical mastectomy on the right and an extended radical mastectomy on the left. A depression is evident in the left parasternal areas, from which the internal mammary lymph nodes were removed. The extended radical mastectomy reduces parasternal recurrences but does not improve survival.

wall and (2) improved the chances of cure. With respect to the former, it is known that metastases in internal mammary nodes enlarge and appear as parasternal recurrences in only 10% of cases in which they are left untreated (Donegan, 1977). If their removal were to prevent this entirely, a 3% reduction in recurrences at this site (0.1 × 30%) would result, or, if used selectively for cases with medial lesions, a somewhat greater reduction would occur. If recurrence at this site were destined to be the first evidence of treatment failure, a small improvement might be seen in disease-free survival. Urban and Marjani (1971) did, in fact, find a reduction in parasternal chest wall recurrences when their extended operations, performed mostly for medial lesions, were matched with radical mastectomies performed at Memorial Hospital, New York City. Five-year disease-free survival, as predicted, was improved when the axilla contained metastases, but overall survival was not improved. Unfortunately, the extended procedure was often supplemented with irradiation, and the time periods were asynchronous.

The first randomized clinical trial compared Dahl-Iversen's extended mastectomy (dissection of both the internal mammary and supraclavicular nodes) with McWhirter's technique of simple mastectomy and postoperative irradiation of all regional lymph nodes. The groups were composed of 335 and 331 patients, and no significant differences were found in crude survival, disease-free survival, or local recurrence (Kaae and Johansen, 1969). Irradiating the peripheral lymph nodes appeared as efficacious as removing them.

The cooperative venture between five cancer centers in Lima, Villejuif, Rome, Milan, and Warsaw randomized 1580 cases of T1, T2, T3a, N0, and N1 cancers between radical mastectomy and radical mastectomy with internal mammary node dissection (IMD); no irradiation was given in any case (Lacour et al., 1976). After 5 years of observation, the survival rates of the two groups were statistically indistinguishable: 69% for RM and 72% for internal mammary node dissection. Survival seemed to be better with internal mammary node dissection in the subgroup of small (T1, T2) medial tumors with axillary metastases (71% for internal mammary node dissection versus 52% for radical mastectomy), but the statistical method for determining this was invalid, and it was balanced by an unexplained advantage for radical mastectomy if tumors of similar size were lateral with normal axillary nodes (87% versus 78%). In 1983, Lacour and coworkers reported the 10-year results of this study using the four centers that continued follow-up (Lima, Villejuif, Milan, and Warsaw) (1453 cases) and found such variation in results between centers that no reliable differences in survival or disease-free survival could be identified either overall or in any subgroup (Lacour et al., 1983). Veronesi and Valagussa (1981) concluded the same in a separate report of the 737 cases accrued for the study at Milan (60.7% and 57% 10-year survivals for radical mastectomy and for internal mammary node dissection, respectively). Of interest was that local-regional recurrences were similar at all sites in the two groups except parasternally, where, as predicted, internal mammary dissection reduced them to 0.3% from an already trivial 3.7% after radical mastectomy. In only nine cases were parasternal recurrences unassociated with other metastases, and in four of these they were permanently controlled with irradiation.

It may be concluded that the surgical removal of internal mammary lymph nodes does not contribute to cure. It does result in a reduction of parasternal recurrences; however, this is an infrequent problem, and irradiation is as effective.

The presence of metastases in the internal mammary nodes has implications for prognosis, and when they remain untreated, metastases add to the problem of regional recurrence. Although the proper treatment of these metastases remains uncertain, their existence is a fact that is difficult to ignore. Some clinicians have suggested biopsy in cases likely to have involvement, particularly if axillary nodes are clinically negative for cancer. Biopsy evidence of the presence of metastases has the same implications for systemic adjuvant therapy as has the existence of metastases in axillary lymph nodes and may justify irradiation to the parasternal area to forestall recurrence at this site (Morrow and Foster, 1981; Veronesi and Valagussa, 1981; and Roseman and James, 1982).

TOTAL MASTECTOMY WITH AXILLARY LYMPH NODE DISSECTION (MODIFIED RADICAL MASTECTOMY)

The term ''modified radical mastectomy,'' or more precisely, total mastectomy and axillary lymph node dissection, refers to operations that spare the pectoralis major muscle while removing en bloc the breast and axillary contents (Fig. 17–34). In the mid-1970s, this procedure became the most popular operation for the treatment of early stages of breast cancer in the United States, and it remains the most viable alternative for women not suited for or not desirous of breast-sparing treatment.

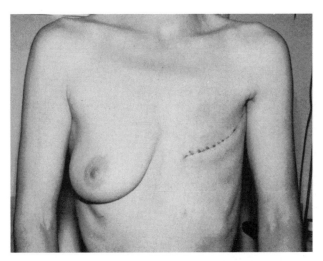

Figure 17–34. Patient with a left modified radical mastectomy. This operation removes the breast and axillary lymph nodes but differs from radical mastectomy in that it preserves the pectoralis major muscle. A "skeletonized" appearance of the chest is avoided, and reconstruction is simplified.

This operation leaves the patient with a more cosmetic result than does the standard radical operation. The pectoralis major muscle accounts for much of the normal contour and softness of the anterior chest wall; its preservation avoids the hollow inferior to the clavicle and the skeletonized appearance of the chest wall so obvious after a radical mastectomy. The patient is left with a stronger arm, and reconstruction of the breast is greatly facilitated. Attachment of a primary tumor to muscle is not a contraindication. When extension to the pectoralis major muscle is discovered, the involved area can be removed with a margin without sacrificing the muscle entirely.

This author's studies with intramammary injection of vital dyes indicate that the lymphatics that traverse the pectoralis major muscle accompany branches of the thoracoacromial vessels and the lateral perforating intercostal vessels. In early stages, lymphatic spread of cancer through these routes is embolic, and there would seem to be no greater chance of directly transecting cancer in these lymphatics than in lymphatics draining to the internal mammary nodes, which are cut. Rotter's nodes are not routinely removed in modified radical mastectomy because they are closely apposed to the acromiothoracic vessels and the lateral anterior thoracic (medial pectoral) nerve, which are essential to preservation of the pectoralis major muscle; otherwise a complete dissection of the axilla can be performed. Two versions of the modified radical mastectomy, differing only in the extent of axillary node dissection, are used. In the first, nodes from axillary Levels I, II, and III are removed; in the other, only nodes from Levels I and II are removed.

Total Mastectomy with Level I, II, and III Axillary Dissection

This operation was developed by Patey at the Middlesex Hospital, London, in 1932 and was adopted in 1936 by

R. S. Handley, who wrote extensively about it (Patey, 1967; and Handley, 1974). The technique has been illustrated by Handley (1972). "The incision begins as a circle two inches clear of the edge of the tumor and is either enlarged by incisions toward the coracoid process and xiphisternum or by transverse incision. The flaps are thin but not actually devoid of fat and are cut back to the midline, the clavicle, the latissimus dorsi and one inch caudad to the breast. The breast is then dissected off the pectoralis major, the pectoral fascia being removed as completely as possible ... the dissection proceeding from the medial to the lateral side" (Handley and Thackray, 1962). A complete axillary dissection is accomplished in continuity, "taking care to preserve the thoraco-acromial artery and the lateral anterior thoracic nerve which accompanies it," to preserve "the continued viability and function of the pectoralis major muscle." "In the removal of the pectoralis minor muscle," Handley (1972) pointed out, "the medial anterior thoracic nerve which penetrates it is necessarily sacrificed. Paralysis of the lateral portion of the pectoralis major results, and therefore ... ; [this portion of the pectoralis major muscle] can be justifiably removed with the specimen." Handley completed the operation with survey biopsies of the internal mammary nodes, and if these, or "more than a few" axillary nodes, contained metastases, irradiation therapy followed the operation.

Results with this operation have been comparable with those achieved with the standard radical operation, although no randomized trial has compared the two (Patey, 1967; Handley, 1969; and Lesnick and Papatestas, 1974). Handley's 10-year crude survival rates were reported by Haagensen in 1974 as 63% for CCC Stage A and 37% for Stage B. Although Haagensen considered them inferior to his own results with radical mastectomy (70% for Stage A and 43% for Stage B), the differences were small.

Handley permitted the author to personally review his cases, and 597 treated with the Patey operation were abstracted and staged retrospectively from the clinical records (Donegan et al., 1970). The operative mortality for the series was 0.2%. The number of cases was reduced to 545 through the exclusion of patients with noninvasive cancers; male patients; and women who were pregnant, who had a previous or simultaneous cancer, or who had any treatment other than postoperative irradiation. Of these, 49.2% had axillary metastases, and 10.2% had metastases in the internal mammary nodes. The results, shown in Table 17–20, compare favorably with those achieved with the radical mastectomy. Local control for at least 5 years was achieved by the Patey operation in 84% compared with 81% for radical mastectomy, suggesting that preservation of the pectoralis major muscle did not engender local recurrence.

The operation designed by Scanlon is an improvement over the Patey operation. It permits a full axillary node dissection without paralyzing the lateral portion of the pectoralis major muscle. Instead of removal of the pectoralis minor muscle, the muscle is divided near its origin on the ribs and lifted up with the pectoralis major muscle; as a result, the medial anterior thoracic nerves are preserved while access to the apical nodes at Level III is provided (Scanlon and Coprini, 1975).

Table 17–20. THE AUTHOR'S REVIEW OF PATEY MODIFIED RADICAL MASTECTOMIES (LEVEL III AXILLARY DISSECTION) PERFORMED BY R. S. HANDLEY (LONDON)

Clinical Stage	No. of Cases	Relative Survival (%)		5-y Local Recurrence (%)
		5 y	10 y	
CCC A	337	83	79	10
B	175	72	48	24
C	27	51	46	34
Pathologic Stage				
Ax−	275	90	82	5
Ax+	264	67	48	27
IM+	56	48	18	45

Note: The cases of R. S. Handley treated by modified radical mastectomy with selective postoperative irradiation are shown staged clinically and pathologically. These results compare favorably with those for other forms of local treatment.
Abbreviation: CCC = Columbia Clinical Classification.

Total Mastectomy with Level I and II Axillary Dissection

Total mastectomy with Level I and II axillary dissection is the operation originally advocated by Auchincloss (1963) and by Madden (1965). The justification for performing this operation is simply that 98.5% of cases with axillary metastases are detected with a dissection of this extent, and that removal of high axillary nodes rarely cures if metastases are present in them. Among 204 carefully cleared radical mastectomy specimens, Auchincloss found 107 in which metastases were present in axillary nodes. Seventy-one of the 107 patients (66%) had not been cured by the operation. Exclusion of 5 patients who died of intercurrent disease left 31 patients living 8 to 10 years later, only 4 of whom had metastases in apical nodes. Theoretically, only 2% of all patients (4 of 204) may have benefited from removal of apical nodes. Pickren and associates (1965) reviewed these same specimens with serial sections and found only one additional high node with occult tumor, leaving the results essentially unchanged.

As described by Auchincloss, the operation consists of a wide removal of the breast followed by an en bloc dissection of the axilla in the following manner: "The fascial investment of the pectoralis major muscle is stripped from the muscle around its lateral edge and, staying in the same plane, with the muscle retracted medially, the fascia covering the pectoralis minor muscle is similarly stripped in order to remove interpectoral nodes. The dissection is then carried upward along the edge of the minor muscle and somewhat posterior to it until the axillary vein is encountered. This is the high point of the axillary dissection and is suitably tagged for later pathological identification. It usually lies approximately 3.0 cm below the clavicle. From this point on, the dissection is performed exactly as would be done in a standard radical mastectomy" (Auchincloss, 1963). Madden (1965) supplemented the axillary dissection with discontinuous removal of nodal tissues from selected sites along the axillary vessels. Dissection around the pectoralis minor muscle should avoid damage to the medial anterior thoracic nerve that penetrates or courses lateral to the muscle.

Two randomized trials have compared modified radical mastectomy with radical mastectomy. Both used axillary dissection limited to Levels I and II and found similar results for both operations, thereby justifying adoption of the more limited, and less deforming, modified radical mastectomy. The first, in Manchester, England, concerned 534 patients with TNM Stage I and II cancers randomized between 1969 and 1976. No treatment but surgery was used until failure was evident. After a median follow-up of 5 years, the 10-year actuarial results indicated no significant differences in survival, disease-free survival, local recurrence, or freedom from distant metastasis between the two treatments (Turner et al., 1981). The second study, performed at the University of Alabama between 1975 and 1978, involved 311 patients (Maddox et al., 1983) with TNM Stages I, II, and IIIA. As randomization was by the patient's year of birth, assignment was not blinded, and those found to have axillary nodes positive for cancer received adjuvant chemotherapy. After a median of 5.5 years, no differences were seen in survival or disease-free survival. However, a trend was noted for increased local recurrence after modified mastectomy. In 1979, a consensus meeting at the NCI concluded that total mastectomy and axillary dissection should replace the Halsted radical mastectomy (NIH Consensus Development Panel, 1979).

Among the physical liabilities of modified mastectomy are numbness and paresthesias of the anterior chest and axilla, phantom breast syndrome in some patients, failure to acquire full shoulder motion in a rare patient, and ipsilateral arm edema of varying degree in approximately 16% of patients.

Evaluation of Modified Radical Mastectomy at the Medical College of Wisconsin and Recommendations for the Extent of Axillary Dissection

Experience with modified radical mastectomy at the Medical College of Wisconsin (MCW) between the years 1969 and 1979 demonstrated its comparability with standard radical mastectomy. Survival and disease-free survival after treatment of TNM Stage I, II, and III carcinomas were not significantly different after observation periods of up to 15 years (Figs. 17–35 and 17–36), nor were significant differences found when comparisons were made by TNM stage

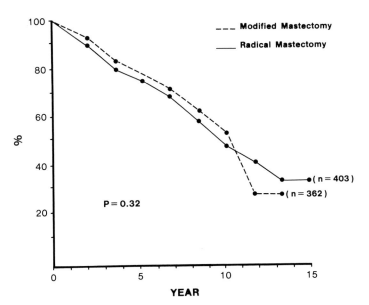

Figure 17-35. Modified and radical mastectomies performed at MCW between 1967 and 1979 resulted in survival rates that were indistinguishable. Irradiation and adjuvant chemotherapy were used selectively.

or by axillary nodal status (Figs. 17–37 to 17–40). Local-regional recurrence increased with time but did not differ overall or when analyzed by stage or by axillary nodal status (Figs. 17–41 to 17–43). Both operations were followed by irradiation or chemotherapy at the discretion of attending physicians.

The modified operations were almost equally divided between those with Level II and those with Level III axillary node dissections, and these two operations served equally well in all situations except one (Figs. 17–44 to 17–46). Local-regional recurrence was significantly higher after a Level II dissection in patients with four or more axillary nodes involved (Fig. 17–47) because of a higher rate of recurrence in the axilla (Table 17–21). The more abbreviated axillary dissection was not as effective in controlling disease in the axilla when it was extensively involved. Therefore, a full axillary dissection (Levels I, II, and III) should be performed if evidence of axillary metastases either clinically or at the time of dissection is present. This recommendation is supported by data from other sources. The Yorkshire Breast Cancer Study Group also reported increased axillary recurrences after limited axillary dissections (Benson and Thorogood, 1986). Based on these findings, the extent of the problem can be projected: Fisher and coworkers (1985) demonstrated that when the axilla remained untreated, it was the first site of failure in an estimated 50% of cases with retained metastases. Although a Level II dissection is satisfactory for detecting metastases, it leaves metastases at Level III unremoved in 18.6% to 41.6% of cases (Pigott et al., 1984; and Veronesi et al., 1987). If metastases are found only at Level I, involved nodes can be expected at Level III in 3.7% to 7.5% of

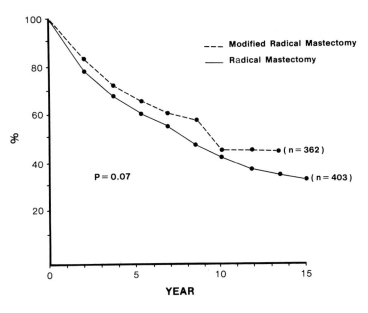

Figure 17-36. Modified and radical mastectomies at MCW between 1967 and 1979 produced disease-free survival rates that were not significantly different. The slight advantage for modified mastectomy may relate to the fact that patients with the prospect of a more favorable outcome were selected for this operation during its introduction.

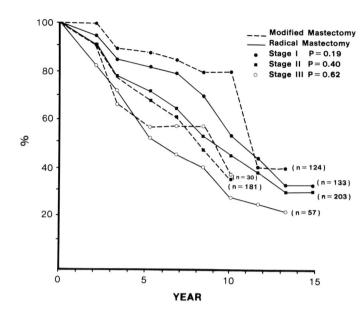

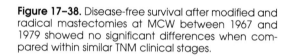

Figure 17–37. No significant difference in survival is evident between patients who underwent modified mastectomies and those who underwent radical mastectomies at MCW when compared by TNM clinical stage. The total number of cases is shown in parentheses.

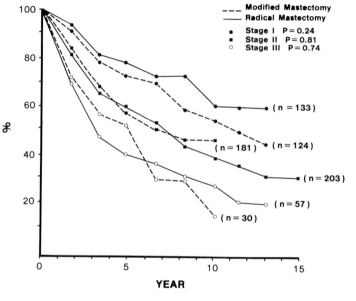

Figure 17–38. Disease-free survival after modified and radical mastectomies at MCW between 1967 and 1979 showed no significant differences when compared within similar TNM clinical stages.

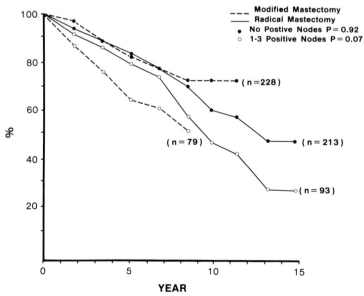

Figure 17–39. Radical and modified mastectomies performed at MCW provided similar survivals when compared by pathologic node category (no nodal metastases and 1 to 3 positive lymph nodes).

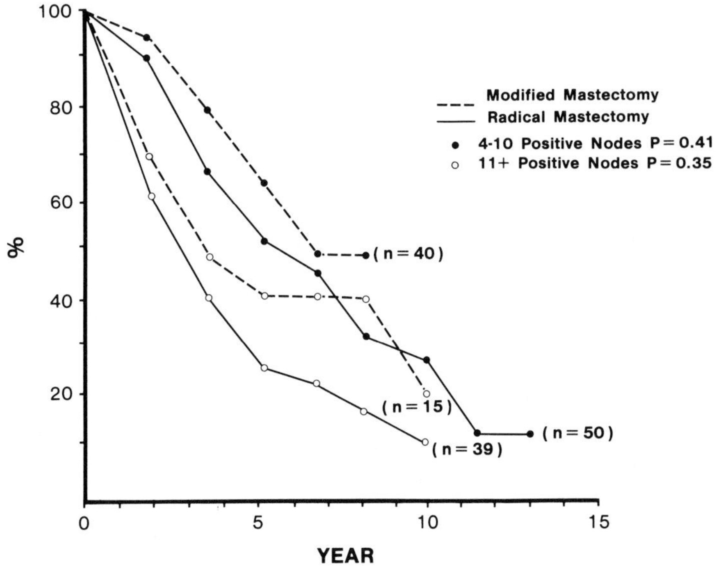

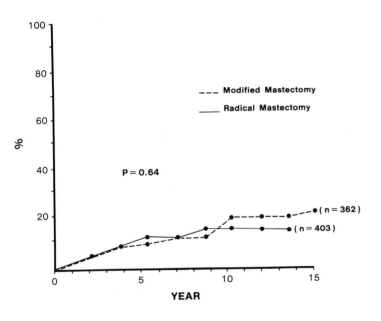

Figure 17-40. Modified and radical mastectomies performed at MCW between 1967 and 1979 resulted in no significant difference in survival when compared by nodal categories (4 to 10 positive nodes and 11 or more positive nodes). During this period, modified mastectomy became the predominant method of surgical treatment, the use of postoperative irradiation declined, and treatment with adjuvant chemotherapy increased.

Figure 17-41. Overall cumulative local-regional recurrence for patients treated with modified versus radical mastectomy at MCW during the 12 years prior to 1979. No significant difference is present.

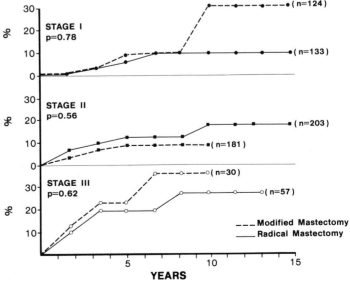

Figure 17-42. Local-regional recurrence after modified and radical mastectomies according to TNM (1988) clinical stage. Cumulative recurrence progressively increases over time and with clinical stage, without a significant difference between the two operations.

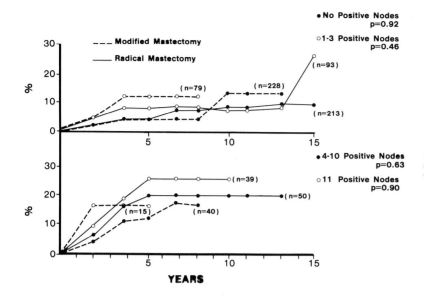

Figure 17-43. Cumulative local-regional recurrence by quantitative axillary node involvement. Recurrence increases progressively with increasing nodal involvement but without a significant difference between the two operations.

cases, and if found only at Level II, they exist at Level III in 66.7% to 82.2% of cases. If both Levels II and III are involved, then unremoved metastases exist at Level III in 42.9% to 61.1% of cases. Axillary recurrences are rare after a complete dissection, so one can expect to prevent axillary failures in from 9% to 20% of patients with metastases (50% of 18.6% to 41.6%) by using a Level III rather than a Level II dissection.

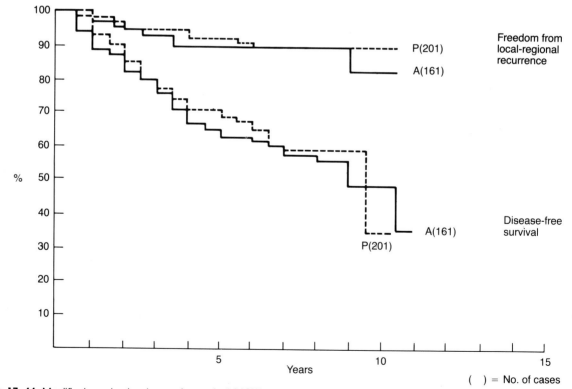

COMPARATIVE PROGNOSIS—TOTAL MASTECTOMY AND LEVEL II AXILLARY DISSECTION (A) VS. TOTAL MASTECTOMY AND LEVEL III AXILLARY DISSECTION (P)

( ) = No. of cases

Figure 17-44. Modified mastectomies performed at MCW were almost equally divided between those with a Level II axillary dissection (A) and those with a Level III axillary dissection (P). Freedom from local-regional recurrence and disease-free survival were indistinguishable.

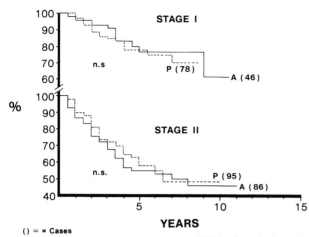

Figure 17–45. Disease-free survival by TNM clinical stage for modified mastectomies with a Level II (A) or Level III (P) axillary dissection. Approximately 80% of patients with Stage I disease were alive and well after 5 years compared with 60% of those with Stage II disease, with no significant difference between the operations. Stage II in this instance omits T3N0 cases.

TOTAL (SIMPLE) MASTECTOMY

"Total mastectomy" has replaced the term "simple mastectomy" to emphasize the objective of completely removing all mammary tissue, something that earlier simple mastectomies often failed to do (Holleb et al., 1965). The procedure for total removal requires flap development as extensive as that for a radical operation combined with removal of some of the lower axillary tissues (Level I) in order to encompass the axillary tail of the breast.

Table 17–21. DISTRIBUTION OF LOCAL-REGIONAL RECURRENCE IN CASES WITH METASTASES IN FOUR OR MORE AXILLARY NODES ACCORDING TO LEVEL OF AXILLARY DISSECTION

Level of Dissection	Site (No. of Cases [%])			
	Skin	*Axillary*	*Supraclavicular*	*Total*
Level II*	10 (56)	5 (28)	3 (17)	18 (100)
Level III†	13 (68)	1 (5)	5 (26)	19 (100)
Level III‡	36 (70)	7 (13)	9 (17)	52 (100)

*Modified radical mastectomy.
†Modified radical mastectomy.
‡Standard radical mastectomy.
Note: Data for surgical cases performed at the Medical College of Wisconsin indicate that recurrence in the axilla is high when an incomplete (Level II) axillary dissection is performed in the presence of extensive axillary metastases.

A number of surgeons have maintained that removal of the breast alone, with or without postoperative irradiation, is appropriate treatment for clinically localized (Stage I) breast cancer (Grace and Moitrier, 1936; McWhirter, 1964; Crile, 1975; and Meyer et al., 1978) and have published favorable results with selected cases treated in this fashion. Total mastectomy without supplemental irradiation for apparently localized cancers poses the question of whether temporary neglect of occult metastases in regional nodes influences the chance of cure. Total mastectomy combined with irradiation of regional lymph nodes is radical in concept and simply raises the issue of whether irradiation of nodes is the equal of their surgical removal (Bond, 1967).

In 1971, the NSABP initiated a prospective randomized clinical trial to address the issues raised by total mastec-

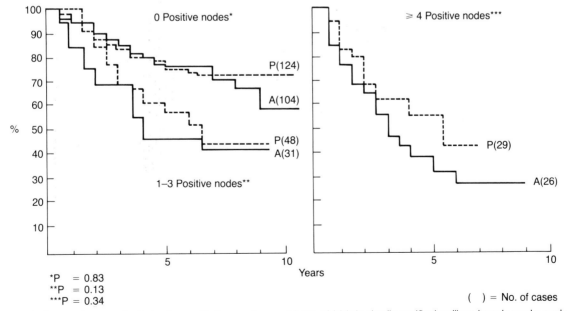

DISEASE-FREE SURVIVAL BY AXILLARY NODAL STATUS—TOTAL MASTECTOMY WITH LEVEL II (A) VS. LEVEL III (P) AXILLARY NODE DISSECTION

*P = 0.83
**P = 0.13
***P = 0.34

( ) = No. of cases

Figure 17–46. Disease-free survival declines with increasing numbers of histologically verified axillary lymph node metastases without a significant difference in results between modified mastectomies with level II or III node dissections.

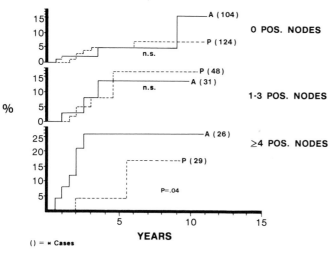

CUMULATIVE LOCAL-REGIONAL RECURRENCE AFTER
TOTAL MASTECTOMY WITH LEVEL II (A)
OR LEVEL III (P) AXILLARY NODE DISSECTION

() = # Cases

Figure 17–47. Local-regional recurrence is higher after a level II node dissection when four or more nodes are involved by metastases, principally because of more frequent recurrences in the axilla. A level III dissection is indicated in cases likely to have involvement of multiple nodes.

tomy. Patients with early cancers confined to the breast (clinical Stage I, but without regard to size) were randomized for treatment with radical mastectomy, total mastectomy alone, or total mastectomy combined with postoperative irradiation to regional lymph nodes (axillary, internal mammary, and supraclavicular). Patients treated initially with total mastectomy alone had an axillary dissection if isolated axillary metastases became apparent. They were not considered treatment failures unless cancer subsequently reappeared.

Beyond including an empirical comparison of three treatment alternatives, the NSABP trial involved certain conceptual questions: (1) If the breast is removed in all cases, are clinically occult metastases in axillary lymph nodes managed as successfully with irradiation as with surgical removal? (2) Does the preservation of clinically uninvolved regional lymph nodes benefit the patient? (3) If occult axillary metastases are not removed initially en bloc with the breast, can they be removed at a later date if they become clinically enlarged without compromising cure?

Patients who presented initially with clinically involved axillary lymph nodes (Stage II) were randomized for treatment with either radical mastectomy (surgical removal of axillary nodes) or total mastectomy and irradiation to axillary and other regional nodes. One thousand seven hundred sixty-five patients entered the study, and in 1985 a report on 1665 eligible patients was made after an average follow-up of 126 months (Fisher et al., 1985*b*). No significant difference was evident in disease-free survival, distant metastasis, or cumulative survival between the three treatment options for clinical Stage I breast cancer. Irradiation reduced regional recurrence but did not improve survival. Eighteen per cent of patients initially treated with total mastectomy alone required subsequent axillary dissection for treatment of progressive metastases as late as 112.6 months after mastectomy (Table 17–22). More than one-half (71%) of those who required a subsequent axillary dissection had a further treatment failure, identifying them as being part of a high-risk group. As it is known that 40% of clinical Stage I patients have occult axillary metastases,

it is of interest that so few patients had tumor progression at this site as the first sign of failure. How many had progression in the axilla after recurrence was detected elsewhere, however, was not reported; thus, whether some regional metastases lie permanently dormant remains uncertain. Noteworthy was a negligible (1.4%) recurrence rate in the axilla after complete axillary dissection in the radical mastectomy group. Also of interest was the failure of regional irradiation, which included the internal mammary nodes, to improve survival.

The two treatment options in Stage II were equally efficacious in terms of survival and disease-free survival. Surgery was more effective than irradiation for controlling clinically enlarged axillary metastases and almost equally

Table 17–22. RECURRENCES, NATIONAL SURGICAL ADJUVANT BREAST PROJECT, B-04 FEBRUARY 1986

	AX −			AX +	
	RM	TMR	TM	RM	TMR
Total Number	362	352	365	292	294
I Local	5%	1.4%	7.1%	7.9%	2.7%
II Regional			18% ←Ax. Salvage*		
Axillary	1.4%	3.1%	1.4%	1.0%	10.5%
Supraclavicular	1.1%	0.3%	2.7%	5.1%	0
Parasternal	0	0	0	0	0
III Distant	27.1%	32.7%	30.1%	37.1%	40.8%

*3 to 117 mo; 71% subsequent failure.

This table shows sites of recurrence after radical mastectomy (RM), total mastectomy and regional irradiation (TMR), and total mastectomy alone (TM), according to the NSABP B-04 protocol. Regional recurrence in the axilla as the first sign of failure appeared in 18% of patients treated with total mastectomy alone. After an axillary lymph node dissection in these cases, total axillary failures do not exceed 1.4%, equivalent to a prophylactic axillary dissection as performed in the RM cases and somewhat better than the 3.1% seen after axillary irradiation. Axillary failures were substantially fewer after radical mastectomy (1%) for clinically involved nodes than after total mastectomy and irradiation of the axilla (10.5%). Supraclavicular recurrences were few in all categories, and no parasternal recurrences were recognized. Distant dissemination was constant despite variations in the method of primary treatment. This study demonstrated that prophylactic removal or irradiation of axillary lymph nodes did not influence the probability of cure.

effective for control of occult axillary metastases in Stage I. Local and supraclavicular recurrences were lowest in both Stages I and II when treatment included irradiation.

This study, more convincingly than any other, casts doubt on the contribution to cure of prophylactic removal or irradiation of regional lymph nodes. It would appear that the case for lymph node dissection must be made on the usefulness of the nodes for pathologic staging and for preventing the progressive growth of regional metastases, two not inconsequential considerations. The study also failed to confirm that preservation of regional nodes retards dissemination of a tumor, as might be expected if they made a significant contribution to immunologic host defense.

The International Multicenter Trial of the Cancer Research Campaign coordinated at King's College Hospital in London also addressed total mastectomy. In this study, 2268 patients in Manchester clinical Stages I and II (i.e., TNM T1 or T2, N0 or N1, M0) were randomized between May 1970 and April 1975 for treatment with total mastectomy followed, in randomly selected cases, by irradiation to the skin flaps and the axillary, supraclavicular, and internal mammary nodes (Murray et al., 1976). After 5 years, patients with Stage I cancers had identical survival rates and freedom from dissemination whether or not they received postoperative irradiation. The same was true for patients with Stage II cancers. The point of greatest interest was that patients in both Stage I and Stage II had significantly higher frequencies of regional and local recurrence if irradiation was not used. This was most common in the axilla (observed in 70% of cases), followed by the chest wall (observed in 35% of cases). Although patients with local and regional recurrence had a poor prognosis, 70% of the local recurrences were successfully controlled by additional treatment. This study further illustrates that treatment (in this case, irradiation) of metastases in regional lymph nodes does prevent their progressive growth but has no impact on survival and dissemination. These results were confirmed by a similar trial with 1022 patients in Manchester, England (Lythgoe and Palmer, 1982). One-third of Stage I (T1-2 N0 M0) patients treated only with total mastectomy had progression in the axilla, and 38% had local recurrence.

It would appear that total mastectomy alone is insufficient to provide optimum local-regional control of invasive breast cancer, principally because of frequent progression of cancer in the axilla. As neglected cancer in axillary nodes progresses during a patient's remaining lifetime in a substantial number of cases, regional control is best achieved by treating it initially and sparing the patient, as far as possible, from repeated subsequent bouts of treatment. Surgical removal and irradiation are equally effective for controlling occult axillary metastases and apparently are equally undistinguished in preventing dissemination of disease in Stages I and II. The advantage of axillary dissection is that it also provides staging information important for accurately determining prognosis and, in some cases, for selecting systemic adjuvant therapy. If delayed treatment of clinically inapparent metastases in regional lymph nodes by either method enhances or jeopardizes chances for cure, it has not been apparent in clinical trials to date.

Total mastectomy results in anesthesia of the skin of the anterior chest. Arm edema is not expected unless irradiation

of regional nodes is added, in which case it may be seen eventually in 5% patients or fewer. Treatment with total mastectomy and irradiation has the advantage of being relatively simple from the surgical standpoint, and it may be all that can be tolerated by some fragile patients, but it combines the most cosmetically objectional aspect of surgery (i.e., removal of the breast) with all of the liabilities of irradiation and provides no information for nodal staging.

It is difficult to find an indication for total mastectomy in the treatment of potentially curable invasive breast cancer or to understand its appeal. It is not a simple matter to remove the entire breast, although it has often been made one with the traditional "simple" mastectomy, which usually results in only partial removal. Since the axilla is not dissected, lymphedema is not expected. As usually practiced, irradiation to the chest and regional nodes follows and is required to reduce local-regional recurrence. Irradiation itself contributes to morbidity, provides less effective control of clinical adenopathy than does axillary dissection, and entails some risk of lymphedema (Harris and Hellman, 1983). The operation may be suitable for patients with large tumors located in the center of the breast who are unable to tolerate an operation of greater extent.

PARTIAL MASTECTOMY (BREAST-CONSERVING OPERATIONS)

The terms that have been used to describe breast conserving operations are varied. When the NSABP began the first clinical trial of breast-conserving surgery in the United States in 1976, the term "segmental mastectomy" seemed appropriate for the operation. But the breast has no true segments, and subsequently, to indicate that a limited excision was acceptable provided that the surgical margins were free of cancer, the NSABP changed the name of the operation to "lumpectomy." This is less than accurate because with extensive use of mammography many of the cancers were found as microcalcifications rather than as a palpable or mammographic lump. The same limitation applies to "tylectomy" (proposed at Guy's Hospital, London), which in Greek means removal of a knot. "Quadrantectomy," the operation used in initial trials in Italy, refers to removal of an entire quadrant of the breast without reference to what is removed, as does "partial mastectomy" or "wide local excision." The term "tumorectomy," used by some, literally means the removal of a swelling, which is often not the case; however, it serves better in the pathologic sense to indicate the removal of a morbid swelling or new growth (i.e., a neoplasm), whatever the manner of discovery. All of the terms seek to indicate an operation that removes a cancer without removing the entire breast and the results of which are cosmetically successful. Although they imply excision of the cancer with operations of varying magnitude, they have not been uniformly performed to ensure that histologically cancer-free surgical margins were obtained.

The attractiveness of partial mastectomy is its cosmetic appeal. Earlier consultation and increased cures might be anticipated if women had a surgical option that provided a better cosmetic outcome than yielded by mastectomy. The objective of breast-conserving operations is retention of a cosmetically acceptable breast without the compromise of local control of a tumor or a patient's prospects for survival. These are the bases for comparison with mastectomy. The extent of axillary dissection is similar for both procedures; the difference lies in how the breast is managed.

Partial mastectomy has undergone intensive study. Central to the issue is the multicentricity of breast cancer. A distinction is sometimes made between multifocality (at multiple sites in the immediate vicinity of the primary tumor in the same quadrant) and multicentricity (additional tumor in other quadrants), but both represent tumor that could potentially escape removal with local resection. Subserial sections of mastectomy specimens show foci of cancer in quadrants remote from the primary tumor in 40% to 50% of cases, the frequency increasing with increases in the number of sections and in the diligence of the search (Qualheim and Gall, 1957; Gallager and Martin, 1969; Fisher et al., 1975a; and Tinnemans et al., 1986). Rosen and colleagues (1975) performed simulated partial mastectomies on 203 mastectomy specimens and related residual tumor to the size of the primary. Unremoved tumor was present in 26% of specimens when the primary tumor was smaller than 2.0 cm in diameter and in 38% when it was larger. Morimoto and associates (1993) examined primary cancers smaller than 2.0 cm in diameter and found cancer that extended more than 2.0 cm from their gross margins in 15% to 20% of the cases. Holland and coworkers (1985) studied 282 mastectomy specimens removed for solitary invasive cancers smaller than 5.0 cm in diameter. Serial 5.0-mm sections were studied both grossly and radiologically, and histologic study of any suspicious sites as well as of random sections was made. The presence of invasive and in situ cancer diminished with increasing distance from the primary tumor and was unrelated to its size (Fig. 17-48A). In 41% of 264 cases with tumors 4.0 cm or less in diameter, in situ or invasive cancer was found at a distance of 2.0 cm from the primary tumor. It was estimated that a margin of resection of 3.0 to 4.0 cm around the primary tumor would have left residual invasive tumor in the breast in 7% to 9% of cases and in situ cancer in an additional 4% to 9%. Margins up to 16.0 cm did not completely eliminate residual cancer. Even small breast cancers detected only with mammography can be locally extensive (Arbutina et al., 1992). Tinnemans and colleagues (1986) reported multicentricity in 47% of 57 nonpalpable invasive carcinomas. Among potential sites of residual tumor is the nipple. Santini and coworkers (1989) found Paget's disease of the nipple in 12% of 1291 mastectomy specimens removed because of invasive carcinoma. The frequency of involvement increased with increases in tumor size and was unsuspected clinically in three-quarters of the cases.

The data from these investigations have important implications for treatment with partial mastectomy. They indicate that the extent of resection is inversely related to the risk of unremoved cancer and, by inference, to cosmetic results. Limited resections with preservation of the nipple are more likely to be cosmetic than are more extensive ones but are also more likely to leave residual cancer unremoved. This dilemma is depicted in Figure 17-48B.

In the 19th century, when breast cancers were large when discovered and irradiation was not available, local excisions regularly failed to cure. Even recent experience with local excision continues to confirm an unacceptably high frequency of recurrence in the breast, particularly if surgical margins are not tumor-free (Lagios et al., 1983; and Tagert et al., 1985). Local excision followed by irradiation, however, serves to reduce the frequency of recurrence in the breast. Supportive historical reference is often made to the early works of Keynes with interstitial implants after local tumor excision (Keynes, 1932). Peters (1970) observed after a review at the Princess Margaret Hospital that the extent of resection appeared to have little influence on local tumor control or survival, provided it was accompanied by comprehensive irradiation.

The literature contains many reports of experience with breast conservation and reports of a number of randomized trials that differed in the selection of patients, the extent of resection, and the technique of irradiation (Table 17-23).

Prospective randomized trials of partial mastectomy first began at Guy's Hospital, London, in 1961. Patients with Manchester clinical Stage I or Stage II (T1 or T2, N0 or N1) cancers were randomized to treatment with either "extended tylectomy" (no assessment of margins histologically) or classic radical mastectomy. Both operations were followed by comprehensive irradiation to regional lymph nodes, and the residual breast of those treated with tylectomy was also irradiated. Patients received doses of irradiation not exceeding 2700 rad to the apex of the axilla or 3800 rad to the remaining breast, which are low by current standards. One hundred seven Stage I patients and 81 Stage II patients were treated and observed for up to 10 years. A significantly higher rate of local recurrence attended local excision in both Stage I and Stage II. Half of the local recurrences after local excision and irradiation occurred in the axilla or supraclavicular areas, but another quarter occurred in the parenchyma (7%) and skin (22%) of the breast. Although the survival of Stage I patients did not differ between the two treatments, the survival of Stage II patients treated with the simpler surgery was significantly shorter.

This study demonstrated that local and regional control of mammary carcinoma was poor if only low doses of radiation were used. Furthermore, poor local regional control in the presence of axillary adenopathy appeared to invite dissemination and death. Because Stage I survival had not suffered, the investigators continued with a second series of 252 Stage I (T1 to T3a, N0 to N1a) cases, and this time conservative treatment resulted not only in poor local control but also in poor survival (Hayward, 1983). The Guy's Hospital trials raised the real possibility that poor local and regional control contributed to ultimate treatment failure in both Stage I and Stage II cases.

In the first Milan trial, which followed in Italy between 1973 and 1980, high-dose irradiation was combined with removal of the entire quadrant of the breast containing the tumor. Seven hundred one patients with small (2.0 cm), localized tumors (TNM Stage I) were randomized between radical mastectomy (later switched to modified mastectomy) and quadrantectomy (no assessment of surgical margins) combined with full axillary dissection (Levels I to III) followed by 5000 rad of radiation to the breast and a 1000-

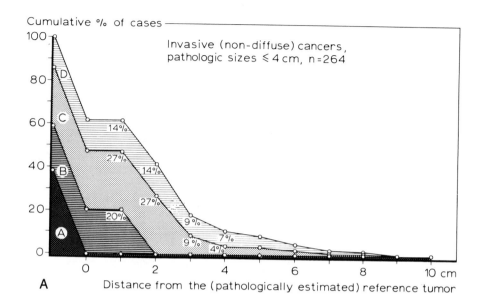

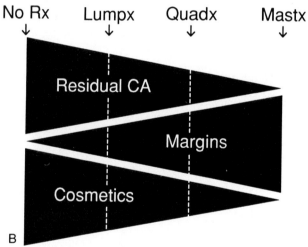

Figure 17–48. *A,* Graph showing the per cent of cases with in situ and invasive carcinoma at various distances from the margins of primary invasive cancers. The anticipated frequency of retained cancer after partial mastectomy decreases with increases in the width of surgical margins. Abbreviations: C = in situ cancer; D = invasive cancer 2.0 cm or more beyond the margin of the tumor. (From Holland, R., Veling, S. H. J., Mravunmac, M., et al.: Histologic multifocality of Tis, T1–2 breast carcinomas. Cancer, *56*:979–990, 1985.) *B,* The surgical dilemma associated with breast conserving treatment of mammary carcinoma is represented by this diagram that depicts the compromise between surgical margins, the likelihood of residual cancer, and surgically related cosmetic results. On the extreme left, no treatment other than biopsy involves minimal or no margins, maximum probability of residual cancer, and optimum cosmetic results. Lumpectomy (LUMPX) with narrow tumor-free margins leaves less residual cancer and little cosmetic compromise. Quadrantectomy (QUADX) provides greater margins and leaves minimal residual cancer but yields less favorable cosmetic results. On the extreme right, mastectomy (MASTX), which removes all breast tissue, provides the greatest margins around the tumor and leaves no residual cancer but is also cosmetically the least desirable. Irradiation of the breast appears to provide a fractional reduction in the frequency of breast recurrence from residual cancer.

Illustration continued on following page

Quadrantectomy versus Mastectomy, Milan I Study

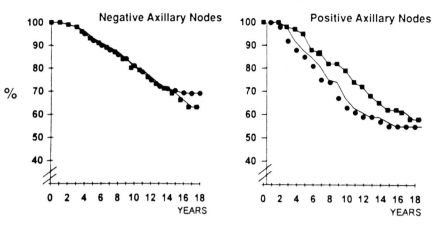

Overall survival in relation to lymph node status
■ = Quadrantectomy + axillary dissection + Rt
C   ● = Halsted mastectomy

Figure 17–48 *Continued C,* Eighteen-year actuarial survivals of women treated with quadrantectomy plus axillary dissection plus breast irradiation versus Halsted mastectomy, shown by axillary node status. Survivals were not significantly different between the two treatments. All patients had invasive carcinomas 2.0 cm or less in diameter. (From Veronesi, U., Luini, A., Galimberti, V., et al.: Conservation approaches for the management of Stage I/II carcinoma of the breast: Milan Cancer Institute trials. World J. Surg., *18*:70–75, 1994).

rad boost to the area of excision. This was called the QUART treatment (*QU*adrantectomy, *A*xillary dissection, and *R*adio-*T*herapy). Adjuvant therapy was inconsistent: initially, patients with axillary metastases were randomized for observation or to receive postoperative irradiation to internal mammary and supraclavicular nodes. After 1976, this was changed to cyclophosphamide, methotrexate, and 5-fluorouracil (CMF) systemic adjuvant chemotherapy (12 cycles) for all patients with pathologically involved axillary lymph nodes, about 26% of the total. It can be conjectured that in each of the two primary treatment groups, about 20 patients received nodal irradiation, 52 received adjuvant chemotherapy, and 278 received no adjuvant therapy. Survival and disease-free survival through 18 years have been statistically indistinguishable between the groups overall and when separated by axillary nodal status (Veronesi et al., 1994). The rate of recurrent or new tumor in the irradiated breast (6.5%) was low but twice as high as that of

Table 17–23. RANDOMIZED TRIALS OF BREAST CONSERVATION AND IRRADIATION VERSUS MASTECTOMY FOR STAGES I AND II INVASIVE BREAST CARCINOMA

Trial	No. of Cases	Tumor Size	Surgical Margins	RT Boost	Breast/Local Recurrence BCT (%)	Mast (%)	Survival BCT (%)	Mast (%)	FU (y)
Guy's*	370	Any	3 cm	No	44	14	60	70	10
Guy's (EORTC)†	399	≤4 cm	Narrow	Yes‡‡	7	7	91	92 AX+	5
							68	73 AX−	
NSABP B-06‡	1855	≤4 cm	Histologically clear	NO	10	8	77	70	8
Milan I§	701	≤2.0 cm	QUART	Yes	4.8	2.3	69	67	18
Milan II§	705	≤ 2.5 cm	QUART vs TART	Yes	5.3		88		7
				Yes	13.3		87		7
Milan III§	567	≤ 2.5 cm	QUART vs QUAD	Yes	0.3		97		3.5
					8.8		84		3.5
NCI‖	247	≤5	Grossly clear	Yes‡‡	12	1	85	79	9
EORTC¶	874	<5 cm	1 cm	Yes‡‡	15	10	60	64	8
Danish BCG**	859	Any	Grossly clear	Yes	3	4	79	82	3
Gustave-Roussy††	179	<2 cm	2 cm	Yes	7	9			10

*Atkins et al., 1972.
†Fentiman, 1990.
‡Fisher et al., 1989.
§Veronesi et al., 1986.
‖Lichter et al., 1992.
¶van Dongen et al., 1992.
**Blichert-Toft et al., 1992.
††Radford and Wells, 1993.
‡‡Interstitial irradiation boost.
Abbreviations: RT = radiation therapy; FU = follow-up; BCT = breast conservation combined with irradiation; Mast = mastectomy AX+ = Axillary Metastases present; AX − = Axillary Metastases Absent; EORTC = European Organization for Research in the Treatment of Cancer; NCI = National Cancer Institute; BCG = Breast Cancer Group; QUAD = quadrantectomy and axillary dissections without breast irradiation; QUART = quadrantectomy, axillary dissection, and breast irradiation; TART = tumorectomy, axillary dissection, and breast irradiation.

chest wall recurrence after mastectomy (2.3%). Primary tumors in the second breast were also slightly more numerous after QUART, but not statistically. Cosmetic results were good or better in 67% of patients treated with QUART.

Since removal of an entire quadrant of the breast and addition of high-dose irradiation did not always provide optimal cosmetic results (Berrino et al., 1987), two additional Milan trials sought to determine whether the extent of resection could be reduced or whether irradiation could be eliminated. The first (Milan II), conducted between 1985 and 1987, addressed slightly larger tumors (up to 2.5 cm in diameter) in 705 patients. Without changing the extent of axillary dissection or breast irradiation, this trial compared quadrantectomy of the breast (QUART) with "tumorectomy" (i.e., tumor removal with a 1.0-cm margin, designated the *TART approach* [*T*umorectomy, *A*xillary dissection, and *R*adio *T*herapy). Not surprisingly, surgical margins were more often involved with tumor in the TART group than in the QUART group (i.e., 16% of cases versus 3%, respectively). Survival at 4 years was identical in the two groups, and patients treated with tumorectomy had better cosmetic results; however, breast recurrence was threefold higher after tumorectomy (7.0%) than after quadrantectomy (2.2%) (Veronesi et al., 1990). In the second

study (Milan III), conducted between 1987 and 1989, quadrantectomy and axillary dissection were used with and without breast irradiation for tumors up to 2.5 cm in diameter in 567 randomized patients. After a short follow-up period, the rate of breast recurrences was substantially higher when irradiation was omitted (8.8% compared with 0.3%, respectively (Veronesi et al., 1993). The three Milan trials demonstrated that, when compared with quadrantectomy and irradiation, any attempt to reduce the extent of resection or to eliminate irradiation therapy is met with an increase in the rate of tumor recurrence in the breast.

The NSABP in the United States extended the lumpectomy approach to patients with Stage I and II tumors up to 4.0 cm in diameter in a randomized trial (Protocol B-06) conducted between 1976 and 1983, and the results further confirmed the need for irradiation if breasts were to be retained (Fisher et al., 1989). Two thousand one hundred sixty-three patients were randomized between modified radical mastectomy or lumpectomy (initially designated "segmental mastectomy") with or without breast irradiation (5000-cGy exposure with no boost). Surgical margins had to be free of tumor. All patients had at least a Level II axillary dissection, and those with nodal metastases received adjuvant chemotherapy (Fig. 17–49). After a mean follow-up period of 80 months, the 9-year survival, disease-

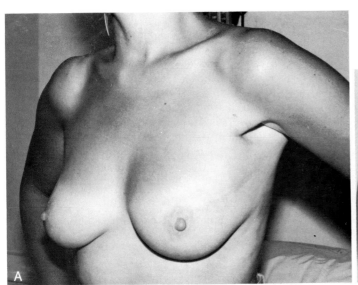

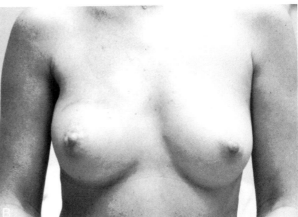

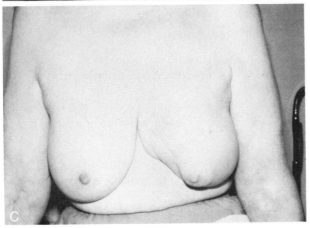

Figure 17–49. Cosmetic results of breast-conserving surgery. *A,* Appearance of a 34-year-old patient treated with breast-conserving lumpectomy, axillary dissection, and breast irradiation 3 years earlier. Patients with small tumors located at the periphery of the breast are likely to have the least disruption of symmetry. *B,* Frontal view of a patient after lumpectomy and irradiation for treatment of a small tumor of the upper outer quadrant of the right breast shows minimal alteration of contours. Also, the axillary scar is not visible. *C,* Removal of a large tumor from the medial side of the breast produced obvious contour deformity.

free survival, and distant disease-free survival did not differ among the three groups (Fisher et al., 1992). However, 88% of lumpectomy patients who received irradiation were free of recurrence in the breast compared with only 57% of those who received no irradiation. It can be estimated from these figures that irradiation of the breast was successful in preventing or delaying growth of occult residual cancer in 72% (31 out of 43) of the patients in whom it was present. Breast recurrences predominated at the site of lumpectomy, implying incomplete tumor removal despite the presence of tumor-free surgical margins. Three factors predisposed to recurrence in the breast: (1) absence of irradiation, (2) poor nuclear grade, and (3) a tumor size of 2.0 cm or greater. Adjuvant chemotherapy (used in node-positive patients) did not improve tumor control in the breast. When irradiation was not used, the rate of failure was equally high with and without chemotherapy. When irradiation was used, the addition of chemotherapy, however, did further reduce the rate of tumor recurrence in the breast. Recurrence in the breast was not considered a local failure, but recurrence in the breast after lumpectomy with irradiation was more frequent than recurrence on the chest wall after mastectomy, 8.1% versus 12.2% (Fisher et al., 1989).

In 1990, it was discovered that fraudulent data had been entered into the B-06 study by one institution, and in 1994 a reanalysis was performed by the EMMES Corporation (Potomac, MD), excluding 354 cases. This reduced the total number in the study to 1527: 492 cases in the total mastectomy (TM) arm, 520 in the lumpectomy (L) arm, and 515 in the lumpectomy plus breast irradiation (LRT) arm. It included a 10-year follow-up (Table 17–24). Cancer reappeared in the treated breast as a first event in 206 cases after lumpectomy alone (38.2% of cases) and in 64 cases after LRT (12.2% of cases), a highly significant difference. Essentially, irradiation reduced breast recurrences expected after lumpectomy alone by 68%. After lumpectomy alone, the rate of breast recurrence was swifter and greater if

Table 17–24. SITES OF RECURRENCE AFTER MASTECTOMY AND AFTER LUMPECTOMY WITH AND WITHOUT IRRADIATION—NSABP PROTOCOL B-06, 10-YEAR RESULTS (revised analysis without St. Luc cases)

	TM + AD	Lump + AD	Lump + AD + RT
Total no. of cases	492	520	515
Recurrences			
Breast (%)	—	38.2	12.2
Local (%)	10.2	7.3*	1.9*
Regional (%)	4.5	8.5	5.1
Distant (%)	23.4	28.9	28.9
Total (%)	39.0	46.0	37.3
Alive and well (%)	50.2	45.2	52.2

(From Stablein, D. M.: A reanalysis of NSABP Protocol B-06. Potomac, MD, The EMMES Corporation, March 30, 1994, pp. 1–22.)
*Secondary failures.
AD = Axillary dissection

axillary nodes contained metastases than if they did not (Fig. 17–50). Salvage mastectomies were performed in approximately one-third of cases with breast recurrence in each the L and LRT arms (i.e., 35.4% and 32.8%, respectively). Overall survival was not significantly different in the three treatment groups, nor was distant disease-free survival, but the lumpectomy group fared poorly in each respect. The lumpectomy group was significantly inferior to the LRT group with respect to disease-free survival (48% versus 56% at 10 years, P = .01) (Fig. 17–51). The basic conclusions were unchanged by the reanalysis and were essentially that LRT provided local tumor control and survival similar to that provided by modified radical mastectomy. The poor results of lumpectomy alone suggest, as did the Guy's Hospital trial, that poor initial local control of the cancer results in a reduced chance of cure.

NSABP B-06 (revised)

Distribution of Time to Ipsilateral Breast Recurrence, Eligible Patients Accepting Treatment Assignment

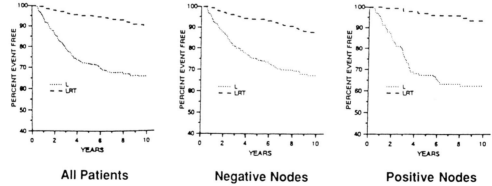

All Patients   **Negative Nodes**   **Positive Nodes**

L = Lumpectomy (520)
LRT = Lumpectomy + breast radiation (515)

Figure 17–50. Ten-year survival free of breast recurrence, overall and by node status, after treatment with lumpectomy and with lumpectomy combined with breast irradiation. Breast recurrence is reduced by 68% when lumpectomy is followed by breast irradiation. (Reproduced with permission from Stablein, D. M.: A reanalysis of NSABP Protocol B06. Potomac, MD, the EMMES Corporation, March 30, 1994, pp. 1–22.)

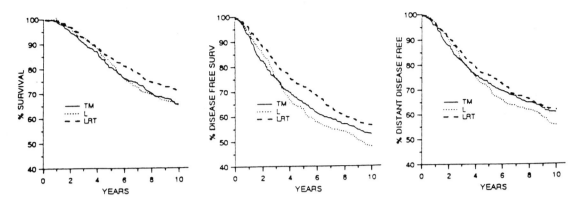

NSABP B-06 (revised)
Event Free Distributions for Eligible Patients Who Accepted Assigned Therapy

TM = Total Mastectomy (492)
L = Lumpectomy (520)
LRT = Lumpectomy + Radiation to Breast (515)

Figure 17–51. Ten-year results of NSABP Protocol B-06 comparing total mastectomy (TM) with lumpectomy (L) and with lumpectomy combined with breast irradiation (L + XRT). Survival, and distant disease-free survival do not differ between TM and TM and L + XRT. (From Stablein, D. M.: A reanalysis of NSABP Protocol B-06. Potomac, MD, The EMMES Corporation, March 30, 1994, pp. 1–22.)

The only other randomized trial comparing mastectomy and lumpectomy combined with irradiation conducted in the United States (237 patients with T1 and T2 tumors treated at the NCI) also revealed a higher local failure rate after lumpectomy and irradiation. Survival was comparable at 5 years, but recurrence in the breast was 12% at 5 years and projected to be 20% at 8 years. Ultimate local regional control, however, appeared similar in the two groups (Lichter et al., 1992).

From the experience to date, it is clear that local tumor resection leaves cancer in the breast in a substantial proportion of patients (inversely related to the width of surgical margins) and that pathologically uninvolved surgical margins are not a guarantee that local extensions of tumor have been encompassed (Carter, 1986). It is also plain that local resection with high-dose breast irradiation results in survival that is comparable to that after mastectomy. Irradiation of the breast does not influence survival; it only serves to reduce recurrence in the breast. In this capacity, it is partly successful; the reduction in recurrence is an estimated 67% to 75% when compared with recurrence rates for patients treated without irradiation. Whether breast recurrence due to locally uncontrolled cancer compromises the chances for cure is unresolved, but some studies suggest that high frequencies do so. It is not as portentous as chest wall recurrence after mastectomy, but the two situations are not comparable. The latter likely reflects the presence of a tumor that was initially more extensive. Patients with breast recurrence fare surprisingly well after salvage mastectomy, having 5-year survivals that exceed 50% (Kurtz et al., 1988; and Osborne et al., 1992) but survivals are inferior to those of patients who remain well, particularly if recurrence occurs early (Clark, 1983; Haffty et al., 1989; and Stotter et al., 1990). Fisher and coworkers (1991) determined that breast recurrence was associated with a three- to fourfold

risk of distant dissemination but considered it a sign of dissemination rather than its cause. The possibility remains, however, that recurrence in the breast is not a trivial event and that it possibly provides some cancers with a second chance to disseminate.

The potential morbidity of lumpectomy and irradiation should be appreciated by both patient and physician. The risk of lymphedema is no less than that expected after mastectomy when a similar axillary dissection is performed (Lichter et al., 1992). The surgical procedure on the breast may result in less than the desired cosmetic result, particularly if the tumor is large. Irradiation therapy requires 5 to 6 weeks of daily visits to complete and is expensive. Mild fatigue is the most frequent side effect. Temporary inflammation of the breast and fibrosis of a portion of the lung are expected and may be attended by a temporary cough (Lipsztein et al., 1985). Breast edema and progressive shrinkage of the breast after irradiation are frequent and obvious side effects (Clarke et al., 1982) (Fig. 17–52*A* and *B*). Less frequent complications include excessive fibrosis of the breast, irradiation pneumonitis, rib fractures, fat necrosis, and pleural effusion (Clark et al., 1983; Prosnitz et al., 1983; and Kisner, 1992). Harris and Hellman (1983) reported mild to severe radiation complications in 14% of patients. Lichter and colleagues (1992) reported postoperative wound infections in 10% to 15% of patients and rib fractures after irradiation in 8%. Inferior cosmetic results may follow concurrent use of chemotherapy and irradiation (Wazer et al., 1992). Irradiation-induced secondary neoplasias (including leukemia and sarcomas) in the field of irradiation are a potential long-term hazard. Some case reports describe the development of angiosarcomas of the irradiated breast (Curtis et al., 1992; Edeiken et al., 1992; and Stokkel and Petersen, 1992). The frequency of radiation-induced cancers is estimated at 1.5% based on past experi-

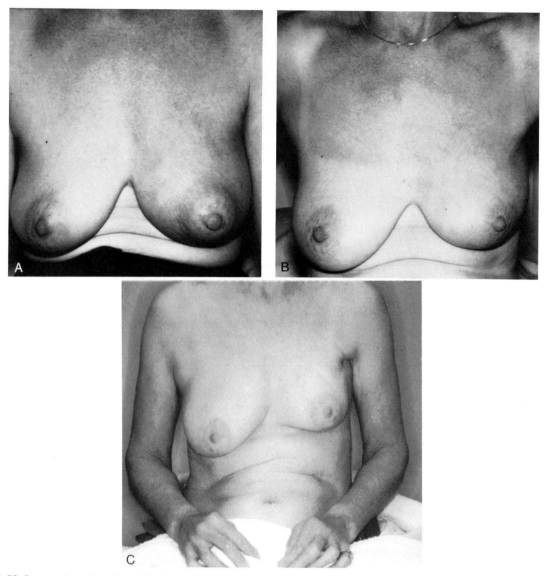

Figure 17–52. Progressive retraction of the breast is a frequent sequel of irradiation. *A,* The appearance of the left breast shortly following segmental mastectomy and irradiation. Mild edema is present, but the size approximates that of the right breast. *B,* The appearance 2.5 years later; there has been obvious shrinkage of the treated breast. *C,* This patient with scleroderma demonstrates marked fibrosis and retraction of the left breast after irradiation. Patients with collagen-vascular diseases are poor candidates for breast conservation because of this problem. This patient's scleroderma developed shortly after treatment.

ence with irradiation of the chest wall after mastectomy (Ferguson et al., 1982). With irradiation of one breast, the opposite breast is exposed to 200 to 2000 cGy of radiation during the course of treatment. Montague (1984) and Veronesi and associates (1994) found no evidence for an increased risk of cancer in the second breast, but Boice and colleagues (1992) reported an elevated risk (relative risk of 1.59) among patients younger than 45 years of age. Although breast preservation is the objective, it is not always achieved. Recurrence in the breast usually requires "salvage" mastectomy, although further local resection is sometimes used (Kurtz et al., 1988a and b; and Veronesi et al., 1990). Mastectomy is occasionally made necessary by the morbid effects of irradiation rather than by recurrence (Durand and Pilleron, 1977).

The time, cost, and potential morbidity of irradiation raise the question of whether it could be omitted in selected cases without the risk of excessive breast recurrence. The issue is unsettled. Some solitary tumors no larger than 2.0 cm in diameter are excised without irradiation at the Cleveland Clinic (Hermann et al., 1993). Researchers in the Uppsala-Orebro Breast Cancer Study Group suggested that irradiation represented overtreatment for 90% of their patients with small tumors. They reported breast recurrences 3 years after "sector resection" in 7.6% of patients with unifocal Stage I tumors (compared with 2.9% in irradiated patients) and speculated that omission of irradiation would require only a few additional salvage procedures. Nemoto and associates (1991) speculated that patients with small tumors and elderly patients might not need irradiation;

however, the number of such patients that they studied was small, and long-term follow-up was not conducted. After a median period of 4 years' duration, no local recurrences were observed among 20 patients with tumors smaller than 1.0 cm in diameter and only 1 among 31 women older than 70 years of age. On the other hand, large trials with longer follow-up periods provide no clues to selection. Small tumor size did not prevent substantial recurrences of breast tumors in the NSABP trial of lumpectomy (Protocol B-06). Twenty-five per cent of unirradiated patients with tumor diameters less than 1.0 cm had breast recurrence at 8 years compared with only 10% of irradiated patients (Fisher et al., 1992a). In a trial of lumpectomy and axillary dissection at the Princess Margaret Hospital (Toronto, Canada), 837 patients were randomized to receive postoperative breast irradiation or no irradiation (Clark et al., 1992). After a median follow-up of 43 months, breast recurrences were diagnosed in 5.5% and 25.7% of patients, respectively. No low-risk group (i.e., one with patients who have less than a 5% chance of relapse in the breast) could be identified among patients who were not irradiated.

Clinical and pathologic discriminants for increased recurrence in the breast are numerous. Failure to irradiate is the most important. Others pertain to recurrence in the irradiated breast. These are not contraindications to breast conservation but may decrease its chances for success. They include:

1. Large tumor size (i.e., larger than 2.0 cm in diameter [Fisher et al., 1992a])

2. Presence of residual gross tumor (Harris et al., 1981)

3. Presence of surgical margins involved with tumor in irradiated (Anscher et al., 1993) or unirradiated patients (Lagios et al., 1993)

4. Presence of narrow surgical margins (Ghossein et al., 1992)

5. Poor histologic differentiation (Fisher et al., 1992a; and Clark et al., 1992)

6. An extensive intraductal component (EIC) (i.e., 25% or more of the tumor is composed of DCIS both within and at the periphery [Eberlein et al., 1990; Vicini et al., 1991; and Veronesi et al., 1993])

7. Presence of multiple macroscopic primary tumors (Leopold et al., 1989; Kurtz et al., 1990; and Wilson et al., 1993)

8. Inordinate delay of irradiation (e.g., longer than 16 weeks [Recht et al., 1991])

9. Young age (less than 40 years), apparently owing to a correlation with poor histologic grade and excessive intraductal component (Kurtz et al., 1990)

10. Invasive lobular histology. Breast recurrences are reported in 11% of patients within 29 months (Martin et al., 1989) and in 13.5% at 5 years (Kurtz et al., 1989). These patients have a more diffuse distribution of cancer. However, higher rates of breast recurrence based on histologic type were not confirmed by Weiss and coworkers (1992).

Not all patients with Stage I or II breast cancer are candidates for breast conservation. Candidates should meet the following criteria:

1. Have a tumor that can be excised with tumor-free surgical margins and not produce a cosmetically unaccept-able breast. Randomized trials have included patients with tumors of up to 5.0 cm in diameter, but much depends on the ratio of breast size to tumor size. Bonadonna and associates (1990) proposed that more patients might be candidates for breast conservation if their tumors were reduced with preoperative chemotherapy.

2. Have a solitary cancer that can be removed with no clinical or mammographic evidence of residual cancer

3. Have no contraindications to irradiation

4. Be motivated for breast conservation

Unsuitable candidates are patients who

1. Have multiple macroscopic cancers

2. Have a large tumor in a small breast, the excision of which makes a cosmetic result superior to mastectomy and reconstruction unlikely

3. Have diffuse, suspicious microcalcifications on mammography

4. Have collagen vascular disease (e.g., scleroderma, rheumatoid arthritis, or lupus erythematosis), in which case a severe reaction to irradiation can be expected (Robertson et al., 1991) (see Fig. 17–52C)

5. Are pregnant, unless the patient is near enough to the time of delivery (third trimester) that irradiation can begin after delivery without entailing a significant delay

6. Have a centrally located tumor for which removal of the nipple is required if a tumor-free margin is to be obtained. Patients with Paget's disease and underlying cancer are in this category. Removal of the nipple and depression of the central region of the breast detract greatly from the cosmetic result, but not all physicians consider this to be a contraindication, particularly if the breast is large and the nipple can be reconstructed (Radford and Wells, 1993; and Williams and Murr, 1993)

7. Have no access to radiation facilities, are unlikely to complete a course of irradiation, are not able to undergo irradiation, or refuse to undergo irradiation therapy

In a number of special circumstances, patients can be managed with breast conservation provided that the usual criteria are satisfied. The presence of bilateral cancers is not a contraindication. Such a patient can be effectively treated, but the technical aspects of irradiating both breasts are more challenging. Precedent is also established for using breast conservation to treat patients with occult carcinoma of the breast that presents as axillary metastases (Kemeny et al., 1986; and Merson et al., 1992). In defense of this practice are the following: no cancer is found in the breasts of many of these patients, irradiation is appropriate for the treatment of subclinical disease, and survival after breast-conserving surgery is similar to that after mastectomy. The presence of breast implants is also not a contraindication to breast conservation, as is discussed in the following section.

Breast Conservation in Patients with Breast Implants

Observations vary about whether women who have breast implants for augmentation present with more advanced cancers than do others who do not have such implants (Silverstein et al., 1988; and Birdsell et al., 1993). However, when otherwise eligible, patients with silicone breast implants have not been excluded from treatment with breast conservation. The principles of complete tumor excision, axillary dissection, and whole-breast irradiation are followed, but experience in the treatment of such patients is scant, follow-up is short, and the ultimate results uncertain. At this point, evaluation is largely confined to assessment of cosmetic results. Investigations show no significant difference in photon or electron dose distribution when a silicone prosthesis and a tissue-equivalent water phantom are irradiated; furthermore, no appreciable effect on the physical properties of prostheses is observed. Thus, standard irradiation techniques and doses can be used in patients with breast prostheses. Most reports include a variety of clinical situations (e.g., irradiation for local recurrence after breast reconstruction, postoperative irradiation after mastectomy and immediate reconstruction, and irradiation for cancers that arise after prophylactic subcutaneous mastectomy in patients with implants or previously augmented breasts) (Halpern et al., 1990; Ryu et al., 1990; and Chu et al., 1992). The complication most often reported is an unsatisfactory cosmetic result due to capsular contracture around the implant, which causes it to become rounded, firm, and retracted upward. Capsular contracture is more frequent (1) if it was noticeable beforehand, (2) in patients receiving high doses of radiation, and (3) in patients with subcutaneous rather than with subpectoral implants. Chu and associates reported good to excellent cosmetic results in 93% of 27 patients after irradiation; Ryu and coworkers noted the same for 67% of 9 patients with at least 2 years of follow-up. Handel and colleagues (1991), however, found results that were less satisfactory in 15 women with previous augmentation. Ten (67%) developed severe capsular contracture within 2 to 40 weeks after completion of irradiation. In four, the symptoms were sufficient to require surgical revision with capsulectomy. This group suggested that women

Survival-Modified Radical Mastectomy vs Lumpectomy by Axillary Node Status (MCW)

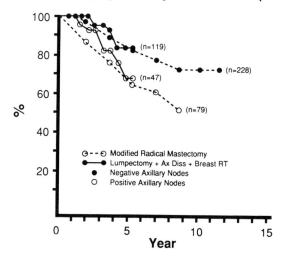

Figure 17–54. Actuarial survivals of patients treated for invasive breast carcinoma at MCW with breast conservation and with modified radical mastectomy, by axillary node status. The 5-year survivals of patients with and without axillary metastases are similar after the two treatments.

with breast augmentation were less than ideal candidates for breast conservation. The author excludes from breast conservation those patients whose tumor reaches the capsule of the implant.

Experience with breast-conserving treatment may vary at different institutions. The author reviewed cases of invasive breast carcinoma treated with partial mastectomy at the MCW and identified 166 cases whose treatment combined wide tumor excision with axillary lymph node dissection and irradiation of the breast. Only 28% had axillary metastases. The overall survival of these selected cases is comparable with that of patients treated with radical mastectomy and with modified radical mastectomy at this institution (Fig. 17–53). The survival of patients with involved and uninvolved axillary nodes is also comparable with that of patients treated with modified radical mastectomy (Fig. 17–54). Four of the patients treated with breast conservation had a recurrence confined to the breast, for a 5-year actuarial breast recurrence rate of 5.5%, which is approximately that reported by others. The recurrences were diagnosed between 1.5 and 2.5 years after treatment was initiated.

Summary

The two principal treatments for Stage I and II breast cancer are (1) total mastectomy with axillary dissection (modified radical mastectomy) and (2) lumpectomy, axillary dissection, and breast irradiation (breast conservation). Many patients are eligible for either treatment and do have a choice. The choice is essentially between experiencing the psychologic and social morbidity due to loss of a breast or enduring the physical and biologic morbidity of treatment with

Survival-Modified Radical Mastectomy vs Radical Mastectomy vs Lumpectomy + AD + RT (MCW)

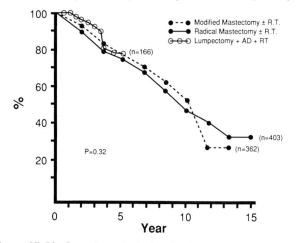

Figure 17–53. Overall survival of patients with invasive breast carcinoma treated at the MCW with breast conservation (partial mastectomy plus axillary node dissection plus breast irradiation), modified radical mastectomy, and radical mastectomy. Survival was comparable among all three treatments.

irradiation. Neither choice is appealing, simple, free of complications, or guaranteed to cure. In 1991, the NCI recommended breast-conserving treatment for women with early breast cancer because survival after such treatment was equivalent to that after mastectomy and because its cosmetic results were superior to those of mastectomy. Cosmetic results are judged to be good to excellent in most cases. In 1990, 25% of operations for breast cancer were partial mastectomies (Osteen et al., 1994). As of 1994, probably one-third of women with Stage I and II breast cancers in the United States receive breast-conserving therapy. Use has gradually increased but shows wide geographic variation. A survey of SEER areas indicated that from 19.6% to 41.5% of women with localized cancers were so treated, with use favoring those younger than 65 and older than 74 years of age (Farrow et al., 1992). Nattinger and coworkers (1992) reviewed Medicare records and found that 12.1% of women older than 65 years of age were treated with breast conservation. Utilization was highest on the east and west coasts of the United States. Elderly patients are less likely than younger ones to undergo irradiation (Lazovich et al., 1991). It is uncertain to what degree patterns of use reflect patient preference, physician bias, economic factors and unsuitable clinical presentations (Tarbox et al., 1992). According to some reports, one-half of patients who are offered breast-conserving treatment do choose it (Wolberg, 1991). Inconvenience and fear of radiotherapy are predominant among the reasons for not choosing such treatment (Tate et al., 1993). With respect to quality of life, psychologic studies have indicated that patients treated with breast conservation have fewer disturbances of their sexual activity and less trouble with clothing and body image problems than do mastectomy patients; however, they require more support to cope with irradiation and enjoy no greater satisfaction with life than do mastectomy patients, provided that both groups of patients had a choice of treatment (Ganz et al., 1992; and Pozo et al., 1992).

LOCALLY AND REGIONALLY ADVANCED CANCERS (TNM STAGE III)

Stage III is a broad spectrum both clinically and prognostically and includes from 10% to 15% of patients seen in most medical centers. The diverse presentation and relative infrequency of Stage III tumors make randomized trials of treatment difficult to accomplish. Most information on Stage III cancers is from pilot studies and studies without controls.

From the practical standpoint, Stage IIIA tumors are technically suitable for mastectomy and, for the most part, can be managed surgically in the same manner as are Stage II cases. Stage IIIB tumors, with some exceptions, are technically inoperable (i.e., the disease cannot be removed from the breast and axilla with tumor-free margins, and surgery is not an initial option). By definition, Stage III excludes patients with demonstrable distant (or supraclavicular) metastases, but the majority of these patients do have occult distant metastases at the outset and require a combination of aggressive local-regional therapy and systemic therapy. The optimal management remains uncertain. As the extent of disease in Stage III patients routinely requires multimodal therapy, questions focus less on the need for radiotherapy, surgery, and chemohormonal therapy than on the intensity of each and their sequence.

The 5-year survival of patients with Stage III tumors ranges from 40% to 65%, depending on the particular presentation (Frank et al., 1992). At MCW, the overall 5-year disease-free survival of 123 cases was 40%, and at 10 years it was 20% (Fig. 17–55). Sheldon and colleagues (1987) reported actuarial survivals of 41% and 23% for 192 cases at 5 and 10 years, respectively, treated at the Joint Center for Radiation Therapy in Boston. The 5-year survival of 118 patients at the Medical College of Virginia was 54% (34% for disease-free survival), and for 41 patients at Parkland Hospital in Dallas it was 46% (Hobar et al., 1988; and Frank et al., 1992).

With respect to prognostic factors, our experience confirms that patients with Stage IIIA disease fare better than do those with Stage IIIB disease and that women with inflammatory cancers have a prognosis that is worse than either of these. The prognosis for operable cases at the MCW was influenced by the number of axillary metastases (Fig. 17–56). Patients with axillary nodes negative for cancer had a 5-year disease-free survival of 65%, and this rate was only slightly lower at 10 years. The favorable survival of node-negative Stage III cases was also observed by Francchia and coworkers (1980), who reported survivals of 82% at 5 years and 75% at 10 years. The presence or absence of grave local signs, as defined by Haagensen, did not influence the survival of node-negative patients. A benefit of initial surgical treatment of operable cases is identification of this favorable group. In addition to substage and extent of axillary node involvement, Frank and associates (1992) found that patients with a tumor greater than 9.0 cm in diameter had poorer survival than did patients with smaller tumors. Estrogen receptor status had no prognostic value, a finding that confirms earlier reports (Ragaz, 1988).

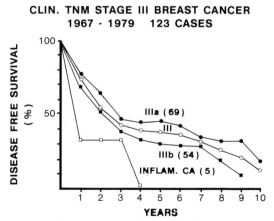

Figure 17–55. Disease-free survival of locally or regionally advanced (Stage III) noninflammatory breast cancers treated at MCW. Stage IIIA tumors, so-called "operable" cases, have a better prognosis than Stage IIIB lesions.

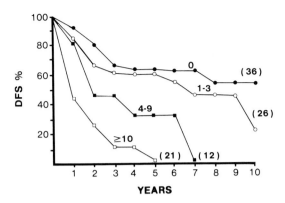

Figure 17–56. The number of involved axillary lymph nodes influences disease-free survival of surgically treated Stage III breast cancer. Despite the advanced clinical stage, patients without axillary metastases are a favorable group, with a 5-year survival of 65%. (Patients treated at the MCW.)

Local-Regional Treatment

Retrospective reviews of multimodality treatment with surgery and irradiation for Stage III tumors have suffered from selection bias and lack of uniform follow-up. Patients for whom mastectomy was selected as initial treatment likely had less local advancement, whereas patients with unresectable tumors were treated initially with irradiation. When irradiation was used initially, patients who subsequently had mastectomy were selected because of their good response to irradiation and failure to develop dissemination.

Reports suggest that irradiation is most effective for patients who do not have gross disease. Rao and coworkers (1982) reported that the local failure rate and the 5-year disease-free survival of patients with Stage III cancers treated with irradiation were influenced by the size of the primary tumor and by the nodal status. Patients with tumors larger than 8.0 cm had a local failure rate of 76%, and those with gross adenopathy had a regional failure rate of 58%. No influence of tumor size or nodal involvement was noted

in patients who received a combination of radiation therapy and mastectomy. Intensive irradiation can produce high levels of local-regional tumor control, but not without morbidity. Management of almost 200 patients with Stage III cancers with irradiation and chemotherapy without mastectomy resulted in local-regional control in 73% of cases at 5 years (actuarial) and in 68% at 10 years (Sheldon et al., 1987). Doses in excess of 6000 cGy were more effective than smaller doses, but significant complications, including severe arm edema and brachial plexopathy, were documented in 8% of patients in the series.

Bedwinek and colleagues (1982) found a marked improvement in local control when mastectomy was used in combination with irradiation, but this analysis was not free of selection bias. Fletcher and coworkers (1980) emphasized the importance of surgically removing gross tumor when possible to improve the results with local-regional irradiation, reporting a local-regional failure rate of only 15% in Stage III patients, excluding those with inflammatory cancer (Fig. 17–57). Survival, however, is not improved by the combination of surgery and irradiation. Arnold and Lesnick (1979) reported the results of radical mastectomy in 229 patients with Stage III breast cancers and found actuarial survival rates of 33% at 5 years and 22% at 10 years. Treatment with preoperative or postoperative irradiation did not lead to survival superior to that of mastectomy alone. Ninety per cent of the patients had recurrence (predominantly systemic) within 10 years, and the results were similar whether irradiation was given preoperatively or postoperatively.

In an analysis of 108 consecutive patients with Stage III breast cancer, Balawajder and colleagues (1983) found that radiation followed by mastectomy improved 5-year local control (80%) but did not alter the probability of remaining free from metastatic disease. Minimum tumor doses of 6000 rad were recommended.

Townsend and coworkers (1985) sought to reduce local recurrence in locally-regionally advanced cases with a combination of initial radiation followed by total mastectomy. Radiation consisted of 4500 to 5000 rad to the breast, chest

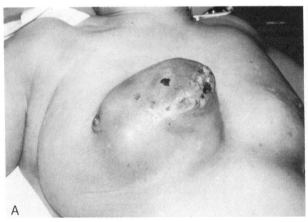
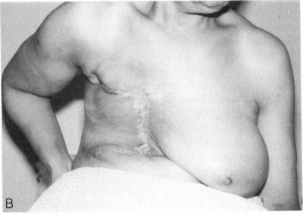

Figure 17–57. *A,* Large Stage III carcinoma of the right breast with ulceration and hemorrhage treated with modified radical mastectomy. *B,* The wound was closed with a rotation skin flap based laterally. Subsequent treatment was with systemic chemotherapy and irradiation of the chest and regional nodes. If tumor-free margins can be obtained, an initial operation that eliminates gross disease can facilitate irradiation and chemotherapy.

wall, and regional lymph nodes over 5 weeks. Fifty-three patients were so treated and followed from 3 to 134 months. Twenty-two patients (41%) developed wound complications. Recurrences were seen in 6 of the 53 patients (11%). Although a significant reduction appeared to occur in local recurrences, there was rapid development of distant dissemination.

Evidence is reasonably good that the combination of resection and irradiation can improve local-regional control in selected cases and can be applied without causing undue morbidity (Duggan, 1991). The sequence of the two modalities is probably not critical unless operability is a factor. Since the objective of an operation must be the clean removal of gross tumor, surgical opportunity is determined either by primary operability or by conversion to operability by initial irradiation or chemotherapy. Careful surgical technique is necessary to minimize postoperative complications in heavily pretreated patients. Sauter and associates (1993) reported complications in 65% of mastectomies that followed chemotherapy and irradiation. Wound infections and delayed wound healing were the most frequent complications.

Systemic Therapy

In one of the first prospective trials of systemic chemotherapy, DeLena and colleagues (1978) demonstrated that the addition of systemic chemotherapy with doxorubicin hydrochloride (Adriamycin) and vincristine both before and after irradiation improved relapse-free survival and total survival of Stage III patients compared with historical controls. Still, local treatment failure was observed in 37.5% of the patients. This led to a randomized study of patients with Stage III tumors in which local irradiation and mastectomy were found equally efficacious in producing local control in operable cases if preceded by systemic chemotherapy (DeLena et al., 1981). In this study, 132 women with operable Stage III carcinomas (not inflammatory) received three cycles of doxorubicin hydrochloride combined with vincristine and then were randomized for (1) radical (or modified) mastectomy or (2) radiation therapy to the breast and regional nodes (6000 rad over 6 weeks). Local treatment was followed by continued chemotherapy to a cumulative dose of 500 mg/m^2 of doxorubicin hydrochloride. In excess of 79% of patients responded to initial chemotherapy. There was no significant difference between the two treatment groups in terms of patterns of treatment failure, median duration of response, and total survival. Local-regional control was achieved in 50% of both groups at 3 years after treatment ended, and survival was a similar 51.7% and 49.1% at 4 years. The study did not address whether the combination of surgery and irradiation would improve local control. Perloff and associates (1988) reported a similar trial in which 87 patients with Stage III tumors rendered operable with combination chemotherapy (cyclophosphamide, doxorubicin hydrochloride, fluorouracil, vincristine, and prednisone [CAFVP]) were randomized to either modified radical mastectomy or to irradiation to the breast and regional nodes. Chemotherapy was continued afterward. Con-

trol of local disease and survival were similar in the two groups.

Shanta and coworkers (1985) treated 521 patients with Stage III breast cancer who were unsuitable for initial surgery. Most of the patients treated earlier had preoperative irradiation followed by radical mastectomy, whereas 109 patients treated between 1976 and 1978 received preoperative concomitant chemotherapy and irradiation and then a modified mastectomy. Tumors became resectable in 68% and 77% of the two groups. All premenopausal patients had a bilateral oophorectomy. Chemotherapy included methotrexate, fluorouracil, and Endoxan. Five-year survival without disease was 45% in the earlier group, in contrast to 64.6% in the group that received systemic chemotherapy. The authors concluded that preoperative chemotherapy added to irradiation distinctly improved the survival of these patients, but the effect was almost entirely in the cases with positive nodes. Hery and colleagues in France (1986) also used induction chemotherapy with three cycles of cyclophosphamide, doxorubicin hydrochloride, fluorouracil, and vincristine (CAFV) followed by local-regional irradiation and then maintenance chemotherapy to treat 25 patients. Response rates of 50% or more were observed in 86% of breast lesions and in 80% of adenopathies. Local recurrences occurred in 24% of the patients, and the survival rate at 4 years was a favorable 55%.

Hortobagyi and coworkers (1983) reported a high rate of complete remission in Stage III cases managed with initial systemic therapy with 5-fluorouracil, doxorubicin hydrochloride, and cyclophosphamide (FAC) in addition to bacille Calmette-Guérin (BCG). This was followed by simple mastectomy or radiotherapy, or a combination of the two, and then by continued chemotherapy. Ninety-four per cent of patients were rendered disease-free, but treatment compliance was poor, and only 32 of 52 patients (62%) completed the full 2 years of treatment. After a median follow-up of 60 months, local recurrences were observed in 21% of patients, and 55% of patients were alive at 5 years.

Aisner and associates (1982) treated 27 patients with inoperable bulky primary tumors initially with three to four courses of chemotherapy (CAF with and without vincristine and prednisone). Seventy-four per cent of patients responded with tumor reduction; 4% had a complete response. Thirty-six per cent of the patients had local recurrence, and after 3 years, 42% of patients with noninflammatory Stage IIIB tumors were alive, approximately that which is generally expected.

Papaioannou and associates (1983) conducted a trial of initial systemic combination chemoendocrine therapy followed by mastectomy with complete axillary dissection and then randomized the patients in the trial to local-regional irradiation followed by 10 additional cycles of chemotherapy and antiestrogen therapy. They encountered numerous complications of chemotherapy, including one death, and reported that local disease control was not enhanced by the addition of irradiation.

Loprinzi and coworkers (1984) reported a pilot study using initial surgery to remove gross disease followed by radiation and non–cross-resistant alternating chemotherapy regimens. Patients had Stages IIIA and IIIB tumors and inflammatory carcinomas. Thirty-two women were treated with initial surgery followed by two courses of induction chemotherapy with CMF ± prednisone ± tamoxifen. Local-regional radiotherapy followed and then randomization to maintenance chemotherapy with the earlier regimen, alternating with doxorubicin hydrochloride or vincristine ± tamoxifen. After a follow-up of 19 to 70 months, the 3-year survival was 65%; median disease-free survival was 29.5 months. Cardiotoxicity was seen in 25% of the patients, and this high frequency was thought to be attributable to the combination of doxorubicin hydrochloride and radiotherapy.

Inflammatory Carcinoma

Inflammatory carcinoma is considered separately among Stage III cancers because of its distinctive presentation and the special challenge it presents to effective treatment; it is staged according to extent but is given special notice in the TNM staging system.

Dermal lymphatic invasion is the pathologic hallmark of inflammatory carcinoma. Clinicians, however, still accept the classic clinical signs of diffuse redness, edema, heat, and general enlargement and induration of the breast as satisfying the diagnosis. Inflammatory carcinoma is found in TNM Stages IIIB and IV and may be of varied histologic type. Emphasis on involvement of dermal lymphatics created some confusion about defining the entity, as cases can be found in which such involvement is present without typical clinical signs, in which it is present with clinical signs, and in which it is not found when the clinical signs are present. Ellis and Teitelbaum (1974) could document no instance of dermal lymphatic invasion in eight patients with inflammatory carcinoma who had lived for 5 years after mastectomy and emphasized the key importance of this finding. However, Lucas and Perez-Mesa (1978) found that prognosis was poor in all three circumstances, although perhaps slightly less so when clinical signs were absent (Fig. 17–58). In the presence of typical clinical signs, the presence or absence of dermal lymphatic invasion appears to have no influence on prognosis. The more reliable histologic feature of inflammatory carcinoma is the regular presence of extensive lymphatic involvement within the breast, which may or may not have reached the dermis (Gallager, 1984).

The results with mastectomy for inflammatory carcinoma are so poor that it has been considered inoperable since the early decades of this century (Lee and Tannenbaum, 1925). Haagensen (1971) reported that none of 20 patients treated with radical mastectomy were cured, and 50% had recurrence on the chest wall. As a consequence, irradiation became the preferred treatment even though it still had little success in permanent control. The work of Chu and associates (1980) is representative, in which a 6% 10-year disease-free survival followed irradiation and 69% of patients had chest wall recurrence. The combination of mastectomy and irradiation achieved minimal improvement (Bozzetti et al., 1981).

Typical results prior to 1965 are seen in the author's experience at EFSCH. Fifty-one patients with this diagnosis

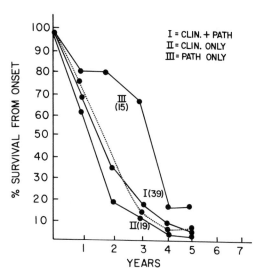

Figure 17–58. The survival of patients with typical clinical signs of inflammatory carcinoma (CLIN) is equally poor whether or not dermal lymphatic invasion can be demonstrated histologically (PATH). Patients with dermal lymphatic invasion but without a characteristic clinical picture have a prognosis that is slightly more favorable. (From Lucas, F. V., and Perez-Mesa, M.: Inflammatory carcinoma of the breast. Cancer, *41*:1595, 1978. Reprinted with permission.)

were seen. They represented approximately 2% of all patients with mammary carcinomas, a proportion generally reported in the literature. All were women with ages ranging from 33 to 86 years; the average age (57 years) was slightly lower than the mean age of patients with noninflammatory cancers (61 years). In no instance was pregnancy associated. The condition was bilateral and simultaneous in two patients (4%). Unilateral disease was marginally more frequent in the right breast (27 cases) than in the left (22 cases), although the eventual involvement of both breasts was not uncommon. Barber and coworkers (1961) reported that 18.9% of cases at the Mayo Clinic eventually involved both breasts.

Patients endured their symptoms for a median period of 3 months before seeking medical attention. Physical findings included characteristic signs of inflammation: 31% of the patients had increased heat, 88% had edema, 84% had erythema, and 75% reported swelling of the breast. Twenty-four per cent demonstrated all of the foregoing, and 53% reported pain in the breast. Forty-two (82%) had axillary adenopathy, and 42% had enlarged supraclavicular lymph nodes. Five patients had been treated with antibiotics for presumed inflammation, and one was treated with excision and drainage for a suspected abscess. Admission white blood cell counts varied from 3900 cells/cm³ to a high of 12,300 cells/cm³. Dermal lymphatic invasion was demonstrated in 64% of the 22 patients who had biopsies of the skin. All had histologic diagnoses except three, who were untreated and who died of clinical cancer within 4 to 7 months. In one case, the primary tumor was a medullary carcinoma. One patient had Paget's disease of the nipple.

Seven patients received no treatment during the entire course of the disease. These individuals survived a median duration of 6.5 months (durations ranged from 4 to 36 months). Two long-term survivors (33 and 36 months) raised the mean survival to 14.3 months. All forms of treatment, both local and systemic, were associated with median survivals (13.5 to 41.5 months) superior to those with no treatment, but with mean survivals only increased by 6 months. The patients who had preoperative radiotherapy followed by radical mastectomy enjoyed an interval from their first sign of disease until death that was no longer than that of those treated with radiotherapy alone, and it was not possible to determine whether the combination provided more permanent local control of cancer than irradiation. One patient treated solely with irradiation was the only 5-year survivor. Systemic therapy with hormones, endocrine ablation, or single-drug chemotherapy did not result in a longer mean clinical course (19.6 months) than did local treatment alone (19.8 months).

Current strategy is a multimodality approach that includes intensive multiagent systemic chemotherapy combined with local-regional irradiation and, in selected cases, mastectomy. The success of initial chemotherapy in producing tumor reduction has reawakened interest in adding mastectomy to irradiation or in using it as the sole local treatment (Wiseman et al., 1982; Morris, 1983; and Israel et al., 1986). Chemotherapy is begun initially and continued after local treatment is completed. Typically it consists of customary regimens of CAF, CMF, CFP, FAC, or CAFVP. Some reduction in tumor mass is achieved in more than 90% of cases, with complete responses ranging from 20% to 72%. After one to three cycles, or after optimum regression, irradiation is begun. If tumor regression is particularly marked, mastectomy may replace or precede irradiation, but in any case, it is reserved for patients with tumors clearly rendered operable. The results achieved with various combinations of multimodality therapy are shown in Table 17–25. Projected survivals are noticeably improved over those that have followed local therapy alone, and local control is also possibly more effective.

This author reviewed 25 cases of inflammatory breast cancer treated since 1967 at MCW (Donegan and Padrta, 1990). Patient ages ranged from 27 to 80 years with a median of 46 years; 30% of the patients were younger than 40 years old. One had bilateral involvement at the time of diagnosis. The median duration of symptoms was 6 weeks, and 20% were treated with antibiotics before diagnosis. The axilla was clinically involved in 75% of cases, and five of the patients already had metastases in bones, lung, or liver. Dermal lymphatic invasion was found in 60 per cent of skin biopsies. Estrogen receptors were measured in 13 cases and were positive in only 4 (33%). Two of six patients had positive progesterone receptors. The overall survival rate of the 25 patients was 20% at 5 years. The 5-year survival of Stage IIIB cases was 24%.

The 20 cases without dissemination had a 5-year survival rate of 24%. Among these, a clinically negative axilla or the absence of a distinct breast mass were good prognostic signs. As expected, dermal lymphatic invasion had no influence on prognosis. Initial treatment for all patients except one included irradiation or mastectomy or both, and most received combination chemotherapy. No influence of mastectomy on survival could be appreciated. Sixteen patients

Table 17–25. RESULTS WITH TREATMENT OF NONDISSEMINATED INFLAMMATORY CARCINOMA

Reference	Years of Treatment	Total No. of Cases	Dermal Lymphatic Invasion	Treatment	Median Survival	5-Year Survival (%)	DFS (%)	Local Recurrence (%)
Barker et al., 1980	1948–1972	69	Unknown	RT ± C				46
McBride and Hortobagyi, 1985	1954–1981	81	Unknown	RT or S ± C				
Chu et al., 1980	1960–1977	62	27%	RT alone	18 mo	14	6	69
Hagelberg et al., 1984	1969–1980	24	100%	C ± RT ± S	26 mo	29		
Knight et al., 1986	1974–1982	18	72%	C + RT → S	23 mo			29
Fastenberg et al., 1985	1973–1981	63	25%	C ± RT ± S	43 mo	40	31	31
Sherry et al., 1985	1976–1983	11	"Most"	C ± RT + S	27 mo	60		
Israel et al., 1986	1978–1983	24	Unknown	C → S → C	46 mo	60	45	29
Noguchi et al., 1988	1972–1985	28	89%	IAC → S* → C		59		
Brun et al., 1988	1978–1982	26		C → RT ± S → C	31 mo	25		50
Donegan and Padrta, 1990	1967–1987	20	65%	C/S/RT	30 mo	24		40
Lamb et al., 1991	1968–1986	65	72%	RT ± C	24 mo	28	17	45
Elias et al., 1991		17		C → S/RT → C	32 mo	18		
Moore et al., 1991	1975–1984	56	100%	C → S → C or S → C or C → RT → C	56 mo	45	37	34
Pisansky et al., 1992	1983–1987	36	61%	C + RT → S → C	30 mo	34	24	43

Abbreviations: C = chemotherapy; S = mastectomy; RT = radiotherapy, DFS = disease-free survival; I = immunotherapy; IAC = intra-arterial chemotherapy.

Note: Five-year survival and freedom from recurrence of patients with inflammatory carcinoma of the breast have been improved by the addition of systemic combination chemotherapy to local treatment. Local recurrence may also have been reduced by the use of mastectomy in selected cases, but this is less certain.

*Intra-arterial chemotherapy and extended radical mastectomy.

received chemotherapy as a component of treatment with a 5-year survival of 20%. The 5-year survival was 40% for eleven patients in whom chemotherapy preceded surgery or irradiation.

A clear improvement in survival compared with earlier experience is evident. This may be because cases are being found earlier or, more likely, because all patients now receive combination chemotherapy. Evaluation of treatment is difficult because inflammatory carcinoma is not entirely homogeneous prognostically. Patients with involvement of the breast alone have more favorable courses than do those with regional node involvement, and the latter do better than patients with distant metastases (McBride and Hortobagyi, 1985; and Sherry et al., 1985). Patients with a discrete mass in the breast likewise have a better prognosis than do those without a mass (Hagelberg et al., 1984). Younger patients (younger than 50 years of age) seem to have a poorer prognosis than older patients (Fastenberg et al., 1985). From the therapeutic standpoint, patients whose tumors undergo complete or partial regression on chemotherapy appear to have a more favorable course than those with no response or progression (Fastenberg et al., 1985).

Other authors have found that these tumors often contain estrogen receptors. Sherry and coworkers (1985) reported them positive in 78% of nine cases, and Hagelberg and colleagues (1984) in 57% of seven cases. Consequently, hormonal therapy (tamoxifen is usually used) is often effective. One of six (17%) of this author's patients responded to castration, 18% of 11 patients responded to androgen therapy, and 1 of 7 patients (14%) responded to estrogen therapy.

Summary

Patients with Stage III breast cancer are a therapeutic challenge and require a coordinated plan of management. In those with tumors that are clearly inoperable, initiation of treatment with systemic therapy has a number of advantages. Tumor response can be evaluated, a considerable number of patients are converted to operable status, and the development of dissemination may be delayed with an improvement in survival (Olson, 1986). Irradiation is the mainstay of local-regional treatment in inoperable cases and can be made more effective by the surgical elimination of gross disease in selected cases either beforehand or afterward. The combination of surgery and irradiation appears to improve the prospects for tumor control within the field of treatment but has no detectable influence on distant failure, control of which depends on effective systemic therapy. Patients show reasonably good compliance with the complicated programs required to treat this stage of the disease (Berger et al., 1988).

DISSEMINATED CARCINOMA (TNM STAGE IV)

These patients have clinically evident distant metastases that involve one or more organ systems. The objective of management is palliation. Regardless of how obvious the

tumor is, a biopsy diagnosis is important in all instances before treatment is initiated. One objective of treatment is to control progressive disease on the chest wall in a manner that does not interfere with systemic therapy. Resection should be relegated to that which expedites radiation or systemic treatment. The simplest surgery is best so that potential complications are avoided. Small tumors are removed for diagnosis, estrogen and progesterone receptor assay, and elimination of gross disease. If removal of a large tumor will simplify the physics of irradiation, this can usually be performed with wide resection. Axillary dissection for extensive and fixed axillary involvement is not a useful procedure, because when surgery is not successful in clearing all disease from the axilla, irradiation to the axilla must be added, and the combination risks considerable morbidity.

A National Survey of the American College of Surgeons on breast cancer indicated that a surprisingly high proportion of women with initial distant dissemination (50.5%) had a modified or radical mastectomy (Wilson et al., 1984). Many of these cases were possibly those in which a postoperative bone scan demonstrated metastases. Appropriate preoperative staging can eliminate this problem; local control can often be achieved with irradiation in these cases rather than adding the burden of a mastectomy.

In a review of 40 cases with distant metastases seen between 1967 and 1979, this author found that only 60% of the patients survived for 1 year, 25% for 3 years, and 5.7% for 5 years. The average age was 64 years, somewhat higher than the age of 59 years of other patients with breast cancer. More than half (53%) were managed with biopsy or segmentectomy followed by local-regional irradiation or systemic therapy. An additional six patients (15%) were managed with a palliative simple mastectomy. The remainder (32.5%) had a total removal of the breast with a variable extent of axillary lymph node dissection. It was not possible to determine the success of local-regional control during the patients' remaining lifetimes, nor is information readily available on this point. Survival was not enhanced by more radical surgical procedures. Younger patients and those with more favorable prognoses had more extensive operations, which may account for a slightly higher 1-year survival (73.6% versus 52%) but 2- and 3-year survivals were virtually identical (42% versus 37% and 26.2% versus 26.4%, respectively). Palliation is a complicated task, and palliative operations should be performed in consultation with other professionals who will be managing the patient so that a coherent plan is followed. Any operation should enhance rather than interfere with other methods of treatment. When performed, operations should not transect gross tumor and should be performed in a manner that ensures prompt healing.

SUMMARY

Prognosis correlates more closely with the stage of the disease at the time of treatment than with the particular form of treatment. Thus, the extent of disease must be considered the ultimate determinant of prognosis. Because several therapeutic alternatives appear to provide virtually identical rates of survival, control of cancer within the field of treatment with least morbidity may be the most meaningful end result of local-regional treatment.

References

Adair, F., Berg, J., Joubert, L., et al.: Long-term follow-up of breast cancer patients: The 30-year report. Cancer, *33*:1145, 1974.

Aisner, J., Morris, D., Elias, E. G., et al.: Mastectomy as an adjuvant to chemotherapy for locally advanced or metastatic breast cancer. Arch. Surg., *117*:882, 1982.

Albert, S., Belle, S., Eckert, D., et al.: Current surgical management of in situ cancer of the female breast. J. Surg. Oncol., *20*:99, 1982.

American Joint Committee on Cancer: Manual for Staging of Cancer. 4th ed. Philadelphia, J. B. Lippincott, 1992, pp. 149–154.

Andersen, J, A.: Lobular carcinoma in situ of the breast. An approach to rational treatment. Cancer, *39*:2597, 1977.

Andreassen, M., Dahl-Iverson, E., and Sorenson, B.: Glandular metastases in carcinoma of the breast: Results of a more radical operation. Lancet, *i*:176, 1954.

Anscher, M. S., Jones, P., Prosnitz, L. R., et al.: Local failure and margin status in early-stage breast carcinoma treated with conservation surgery and radiation therapy. Ann. Surg., *218*:22–28, 1993.

Arbutina, D. R., Crus, B. K., Harding, C. T., et al.: Multifocality in the earliest detectable breast carcinomas. Arch. Surg., *127*:421–423, 1992.

Arnold, D. J., and Lesnick, G. J.: Survival following mastectomy for stage III breast cancer. Am. J. Surg., *137*:362, 1979.

Atkins, H., Hayward, J. L., Klugman, D. J., et al.: Treatment of early breast cancer: A report after ten years of a clinical trial. Br. Med. J., *2*:423, 1972.

Attiyeh, F. F., Jensen, M., Huvos, A. G., et al.: Axillary micrometastasis and macrometastasis in carcinoma of the breast. Surg. Gynecol. Obstet., *144*:839, 1977.

Auchincloss, H.: Significance of location and number of axillary metastases in carcinoma of the breast: A justification for a conservative operation. Ann. Surg., *158*:37, 1963.

Baker, R. R., Holmes, E. R., Alderson, P. O., et al.: An evaluation of bone scans as screening procedures for occult metastases in primary breast cancer. Am. Surg., *186*:363, 1977.

Baird, R. M., Worth, A., Hislop, F.: Recurrence after lumpectomy for comedo-type intraductal carcinoma of the breast. Am. J. Surg., *159*:479–481, 1990.

Balawajder, I., Antich, P. P., and Boland, J.: An analysis of the role of radiotherapy alone and in combination with chemotherapy and surgery in the management of advanced breast carcinoma. Cancer, *51*:574, 1983.

Barber, K. W., Jr., Dockerty, M. B., and Clagett, O. T.: Inflammatory carcinoma of the breast. Surg. Gynecol. Obstet., *112*:406, 1961.

Barker, J. L., Montague, E. D., and Peters, L. J.: Clinical experience with irradiation of inflammatory carcinoma of the breast with and without elective chemotherapy. Cancer, *44*:625, 1980.

Bassett, L. W., Giullano, A. E., and Gold, R. H.: Staging for breast carcinoma. Am. J. Surg., *157*:250–255, 1989.

Beahrs, O. H.: Staging of cancer. C. A. Cancer J. Clin., *41*:121–125, 1991.

Bedwani, R., Vana, J., Rosner, D., et al.: Management and survival of female patients with "minimal" breast cancer: As observed in the long-term and short-term surveys of the American College of Surgeons. Cancer, *47*:2769, 1981.

Bedwinek, J., Rao, D. V., Perez, C., et al.: Stage III and localized stage IV breast cancer: Irradiation alone vs irradiation plus surgery. Int. J. Radiation Oncol. Biol. Phys., *8*:31, 1982.

Benson, E. A., and Thorogood, J.: The effect of surgical technique on local recurrence rates following mastectomy. Eur. J. Surg. Oncol., *12*:267–271, 1986.

Berg, J. W.: The significance of axillary node levels in the study of breast carcinoma. Cancer, *8*:776, 1955.

Berger, D., Braverman, A., Sohn, C. K., and Morrow, M.: Patient compliance with aggressive multimodal therapy in locally advanced breast cancer. Cancer, *61*:1453–1456, 1988.

Berrino, P., Campora, E., and Peirlurgi, S.: Post quadrantectomy breast deformities: Classification and techniques of surgical correction. Plast. Reconstr. Surg., *79*:567–572, 1987.

Birdsell, D. C., Jenkins, H., and Berkel, H.: Breast cancer diagnosis and survival in women with and without breast implants. Plast. Reconstr. Surg., *92*:795–800, 1993.

Black, M. M., Barclay, T. H. C., and Hankey, B. F.: Prognosis in breast cancer utilizing histology characteristics of the primary tumor. Cancer, *36*:2048, 1975.

Blevins, P. K.: Subcutaneous mastectomy and breast replacement: Its role in the treatment of benign, premalignant, and malignant breast disease. Am. Surgeon, *47*:281, 1981.

Blichert-Toft, M., Rose, C., Andersen, J. A., et al.: Danish randomized trial comparing breast conservation therapy with mastectomy: Six years of life-table analysis. Monogr. J. Natl. Cancer Inst., *11*:19–25, 1992.

Bloom, H. J. G.: Survival of women with untreated breast cancer—past and present. *In* Forrest, A. P. M., and Kunkler, P. B. (Eds.): Prognostic Factors in Breast Cancer. Baltimore, Williams & Wilkins, 1968, p. 3.

Bloom, H. J. G., Richardson, W. W., and Harries, E. J.: Natural history of untreated breast cancer (1805–1933). Comparison of untreated and treated cases according to histologic grade of malignancy. Br. Med. J., *2*:213, 1962.

Boice, J. D., Jr., Harvey, E. B., Buettner, M., et al.: Cancer in the contralateral breast after radiotherapy for breast cancer. N. Engl. J. Med., *326*:781–785, 1992.

Bonadonna, G., Veronesi, U., Brambilla, C., et al.: Primary chemotherapy to avoid mastectomy in tumors with diameters of three centimeters or more. J. Natl. Cancer Inst., *82*:1539–1545, 1990.

Bond, W. H.: The influence of various treatments of survival rates in cancer of the breast. *In* Jarrett, A. A. (Ed.): The Treatment of Carcinoma of the Breast. Amsterdam, Excerpta Medica Foundation, 1967, p 24.

Boova, R. S., Bonanni, R., and Rosato, F. E.: Patterns of axillary nodal involvement in breast cancer: Predictability of level one dissection. Ann. Surg., *196*:642, 1982.

Bornstein, B. A., Recht, A., Connolly, J. L., et al.: Results of treating ductal carcinoma in situ of the breast with conservative surgery and radiation therapy. Cancer, *67*:7–13, 1991.

Bosari, S., Lee, A. K. C., Viale, G., et al.: Abnormal p53 immunoreactivity and prognosis in node-negative breast carcinoma with long-term follow-up. Virchows Arch. A. Pathol. Anat. Histopathol., *421*:291–295, 1992.

Bozzetti, F., Saccozzi, R., DeLena, M., et al.: Inflammatory cancer of the breast: Analysis of 14 cases. J. Surg. Oncol., *18*:355, 1981.

Brar, H. S., Sisley, J. F., and Johnson, R. H.: Value of preoperative bone and liver scans and alkaline phosphatase in the evaluation of breast cancer patients. Am. J. Surg., *165*:221–224, 1993.

Brun, B., Otmezouine, Y., Feuilhade, F., et al.: Treatment of inflammatory breast cancer with combination chemotherapy and mastectomy versus breast conservation. Cancer, *61*:1096–1103, 1988.

Bucalossi, P., Veronesi, U., Zinge, L., et al.: Enlarged mastectomy for breast. A. J. R. Am. J. Roentgenol., *111*:119, 1971.

Bur, M. E., Zimmarowski, J. J., Schnitt, S. J., et al.: Estrogen receptor immunohistochemistry in carcinoma in situ of the breast. Cancer, *69*:1171–1181, 1992.

Caceres, E.: An evaluation of radical mastectomy and extended radical mastectomy for cancer of the breast. Surg. Gynecol. Obstet., *125*:337, 1967.

Caceres, E.: Incidence of metastases in the internal mammary chain in operable cancer of the breast. Surg. Gynecol. Obstet., *108*:715, 1959.

Cahan, W. G., and Castro, E. B.: Significance of a solitary lung shadow in patients with breast cancer. Ann. Surg., *181*:137, 1975.

Carter, D.: Margins of "lumpectomy" for breast cancer. Hum. Pathol., *17*:330–332, 1986.

Carter, C. L., Allen, C., and Henson, D. E.: Relation of tumor size, lymph node status, and survival in 24,730 breast cancer cases. Cancer, *63*:181–187, 1989.

Carter, D., and Smith, R. L.: Carcinoma in situ of the breast. Cancer, *40*:1189, 1977.

Casey, J. J., Stempel, B. G., Scanlon, E. F., et al.: The solitary pulmonary nodule in the patient with breast cancer. Surgery, *96*:801, 1984.

Castagna, J., Benfield, J. R., Yamada, H., et al.: The reliability of liver scans and function tests in detecting metastases. Surg. Gynecol. Obstet., *134*:463, 1972.

Charkes, N. D., Malmud, L. S., Caswell, T., et al.: Preoperative bone scans. Use in women with early breast cancer. J.A.M.A., *233*:516, 1975.

Chu, F. C. H., Kaufmann, T. P., Dawson, G. A., et al.: Radiation therapy of cancer in prosthetically augmented or reconstructed breasts. Radiology, *185*:429–433, 1992.

Chu, A. M., Wood, W. C., and Doucette, J. A.: Inflammatory breast carcinoma treated by radical radiotherapy. Cancer, *45*:2730, 1980.

Ciatto, S., Pacini, P., Axxini, V., et al.: Preoperative staging of primary breast cancer: A multicenter study. Cancer, *61*:1038–1040, 1988.

Citrin, D. L., Furnival, C. M., Bessent, R. G., et al.: Radioactive technetium phosphate bone scanning in preoperative assessment and follow-up study of patients with primary cancer of the breast. Surg. Gynecol. Obstet., *143*:360, 1976.

Clark, C. P., Foreman, M. L., Peters, G. N., et al.: Efficacy of perioperative liver function tests and ultrasound in detecting hepatic metastasis in carcinoma of the breast. Surg. Gynecol. Obstet., *167*:510–514, 1988.

Clark, G. M., Mathieu, M-C., Owens, M. A., et al.: Prognostic significance of S-phase fraction in good-risk node-negative breast cancer patients. J. Clin. Oncol., *10*:428–432, 1992.

Clark, R. M.: Alternatives to mastectomy—the Princess Margaret Hospital experience. *In* Harris, J. R., Hellman, S., and Silen, W. (Eds.): Conservative Management of Breast Cancer. Philadelphia, J. B. Lippincott, 1983, pp. 35–46.

Clark, R. M., McCulloch, P. B., Levine, M. N., et al.: Randomized clinical trial to assess the effectiveness of breast irradiation following lumpectomy and axillary dissection for node-negative breast cancer. J. Nat. Cancer Inst., *84*:683–689, 1992.

Clarke, D., Curtis, J. L., Martinez, A., et al.: Fat necrosis of the breast simulating recurrent carcinoma after primary radiotherapy in the management of early stage breast carcinoma. Cancer, *52*:442–445, 1983.

Clarke, D., Martinez, A., Cox, R. S., et al.: Breast edema following staging axillary node dissection in patients with breast carcinoma treated by radical radiotherapy. Cancer, *49*:2295, 1982.

Cody, H. S., III, Egeli, R. A., and Urban, J. A.: Rotter's node metastases: Therapeutic and prognostic considerations in early breast carcinoma. Ann. Surg., *199*:266, 1984.

Colizza, S., Lupattelli, R., DeFazio, S., et al.: Hepatic staging in operable breast cancer: A reappraisal from a prospective study. J. Surg. Oncol., *30*:113–115, 1985.

Crile, G. Jr.: Results of conservative treatment of breast cancer at ten and 15 years. Ann. Surg., *181*:26, 1975.

Curtis, R. E., Boice, J. D., Stovall, M., et al.: Risk of leukemia after chemotherapy and radiation treatment for breast cancer. N. Engl. J. Med., *326*:1745–1751, 1992.

Cutler, S. J.: Classification and extent of disease in breast cancer. Semin. Oncol., *1*:91, 1974.

Cutler, S. J., Asire, A. J., and Taylor, S. G., III: Classification of patients with disseminated cancer of the breast. Cancer, *24*:861, 1969.

Dahl-Iversen, E., and Tobiassen, T.: Radical mastectomy with parasternal and supraclavicular dissection for mammary carcinoma. Ann. Surg., *170*:889, 1969.

Daland, E. M.: Untreated cancer of the breast. Surg. Gynecol. Obstet., *44*:264, 1927.

Danforth, D. N., Jr., Findlay, P. A., McDonald, H. D., et al.: Complete axillary lymph node dissection for stage I-II carcinoma of the breast. J. Clin. Oncol., *4*:655, 1986.

Davies, G. C., Millis, R. R., and Hayward, J. L.: Assessment of axillary lymph node status. Ann. Surg., *192*:148, 1980.

Davis, N., and Baird, R. M.: Breast cancer in association with lobular carcinoma in situ. Clinicopathologic review and treatment recommendation. Am. J. Surg., *147*:641, 1984.

Davis, R. P., Nora, P. F., Kooy, R. G., et al.: Experience with lobular carcinoma of the breast: Emphasis on recent aspects of management. Arch. Surg., *114*:485–488, 1979.

DeLena, M., Romero, A., Rabinovich, M., et al.: Metastatic pattern and DNA ploidy in stage IV breast cancer at initial diagnosis. Am. J. Clin. Oncol., *16*:245–249, 1993.

DeLena, M., Varini, M., Zucali, R., et al.: Multimodal treatment for locally advanced breast cancer: Results of chemotherapy-radiotherapy versus chemotherapy-surgery. Cancer Clin. Trials, *4*:229, 1981.

DeLena, M., Zucali, R., Viganotti, G., et al.: Combined chemotherapy-radiotherapy approach in locally advanced (TIIb-TIVMO) breast cancer. Cancer Chemother. Pharmacol., *1*:53, 1978.

deWaard, F.: Breast cancer incidence and nutritional status with particular reference to body weight and height. Cancer Res., *35*:3351, 1975.

Diel, I. J., Kaufmann, M., Goemer, R., et al.: Detection of tumor cells in bone marrow of patients with primary breast cancer: A prognostic factor for distant metastasis. J. Clin. Oncol., *10*:1534–1539, 1992.

DiStefano, A., Tashima, C. K., Yap, H. Y., et al.: Bone marrow metastases

without cortical bone involvement in breast cancer patients. Cancer, *44*:196, 1979.

Donegan, W. L.: Mastectomy in the primary management of invasive mammary carcinoma. *In* Hardy, J. D. (Ed.): Advances in Surgery. Vol. 6. Chicago, Year Book Medical Publishers, 1972, p. 1.

Donegan, W. L.: Patterns and prognosis of advanced breast carcinoma. Missouri Med., *67*:853, 858, 1970.

Donegan, W. L.: Prognostic factors: Stage and receptor stratus in breast cancer. Cancer, *70*:1755–1764, 1992.

Donegan, W. L.: Symposium—Recent trends in the management of breast cancer: 1. Carcinoma in situ of the breast. Can. J. Surg., *35*:361–365, 1993*b*.

Donegan, W. L.: The influence of untreated internal mammary metastases upon the course of mammary cancer. Cancer, *39*:533, 1977.

Donegan, W. L.: Treatment of breast cancer in the elderly. *In* Yancik, R., et al. (Eds.): Perspectives on Prevention and Treatment of Cancer in the Elderly. New York, Raven Press, 1983, p. 83.

Donegan, W. L., Hartz, A. J., and Rimm, A. A.: The association of body weight with recurrent cancer of the breast. Cancer, *41*:1590, 1978.

Donegan, W. L., and Padrta, B.: Combined therapy for inflammatory breast cancer. Arch. Surg., *125*:578–582, 1990.

Donegan, W. L., and Perez-Mesa, C. M.: Lobular carcinoma—an indication for elective biopsy of the second breast. Ann. Surg., *176*:178, 1972.

Donegan, W. L., Stine, S. B., and Samter, T. G.: Implications of extracapsular nodal metastases for treatment and prognosis of breast cancer. Cancer, *72*:778–782, 1993*a*.

Donegan, W. L., Sugarbaker, E. D., Handley, R. S., et al.: The Management of Primary Operable Breast Cancer: A Comparison of Time-Mortality Factors After Standard, Extended, and Modified Radical Mastectomy. Sixth National Cancer Conference Proceedings. Philadelphia, J. B. Lippincott Co., 1970, pp. 135–143.

Duggan, D.: Local therapy of locally advanced breast cancer. Oncology, *5*:68–74, 1991.

Durand, J. C., and Pilleron, J. P.: Cancer of the breast, limited excision followed by radiation: Therapy and results in 150 cases treated at the Curie Foundation, 1960 to 1970. Bull. Cancer (Paris), *64*:611, 1977.

Eberlein, T. J., Connolly, J. L., Schnitt, S. J., et al.: Predictors of local recurrence following conservative breast surgery and radiation therapy. Arch. Surg., *125*:771–777, 1990.

Edeiken, S., Russo, D. P., Knecht, J., et al.: Angiosarcoma after tylectomy and radiation therapy for carcinoma of the breast. Cancer, *70*:544–547, 1992.

Eldar, S., Meguid, M. M., and Beatty, J. D.: Cancer of the breast after prophylactic subcutaneous mastectomy. Am. J. Surg., *148*:692, 1984.

El-Domeiri, A. A., and Shroff, S.: Role of preoperative bone scan in carcinoma of the breast. Surg. Gynecol. Obstet., *142*:722, 1976.

Elias, E. G., Vachon, D. A., Didolkar, M. S., et al.: Long-term results of a combined modality approach in treating inflammatory carcinoma of the breast. Am. J. Surg., *162*:231–235, 1991.

Ellis, D. L., and Teitelbaum, S. L.: Inflammatory carcinoma of the breast: A pathologic definition. Cancer, *33*:1045, 1974.

Farrow, D. C., Hunt, W. C., and Samet, J. M.: Geographic variation in the treatment of localized breast cancer. N. Engl. J. Med., *326*:1097–1101, 1992.

Fastenberg, N. A., Buzdar, A. U., Montague, E. D., et al.: Management of inflammatory carcinoma of the breast: A combined modality approach. Am. J. Clin. Oncol., *8*:134, 1985.

Feinstein, A. R., Sosin, D. M., and Wells, C. K.: The Will Rogers phenomenon: Stage migration and new diagnostic technologies as a source of misleading statistics for survival in cancer. N. Engl. J. Med., *312*:1604–1608, 1985.

Felix, E. L., Bagley, D. H., Sindelar, W. F., et al.: The value of the liver scan in preoperative screening of patients with malignancies. Cancer, *38*:1137, 1976.

Fentiman, I. S.: Detection and Treatment of Early Breast Cancer. Philadelphia, J. B. Lippincott, 1990, pp. 79–80.

Fentiman, I. S., Lavelle, M. A., Caplan, D., et al.: The significance of supraclavicular fossa node recurrence after radical mastectomy. Cancer, *57*:908, 1986.

Ferguson, D. J., Meier, P., Karrison, T., et al.: Staging of breast cancer and survival rates: No assessment based on 50 years of experience with radical mastectomy. J.A.M.A., *248*:1337, 1982.

Fisher, B.: Some thoughts concerning the primary therapy of breast cancer: A multidisciplinary approach. Recent Results Cancer Res., *57*:150–163, 1976.

Fisher, B., Anderson, S., Fisher, E. R., et al.: Significance of ipsilateral breast tumor recurrence after lumpectomy. Lancet, *338*:327–331, 1991.

Fisher, B., Bauer, M., Margolese, R., et al.: Five-year results of a randomized clinical trial comparing total mastectomy and segmental mastectomy with or without radiation in the treatment of breast cancer. N. Engl. J. Med., *312*:665, 1985*a*.

Fisher B., Costantino, J., Redmond, C., et al.: Lumpectomy compared with lumpectomy and radiation therapy for the treatment of intraductal breast cancer. N. Engl. J. Med., *328*:1581–1586, 1993.

Fisher, B., and Redmond, C.: Lumpectomy for breast cancer: An update of the NSABP experience. Monogr. J. Natl., Cancer Inst., *11*:7–13, 1992*a*.

Fisher, B., Redmond, C., Fisher, E. R., et al.: Ten-year results of a randomized clinical trial comparing radical mastectomy and total mastectomy with or without radiation. N. Engl. J. Med., *312*:674–681, 1985.

Fisher, B., Redmond, C., Poisson, R., et al.: Eight-year results of a randomized clinical trial comparing total mastectomy and lumpectomy with or without irradiation in the treatment of breast cancer. N. Engl. J. Med., *320*:822–928, 1989.

Fisher, B., Slack, N., Katrych, D., et al.: Ten year follow-up results of patients with carcinoma of the breast in a cooperative clinical trial evaluating surgical adjuvant chemotherapy. Surg. Gynecol. Obstet., *140*:528, 1975*b*.

Fisher, B., and Slack, N. H.: Number of lymph nodes examined and the prognosis of breast carcinoma. Surg. Gynecol. Obstet., *131*:79, 1970.

Fisher, B., Wolmark, N., Bauer, M., et al.: The accuracy of clinical nodal staging and of limited axillary dissection as a determinant of histologic nodal status in carcinoma of the breast. Surg. Gynecol. Obstet., *152*:765, 1981.

Fisher, E. R., Costantino, J., Fisher B., et al.: Pathologic findings from the National Surgical Adjuvant Breast Project (Protocol 4). Cancer, *71*(Suppl.):2141–2150, 1992*b*.

Fisher, E. R., Gregorio, R. M., Fisher, B., et al.: The pathology of invasive breast cancer: A syllabus derived from findings of the National Surgical Adjuvant Breast Project (Protocol No. 4). Cancer, *36*:1, 1975*a*.

Fisher, E. R., Gregorio, R. M., Redmond, C., et al.: Pathologic findings from the National Surgical Adjuvant Breast Project (Protocol No. 4). Am. J. Clin. Pathol., *65*:439–444, 1976.

Fisher, E. R., Leeming, R., Anderson, S., et al.: Conservative management of intraductal carcinoma (DCIS) of the breast. J. Surg. Oncol., *47*:139–147, 1991.

Fletcher, G. H., Montague, E. D., Tapley, N. D., et al.: Radiotherapy in the management of nondisseminated breast cancer. *In* Fletcher, G. H. (Ed.): Textbook of Radiotherapy. 3rd ed. Philadelphia, Lea & Febiger, 1980, p. 527.

Foley, W. D., Berland, L. L., Lawson, T. L., et al.: Contrast enhancement technique for dynamic hepatic computed tomographic scanning. Radiology, *147*:797–803, 1983.

Foote, F. W., Jr., and Stewart, F. W.: Lobular carcinoma in situ: A rare form of mammary cancer. Am. J. Pathol., *17*:491, 1941.

Forber, J. E.: Incurable cancer. Ministry of Health Reports on Public Health and Medical Subjects, No. LXVI. London, His Majesty's Stationery Office, 1931.

Forrest, A. P. M., Stewart, H. J., Roberts, M. M., et al.: Simple mastectomy and axillary node sampling (pectoral node biopsy) in the management of primary breast cancer. Ann. Surg., *196*:371, 1982.

Francchia, A. A., Evans, J. F., and Eisenberg, B. L.: Stage III carcinoma of the breast: A detailed analysis. Ann. Surg., *192*:705, 1980.

Frank, J. L., McClish, K. K., Dawson, K. S., et al.: Stage III breast cancer: Is neoadjuvant chemotherapy always necessary? J. Surg. Oncol., *49*:220–225, 1992.

Frykberg, E. R., Santiago, F., Betsill, W. L., Jr., et al.: Lobular carcinoma in situ of the breast. Surg. Gynecol. Obstet., *164*:285–301, 1987.

Galasko, C. S. B.: The significance of occult skeletal metastases, detected by skeletal scintigraphy, in patients with otherwise apparently "early" mammary carcinoma. Br. J. Surg., *62*:694, 1975.

Gallager, H. S.: Pathologic types of breast cancer: Their prognoses. Cancer, *53*:623, 1984.

Gallager, H. S., and Martin, J. E.: The study of mammary carcinoma by mammography and a whole organ sectioning—early observations. Cancer, *23*:855, 1969.

Gallager, H. S., and Martin, J. E.: An orientation to the concept of minimal breast cancer. Cancer, *28*:1505, 1971.

Gallagher, W. J., Koerner, F. C., and Wood, W. C.: Treatment of intraductal carcinoma with limited surgery: Long-term follow-up. J. Clin. Oncol., *7*:376–380, 1989.

Ganz, P. A., Schag, A. C., Lee, J., et al.: Breast conservation versus mastectomy. Cancer, *69*:1729–1738, 1992.

Gapinski, P. V., and Donegan, W. L.: Estrogen receptors and breast cancer: Prognostic and therapeutic implications. Surgery, *88*:386, 1980.

Gasparioni, G., Bevilacqua, P., Pozza, F., et al.: Value of epidermal growth factor receptor status compared with growth fraction and other factors for prognosis in early breast cancer. Br. J. Cancer, *66*:970–976, 1992.

Ghossein, N. A., Alpert, S., Barba, J., et al.: Breast cancer: Importance of adequate surgical excision prior to radiotherapy in the local control of breast cancer in patients treated conservatively. Arch. Surg., *127*:411–415, 1992.

Gibbons, J., Holleb, A. I., and Farrow, J. H.: An evaluation of routine preoperative skeletal survey for the patient with operable breast cancer. N. Y. State J. Med., *61*:4219, 1961.

Gion, M., Mione, R., Nescimben, O., et al.: The tumor associated antigen CA 15.3 in primary breast cancer: Evaluation of 667 cases. Cancer, *63*:809–813, 1991.

Giordano, J. M., and Klopp, C. T.: Lobular carcinoma in situ: Incidence and treatment. Cancer, *31*:105–109, 1973.

Goodwin, J. S., Samet, J. M., and Key, C. R.: Stage at diagnosis of cancer varies with the age of the patient. J. Am. Geriat. Soc., *34*:20–26, 1986.

Grace, E. J., and Moitrier, W. Jr.: Simple mastectomy with x-ray in the treatment of cancer of breast. N. Y. State J. Med., *26*:1, 1936.

Greenough, R. B., Simmons, C. C., and Barney, J. D.: The results of operations for cancer of the breast at the Massachusetts General Hospital from 1894 to 1904. Am. Surg. Assoc., *25*:80, 1907.

Greenwood, M.: The natural history of cancer. Ministry of Health Reports on Public Health and Medical Subjects, No. XXVI, London, His Majesty's Stationery Office, 1926.

Haagensen, C. D.: Diseases of the Breast. Philadelphia, W. B. Saunders, 1971, pp. 426, 582, 637, 642.

Haagensen, C. D.: Diseases of the Breast. 3rd ed. Philadelphia, W. B. Saunders, 1986, pp. 192–241.

Haagensen, C. D., and Bondian, C.: A personal experience with Halsted's radical mastectomy. Ann. Surg., *199*:143, 1984.

Haagensen, C. D., and Stout, A. P.: Carcinoma of the breast: Criteria for operability. Ann. Surg., *118*:859, 1032, 1943.

Haagensen, C. D., Cooley, E., Miller, E., et al.: Treatment of early mammary carcinoma: A cooperative international study. Ann. Surg., *170*:875, 1969.

Haagensen, C. D., Lane, N., and Bodian, C.: Coexisting lobular neoplasia and carcinoma of the breast. Cancer, *51*:1468, 1983.

Haagensen, C. D., Lane, N., Lattes, R., et al.: Lobular neoplasia (so-called lobular carcinoma in situ) of the breast. Cancer, *42*:737, 1978.

Haffty, B. G., Goldberg, N. B., Rose, M., et al.: Conservative surgery with radiation therapy in clinical Stage I and II breast cancer. Arch. Surg., *124*:1266–1270, 1989.

Hagelberg, R. S., Jolly, P. C., and Anderson, R. P.: Role of surgery in the treatment of inflammatory breast carcinoma. Am. J. Surg., *148*:125, 1984.

Halpern, J., McNeese, M. D., Kroll, S. S., et al.: Irradiation of prosthetically augmented breasts: A retrospective study of toxicity and cosmetic results. Int. J. Radiat. Oncol. Biol. Phys., *18*:189–191, 1990.

Halsted, W. S.: The results of operations for the cure of cancer of the breast performed at the Johns Hopkins Hospital from June 1889 to January 1894. Johns Hopkins Hosp. Rep., *4*:297, 1894–1895.

Halsted, W. S.: A clinical and histological study of certain adenocarcinomas of the breast: And a brief consideration of the supraclavicular operation and of the results of operations for cancer of the breast from 1889–1898 at the Johns Hopkins Hospital. Trans. Am. Surg. Assoc., *16*:144, 1898.

Halsted, W. S.: Developments in the skin grafting operation for mammary carcinoma. Trans. Am. Surg. Assoc., *30*:287, 1912.

Handel, N., Lewinsky, B., Silverstein, M. J., et al.: Conservation therapy for breast cancer following augmentation mammaplasty. Plast. Reconstr. Surg., *87*:873–878, 1991.

Handley, R. S.: A surgeon's view of the spread of breast cancer. Cancer, *24*:1231, 1969.

Handley, R. S.: Modified radical mastectomy. *In* Nora, P. F. (Ed.): Operative Surgery—Principles and Techniques. Philadelphia, Lea & Febiger, 1972, p. 198.

Handley, R. S.: Techniques of surgical treatment. *In* Atkins, H. (Ed.): The Treatment of Breast Cancer. Baltimore, University Park Press, 1974, p. 49.

Handley, R., Patey, D., and Hand, B.: Excision of the internal mammary chain in radical mastectomy. Results of 57 cases. Lancet, *i*:457, 1956.

Handley, R. S., and Thackray, A. C.: Conservative and radical mastectomy (Patey's operation). Ann. Surg., *157*:162, 1962.

Handley, R. S., and Thackray, S. G.: Internal mammary lymph chain in carcinoma of the breast. Study of 50 cases. Lancet, *ii*:276, 1949.

Handley, W. S.: Parasternal invasion of thorax in breast cancer and its suppression by use of radium tubes as operative precaution. Surg. Gynecol. Obstet., *45*:721, 1927.

Harris, J. R., and Hellman, S.: Primary radiation therapy for early breast cancer. Cancer, *52*:2547–2552, 1983.

Hayward, J. L.: The Guy's hospital trials on breast conservation. *In* Harris, J. R., Hellman, S., and Silen, W. (Eds.): Conservative Management of Breast Cancer: New Surgical and Radiotherapeutic Techniques. Philadelphia, J. B. Lippincott, 1983, p. 77.

Henderson, I. C., and Canellos, G. P.: Cancer of the breast: The past decade. N. Engl. J. Med., *302*:17, 1980.

Henson, D. E., Ries, L., Freedman, L. S., et al.: Relationship among outcome, stage of disease, and histologic grade for 22,616 cases of breast cancer. Cancer, *68*:2142–2149, 1991.

Hermann, R. E., Esselstyn, C. B., Jr., Grundfest-Broniatowski, S., et al.: Partial mastectomy without radiation is adequate treatment for patients with Stages 0 and I carcinoma of the breast. Surg. Gynecol. Obstet., *177*:247–253, 1993.

Hery, M., Namer, M., Moro, M., et al.: Conservative treatment (chemotherapy/radiation) of locally advanced breast cancer. Cancer, *57*:1744, 1986.

Hobar, P. C., Jones, R. C., Schouten, J., et al.: Multimodality treatment of locally advanced breast carcinoma. Arch. Surg., *123*:951–955, 1988.

Hoffman, H. C., and Marty, R.: Bone scanning: Its value in the preoperative evaluation of patients with suspicious breast masses. Am. J. Surg., *124*:194, 1972.

Holland, R., Hendriks, J. H. C. L., Verbeek, A. L. M., et al.: Extent, distribution, and mammographic/histological correlations of breast ductal carcinoma in situ. Lancet, *335*:519–522, 1990.

Holland, R., Veling, S. H. J., Mravunmac, M., et al.: Histologic multifocality of Tis, T1-2 breast carcinomas. Cancer *56*:979–990, 1985.

Holleb, A. I., Montgomery, R., and Farrow, J. H.: Hazard of incomplete simple mastectomy. Surg. Gynecol. Obstet., *121*:819, 1965.

Hortobagyi, G. N., Blumenschein, G. R., Spanos, W., et al.: Multimodal treatment of locoregionally advanced breast cancer. Cancer, *51*:763, 1983.

Host, H., and Lund, E.: Age as a prognostic factor in breast cancer. Cancer, *57*:2217, 1986.

Hunter, R. L., Ferguson, D. J., and Coppleson, L. W.: Survival with mammary cancer related to the interaction of germinal center hyperplasia and sinus histiocytosis in axillary and internal mammary lymph nodes. Cancer, *36*:528, 1975.

Hutter, R. V. P.: The management of patients with lobular carcinoma in situ of the breast. Cancer, *53*:798, 1984.

Hutter, R. V. P., and Foote, F. W. Jr.: Lobular carcinoma in situ: Long-term follow-up. Cancer, *24*:1081–1085, 1969.

Ingle, J. N., Tormey, D. C., and Tan, H. K.: The bone marrow examination in breast cancer. Diagnostic considerations and clinical usefulness. Cancer, *41*:670, 1978.

Israel, L., Breau, J. L., Goguel, B., et al.: Impact of post mastectomy irradiation on survival and recurrence rates: A retrospective study comparing 345 irradiated and 432 nonirradiated patients between 1972 and 1984. Proceedings of ASCO, *5*:58, 1986.

Joensuu, H., Toikkanen, S., Klemi, P. J.: DNA index and S-phase fraction and their combinations as prognostic factors in operable ductal breast carcinoma. Cancer, *66*:331–340, 1990.

Johnson, H., Masood, S., Belluco, C., et al.: Prognostic factors in node-negative breast cancer. Arch. Surg., *127*:1386–1391, 1992.

Kaae, S., and Johansen, H.: Simple mastectomy plus postoperative irradiation by the method of McWhirter for mammary carcinoma. Ann. Surg., *170*:805, 1969.

Kay, S.: Evaluation of Rotter's lymph nodes in radical mastectomy specimens as a guide to prognosis. Cancer, *18*:1441, 1965.

Kemeny, M. M., Rivera, D. E., Terz, J. J., et al.: Occult primary adenocarcinoma with axillary metastases. Am. J. Surg., *152*:43, 1986.

Kemeny, N., and Schneider, A.: Regional treatment of hepatic metastases and hepatocellular carcinoma. Curr. Probl. Cancer, *13*:197–283, 1989.

Keynes, G.: Radium treatment of breast cancer. Br. J. Surg., *19*:415, 1932.

Khansur, T., Haick, A., Patel, B., et al.: Evaluation of bone scan as a screening work-up in primary and local-regional recurrence of breast cancer. Am. J. Clin. Oncol., *10*:157–170, 1987.

Kinne, D. W., Petrek, J. A., Osborne, M. P., et al.: Breast carcinoma in situ. Arch. Surg., *124*:33–36, 1989.

Kinne, D. W.: Controversies in primary breast cancer management. Am. J. Surg., *166*:502–508, 1993.

Kisner, W. H.: Multiple spontaneous rib fractures secondary to osteoradionecrosis. Contemp. Surg., *40*:22–24, 1992.

Klamer, T. W., Donegan, W. L., and Max, M. H.: Breast tumor incidence in rats after partial mammary resection. Arch. Surg., *118*:933, 1983.

Knight, C. D., Jr., Martin, J. K., Jr., Welch, J. S., et al.: Surgical considerations after chemotherapy and radiation therapy for inflammatory breast cancer. Surgery, *99*:385–1986.

Knight, W. A., III, Livingston, R., Gregory, E., et al.: Estrogen receptor as an independent prognostic factor for early recurrence in breast cancer. Cancer Res., *37*:4669, 1977.

Komaki, R., Donegan, W. L., Manoli, R., et al.: Prognostic value of pretreatment bone scans in breast carcinoma. A.J.R. Am. J. Roentgenol., *132*:877, 1979.

Kurtz, J. M., Amalric, R., Brandone, H., et al.: Results of salvage surgery for mammary recurrence following breast conserving therapy. Ann. Surg., *207*:347–351, 1988*a*.

Kurtz, J. M., Amalric, R., Brandone, H., et al.: Results of wide excision for mammary recurrence after breast conserving therapy. Cancer, *61*:1969–1972, 1988*b*.

Kurtz, J. M., Jacquemier, J., Amalric, R., et al.: Breast-conserving therapy for macroscopically multiple cancers. Ann. Surg., *212*:35–44, 1990*a*.

Kurtz, J. M., Jacquemier, J., Amalric, R., et al.: Why are local recurrences after breast-conserving therapy more frequent in younger patients? J. Clin. Oncol., *8*:591–698, 1990*b*.

Kurtz, J. M., Jacquemier, J., Torhorst, J., et al.: Conservation therapy for breast cancers other than infiltrating ductal carcinoma. Cancer, *63*:1630–1635, 1989.

Kusama, S., Spratt, J. S., Donegan, W. L., et al.: The gross rates of growth and human mammary carcinoma. Cancer, *30*:594, 1972.

Lacour, J., Bucalossi, P., Caceres, E., et al.: Radical mastectomy versus radical mastectomy plus internal mammary dissection. Cancer, *37*:206, 1976.

Lacour, J., Le, M., Caceres, E., et al.: Radical mastectomy versus radical mastectomy plus internal mammary dissection. Cancer, *51*:1941, 1983.

Lagios, M. D.: Ductal carcinoma in situ: Pathology and treatment. Surg. Clin. North Am., *70*:853–871, 1990.

Lagios, M. D., Margolin, F. R., Westdahl, P. R., et al.: Mammographically detected duct carcinoma in situ. Cancer, *63*:1618–1624, 1989.

Lagios, M. D., Richards, V. E., Rose, M. R., et al.: Segmental mastectomy without radiotherapy: Short-term follow-up. Cancer, *52*:2173, 1983.

Lagios, M. D., Westdahl, P. R., Margolin, F. R., et al.: Duct carcinoma in situ: Relationship of extent of noninvasive disease to the frequency of occult invasion, multicentricity, lymph node metastases, and short-term treatment failures. Cancer, *50*:1309, 1982.

Lamb, C. C., Berlein, T. J., Parker, L. M., et al.: Results of radical radiotherapy for inflammatory breast cancer. Am. J. Surg. *162*:236–242, 1991.

Lambird, P. A., and Shelley, W. M.: The spatial distribution of lobular in situ mammary carcinoma. J.A.M.A., *210*:689, 1969.

Laroye, G. J., and Minkin, S.: The impact of mitotic index on predicting outcome in breast carcinoma: A comparison of different counting methods in patients with different lymph node stains. Mod. Pathol., *4*:456–460, 1991.

Lattes, R.: Lobular neoplasia (lobular carcinoma in situ) of the breast—a histological entity of controversial clinical significance. Pathol. Res. Pract., *166*:415, 1980.

Lazovich, D., White, E., Thomas, D. B., et al.: Underutilization of breast-conserving surgery and radiation therapy among women with Stage I or II breast cancer. J. Am. Med. Assoc., *266*:3433–3438, 1991.

Lee, A. K. C., DeLellis, R. A., Silverman, M. L., et al.: Prognostic significance of peritumoral lymphatic and blood vessel invasion in node-negative carcinoma of the breast. J. Clin. Oncol., 8:1457–1465, 1990.

Lee, B. J., and Stubenbord, J. G.: Clinical index of malignancy for carcinoma of the breast. Surg. Gynecol. Obstet., 47:812, 1928.

Lee, B. J., and Tannenbaum, N. E.: Inflammatory carcinoma of the breast. Surg. Gynecol. Obstet., 75:580, 1925.

Lee, Y. T.: Bone scanning patients with early breast carcinoma: Should it be a routine staging procedure? Cancer, 47:486–495, 1981.

Lee, Y. T.: Delayed cutaneous hypersensitivity, lymphocyte count, and blood tests in patients with breast carcinoma. J. Surg. Oncol., 27:135, 1984.

Lennington, W. J., Jensen, R. A., Dalton, L. W., et al.: Ductal carcinoma in situ of the breast: Heterogeneity of individual lesions. Cancer, 73:118–124, 1993.

Leone, B. A., Romero, A., Rabinovich, M. G., et al.: Stage IV breast cancer: Clinical course and survival of patients with osseous versus extraosseous metastases at initial diagnosis. Am. J. Clin. Oncol., 11:618–622, 1988.

Leopold, K. A., Recht, A., Schnitt, S. J., et al.: Results of conservative surgery and radiation therapy for multiple synchronous cancers of one breast. Int. J. Radiat. Oncol. Biol. Phys., 16:11–16, 1989.

Lesnick, G. J., and Papatestas, A.: Results of treatment of stage I and stage II primary carcinoma of the breast by modified radical mastectomy with preservation of the pectoralis major muscle (Patey's operation). Abstract for the XI International Cancer Congress, Florence, Italy, October 20–26, 1974.

Lewi, H. J., Roberts, M. M., Donaldson, A. A., et al.: The use of cerebral computer-assisted tomography as a staging investigation of patients with carcinoma of the breast and malignant melanoma. Surg. Gynecol. Obstet. 151:385, 1980.

Lichter, A. S., Lippman, M. E., Danforth, D. N., et al.: Mastectomy versus breast-conserving therapy in the treatment of Stage I and II carcinoma of the breast: A randomized trial at the national cancer institute. J. Clin. Oncol., 10:976–983, 1992.

Lipsztein, R., Dalton, J. F., and Bloomer, W. D.: Sequelae of breast irradiation. J. Am. Med. Assoc. 263:3582–3584, 1985.

Livingston, S., and Arlen, M.: The extended extrapleural radical mastectomy. Ann. Surg., 179:260, 1974.

Loprinzi, C. L., Carbone, P. P., Tormey, D. C., et al.: Aggressive combined modality therapy for advanced local-regional breast carcinoma. J. Clin. Oncol., 2:157, 1984.

Lucas, F. V., and Perez-Mesa, C.: Inflammatory carcinoma of the breast. Cancer, 41:1595, 1978.

Lythgoe, P. J., and Palmer, K. M.: Manchester regional breast study—5 and 10 year results. Br. J. Surg., 69:693, 1982.

Madden, J. L.: Modified radical mastectomy. Surg. Gynecol. Obstet., 121:1221, 1965.

Maddox, W. A., Carpenter, J. T., Laws, H. L., et al.: A randomized prospective trial of radical (Halsted) mastectomy versus modified radical mastectomy in 311 breast cancer patients. Ann. Surg., 198:207, 1983.

Mambo, N. C., and Gallager, H. S.: Carcinoma of the breast: The prognostic significance of extranodal extension of axillary disease. Cancer, 39:2280, 1977.

Margottini, M., and Bucalossi, P.: Le metastasi linfoghian dolari mammarie interne nel cancro della mammella. Oncologia, 23:70, 1949.

Martin, M. A., Welling, R. E., and Strobel, S. L.: Infiltrating lobular carcinoma of the breast treated with segmental and modified radical mastectomy. J. Surg. Oncol., 41:117–120, 1989.

Matas, R.: Personal experience with remarks of the operative treatment of cancer of the breast—discussion. Trans. Am. Surg. Assoc., 16:144, 1898.

McBride, C. M., and Hortobagyi, G. N.: Primary inflammatory carcinoma of the female breast: Staging and treatment possibilities. Surgery, 98:792, 1985.

McCready, D. R., Hortobagyi, G. N., Kau, S. W., et al.: The prognostic significance of lymph node metastases after preoperative chemotherapy for locally advanced breast cancer. Arch. Surg., 124:21–25, 1989.

McDivitt, R. W., Hutter, R. V. P., Foote, F. W. Jr., et al.: In situ lobular carcinoma: A prospective follow-up study indicating cumulative patient risks. J.A.M.A., 201:96, 1967.

McDivitt, R. W., Stewart, F. W., and Berg, J. W.: Tumors of the breast. In Atlas of Tumor Pathology. Washington, D.C., Armed Forces Institute of Pathology, 1968.

McGuire, W. L., and Clark, G. M.: Prognostic factors and treatment decisions in axillary node-negative breast cancer. N. Engl. J. Med., 326:1756–1761, 1992.

McGuire, W. L., Tandon, A. K., Allred, C., et al.: How to use prognostic factors in axillary node-negative breast cancer patients. J. Nat. Cancer Inst., 82:1006–1015, 1990.

McWhirter, R.: Should more radical treatment be attempted in breast cancer? Caldwell Lecture, 1963. A.J.R. Am. J. Roentgenol., 92:3, 1964.

Merson, M., Andreola, S., Galimberti, V., et al.: Breast carcinoma presenting as axillary metastases without evidence of a primary tumor. Cancer, 70:504–508, 1992.

Meyer, A. C., Smith, S. S., and Potter, M.: Carcinoma of the breast. A clinical study. Arch. Surg., 113:364, 1978.

Meyer, J. S., and Province, M.: Proliferation index of breast carcinoma by thymidine labeling: Prognostic power independent of stage, estrogen and progesterone receptors. Breast Cancer Res. Treat., 12:191–204, 1988.

Meyer, K. K.: Radiation-induced lymphocyte-immune deficiency: A factor in the increased visceral metastases and decreased hormonal responsiveness of breast cancer. Arch. Surg., 101:114, 1970.

Meyer, W.: Carcinoma of the breast: Ten years' experience with my method of radical operation. J.A.M.A., 45:297, 1905.

Montague, E. D.: Conservation surgery and radiation therapy in the treatment of operable breast cancer. Cancer, 53:700, 1984.

Moore, M. P., Ihde, J. K., Crowe, J. P. Jr., et al.: Inflammatory breast cancer. Arch. Surg., 125:304–306, 1991.

Morimoto, T., Okazaki, K., Komaki, K., et al.: Cancerous residue in breast-conserving surgery. J. Surg. Oncol., 52:71–76, 1993.

Morris, D. M.: Mastectomy in the management of patients with inflammatory breast cancer. J. Surg. Oncol., 23:255, 1983.

Morrow, M., and Foster, R. S. Jr.: Staging of breast cancer: A new rationale for internal mammary node biopsy. Arch. Surg., 116:748, 1981.

Mueller, C. B.: Stage II breast cancer is not simply a late Stage I. Surgery, 104:631–638, 1988.

Muir, R.: The evolution of carcinoma of the mamma. J. Pathol., Bacteriol., 52:155, 1941.

Murray, J. G., Mitchell, J. S., Gresham, G. A.: Management of early cancer of the breast: Report on an international multicentre trial supported by the Cancer Research Campaign. Br. Med. J., 1:1035, 1976.

Muss, H. B., White, D. R., and Cowan, R. J.: Brain scanning in patients with recurrent breast cancer. Cancer, 38:1574, 1976.

Myers, R. E., Sutherland, D. J., Meakin, J. W., et al.: Prognostic value of CEA in breast cancer patients (Abstract). Proc. Am. Assoc. Cancer Res. Am. Soc., 19:148, 1978.

Nathanson, I. T., and Welch, C. E.: Life expectancy and incidence of malignant disease: Carcinoma of the breast. Am. J. Cancer, 28:40, 1936.

Nattinger, A. B., Gottlieb, M. S., Veum, J., et al.: Geographic variation in the use of breast-conserving treatment for breast cancer. N. Engl. J. Med., 325:1102–1107, 1992.

Nemoto, T., Patel, J. K., Rosner, D., et al.: Factors affecting recurrence in lumpectomy without irradiation for breast cancer. Cancer, 67:2079–2082, 1991.

Nemoto, T., Vana, J., Bedwani, R. N., et al.: Management and survival of female breast cancer: Results of a national survey by the American College of Surgeons. Cancer, 45:2917–2924, 1980.

NIH Consensus Development Panel: Treatment of primary breast cancer. N. Engl. J. Med., 301:340, 1979.

Noguchi, M., Koyasaki, N., Ohta, N., et al.: Internal mammary nodal status is a more reliable prognostic factor than DNA ploidy and c-erb B$_2$ expression in patients with breast cancer. Arch. Surg., 128:242–246, 1993.

Noguchi, S., Miyauchi, K., Nishizawa, Y., et al.: Management of inflammatory carcinoma of the breast with combined modality therapy including intraarterial infusion chemotherapy as an induction therapy. Cancer, 61:1483–1291, 1988.

Olson, J. E.: Breast cancer: Stage III disease. Current Concepts Oncol., 8:17, 1986.

Osborne, C. K.: Prognostic factors in breast cancer. P.P.O. Updates 4:1–11, 1990.

Osborne, M. P., Borgen, P. T., Wong, G. Y., et al.: Salvage mastectomy for local and regional recurrence after breast-conserving operation and radiation therapy. Surg. Gynecol. Obstet., *174*:189–194, 1992.

Osteen, R. T., Cady, B., Chmiel, J. S. et al.: 1991 National Survey of Carcinoma of the Breast of the Commission on Cancer. J. Am. Coll. Surg., *178*:213–219, 1994.

Ozello, L., and Sanpitak, P.: Epithelial-stromal junction in intraductal carcinoma of the breast. Cancer, *26*:1186, 1970.

Page, M.: President's address. Proc. R. Soc. Med., *41*:121, 1948.

Papaioannou, A. N., and Urban, J. A.: Scalene node biopsy in locally advanced primary breast cancer of questionable operability. Cancer, *17*:1006, 1964.

Papaioannou, A., Lissaios, B., Vsilaros, S., et al.: Pre- and postoperative chemoendocrine treatment with or without postoperative radiotherapy for locally advanced breast cancer. Cancer, *51*:1284, 1983.

Papatestas, A. E., Lesnick, G. J., Genkins, G., et al.: The prognostic significance of peripheral lymphocyte counts in patients with breast carcinoma. Cancer, *37*:164, 1976.

Patey, D. H.: A review of 146 cases of carcinoma of the breast operated on between 1930 and 1943. Br. J. Cancer, *21*:260, 1967.

Pavrosky, J., Tersip, L., and Palecek, L.: Results of radical operation for mammary gland carcinoma with revision of the parasternal space. Int. Surg., *51*:509, 1969.

Pearlman, A. W.: Breast cancer—influence of growth rate on prognosis and treatment evaluation: A study based on mastectomy scar recurrences. Cancer, *38*:1826, 1976.

Pearlman, N. W., Guerra, O., and Fracchia, A. A.: Primary inoperable cancer of the breast. Surg. Gynecol. Obstet., *143*:909, 1976.

Perloff, B., Lesnick, G. J., Karzun, F., et al.: Combination chemotherapy with mastectomy or radiotherapy for Stage III breast carcinoma: A Cancer and Leukemia Group B Study. J. Clin. Oncol., *6*:261–269, 1988.

Peters, M. V.: Radiation therapy in the management of breast cancer. Proceedings of the Sixth National Cancer Conference. Philadelphia, J. B. Lippincott, 1970, p. 163.

Phillips, A. J.: A comparison of related and untreated cases of cancer of the breast. Br. J. Cancer, *13*:20, 1959.

Pickren, J. W., Rube, J., and Auchincloss, H. Jr.: Modification of conventional radical mastectomy: A detailed study of lymph node involvement and follow-up information to show its practicality. Cancer, *18*:942, 1965.

Pigott, J., Nichols, R., Maddox, W. A., et al.: Metastases to the upper levels of the axillary nodes in carcinoma of the breast and its implications for nodal sampling procedures. Surg. Gynecol. Obstet., *158*:255, 1984.

Pisansky, T. M., Schaid, D. J., Loprinzi, C. L., et al.: Inflammatory breast cancer: Integration of irradiation, surgery, and chemotherapy. Am. J. Clin. Oncol., *15*:376–387, 1992.

Portmann, U. V.: Clinical and pathologic criteria as a basis for classifying cases of primary cancer of the breast. Cleveland Clin. Q., *10*:41, 1943.

Powers, R. W., O'Brien, P. H., and Kreutner, A. Jr.: Lobular carcinoma in situ. J. Surg. Gynecol., *13*:269, 1980.

Pozo, C. P., Carver, C. S., Noriego, V., et al.: Effects of mastectomy versus lumpectomy on emotional adjustment to breast cancer: A prospective study of the first year postsurgery. J. Clin. Oncol., *10*:1292–1298, 1992.

Prosnitz, L. R., Goldenberg, I. S., Harris, J. R., et al.: Radiotherapy for carcinoma of the breast instead of mastectomy. An update. Front. Radiat. Ther. Oncol., *17*:69, 1983.

Prudente, A.: L'amputation inter-scapulo-mammothoracique (technique et resultats). J. Chir., *65*:729, 1949.

Qualheim, R. E., and Gall, E. A.: Breast carcinomas with multiple sites of origin. Cancer, *10*:460, 1957.

Radford, D. M., and Wells, S. A. Jr.: Surgical techniques in breast conservation. Adv. Surg., *26*:1–27, 1993.

Raffl, A. B.: The use of negative pressure under skin flaps after radical mastectomy. Ann. Surg., *136*:1048, 1952.

Ragaz, J.: Management of Stage III breast cancer—any progress? Rev. Endocrine-Related Cancer, *28*:5–12, 1988.

Rao, D. V., Bedwinek, J., Perez, C., et al.: Prognostic indicators in stage III and localized stage IV breast cancer. Cancer, *50*:2037, 1982.

Recht, A., Come, S. E., Felman, R. S., et al.: Integration of conservative surgery, radiotherapy, and chemotherapy for the treatment of early-stage, node-positive breast cancer: Sequencing, timing, and outcome. J. Clin. Oncol., *9*:1662–1667, 1991.

Recht, A., Danoff, B. S., Solin, L. J., et al.: Intraductal carcinoma of the breast: Results of treatment with excisional biopsy and irradiation. J. Clin. Oncol., *3*:1339, 1985.

Ridell, B., and Landys, K.: Incidence and histopathology of metastases of mammary carcinoma in biopsies from the posterior iliac crest. Cancer, *44*:1782, 1979.

Riesco, A.: Five-year cancer cure: Relation to total amount of peripheral lymphocytes and neurophils. Cancer, *25*:135, 1970.

Robbins, G. F., Knapper, W. H., Barrie, J., et al.: Metastatic bone disease developing in patients with potentially curable breast cancer. Cancer, *29*:1702, 1972.

Robert, N. J.: Biologic indicators of prognosis in breast cancer. Hosp. Pract., *25*:93–102, 1990.

Robertson, J. M., Clarke, D. H., Pevzner, M. M., et al.: Breast conservation therapy: Severe breast fibrosis after radiation therapy in patients with collagen vascular disease. Cancer, *68*:502–508, 1991.

Roseman, J. M., and James, A. G.: The significance of the internal mammary lymph nodes in medially located breast cancer. Cancer, *50*:1426–1429, 1982.

Rosen, P. P., Braun, D. W. Jr., Lyngholm, B., et al.: Lobular carcinoma in situ of the breast: Preliminary results of treatment by ipsilateral mastectomy and contralateral breast biopsy. Cancer, *47*:813–891, 1981.

Rosen, P. P., Fracchia, A. A., Urban, J. A., et al.: "Residual" mammary carcinoma following simulated partial mastectomy. Cancer, *35*:739, 1975.

Rosen, P. P., Lesser, M. L., Kinne, D. W., et al.: Discontinuous or "skip" metastases in breast carcinoma: Analysis of 1228 axillary dissections. Ann. Surg., *197*:276, 1983.

Rosen, P. P., Lieberman, P. H., Braun, D. W. Jr., et al.: Lobular carcinoma in situ of the breast: Detailed analysis of 99 patients with average follow-up of 24 years. Am. J. Surg. Pathol., *2*:225, 1978.

Rosen, P. P., Saigo, P. E., Braun, D. W., et al.: Axillary micro- and macrometastases in breast cancer. Ann. Surg., *194*:585–591, 1981.

Rosen, P. P., Senie, R., Schottenfeld, D., et al.: Noninvasive breast carcinoma. Frequency of unsuspected invasion and implications of treatment. Ann. Surg., *189*:377, 1979.

Rosner, D., Bedwani, R. N., Vana, J., et al.: Noninvasive breast carcinoma. Results of a national survey by the American College of Surgeons. Ann. Surg., *192*:139, 1980.

Rosner, D., Lane, W. W., and Penetrante, R.: Ductal carcinoma in situ with microinvasion. Cancer, *67*:1498–1503, 1991.

Rubens, J. R., Lewandrowski, K. B., Kopans, D. B., et al.: Medullary carcinoma of the breast. Arch. Surg., *125*:601–604, 1990.

Ryu, J., Yahalom, J., Shank, B., et al.: Radiation therapy after breast augmentation or reconstruction in early or recurrent breast cancer. Cancer, *66*:844–847, 1990.

Santini, D., Taffurelli, M., Gelli, M. C., et al.: Neoplastic involvement of nipple-areolar complex in invasive breast cancer. Am. J. Surg., *158*:399–403, 1989.

Sariego, J., Kerstein, M. D., and Matsumoto, T.: Inaccurate staging in clinically node-negative breast cancer patients. Contemp. Surg., *43*:207–211, 1993.

Sauter, E. R., Eisenberg, B. L., Hoffman, J. P., et al al.: Postmastectomy morbidity after combination preoperative irradiation and chemotherapy for locally advanced breast cancer. World J. Surg., *17*:237–242, 1993.

Savlov, E. D., Wittliff, J. L., Hilf, R., et al.: Correlations between certain biochemical properties of breast cancer and response to therapy: A preliminary report. Cancer, *33*:303, 1974.

Scanlon, E. F., and Caprini, J. A.: Modified radical mastectomy. Cancer, *35*:710, 1975.

Schnitt, S. J., Connolly, J. L., Harris, J. R., et al.: Pathologic predictors of early local recurrence in stage I and II breast cancer treated by primary radiation therapy. Cancer, *53*:1049–1057, 1984.

Schnitt, S. J., Silen, W., Sadowsky, N. L., et al.: Ductal carcinoma in situ (intraductal carcinoma) of the breast. N. Engl. J. Med., *318*:898–902, 1988.

Schottenfeld, D., Nash, A. G., Robbins, G. F., et al.: Ten-year results of the treatment of primary operable breast carcinoma: A study of 304 patients evaluated by the TNM system. Cancer, *38*:1001, 1976.

Schuh, M. E., Nemoto, T., Penetrante, R. B., et al.: Intraductal carcinoma: Analysis of presentation, pathologic findings, and outcome of disease. Arch. Surg. *121*:1303–1307, 1986.

Schwartz, G. F., D'Ugo, D. M., and Rosenberg, A. L.: Extent of axillary dissection preceding irradiation for carcinoma of the breast. Arch. Surg. *121*:1395–1398, 1986.

Schwartz, G. F., Patchefsky, A. S., Feig, S. A., et al.: Clinically occult breast cancer. Multicentricity and implications for treatment. Ann. Surg., *191*:8, 1980.

Schwartz, G. F., Patchefsky, A. S., Finkelstein, S. E., et al.: Nonpalpable in situ ductal carcinoma of the breast: Predictors of multicentricity and microinvasion and implications for treatment. Arch. Surg. *124*:29–32, 1989.

Schwartz, F. F., Finkel, G. C., Garcia, J. C., et al.: Subclinical ductal carcinoma in situ of the breast. Cancer, *70*:2468–2474, 1992.

Sears, H. F., Gerber, F. H., Sturtz, D. L., et al.: Liver scan and carcinoma of the breast. Surg. Gynecol. Obstet., *140*:409, 1975.

Senofsky, G. M., Moffat, F. L., Davis, K., et al.: Total axillary lymphadenectomy in the management of breast cancer. Arch. Surg., *126*:1136–1142, 1991.

Shanta, V., Krishnamurthi, S., Sastry, D. V. L. N., et al.: Multimodal approach in the therapy of stage III female breast cancer. J. Surg. Oncol., *28*:134, 1985.

Sheldon, T., Hayes, D. F., Cady, B., et al.: Primary radiation therapy for locally advanced breast cancer. Cancer Arch. Surg., *60*:1219–1225, 1987.

Sherry, M. M., Johnson, D. H., Page, D. L., et al.: Inflammatory carcinoma of the breast. Clinical review and summary of the Vanderbilt experience with multimodality therapy. Am. J. Med., *79*:355, 1985.

Silverstein, M. J., Gierson, E. D., Waisman, J. R., et al.: Axillary lymph node dissection for Tla breast carcinoma: Is it indicated? Cancer, *73*:664–667, 1994.

Silverstein, M. J., Handel, N., Gemagami, P., et al.: Breast cancer in women after augmentation mammoplasty. Arch. Surg., *123*:681–685, 1988.

Silverstein, M. J., Waisman, J. R., Gamagami, P., et al.: Intraductal carcinoma of the breast (208 cases). Cancer, *66*:102–108, 1990.

Silverstein, M. J., Waisman, J. R., Gierson, E. D., et al.: Radiation therapy for intraductal carcinoma. Arch. Surg., *125*:424–428, 1991.

Sklaroff, R. B., and Sklaroff, D. M.: Bone metastases from breast cancer at the time of radical mastectomy as detected by bone scan. Eight-year follow-up. Cancer, *38*:107, 1976.

Smith, J. A., III, Gamez-Araujo, J., Gallagher, H. S., et al.: Carcinoma of the breast: Analysis of total lymph node involvement versus level of metastasis. Cancer, *39*:527, 1977.

Smithers, D. W., Rigby-Jones, P., Galton, D. A. G., et al.: Cancer of the breast: A review. Br. J. Radiol. (Suppl. No. 4), 1, 1952.

Solin, L., Recht, A., Fourquet, A., et al.: Ten-year results of breast-conserving surgery and definitive irradiation for intraductal carcinoma (ductal carcinoma in situ) of the breast. Cancer, *68*:2387–2344, 1991.

Spratt, J. S.: Realities of breast cancer control, public expectations and the law. Surg. Oncol. Clin. North Am., *3*:25–44, 1994.

Stablein, D. M.: A reanalysis of NSABP Protocol BO6. Potomac, MD, The EMMES Corporation, March 30, 1994, pp. 1–22.

Steinthal, C. F.: Zur Dauerheilung des Brustkrebses. Beitr. z klin. Chir., *47*:226, 1905.

Stokkel, M. P. M., and Petersen, J. L.: Angiosarcoma of the breast after lumpectomy and radiation therapy for adenocarcinoma. Cancer, *69*:2965–2968, 1992.

Stotter, A. T., Atkinson, E. N., Fairston, B. A., et al.: Survival following locoregional recurrence after breast conservation therapy for cancer. Ann. Surg., *212*:166–172, 1990.

Sugarbaker, P. H., Beard, J. O., and Drum, D. E.: Detection of hepatic metastases from cancer of the breast. Am. J. Surg., *133*:531, 1977.

Sunshine, J. A., Moseley, H. S., Fletcher, W. S., et al.: Breast carcinoma in situ: A retrospective review of 112 cases with a minimum 10 year follow-up. Am. J. Surg., *150*:44–51, 1985.

Swain, S. M.: Lobular carcinoma in situ: Incidence, presentation, guidelines to treatment. Oncology, *3*:35–51, 1989.

Tagert, R., Bratherton, D., Hartley, L., et al.: Partial mastectomy alone in early breast cancer. Br. Med. J., *290*:434, 1985.

Tarbox, B. B., Rockwood, J. K., and Abernathy, C. M.: Are modified radical mastectomies done for T1 breast cancers because of surgeon's advice or patient's preference? Am. J. Surg. *164*:417–422, 1992.

Tartter, P. I., Papatestas, A. E., Iannovich, L., et al.: Cholesterol and obesity as prognostic factors in breast cancer. Cancer, *47*:2222, 1981.

Tate, P. S., McGee, E. M., Hopkins, S., et al.: Breast conservation versus mastectomy: Patient preferences in a community practice in Kentucky. J. Surg. Oncol., *152*:213–216, 1993.

Temple, W. J., Jenkins, M., Alexander, F., et al.: Natural history of in situ breast cancer in a defined population. Ann. Surg., *210*:653–657, 1989.

The Uppsala-Orebro Breast Cancer Study Group: Sector resection with or without postoperative radiotherapy for Stage I breast cancer: A randomized trial. J. Nat. Cancer Inst., *82*:277–282, 1990.

Tinnemans, J. G. M., Wobbes, T., van der Sluis, R. F., et al.: Multicentricity in nonpalpable breast carcinomas and its implications for treatment. Am. J. Surg., *151*:334–338, 1986.

Toikkanen, S., Helin, K. H., Isola, J., et al.: Prognostic significance of *HER-2* oncoprotein expression in breast cancer: A 30 year follow-up. J. Clin. Oncol., *10*:1044–1048, 1992.

Tomin, R., and Donegan, W. L.: Screening for recurrent breast cancers—Its effectiveness and prognostic value. J. Clin. Oncol., *5*:62–67, 1987.

Townsend, C. M., Abston, S., and Fish, J. C.: Surgical adjuvant treatment of locally advanced breast cancer. Ann. Surg., *201*:604, 1985.

Turner, L., Swindell, R., Bell, W. G. T., et al.: Radical versus modified radical mastectomy for breast cancer. Ann. R. Coll. Surg. Engl., *63*:239, 1981.

Urban, J. A., and Marjani, M. A.: Significance of internal mammary lymph node metastases in breast cancer. A.J.R. Am. J. Roentgenol., *111*:130, 1971.

Valagussa, P., Bonadonna, P., and Veronesi, U.: Patterns of relapse and survival following radical mastectomy: Analysis of 716 consecutive patients. Cancer, *41*:1170, 1978.

van Dongen, J. A., Bartelink, H., Gentiman, I. S., et al.: Randomized clinical trial to assess the value of breast-conserving therapy in stage I and II breast cancer, EORTC 10801 trial. Monogr. J. Natl. Cancer Inst., *11*:15–18, 1993.

Veronesi, U., Banti, A., Del Vecchio, M., et al.: Comparison of Halsted mastectomy with quadrantectomy, axillary dissection and radiotherapy in early breast cancer: Long-term results. Eur. J. Cancer Clin. Oncol., *22*:1085–1089, 1986.

Veronesi, U., Cascinelli, N., Greco, M., et al.: Prognosis of breast cancer patients after mastectomy and dissection of internal mammary nodes. Ann. Surg., *202*:702–707, 1985.

Veronesi, U., Luini, A., Del Vecchio, M., et al.: Radiotherapy after breast-preserving surgery in women with localized cancer of the breast. N. Engl. J. Med., *328*:1587–1591, 1993.

Veronesi, U., Luini, A., Galimberti, V., et al.: Conservation approaches for the management of Stage I/II carcinoma of the breast. Milan Cancer Institute trials. World J. Surg., *18*:70–75, 1994.

Veronesi, U., Rilke, F., Luini, A., et al.: Distribution of axillary node metastases by level of invasion: An analysis of 539 cases. Cancer, *59*:682–687, 1987.

Veronesi, U., and Valagussa, P.: Inefficacy of internal mammary nodes dissection in breast cancer surgery. Cancer, *47*:170, 1981.

Veronesi, U., Volterrani, F. Luini, A., et al.: Quandrantectomy versus lumpectomy for small size breast cancer. Eur. J. Cancer, *26*:671–673, 1990.

Vicini, F. A., Eberlein, T. J., Connolly, J. L., et al.: The optimal extent of resection for patients with stages I or II breast cancer treated with conservative surgery and radiotherapy. Ann. Surg., *214*:200–205, 1991.

Von Rueden, D. G., and Wilson, R. E.: Intraductal carcinoma of the breast. Surg. Gynecol. Obstet., *158*:105, 1984.

Wade, P.: Untreated carcinoma of breast: Comparison with results of treatment of advanced breast carcinoma. Br. J. Radiol., *19*:272, 1946.

Wangensteen, O. H.: Remarks upon a more radical operation for breast cancer. Ann. Surg., *130*:315, 1949.

Wangensteen, O. H.: Further experiences with a cervicoaxillary mediastinal dissection for cancer of the breast. Ann. Surg., *132*:839, 1950.

Wangensteen, O. H.: Another look at super-radical operation for breast cancer. Surgery, *41*:857, 1957.

Wangensteen, O. H., Lewis, F. J., and Arhelger, S. W.: The extended or super-radical mastectomy for carcinoma of the breast. Surg. Clin. North Am., *36*:1051, 1956.

Wazer, D. E., Dipetrillo, T., Schmidt-Ullrich, R., et al.: Factors influencing cosmetic outcome and complication risk after conservative surgery and radiotherapy for early-stage breast carcinoma. J. Clin. Oncol., *10*:356–363, 1992.

Webber, B. L., Heise, H., Neifeld, J. P., et al.: Risk of subsequent contralateral breast carcinoma in a population of patients with in-situ breast carcinoma. Cancer, *47*:2928, 1981.

Weidner, N., Semple, J. P., Welch, W. R., et al.: Tumor angiogenesis and metastasis: correlation in invasive breast carcinoma. N. Engl. J. Med., *324*:1–8, 1991.

Weisberg, L. A.: The computed tomographic findings in intracranial metastases due to breast carcinoma. Comput. Radiol., *10*:297–306, 1986.

Weiss, M. C., Fowble, B. L., Sohn, L. J., et al.: Outcome of conservative therapy for invasive breast cancer by histologic subtype. Int. J. Radiat. Oncol. Biol. Phys., *23*:941–947, 1992.

Wheeler, J. E., Enterline, H. T., Roseman, J. M., et al.: Lobular carcinoma in situ of the breast. Cancer, *34*:554, 1974.

Wiener, S. N., and Sachs, S. H.: An assessment of routine liver scanning in patients with breast cancer. Arch. Surg., *113*:126, 1978.

Wilkinson, E. J., Hause, L. L., Hoffman, R. G., et al.: Occult axillary lymph node metastases in invasive breast carcinoma: Characteristics of the primary tumor and significance of the metastases. Pathol. Annu., *17*:67–91, 1982.

Williams, M. D., and Murr, P. C.: Paget's disease of the breast: Is breast-conservation therapy appropriate? Surgical Rounds, July 1993, pp. 521–527.

Wilson, L. D., Beinfield, M., McKhann, C. F., et al.: Conservative surgery and radiation in the treatment of synchronous ipsilateral breast cancers. Cancer, *72*:137–142, 1993.

Wilson, R. E., Donegan, W. L., Mettlin, C., et al.: The 1982 national survey of carcinoma of the breast in the United States by the American College of Surgeons. Surg. Gynecol. Obstet., *159*:309, 1984.

Windeyer, B. W.: Cancer of the breast. A.J.R. Am. J. Roentgenol., *62*:345, 1949.

Wiseman, C., Jessup, J. M., Smith, T. L., et al.: Inflammatory breast cancer treated with surgery, chemotherapy and allogeneic tumor cell/BCG immunotherapy. Cancer, *49*:1266, 1982.

Wolberg, W. H.: Surgical options in 424 patients with primary breast cancer without systemic metastases, Arch. Surg., *126*:817–820, 1991.

Wong, J. H., Kopald, K. H., and Morton, D. L.: The impact of microinvasion on axillary node metastases and survival in patients with intraductal breast cancer. Arch. Surg., *125*:1298–1302, 1990.

Wyatt, J., Sugarbaker, E., and Stanton, M.: Involvement of internal mammary lymph nodes in carcinoma of the breast. Am. J. Patho., *31*:143, 1955.

Young, J. O., Sadowsky, N. L., Young, J. W., et al.: Mammography of women with suspicious breast lumps. Arch. Surg., *121*:807, 1986.

Zafrani, B., Fourquet, A., Vilcoq, J. R., et al.: Conservative management of intraductal breast carcinoma with tumorectomy and radiation therapy (Abstract). Int. J. Radiation Oncol. Biol. Phys., *10*(Suppl. 2):140, 1984.

Zeman, R. K., Paushter, D. M., Schiebler, M. L., et al.: Hepatic imaging: Current status. Radiol. Clin. North Am., *23*:473, 1985.

Zippin, C.: Comparison of the International and American systems for the staging of breast cancer. J. Natl. Cancer Inst., *36*:53, 1966.

18 *Surgical Management*

John S. Spratt
William L. Donegan

The natural history of breast cancer is influenced favorably by a number of surgical procedures. Certain minor procedures are required for histologic diagnosis. These include core needle biopsy and open biopsy of the breast as well as excisional biopsy of regional lymph nodes. Therapeutic procedures include (1) removal of the breast either entirely or in part; (2) removal of regional lymph nodes, principally the axillary nodes; and (3) other operations for palliation or that facilitate nonsurgical treatment. These include oophorectomy, skin grafting, and establishment of venous access. This chapter discusses these operations as well as their indications and potential complications. Other chapters in this book address orthopedic, reconstructive, and thoracic procedures.

PREOPERATIVE PREPARATION

These operations are rarely performed as emergency procedures. Their elective nature permits optimum preoperative preparation. Such preparation should include appropriate staging, correction of concomitant problems to reduce surgical risk, consultation with specialists in other disciplines when advisable, discussion of alternatives with the patient, and obtaining informed consent. When hospitalization is necessary, preoperative testing and preparation are accomplished on an outpatient basis before admission (Edwards et al., 1988).

TIMING OF OPERATIONS

Some considerations relate to the timing of operations. First, when a biopsy is indicated, there is little reason to advise its delay. A negative biopsy result relieves the burden of continuing suspicion; a positive result expedites treatment. Second, when a biopsy demonstrates the presence of cancer, a period sufficient to permit staging and consultations is necessary. A delay of 2 or 3 weeks between biopsy and the initiation of definitive treatment (a "two-step" procedure) has no demonstrable influence on prognosis (Fisher et al., 1985; and Abramson, 1989). This fact permits the economy of an outpatient biopsy procedure, with preparations for treatment made only when therapy is necessary. Nevertheless, it is unwise to delay treatment unnecessarily. In some instances, such as when the presence of cancer is highly likely and preparations are complete, performing diagnosis and treatment at one operation (a

"one-step" procedure) may be mutually agreed upon by the patient and the surgeon.

When a mastectomy is planned, the option of breast reconstruction and its timing needs to be discussed with the patient preoperatively. The decision to be made is whether reconstruction is to be delayed or whether immediate reconstruction is to be performed at the time of mastectomy. If the patient is interested in reconstruction, delaying it for 4 to 6 months after mastectomy has some advantages. Postponement simplifies the initial decisions that must be made by the patient during a time of stress. It allows the first priority (i.e., treatment of the cancer) to be addressed on schedule and eliminates the risk of interruption or delay from the potential complications of the added surgical procedure. It also provides the patient an opportunity to consult at leisure with more than one plastic surgeon and to consider the several reconstructive options that are available. However, a growing number of surgeons advocate immediate reconstruction, pointing out that it avoids the need for a separate operation and has psychologic advantages for the patient that outweigh the risks of the additional surgery.

Whether operations on young women with breast cancer should coincide with a particular phase of the menstrual cycle is an unsettled issue. Laboratory studies indicate that operations on rodents during periods of unopposed estrogen stimulation (i.e., early or late in the estrus cycle) are followed by increased metastasis of implantable tumors (Hrushesky et al., 1988, 1989; and Ratajczak et al., 1988). A rationale is found in the demonstration that natural killer cell cytotoxicity is reduced in mice that have high estrogen levels (Hanna and Schneider, 1983). The clinical application of this finding is uncertain. In retrospective studies, attempts to confirm a relationship between operations conducted during a particular phase of the menstrual cycle and the prognosis of women with breast cancer have proved contradictory and inconclusive (Spratt et al., 1993; and Donegan and Shah, 1993). Perioperative influences on natural killer cell activity and on hormonal milieu are subjects of continuing investigation (Pollock, 1987; Uchida et al., 1982; and Fentiman et al., 1988).

BLOOD TRANSFUSIONS

The potentially adverse effects of blood transfusions have considerably reduced their use in operations for breast cancer. The risks of sensitization and transmission of disease (e.g., hepatitis and the human immunodeficiency virus

[Cummings et al., 1989]) are reasons for exercising prudence; in addition, transfusions possibly interfere with wound healing (Tadros et al., 1992). More relevant to oncology, the undesirable effects of blood transfusion include immunosuppression, which may have implications for the spread of cancer. The immunosuppressive effects of blood transfusion are well documented and are additive to those associated with the trauma of an operation. Operations themselves cause a variety of reversible immunologic disturbances that provide an opportunity for bacterial pathogens to enter the patient and that may potentially promote tumor cell metastasis. Circulating numbers of all T-lymphocyte subpopulations decrease following an operation, and approximately 1 week is required for their recovery; the degree and duration of immune depression are related to the magnitude of trauma (Lennard et al., 1985). Recovery of cellular immunity is more rapid than that of plasma reactants.

Transfusion of whole blood is known to impair cell-mediated immunity. Documented effects of transfused homologous blood products include an increase in the number of suppressor T-cells, a decrease in natural killer cell function, and a reduction in the function of macrophages and monocytes (Blumberg and Heal, 1989). Induction of anti-idiotypic antibodies known to suppress recognition of allogeneic antigens has been observed as have decreases in the alloreactivity of mononuclear cells in mixed lymphocyte culture. An associated clinical observation is improved survival of renal allografts in transfusion recipients (Fuller et al., 1982). That immunomodulation contributes to the potential for tumor growth and metastasis has been demonstrated in animal models. The metastatic ability of chemically induced mammary carcinomas in rats is influenced by the competence of host immunity (Kim, 1986). Transfusion of allogeneic blood in Wistar rats reduces lymphocyte reactivity and increases the growth of inoculated 3-methylcholanthrene–induced sarcomas (Francis and Shenton, 1981). The same effect is not seen with infusion of saline or syngeneic blood.

Whether perioperative blood transfusion affects the prognosis of patients with breast cancer remains unresolved. Tartter and coworkers (1985) compared the disease-free survival following mastectomy in patients who had received perioperative transfusions and those who had not. The two groups, which comprised a total of 169 patients, were comparable for type of mastectomy, hemoglobin level at discharge, cancer stage, and age. Survivorship at 1 year was 77% for those who received transfusions compared with 94% for those who did not. By contrast, Foster and colleagues (1984) conducted a similar study of 226 patients treated with mastectomy and were unable to confirm an adverse effect on prognosis associated with perioperative transfusions. Crowe and associates (1989) conducted a study of 812 patients with Stage I and Stage II breast cancers. The prognosis of patients with Stage II disease was not affected by perioperative transfusions; however, for those with Stage I cancers, the prognosis was compromised significantly.

The real and potential risks of blood transfusions have led to the undertaking of more precautions in blood banking and have emphasized the medicolegal implications of elective transfusions. The use of predeposited homologous blood is a relatively safe option when the need for transfusion can be anticipated (Toy et al., 1987; and The National Blood Resource Education Program Expert Panel, 1990). Informed consent for transfusion is also obtained whenever possible. In addition, the risks of transfusion have encouraged the use of surgical techniques that minimize blood loss and the need for transfused blood products (Waymack et al., 1986). With careful anatomic dissection and meticulous hemostasis, blood loss can be kept at a minimum so that transfusion of blood or blood products is required infrequently.

Indications for transfusion are being reassessed. Historically, maintenance of the hemoglobin level was used as justification for transfusion. The belief that a level of 10 g/dL or greater is required before elective surgery can be performed is a misconception (Zander, 1990). The oxygen transfer and carrying capacity of the blood, the amount of blood loss, and the patient's physiologic response to the loss should dictate transfusion needs. During an operation, the anesthesiologist has the capacity to monitor blood loss and oxygen carrying capacity of the blood. Relatively low hemoglobin levels can be tolerated, particularly by young patients, if the intravascular volume is adequately restored with electrolyte solutions. Postoperatively, administration of oral iron supplements to patients helps to reconstitute normal levels of hemoglobin. Erythropoietin administration is also an option (Dudrick et al., 1985). Until the question of whether transfusions promote tumor spread in humans is resolved, some have recommended the use of washed packed red blood cells or of washed frozen red blood cells when oxygen carrying capacity of the blood must be increased (Gantt, 1981).

Phlebotomy for diagnostic laboratory testing may result in blood loss sufficient to cause anemia and, hence, contributes to transfusion requirements. Smoller and Kruskall (1986) reported that patients in intensive care units with arterial lines have an average of 944 mL of blood loss per hospital stay that is attributable to phlebotomy. Among the 36 patients they studied, blood loss from phlebotomy contributed to the need for transfusion in 17. Routine phlebotomy orders that are not always appropriate and automated laboratory techniques contribute to patient blood loss. Blood-conserving procedures (e.g., pediatric sampling and batched collection) considerably reduce waste. Capillary tube sampling from finger sticks can often replace phlebotomy. Sound justification should exist for ordering each laboratory test that requires blood collection.

PROPHYLACTIC ANTIBIOTICS

The administration of preoperative antibiotics decreases the frequency of infections in patients following mastectomy. Platt and colleagues (1990) found that a single intravenous dose of cefonicid (a long-acting, beta-lactamase–resistant cephalosporin) administered 30 minutes preoperatively reduced infections after all types of breast operations from 12.2% (in 37 of 303 patients receiving a placebo) to 6.6% (in 20 of 303 of those receiving the antibiotic). Seventy-five per cent of wound infections and 72% of infections of all types occurred after patients left the hospital. Platt and colleagues concluded that the use of antibiotics reduced the occurrence of all infections by 48%. They also estimated that their use would prevent 56% of all infections as well as 23 wound infections and 16 urinary tract infections per 1000 patients. Urinary tract infections may have been associated with urethral catheterization. Since catheter-associated urinary tract infection remains the most frequently acquired nosocomial infection, the authors never catheterize patients electively for surgery of the breast. The effect of prophylactic antibiotic use in preventing infections in uncomplicated elective operations is greatest when the antibiotics are given preoperatively as opposed to intraoperatively or postoperatively (Classen et al., 1992). Beatty and coworkers (1983) reported a clean wound infection rate of 8.2% after mastectomy in 294 patients. The rate varied considerably as a function of the type and timing of diagnostic biopsy. The lowest rate of infection (3.2%) followed needle aspiration biopsies. With one-step incisional biopsy and mastectomy, the rate of infection increased to 5.3%. It was even higher (12.4%) when mastectomy did not immediately follow open biopsy (i.e., a two-step procedure). The rate of infections was highest when mastectomy occurred 4 to 7 days after open biopsy. These rates appear to be high; however, the presence of hematomas, drains, and infections in biopsy incisions may well contribute to subsequent infections, and efforts should be made to avoid them when biopsy is performed. The use of prophylactic antibiotics is useful, particularly in patients with conditions that predispose them to infection. Patients should be examined at intervals of several days after leaving the hospital to detect and abort possible delayed infections.

For patients predisposed to bacterial endocarditis, the recommendations of the American Heart Association should be followed (Dajani et al., 1990). Prophylactic antibiotics are specifically recommended for patients with prosthetic cardiac valves, previous history of bacterial endocarditis, most congenital cardiac malformations, rheumatic and acquired valvular dysfunctions, hypertrophic cardiomyopathy, and mitral valve prolapse or regurgitation. Oral prophylaxis with amoxicillin is recommended 1 hour before the procedure (3 g) and 6 hours after the procedure (1.5 g). For patients allergic to amoxicillin, erythromycin ethylsuccinate (800 mg) or erythromycin stearate (1 g) is administered orally 2 hours before the start of the procedure; 6 hours later, one-half the initial dose is given. Clindamycin may be used in place of erythromycin (300 mg orally 1 hour before the procedure and one-half of this dose 6 hours later). Consultation with a cardiologist is also helpful in managing patients at risk.

BREAST BIOPSY

Indications

The presence of a palpable mass confirmed as solid by needle aspiration or ultrasound or the presence of a suspicious lesion on mammography are the two principal indications for biopsy. Less frequently, suspicious nipple changes, nipple discharge, signs of inflammation, or skin retraction are indications. An accurate diagnosis requires close collaboration between the surgeon, diagnostic radiologist, and pathologist.

Core Needle Biopsy

Hand-Held Core Biopsy Needle. Tissue samples from palpable solid masses are easily obtained for histologic diagnosis with Tru-Cut disposable biopsy needles (Baxter Healthcare Corporation, Pharmacal Division, Valencia, CA) (Cusick et al., 1990). Biopsy of such masses is an office procedure that is performed using local anesthesia. Needle biopsy is restricted to the assessment of tumors that are larger than 2 cm in diameter and are not deeply situated in the breast. Selection of small and mobile masses increases the chance of obtaining a false-negative result. The technique for use of the needle is explained in the package insert and is illustrated in Figure 18–1. After injection of a local anesthetic, a small skin incision is made using sterile technique with a No. 11 blade at the point selected for needle entry. The surgeon must guard against penetrating the pleura, pricking the lung, and producing a pneumothorax. Whenever possible, the needle shaft should remain tangential to the surface of the thorax. The mass is stabilized during entry. One or two cores of tissue are taken and placed in fixative for permanent section or in saline for frozen section. Pressure is applied to the biopsy site for several minutes afterward, and a sterile dressing is applied. If a diagnosis of cancer cannot be made by the pathologist, an open biopsy is required. Open biopsy is performed in those patients who do not meet the criteria for core needle biopsy.

Stereotactic Core Needle Biopsy. The recent availability of stereotactic core needle biopsy equipment makes it possible to obtain histologic samples of nonpalpable lesions found on mammography alone (Hoeffken and Vaillant, 1985; and Parker et al., 1991). This technique employs local anesthesia and a specially designed table on which the patient lies prone with the breast hanging dependently through an aperture. The breast is compressed, and two radiographic images are made of it at angles. Using the trigonometry of right angles and a computer program, it can be determined how far into the still compressed breast a mounted, 14-gauge core biopsy needle is to be advanced in order to precisely engage the lesion (Figure 18–2). This can be achieved with an accuracy in millimeters. With the tip of the needle at the lesion, a core sample is obtained using a spring-loaded mechanism. This device prevents displacement of the lesion, which might occur if the needle were advanced slowly. Only a small stab wound on the breast large enough to introduce the needle is necessary. The sample permits a histologic diagnosis; therefore, a diagnosis of cancer is secure. The potential advantage is that a negative result may avoid the need for localization and open biopsy as well as the resultant scar and added expense that these entail. The procedure is subject to a small risk of sampling error. Preliminary indications are that 96% of cancers are correctly identified. Evaluation with wider clinical use will answer more completely questions about the technique's sensitivity, specificity, and overall accuracy.

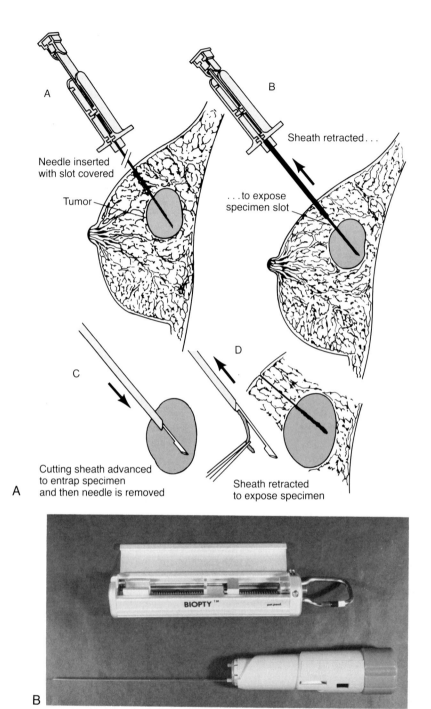

Figure 18–1. Core needle biopsy. *A,* The biopsy is taken under local anesthesia. A small incision, the width of the needle shaft, is made, and the shaft is inserted into the breast until the needle passes into the mass that is to be biopsied. The sheath is then retracted to expose the specimen slot, after which it is advanced to shear the specimen from surrounding tissues. In an alternative technique, the needle shaft is advanced into the breast until its tip meets the mass. The obturator alone is advanced into the mass, and the sheath is then slipped forward over it to entrap the specimen. The needle is removed, and gentle pressure is applied on the biopsy site for hemostasis. The specimen is delivered by retracting the sheath of the needle and picking it from the slot or washing it into a specimen cup with a bit of saline. Its size is adequate for a frozen section examination and for permanent sections but not for quantitative sex steroid analysis. Care is taken to avoid penetration of the pleural cavity, approaching tumors with the needle tangential to the chest wall.

B, Two automated core needle biopsy instruments are pictured, both of which are spring powered. Above is the reusable Biopty instrument by Radiplast AB of Uppsala. Below is the Monopty instrument available from Baird made for single use.

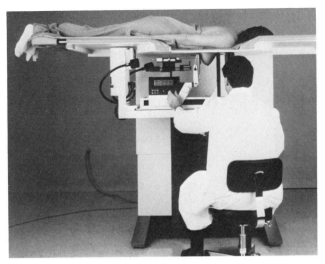

Figure 18–2. The steriotactic core needle biopsy apparatus allows histologic samples to be obtained from nonpalpable breast lesions by using multiple view mammography and a computer program to guide the biopsy needle. (Courtesy of J. Ziebart of Delta Medical Systems, Inc., Broofield, WI.)

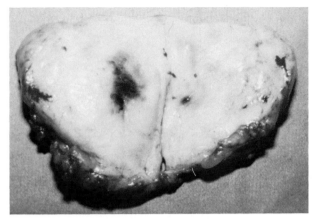

Figure 18–3. A biopsy specimen identified with a spot of methylene blue dye. Injection of the dye preoperatively into small or vaguely palpable masses contributes to accurate removal. If the spot is not found in the specimen, the lesion is unlikely to have been removed.

Open Biopsy

General Considerations. Open biopsies are routinely performed on an outpatient basis with sedation and local anesthesia. Ideally, they are done in a fully equipped operating room. Of primary importance is the collection of diagnostic tissue. If the suspicion of cancer was sufficiently great to indicate biopsy, the surgeon is obligated to accurately remove the lesion that gave rise to the suspicion, even if more than one attempt is required.

An incisional biopsy (a sample) of large tumors is usually satisfactory if it produces a diagnosis of cancer. For small lesions, excisional biopsies (complete removals) are performed; a margin of normal tissue is also excised if cancer is strongly suspected. Clear margins around small cancers may obviate the need for a further operation on the breast if the patient is treated with breast conservation (Fisher, 1985). Occasionally, small or vague masses that are palpable preoperatively cannot be readily identified after the incision is made. Injecting them with methylene blue preoperatively can be helpful when this problem is anticipated (Figure 18–3). During biopsy, the surgeon should try to avoid opening the deep pectoral fascia, which theoretically could contaminate a potential future plane of dissection between the deep pectoral fascia and the anterior surface of the pectoralis major muscle. Deep cancers may extend to the deep pectoral fascia.

Special situations sometimes pertain. When changes in the skin suggest the presence of inflammatory cancer, a sample of the involved skin is included for histologic study. A biopsy of the skin of the nipple should be performed if changes suggest Paget's disease (Figure 18–4). Occasionally, the surgeon encounters an abscess during biopsy. Such abscesses may be cancers with a necrotic center or areas of infection associated with a cancer. Rather than being content with mere drainage, the surgeon should secure a biopsy specimen of the wall of the abscess. Broad-spectrum antibiotics are administered until the results of bacterial staining, culturing (aerobic and anaerobic), and histologic studies have been obtained. When sensitivities are reported, more specific antibiotics can be used.

Technique. The location of an incision for open biopsy is determined by a number of considerations. Incisions should be placed directly over masses, particularly if the masses are likely to be malignant. They should lie within the bounds of a subsequent operation if one is required. Since a mastectomy is the most extensive procedure that may be necessary, incisions are best located centrally and in a transverse or diagonal plane. Radial incisions on the upper or lower part of the breast are neither cosmetic nor easily encompassed (Figure 18–5).

Because most biopsies are for benign conditions and will leave a scar, due consideration should be given to cosmetic results. The most cosmetic incision is circumareolar. The least obvious scars develop with incisions that follow the lines of cutaneous tension. In the supine position, these lines are concentric with the nipple. The situation is

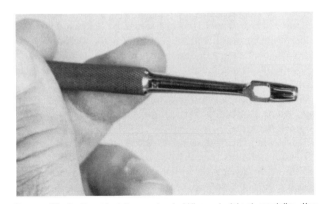

Figure 18–4. Punch biopsy tool. When twisted rapidly, the sharp round end of the instrument cuts a full thickness plug of skin. It is useful for sampling lesions of the nipple and skin. Disposable models are available.

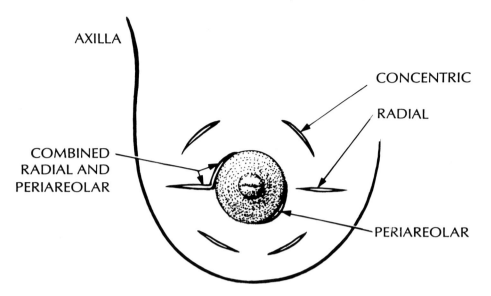

AXILLA

CONCENTRIC

RADIAL

COMBINED
RADIAL AND
PERIAREOLAR

Figure 18–5. Incisions for biopsy of the breast lie within the bounds of a possible future mastectomy and follow principles described in the text.

PERIAREOLAR

INCISIONS FOR BREAST BIOPSY

changed when the patient is in the upright position, in which gravitational stress on a heavy breast is radial to the nipple and most evident medially and laterally. It is also advisable to avoid placing incisions within 2 cm of the midline of the chest, since keloid formation is frequent in this area. Rather than make new scars, incisions are made through old scars if these scars are located in areas appropriate for biopsy. Normal subcutaneous tissue should not be excised; it is needed for cosmetic closure. Likewise, normally appearing fat should not be needlessly removed from the breast, as it contributes to the breast's volume and shape. Such fat is moved aside and not devitalized during dissection. In general, if a para-areolar incision is not feasible, incisions concentric with the nipple are best made in the upper and lower hemispheres of the breast; radial incisions are best made directly medial or lateral. Incision in the lower hemisphere is more problematic. Concentric incisions are usually best, but if considerable skin must be removed, radial incisions avoid downward displacement of the nipple.

The patient is positioned supine with the thorax elevated on the side to be biopsied. The ipsilateral arm is abducted to the side on an arm board. During the procedure, the patient monitoring includes pulse oximetry, blood pressure measurement, and continuous electrocardiography. Diazepam (Valium) is administered intravenously by slow injection (usually 10 mg) and ordinarily provides suitable sedation. It is given before the skin preparation and during the procedure, as needed. The skin is prepared with povidone-iodine (Betadine).

The anticipated incision is marked on the skin before the local anesthetic is injected. A local anesthetic that contains no epinephrine and to which the patient is not allergic is used (e.g., 1% lidocaine, or a mixture consisting of a 1:1 ratio of 1% lidocaine and 0.5% bupivacaine). The initial intradermal wheal is made using a 25- or 30-gauge needle. A small needle causes little or no discomfort to the patient.

Adding sodium bicarbonate solution to the anesthetic solution (1:9) further reduces discomfort by neutralizing the drugs' acidity. The dermal wheal is made along the length of the planned incision; the subcutaneous tissue is also infiltrated. Pinching the skin with a forceps is performed to test for adequate anesthesia. Then, the incision is made. After a pause to secure dermal and subcutaneous bleeders, it is extended down to the glandular tissue. No subcutaneous tissue is removed. The glandular tissue is separately innervated, and infiltration of anesthetic about the periphery of the target tissue is necessary before further dissection is undertaken. A "Z" stitch with 2-0 silk is used to secure the tissue and is used as a tenaculum. The tumor is then dissected sharply away from the surrounding tissues. Electrocautery is adequate for small bleeders. Ligatures are occasionally necessary and are placed about bleeding points with a medium-sized cutting needle. Figure 18–6 illustrates excisional biopsy of a small mass. If the tumor is large, only an incisional biopsy may be performed, but if a diagnosis of cancer is not forthcoming, the entire mass is removed. The specimen is placed immediately on crushed ice for transport to the pathologist.

Closure of the parenchymal defect is optional. If it is not closed, a small collection of fluid or blood may be anticipated; on the other hand, closure can result in undesirable distortion of the breast. No drains are needed, but hemostasis must be absolute. The subcutaneous tissue is closed with interrupted absorbable sutures. A running subcuticular suture of absorbable material is used to close the skin, and Steri-Strips are applied (after application of benzoin solution to the skin). A sterile, padded dressing secured with foam tape reduces breast motion and discomfort to the patient as does wearing a brassiere for several days. The tape must not be stretched taut, as this causes blistering of the skin; also, tape should not be placed directly on the nipple. The dressing is left in place for several days or until the patient's scheduled return to the office. The patient is

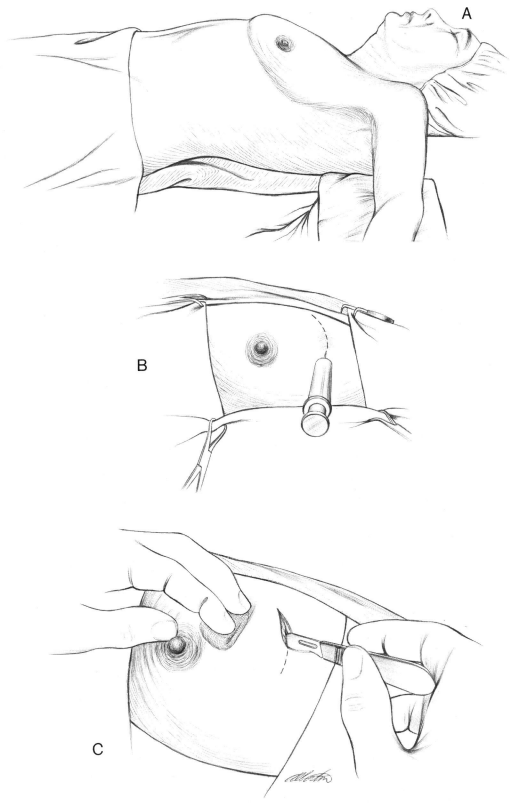

Figure 18–6. Technique for surgical biopsy of the breast. See text for details. *A,* Position of the patient. *B,* Local anesthesia. *C,* The incision.

Illustration continued on following page

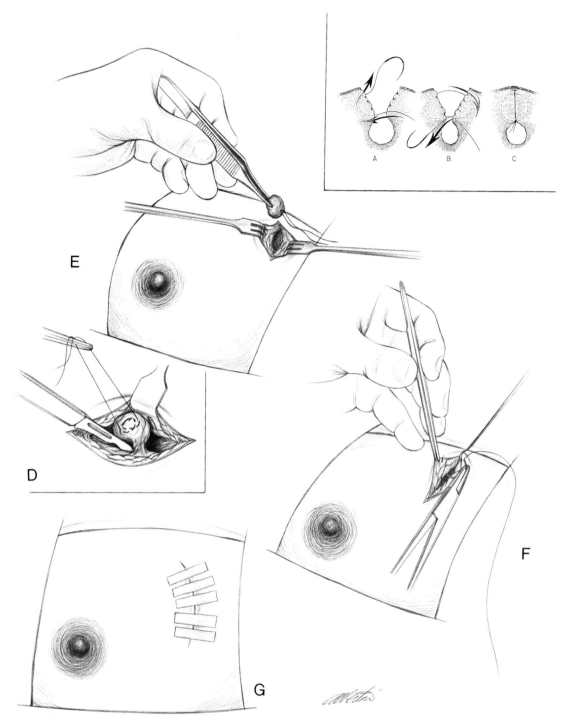

Figure 18–6 *Continued D*, Dissection. *E*, Removal of mass. *F*, Closure of subcutaneous tissue. *G*, Skin closed.

given written instructions and a prescription for analgesia, and an appointment for a follow-up visit is scheduled (Table 18–1).

Pathologic Considerations. A decision regarding frozen section is best left to the pathologist. With large lesions, frozen sections can permit an immediate diagnosis. Small or occult lesions may be best submitted entirely for permanent sections. Estrogen and progesterone receptor assays should be obtained on cancers (Table 18–2). Currently,

cytokinetic studies are also requested (e.g., S-phase fraction, ploidy, and DNA index analyses). Because estrogen and progesterone receptor assays have prognostic value and are considered in the selection of adjuvant therapy, care in handling tissues is important. The values obtained from preoperative biopsies and from tumors removed with mastectomy are not significantly different provided that the tissue is kept cold after removal and frozen rapidly (Bridges et al., 1983). Since the intraoperative period of devascular-

Table 18–1. INSTRUCTIONS FOR PATIENTS AFTER BREAST BIOPSY

1. Wear a brassiere for 3 days; it improves comfort and promotes healing.
2. Keep the bandage and incision dry for 1 week.
3. Take pain medication as needed. A prescription will be provided before you leave the hospital.
4. Schedule an office visit for 1 week from the date of biopsy.
5. The bandage can be removed after 4 days, but not the tapes on the incision. The tapes stay on for 7 days.
6. Call the office between 9:00 AM and 5:00 PM if you have problems (e.g., fever, increasing pain, or blood on the bandages).
7. If a problem arises at other times, go to the emergency room.

ization is not critical, it is not necessary to remove tumor tissue in advance of mastectomy specifically for this purpose. If cautery is used for dissection, care must be exercised to stay clear of the tissue to be analyzed. The heat of cautery kills tissue and may cause falsely low receptor values (Rosenthal, 1979).

Needle-Localized Open Biopsy

The procedure for open biopsy is modified if the objective is to remove a nonpalpable mammographically identified abnormality: needle localization is performed immediately before biopsy, and the patient arrives in the operating room with the localizing needle in place. The patient is accompanied by the localizing mammograms and the written observations of the mammographer. The incision follows natural skin lines, with the localizing wire entry site at the midpoint of the incision. An incision is made through the skin to the parenchyma. At the site where the wire enters the parenchyma, the glandular tissue is exposed in the plane between it and the subcutaneous fat, and stay sutures are placed in the parenchyma. These sutures are used for traction as the scalpel or cautery device is used to core out the cylindrical tract of tissue around the wire. If the spot technique of localization is used (which employs dye rather than a wire), the procedure is similar. At the point where the dye enters the glandular tissue, a strong stay suture is placed, and the tract of visible dye is dissected out with a surrounding core of glandular tissue to an appropriate depth. The diameter of the cylinder should be great enough to allow a margin of normal breast tissue around the lesion.

The specimen goes immediately to the radiologist for a radiograph of the specimen, which is compared with the original mammograms to confirm that the suspicious area has been removed; the surgeon is then notified regarding the results. If the lesion is not in the specimen radiograph, further tissue may be removed and similarly examined. Needle localization biopsy is successful in removing nonpalpable lesions in 86.4% to 100% (average = 97.6%) of cases (Reid et al., 1990). Between 10.7% and 30% of lesions prove to be cancers (approximate median = 18%) (Blichert-Toft et al., 1982; Proudfoot et al., 1986; and Meyer et al., 1990). With a marker in place to indicate the site of interest, the specimen and specimen radiographs are relayed to the pathologist for histologic section. Lesions requiring needle localization are frequently small and are best processed by permanent section, as frozen section risks loss of critical tissue. If cancers are diagnosed after fixation or are too small for biochemical hormone receptor analysis,

Table 18–2. HANDLING OF TUMOR BIOPSY SPECIMEN FOR BIOCHEMICAL STEROID RECEPTOR ANALYSIS

1. Receptor assays may be performed on primary tumors or metastatic lesions of all types. If requests for both are submitted, specimens must be identified separately.
2. Receptors are heat labile. A biopsy specimen should be transferred from the operation site on ice and handled at room temperature as little as possible. If the specimen is taken as part of the frozen section at diagnosis, keep it frozen. If the specimen is to come from the mastectomy specimen, the breast should be delivered directly to the pathologist who must excise promptly an aliquot of cancer to be placed on ice and sent for hormone receptor assays.
3. The specimen must be transported and stored dry. Hypertonic saline solutions interfere with some of the assay methods. *Formalin destroys receptors.* Sterility is not important.
4. The amount of material required is about 0.3 to 0.5 cm³ of solid tumor, trimmed of excess fat and of necrotic and connective tissues. These constituents add undesirable elements to the binding reaction. If the specimen weighs more than 0.4 g, the pathologist should divide the specimen into smaller portions before freezing. (Extra specimens are used for back-up.) Assays should not be performed on specimens for which no histologic confirmation is made.
5. Specimens may be frozen in the cryostat or ultrafreezer, or in liquid nitrogen. Store and transport dry, preferably in a clean plastic container. Use a waterproof marking pen to identify container. Do not use tapes and stickers that are easily detached at low temperatures. Do not include identifying slips in containers if they will be in contact with the specimen. If sent to the Hormone Receptor Laboratory by commercial carrier, the specimen must be packed with sufficient dry ice to last until delivery.
6. Accompanying papers must include the following:
   a. Patient's name, sex, age, hospital, and accession or admission number
   b. Surgery date and surgery number
   c. Requesting physician's name
   d. Pathologist's name
   e. Kinds of assays requested
   f. Billing address
7. Also submit other information regarding the patient's history, especially any previous hormone therapy that might influence steroid receptor levels. Pregnancy status must be stated for the same reason.
8. Mark outside clearly: BIOLOGICAL SPECIMEN; REFRIGERATE IMMEDIATELY; RUSH.

(Courtesy of James L. Wittliff, M.D.)

assay with immunocytochemical techniques is necessary. Postoperative care includes routine mammography of the breast 2 to 3 months after the biopsy to document that the target tissue has been removed and to provide a new baseline mammogram.

Microdochectomy

Microdochectomy is an open biopsy technique designed to discretely remove a ductal system (Locker et al., 1988; and Choudhury et al., 1989). It is used to investigate localized nipple discharge when no lesion is palpable or seen on mammography. Previous ductography may have demonstrated a filling defect, but this is not necessary. The procedure can be performed with the patient under local anesthesia. Caution is taken not to deplete the discharge with excessive examination prior to the operation.

The patient is sedated, and after the surgical field has been prepared and draped, the discharging duct is identified by gentle pressure in an area that produces a small bead of discharge. The duct is then cannulated by introduction of a small (size 3-0) lacrimal probe that has been placed through the plastic sheath of a No. 22 Angiocath (Fig. 18–7). Wearing a magnifying loupe during this part of the procedure is helpful. When the lacrimal probe has passed a few millimeters into the duct, the plastic sheath is advanced over it and the probe is removed, leaving the angiocatheter in the duct. Correct location is checked by pressing to ascertain whether the discharge appears elsewhere. A small (1-mL capacity) syringe filled with methylene blue solution is attached to the hub of the angiocatheter, and 0.4 to 0.6 mL of the solution is gently injected; care is taken not to rupture the duct with excessive pressure. Complete filling is promoted by continuing to inject as the catheter is removed. Any spill is washed away with saline or alcohol solution. After the duct has been stained, it can be easily identified during the operation.

After a local anesthetic is introduced, a para-areolar incision is made on the side corresponding to the location of the duct, and the areola is elevated in a subdermal plane until the ductal system under the nipple is reached. The blue duct is identified, isolated, ligated to avoid spillage, and transected just beneath the nipple. The duct and its entire system (dyed blue) is carefully dissected and removed, yielding a cone-shaped specimen with the ligated major duct at its apex. The specimen is submitted for pathologic examination with the description ''discharging ductal system,'' so as to alert the pathologist to the problem. It is particularly important to remove only the offending ductal system in premenopausal women so that the capacity to lactate is preserved. In postmenopausal women, this is not as important. In both instances, failure to remove the lesion accurately eliminates the symptom (i.e., the discharge) but allows a potentially dangerous lesion to progress occultly.

After complete hemostasis is obtained, the incision is closed without the suturing of the glandular tissue or the use of drains. Interrupted absorbable sutures are used to approximate the thin layer of subcutaneous tissue, and the dermis is closed with a fine, running subcuticular suture of absorbable material. Steri-Strips are applied to the skin, and the incision is covered with a soft, sterile dressing.

Complications of Open Biopsy

Complications of open biopsy are infrequent and rarely serious. They are minimized by adherence to aseptic technique and by scrupulous hemostasis. The most frequent complications are hematomas and infections. The delayed appearance of both may be increased by the use of epinephrine in the anesthetic. The authors do not use epinephrine. Pneumothorax is also possible.

Expanding hematomas occur within the first 24 hours after surgery and indicate continuing or delayed hemorrhage. Swelling of the breast, discomfort, and bloody incisional drainage are the signs of a hematoma. Appropriate treatment consists of reopening the wound under sterile conditions, the evacuation of blood, and the ligation of bleeding vessels in the operating room. The wound is reclosed with or without open drainage, depending on the circumstances. Oral antibiotics are prescribed. Stable hematomas are generally found at a follow-up visit as fluctuant fullness at the biopsy site often associated with dependent ecchymosis. The liquefied blood is aspirated with a needle using sterile technique as completely as possible on one or more occasions without reopening the wound; otherwise, healing is generally uncomplicated. If left untreated, a sizeable hematoma will eventually efface the overlying skin and drain spontaneously through the incision, risking infection and a poor cosmetic result.

Infections are caused by skin bacteria (usually staphylococci or streptococci) and are signaled by the presence of local pain and erythema. If pus is evident by drainage or fluctuance or is found on aspiration, the wound is opened, specimens are obtained for culture, and antibiotics are administered. The site is allowed to heal secondarily. If the signs are mild and an abscess is not evident, the prescription of warm soaks and antibiotics in addition to careful follow-up may be sufficient for resolution.

Pneumothorax during biopsy is due to accidental penetration of the anesthetic needle (or localizing wire) through a rib space that results in injury to the lung. The most common symptom of pneumothorax is sudden onset of chest pain that persists after the needle is withdrawn (Gately et al., 1991). Pain typically is experienced at the tip of the shoulder when the patient is upright; the patient may also complain of dyspnea. These symptoms should be evaluated immediately with radiography of the chest. Most cases of pneumothorax can be treated with simple aspiration and close observation; however, placement of a chest tube is occasionally required. Significant bleeding is unusual.

LYMPH NODE BIOPSY

The removal of lymph nodes for diagnosis is largely confined to the excision of a palpably enlarged axillary node when no primary cancer can be found in the breast; for staging, it is limited to the excision of an enlarged supracla-

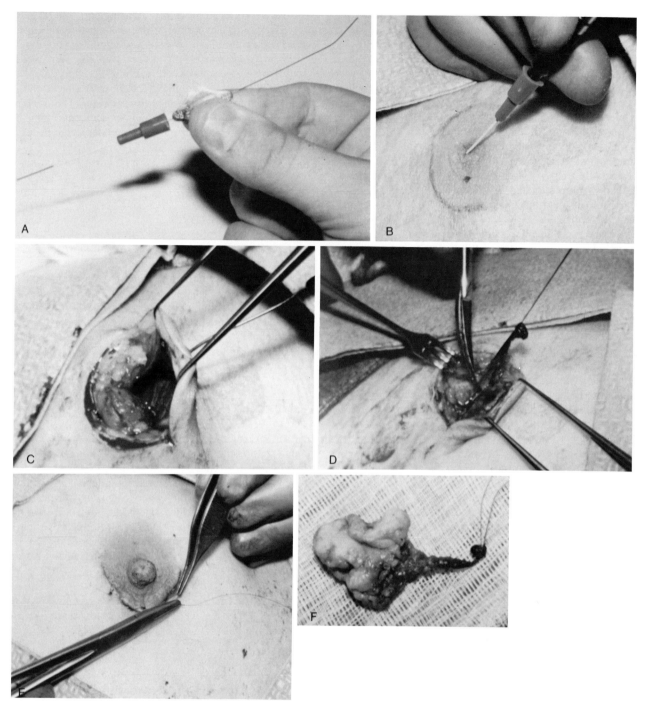

Figure 18–7. Technique for microdochectomy of a discharging duct. *A,* Lacrimal probe threaded through a No. 22 Angiocath sheath for cannulation of the discharging duct. After the probe is in the duct, the sheath is advanced over it, and the probe is removed, leaving the catheter in the duct. *B,* Methylene blue is injected into the duct through the catheter. The planned incision is marked at the areolar margin. *C,* The nipple is elevated in a subdermal plane to expose the stained duct. The lacrimal probe has been reintroduced in this case, but this is not necessary. *D,* The ductal system is dissected from the surrounding tissues. *E,* The incision is closed without drainage. *F,* The surgical specimen is shown with the apex marked with a ligature.

vicular or contralateral axillary node. These procedures are performed with local anesthesia, and the entire node is removed intact if possible. Incisions are placed in skin lines and are closed cosmetically without drainage.

Axillary incisions are placed two fingerbreadths below the most superior axillary fold and parallel to it. Deep to

the axillary fascia, an enlarged node can easily be felt and freed from the surrounding loose areolar tissues. Dissection is maintained close to the node, and care is taken not to injure the long thoracic and thoracodorsal nerves and the intercostobrachial nerve, all of which are in the vicinity of the axillary vein.

Adenopathy in the prescalene area lies deep to the platysma. Exposure is limited, and involved nodes are often matted. Biopsy is tedious, even for the experienced surgeon. Nearby structures at risk of damage include the internal jugular vein, recurrent laryngeal nerve, vagus nerve, phrenic nerve, and the thoracic duct, or the right lymphatic duct. Persistent postoperative lymphoceles are a vexing complication of injury to the lymphatic duct and often require reoperation for ligation of the duct.

Adenopathy in the posterior triangle of the neck tends to follow the course of the spinal accessory nerve, which crosses the triangle. Damage to this nerve by the unwary surgeon is not immediately apparent but eventually results in atrophy of the trapezius muscle and a debilitating shoulder drop.

Biopsy of an internal mammary node may also be performed for staging purposes either during mastectomy or if involvement is suggested by clinical findings or imaging. The internal mammary nodes contain metastases in from 4.5% to 26% (mean = 7.6%) of operable cases with tumors in the medial side of the breast when the axillary nodes are not involved (Morrow and Foster, 1981). Prognostic implications are similar to those for axillary metastases. Potential candidates are patients with an invasive carcinoma positioned medially in the breast and with axillary nodes that are clinically negative for cancer. The procedure is illustrated in Figure 18–8.

While the patient is under general anesthesia, a transverse skin incision is made at the first or second rib space near the sternal border to expose the pectoralis major muscle. When this procedure is performed in conjunction with either total or partial mastectomy, no extra skin incision is required, as the muscle is already exposed. The pectoralis major muscle is split in the direction of its fibers and, with avoidance of the anterior perforating vessels, the intercostal muscles are progressively transected to expose the internal mammary artery and vein, which lie just superficial to the pleura. Nodes lie in the fatty tissue surrounding these ves-

sels and are obtained by gently ''teasing out'' the fat extrapleurally. Since the normal nodes are very small, an enlarged node is usually obvious. The pectoralis major muscle is reapproximated over the defect, and the skin closed. Troublesome hemorrhage can be controlled through occlusion of the internal mammary vessels with a steel clip. A chest radiograph is obtained postoperatively. The principal complication is pneumothorax due to accidental puncture of the pleura; however, if the lung is undamaged, pneumothorax is not progressive.

MASTECTOMY

Total Mastectomy

Total mastectomy is the removal of the entire mammary gland. It is used to treat large sarcomas of the breast and multicentric ductal carcinoma in situ that has a low risk for occult invasion. It is also the appropriate operation for prophylaxis against future breast cancer (e.g., as an option bilaterally for women at high risk, such as those with lobular carcinoma in situ). Subcutaneous mastectomy is not an adequate procedure for this purpose (Goodnight et al., 1984).

Technique

The patient is in the supine position with the ipsilateral arm on an arm board. The legs are fitted with long elastic hose and elevated to a plane that is level with the atrium so as to avoid stagnation of venous blood in the legs and to reduce the risk of pulmonary embolism (Sabiston, 1981). If desired, the side on which the operation is to be performed can be elevated with a pad placed beneath the upper back. The skin is prepared and draped with sterile technique. The ipsilateral arm is wrapped and included in the sterile field.

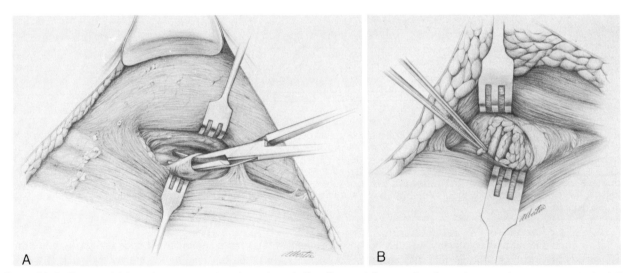

A   B

Figure 18–8. Biopsy of internal mammary lymph nodes. *A,* The fibers of the pectoralis major muscle are separated at the intercostal space selected for biopsy, and fibers of the intercostal muscles are progressively elevated with a clamp and divided. *B,* Nodes are teased out from around the internal mammary artery and vein with the fatty tissue. In closing, the muscles are not resutured.

The anticipated extent of flap development is marked on the skin. This line follows the clavicle to the anterior midline; it then passes inferiorly along the midline of the sternum. It courses laterally parallel to and 4.0 cm distal to the inframammary fold until the anterior border of the latissimus dorsi muscle is encountered. Then, it follows superiorly to the axilla, continues along the superior axillary fold, and finally joins the line of the clavicle at the deltopectoral triangle. Dissection beyond this line is unnecessary and only jeopardizes viability of the flaps. The skin incision is a diagonal ellipse that includes the areola and any biopsy incisions and that extends from the upper midaxillary line to the lower anterior midline. It is arranged to provide a minimum margin of 4.0 cm beyond any palpable tumor. Smoothly tapering skin flaps are developed from the incision to the peripheral line that was previously marked where the flap reaches full thickness. The breast and deep pectoral fascia are then dissected en bloc off the pectoralis major muscle and upper abdominal fascia, usually in a medial to lateral direction. Hemostasis is achieved chiefly with cautery. No attempt is made to remove axillary lymph nodes, but any breast tissue extending into the axilla is included with the specimen. Drainage catheters are placed medially and laterally in the wound and exit through the skin beyond the lower flap. Drainage through the axillary skin is avoided because of its high indigenous bacteria count. The catheters are attached to portable suction reservoirs. An airtight skin closure is required. Skin edges are approximated with absorbable subcutaneous sutures of 3-0 size. Staples or sutures may be used to close the skin. A subcuticular closure is the more cosmetic. The incision and catheter exit sites are dressed with gauze that is held in place with tape and a soft brassiere (Figure 18–9). Each suction catheter remains in place until its 24-hour drainage volume is less than 30 mL (usually by the 5th to the 7th postoperative day). Patients leave the hospital within 1 to 3 days with the catheters in place after being instructed as to how to measure and record the drainage at home.

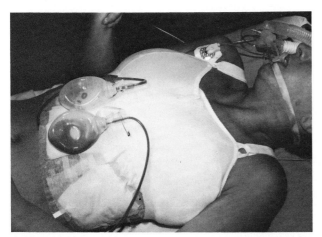

Figure 18–9. A soft brassiere with Velcro fasteners that is used to hold dressings in place on the incision after mastectomy or breast-conserving operations provides gentle pressure and avoids the need for tape. The portable suction reservoirs may be attached as shown.

Modified Radical Mastectomy (Total Mastectomy with Axillary Lymph Node Dissection)

This operation removes the entire breast and the axillary lymph nodes en bloc but not the pectoralis major muscle. By 1976, it had replaced the Halsted radical mastectomy as the most frequent operation performed in the United States for nondisseminated breast carcinoma. It can be followed by immediate or delayed reconstruction of the breast. Modified radical mastectomies vary mainly with respect to the extent of axillary dissection (Figure 18–10 identifies node levels). A low (Level 1) dissection is appropriate for patients with large or extensive in situ ductal carcinomas who are at some risk of occult invasion. For patients with invasive carcinomas, the lymph node dissection encompasses at least Levels I and II. If lymph nodes are involved clinically or pathologically, Level III lymph nodes are also included. Rotter's nodes, which lie along the thoracoacromial vessels on the underside of the pectoralis major muscle, are not removed routinely, but they can be dissected out as a separate specimen.

Technique

The patient is positioned supine. The entire anterior thorax, the abdomen above the umbilicus and the ipsilateral axilla, the shoulder, and the upper extremity peripheral past the elbow are prepared antiseptically (Fig. 18–11). Draping is performed so that the arm can be manipulated during the operation (Fig. 18–12). The anticipated extent of flap dissection is marked on the skin, and the skin incision and skin flap dissection proceed as described for total mastectomy As the breast is dissected off the pectoralis major muscle, a deep-lying cancer may be found to adhere to the muscle, or a previous biopsy cavity may be seen to have reached or entered the muscle. In these instances, the involved part of the muscle is included en bloc with the breast. This most often occurs laterally and simply involves removal of the lateral margin of the muscle.

For a Level I axillary dissection, nodes inferior to the axillary vein and lateral to the pectoralis minor muscle are removed with the breast. With a Level I and II dissection, the pectoralis minor muscle is retracted upward and medially to permit removal of the nodes beneath it as well. To also remove Level III nodes by the usual axillary route, the pectoralis minor muscle must be removed or divided. Patey (Patey, 1948; and Handley, 1965) totally excised the pectoralis minor muscle along with branches of the medial anterior thoracic nerve, which penetrates it. This paralyzes the lateral half of the pectoralis major muscle, and the result of this paralysis is cosmetically undesirable. The Scanlon variation of this procedure is preferred (Scanlon and Caprini, 1975). It divides the pectoralis minor muscle near its origin distal to the medial anterior thoracic nerve branches, thereby preserving the innervation of the pectoralis major muscle. An alternative approach to axillary dissection used selectively by one of the authors of this chapter (JSS) is as follows: when the breast has been reflected laterally, result-

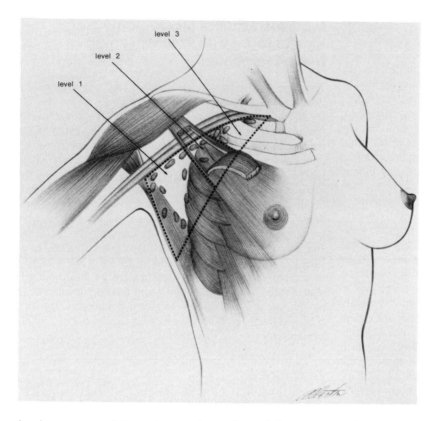

Figure 18–10. Surgical grouping of axillary nodes. Axillary nodes are divided into three levels as determined by their relationship to the pectoralis minor muscle. Level 1 (I) nodes are lateral to the pectoralis minor muscle. Level 2 (II) nodes are behind (deep to) the pectoralis minor muscle, and Level 3 (III) nodes are medial to the pectoralis minor muscle. Surgeons should indicate the levels that are removed with an axillary dissection.

ing in exposure of the entire anterior surface of the pectoralis major muscle, the avascular natural cleavage between the clavicular and the sternal portion of the pectoralis major muscle is opened for its entire length. Interpectoral nodes are seen in the fat about the nerves and vessels traversing this space. The node-bearing fat may be dissected away from the nerves, leaving them intact. Then, the pectoralis minor muscle may be transected at its origin on the chest wall, leaving enough muscle on the ribs to hold sutures when the pectoralis minor muscle is reapproximated. The divided pectoralis minor muscle is then rotated cephalad on its intact insertion. This tends to stretch out and expose the multiple muscular nerve branches traveling to both the major and minor pectoral muscles. With this exposure, complete axillary lymph node dissection may be performed by teasing fat and fascia away from nerves; in this way, good

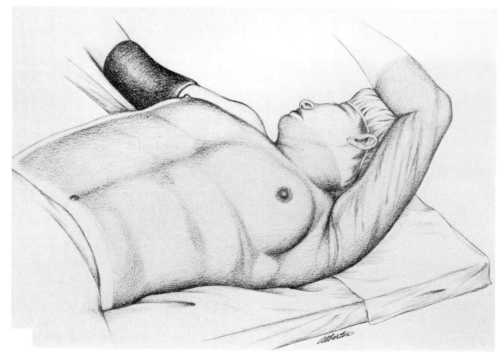

Figure 18–11. Extent of skin preparation for mastectomies.

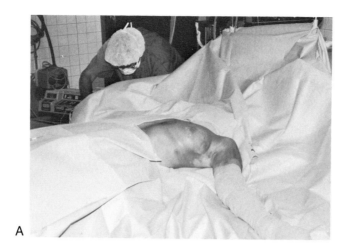

A

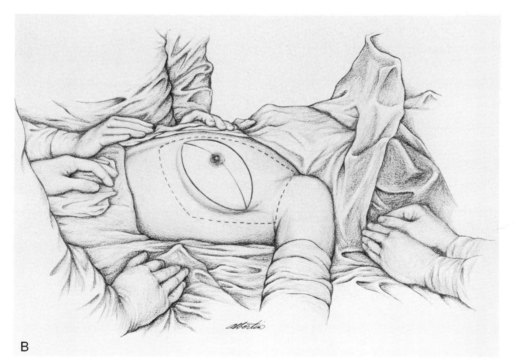

B

Figure 18–12. Technique of modified radical mastectomy. *A,* The upper extremity is draped so that it can be conveniently manipulated during the operation. *B,* An elliptical incision is outlined on breast. The *dotted line* indicates the planned extent of flap development. The area of anticipated skin flap dissection is encompassed by a line at the midline of the sternum, along the inferior border of the clavicle, following the course of the cephalic vein in the deltopectoral groove, across the axillary fold, along the latissimus dorsi laterally, and rejoining the midline inferiorly along the course of a line two fingerbreadths below the inframammary fold. A diagonal incision is fashioned, which reaches the midline anteriorly and to the lateral edge of the breast laterally. It encompasses the nipple, the tumor site, and any previous biopsy incisions. The upper and lower lines of the incision are deliberately made of equal length by measuring with a silk ligature so that the incision can be closed smoothly and without corrugations.

Illustration continued on following page

function of the pectoral muscles is ensured. Care is taken during the axillary dissection to preserve the long thoracic, thoracodorsal, and, if possible, the intercostobrachial nerves. The thoracodorsal vessels may also be preserved.

When the operation is complete, closed suction drainage catheters are placed in the wound—one medially, and the other in the axilla. The catheters are tunneled subcutaneously for several centimeters beyond the base of the lower flap before they exit the skin and are attached to portable suction reservoirs. If excess skin is present in the axillary region, it is trimmed to prevent redundancy. If the patient undergoing the operation is obese, it may be necessary to carry the excision beyond the posterior axillary line to accomplish this step. The wound is closed primarily with subcutaneous sutures and a subcuticular skin suture. Dressings are placed on the catheter exit sites and on the incision. The use of tape can be reduced by holding the dressings on the incision in place with a soft, fitted brassiere.

Text continued on page 466

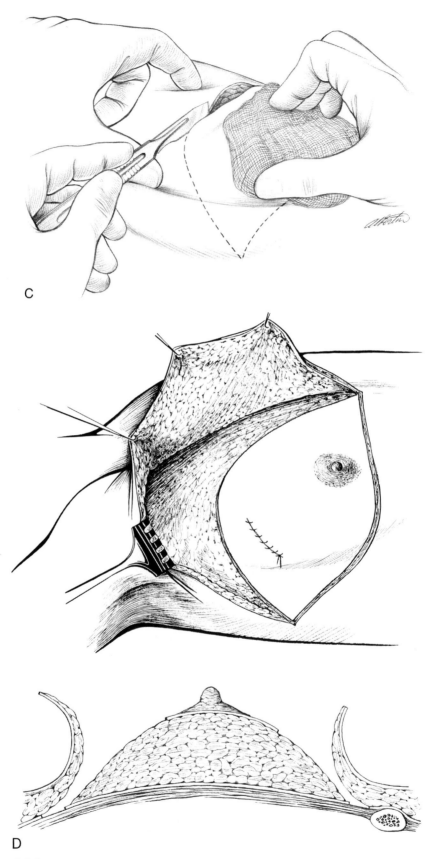

C

D

Figure 18–12 *Continued C,* The initial incision is made just through the skin so that the underlying fatty tissue bulges but is not incised. *D,* Superior and inferior skin flaps are raised, the former up to the lower border of the clavicle and the deltopectoral groove, and the latter to the border previously marked. Flaps are relatively thin so that no breast tissue remains on the flaps. They are retracted with skin hooks to avoid damaging and devitalizing the fatty tissue and are raised smoothly and with gentle tapering toward the base so that the blood supply from the periphery is not interrupted.

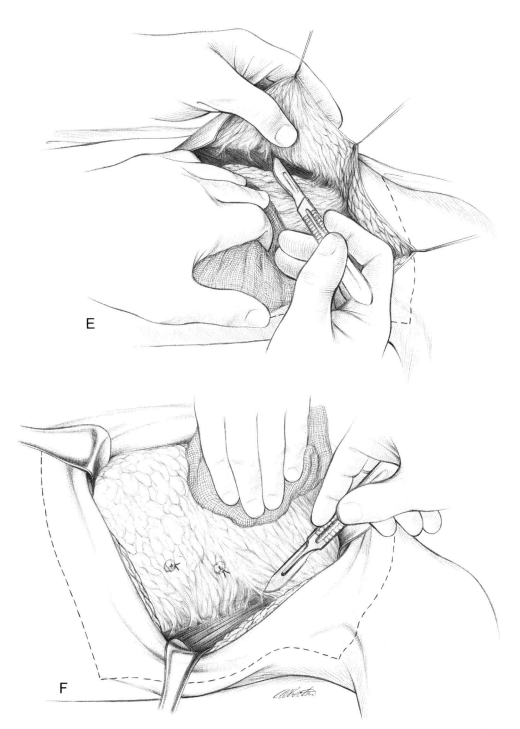

E

F

Figure 18–12 *Continued E,* At the free margin of the flap, approximately 0.5 cm or less of subcutaneous fat is left on the flap and this gradually thickens as the dissection proceeds toward the periphery until full thickness is reached at the lateral boundary. An important technique for continuous monitoring of flap thickness is for the surgeon's left hand to be placed behind the flap directly opposite the dissecting scalpel as shown here. An assistant's hand retracts the specimen. In this figure, the medial flap has been raised to the midline of the sternum. *F,* The lateral flap is raised to the anterior border of the latissimus dorsi muscle. Lateral perforating vessels are secured with ligatures in the process. The distal end of the latissimus is exposed to the limit of the lower flap. Toward the axilla, it is exposed until its tendinous portion becomes evident or to the level of the border of the pectoralis major muscle. In the process, the axillary flap is elevated from the underlying tissues. If the intercostobrachial nerve is to be preserved, the dissection toward the axilla is more limited in order to avoid accidental damage to the nerve.

Illustration continued on following page

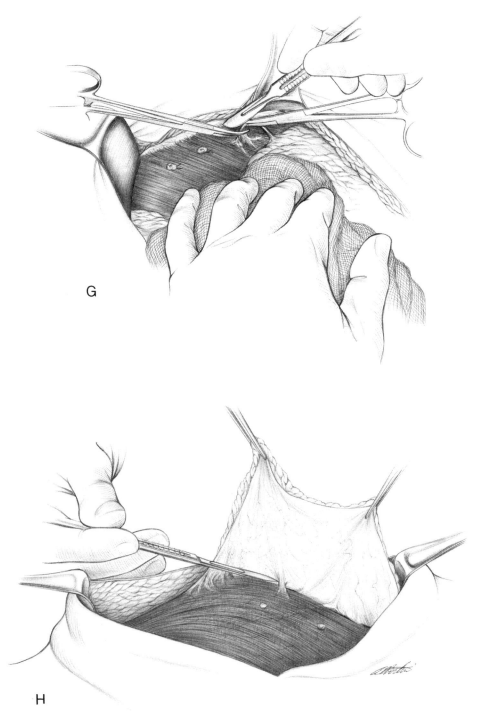

G

H

Figure 18–12 *Continued G,* Turning back to the medial side of the chest, the breast and deep pectoral fascia are elevated off the pectoralis major muscle, and the dissection proceeds from medial to lateral, securing the anterior perforating vessel in the process with clamps and ligatures of absorbable suture. *H,* Here, the deep fascia is shown raised off the pectoralis major muscle and the dissection approaching its lateral border. At the lower end, beyond the insertion of the pectoralis major, the deep fascia of the upper abdominal muscles is left intact and only the overlying tissues are included with the specimen.

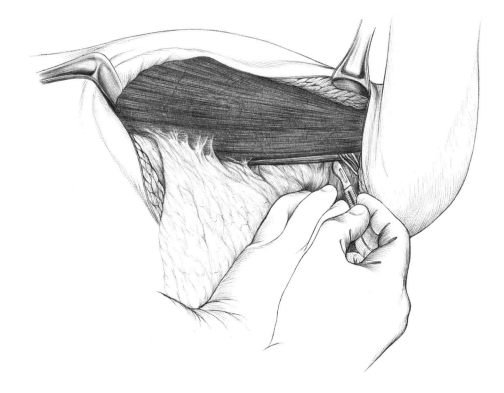

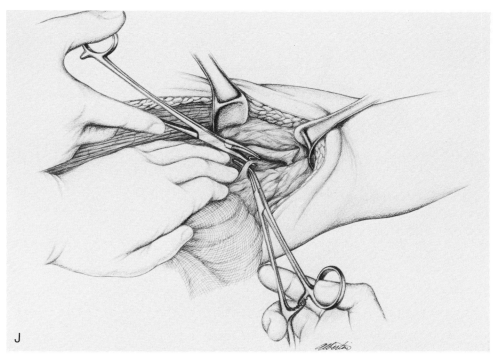

Figure 18–12 *Continued I,* The specimen is gradually dissected from the lateral margin of the pectoralis major muscle, and the shoulder is extended to relax this muscle so that the pectoralis minor can be exposed. The border of the pectoralis minor muscle is cleaned, taking care to preserve the medial anterior thoracic nerve (and accompanying vessels) that innervates the lateral portion of the pectoralis major muscle. These structures are shown here just superior to the scalpel. *J,* The axillary vein is exposed, and minor tributaries are divided between steel clips.

Illustration continued on following page

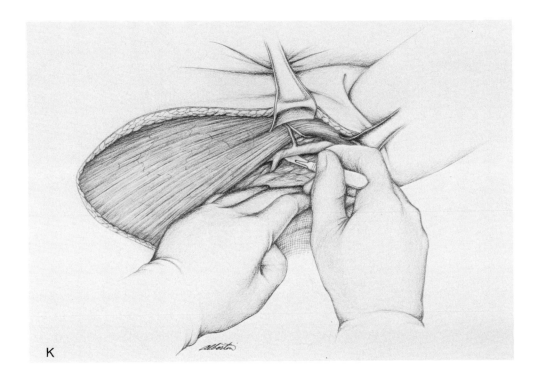

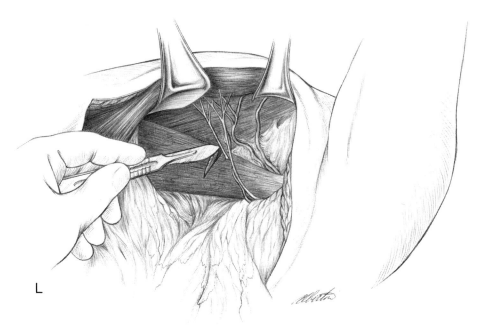

Figure 18–12 *Continued K,* The axillary vein is exposed from the latissimus dorsi to the pectoralis minor muscle. The external mammary vein (shown coursing inferiorly) and the accompanying artery are divided. The medial anterior thoracic nerve and vein (coursing upward) are protected. *L,* With the pectoralis major muscle retracted, the pectoralis minor muscle is divided distal to the medial anterior thoracic nerve and its branches, which course lateral to, and frequently through, the substance of the pectoralis minor muscle. More deeply in the wound arising medial to the pectoralis minor muscle and spreading on the posterior side of the pectoralis major are seen the lateral anterior thoracic nerve and the accompanying thoracoacromial vessels. These vessels and nerves are also protected during the dissection. Along their course lie Rotter's interpectoral lymph nodes in fat. These nodes may be removed by carefully defatting the nerves and vessels traversing the space between pectoralis minor and pectoralis major muscles.

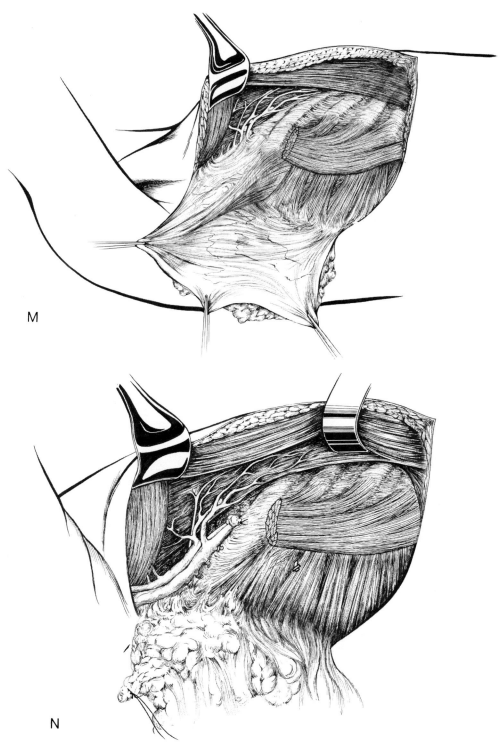

M

N

Figure 18–12 *Continued M,* With the pectoralis minor muscle divided, the upper portion is retracted on its insertion, and the axillary vein is exposed. The entire contents of the axilla to its apex, where the axillary vein crosses the first rib, can be cleaned of fatty node-bearing tissue. *N,* Dissection of the axilla proceeds from medial to lateral with the tissues of the apex marked with a ligature for the orientation of the pathologist. Branches of the axillary vein coursing into the specimen are divided between hemoclips; the ligated apical lymphatics, still in continuity with the axillary contents, are shown laterally. The preserved lateral anterior thoracic nerve and the thoracoacromial vessels are shown spreading on the underside of the pectoralis major muscle. Some of Rotter's nodes are also visible. In this case, the intercostobrachial nerve appearing at the second intercostal space has been sacrificed and is shown secured by a clip. Three to four centimeters more lateral, the surgeon can anticipate encountering the long thoracic nerve, which will appear in fatty tissues just off the chest wall and will course inferiorly and superiorly, crossing deep to the axillary artery and vein.

Illustration continued on following page

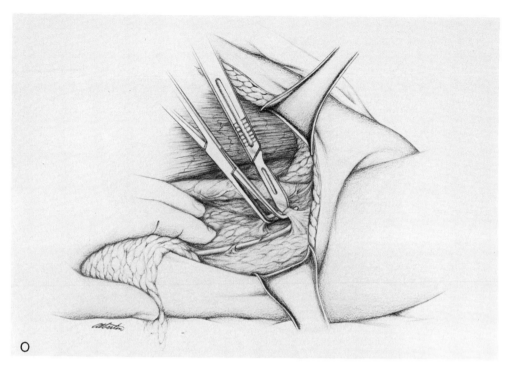

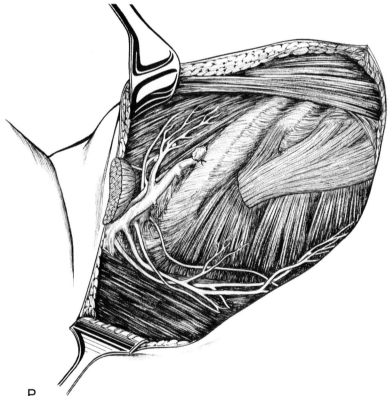

Figure 18–12 *Continued O,* In this figure, a technique is shown for freeing the intercostobrachial nerve when it is preserved. *P,* The axillary tissues are dissected off the subscapularis and latissimus dorsi muscles and finally off the border of the latissimus dorsi muscle, preserving in the process the long thoracic nerve, shown here lying along the serratus anterior muscle, as well as more lateral to it the thoracodorsal nerve, which innervates the latissimus dorsi accompanying the thoracodorsal vessels. It should be appreciated that this nerve appears from beneath the axillary vein and crosses laterally, usually superficial to the thoracodorsal vessels. Both the long thoracic nerve and the thoracodorsal nerve arise from the brachial plexus. The intercostobrachial nerve, which crosses the axilla from medial to lateral superficial to other structures, has not been preserved in this case. It is not necessary to reconstitute the pectoralis minor muscle, although it can be done. A contracted mass of muscle may be confused as a recurrence of tumor. Also, with healing, it may resume its normal musculoskeletal function.

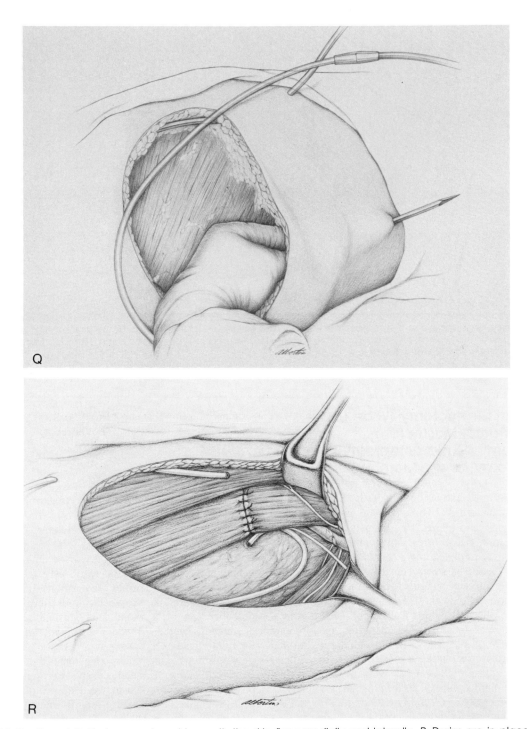

Figure 18–12 *Continued Q,* Drains are placed beneath the skin flaps medially and laterally. *R,* Drains are in place, and the pectoralis minor muscle has been resutured. Resuturing is facilitated by depressing the shoulder to bring the ends of the muscle into contact. The long thoracic and thoracodorsal nerves are shown appearing from beneath the axillary vein; the intercosto-brachial nerve, shown crossing them in this figure, is intact.

Illustration continued on following page

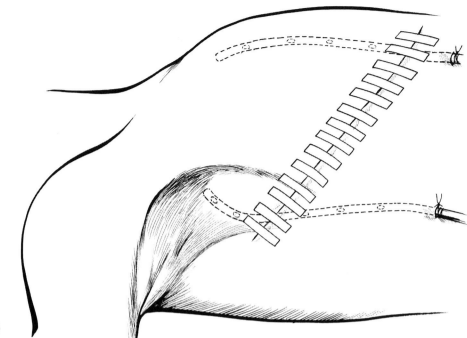

Figure 18–12 *Continued S,* The incision is closed with absorbable sutures to the subcutaneous tissues followed by a continuous subcuticular suture of absorbable fine suture and Steri-Strips. Alternatively, skin clips may be used in place of the subcuticular layer. A light dressing is applied to the incision and the catheter exit sites. A pad of fluffed gauze in the axilla stabilizes the skin. The arm is not restricted. Drainage from each suction catheter is measured separately, and each is removed when the drainage has fallen to less than 30 mL per 24 hours.

Segmental Mastectomy (Wide Local Excision, Partial Mastectomy, Lumpectomy, Quadrantectomy, Tumorectomy, and Tylectomy)

Breast-conserving operations for cancer have many labels and are not standardized. Their purpose is to provide a cosmetic alternative to mastectomy for patients with breast cancer that is in its early stages. The common objective of these operations is complete removal of the primary tumor while leaving the breast still acceptable from the cosmetic standpoint. The surgical margins around the tumor should be free of cancer histologically. The operations are accompanied by an axillary dissection and are followed by therapeutic irradiation of the breast. The operations are appropriate for treatment of localized ductal carcinoma in situ and of invasive carcinomas that are less than 4.0 cm in diameter and without extensive clinical involvement of the axilla. Standard contraindications to performing these operations include (1) the presence of poorly defined tumors; (2) the presence of multiple primary tumors; (3) pregnancy; (4) previous irradiation to the chest; (5) the presence of central tumors with involvement of the nipple; (6) the unavailability of facilities for radiation therapy; and (7) when a reasonable cosmetic result cannot be anticipated. The presence of an invasive carcinoma with an extensive intraductal component is considered a relative contraindication by some clinicians. If a previous excisional biopsy has resulted in

surgical margins that are histologically free of cancer, re-excision of the tumor site is not necessary.

Technique

The patient is prepared and draped to permit access to both the breast and the axilla (Fig. 18–13). The skin incision is made directly over the tumor following lines of dermal tension and includes any previous biopsy incision. In the upper breast, these lines are curvilinear and concentric with the nipple; medially and laterally, they are radial. In the lower hemisphere, the lines are curvilinear; however, when more than minimal skin excision is necessary, they are probably best made radial to avoid displacing the nipple downward. Neither skin nor subcutaneous tissue is routinely removed except when it is necessary to encompass a previous biopsy incision or extension of the tumor. No flaps are raised, and subcutaneous tissue is preserved as much as possible. Excision down to the deep pectoral fascia is not necessary unless required for establishment of a cancer-free margin. The tumor is excised sharply, preferably with a scalpel (the use of cautery can impair the histologic evaluation of margins). Generally, the tumor is removed along with 1 or 2 cm of normal surrounding tissue (approximately the breadth of one finger). Increasingly wide excision improves the prospects of obtaining a histologically normal margin but also increases the risk of producing deformity of the breast.

Text continued on page 472

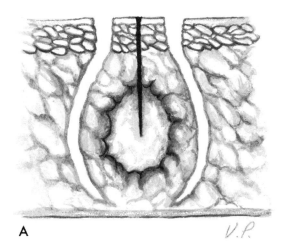

A

Figure 18-13. *A,* Schematic cross-section of the technique for thera-peutically excising a primary tumor mass that has been previously biopsied. The incisional biopsy tract is shown extending as a vertical line from the skin into the tumor. A modest amount of skin and subcu-taneous tissue is removed around the biopsy incision. At the junction between subcutaneous tissue and breast tissue, the excision is wid-ened to encompass the tumor mass with a margin of tissue that is palpably and visibly normal. The excision extends to, but not neces-sarily through, the deep pectoral fascia. If the tumor is small and has not previously been biopsied, this procedure can be performed as both an excisional biopsy and a therapeutic removal of the primary tumor. In this case, no skin or subcutaneous tissue is removed. Imme-diate examination by a pathologist to ensure that all margins are free of neoplasm is desirable. If margins are not free, a wider removal may be possible. If not, removal of the breast may be more effective than radiotherapy. *B,* Incisions for tumorectomy. In the upper hemisphere of the breast, they are transverse and curvilinear, following the skin lines. For deep-lying central tumors, a para-areolar incision may be used. Radial incisions in the lower hemisphere of the breast preserve the distance between the nipple and the inframammary fold and prevent downward displacement of the nipple. Curvilinear incisions in the lower hemisphere are preferred if excision of skin and tissue is not extensive. The incision for a tumorectomy is kept separate from that of an axillary dissection.

Illustration continued on following page

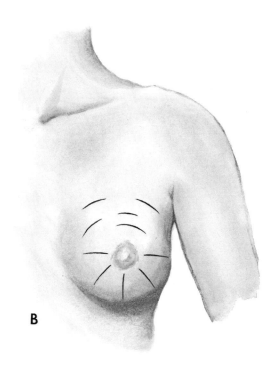

B

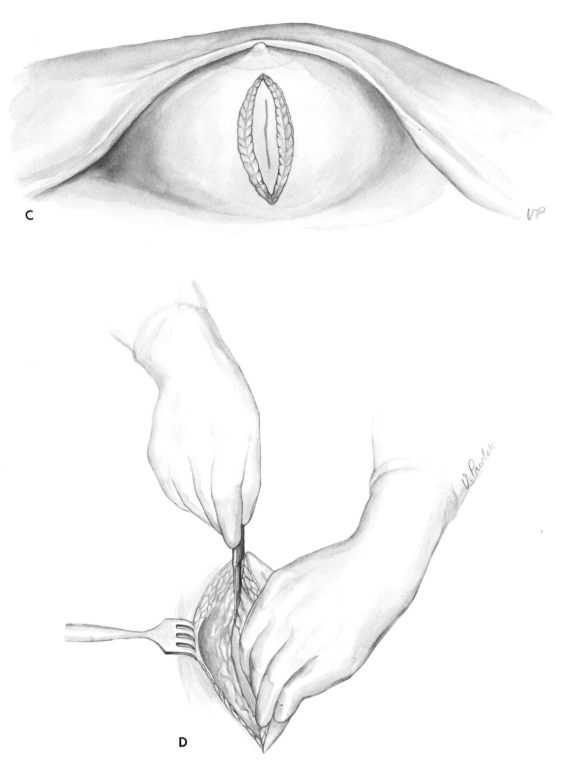

C

D

Figure 18-13 *Continued C,* Tumorectomy and axillary dissection are usually performed at the same operation, and the breast and axilla are prepared simultaneously. Tumorectomy is performed first; during this part of the procedure, the area of the axillary dissection is draped out of the field and is exposed later. This figure shows the initial incision around a previous biopsy incision. If estrogen and progesterone receptors were not obtained initially, the residual tumor in the breast may be assayed at this time. The initial incision extends around the previous biopsy incision and partially or totally through the subcutaneous tissue. Care is taken not to encounter the tumor mass or to break into the previous biopsy cavity. This tumor was in the lateral portion of the breast, and a radial excision was therefore performed. When possible, the incision avoids the areola. *D,* Once through the subcutaneous tissue, the incision is widened to ensure a tumor-free margin and is carried down to the pectoral fascia on one side. At this level, the deep margin is developed either deep to or superficial to the pectoral fascia.

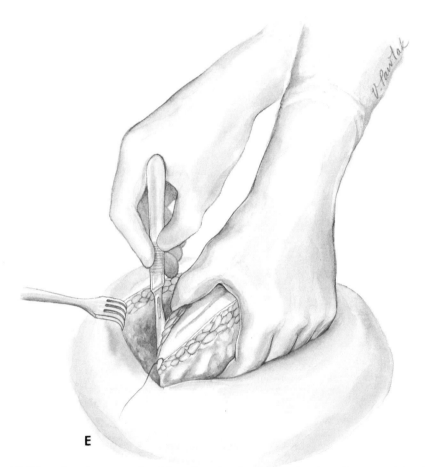

E

Figure 18–13 *Continued E,* When the deep margin of the dissection has been developed on one side of the involved area, fingers of the left hand are inserted beneath the tumor, lifting it, and using the thumb and tips of the fingers to identify a normal margin on the opposite side, which is then dissected. Silk sutures are placed at the margins of the specimen to identify its lateral and superior margins for the pathologist. The pathologist examines the specimen immediately and informs the surgeon whether margins are inadequate so that an additional margin of tissue can be removed if necessary at this point.

Illustration continued on following page

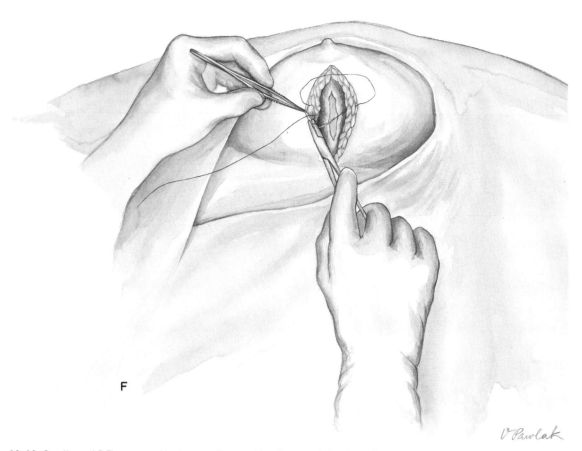

F

Figure 18–13 *Continued F,* The wound is shown after excision is complete. A portion of the deep fascia has been removed at the bottom of the wound with the specimen. It is not only unnecessary but undesirable to approximate breast tissue, as approximation distorts the contour of the breast. After meticulous hemostasis, it is usually unnecessary to use drains, but if the defect is large, a small closed drainage catheter that exits at a distance from the incision is used. The closure involves only the subcutaneous tissue and skin. The underlying cavity fills with serum, which is eventually absorbed and replaced with scar. The subcutaneous layer is closed with interrupted inverted sutures of 3–0 chromic catgut.

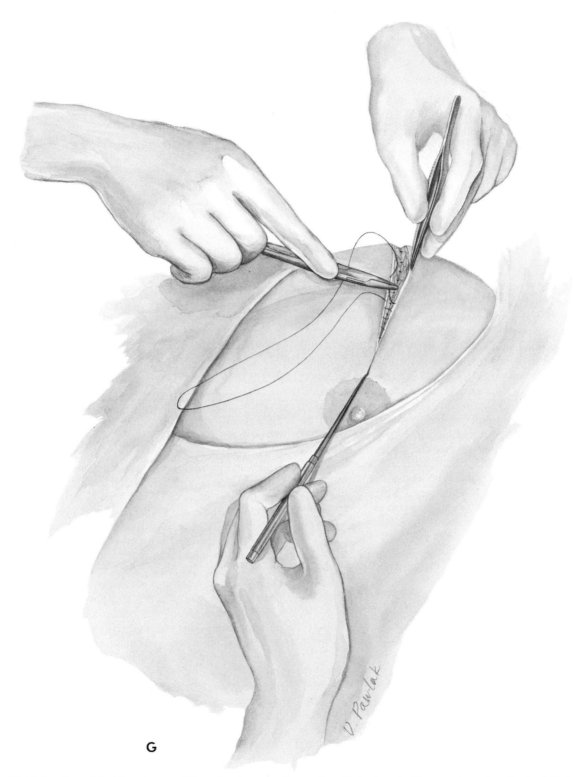

G

Figure 18–13 *Continued G,* After closure of the subcutaneous tissues, the skin is closed with a running subcuticular 4–0 absorbable suture. A skin hook at one or both ends is used to provide tension and facilitate suturing.

Illustration continued on following page

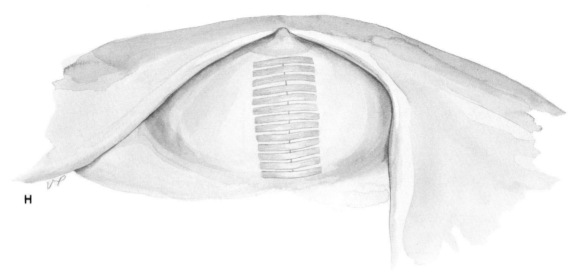

H

Figure 18–13 *Continued H,* Closure is completed by applying benzoin to the skin followed by Steri-Strips, which are left in place for 7 to 8 days. Induration at the site of excision will persist for 3 to 4 months as a result of the healing reaction. The tissue subsequently softens. An axillary dissection immediately follows this procedure. When it is completed, a light dressing is applied, and the patient wears a brassiere for several days to provide support for the breast and to improve comfort.

The specimen is oriented for the pathologist by placing sutures on it to identify the medial, superficial, and cephalic margins. It is submitted in ice and examined immediately by the pathologist both grossly and histologically. The surfaces are stained by the pathologist before sectioning so that surgical margins are evident histologically, and the surgeon is notified of the results. If a margin is involved, its location is specified so that the surgeon can remove additional tissue from the site, if feasible. The specimen is again oriented for the pathologist so that the new surgical margin can be assessed. With the persistent removal of margins that test positive for cancer, a point may be reached at which a cosmetic outcome is not possible and a mastectomy is preferable.

If hemostasis is complete, closure may be performed without drainage. However, if the resection is sizeable, a small (No. 10 French) suction drain is placed in the wound and exited from the breast separately, and it is removed on the 2nd postoperative day. The breast tissue is not closed with sutures. The subcutaneous tissue is closed with interrupted absorbable sutures, and the skin with a fine, absorbable subcuticular suture and with Steri-Strips.

Axillary Lymph Node Dissection

Axillary lymph node dissection permits pathologic staging of regional nodes and largely prevents recurrence of cancer in the axilla. It makes possible the most accurate assessment of prognosis and influences decisions regarding adjuvant therapy. It accompanies segmental mastectomy for the treatment of all invasive carcinomas and of in situ ductal carcinomas if nodal metastasis is likely.

Technique

A separate incision is used when axillary dissection is performed in conjunction with segmental mastectomy (Fig. 18–14). An incision that follows the natural skin creases of the axilla and one that is not apparent in the frontal view is preferred. Thus, the incision runs about two fingerbreadths below and parallel to the upper axillary fold, and it travels from the lateral border of the pectoralis major muscle anteriorly to the anterior border of the latissimus dorsi muscle posteriorly. Skin flaps are developed in the plane of the axillary fascia. The superior flap is of uniform thickness and is developed to the superior axillary fold. The inferior flap tapers distally for 3 to 4 cm toward (but not reaching) the chest wall. Then, in succession, the lateral borders of the pectoralis major and pectoralis minor muscles are exposed anteriorly (identifying and preserving the medial anterior thoracic nerve), the border of the latissimus dorsi muscle posteriorly, and the axillary vein superiorly. The axillary vein is exposed along its length from the latissimus dorsi muscle to the lateral border of the pectoralis minor muscle (for a Level I dissection), to the medial border of the pectoralis minor muscle (for a Level II dissection), or to where it crosses the first rib (for a Level III dissection). Inferior branches are divided between clips. The subscapular and thoracodorsal vessels are preserved. Node-bearing tissues of the axilla are divided at the appropriate level and tagged at the apex for identification by the pathologist. These tissues are dissected laterally off the chest wall while care is taken to expose and protect the intercostobrachial nerve, the long thoracic nerve, and the thoracodorsal nerve (in this order) (Fig. 18–15). The axilla is drained with closed suction until daily drainage volume totals are less

Text continued on page 478

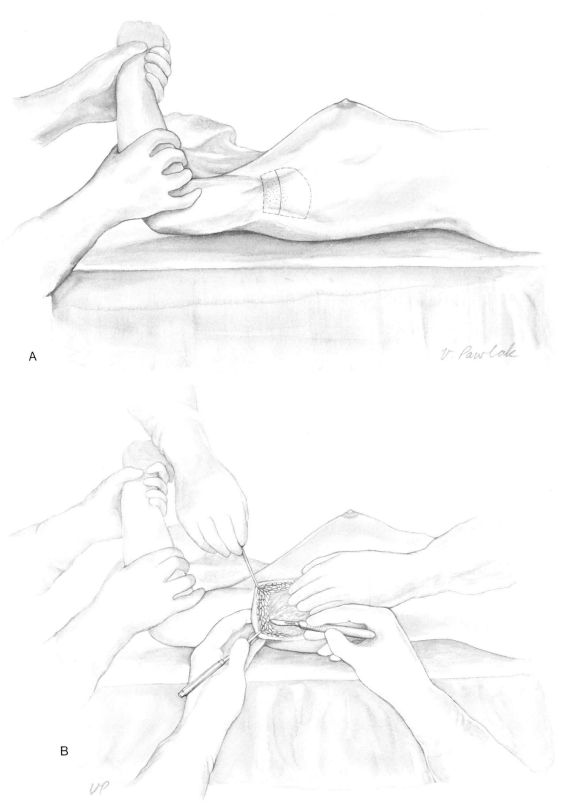

A

B

Figure 18–14 *A,* The incision for an axillary dissection is made transversely in the skin lines two fingerbreadths below the axillary fold and extends from the border of the pectoralis major muscle to the latissimus dorsi muscle. The incision is ordinarily just within the hairline. The extent of flap development is shown by the *dotted line* in the figure. *B,* The initial incision extends through the skin and subcutaneous tissue, and flap development is at the level of the axillary fascia. Flaps are developed with sharp dissection, using skin hooks to retract the skin edges. Uniform thickness of the flap is ensured by keeping the fingers of the surgeon's retracting hand exactly opposite the dissecting scalpel. The lower flap is thicker and tapers gradually toward the chest wall.

Illustration continued on following page

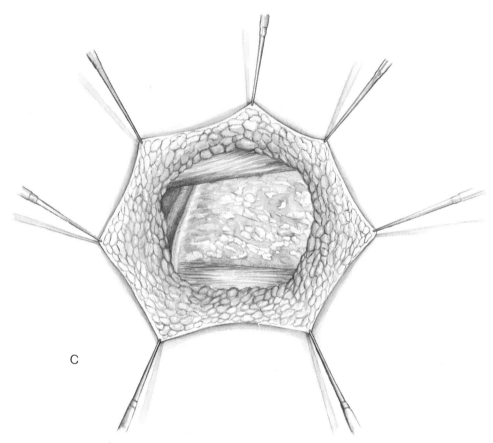

C

Figure 18–14 *Continued C,* With the skin flaps elevated, the anterior border of the dissection exposes the lateral border of the pectoralis major muscle. Posteriorly, the latissimus dorsi muscle is exposed, and superiorly, the axillary vein.

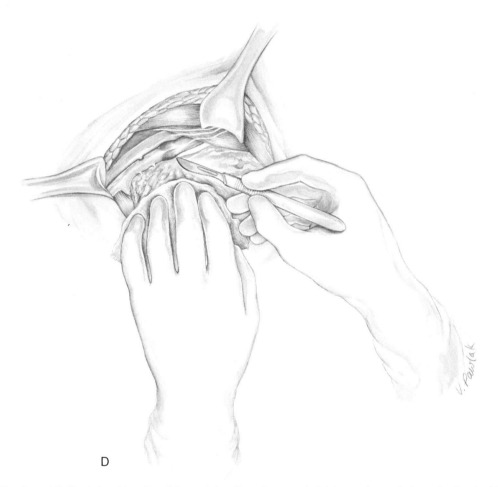

D

Figure 18–14 *Continued D,* The lateral border of the pectoralis major muscle is cleaned superiorly and retracted to expose the lateral border of the pectoralis minor. Crossing the latter, the medial anterior thoracic nerve and its accompanying vessels are found. These are preserved to maintain innervation to the lateral third of the pectoralis major muscle. These vessels are traced deeply and followed to their origin from the axillary vein, which is then cleaned from medial to lateral, the inferior tributaries being divided between hemoclips. The subscapular vessels, which disappear posteriorly between the subscapular and latissimus dorsi muscles and give rise to the circumflex scapular and thoracodorsal vessels, are left intact.

Illustration continued on following page

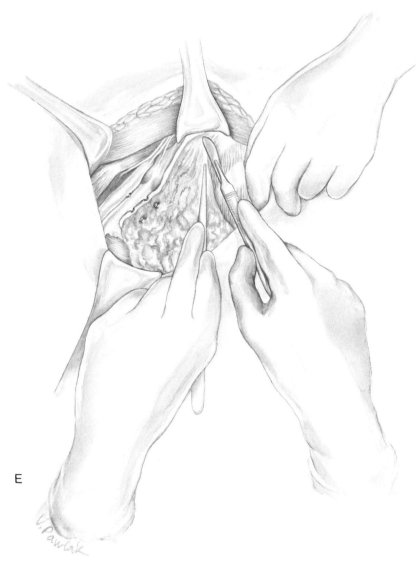

E

Figure 18–14 *Continued E,* With the shoulder flexed, adducted, and internally rotated, the pectoral muscles are relaxed, allowing them to be retracted medially and upward, exposing the axillary contents to the level of the medial border of the pectoralis minor muscle. This permits the surgeon to remove all Level II lymph nodes as well as those at axillary Level I. Here, the surgeon has reached the apex of the dissection. This point is marked with a silk ligature for orientation for the pathologist. All of the fatty tissues and lymph nodes of the axilla from this point laterally and inferior to the axillary vein are dissected off the chest wall as the specimen. The next major structure to be encountered is the intercostobrachial nerve, which appears with accompanying vessels in the second intercostal space. The advantage of sparing this nerve, when possible, is that sensation is preserved to the inner side of the upper arm (Temple and Ketcham, 1985). The nerve also serves as a landmark, indicating that the long thoracic nerve to the serratus anterior muscle will be encountered only 2 to 3 cm further laterally.

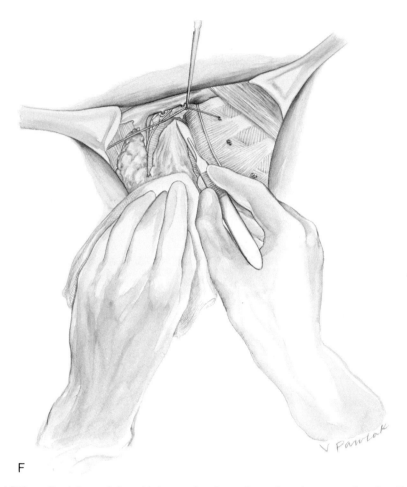

F

Figure 18–14 *Continued F,* Here, the intercostobrachial nerve has been traced and preserved, as has the long thoracic nerve. Dissection is never performed medial to the latter, as this will destroy the small slips that innervate the serratus anterior muscle. The dissection proceeds lateral to it until the fascia of the subscapularis muscle is incised. The thoracodorsal nerve, which curves laterally in the fatty tissues, is identified, and the node-bearing tissue inferior to the axillary vein, between the long thoracic nerve medially and the thoracodorsal nerve laterally, is dissected off the fascia of the subscapularis muscle from above downward en bloc with the specimen.

Illustration continued on following page

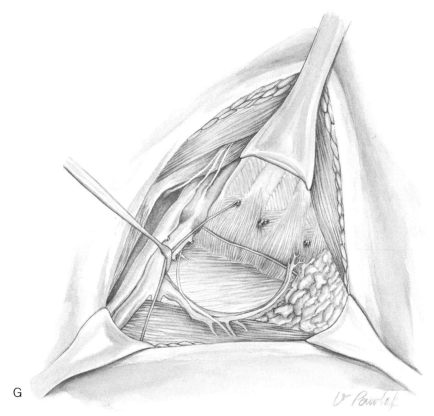

G

D Bawloj

Figure 18–14 *Continued G,* Here, the node-bearing tissue has been removed both medial and lateral to the thoracodorsal vessels and detached and removed from the fat and breast tissues attached to it inferiorly. Noteworthy is that the thoracodorsal nerve, after joining the vessels of the same name, crosses superficial to them laterally to innervate the latissimus dorsi, a point that should be kept in mind during the dissection. Furthermore, the nerve to the subscapularis muscle, shown here just beneath the axillary vein, is sometimes encountered during removal of the specimen from the fascia of this muscle and should be preserved. Also noteworthy is that the thoracodorsal vessels divide into branches that supply the latissimus dorsi and into those coursing medially into the chest wall. There is no need to interrupt either in the dissection. Damage to the long thoracic nerve produces an unsightly "winged" scapula. Damage to the thoracodorsal nerve paralyzes the latissimus dorsi muscle, which extends, adducts, and internally rotates the humerus, making it difficult for the patient to reach to her back. A single closed suction drain is placed in the incision, looping gently forward inferior to the axillary vein. It should not impinge on the vein. It exits through a stab wound 8 to 10 cm inferior to the base of the lower flap. Irrigation of the wound with warm saline removes loose fat and tissue particles.

than 30 mL. A No. 15 French round fluted drain is used for this purpose. It is curved anteriorly into the wound and exited low on the lateral chest wall. The wound is closed with subcutaneous sutures and a subcuticular suture to the skin.

Standard ("Halsted") Radical Mastectomy

This operation removes en bloc the breast, axillary lymph nodes, and pectoralis major and minor muscles. It routinely accomplishes a Level III axillary node dissection and removes Rotter's nodes. Radical mastectomy was the principal treatment for breast cancer in the United States until the mid-1970s, but by 1990 it was being performed in only 0.4% of patients (Osteen et al., 1994). It results in conspicuous deformity of the chest and is now reserved only for locally advanced cases of breast cancer, such as when a tumor extensively involves the pectoralis major muscle or

when a primary tumor is associated with extensive axillary metastases.

Technique

The patient is positioned on the operating table with the side on which the mastectomy is to be performed adjacent to the edge of the table. The ipsilateral arm is abducted. The field is prepared and draped to allow mobility of the upper extremity. The incision and skin flap development are the same as those for a total or modified radical mastectomy. When the periphery of the flaps is reached, the insertion of the pectoralis major muscle is transected in its tendinous portion, and the few vessels encountered are secured. The muscle is dissected away from the cephalic vein. The vessels and nerves that enter the superior margin and deep surface of the muscle are transected and ligated (Fig. 18–16 *A* and *B*). The clavipectoral fascia is then incised near the coracoid process, and the insertion of the pectoralis

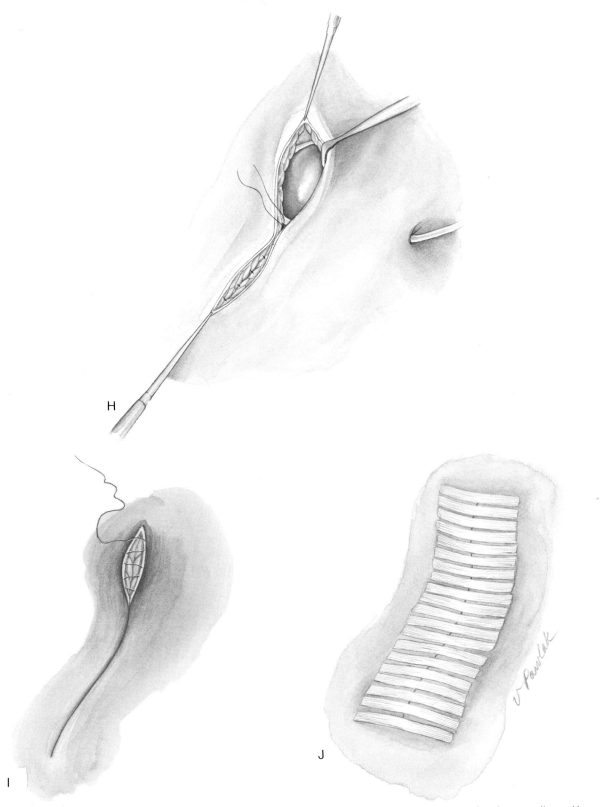

Figure 18–14 *Continued H,* The incision is closed with interrupted 3–0 catgut or Dexon sutures to the subcutaneous tissue. Here, the closed suction drain is shown in place. *I,* Closure of the skin is accomplished with a continuous subcuticular 5–0 absorbable suture. *J,* The skin closure is completed with application of Steri-Strips and a light dressing. No arm exercises are begun until the drains are out. Steri-Strips are removed on the 10th or 12th postoperative day.

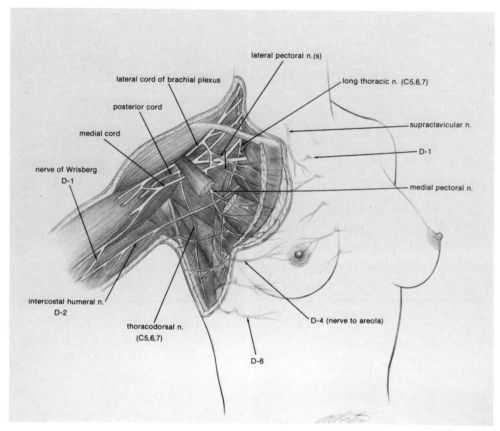

Figure 18–15. Major nerves encountered during axillary node dissections. Note the relationship between the intercostobrachial, long thoracic, and thoracodorsal nerves.

minor muscle is transected (see Fig. 18–16C). When this muscle has been folded inferiorly, its blood and nerve supplies can be identified for division and ligation. Dissection of the axilla is technically much simpler if at this time the pectoral muscles are transected at their origins; this permits the entire specimen to fall laterally and places traction on the axillary tissues. The pectoralis major muscle is first detached from the clavicle. A tunnel can be established digitally between the origin of the muscle and the anterior portion of the chest wall. Removing only the sternal portion of the muscle by splitting it in the direction of its fibers and by leaving the clavicular portion intact is an option. The sternal origin of the muscle contains the anterior perforating vessels from the internal mammary vessels, and these vessels must be secured as the origin is transected. When a cancer is present deep in the lower inner quadrant, the upper rectus sheath is included in the en bloc removal. The pectoralis major muscle is reflected off the loose fascia of the chest wall. When the origin of the pectoralis minor muscle from the third to the fifth ribs has been reached, the muscle is divided. After mobilizing the specimen from the serratus anterior muscle, it falls laterally to expose the axilla. Fascia enveloping the axillary vein and artery is now under tension (Fig. 18–17). The axillary vein is exposed and cleaned from beneath the clavicle medially to the latissimus dorsi muscle laterally. Venous tributaries from the breast and axilla are ligated as they enter the vein; the subscapular vessels are spared. Appearing on the lateral

chest wall beneath the axillary vein is the nerve to the serratus anterior muscle (the long thoracic nerve); the specimen is freed from this nerve, with special care taken so as not to injure it (Fig. 18–18A). Appearing from beneath the axillary vein at a more lateral point is the thoracodorsal nerve, which joins the thoracodorsal vessels on its course to the latissimus dorsi muscle. This nerve is also preserved. Laterally, the axillary fat containing the lymphatics from the arm is transected over the tendon of the latissimus dorsi muscle. The fat is then reflected medially to expose the subscapular muscle. Caution is exercised to avoid injuring the nerve to this muscle, which lies on the muscle's surface. The axillary contents are mobilized inferiorly by dividing and securing the remaining vessels along the margin of the latissimus dorsi muscle; the specimen is then removed (see Fig. 18–18B). Two suction catheters are placed, and the wound is closed as described earlier for modified radical mastectomy.

Internal Mammary Lymph Node Dissection with Mastectomy (Extended Radical Mastectomy)

The internal mammary lymph nodes are a frequent site of metastasis from breast cancer. This once led to their routine removal as an extension of radical mastectomy. Controlled studies indicate that such removal reduces parasternal re-

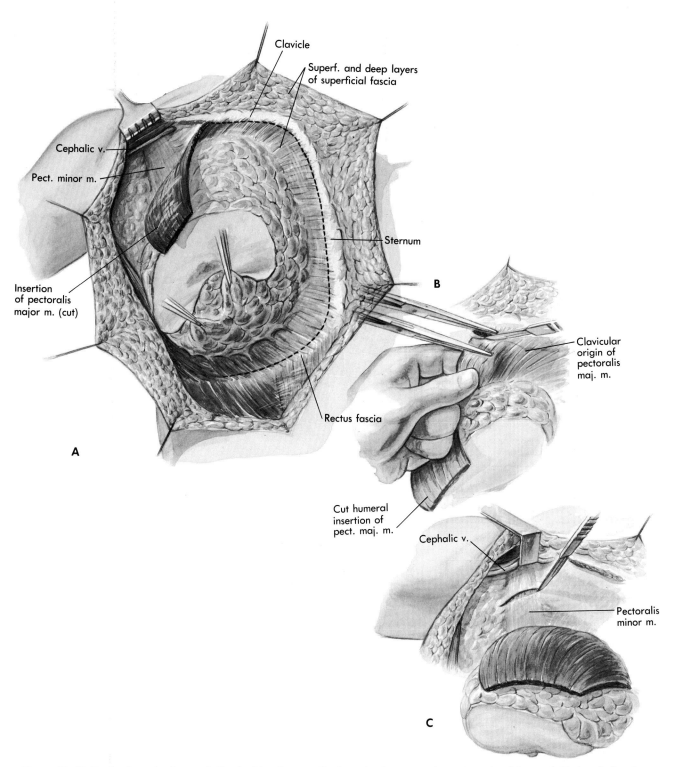

Figure 18–16. Radical mastectomy. *A,* The incision for a radical mastectomy requires a margin of 4 cm of skin in all directions around the palpable margin of the cancer, including the areola. Cutaneous flaps are elevated in a relatively avascular plane between the dermis and the superficial layer of superficial fascia to the midline of the sternum, the clavicle, the deltopectoral groove containing the cephalic vein, the insertion of the pectoralis major muscle, the latissimus dorsi muscle, and across the lower thorax at the level of the rectus sheath. At this periphery, the superficial and deep layers of superficial fascia and the panniculus between them are incised down to the underlying deep fascia and muscles. *B,* The pectoralis major muscle is separated from the humerus at its tendinous insertion, and the upper belly is folded caudally to its clavicular origin. As this is done, muscular branches of the acromiothoracic artery and the nerve to the pectoralis major muscle will be ligated and transected. As the clavicular origin of the muscle is approached, this is transected between clamps. Subsequently, the muscle ends are suture ligated. *C,* The clavipectoral fascia overlying the pectoralis minor muscle is incised. Subsequently, the muscle will be transected near the coracoid process. As it is folded caudally, its blood and nerve supply are similarly ligated and transected. The fascia is separated from the thoracic wall medially, and the origins of the pectoralis minor muscle on the third, fourth, and fifth ribs are identified and transected.

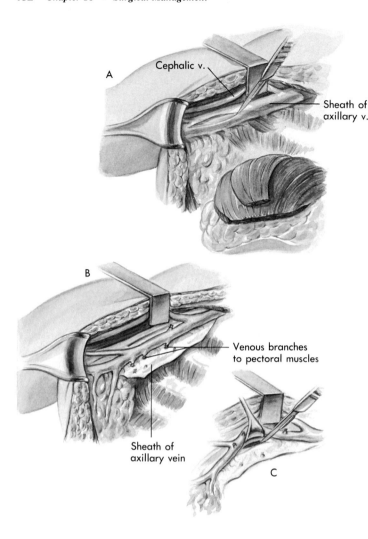

Figure 18–17. Radical mastectomy *Continued. A,* The sheath of the axillary vein is incised near its upper margin and is reflected inferiorly off the vein. As the sheath is reflected, individual venous branches are ligated and transected on the venous side of the sheath. *B,* This reflection is carried out over the entire length of the axillary vein from the clavicle to the tendon of the latissimus dorsi muscle. *C,* The thin sheath of the vein is transected a second time along the dorsal caudal surface of the vein to continue the en bloc mobilization of the axillary contents.

currences of cancer but achieves no increase in the rate of cure (Veronesi and Valagussa, 1981; and LaCour et al., 1983). Radiotherapy is also effective in reducing parasternal recurrences when a patient's risk for this problem is high. At present, extended radical mastectomy is rarely employed in the United States, but it is still used in some parts of the world.

Technique

For resection of the internal mammary lymph nodes en bloc with radical mastectomy, the skin incision is fashioned so that it does not cross the anticipated chest wall defect; after the skin flaps are raised, the origin of the pectoralis major muscle is left in continuity with the portion of the chest wall to be resected. At the first intercostal space, the medial fibers of the pectoralis major muscle are split, and the intercostal muscles are divided from the sternal border to about 3 cm laterally. This exposes the internal mammary vessels, which are ligated and divided (Fig. 18–19A). A similar maneuver is performed in the fifth intercostal space. Deep to the pectoralis major muscle, a tunnel is established digitally just lateral to the muscle's origin. A Lebsche sternal knife is inserted into the first interspace, tapped to the

midsternum, directed down the middle of the sternum until the fifth interspace is reached, and then turned into this space. The chondral portion of the second, third, fourth, and fifth ribs are transected just lateral to the origin of the pectoralis major muscle along the previously established tunnel, with care taken to secure the intercostal vessels along the lower margin of each rib. Throughout this dissection, the underlying pleura is included. The entire internal mammary lymph node chain adherent to the under surface of the resected chest wall will have been removed en bloc (see Fig. 18–19B). To manage the pneumothorax, a medial catheter is placed through the skin distal to the lower skin flap and lies in the chest wall defect. When the remainder of the operation is complete, the skin is securely closed, and both medial and lateral catheters are connected to a source of closed suction.

SKIN GRAFTING

Skin grafting is infrequently needed with mastectomy. Primary closure is routine, except possibly in patients with locally advanced carcinomas, but even in these patients local flaps provide a more secure and cosmetic closure. When skin grafting is necessary, small defects can be

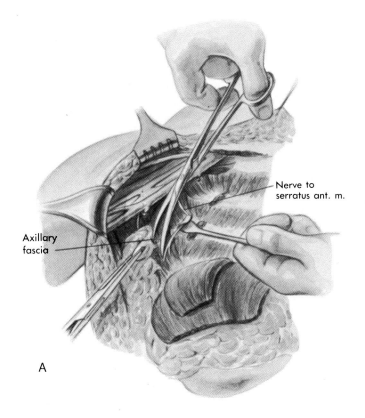

Nerve to
serratus ant. m.

Axillary
fascia

A

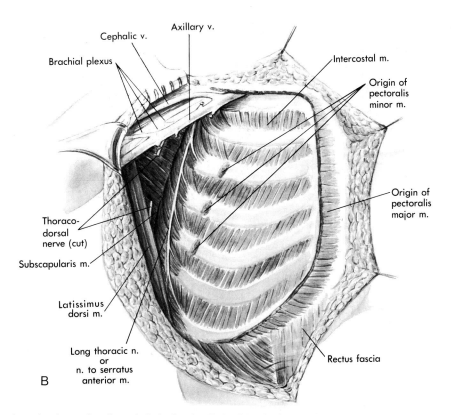

Cephalic v.

Axillary v.

Brachial plexus

Intercostal m.

Origin of
pectoralis
minor m.

Origin of
pectoralis
major m.

Thoraco-
dorsal
nerve (cut)

Subscapularis m.

Latissimus
dorsi m.

Long thoracic n.
or
n. to serratus
anterior m.

Rectus fascia

B

Figure 18–18. Radical mastectomy *Continued. A,* As the fascia is dissected away from the undersurface of the axillary vein and from the intercostal muscles, the nerves to the latissimus dorsi and serratus anterior muscles are seen. The more medial nerve to the serratus anterior muscle is separated from the axillary fascia throughout its length from the axillary vein to the insertion into the muscle. *B,* Appearance of the surgical defect existing after completion of a radical mastectomy. The thoracodorsal nerve is shown excised. Although this is an option when the axilla is heavily involved, excising this nerve is not routine.

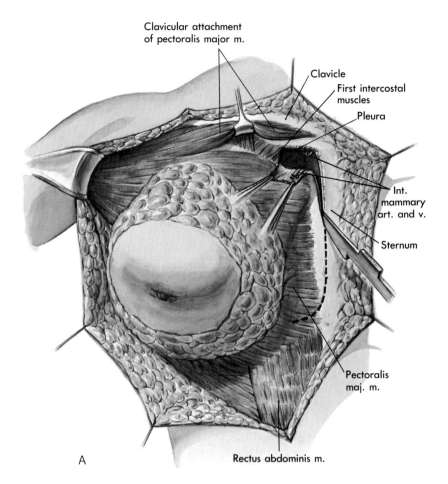

Clavicular attachment
of pectoralis major m.

Clavicle
First intercostal
muscles
Pleura

Int.
mammary
art. and v.

Sternum

Pectoralis
maj. m.

A

Rectus abdominis m.

Figure 18–19. Extended radical mastectomy. *A,* When the internal mammary lymph node chain is to be resected, the medial end of the clavicular attachment of pectoralis major muscle is either retracted superiorly and preserved along with the remaining clavicular head of the muscle, as in this illustration, or is reflected inferiorly along with the detached clavicular origin of the muscle. The intercostal muscles are then incised along the upper margin of the first interspace, and the internal mammary artery and vein are ligated and transected near the upper margin of the interspace. A similar maneuver is performed through the intercostal muscles at the lower margin of the fifth interspace. The Lebsche sternal knife is then inserted into the interspace, is tapped to about midsternum, and is then directed inferiorly down the midline, turning laterally into the fifth interspace. A tunnel is established by blunt digital dissection deep to the pectoralis major muscle and just lateral to its sternal insertion. The second, third, fourth, and fifth ribs and the intervening intercostal muscles are then transected in this tunnel with either straight bone-cutting forceps or heavy scissors. The pleura and the underlying areolar tissues are taken with this segment of thoracic wall.

closed with a defatted, full-thickness graft trimmed from a redundant part of the skin flap, usually laterally. The suction catheters are placed as usual, and the margins of the skin flaps are sutured to the underlying muscle with interrupted silk sutures to make the space between the flaps airtight. The silk sutures are left long. The skin graft is placed on the defect and sutured to the margin with continuous fine silk or staples. The long tails of the silk sutures at the margin are tied firmly over a bulky gauze dressing that holds a shaped piece of Telfa or gauze against the graft. This gauze mold holds the graft firmly pressed against the chest wall. By the fifth postoperative day, the sutures can be cut and the dressing removed. The surface of the graft can be covered with a light dressing to protect it from abrasion.

For a split-thickness graft, the circumference of one thigh from below the knee to the groin is prepared and draped.

Grafts are then cut with a dermatome with its micrometer scale set to 15 one-thousands of an inch. A thinner cutting can be made, but rarely one less than 12 one-thousands of an inch. Only the anterior or lateral thigh are used as donor sites. After capillary bleeding has ceased and the site is blotted dry, fine bacteriostatic impregnated gauze or Telfa is applied to the donor site. This is held in place with a circumferential dressing. Several days later, the dressing is removed down to the fine gauze or Telfa, and this is left undisturbed until it comes off spontaneously in about 2 weeks.

POSTOPERATIVE MANAGEMENT

Hospitalization for mastectomy or breast conserving operations has an average duration of only 2 or 3 days (Orr et

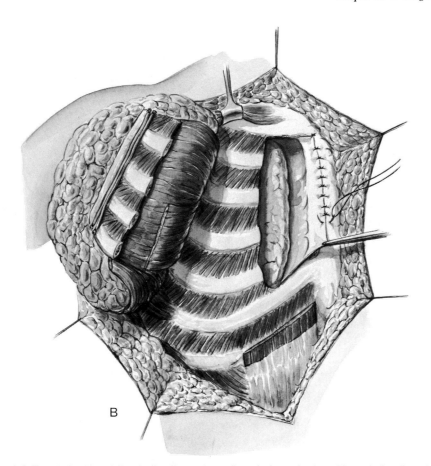

B

Figure 18–19 *Continued. B,* The defect persisting in the thoracic wall and pleura is closed by suturing the pleura to the thoracic wall around the periphery. Holes are made in the rib ends and sternum, and sutures of No. 1 chromic catgut are passed through the holes. These are tied across the defect with the chest wall compressed medially to reduce the size of the defect. A suction catheter is then placed through a stab wound in the lower medial flap with the tip of the catheter lying in the upper end of the defect. The medial flap is then pulled across the defect and is sutured firmly to the intercostal muscles on the lateral side of the defect. The lungs are kept at near full inflation as the defect is closed. The medial catheter is attached immediately to suction. In our experience, a separate chest tube through the lateral thoracic wall leading to water-sealed drainage has not been necessary.

al., 1987). Before the patient leaves the hospital, oral analgesics are supplied, a request is made for a visit by an American Cancer Society Reach to Recovery volunteer (if the patient agrees to such a visit), and the patient or a relative is taught to manage the closed suction drains. This management involves periodically emptying the reservoirs and recording the amount of drainage. Arrangements to have a nurse visit the patient to do this may be necessary in some cases. Each drain remains in place until the volume of the reservoirs is less than 30 mL per 24 hours. The medial drain usually can be removed before the patient leaves the hospital, and the lateral (axillary) drain within 1 to 2 weeks after discharge. After both drains are out, shoulder exercises are begun. With proper instruction, patients are almost always able and willing to perform these exercises themselves (Table 18–3). Progress is followed with weekly measurements, and if range of motion has not returned to normal within 4 weeks, a referral is made for physical therapy. Also, baseline circumferential measurements for future reference are made of the arms at points 15 cm proximal and distal to the elbow. When the mastec-

tomy incision, or skin and axillary incisions, are healed (in 8–10 days), the adhesive skin strips are removed and the patient may bathe the sites. The patient is then fitted with a breast prosthesis. Toward the end of the first month following surgery, plans are completed for systemic adjuvant therapy and for radiation therapy (if needed). Decisions are also made regarding a long-term follow-up program and about who will be responsible for it. Finally, the option and timing of breast reconstruction are again discussed with the patient.

COMPLICATIONS OF MASTECTOMY

Mortality

Mastectomy has become a very safe operation. Budd and coworkers (1978) reported no deaths among 146 consecutive mastectomy patients aged 34 to 88 years. In 1979, the operative mortality was 0.4% among cases of breast cancer reported to the Surveillance Epidemiology and End Results

Table 18–3. SHOULDER EXERCISES

1. You have reached the point in your recovery where you may begin performing shoulder exercises. You can be referred to a physical therapist if you wish, but with the exercise program that follows most everyone is able to do the job themselves. The only joint that needs limbering after mastectomy is the shoulder joint, and exercises are designed specifically to do this. Exercising other joints and the hand is needless. Raising the arm over the head is the motion most limited, so restoring this motion is the principal target of the exercises.
2. You will not damage the surgical area. Stretching the underarm may be uncomfortable, but it is not going to pull anything apart. Mild discomfort can be expected as the price of progress.
3. Do the exercises three or four times each day for about 5 minutes each time. Mark your progress with a pencil on a strip of tape mounted on the wall. Try to exceed the previous mark each session.
4. The three exercises you should do at each session are:
    a. Face the wall, and with your forehead against it reach as high on the wall as possible with both hands. Walk up the wall with your fingers. When you reach the highest point that you can without undue discomfort, hold it there a few seconds before coming back down. Repeat this several times.
    b. Turn sideways to the wall (face along the wall rather than at it) and walk up the wall with your fingers to the highest point you can reach. Move it closer to the wall if necessary. Repeat this several times.
    c. Place a rope, belt, or scarf up over a shower curtain rod or the top of a door. Grasp the ends with each hand and alternately pull up and down on the ends. When one arm pulls down, it will pull the other one up and elevate the shoulder. Do this for a short period.
5. Do the exercises regularly for best results. Your range of motion will be measured initially (baseline) and at each subsequent visit to document progress for the record. Shoulder motion can be expected to be back to normal within 1 month after surgery. In the occasional case that is not, referral for physical therapy will be arranged.

(SEER) program of the National Cancer Institute (Schneiderman and Axtell, 1979). More recently, a review of 715 consecutive cases of patients treated with modified or radical mastectomy at a community teaching hospital revealed that only two deaths (0.3%) had occurred within the first postoperative month (Donegan, 1983). Neither of the two deaths was directly related to the operation. Mortality is related to comorbid conditions and is concentrated in the elderly. In the latter study, the death rate within 1 month of surgery was 0.2% for patients under the age of 65 years, 0.4% for those older than 65 years, and 3.5% for those over the age of 80 years. The author (WLD) has treated 413 consecutive patients with mastectomy or breast conservation without a perioperative death.

Infections

Wound infections occur in from 4% to 18% of mastectomy patients (Vinton et al., 1991). With attention devoted to aseptic technique, the careful development of viable skin flaps, and the use of prophylactic antibiotics, infections after mastectomy are not frequent. When infections do occur, they are usually due to skin contaminants, notably *Staphylococcus aureus*. Prompt antibiotic therapy is necessary to avoid progressive loss of the skin flaps. Infections cause little discomfort because the skin at the mastectomy site has been denervated by the operation. Infections begin with erythema of the skin edges, which is often associated with a mild temperature rise or an initial spike. What may appear to be delayed flap necrosis is usually infection. Infection can quickly progress to necrosis of the flap and to dehiscence of the mastectomy closure. At the first sign of erythema, treatment with antibiotics is begun. The development of pus beneath the flaps requires opening of the wound, débridement of the necrotic tissue, the application of wet dressings, and dependent drainage. With prompt attention, serious infections can be brought rapidly under control with minimal loss of tissue. Occasionally, a coun-

terincision at the base of the inferior flap is necessary to permit dependent drainage (Fig. 18–20). The granulating wound can be cared for at home with gentle bathing, hydrogen peroxide rinses, and the application of light dressings. Eventual healing with only moderate widening of the scar can be anticipated; only occasionally is surgical wound closure or skin grafting required.

Hematoma

Closed suction drainage after mastectomy is designed to prevent the collection of blood and serum beneath the skin flaps. Hematoma formation is a sign of brisk hemorrhage or of suction catheter malfunction. Hematomas large enough to elevate a skin flap and to threaten its adherence

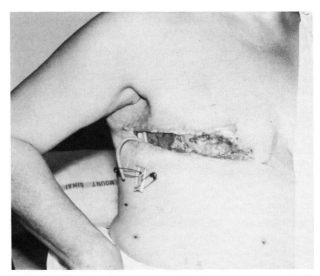

Figure 18–20. Mastectomy wound is shown open and débrided after postoperative infection with skin necrosis. A counterincision provides dependent drainage for the lower flap.

to the underlying tissues generally result in delayed healing and are best managed by returning the patient to the operating room for evacuation of the hematoma under sterile conditions. Bleeding points are secured, and the skin flaps are reclosed. If performed gently, this procedure is possible with sedation and local anesthesia.

Seromas and Lymphoceles

Seromas and lymphoceles under the skin flaps are one of the more frequent complications of mastectomy and of axillary dissection. They are detected by ballottement of the flaps. If left untreated, they prevent adherence of the flaps to the chest and can stretch the overlying skin. At the lateral margin of an axillary dissection, most of the afferent lymphatics from the upper extremity are transected. Their open ends spill lymph directly into the wound. This can be prevented to some extent by ligating the bundles of fatty tissues about the axillary vein at the lateral side of the axilla during the operation (Spratt et al., 1965). Excessive motion of the arm also promotes the flow of lymph. For this reason, exercises are delayed until the closed suction catheters have been removed; however, use of the arm is not otherwise restricted before that time (Lotze et al., 1981). Drainage immediately after mastectomy consists of blood and serum, but it gradually becomes serous and ultimately consists of lymph from severed lymphatics. The fluid may continue to accumulate after suction via the catheters has been discontinued. The problem is likely to occur in patients who have a large amount of drainage. Seromas and lymphoceles requiring one or more needle aspirations were seen in 53% of patients following mastectomy at the Medical College of Wisconsin, and in a few of these, fluid collections persisted for many months (Tadych and Donegan, 1987). The frequency of seroma and lymphocele occurrence is directly related to the amount of drainage at the time of catheter removal. This frequency can be reduced to 11% by delaying removal until drainage is less than 30 mL per 24 hours (Fig. 18–21). Suction catheters need not be removed in

haste; after receiving instruction in their management and with antiseptic dressings securely in place at drain exit sites, patients may be discharged from the hospital to care for them at home. The dressings are changed and the sites inspected every several days at office visits.

Lymphoceles can be managed simply with periodic percutaneous aspirations until lymphatics seal and accumulation stops. In some patients, a smooth-walled capsule that prevents resolution develops. In these cases, open drainage provides a prompt solution to the problem. A small drain is placed into the cavity through an incision at the most dependent margin of the collection, and dressings are changed as necessary. Granulations appear promptly, and the cavity closes, usually in less than 2 weeks. If infection of the collection occurs during aspirations, open drainage will also be required. Rarely, a permanent lymph fistula develops; such a fistula requires excision of its tract with closure (Kinmonth, 1982).

Neuropathies

A temporary sensory and motor neurapraxia of the upper extremity can follow an apparently uneventful mastectomy. This neurapraxia is immediate and of varying severity, ranging from mild tingling in the fingers to motor weakness and dysesthesia of the entire arm in a sleeve distribution (Fig. 18–22). Budd and coworkers (1978) reported the incidence as 0.7%. The problem may result from inadvertent stretching of the brachial plexus during the operation. Hence, pulling on the arm during skin preparation, retraction of the brachial plexus during dissection, and manipulation of the shoulder into extreme positions are avoided. Patients can be reassured that the problem is temporary and that complete recovery can be expected within several weeks. Physical therapy may be helpful in the interim to maintain range of motion of the arm.

Injury to the long thoracic nerve of a patient results in paralysis of the serratus anterior muscle and in hypermobility of the scapula (the so-called "winged scapula"), which

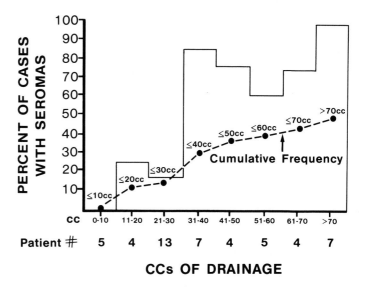

Figure 18–21. The frequency of seroma formation after drainage catheter removal is directly related to the 24-hour drainage volume immediately prior to removal. This correlation is based on experience with 49 patients treated with modified mastectomy at the Medical College of Wisconsin. (From Tadych, K., and Donegan, W. L.: Postmastectomy seromas and wound drainage. Surg. Gynecol. Obstet., *165*:483, 1987. By permission of Surgery, Gynecology & Obstetrics.)

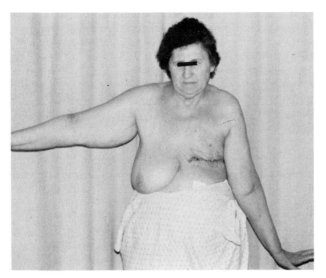

Figure 18–22. Neurapraxia of the left arm following mastectomy. This is a temporary condition of uncertain cause that involves motor and sensory function. Complete recovery can be expected within a few weeks.

does not remain closely applied to the thoracic wall (Fig. 18–23*A*). The deformity can be exaggerated by having the patient extend her arms in front of her or by having her lean forward with her hands against a wall. Each of these positions pushes the scapula dorsally, allowing its prominence to become evident. If the nerve has been transected, the deformity is permanent. If the nerve is known to be intact, one can expect the return of normal muscle tone within a few weeks.

Injury to the thoracodorsal nerve paralyzes the latissimus dorsi muscle. This muscle extends, internally rotates, and adducts the humerus. The functional deficit most frequently noticed by a patient is an inability to reach posteriorly as high up on her back as was possible for her before surgery (see Fig. 18–23*B*). The latissimus dorsi muscle also covers the tip of the scapula and helps to keep it closely applied against the thorax. Thus, as the muscle atrophies, the tip of the scapula may become more prominent.

Excision of the intercostobrachial nerve, the anterior ramus of the second thoracic nerve that supplies cutaneous sensation to the inner side of the upper arm, causes numbness and dysesthesias in its distribution (Teicher et al., 1982; and Temple and Ketchum, 1985). The sensations are variously interpreted as swelling or aching. When this nerve is absent or attenuated, sensation to the inner arm is supplied by the first thoracic nerve via the nerve of Wrisburg. Disagreeable sensations more frequently are related to the desensitized area in the axilla and lateral to the scapula owing to transection of segmental cutaneous nerves necessary in the course of the operation. A typical pattern can be demonstrated on the skin that is insensitive to touch or pin prick (Fig. 18–24). To the patient, this area feels swollen and tight and may ache. Complaints include formication or itching sensations that are not relieved by scratching. Patients misinterpret these symptoms as ominous but should be reassured that they are a sequela of the operation and will gradually become less noticeable. The size of the desensitized area does diminish with time.

The medial anterior thoracic nerve (lateral pectoral nerve) supplies motor function to the lateral half of the pectoralis major muscle. Injury to this nerve, most likely where it crosses the pectoralis minor muscle laterally, causes atrophy of the denervated part of the muscle. This detracts from the cosmetic results of the modified radical mastectomy (Scanlon, 1981).

The *phantom breast syndrome* is analogous to the phantom limb syndrome seen after amputation of a limb. It occurs frequently but may not be mentioned by a patient unless an inquiry is made. Typically, patients perceive that the removed breast is still present following mastectomy and, in some patients, that it causes pain (Jamison et al., 1979; Aitken and Minton, 1983; Staps et al., 1985; and Karydas et al., 1986). If the symptom is distressing to a patient, the prescription of tricyclic antidepressants may be helpful.

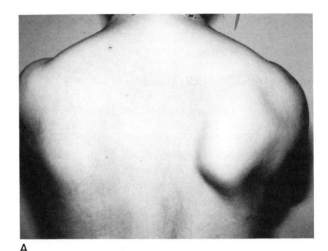

A

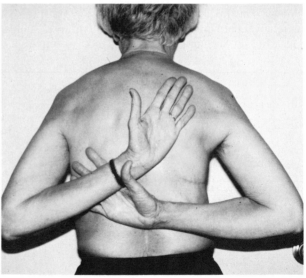

B

Figure 18–23. *A*, A "winged" scapula. Damage to the long thoracic nerve results in paralysis of the serratus anterior muscle and an unstable scapula. *B*, Disability resulting from injury to the thoracodorsal nerve is similar to that shown in this patient who has a nonfunctioning latissimus dorsi muscle. The hand on the injured (right) side cannot be placed as high on the back as that on the uninjured side.

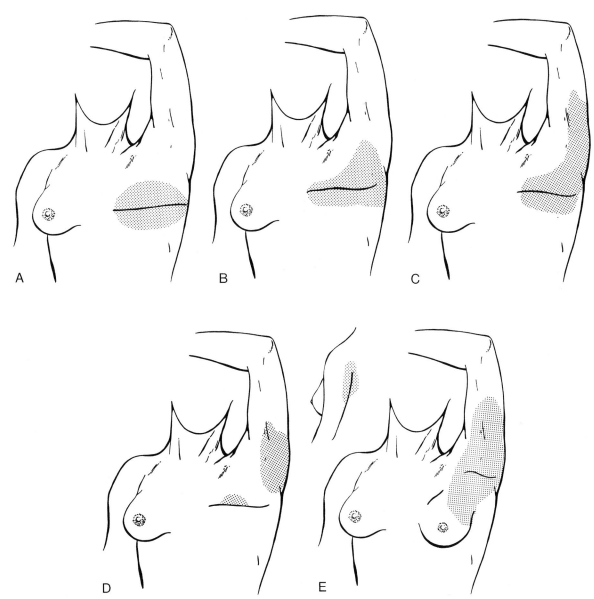

Figure 18–24. Patterns of cutaneous anesthesia *(shaded areas)* immediately following various operations on the breast. These are illustrated on the author's (WLD) cases as areas insensitive to touch and pin-prick. Paresthesias can be expected within the insensitive areas, and patients may be reassured that they are not unusual and can be expected to diminish with time. The insensitive area is larger if an axillary lymph node dissection is included with the mastectomy and even larger if the intercostobrachial nerve cannot be preserved. *A*, Total mastectomy (no axillary lymph node dissection). *B*, Modified radical mastectomy with preservation of the intercostobrachial nerve. *C*, Modified radical mastectomy with removal of the intercostobrachial nerve. The area of anesthesia extends for a long distance along the inner side of the arm. *D*, Case *C*, 1 year following the operation, shows that the insensitive areas are smaller because of regeneration of sensory nerves. Because the intercostobrachial nerve has a long course and regrowth is unlikely, the area of anesthesia on the inner side of the arm is persistent. *E*, Segmental mastectomy and axillary lymph node dissection without preservation of the intercostobrachial nerve. Hughes and coworkers (1989) indicate that a large branch of the intercostobrachial nerve goes to the upper outer quadrant of the breast so the area of anesthesia on the breast shown here can probably be reduced by sparing of the nerve.

Frozen Shoulder

Abduction of the ipsilateral shoulder is temporarily compromised after axillary dissection. Restoration to the full range of motion is accomplished in almost all instances by routine physical therapy or by a prescribed program of shoulder exercises. With diligence, this goal is reached well within 1 month of the operation. Capsular contracture and a frozen shoulder are unusual but can result from failure to exercise because of discomfort or lack of motivation on the part of the patient. As long as progress is being made, physical therapy should be continued with the expectation of ultimate success; if not, an orthopedic consultation is necessary.

Lymphedema of the Upper Extremity

Lymphedema of the upper extremity is perhaps the most distressing complication of axillary node dissection, and it continues to be a vexing problem. To date, no completely effective treatment for it is available.

Lymphatic Anatomy of the Extremity. The lymphatic system of the extremities consists of two major portions: (1) a complex system of intercommunicating capillaries and vessels that conducts lymph from the periphery and empties it centrally into the venous system; and (2) the lymph nodes, which are interspersed along the lymphatic channels and serve various functions, including filtration, lymphocyte production, and antibody production. Lymph nodes tend to cluster in fatty tissue near the bifurcation of great veins between layers of fascia. The fluid circulating in the tissue spaces between the cells is distinguished from the lymph, which is the fluid contained within lymphatic vessels.

Lymph circulates through the skin and other tissues by means of a system of closed vessels (Gray, 1939; Butcher and Hoover, 1955; Rusznyak et al., 1960; and Spratt et al., 1965). The cutaneous lymphatic circulation arises in the subepithelial region of the dermis as a superficial plexus of capillaries with blind-ended papillae extending upward toward the epidermis. This plexus is valveless and is continuous over the entire surface of the body. There are no lymphatic vessels in the epidermis. The subepithelial plexus is connected by oblique and vertical trunks to a system of larger lymphatic vessels in the subdermal region. The walls of the vessels of the superficial or subepithelial capillary plexus are composed of endothelium alone. There is no differentiation into adventitia or muscularis. The subdermal plexus is a system of collecting radicles that contain valves to ensure unidirectional flow. Lymph flows from the subdermal plexus into a subcutaneous plexus, the major lymph trunks conducting fluid from the periphery. In addition to valves, the vessels of the subcutaneous plexus contain a muscular layer that converts the process of lymph drainage at this level from a completely passive one into a partially active one. It is this system of lymphatic vessels in the subcutaneous tissue that carries the lymph to the regional nodes. There is a system of deep lymphatics (i.e., deep to the muscular fascia) that is much less extensive than the superficial system. This deep system drains the large mus-

cular compartments, but the largest portion of the deep drainage of lymph by volume comes from the joints and the synovial tissues. Lymphatics are sparse within the muscles. Relatively few channels pass through the deep fascia to connect the superficial system with the deep system. Flow between these two systems is normally from the deep system to the superficial system, the opposite of the normal venous drainage. The most significant connection is at the level of the regional lymph nodes, where both systems join to form a common trunk. Thus, each system—the superficial and the deep—functions independently of the other in the usual circumstances.

Although the vessels in the subcutaneous system branch and reanastomose with each other, their caliber remains approximately that of a 27-gauge needle and seldom increases as the vessels proceed proximally. Valves with paired cusps are located at regular intervals in the system. Distal in each valve is a small constriction, and proximal to each valve a small dilatation of the lumen is present. Bypass channels exist for any particular lymph node or group of nodes, allowing lymph to continue on to the next, higher node group. As a result of the function of the valves in the main lymphatics, flow of lymph remains unidirectional; retrograde lymphatic metastases occur only when proximal lymphatics are blocked and become dilated to a degree that makes the valves incompetent. The system of channels and nodes is without specific anatomic demarcation. For convenience of description, lymph nodes are artificially divided into groups that are named by their anatomic surroundings. This grouping gives the impression of discontinuous node groups, each of which drains separate anatomic regions. Although the lymph from certain regions does drain primarily into specific nodes, the continuity of the system must be kept in mind. The risk for lymphedema of the arm arises because lymphatics from the breast and the upper extremity converge in the axillary lymph nodes. Conditions are created for the development of lymphedema whenever major lymphatics in the axilla are interrupted by lymph node dissection, irradiation, or the uncontrolled progression of cancer. Based on the clearance of radioactive iodine–labeled albumen from subcutaneous tissues, Ju and coworkers (1954) estimated that radical mastectomy reduced lymph flow from the upper extremity by 48%. The reduc-

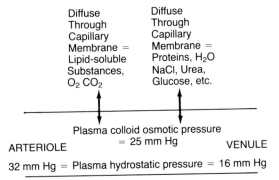

Figure 18–25. Diagram of factors considered in the Starling hypothesis. Considerable variation in the recorded pressure may exist. (U. of L. Medical illustrations No. 13685–1.) (Adapted from Stillwell, G. K.: Treatment of postmastectomy lymphedema. Mod. Treat., 6:396, 1959.)

tion leaves some patients with lymphatic insufficiency or only borderline function.

Physiology of Lymphedema. The formation of lymphedema is explained by Starling's hypothesis (1898) concerning the movement of water between the blood vessels and tissue spaces (Fig. 18–25). As indicated by the protein content of thoracic duct lymph, a considerable fraction of plasma protein normally enters tissue spaces. With injury, infection, capillary rupture, or obstruction to outflow of lymph or venous blood and with arteriolar dilation from heat or exercise, protein leakage into the tissues is accelerated. The increased protein content in the tissues increases the osmotic pressure, drawing more water into tissue spaces. Concomitant stretching of skin and subcutaneous tissues reduces the hydrostatic pressure produced by their normal turgor. Even after edema fluid is removed, this turgor may remain reduced, increasing susceptibility to reaccumulation of fluid.

Untreated lymphedema inexorably progresses from a reversible pitting phase through phases of subcutaneous fibrosis with nonpitting edema and on to fibrokeratotic skin changes called *elephantiasis*. The progress is subtle, but when fibrosis occurs, it is permanent. Fibrosis results from organization of excess protein-containing lymph by fibroblasts. The weight of a neglected lymphedematous arm can become so great that it dislocates the shoulder and stretches the brachial plexus until the arm is completely denervated (Fig. 18–26, A–D). Lymphangiosarcoma is an infrequent but usually fatal complication of chronic lymphedema.

Prevention. Prevention is of great importance because lymphedema is usually progressive and permanent. The best prevention is avoidance of axillary dissection or axillary irradiation without clear justification, and particularly both in combination (Treves, 1957). Otherwise, prevention is best accomplished by educating the patient about the cause and consequences of lymphedema and the susceptibility of the extremity to infection. Evidence exists that cellular immunity of the arm is impaired (Stark et al., 1960; Schick et al., 1976). Instruction begins preoperatively by informing the patient that permanent enlargement of the arm is a possible consequence of treatment. The risk is similar (10–20%) whether axillary dissection is performed in conjunction with mastectomy or breast conservation. When it does occur it is generally only slight or moderate.

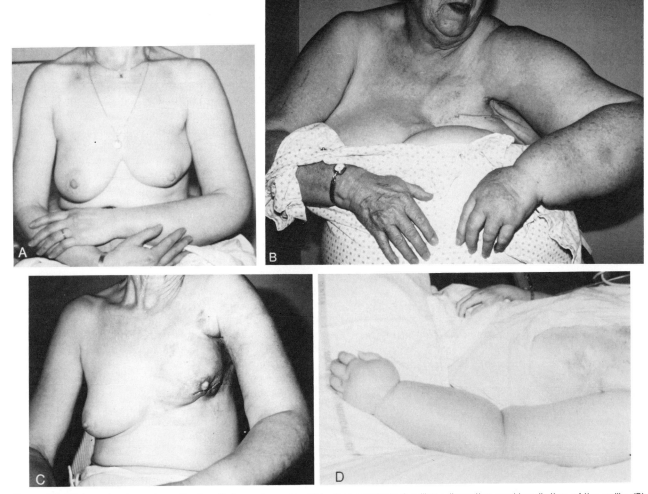

Figure 18–26. Lymphedema in patients with breast cancer (A), after combined axillary dissection and irradiation of the axilla (B) and after radical mastectomy (C) due to progressive cancer in the axilla. D, Advanced lymphedema after mastectomy. The weight of the arm caused subluxation of the shoulder and paralysis of the arm.

Instruction continues postoperatively with the lifelong need to protect the extremity from trauma, infections, overheating (e.g., sunburn), and excessive exercise (Table 18–4) The ipsilateral arm is not used for blood pressures, intravenous fluid administration or phlebotomies, nor is the subclavian vein on the ipsilateral side used as access for central venous lines. Even minor injuries are treated promptly with antiseptics and protection.

Lymphedema may occur early or late and often without an obvious precipitating event. The frequency of lymphedema occurrence is related to the extent of axillary dissection (a Level I dissection is rarely followed by lymphedema) and is increased by the combination of axillary dissection and irradiation of the axilla. A study by one of the authors (WLD) indicates that the period of greatest risk is the first 3 years after axillary dissection (Figs. 18–27 and 18–28). Onset of lymphedema in conjunction with a severe infection of the arm is not infrequent (see Fig. 18–29*A* and *B*). The patient who presents with enlargement of the arm should be examined for infection, for recurrent cancer in the axilla and supraclavicular areas, and for signs of venous thrombosis. Routine venograms, however, rarely show thrombosis of the axillary or subclavian vein unless there are other reasons to suspect it.

Some researchers have quantified lymphedema based on comparisons of the volume of one upper extremity with that of the opposite upper extremity. Tracy and coworkers (1961) considered an increase in volume of less than 150 mL insignificant, of 150 to 600 mL slight, of 400 to 750 mL moderate, and of greater than 750 mL severe. Others

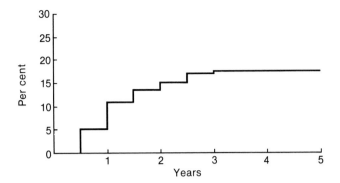

Figure 18–27. Cumulative frequency of lymphedema following 212 axillary node dissections. Most cases develop within the first three postoperative years.

have based estimates on per cent increases in volume (Stillwell, 1959). A less precise but more convenient means for evaluating and following the course of lymphedema is the recording of periodic circumferential measurements of the extremity and their comparison with those of the opposite member. Fifteen centimeters proximal and distal to the olecranon are convenient points for measurement of circumference.

Treatment. Obvious infection is brought under control with the use of antibiotics, arm rest, and arm elevation; possible occult infection is also treated with antibiotics. Patients subject to recurrent bouts of infection should have antibiotics (e.g., penicillin, cephalosporin, or ciprofloxacin) in their possession so that they are able to start treatment immediately when they first observe a sign of infection.

Treatment of persistent edema is a coordinated program of elevation of the arm, periodic pneumatic or manual massage, elastic compression, and moderate exercise (Vasudevan and Melvin, 1979). Benefit is obtained only as long as the program is continued. If edema is any more than slight, patients are fitted with an elastic sleeve that is worn on a schedule to minimize swelling. If a patient's hand swells, an elastic gauntlet is also worn. Massage, performed from distal to proximal, is helpful but is labor-intensive. It is most convenient when practiced by the patient herself. Multichambered sequential pneumatic compression pumps are very effective in reducing edema prior to the fitting of a patient with an elastic sleeve and, when used on a regular schedule, help to control the problem (Richmand et al., 1985). Care must be exercised, as efforts to remove edema with too much pressure can rupture lymphatics and further deplete their number.

Surgical procedures to correct this problem are designed either to remove the edematous tissue or to provide a means for obstructed lymph to reach unobstructed lymphatics or the venous system. Lymphatics do regenerate across linear incisions after transection (Reichert, 1926; Butcher and Hoover, 1955; and Howard et al., 1964). Butcher and Hoover demonstrated bridging of superficial lymphatics across linear incisions by the 15th day after transection with healing by first intention. Infection, delayed wound healing, excessive scarring, irradiation, and the persistence of cancer all delay or permanently prevent this bridging process.

Table 18–4. CARE OF THE ARM AFTER MASTECTOMY

During your breast surgery, lymph nodes were removed from your axilla (armpit) on that same side. Usually this causes no problem. But fluid can accumulate in the arm as a result of the change in lymph flow. Infections, injuries, strains, or constrictions around the arm can cause swelling or worsen it. Therefore, it is necessary for you to take precautions to prevent infection and injury.

Suggestions:
1. Do not wear tight jewelry or clothing that is constricting.
2. Avoid cutting or pulling cuticles or hangnails on the involved side.
3. Wear padded gloves when cooking or baking to avoid burns.
4. Use the other arm to carry purse, suitcase, or heavy packages.
5. Avoid sunburn of the arm. Cover with clothing or use a strong sunscreen.
6. Wash cuts, scrapes, and insect bites immediately with soap and water, and apply an antiseptic. If redness or swelling develop, call your doctor or nurse.
7. Make sure blood pressure is taken on your other arm.
8. Make sure injections, vaccinations, and blood sampling is done on your other arm unless recommended otherwise by a physician or nurse who knows that you have had breast surgery.
9. Wear protective gloves when washing dishes or doing other work (e.g., housework or gardening).
10. Do not move heavy objects by yourself. Find someone to help you.

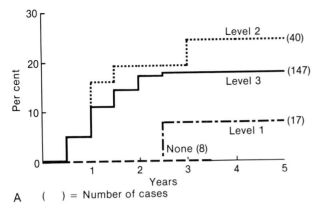 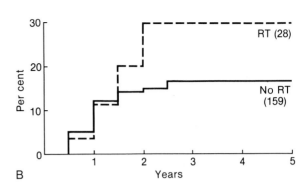

A ( ) = Number of cases
B

Figure 18-28. *A,* Cumulative frequency of lymphedema following mastectomy related to the level of axillary node dissection. Lymphedema is unusual after no node dissection and infrequent after a Level 1 node dissection. It is equally frequent after a Level 2 or Level 3 node dissection. *B,* The frequency of lymphedema is increased in patients who had regional irradiation after axillary dissection. (Data for patients with Level 2 or 3 axillary dissection only. RT = radiation treatment.)

Operations to correct this problem are many, but they have a history of failure (Thompson, 1967). Among them are implantation of subcutaneous threads or tubes, which provide conduits back to the trunk; burying of dermis flaps (i.e., invagination of de-epithelialized dermis into the muscular compartment to make possible connection with deep lymphatics [Kinmonth, 1982]); rotation of skin or myocutaneous flaps from the trunk into the arm (Medgyesi, 1983); extension of a pedicle of omentum into the arm (Goldsmith et al., 1968); and excision of all edematous subcutaneous tissue and using the skin for split grafts back on the fascia of the muscles (Charles's operation). The most physiologically appealing procedure is the surgical creation of direct lymphovenous anastomoses in the arm, but such anastomoses are plagued with early closure (O'Brien and Shafiroff, 1979; and Savage, 1985).

Continued education of patients about the prevention of lymphedema, the performance of baseline and periodic measurements of the patient's extremity, expeditious treatment of infections, and optimum management of chronic edema are integral parts of continuing care.

OOPHORECTOMY

As first demonstrated by Beatson in 1896, oophorectomy in menstruating women can provide temporary regression of metastatic breast cancer. Its role as an adjuvant to primary treatment is less well established (Tengrup et al., 1986; and Early Breast Cancer Trialists Collaborative Group, 1992). Oophorectomy has fallen into disuse in favor of pharmacologic methods of reducing estrogen stimulation, most notably, with the synthetic antiestrogen drug tamoxifen. Pharmacologic methods offer similar response rates and avoid the need for an operation, and their effects are reversible. Nevertheless, oophorectomy is occasionally useful when pharmacologic methods are not feasible, have failed, or have ceased to be effective (Planting et al., 1985; Ingle et al., 1986; and Sawka et al., 1986). Its usefulness is not reduced by prior chemotherapy (Conte et al., 1989). Patients who respond to oophorectomy generally live longer than those who do not.

Objective response rates of 6 months or longer range from 20% to 48%, depending on patient selection. Circum-

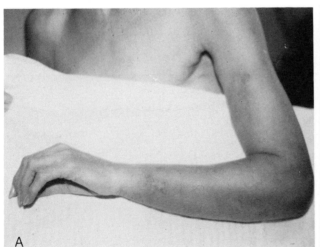 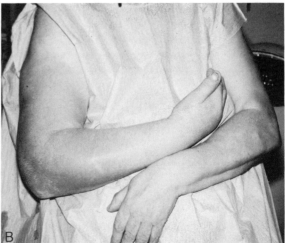

Figure 18-29. *A,* Infection of the arm after mastectomy with axillary dissection. *B,* The arm is less resistant to infection after axillary dissection, and infections may result in chronic lymphedema.

stances that favor a response are the presence of estrogen receptor–positive tumors, well-differentiated tumors, a long disease-free interval, and soft tissue or bone metastases. Patients with symptomatic pulmonary metastases, extensive hepatic or central nervous system metastases, or an estrogen receptor–negative tumor are generally not candidates for oophorectomy.

Technique

The operation is performed with laparotomy or laparoscopically with the patient under general anesthesia. For the open technique, a low midline incision, or a more cosmetic low transverse (Pfannenstiel) incision is used. After the peritoneum has been entered, a self-retaining retractor is used for exposure. The patient is placed in the Trendelenburg position, and the intestines are packed upwards in the abdomen where they are retained with a retractor. The bladder (emptied preoperatively with a catheter) and the uterus are retracted anteriorly, and the ovary is grasped with a Babcock clamp. The mesovarium is perforated through its transparent center, and clamps are placed wide of the ovary on both sides. These bundles, which contain the ovarian artery laterally and the ligament of the ovary on the medial side, are transected and suture-ligated with heavy silk suture after the ovary has been removed. By staying close to the ovary, the ureters are avoided. If the presence of adhesions or the patient's anatomy requires concomitant removal of the fallopian tubes, the distal portion of the infundibulopelvic ligament, which contains the ovarian vessels, is encompassed by incising the peritoneum on either side of it and passing a right-angle clamp beneath it, with care taken not to include the underlying ureter. The ligament is ligated with heavy, nonabsorbable suture and also suture ligated; it is then divided. The fallopian tube and ligament of the ovary are clamped at their juncture with the uterus, divided, and ligated with silk suture. With the major vessels and ligaments secured, the remaining tissues attached to the tube and ovary are carefully transected, and the ovary and tube are removed. Both ovaries are removed in similar fashion. Blood loss is minimal. The bowel is replaced in the pelvis, and the incision is closed with stout, interrupted nonabsorbable sutures to the musculofascial layers. The skin is closed with a subcuticular suture, and a dressing is applied. Postoperatively, nasogastric decompression is not necessary. A bloody vaginal discharge may follow the operation, as hormonal support of the endometrium is lost. Hot flashes can be expected, and osteoporosis is a long-term risk.

ADRENALECTOMY

Bilateral adrenalectomy is an effective palliative procedure for breast cancer and traditionally served as secondary endocrine therapy if a previous oophorectomy was successful. At present it is rarely performed because the same effects can be achieved medically with the use of aminoglutethimide and hydrocortisone, and on some regimens, with use of aminoglutethimide alone (Cocconi et al., 1992). The introduction of aromatase inhibitors has also changed the treatment strategy from one of eliminating the adrenal substrate for estrogen production to one of blocking its conversion to estrogen. Adrenalectomy is a major operation and entails a permanent commitment on the part of the patient to corticosteroid replacement. It may be indicated in unusual circumstances when medical endocrine therapy is not feasible because of intolerable side effects. High levels of tumor estrogen and progesterone receptors and a previous objective response to ovarian ablation are the best predictors of a useful response.

Preoperative preparation of the patient and postoperative care are critical to the success of adrenalectomy. Replacement therapy is begun preoperatively and must be ensured postoperatively. Patients who are unreliable or who do not have easy access to medical care are not suitable candidates for the operation. Maintenance is almost always possible with the administration of cortisone acetate, 25 mg twice daily, as well as a daily intake of 3.0 g of salt. Rarely, a patient requires fludrocortisone acetate (Florinef) in doses of 0.05 mg to 0.1 mg daily to maintain electrolyte balance. A replacement schedule is given in Table 18–5. Extreme weakness, nausea and vomiting, elevated temperature, rapid weight loss, and hypotension are signs of adrenal insufficiency. Added stress may require additional daily cortisone

Table 18–5. REPLACEMENT SCHEDULE FOR BILATERAL TOTAL ADRENALECTOMY*

Day	Medication	Route
Day before operation	50 mg cortisone twice or 100 mg hydrocortisone sodium succinate (Solu-Cortef) at 6 PM	Orally Intravenous
Day of operation	100 mg Solu-Cortef prior to operation, 100 mg during surgery and 50 mg every 4 h thereafter	Intravenous
1st postoperative day	100 mg Solu-Cortef every 8 h	Intravenous
2nd postoperative day	50 mg Solu-Cortef every 6 h	Intravenous
3rd postoperative day	50 mg Solu-Cortef every 12 h	Intravenous
4th postoperative day	25 mg Solu-Cortef every 8 h or 25 mg cortisone every 8 h	Intravenous Orally
5th postoperative day	25 mg cortisone every 12 h	Orally
Maintenance	25 mg cortisone twice a day	Orally

*Diet to include 3.0 g of sodium chloride daily. Supplementation with fludrocortisone acetate may be necessary if electrolyte balance is not maintained.

administration. Acute crises may necessitate hospitalization of patients as well as intensive therapy with intravenous saline and corticosteroids.

Technique

The adrenal glands are removed by means of an anterior or posterior approach. The anterior approach is advantageous because both adrenal glands can be removed through a single incision and because the approach allows the abdomen to be explored to evaluate the extent of disease (Figs. 18–30 to 18–33). The posterior approach offers a smaller risk of ileus and a faster recovery. By either route, the operation is greatly facilitated by the use of long instruments and of steel clips (hemoclips) for hemostasis. Considerable care is required in dissection. One is well advised to ''dissect the patient away from the adrenal gland'' rather than to dissect the adrenal gland from the patient. Approached anteriorly, the incision either extends transversely across the upper abdomen or vertically along the upper midline. The right adrenal gland is removed first because it is the more difficult of the two to excise. The hepatic flexure of the colon is reflected inferiorly. The peritoneum lateral to the second part of the duodenum is incised, and the duodenum is reflected medially in a Kocher maneuver. The peritoneal incision is extended over the upper pole of the right kidney, and a right-angled flap is turned laterally and superiorly, exposing the fatty areolar tissue close to the vena cava. This tissue is gently teased away from the vena cava and the right renal vein. The dark golden color of the adrenal gland is distinct from that of the surrounding fat. When the gland is identified, it is teased from the renal vein

and vena cava to expose the adrenal vessels, particularly the large, short vein that directly enters the vena cava. These vessels are individually secured with hemoclips and then transected. The medial side of the adrenal gland is intimately attached to the vena cava and frequently extends behind it. When the medial margin has been freed, the remainder is relatively avascular, and removal of the gland is completed. On the left side, the adrenal gland is approached by incising the peritoneum lateral to the descending colon and the splenic flexure and by reflecting the colon medially. In the retroperitoneal space, the colon and pancreas are reflected off the left kidney until the tissues adjacent to the aorta above the upper pole are exposed. The adrenal gland is located in this fatty tissue. The gland can also be approached through the lesser sac by elevating the pancreas. Its vasculature is identified and transected between hemoclips, and the gland is removed. The largest vein of the left adrenal gland is long and enters the left renal vein. After careful hemostasis has been accomplished, the abdominal incision is closed using interrupted nonabsorbable sutures to the musculofascial layers and staples or sutures to the skin.

The posterior approach through bilateral lumbar incisions is advantageous in obese patients and in those who have had previous abdominal operations or who have abdominal carcinomatosis (Egdahl and Melby, 1972) (Fig. 18–34). The patient is placed in the jackknife position to flatten the back. The incisions extend from the iliac crest to the 10th rib and run 6 to 7 cm lateral to the midvertebral line. The lumbar fascia is incised, and the 12th rib is freed from its periosteal sheath and resected, preserving the 12th intercostal nerve. Damage to this nerve is uncomfortable for the patient, as it produces a persistent beltlike distribution of

Text continued on page 500

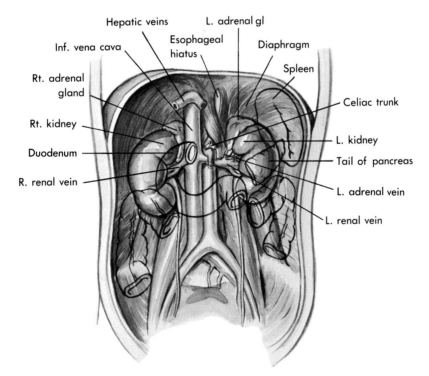

Figure 18–30. The relationship of the adrenal glands to other abdominal organs and the vena cava can be appreciated in this perspective.

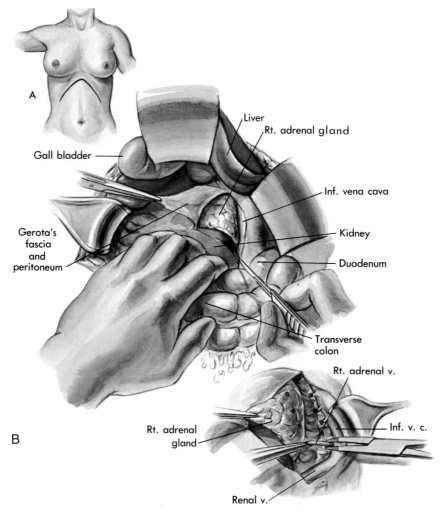

Figure 18–31. Either a transverse incision parallel to and about 1 inch below the costal margins (A) or preferably a high straight transverse incision can be used to approach the adrenal glands. If the ovaries are also to be removed, a single vertical midline incision is advantageous.

B, The right adrenal gland is taken first. The hepatic flexure of the colon is reflected inferiorly, and the duodenum is reflected medially. The kidney is manually retracted caudally. The flap of Gerota's fascia is incised and elevated lateral to the vena cava and above the upper pole of the kidney. The fatty areolar tissue investing the adrenal and kidney is teased away from the vena cava down to and along the upper margin of the right renal vein. As this is done, the veins and arteries bridging across to the adrenal gland are encountered. These are doubly occluded with hemoclips and transected between the clips as they are identified. Occasionally, a vein leaves the adrenal gland from its upper pole, and this must be dissected under direct vision. With the aforementioned complete, the gland can be dissected from its bed without further concern about significant hemorrhage.

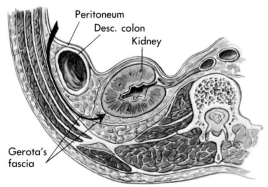

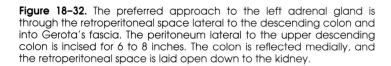

Figure 18–32. The preferred approach to the left adrenal gland is through the retroperitoneal space lateral to the descending colon and into Gerota's fascia. The peritoneum lateral to the upper descending colon is incised for 6 to 8 inches. The colon is reflected medially, and the retroperitoneal space is laid open down to the kidney.

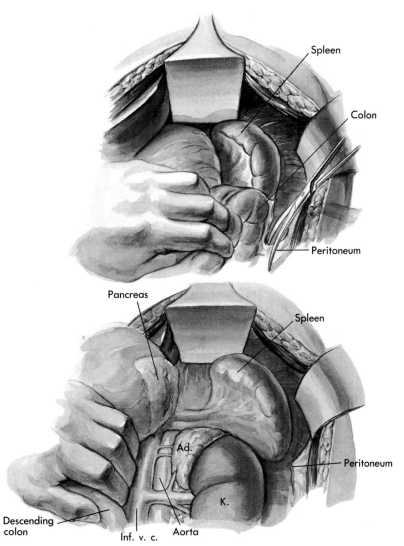

Figure 18–33. The steps described in Figure 18–31 are being carried out in this illustration. The left adrenal gland is more accessible than the right. The vasculature is transected between hemoclips.

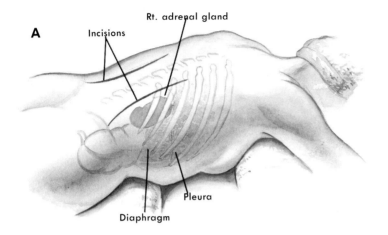

A

Incisions

Rt. adrenal gland

Pleura

Diaphragm

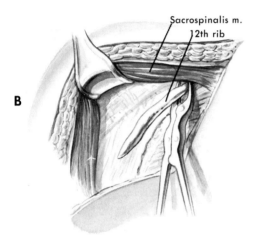

B

Sacrospinalis m.

12th rib

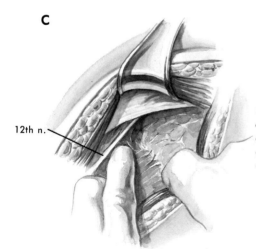

C

12th n.

Pleura being freed from
diaphragm. Surgeon's fingers
are exploring the adrenal
gland beneath the
diaphragmatic fibers.

Figure 18–34. The posterior surgical approach for removal of the adrenal glands is illustrated in these figures. Indications for adrenalectomy and for the posterior approach are discussed in the text.

A, General endotracheal anesthesia is induced with the patient in the supine position, and the patient is then turned and placed in the prone ``jackknife'' position. The patient's knees are slightly flexed to prevent venous stagnation, and supports are placed under the shoulders and hips to permit effective ventilation. The center of the operating table is elevated in order to flatten the normal lumbar curve. A curvilinear incision is made approximately 5 cm lateral to the spinous processes of the vertebrae, extending from the level of the 10th rib to the level of the superior border of the posterior iliac crest.

B, The incision is extended through the subcutaneous tissues and through the posterior lamella of the lumbodorsal fascia medial to the border of the latissimus dorsi muscle. This exposes the sacrospinalis muscle on the medial side of the wound. The sacrospinalis muscle is perforated by small blood vessels and posterior lumbar nerves, which must be secured and divided. The sacrospinalis muscle is retracted medially, and the 12th rib is resected subperiosteally, with care taken not to enter the subjacent pleural cavity.

C, The middle lamella of the lumbodorsal fascia is divided in the direction of the incision, and the pleural reflection is pushed superiorly out of harm's way. The quadratus lumborum muscle is evident laterally.

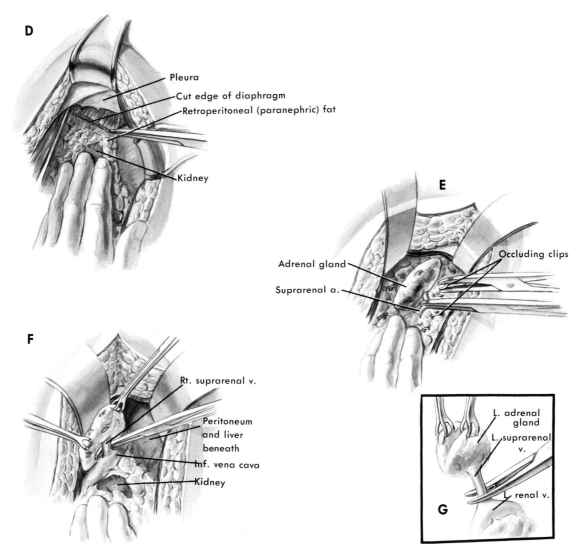

Figure 18–34 *Continued D,* The transversalis fascia, the lower fibers of the diaphragm, and the posterior layer of Gerota's fascia are divided, and the perinephric fat is separated to expose the kidney. The kidney is manually depressed to facilitate exposure of the adrenal gland.

E, Within the fatty tissues at the superior pole of the kidney (and closely applied to the inferior vena cava on the right side), the adrenal gland is easily distinguished from the surrounding fat by its bright golden color. With gentle dissection, the adrenal gland is mobilized from the surrounding fat, while the multiple small vessels that enter it are secured with metal clips. This greatly facilitates the dissection. The arteries are small and multiple, whereas the adrenal vein is usually large and solitary.

F, The adrenal vein is carefully isolated. The vein of the left adrenal gland enters the renal vein, whereas that of the right adrenal is considerably shorter and enters the inferior vena cava directly. It is important to secure the vein prior to dividing it. Substantial bleeding follows accidental division of the right adrenal vein, and blind attempts to control it are ill-advised, as they can result in damage to the vena cava with even more profuse bleeding. If heavy bleeding occurs, local digital compression of the vena cava or a period of packing usually permits the field to be cleared long enough for the vessel to be secured precisely.

G, The adrenal vein is secured with metal clips prior to its division, and it is transected several millimeters from the clip in order to leave a secure cuff of vessel. The adrenal gland must be removed in its entirety, as must any accessory adrenal tissue that is found in the operative field.

When the operation is completed on one side, moist gauze is placed in the wound, and it is covered while the operation is performed on the second side. At the end of the operation, both wounds are inspected for hemostasis and irrigated with saline. The incisions are closed in layers using stout, nonabsorbable, interrupted sutures and no drains. The skin is closed with interrupted sutures of fine nylon, and a dressing is applied. The sutures are not removed for 2 weeks, since earlier removal can result in separation of the skin edges. If the pleura is opened during the dissection, the lung is re-expanded by placing a suction catheter into the pleural cavity through a defect and by withdrawing it as the pleura is closed. An indwelling chest tube with water-sealed drainage is ordinarily not necessary. Patients tolerate adrenalectomy by the posterior approach very well; postoperative ileus is minimal, and recovery is rapid.

paresthesia. The transveralis fascia and renal fascia are incised to expose the kidney, and the pleura is reflected away from the diaphragm without being opened. The pleura is held cephalad with a retractor while the diaphragm is opened for digital exploration of the suprarenal space. Next, the adrenal gland is found in the fatty tissue and dissected from its attachments. The last attachments medially are its vascular connections. As they are encountered, arteries and veins are occluded proximally and distally with clips and then divided. The incision is closed in layers with strong, nonabsorbable sutures. The technique for removal of the other adrenal gland is similar.

RESECTION AND REGIONAL CHEMOTHERAPY FOR HEPATIC METASTASES

Metastasis to the liver from breast cancer is an ominous development. Fewer than 28% of patients with this complication survive for longer than 1 year. A solitary hepatic metastasis or metastases isolated to the liver are uncommon; hence, experience with local and regional treatment is limited.

Resection. Resection of hepatic metastases from carcinoma of the breast is possible only occasionally and has been documented in only a few case reports. Foster (1978) found only five such cases in a large survey. The only operative death occurred after resection of a large solitary metastasis of the left lateral hepatic segment that appeared 17 years after mastectomy. Three of the five patients died 6, 8, and 12 months after resection. One was alive 3 months after resection with known residual cancer. Although the experience with hepatic resection for breast cancer is not encouraging, an occasional patient with an isolated, limited metastasis from a tumor with an indolent pattern of behavior may be a candidate.

Regional Chemotherapy. Progressive metastases isolated to the liver and resistant to systemic therapy have occasionally been treated with hepatic artery infusion (HAI) chemotherapy. The drugs used are those with proven activity against breast cancer. Partial responses have been reported, but complete remissions have not, and without controls the true impact of this treatment remains unknown. A sustained effort to control hepatic metastases was initiated by the late J. P. Minton, and the results of his work were reported by his successors (Schneebaum et al., 1993). Schneebaum and associates reported on 74 cases treated with "aggressive" regional chemotherapy. Among 40 who had only hepatic metastases, 18 were treated by surgical resection with or without chemotherapeutic drugs infused through the hepatic artery or portal vein. Twenty-two received systemic therapy. Median survival for the group with regional treatment was 17 months; this is significantly longer than the 5-month median survival of the patients who were treated systemically. They concluded that a small percentage of breast cancer patients with metastatic breast cancer confined to the liver might benefit from regional therapy. Two such patients were treated in this manner by the author (WLD).

Case History 1

A 39-year-old woman's inflammatory breast cancer was controlled locally with irradiation and combination chemotherapy that included cyclophosphamide, doxorubicin, methotrexate, vincristine, tamoxifen, and prednisone; however, hepatic metastases in the patient progressed relentlessly. At laparotomy, a catheter was placed in the hepatic artery via the gastroduodenal artery, the liver was biopsied, and the ovaries and gallbladder were removed. Metastases were isolated to the liver. She received HAI with continuous fluorouracil (300 mg per 24 h) and three 48-hour infusions of mitomycin C (10 mg/m²) during a period of 8 months. Hepatic metastases showed partial regression on computed tomography of the abdomen, and the patient's liver functions improved; however, progression of tumor in the breast after 5 months and the appearance of brain metastases after 7 months required that the patient receive additional therapy. The patient survived for 9 months after initiation of HAI.

Case History 2

A 37-year-old woman with hepatic metastases resistant to systemic combination chemotherapy was treated with HAI through a catheter implanted at laparotomy. As with the patient discussed in Case History 1, no metastases were found elsewhere. A schedule of continuous fluorouracil administration supplemented with intermittent injections of doxorubicin was implemented. Serial computed tomography demonstrated necrosis of lesions in the liver. The patient survived 26 months after initiation of HAI.

These cases illustrate that HAI can produce objective regression of hepatic metastases when other measures fail, but HAI's influence on survival is uncertain.

ANGIOACCESS

Dependable access to major central veins is an increasingly frequent need of patients with breast cancer (Groeger et al.,

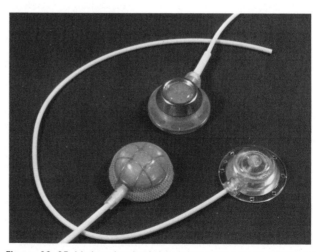

Figure 18–35. Various implantable intravenous ports attached to central venous catheters. After the catheter is introduced, the port is placed in the subcutaneous tissues of the anterior chest. The port provides reliable long-term intravenous access by percutaneous needle puncture.

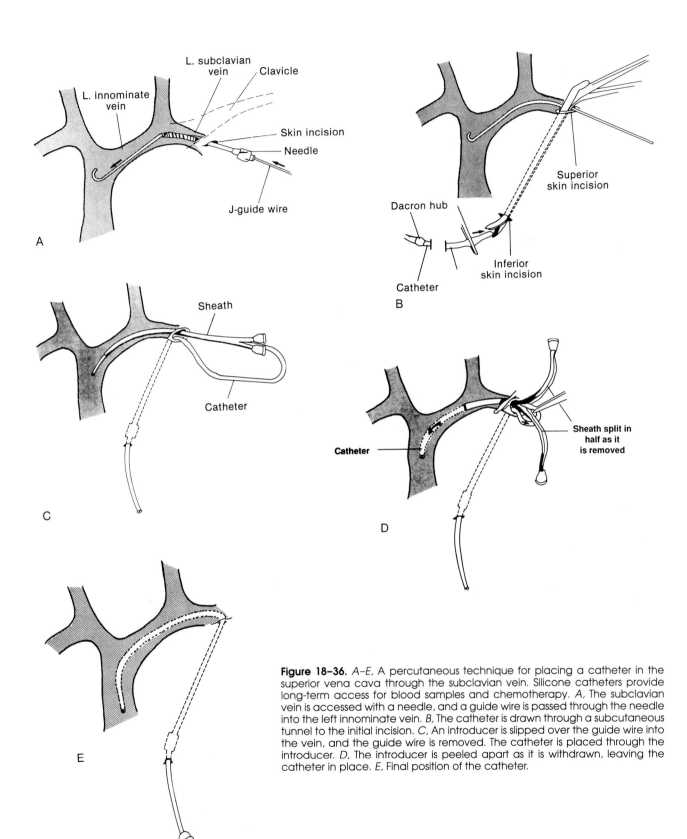

Figure 18–36. *A–E,* A percutaneous technique for placing a catheter in the superior vena cava through the subclavian vein. Silicone catheters provide long-term access for blood samples and chemotherapy. *A,* The subclavian vein is accessed with a needle, and a guide wire is passed through the needle into the left innominate vein. *B,* The catheter is drawn through a subcutaneous tunnel to the initial incision. *C,* An introducer is slipped over the guide wire into the vein, and the guide wire is removed. The catheter is placed through the introducer. *D,* The introducer is peeled apart as it is withdrawn, leaving the catheter in place. *E,* Final position of the catheter.

1991). It is most frequently indicated to permit adjuvant or palliative chemotherapy when peripheral veins are inadequate or have become exhausted. Less often, it is needed for nutrition or prolonged antibiotic administration. Catheters implanted for this purpose can be maintained for prolonged periods and avoid the risk of tissue necrosis from extravasation of corrosive drugs. The specially designed silicone catheters are implanted by means of an open operation or by percutaneous techniques and are accessed either via an implanted subcutaneous port (Fig. 18–35) or by leaving the distal end of the catheter exposed externally. Implantation is an outpatient procedure and is performed using local anesthesia under sterile operating room conditions. An important objective is to place the tip of the catheter in the superior vena cava short of the right atrium so that the drug is immediately diluted and does not cause thrombosis and so that the tip of the catheter does not irritate the heart. Access to the vena cava using percutaneous techniques is gained through the subclavian vein or the internal jugular vein. Alternatively, these veins, as well as the cephalic vein or external jugular vein, can be approached through open incisions. When the internal jugular vein is to be used, the vein on the right side provides the most direct access to the vena cava. Fields of irradiation or of anticipated irradiation are avoided as entry sites as are areas on which recurrent cancer is encroaching or is likely to encroach. Access is also made on the side opposite to an axillary dissection, as infection or venous thrombosis invites lymphedema of the arm (Lokich et al., 1985). If one lung is already compromised, the side that it is on is chosen as the side of entry in an effort to avoid exposing the remaining lung to the risk of pneumothorax. The explicit directions provided with each of the many catheters manufactured for this purpose are followed; and, to avoid malpositioning the catheter, its position is visualized during the procedure using a portable C-arm fluoroscopy apparatus.

The principal operative hazards with percutaneous techniques are pneumothorax and mediastinal hemorrhage (Takasugi and O'Connell, 1988). A postoperative chest radiograph is always obtained both to detect any pneumothorax that may need treatment and to document correct positioning of the catheter tip. Rarely, catheters break or segments of them are sheared off and embolize to the heart. These segments can be retrieved using interventional radiologic techniques (Franey et al., 1988). Repair kits to repair damage to exposed parts of a catheter are available. The most troublesome long-term complication is catheter-related infection. This is minimized by maintaining meticulous aseptic technique during insertion and during injection and by continuing antiseptic care of the exit site. The use of large, multilumen catheters and exposed catheters is attended by a higher risk of infection than is the use of small, single-lumen catheters and implanted ports (Parsa et al., 1989). A technique for percutaneous catheter placement via the subclavian vein is shown in Figure 18–36A–E).

SUMMARY

In this chapter, a variety of surgical techniques for the diagnosis and treatment of breast cancer have been re-

viewed. With their judicious use, many patients can be made more comfortable, many others can be given long periods of symptom-free survival, and some experience personal cures of their cancers.

References

Abramson, D. J.: Outpatient breast biopsy—Delayed mastectomy: A review. Contemp. Surg., *34*:2530, 1989.

Aitken, D. R., and Minton, J. P.: Complications associated with mastectomy. Surg. Clin. North Am., *63*:1331, 1983.

Beatson, G. T.: On the treatment of inoperable cases of carcinoma of the mamma. Lancet, *2*:104–107, 162–165, 1896.

Beatty, J. D., Robinson, G. V., Zaia, J. A., et al.: A prospective analysis of nosocomial wound infection after mastectomy. Arch. Surg., *118*:1421, 1983.

Blichert-Toft, M., Dyreborg, U., Bogh, L., et al.: Nonpalpable breast lesions: Mammographic wire-guided biopsy and radiologic-histologic correlation. World J. Surg., *6*:119–125, 1982.

Blumberg, N., and Heal, J. M.: Transfusion and recipient immune function. Arch. Pathol. Lab. Med., *113*:246–253, 1989.

Bridges, K. G., Keshgegian, A. A., Kumar, H. A. M., et al.: Influence of surgical technique on estrogen progesterone determinations in breast cancer. Cancer, *51*:2317, 1983.

Budd, D. C., Cochran, R. C., Sturtz, D. L., et al.: Surgical morbidity after mastectomy operations. Am. J. Surg., *135*:218–220, 1978.

Butcher, H. R., and Hoover, A. L.: Abnormalities of human superficial cutaneous lymphatics associated with stasis ulcers, lymphedema, scar and cutaneous autografts. Ann. Surg., *142*:663, 1955.

Choudhury, A., Wengert, P. A. Jr., and Smith, J. S.: A new surgical localization technique for biopsy in patients with nipple discharge. Arch. Surg., *124*:874–875, 1989.

Classen, D. C., Evans, R. S., Pestotnik, S. L., et al.: The timing of prophylactic administration of antibiotics and the risk of surgical wound infection. N. Engl. J. Med., *326*:281–286, 1992.

Cocconi, G., Bosagni, G., Ceci, G., et al.: Two-dose aminoglutethimide with and without hydrocortisone replacement as a first line endocrine treatment in advanced breast cancer: A prospective randomized trial of the Italian Oncology Group for Clinical Research. J. Clin. Oncol., *10*:984–989, 1992.

Conte, C. C., Nemoto, T., Rosner, D., et al.: Therapeutic oophorectomy in metastatic breast cancer. Cancer, *64*:150–153, 1989.

Crowe, J. P., Gordon, N. H., Fry, D. E., et al.: Breast cancer survival and perioperative blood transfusion. Surgery, *106*:836–841, 1989.

Cummings, P. D., Wallace, E. L., Schorr, J. B., et al.: Exposure of patients to human immunodeficiency virus through the transfusion of blood components that test antibiotic-negative. N. Engl. J. Med., *321*:941–946, 1989.

Cusick, J. D., Doran, J., Jaecks, R. D., et al.: The role of Tru-Cut needle biopsy in the diagnosis of carcinoma of the breast. Surg. Gynecol. Obstet., *170*:407–410, 1990.

Dajani, A. S., Bisno, A. L., Chung, K. J., et al.: Prevention of bacterial endocarditis. J. A. M. A., *264*:2919–2922, 1990.

Donegan, W. L.: Treatment of breast cancer in the elderly. *In* Yancik, R., Carbone, P. P., Patterson, W. B., et al. (Eds.): Perspectives on Prevention and Treatment of Cancer in the Elderly. New York, Raven Press, 1983, pp. 83–96.

Donegan, W. L., and Shah, D.: Prognosis of patients with breast cancer related to the timing of operation. Arch. Surg., *128*:309–313, 1993.

Dudrick, S. J., O'Donnell, J. J., Raleigh, D. P., et al.: Rapid restoration of red blood cell mass in severely anemic surgical patients who refuse transfusion. Arch. Surg., *120*:721–727, 1985.

Early Breast Cancer Trialists Collaborative Group: Systemic treatment of early breast cancer by hormonal, cytotoxic, or immune therapy. Lancet, *339*:2–85, 1992.

Edwards, M. J., Broadwater, J. R., Bell, J. L., et al.: Economic impact of reducing hospitalization for mastectomy patients. Ann. Surg., *208*:330–336, 1988.

Egdahl, R. H., and Melby, J. C.: Bilateral adrenalectomy for metastatic breast cancer. Hosp. Pract., August 1972, p. 79.

Fentiman, I. S., Brame, K., Chaudary, M. A., et al.: Perioperative bromocriptine adjuvant treatment for operable breast cancer. Lancet, *i*:609–610, 1988.

Fisher, B.: Reappraisal of breast biopsy prompted by the use of lumpectomy. J. A. M. A., *253*:3585–3588, 1985.

Fisher, E. R., Sass, R., and Fisher, B.: Biologic considerations regarding the one and two step procedures in the management of patients with invasive carcinoma of the breast. Surg. Gynecol. Obstet., *161*:245–249, 1985.

Foster, J. H.: Survival after liver resection for secondary tumors. Am. J. Surg., *135*:389, 1978.

Foster, R. S. Jr., Foster, J. C., and Costanza, M. C.: Blood transfusions and survival after surgery for breast cancer. Arch. Surg., *119*:1138, 1984.

Francis, D. M. A., and Shenton, B. K.: Blood transfusion and tumor growth: Evidence from laboratory animals. Lancet, *ii*:871, 1981.

Franey, T., DeMarco, L. C., Geiss, A. C., et al.: Catheter fracture and embolization in a totally implanted venous access catheter. J. P. E. N. J. Parenter. Enteral Nutr., *12*:528–530, 1988.

Fuller, T. C., Burroughs, J. C., Delmonico F. L., et al.: Influence of frozen blood transfusions on renal allograft survival. Transplant Proc., *14*:293, 1982.

Gantt, C. L.: Red blood cells from cancer patients. Lancet, *ii*:363, 1981.

Gately, C. A., Maddox, P. R., and Mansel, R. E.: Pneumothorax: Complication of fine needle aspiration of the breast. Br. Med. J., *303*:627–628, 1991.

Goldsmith, H. S., De Los Santos, R., and Beattie, E. J. Jr.: Omental transposition in the control of chronic lymphedema. J. A. M. A., *203*:117, 1968.

Goodnight, J. E. Jr., Quagliana, J. M., and Morton, D. L.: Failure of subcutaneous mastectomy to prevent the development of breast cancer. J. Surg. Oncol., *26*:198–201, 1984.

Gray, J. H.: The relation of lymphatic vessels to the spread of cancer. Br. J. Surg., *26*:462, 1939.

Groeger, J. S., Lucas, A. B., and Colt, D.: Venous access in the cancer patient. PPO Updates, *5*:1–14, 1991.

Handley, R. S.: The technique and results of conservative radical mastectomy (Patey's operation). Prog. Clin. Cancer, *1*:462, 1965.

Hanna, N., and Schneider, M.: Enhancement of tumor metastasis and suppression of natural killer cell activity by β-estradiol treatment. J. Immunol., *30*:974–980, 1983.

Hoeffken, W., and Vaillant, W.: Stereotactic tru-cut biopsy of nonpalpable lesions in mammography. *In* Zander, J., and Baltzer, J. (Eds.): Early Breast Cancer: Histopathology, Diagnosis, and Treatments. New York, Springer-Verlag, 1985, pp. 212–218.

Howard, J. M., Danese, C., and Laine, J. B.: Experimental lymphatic anastomosis. J. Cardiovasc. Surg., *5*:694, 1964.

Hrushesky, W. J. M., Bluming, A. Z., Gruber, S. A., et al.: Menstrual influence on surgical cure of breast cancer. Lancet, *ii*:949–952, 1989.

Hrushesky, W. J. M., Gruber, S., Sothern, R. B., et al.: Natural killer cell activity: Age, estrous and circadian-stage dependence and inverse correlation with metastatic potential. J. Natl. Cancer Inst., *80*:1232–1237, 1988.

Hughes, L. E., Mansel, R. E., Webster, D. J. T.: Benign Disorders and Diseases of the Breast. Philadelphia, Baillière Tindall, 1989, p. 9.

Ingle, J. N., Krook, J. E., Green, S. J., et al.: Randomized trial of bilateral oophorectomy versus tamoxifen in premenopausal women with metastatic breast cancer. J. Clin. Oncol., *4*:178, 1986.

Jamison, K., Wellisch, D. K., Katz, R. L., et al.: Phantom breast syndrome. Arch. Surg., *114*:93, 1979.

Ju, D. M. C., Blakemore, A., Stevenson, T. W.: A lymphatic function test. Surg. Forum, *5*:607, 1954.

Karydas, I., Fentiman, I. S., Habib, F., et al.: Sensory changes after treatment of operable breast cancer. Breast Cancer Res. Treat., *8*:55–59, 1986.

Kim, U.: Pathogenesis and characteristics of spontaneously metastasizing mammary carcinomas and the general principle of metastasis. J. Surg. Oncol., *33*:151–165, 1986.

Kinmonth, J. B.: The Lymphatics: Lymphography and Diseases of the Chyle and Lymph Systems. 2nd ed. London, Edward Arnold, 1982, p. 162.

LaCour, J., Le, M., Caceres, E., et al.: Radical mastectomy versus radical mastectomy plus internal mammary dissection. Cancer, *51*:1941, 1983.

Lennard, T. W. J., Shenton, B. K., Borzotta, A., et al.: The influence of surgical operations on components of the human immune system. Br. J. Surg., *72*:771–776, 1985.

Locker, A. P., Falea, M. H., Ellis, I. O., et al.: Microdochectomy for single-duct discharge from the nipple. Br. J. Surg., *75*:700–701, 1988.

Lokich, J. J., Bothe, A. Jr., Benotti, P., et al.: Complications and management of implanted venous access catheters. J. Clin. Oncol., *3*:710–717, 1985.

Lotze, M. T., Duncan, M. A., Gerber, L. H., et al.: Early versus delayed shoulder motion following axillary dissection. Ann. Surg., *193*:288, 1981.

Medgyesi, S.: A successful operation for lymphedema using a myocutaneous flap as a "wick." Br. J. Plast. Surg., *36*:64–66, 1983.

Meyer, J. E., Eberlein, T. J., Stomper, P. C., et al.: Biopsy of occult breast lesions. Analysis of 1261 abnormalities. J. A. M. A., *263*:2341–2343, 1990.

Morrow, M., and Foster, R. S. Jr.: Staging of breast cancer: A new rationale for internal mammary node biopsy. Arch. Surg., *116*:748, 1981.

The National Blood Resource Education Program Expert Panel: The use of autologous blood. J. A. M. A., *263*:414–417, 1990.

O'Brien, B. M., and Shafiroff, B. B.: Microlymphaticovenous and resectional surgery in obstructive lymphoedema. World J. Surg., *3*:3–15, 1979.

Orr, R. K., Ketcham, A. S., Robinson, D. S., et al.: Early discharge after mastectomy. Am. Surg., *53*:161–163, 1987.

Osteen, R. T., Cady, B., Chmiel, J. S. et al.: 1991 National Survey of Carcinoma of the Breast of the Commission on Cancer. J. Am. Coll. Surg., *178*:213–219, 1994.

Parker, S. H., Lovin, J. D., Jobe, W. E., et al.: Nonpalpable breast lesions: Stereotactic automated large core biopsies. Radiology, *180*:403–407, 1991.

Parsa, M. H., Tabora, F., and Al-Sawwaf, M.: Vascular Access Techniques. *In* Shoemaker, W. C. (Ed.): Textbook of Critical Care. 2nd ed. Philadelphia, W.B. Saunders, 1989, p. 144.

Patey, D. H., and Dyson, W. H.: The prognosis of carcinoma of the breast in relation to the type of operation performed. Br. J. Cancer, *2*:7, 1948.

Planting, A. S. T., Figusch, J. A., Wijst, J. B., et al.: Tamoxifen therapy in premenopausal women with breast cancer. Cancer Treat. Res., *69*:363, 1985.

Platt, R., Zaleznik, D. F., Hopkins, C. C., et al.: Perioperative antibiotic prophylaxis for herniorrhaphy and breast surgery. N. Engl. J. Med., *322*:153–160, 1990.

Pollock, R. E., Lotzova, E., Stanford, S. D., et al.: Effect of surgical stress on murine natural killer cell cytotoxicity. J. Immunol., *138*:171–178, 1987.

Proudfoot, R. W., Mattingly, S., Stelling, C. B., et al.: Nonpalpable breast lesions: Wire localization and excisional biopsy. Am. Surg., *52*:117–121, 1986.

Ratajczak, H. V., Sothern, R. B., and Hrushesky, W. J. M.: Estrus influence on surgical cure of mouse breast cancer. J. Exp. Med., *168*:88–96, 1988.

Reichert, F. L.: The regeneration of lymphatics. Arch. Surg., *13*:871, 1926.

Reid, S. E. Jr., Scanlon, E. F., Bernstein, J. R., et al.: An alternative approach to nonpalpable breast biopsies. J. Surg. Oncol., *44*:93–96, 1990.

Richmand, D. M., O'Donnell, T. E. Jr., and Zelikovski, A.: Sequential pneumatic compression for lymphedema. Arch. Surg., *120*:1116–1119, 1985.

Rosenthal, L. J.: Discrepant estrogen receptor protein levels according to surgical technique. Am. J. Surg., *138*:680, 1979.

Rusznyak, I., Mihaly, F., and Szabo, G.: Lymphatics and lymph circulation. New York, Pergamon Press, 1960.

Sabiston, D. C.: Pulmonary embolism. *In* Sabiston, D.C. Jr. (Ed.): Davis-Christopher Textbook of Surgery. 12th ed. Philadelphia, W.B. Saunders, 1981, p. 1839.

Savage, R. C.: The surgical management of lymphedema. Surg. Gynecol. Obstet., *160*:283–289, 1985.

Sawka, C. A., Pritchard, K. I., Paterson, A. H., et al.: Role and mechanism of action of tamoxifen in premenopausal women with metastatic breast carcinoma. Cancer Res., *46*:3152, 1986.

Scanlon, E. F.: The importance of the anterior thoracic nerves in modified radical mastectomy. Surg. Gynecol. Obstet., *152*:789–791, 1981.

Scanlon, E. F., and Caprini, J. A.: Modified radical mastectomy. Cancer, *35*:710, 1975.

Schick, P. M., Shabot, M. K. M., Block, J. B., et al.: Local delayed cutaneous hypersensitivity reactions in breast cancer patients with and without removal of axillary lymph nodes. Am. J. Surg., *132*:40–45, 1976.

Schneebaum, S., Walker, M. J., Young, D., et al.: The regional treatment of liver metastases from breast cancer. J. Surg. Oncol., *55*:26–31, 1994.

Schneiderman, M. A., Axtell, L. M.: Deaths among female patients with carcinoma of the breast treated by a surgical procedure only. Surg. Gynecol. Obstet., *148*:193–195, 1979.

Smoller, B. R., and Kruskall, M. S.: Phlebotomy for diagnostic laboratory tests in adults: Patterns of use and effect on transfusion requirements. N. Engl. J. Med., *314*:1233, 1986.

Spratt, J. S. Jr., Shieber, W., and Dillard, B. M.: Anatomy and Surgical Technique of Groin Dissection. St. Louis, C.V. Mosby, 1965.

Spratt, J. S., Zirnheld, J., and Yancey, J.: Breast Cancer Detection Demonstration Project data can determine whether the prognosis of breast cancer is affected by the time of surgery during the menstrual cycle. J. Surg. Oncol. *53*:4–9, 1993.

Staps, T., Hoogenhout, J., and Wobbes, T.: Phantom breast sensations following mastectomy. Cancer, *56*:2898–2901, 1985.

Stark, R. B., Dwyer, E. M., and DeForest, M.: Effect of surgical ablation of regional lymph nodes on survival of skin homografts. Ann. N. Y. Acad. Sci., *89*:140–148, 1960.

Starling, E. H.: On absorption of fluid from connective tissue spaces. J. Physiol., *19*:312, 1898.

Stillwell, G. K.: Treatment of postmastectomy lymphedema. Mod. Treat., *6*:396, 1959.

Tadros, T., Wobbes, T., and Hendriks, T.: Blood transfusion impairs the healing of experimental intestinal anastomoses. Ann. Surg., *215*:276, 1992.

Tadych, K., and Donegan, W. L.: Postmastectomy seromas and wound drainage. Surg. Gynecol. Obstet., *165*:483–487, 1987.

Takasugi, J. K., and O'Connell, X. T.: Prevention of complications in permanent central venous catheters. Surg. Gynecol. Obstet., *165*:6–11, 1988.

Tartter, P. I., Burrows, L., Papatestas, A. E., et al.: Perioperative blood transfusion has prognostic significance for breast cancer. Surgery, *97*:225, 1985.

Teicher, I., Poulard, B., and Wise, L.: Preservation of the intercostobrachial nerve during axillary dissection for carcinoma of the breast. Surg. Gynecol. Obstet., *155*:891–892, 1982.

Temple, W. J., and Ketcham, A. S.: Preservation of the intercostobrachial nerve during axillary dissection for breast cancer. Am. J. Surg., *150*:585–588, 1985.

Tengrup, I., Nittby, L. T., and Landberg, T.: Prophylactic oophorectomy in the treatment of carcinoma of the breast. Surg. Gynecol. Obstet., *162*:209,1986.

Thompson, N.: The surgical treatment of chronic lymphoedema of the extremities. Surg. Clin. North Am., *47*:445, 1967.

Toy, P. T. C. Y., Strauss, R. G., Stehling, L. C., et al.: Predeposited autologous blood for elective surgery: A national multicenter study. N. Engl. J. Med., *316*:517–520, 1987.

Tracy, G. D., Reeve, T. S., Fitzsimons, E., et al.: Observations on the swollen arm after radical mastectomy. N. Z. J. Surg., *30*:204, 1961.

Treves, N.: Evaluation of the etiological factors of lymphedema following radical mastectomy. Cancer, *10*:444, 1957.

Uchida, A., Kolb, R., and Micksche, M.: Generation of suppressor cell activity in cancer patients after surgery. J. Natl. Cancer Inst., *68*:735, 1982.

Vasudevan, S. V., and Melvin, J. L.: Upper extremity edema control: Rationale of the techniques. Am. J. Occup. Med., *33*:520–523, 1979.

Veronesi, U., and Valagussa, P.: Inefficacy of internal mammary node dissection in breast cancer surgery. Cancer, *47*:170, 1981.

Vinton, A. L., Traverso, L. W., and Jolly, P. C.: Wound complications after modified radical mastectomy compared with tylectomy with axillary lymph node dissection. Am. J. Surg., *161*:584–588, 1991.

Waymack, J. P., Rapien, J., Garnett, D., et al.: Effect on transfusions on immune function in a traumatized animal model. Arch. Surg., 121:50, 1986.

Wilson, R. E., Donegan, W. L., Mettlin, C., et al.: The 1982 national survey of carcinoma of the breast in the United States by the American College of Surgeons. Surg. Gynecol. Obstet., *159*:309–318, 1984.

Zander, H. L.: Preoperative hemoglobin requirements. Anesth. Clin. North Am., *8*:471–480, 1990.

19

Definitive, Adjuvant, and Palliative Radiation Therapy for Mammary Cancer

J. Frank Wilson
James D. Cox

The remarkable speed with which ionizing radiation was recognized as a highly potent agent against breast cancer shortly after the discovery of x-rays in 1895 was fortuitous (Hodges, 1964). By 1905, the first radiologic textbooks recommended radiation therapy for locally advanced, unresectable primary breast carcinoma or for patients who categorically refused surgery. Despite this early application, subsequent progress toward definition of the optimal role of irradiation in breast cancer management was achieved slowly. Medical opinion concerning acceptable treatment options changed little until the Halstedian precepts of "en bloc" surgical dissection were successfully challenged in a series of modern clinical trials. First tentative attempts to exploit more fully the powerful new technique as an adjuvant to radical mastectomy did not occur until the 1930s. The lack of good quality, highly controllable radiation delivery systems until the late 1950s hampered investigators, and it took nearly another 20 years to fully recognize the regularity with which irradiation is capable of eradicating cancer cell aggregates depending on their size and the radiation doses employed (Fletcher, 1985).

Although it is now generally accepted that radiation doses of 45 to 50 grays (Gy) (1 Gy = 100 rad) are sufficient to eliminate subclinical deposits of cancer cells 90% to 95% of the time (Fletcher, 1974), gross tumor masses are likely to be controlled only when substantially larger doses are administered (Arriagada et al., 1985) (see Table 19–4). Primary or metastatic masses a few centimeters in diameter or larger are likely to require doses that approach or even exceed the radiation tolerance of normal tissues in the area. Therefore, the therapeutic ratio is enhanced when irradiation must contend only with microscopic disease. In this circumstance, moderately intense, well-tolerated doses of irradiation yield a high probability of tumor control, yet the incidence of associated late treatment sequelae will be minimal or nil. Practical applications of these fundamental radiobiologic principles in current strategies for optimal use of irradiation in the management of breast carcinoma will be apparent in the following discussion.

Modern techniques of breast-conserving treatment represent the ultimate clinical extension of the radiobiologic principles just mentioned, as with this approach all gross tumor is excised from the breast prior to administering irradiation in doses appropriate for subclinical residuae. In this manner, not only is a high rate of tumor control achieved, but in addition maximal esthetic and functional preservation is afforded the patient.

Skillfully applied radiation therapy is becoming increasingly indispensable in the management of breast cancer, depending on multiple clinicopathologic factors, including the stage of disease, histopathologic findings, extent of surgery, and the patient's preferences. These and other factors must be weighed carefully in each case, to select patients for treatment and to correctly tailor the irradiation to the individual need. The following discussion will review the rationale and results of the currently recommended uses of radiation therapy in the management of patients with breast cancer.

BREAST CONSERVING TREATMENT OF EARLY INVASIVE BREAST CANCER

The seemingly new concept of treating breast cancer with limited surgery followed by irradiation can actually be traced to its origins in the work of a few early pioneers. Although the British surgeon Keynes (1929) reported gratifying results with extensive radium needle implantations in the breast and nodal areas with occasional tumorectomy, this particular approach was never widely practiced and ultimately was abandoned. It was, more precisely, the explorations of several individuals working with external beam irradiation in Europe and Canada that, by the late 1960s, demonstrated the curative potential of conservative therapy for breast cancer (Baclesse, 1959; Rissanen, 1969; Peters, 1976; Spitalier et al., 1986; and Clark et al., 1987). Aided by rapid technologic development in radiation therapy delivery systems, many other groups then began to expand the clinical experience. Retrospective series that reflect the large worldwide success with conservative breast treatment for Stages I and II breast cancer, are summarized in Table 19–1. These long-term results are remarkable for the consistent demonstration of high local-regional control rates and corresponding survival figures, which are comparable to those reported in mastectomy series.

Ultimately, well-designed and well-executed prospective randomized trials comparing breast conservation therapy to

Table 19–1. LONG-TERM RESULTS OF BREAST CONSERVATION THERAPY

Investigators, Year	Patients (N)	Maximum Primary Tumor Size (cm)	10-Year Survival (%)		Breast Recurrence Rate (%) at 10 Years
			Disease-Free	*Overall*	
Fowble et al., 1991	697	5	73	83	18
Haffy et al., 1989	278	5	—	67	20
Stotter et al., 1989	490	5	—	74*	19
Veronesi et al., 1990	1232	2	—	78	8
Harris et al., 1990	525	5	—	70*	
Leung et al., 1986	493	5	67	68	10
Dubois et al., 1988	392	5	63	78	16
Zafrani et al., 1989	434	†	—	86	11
Amalric et al., 1983	274	5	74	—	
Delouche et al., 1987	410	5	—	63	

(Modified and reprinted from Winchester, D. P., and Cox, J. D.: Standards for breast-conservation treatment. CA Cancer J. Clin., 42:133–162, 1992.)
*Estimated from curves.

mastectomy have clearly demonstrated the equivalence of the two treatments for appropriately selected patients with early breast cancer. Long-term results after 8 to 10 years' follow-up reveal no significant difference in overall survival, disease-free survival, or local-regional control between the two arms in any of the trials (Table 19–2).

Based in part on such evidence, a National Institutes of Health Consensus Conference in 1990 concluded, "breast conservation treatment is an appropriate method of primary therapy for the majority of women with Stage I and II breast cancer, and is *preferable* because it provides survival equivalent to total mastectomy and axillary dissection while preserving the breast."

Despite this stance, recent studies reveal apparent underutilization of breast conservation treatment in patients with early breast cancer in the United States (Osteen et al., 1992). Marked geographical variation in the frequency of use is noted, ranging from 3.5% to 21.2% in various states (Nattinger et al., 1992). Utilization rates have been particularly low for women aged 65 and older and for black women in some areas (Farrow et al., 1992). Further research to precisely determine appropriate utilization rates of

breast conservation therapy as well as educational initiatives to ensure full professional and public awareness of this treatment option are needed. Accordingly, a practice standard for breast conservation treatment developed with the sponsorship and endorsement of four leading national professional organizations concerned with breast cancer was recently published and should be an influential new benchmark (Winchester et al., 1992).

Breast-sparing therapy is not, however, a panacea for all women with breast cancer. Cooperative multidisciplinary approaches to patient selection and to treatment implementation are key to obtaining optimal results. The most suitable candidates are women with relatively small (≤5 cm) single primary tumors, regardless of histologic subtype. Associated inflammatory changes or tumor extension to the skin or chest wall precludes conservative therapy. Other detailed clinical and mammographic findings must also be assessed in each case to identify patients in whom the parallel treatment aims of achieving local-regional tumor control and leaving the breast in a nearly normal state posttherapeutically can be met. Tumor-related contraindications to breast conserving therapy include diffuse microcalcifica-

Table 19–2. RESULTS OF SIX MODERN PROSPECTIVE TRIALS OF BREAST-CONSERVING SURGERY

Trial (Investigators)	Patients (N)	Maximum Primary Tumor Size (cm)	Surgical Technique*	Radiation Dose: Breast/ Boost (Gy)	Disease-Free Survival (%)		Overall Survival Rate (%)	
					Irradiation	*Mastectomy*	*Irradiation*	*Mastectomy*
NSABP (Fisher et al., 1989)	1,219	4	WE	50/000	59	58	76	71
Milan (Veronesi et al., 1986)	701	2	Q	50/10	77	76	79	78
Institut Gustave Roussy (Sarazin et al., 1989)	179	2	WE	45/15	65	56	78	79
EORTC (Van Dongen et al., 1990)	903	5	WE	50/25	—	—	—	—
Danish (Blichert-Toft et al., 1988)	619	No limit	WE	50/10–25	70	66	79	82
NCI (Lichter et al., 1992b)	237	5	WE	45–50/15–20	66	76	85	79

(Modified and reprinted from Winchester, D. P., and Cox, J. D.: Standards for breast-conservation treatment. CA Cancer J. Clin., 42:133–162, 1992.)
Abbreviations: WE, wide excision; Q, quadrantectomy.

tions on mammography, the presence of multiple gross lesions, and either grossly positive or diffusely positive microscopic margins of tumor excision that cannot be rendered negative by re-excision without producing excessive deformity of the breast. These factors are highly predictive of a large residual tumor burden in the breast and are associated with an unacceptably high rate of local recurrence following conservative treatment. Solin and associates (1991a) clearly demonstrated that patients with only focally positive or close excision margins can be successfully treated without decrement in local control. In most series young age or the presence of certain other histopathologic features, particularly the presence of an extensive intraductal cancer component, are associated with increased risk of breast recurrence (McCormick, 1992). In any event, the risk is not so high in these circumstances as to contraindicate conservative treatment if adequate tumor excision is performed (Fourquet et al., 1989; and Solin et al., 1989). Patients of advanced age or with large or pendulous breasts should not be excluded from conservative management, but special radiotherapeutic techniques may be required to obtain optimal results (Gray et al., 1991). Host factors that contraindicate conservative breast management include pregnancy during irradiation, underlying collagen vascular disease (Fleck, 1989; and Robertson, 1991), and patient preference for mastectomy.

Whether wide local excision (tylectomy), segmental resection, or some other surgical approach is used to extirpate the primary mass from the breast, the goals of esthetic and functional preservation must be borne in mind. Ideally the operation removes the mass along with a narrow margin of breast tissue without significantly deforming the breast. Particular care must be taken to avoid excessive surgical distortion if the breast is small or if the primary lesion is positioned in the medial aspect of the breast. Use of the smallest possible incision, respecting normal skin lines and placed directly over the lesion to avoid "tunneling," is recommended. Meticulous hemostasis and preservation of the fat layer overlying the breast tissue are essential to obtaining optimal results.

Dissection of the lateral axilla (Levels I and II) before irradiation is recommended for determination of axillary lymph node status to establish prognosis and often to select patients for adjuvant systemic therapy. Complete axillary dissection is unnecessary since "skip" metastases to the highest level of the axilla are rare if an adequate number of Level I and II nodes are examined and found to be uninvolved (Danforth et al., 1986; Veronesi et al., 1987; and Kiricuta et al., 1992). If involved lymph nodes are recovered, elective irradiation of the apical axillary and supraclavicular nodal areas is justifiable, but this supplementary irradiation is unnecessary if the nodes are negative (Recht et al., 1991b; and Solin, 1992).

Although complete axillary dissection provides a somewhat more accurate assessment than limited dissection, distressing breast or arm edema, the most common major morbidity associated with breast conservation treatment, is much more likely to occur. Clarke and associates (1982) noted a 79% incidence of breast lymphedema after staging axillary dissection and breast irradiation. In contrast, Rose and colleagues (1983) observed only occasional mild breast

edema and no arm complications following low axillary dissection that stopped short of the axillary vein. Risk of breast or arm edema is increased by the addition of regional node irradiation and is radiation dose dependent (Dewar et al., 1987; and Solin, 1992).

Once adequate healing has occurred, usually 10 to 14 days following the surgical procedures, radiation therapy is begun. All remaining breast tissue is irradiated via opposed medial and lateral tangential portals, which parallel the arc of the chest wall at depth and encompass a thin volume of the underlying lung. The margins of these fields are precisely matched with those of the supplementary fields, if any, used to irradiate the peripheral nodal regions (Lichter et al., 1992a). A total dose to the target areas of 45 to 50 Gy is administered in 5 to 5½ weeks. A boost dose of an additional 10 to 20 Gy directed to the operative bed in the breast is usually also administered, either with electron beam irradiation or by temporary interstitial implantation of radioactive sources (iridium 192).

Boosting of either type was usually employed in single-institution series and in five of the six prospective trials cited earlier (Tables 19–1, 19–2). Supporting theoretical arguments for this dose augmentation are that any residual tumor cell aggregates are most likely to lie close to the surgical bed and may be relatively protected by hypoxic conditions in the area. Most breast recurrences are in fact detected close to the site of the original tumor (Kurtz and Spitalier, 1990). Although a local recurrence rate of only 10% without boosting was observed in the National Surgical Adjuvant Breast Project (NSABP) trial (Fisher et al., 1989), surgical margins in other series frequently have not been as complete as in this group study. Therefore, until prospective studies clearly identify any existing subsets of patients, the practice should continue routinely, especially when there is the least doubt concerning the adequacy of the tumor removal.

Esthetically satisfactory end results of conservative therapy for early stage breast cancer have been observed in all reports (Table 19–3, Fig. 19–1). Approximately 65% to 95% of patients have a good to excellent result using observer-based scoring systems (Delouche et al., 1987; and Pierquin et al., 1991). Poor or unacceptable results are described in no more than 5% to 10% of patients. Cosmetic status of the breast does not deteriorate appreciably over time, owing to evolution of late radiation changes in the breast (Olivotto et al., 1989). Moreover, patient self-evaluation indicates that most women are satisfied with the posttherapeutic status of their breast and consistently rate the results higher than do other observers. Few would consider alternative treatment options for contralateral breast carcinoma (Dubois et al., 1990; Matory et al., 1990; and Patterson et al., 1985). Studies that have examined the impact of treatment on quality of life reveal a better-preserved body image and less chance of sexual dysfunction with breast conservation than with mastectomy (McCormick et al., 1989; and Kiebert et al., 1991). Most treatment-related morbidity is avoidable, and adherence to established technical principles of conservative surgery and radiotherapy yields optimal cosmetic results (Van Limbergen et al., 1989; and Winchester et al., 1992). The overall incidence of complications other than breast or arm edema (i.e., pericarditis,

Table 19–3. LOCAL EXCISION AND RADIOTHERAPY FOR DUCTAL CARCINOMA IN SITU

Investigators	Patients (N)	Follow-up (mo)	Recurrences					Survival (%)
			Number	5-Year (%)	10-Year (%)	Crude (%)	Invasive	
Fisher et al., 1986	29	39 (?)	2	—	—	7	24	100%
Kurtz et al., 1989	44	61 (?)	3	4	—	7	3/3	98%
Solin et al., 1990a	51	68 (25–126)	5	6	—	10	2/5	98%
Stotter et al., 1990	42	92 (12–208)	4	—	—	9.5%	4/4	93%
Bornstein et al., 1991	38	81 (35–155)	8	8	27	21	5/8	—
Fourquet et al., 1992	67	104 (14–220)	7	5	10	10	5/7	98%

(Modified from Fourquet, A., Zafrani, B., Campana, J.-C. D., and Vilcoq, J. R.: Breast-conserving treatment of ductal carcinoma in situ. Radiat. Oncol., 2:116–124, 1992.)

brachial plexopathy, rib fracture, pneumonitis) is less than 2% to 3% (Fowble et al., 1991; and Kurtz and Miralbell, R. 1992).

Increasing use of adjuvant chemotherapy in both premenopausal and postmenopausal node-positive and high-risk node-negative patients is problematic relative to its integration with conservative breast treatment. Although patients' ability to tolerate optimal doses of multiagent chemotherapy is not significantly compromised by standard irradiation (Lippman et al., 1984), inferior cosmetic results and more complications are observed in patients who receive chemotherapy, particularly when certain drugs (doxorubicin, methotrexate) are administered concurrently with irradiation (Abner et al., 1991; and Lingos et al., 1991). Adverse effects of chemotherapy on cosmetic results generally are not so serious as to prohibit integration of chemotherapy when indicated (Danoff et al., 1983; and Ray et al., 1983). Competing rationales for delaying either the irradiation or the chemotherapy until the other is completed are conceptually less satisfactory than concurrent or alternating regimens. Of particular concern is recent evidence suggesting an unacceptably high rate of breast recurrence when irradia-

tion is not initiated within 16 weeks postoperatively (Recht et al., 1991a).

BREAST CONSERVING TREATMENT OF NONINVASIVE BREAST CANCER

Large-scale mammographic screening for breast cancer has resulted in a dramatic increase in the detection of cases of ductal carcinoma in situ (DCIS). Correspondingly, the typical clinical presentation of this disease has shifted so that the majority of cases present as abnormal calcifications detectable only on mammography rather than as a palpable breast mass. This must be taken into account in comparing recent treatment results with historical data. In many practices, cases of DCIS already constitute more than 20% of all breast cancers presenting for management, as compared with only a few per cent a decade ago (Rosner et al., 1980; and Wilson et al., 1992).

Mastectomy is highly curative of DCIS but is a more aggressive treatment than is required for early invasive breast cancer. Breast-sparing treatment of DCIS is a valid

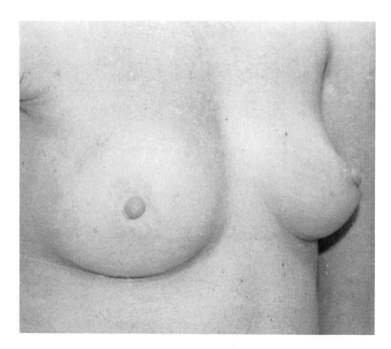

Figure 19–1. Esthetic results at 3 years in a 55-year-old woman treated by excisional biopsy, external beam irradiation (5000 cGy), and boost by electron beam (1000 cGy) for a T1N0M0 (UOQ right breast).

but controversial treatment option for carefully selected patients who desire breast conservation (Solin et al., 1990*a,b*). Candidates for conservative treatment include patients with small, unifocal lesions, negative margins of tumor excision, and no evidence of residual calcifications on postbiopsy mammography (Fowble, 1989). Surgical and radiotherapeutic techniques described earlier for conservative management of invasive breast cancer are appropriate, except that axillary lymph node dissection is unnecessary (Silverstein et al., 1987; and Lagios, 1990). The rationale for implementing breast irradiation following wide local excision of DCIS is to eradicate occult residual carcinoma in the vicinity of the index lesion as well as any neoplastic foci elsewhere in the breast (Holland et al., 1985). A large prospective trial (NSABP B-17) to test this rationale compared outcomes of lumpectomy alone and lumpectomy combined with breast irradiation (Fisher et al., 1993). The early results of this particular study are similar to those of a more mature previous NSABP trial (Fisher et al., 1986). Although the study (NSABP B-06) was designed for patients with invasive breast cancer, subsequent pathologic review revealed that 78 patients with carcinoma in situ had been entered in the study. The rate of local recurrence for patients who underwent wide excision alone was 23%, compared with 7% in patients following wide excision and irradiation.

Reported series of conservative surgery and irradiation for DCIS indicate breast recurrence rates ranging from 4% to 21% (Table 19–4). No more than 5% of all patients experience distant failure (Solin et al., 1990*a;* Bornstein et al., 1991; and Kuske et al., 1992). These retrospective studies have been criticized for nonuniformity of patient material (inclusion of large lesions, incomplete excision) and too short follow-up to fully validate conservative treatment. Responding to this critique, a group of nine U.S. and European institutions recently reported results in 259 women treated with breast-conserving surgery and definitive irradiation for DCIS and followed for a minimum of 5 years (Solin et al., 1991*b*). The 10-year disease-free survival rate was 97% in these patients and the 10-year actuarial rate of local recurrence, 16%; though 24 of the 28 patients who developed breast recurrence were salvaged by additional treatment. Therefore, a high rate of successful salvage treatment results in an ultimate cure rate equivalent to that reported in mastectomy series with the vast majority of patients (84%) retaining their breast. Unless even longer follow-up of such series or new results from ongoing trials eventually reveal inferior survival in selected patients with DCIS who receive conservative surgery and irradiation, it will become an established treatment option.

Vigilant long-term follow-up of patients treated conservatively for DCIS is mandatory. Breast recurrences are commonly detected more than 5 years after treatment for DCIS, and about one-half of these recurrences are invasive lesions. Certain pathologic subtypes (e.g., comedo-type necrosis, high nuclear grade) or bloody nipple discharge at presentation may predict a high rate of local recurrence (Lagios, 1990; Silverstein et al., 1991; and Fourquet et al., 1992). Additional data are needed to clarify these risks, but it is doubtful that any negative influence of such factors will be significant enough to contraindicate conservative treatment if initial tumor excision is adequate. Prospective trials are ongoing to determine whether tamoxifen can prevent recurrences or the development of new neoplastic foci in the breast following conservative surgery alone or with breast irradiation. Eventual results of these studies may greatly alter future management of the growing number of women with DCIS.

Postoperative Irradiation

Numerous retrospective and prospective studies have demonstrated that adequate irradiation following total, modified

Table 19–4. RANDOMIZED TRIALS OF POSTOPERATIVE RADIOTHERAPY AFTER RADICAL MASTECTOMY

Study	Patients (N)	Areas Treated	Follow-up (yr)	Local Control	Relapse-Free Survival	Survival	Comments
Manchester I (Palmer et al., 1985)	720	Chest wall, axilla	20–30	+		0	Randomization not strict, ortho-voltage RT
Manchester II (Ribeiro, 1987)	741	Regional lymph nodes	20–30	+		0	
NSABP (Fisher et al., 1970)	Radiation therapy = 91; control = 235	Regional lymph nodes	5	+	0	0	Randomization not strict, short follow-up
Oslo I (Host et al., 1986)	546	Chest wall, regional nodes	> 11	+	0	0	Ortho-voltage
Oslo II (Host et al., 1986)	542	Regional lymph nodes	> 11	+ +	+ Stage II	0	Super-voltage
Stockholm (Wallgren et al., 1986)	644	Chest wall, regional nodes	8–14	+ +	+	0	

(Modified with permission from Harris, J. R., and Hellman, S.: Put the "Hockey Stick" on ice. Int. J. Radiation Oncol. Biol. Phys., *15*:497–499, 1988. Copyright 1988, Pergamon Press Ltd.)
Symbols: 0, no improvement; +, some improvement; + +, large improvement with use of postoperative radiotherapy.

radical or radical mastectomy for breast carcinoma significantly reduces the incidence of subsequent local and regional recurrence (Paterson and Russell, 1959; Fisher et al., 1970; Host et al., 1986; Fletcher et al., 1989; and Rutqvist et al., 1989). This major advantage is readily provided by employing any of several acceptable treatment techniques to administer moderate doses of 45 to 50 Gy to the regional lymphatics and tissues of the chest wall (Toonkel et al., 1982). Adjunctive irradiation has generally been recommended for patients with dense axillary lymph node involvement (more than four involved nodes) or a large primary lesion (>5 cm). Other indications include tumor involvement of the skin or chest wall and inadequate surgical margins. Elective irradiation alone prevents local or regional recurrence in all but 5% to 10% of patients at risk for such recurrences (Fletcher, 1984).

Whether the improved local and regional control of breast carcinoma consequent to postoperative irradiation is also associated with a reduction in distant metastasis and better rates of survival is an unresolved question. Several randomized trials frequently cited as evidence that irradiation does not provide such benefits are in fact representative of many early trials in which the radiation technique or dosages were deficient (Paterson and Russell, 1959; and Cancer Research Campaign, 1976). It is axiomatic that a reduced incidence of distant metastasis and improved survival could be expected only in patients whose disease was not already disseminated before their initial treatment and in whom uncontrolled clinically occult local or regional disease would give rise to systemic spread. Therefore, these gains from postoperative irradiation would be demonstrable only in a subgroup—perhaps a small one—of appropriately treated patients in whom these conditions existed. Long-term follow-up data from large retrospective series and well-regarded clinical trials continue to emerge addressing this premise and seeking to identify this subgroup (Tubiana et al., 1986; and Fletcher et al., 1989). For example, multivariate analysis of a retrospective series of 1159 axillary node–positive patients, by investigators at the Institut Gustave Roussy recently suggested evidence of reduced risk of metastasis and improved survival for patients with medial breast tumors whose treatment included the internal mammary chain (Arriagada et al., 1988; and Lê et al., 1990). Even more recently, joint analysis of long-term results from the Oslo and Stockholm trials (Host et al., 1986; Rutqvist et al., 1989; and Auqier et al., 1992) was performed to provide as much statistical power as possible for evaluating postoperative irradiation. Significant reduction of distant metastasis with radiation ($P < .01$) and an overall survival difference favoring irradiated patients that corresponded with a 22% relative reduction of deaths of borderline significance ($P < .06$) were found; however, in this analysis the benefit was independent of the position of the primary lesion in the breast. There was no benefit among axillary node–negative patients. At the least, these data appear to confirm that locoregional irradiation can prevent distant dissemination of disease in some node-positive patients with breast cancer and are persuasive evidence that to categorically assume that all such patients have systemic disease from the time of diagnosis is erroneous.

Postmastectomy adjuvant chemotherapy alone does not decrease the incidence of local and regional recurrence when compared with mastectomy alone. Fowble and associates (1988b) analyzed risk factors in 627 node-positive patients who received adjuvant chemotherapy alone in Eastern Cooperative Oncology Group (ECOG) studies and identified a subgroup of patients (four or five involved nodes, tumor size 7.5 cm) whose risk of an isolated local-regional recurrence equals or exceeds the likelihood of distant metastases. They argue that it is this subset of patients that may stand to enjoy a survival benefit from postoperative irradiation, and they have reported encouraging survival data in a similar group of patients treated at their institution (Fowble et al., 1988a,b). This and other studies demonstrating improved local-regional control and disease-free survival with the addition of postoperative irradiation to adjunctive systemic chemotherapy argue strongly for its implementation in patients at high risk for local-regional recurrence (Griem et al., 1987; Rivkin et al., 1989; and Sykes et al., 1989).

Significantly increased risk of death due to ischemic heart disease is reported in some patients who received postoperative irradiation as the only adjunctive treatment in the Oslo and Stockholm trials (Host et al., 1986; and Rutqvist et al., 1992). However, this treatment-related morbidity was confined to subsets of patients in whom the biologic dose of radiation to the heart was unusually large and the cardiac volume irradiated was large as well. These dosimetric problems are avoidable with sophisticated radiotherapy techniques, but the need to confine the use of adjunctive irradiation to the patients most likely to benefit from it is underscored. This is particularly true considering the frequent use of cardiotoxic chemotherapy to treat patients with breast cancer.

Preoperative Irradiation

Preoperative irradiation converts a significant proportion of borderline resectable primary breast masses to full resectability; however, this approach is now seldom considered. Dramatic reduction in the expected incidence of axillary lymph node involvement and of extranodal tumor extension is observed following preoperative irradiation (Table 19–5).

Retrospective and prospective studies of irradiation administered as a preoperative adjunct to radical mastectomy demonstrate that it is at least as effective as postoperative irradiation in securing local and regional control of breast cancer. Long-term follow-up of the Swedish trial (Rutqvist et al., 1992), which compared preoperative or postoperative irradiation combined with modified radical mastectomy to mastectomy alone reveals survival benefit of borderline significance for irradiated patients. There is no significant difference between the two irradiated groups. Whether any of the theoretical advantages of preoperative irradiation were realized, including potential reduction in the release of viable malignant clonogens into the systemic circulation during surgical manipulation, has not been clarified by this or any other trial to date.

Seeking to extend the benefits of breast conservation therapy to selected patients with locally advanced breast

Table 19–5. INCIDENCE OF AXILLARY LYMPH NODE METASTASES AND EXTRANODAL TUMOR EXTENSION FOLLOWING PREOPERATIVE IRRADIATION

Investigator	Clinical Axillary Status	Prevalence of Histologically Positive Nodes (%)		Prevalence of Extranodal Tumor (%)	
		Surgery Only	*With Preoperative Radiation*	*Surgery Only*	*With Preoperative Radiation*
Wallgren (1978)	—	37 (238/638)	21 (65/306)	52	19
Rodger (1983)	N –	44 (396/895)	12 (10/87)	10	5
	N +	64 (711/324)	35 (124/355)		

cancer, Calitchi and associates (1991) have exploited preoperative irradiation (45 Gy) to reduce the tumor bulk of large T2 and T3 primary lesions. In 74 of 138 patients thus treated (54%), the breast tumors regressed to a clinical status that allowed completion of conservative treatment. Adjuvant chemotherapy was administered only after all surgery and irradiation was completed. Promising early results of this approach suggest a potential new role for preoperative irradiation in breast cancer treatment.

RADIATION THERAPY OF LOCAL-REGIONAL RECURRENCES

Evidence that the development of apparently isolated local-regional recurrence of breast carcinoma following mastectomy almost inexorably heralds the subsequent appearance of systemic metastases should not deter implementation of aggressive radiation therapy for such disease. Major palliation for the duration of the patient's remaining life can be secured frequently enough to justify its routine use. The lower ultimate incidence of distressing local-regional symptoms following aggressive irradiation suggests that it may be justified even for patients with asymptomatic local-regional recurrences who already have identifiable distant metastases (Bedwinek et al., 1983). Overall, only about one fourth of patients who develop local-regional recurrence survive 10 years; however, significantly better long-term

survival rates are observed in patients whose recurrences are controlled by irradiation than in patients who have uncontrolled disease (Chu et al., 1984a,b; and Chen et al., 1985) (Fig. 19–2).

Although in some subsets of patients local control rates as high as 78% with a corresponding 5-year disease-free survival rate of 59% have been reported following irradiation of local-regional recurrences, even this modest success rate is highly dependent on a favorable case mix and the adequacy of the irradiation (Chen et al., 1985; and Schwaibold et al., 1991). Overall, however, not more than half of all patients with chest wall recurrences come to medical attention early enough to be treated successfully or in fact to have their disease controlled. Because the majority of patients with locally progressive disease ultimately are functionally compromised by it, this finding underscores the necessity of an aggressive approach (Bedwinek et al., 1981). Most failures following irradiation can be attributed to inadequate radiation doses or failure to use large enough fields to encompass the areas of gross involvement with wide margins. Routinely irradiating the peripheral lymphatics in addition to the chest wall for local recurrences is associated with improved long-term survival (Toonkel et al., 1983; Bedwinek, 1990; and Halverson et al., 1990). Local control rates are inversely proportional to the number and size of the recurrences treated. Doses of at least 6000 rad are required to control recurrent masses 1 to 3 cm in diameter (Bedwinek et al., 1981). For more voluminous

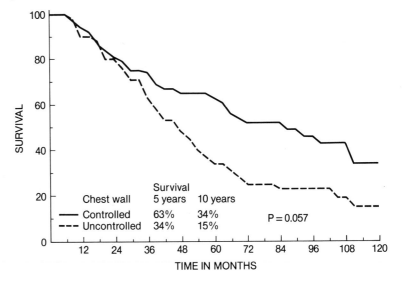

Figure 19–2. Five- and 10-year survival of 106 patients treated at M. D. Anderson Hospital between January 1956 and December 1981 for chest wall recurrence of carcinoma of the breast. The survival rates of patients whose chest wall recurrences were controlled by irradiation are compared with those who failed treatment. (From Chen, K.K., Montague, E.D., and Oswald, M.J.: Results of irradiation in the treatment of locoregional breast cancer recurrence. Cancer, 56:1269, 1985. Reprinted with permission.)

	Survival	
Chest wall	5 years	10 years
—— Controlled	63%	34%
---- Uncontrolled	34%	15%

P = 0.057

cancers, doses must be pushed upward to the limits of normal tissue tolerance. Surgical excision of any accessible macroscopic disease before irradiation enhances local-regional control and is recommended even for small chest wall nodules (Stadler and Kogelnik, 1987). Factors associated with poorer prognosis despite appropriate irradiation include simultaneous nodal and chest wall recurrence, advanced initial disease stage, and a short disease-free interval from the time of initial therapy (Patanaphan et al., 1984; and Halverson et al., 1992a). Results of systemic chemotherapy alone for locally or regionally recurrent breast cancer are inferior to those achieved with irradiation; however, potential enhancement of local control and survival when chemotherapy or hormonal therapy has been used in combination with irradiation has been observed and deserves further evaluation (Janjan et al., 1986; and Halverson et al., 1992b). The argument for *elective* postoperative irradiation in patients at high risk for local-regional recurrences is reinforced when the difficulties encountered in controlling such disease once it is allowed to become clinically apparent are considered.

RADIATION THERAPY OF LOCALLY ADVANCED BREAST CARCINOMA

Locally advanced carcinoma of the breast (AJC-UICC Stage III or IV) includes a wide spectrum of disease presentations. A complete description of the individualized therapy called for in each of these circumstances is beyond the confines of this discussion. Occult distant metastases that eventually become manifest in a large proportion of advanced-stage patients carry a poor prognosis, but, since many of these patients survive for long periods, a paramount goal in such cases is to provide treatment that maximizes the probability that they will be free of symptomatic local-regional disease. To maintain a satisfactory quality of life, distressing treatment sequelae must be kept to a minimum. In this regard, the radiobiologic principles and potential increased toxicity associated with multimodal treatment discussed in preceding sections of this chapter come under consideration.

Whether the local-regional disease is technically resectable or categorically unresectable is the principal determinant of treatment recommendations for locally advanced breast cancer. Radical radiation therapy alone for unresectable breast cancer yields local tumor control rates usually in the range of 30% to 70%. Corresponding 5-year survival figures in the 10% to 30% range have been reported. Arriagada and coworkers (1985) analyzed the results of treating 463 patients with breast cancer with radiation therapy alone. The findings emphasize that the success of such therapy depends on two factors: tumor size and radiation dose to the tumor (Table 19–6). Radiation dose, the single most significant independent factor, produced as much as a 10-fold increase in the probability of local tumor control, compared with a twofold decrease for tumor size. The point is that for tumor masses of the size usually associated with the locally advanced categories (>5 cm diameter), radiation doses likely to result in tumor control must be so large that severe treatment-related sequelae often can be expected.

Table 19–6. THREE-YEAR LOCAL CONTROL RATES FOLLOWING RADIATION THERAPY ALONE FOR PRIMARY BREAST CARCINOMAS ACCORDING TO TOTAL RADIATION DOSE AND TUMOR SIZE

Tumor Dose (Gy)	Tumor Size (%)			
	4 cm	6 cm	8 cm	> 8 cm
>40–50	25	24	5	0
>50–60	59	46	36	17
>60–70	—	—	28	21
>70–80	81	71	61	36
>80	100	66	79	50

(Modified from Arriagada, R., Mouriesse, H., Sarrazin, D., et al.: Radiotherapy alone in breast cancer. I. Analysis of tumor parameters, tumor dose, and local control: The experience of the Gustave-Roussy Institute and The Princess Margaret Hospital. Int. J. Radia. Oncol. Biol. Phys., 11:1751, 1985.)

For example, Spanos and colleagues (1980) reported a 24% rate of late soft tissue necrosis and severe fibrosis in response to doses in excess of 8000 rad when patients lived long enough to develop these complications. Therefore, technically resectable advanced breast cancer is approached more effectively if excisional biopsy or mastectomy, with or without axillary dissection, is performed before irradiation (Bedwinek et al., 1982; and Strom et al., 1991).

Multiagent chemotherapy or hormonal and chemotherapy administered as a neoadjuvant in the management of locally advanced breast cancer results in a high rate (60–90%) of partial or complete tumor response. The large majority of technically unresectable carcinomas convert to a status of full resectability, and the need for effective local-regional treatment measures is not precluded by the induction regimen. The best local-regional control rates are achieved in patients who receive chemotherapy, mastectomy, and radiation therapy (Klefström, et al., 1987; Hortobagyi et al., 1988; and Graham et al., 1991). Breast conserving treatment has been feasible in selected patients who demonstrate adequate response to induction chemotherapy, but further evaluation of this approach is required (Pierce et al., 1992). Further investigation is needed to determine optimal sequencing of currently available therapeutic modalities for locally advanced breast cancer, but especially to develop new, more effective systemic measures (Dorr et al., 1989). The role of adjunctive irradiation in the management of resectable advanced breast carcinomas has been further considered in earlier sections.

The prognosis of patients with inflammatory breast cancer has improved much during the last decade with combined modality therapy (Jaiyesimi et al., 1992). Rates of local-regional control as high as 85% to 95% and improved disease-free and overall survival compared to historical data are reported, depending on tumor response to treatment (Fields et al., 1989). With aggressive management, approximately 35% to 55% of all patients with inflammatory breast cancer can now expect to survive at least 5 years. At present, a preferred treatment sequence for inflammatory carcinoma is induction chemotherapy followed by mastectomy or radiation therapy, or both, in combination with additional chemotherapy. Here again, additional research is needed to identify optimal integration of these modalities. Altered radiation fractionation schedules (hyperfractionation, accelerated fractionation) that allow rapid escalation of radiation dose without increasing normal tissue damage may prove particularly advantageous for this typically fast-growing form of breast cancer (Thoms et al., 1989).

RADIATION THERAPY OF DISTANT METASTASES

A large proportion of patients with cancer of the breast develop distant metastases, which produce distressing symptoms and eventually become life threatening. Radiation therapy is the most effective means of providing symptomatic relief. Such treatment is not undertaken with the expressed purpose of prolonging survival, though, in individual patients, eradication of a tumor that is impinging on a vital structure may have that effect. Two of the most common sites of distant metastasis are the skeletal system and the central nervous system. Data are available that permit realistic expectation of the beneficial effects of radiation therapy.

Skeletal Metastasis

Prospective studies of radiation therapy for skeletal metastasis have been conducted by the Radiation Therapy Oncology Group (RTOG) (Tang et al., 1982; and Blitzer, 1985). In these studies, patients with metastases from tumors arising in many different anatomic sites—and, consequently, with many different histopathologic diagnoses—were treated in a consistent manner. The vast majority had metastases from carcinomas of the breast, lung, or prostate.

Approximately 1000 patients were studied. The results showed that 90% of those who had moderate to severe pain experienced some relief, and more than half had complete disappearance of pain. Results were the same whether there were solitary or multiple sites of symptomatic metastases. Metastases in pelvic bones required a longer time for maximum relief of symptoms than other sites of involvement. Patients with carcinomas of the breast and prostate experienced relief of pain more frequently than those with carcinomas of the lung and other malignant tumors; they also experienced a longer period of symptomatic relief.

The aim of palliative irradiation is to provide the most rapid, complete, and durable relief of symptoms possible. A brief course of treatment is desirable, so that the patient is inconvenienced as little as possible. It is important that there be few short-term side effects, and it is imperative to have a very low risk of late sequelae. However, duration of the palliation depends on administration of a total dose of radiation sufficient to eradicate the tumor, or at least to reduce it to the smallest number of clonogenic cells compatible with a low probably of adverse effects. In practice, palliative courses of radiation therapy last 2 to 3 weeks. In special circumstances, it can be advantageous to treat for longer or shorter periods. Additional clinical studies are needed to precisely determine the effect of radiation dose

and response duration in patients with a relatively long life expectancy (Bates et al., 1992).

At the extreme of short courses of palliative radiation therapy are single treatments. They are, in general, associated with more rapid relief of symptoms, but the duration of palliation is briefer. The presence of multiple symptomatic skeletal metastases may justify half-body irradiation in a single dose. RTOG studies of wide-field irradiation have defined the feasibility and effectiveness of this approach (Salazar et al., 1986). Upper half-body irradiation is associated with moderately acute symptoms that can be prevented by hydration, corticosteroids, and antiemetics; thus, it requires hospitalization. Radiation pneumonitis may result if the single dose is excessive. Somewhat larger doses may be given with middle and lower half-body irradiation. Doses used with half-body treatments are approximately two to four times those used in a course of fractionated radiation therapy (i.e., 6 to 10 Gy versus 2.5 to 4 Gy). Hemibody irradiation results in pain relief in more than 70% of all patients treated, and half of all responders experience relief within 48 hours. Adding hemibody irradiation to local field irradiation delays the appearance of new metastases and reduces the subsequent need for retreatment (Poulter et al., 1992). The bone-seeking radioisotope strontium 89 is undergoing extensive re-evaluation in clinical trials and is likely to enter the radiotherapeutic armamentarium of palliative options for osseous metastases (Montebello and Harton-Eaton, 1989; and Bates et al., 1992).

Metastasis to the Central Nervous System

Carcinoma of the breast may compromise the central nervous system in several ways. The most common problem is metastasis to the parenchyma of the brain, but involvement of the vertebrae with secondary pressure on the spinal cord or nerve roots, extradural metastasis, leptomeningeal carcinomatosis, and even intramedullary metastasis may be observed.

The RTOG has undertaken large-scale, prospective trials of palliative irradiation for brain metastases. The investigators have documented the effectiveness of radiation therapy in relieving symptoms (Coia, 1992*b*). Table 19–7 shows

Table 19–7. RELIEF BY RADIATION THERAPY OF SPECIFIC NEUROLOGIC SYMPTOMS FROM BRAIN METASTASIS

Symptom	Patients (N)	Complete Relief (%)	Rate of Overall Relief (Complete and Partial) (%)
Seizures	327	72	85
Headache	982	60	82
Impaired mentation	780	44	70
Cerebellar dysfunction	477	45	69
Motor loss	910	35	67
Cranial nerve symptoms	459	42	65

the frequency with which palliation of specific neurologic symptoms is achieved. Complete relief is achieved in 35% to 72%, and some benefit is derived from radiation therapy in 65% to 85% of patients. Seizure, both major motor and focal in type, as well as headache, are most consistently relieved, but substantial benefit is seen in the majority of patients with any of the common symptoms. Short courses of radiation (20 Gy in 2 weeks) are generally as effective as more prolonged courses (Coia et al., 1992a).

Back pain and neurologic symptoms and signs may herald the onset of paraplegia caused by metastases from carcinoma of the breast. Computed tomographic myelography or magnetic resonance imaging usually demonstrates the level of the block and whether the impingement on the spinal cord is the result of an extradural tumor or of vertebral collapse and mechanical compromise. In the former case, immediate institution of radiation therapy may alleviate neurologic symptoms without need for decompressive laminectomy. If there is mechanical compromise, laminectomy is usually necessary. Paraplegia that is completely established can still be reversed, but the longer the period of complete paralysis, the lower is the probability of reversing it.

Carcinomatous meningitis is rarely treated effectively with radiation therapy alone. However, irradiation of the base of the skull can reverse distressing cranial nerve abnormalities, and cranial irradiation may be combined with intrathecal administration of cytotoxic chemotherapeutic agents to achieve palliation.

Thoracic Metastases

Intrathoracic spread of mammary cancer is not rare. Secondary involvement of the mediastinum following metastasis to the internal mammary nodes is perhaps far more common than was previously appreciated. Hemoptysis, dyspnea, and even superior vena caval obstruction may occur. Each of these symptoms is consistently reversed by mediastinal irradiation. Pleural effusion, however, cannot be palliated with radiation therapy because it would be necessary to deliver large doses to the entire pleura, which secondarily would produce radiation pneumonitis and scarring, and possibly greater pulmonary compromise than that resulting from the effusion.

Hepatic Metastases

The only indication for palliative irradiation of patients with hepatic metastases from cancer is abdominal pain. Little, if any, benefit is derived from irradiation for abnormal hepatic function or hepatomegaly, but pain resulting from stretching of the capsule of the liver is completely relieved in more than half of patients treated (Leibel et al., 1987).

SIDE EFFECTS OF RADIATION THERAPY

There is a low probability of adverse effects from well-controlled radiation therapy for carcinoma of the breast. The skin of the breast irradiated following excisional biopsy, or that of the chest wall following mastectomy, frequently shows gradual reddening during the third and fourth weeks of treatment. Unless there is a specific need to have a maximal dose of radiation at the surface, most techniques for irradiating the breast or chest wall produce dry desquamation but infrequently cause a moist reaction. In patients with locally advanced mammary tumors with involvement of the skin or inflammatory changes, it may be necessary to have a maximal effect on the surface. Moist desquamation will result and then will heal in a predictable manner in the weeks following completion of irradiation.

Late cutaneous sequelae from radiation therapy include hypochromia, atrophy, and telangiectasia, usually confined to regions that required a maximal dose to the surface of the skin. Patients who receive boost irradiation to the site of the original tumor by means of interstitial implantation of radioactive sources or by high-energy electron beam may have slightly increased skin sequelae confined to the treated area.

Because it is impossible to irradiate the entire thickness of the chest wall without irradiating the adjacent anterior portion of the lung, scarring may be demonstrable in chest radiographs months or years after treatment. Similarly, irradiation of the internal mammary and supraclavicular regions may result in pulmonary effects. Infrequently, symptomatic radiation pneumonitis may occur, which is manifested by cough, fever, and dyspnea. Symptomatic treatment is indicated until the inflammatory changes resolve spontaneously over a period of several weeks. In the rare case of severe symptoms, corticosteroids may be indicated.

Effects on other organs are so infrequent as to be well beyond the scope of this chapter. The interested reader is referred to review articles on the subject (Rubin, 1984; and Cox et al., 1986). It is worth mentioning that a variety of cytotoxic drugs may enhance the side effects of ionizing radiations. Most notable are doxorubicin, dactinomycin, and methotrexate. Both acute and late sequelae may be accentuated by the simultaneous administration of such drugs and radiation therapy. In general, there is little interaction with regard to effects on normal tissues when there is at least a 2-week interval between the administration of drugs and ionizing radiation.

It is well recognized that ionizing radiation is carcinogenic. This fact has been emphasized by some authors as an argument for avoiding radiation therapy in the management of patients with cancer of the breast. However, data derived from whole-body exposures to radiation far different in character from the high-energy photons and electrons used in the treatment of patients with cancer have little bearing on the risk of carcinogenesis following therapeutic applications of carefully focused radiations. Radiotherapy contributes little to the already substantial risk of development of carcinoma in the contralateral breast and should not be a factor in the selection of treatment methods (Boice et al., 1992). There are case reports suggesting that sarcomas arising in the chest wall result from prior irradiation, but the frequency is so low as to approximate the risk of lymphangiosarcoma arising in the chronically lymphedematous arm after axillary dissection (Givens et al., 1989).

Studies such as that of Ferguson and associates (1984), which describe late effects of primitive treatments (conventional x-rays of 1.5 and 3 mm of copper half-value layer administered over 3 to 5 months), have little if any relevance to contemporary radiation therapy. Conclusions from these experiences are no more valid than those from surgery prior to antibiotics and modern anesthesia.

SUMMARY

Radiation therapy has a key role in the management of a major proportion of all women with mammary carcinoma. Conservative breast treatment is established as the preferred treatment for early invasive breast cancer, affording patients high levels of esthetic and functional preservation. Selected patients with DCIS may also be offered conservative therapy.

Adjunctive irradiation is well justified in selected patients at high risk for local-regional recurrence following mastectomy, regardless of the use of systemic adjuvants. Combinations of surgery, radiation therapy, and chemotherapy have improved the prognosis of patients with locally advanced and inflammatory breast cancer, but further research is needed to identify optimal integration of these modalities. The benefits of irradiation to nearly all patients with local-regional recurrence or distant metastases are indisputable. Side effects of well-controlled irradiation are predictable and relatively mild. New educational initiatives should ensure proper utilization of irradiation in the management of the growing number of women diagnosed with breast cancer.

References

Abner, A., Recht, A., Vicini, F., et al.: Cosmetic results after conservative surgery and radiation and chemotherapy for early breast cancer. Int. J. Radiat. Oncol. Biol. Phys., *21*:331, 1991.

Amalric, R., Santamaria, F., Robert F., et al.: Conservation therapy of operable breast cancer—results at five, ten, and fifteen years in 2216 consecutive cases. *In* Harris, J., Hellman, S., and Silen, W. (Eds.): Conservative Management of Breast Cancer, New Surgical and Radiotherapeutic Techniques. Philadelphia, JB Lippincott, 1983, p.15.

Arriagada, R., Mouriesse, H., Sarrazin, D., et al.: Radiotherapy alone in breast cancer. I. Analysis of tumor parameters, tumor dose, and local control: The experience of the Gustave-Roussy Institute and The Princess Margaret Hospital. Int. J. Radiat. Oncol. Biol. Phys., *11*:1751, 1985.

Arriagada, R., Lê, M. G., Mouriesse, H., et al.: Long-term effect of internal mammary chain treatment. Results of a multivariate analysis of 1195 patients with operable breast cancer and positive axillary nodes. Radiother. Oncol., *11*:213, 1988.

Auqier, A., Rutqvist, L. E., Host, H., et al.: Post-mastectomy megavoltage radiotherapy: The Oslo and Stockholm trials. Eur. J. Cancer, *28*:433, 1992.

Baclesse, P.: Roentgentherapy alone in cancer of the breast. Acta Un. Int. Cancre, *15*:1023, 1959.

Bates, T., Yarnold, J. R., Blitzer, P., et al.: Bone metastasis consensus statement. Int. J. Radiat. Oncol. Biol. Phys., *23*:215, 1992.

Bedwinek, J.: Radiation therapy of isolated local-regional recurrence of breast cancer: Decisions regarding dose, field size, and elective irradiation of uninvolved sites. Int. J. Radiat. Oncol. Biol. Phys., *19*:1093, 1990.

Bedwinek, J. M., Fineberg, B., Lee, J., et al.: Analysis of failures following local treatment of isolated local-regional recurrence of breast cancer. Int. J. Radiat. Oncol. Biol. Phys., *7*:581, 1981.

Bedwinek, J. M., Munro, D., and Fineberg, B.: Local-regional treatment of patients with simultaneous local-regional recurrence and distant metastases following mastectomy. Am. J. Clin. Oncol., *6*:295, 1983.

Bedwinek, J., Venkata, R., Perez, C., et al.: Stage III and localized Stage IV breast cancer: Irradiation alone vs. irradiation plus surgery. Int. J. Radiat. Oncol. Biol. Phys., *8*:31, 1982.

Blichert-Toft, M., Brincker, H., Andersen, J. A., et al.: A Danish randomized trial comparing breast-preserving therapy with mastectomy in mammary carcinoma: Preliminary results. Acta Oncol., *27*:671–677, 1988.

Blitzer, P. H.: Reanalysis of the RTOG study of the palliation of symptomatic osseous metastases. Cancer, *55*:1468, 1985.

Boice, J. D., Harvey, E. B., Blettner, M., et al.: Cancer in the contralateral breast after radiotherapy for breast cancer. N. Engl. J. Med., *326*:781, 1992.

Bornstein, B. A., Recht, A., Connolly, J. L., et al.: Results of treating ductal carcinoma in situ of the breast with conservative surgery and radiation therapy. Cancer, *67*:7, 1991.

Calitchi E., Otmezguine, Y., Feuilhade, F., et al.: External irradiation prior to conservative surgery for breast cancer treatment. Int. J. Radiat. Oncol. Biol. Phys., *21*:325, 1991.

Cancer Research Campaign: Management of early cancer of the breast. Report on an international multicentre trial supported by the Cancer Research Campaign. Br. Med. J., *1*:1035, 1976.

Chen, K. K., Montague, E. D., and Oswald, M. J.: Results of irradiation in the treatment of locoregional breast cancer recurrence. Cancer, *56*:1269, 1985.

Chu, A. M., Cope, O., Doucette, J., et al.: Non-metastatic locally advanced cancer of the breast treated with irradiation. Int. J. Radiat. Oncol. Biol. Phys., *10*:2299, 1984*a*.

Chu, A. M., Cope, O., Russo, R., et al.: Patterns of local-regional recurrence and results in Stages I and II breast cancer treated by irradiation following limited surgery. Am. J. Clin. Oncol., *7*:221, 1984*b*.

Clark, R. M., Wilkinson, R. H., Miceli, P. N., et al. Breast cancer: experiences with conservation therapy. Am. J. Clin. Oncol. *10*:461, 1987.

Clarke, D., Martinez, A., Cox, R. S., et al.: Breast edema following staging axillary node dissection in patients with breast carcinoma treated by radical radiotherapy. Cancer, *49*:2295, 1982.

Coia, L. R.: The role of radiation therapy in the treatment of brain metastases. Int. J. Radiat. Oncol. Biol. Phys., *23*:229, 1992*a*.

Coia, L. R., Aaronson, N., and Linggood, R.: A report of the consensus workshop panel on the treatment of brain metastases. Int. J. Radiat. Oncol. Biol. Phys., *29*:223, 1992*b*.

Cox, J. D., Byhardt, R. W., Wilson, J. F., et al.: Complications of radiation therapy and factors in their prevention. World J. Surg., *10*:171, 1986.

Danforth, D. M., Findlay, P. A., McDonald, H. D., et al.: Complete axillary lymph node dissection for Stage I–II carcinoma of the breast. J. Clin. Oncol., *4*:655, 1986.

Danoff, B. F., Goodman, R. L., Glick, J. H., et al.: The effect of adjuvant chemotherapy on cosmesis and complications in patients with breast cancer treated by definitive irradiation. Int. J. Radiat. Oncol. Biol. Phys., *9*:1625, 1983.

Delouche, G., Bachelot, F., Premont, M., et al.: Conservation treatment of early breast cancer: Long-term results and complications. Int. J. Radiat. Oncol. Biol. Phys., *13*:29, 1987.

Dewar, J., Sarrazin, D., Benhamou, S., et al.: Management of the axilla in conservatively treated breast cancer: 592 patients treated at Institute Gustave-Roussy. Int. Radiat. Oncol. Biol. Phys., *13*:475, 1987.

Dorr, F. A., Bader J., and Friedman, M. A.: Locally advanced breast cancer current status and future directions. Int. J. Radiat. Biol. Phys., *16*:775–784, 1989.

Dubois, J. B., Gary-Bobo, J., Pourquier, H., et al.: Tumorectomy and radiotherapy in early breast cancer: A report on 392 patients. Int. J. Radiat. Oncol. Biol. Phys., *15*:1275–1282, 1988.

Dubois, J. B., Saumon-Reme, M., Gary-Bobo, J., et al.: Tumorectomy and radiation therapy in early breast cancer: A report on 392 patients. Radiology, *175*:867, 1990.

Farrow D. C., Hunt W. C., and Samet J. M.: Geographic variation in the treatment of localized breast cancer. N. Engl. J. Med., *326*:1097, 1992.

Ferguson, D. J., Sutton, H. G. Jr., and Dawson, P. J.: Late effects of adjuvant radiotherapy for breast cancer. Cancer, *54*:2319, 1984.

Fields, J. N., Perez, C. A., Kuske, R. R., et al.: Inflammatory carcinoma of the breast: Treatment results on 107 patients. Int. J. Radiat. Oncol. Biol. Phys., *17*:249–255, 1989.

Fisher, B., Costantino, J., Redmond, C., et al.: Lumpectomy compared with lumpectomy and radiation therapy for the treatment of intraductal breast cancer. N. Engl. J. Med., *328*:1561–1586, 1993.

Fisher, B., Redmond, C., Poisson, R., et al.: Eight-year results of a randomized clinical trial comparing total mastectomy and lumpectomy with or without irradiation in the treatment of breast cancer. N. Engl. J. Med., *320*:822, 1989.

Fisher, E. R., Sass, R., Fisher, B., et al.: Pathologic findings from the National Surgical Adjuvant Breast Project (protocol 6). I. Intraductal carcinoma (DCIS). Cancer, *57*:197, 1986.

Fisher, B., Slack, N., Cavanaugh, R. J., et al.: Postoperative radiotherapy in the treatment of breast cancer. Results of the NSABP clinical trial. Ann. Surg., *172*:711, 1970.

Fleck, R., McNeese, M. D., Ellerbroek, N. A., et al.: Consequences of breast irradiation in patients with pre-existing collagen vascular diseases. Int. J. Radiat. Oncol. Biol. Phys., *17*:829, 1989.

Fletcher, G. H.: Clinical dose response curve of subclinical aggregates of epithelial cells and its practical application in the mangement of human cancer. *In* Friedman, M. (Ed.): Biological and Clinical Cases of Radiosensitivity. Springfield, IL, Charles C Thomas, 1974, p. 485.

Fletcher, G. H.: The enigma of breast cancer. *In* Ames F.C., Blumenschein, G.R., and Montague, E.D. (Eds): Current Controversies in Breast Cancer. Austin, University of Texas Press, 1984, pp. 139–147.

Fletcher, G. H.: History of irradiation in the primary management of apparently regionally confined breast cancer. Int. J. Radiat. Oncol. Biol. Phys., *11*:2133–2142, 1985.

Fletcher, G. H., McNeese, M. D., and Oswald, M. J.: Long-range results for breast cancer patients treated by radical mastectomy and postoperative radiation without adjuvant chemotherapy: An update. Int. J. Radiat. Oncol. Biol. Phys., *17*:11, 1989.

Fourquet, A., Campana, F., Zafrani, B., et al.: Prognostic factors of breast recurrence in the conservative management of early breast cancer: A 25-year follow-up. Int. J. Radiat. Oncol. Biol. Phys., *17*:719, 1989.

Fourquet, A., Zafrani, B., Campana F., et al.: Breast-conserving treatment of ductal carcinoma in situ. Semin. Radiat. Oncol. *2*:116–124, 1992.

Fowble, B.: Intraductal noninvasive breast cancer: A comparison of three local treatments. Oncology, *3*:51, 1989.

Fowble, B., Glick, J., and Goodman, R.: Radiotherapy for the prevention of local-regional recurrence in high risk patients post mastectomy receiving adjuvant chemotherapy. Int. J. Radiat. Oncol. Biol. Phys., *15*:627, 1988a.

Fowble, B., Gray, R., Gilchrist, K., et al.: Identification of a subgroup of patients with breast cancer and histologically positive axillary nodes receiving adjuvant chemotherapy who may benefit from postoperative radiotherapy. J. Clin. Oncol., *6*:1107, 1988b.

Fowble, B. L., Solin, L. J., Schultz, D.J., et al.: Ten-year results of conservative surgery and irradiation for stage I and II breast cancer. Int. J. Radiat. Oncol. Biol. Phys., *21*:269–277, 1991.

Givens, S. S., Ellerbroek, N. A., Butler, J. J., et al: Angiosarcoma arising in an irradiated breast: A case report and review of the literature. Cancer, *64*:2214, 1989.

Graham, M. V., Perez, C. A., Kuske, R. R., et al.: Locally advanced (noninflammatory) carcinoma of the breast: Results and comparison of various treatment modalities. Int. J. Radiat. Oncol. Biol. Phys., *21*:311, 1991.

Gray, J. R., McCormick, B., Cox, L., et al.: Primary breast irradiation in large-breasted or heavy women: Analysis of cosmetic outcome. Int. J. Radiat. Oncol. Biol. Phys., *21*:347, 1991.

Griem, K. L., Henderson, I. C., Gelman, R., et al.: The 5-year results of a randomized trial of adjuvant radiation therapy after chemotherapy in breast cancer patients treated with mastectomy. J. Clin. Oncol., *5*:1546, 1987.

Haffty, B. G., Goldberg, N. B., Fischer, D., et al.: Conservative surgery and radiation therapy in breast carcinoma: Local recurrence and prognostic implications. Int. J. Radiat. Oncol., Biol. Phys., *17*:727, 1989.

Halverson, K. J., Perez, C. A., Kuske, R. R., et al.: Isolated local-regional recurrence of breast cancer following mastectomy: Radiotherapeutic management. Int. J. Radiat. Oncol. Biol. Phys., *19*:851, 1990.

Halverson, K. J., Perez, C. A., Kuske, R. R., et al.: Locoregional recurrence of breast cancer: A retrospective comparison of irradiation alone versus irradiation and systemic therapy. Am. J. Clin. Oncol., *15*:93, 1992a.

Halverson, K. J., Perez, C. A., Kuske, R. R., et al.: Survival following locoregional recurrence of breast cancer: Univariate and multivariate analysis. Int. J. Radiat. Oncol. Biol. Phys., *23*:285, 1992b.

Harris, J. R., and Hellman, S.: Pat the "Hockey Stick" on ice. Int. J. Radiat. Oncol. Biol. Phys., *15*:497–499, 1988.

Harris, J. R., and Schnitt, S. J.: Is radiotherapy as curative as mastectomy for patients with ductal carcinoma in situ? Int. J. Radiat. Oncol. Biol. Phys., *19*:1091, 1990.

Hodges, P. C.: The Life and Times of Emil H. Grubbe. Chicago, The University of Chicago Press, 1964.

Holland, R., Veling, S. H. J., Mravunac, M., et al.: Histologic multifocality of TIS, T1–2 breast carcinomas. Cancer, *56*:979, 1985.

Hortobagyi, G. N., Ames, F. C., Buzdar, A. U., et al.: Management of stage III primary breast cancer with primary chemotherapy, surgery, and radiation therapy. Cancer, *62*:2507, 1988.

Host, H., Brennhovd, I. O., and Loeb, M.: Postoperative radiotherapy in breast cancer—long-term results from the Oslo study. Int. J. Radiat. Oncol. Biol. Phys., *12*:727–732, 1986.

Jaiyesimi, I. A., Buzdar, A. U., and Hortobagyi, G.: Inflammatory breast cancer: A review. J. Clin. Oncol., *10*:1014, 1992.

Janjan, N. A., McNeese, M. D., Buzdar, A. U., et al.: Management of locoregional recurrent breast cancer. Cancer, *58*:1552, 1986.

Keynes, G.: The treatment of primary carcinoma of the breast with radium. Acta Radiol. *10*:293, 1929.

Kiebert, G. M., de Haes, J. C. J. M., and van de Velde, C. J. H.: The impact of breast-conserving treatment and mastectomy on the quality of life of early-stage breast cancer patients: A review. J. Clin. Oncol., *9*:1059, 1991.

Kiricuta, C. I., and Tausch, J.: A mathematical model of axillary lymph node involvement based on 1446 complete axillary dissections in patients with breast carcinoma. Cancer, *69*:2496, 1992.

Klefström, P., Gröhn, P., Heinonen, E., et al.: Adjuvant postoperative radiotherapy, chemotherapy, and immunotherapy in stage III breast cancer. Cancer, *60*:936, 1987.

Kurtz, J. M., and Miralbell, R.: Radiation therapy and breast conservation: Cosmetic results and complications. Semin. Radiat. Oncol., *2*:125, 1992.

Kurtz, J. M., and Spitalier, J-M.: Local recurrence after breast-conserving surgery and radiotherapy: What have we learned? Int. J. Radiat. Oncol. Biol. Phys., *19*:1087, 1990.

Kurtz, J. M., Jacquemier, J., Torhorst, J., et al.: Conservation therapy for breast cancers other than infiltrating ductal carcinoma. Cancer, *63*:1630, 1989.

Kuske, R., Bean, J. M., Garcia, D. M., et al.: Breast-conserving therapy for intraductal carcinoma of the breast. Int. J. Radiat. Oncol. Biol. Phys., *26*:391–396, 1993.

Lagios, M. D.: Duct carcinoma in situ. Surg. Clin. North Am., *70*:853, 1990.

Lê, M., Arriagada, R., Vathaire, F., et al.,: Can internal mammary chain treatment decrease the risk of death for patients with medial breast cancers and positive axillary lymph nodes? Cancer, *66*:2313, 1990.

Leibel, S. A., Pajak, T. F., Massullo, V., et al.: A comparison of misonidazole sensitized radiation therapy to radiation therapy alone for the palliation of hepatic metastases: Results of a radiation therapy oncology group randomized prospective trial. Int. J. Radiat. Oncol. Biol. Phys., *13*:1057, 1987.

Leung, S., Otmezguine, Y., Calitchi, E., et al.: Locoregional recurrences following radical external beam irradiation and interstitial implantation for operable breast cancer: A twenty-three year experience. Radiother. Oncol., *5*:1, 1986.

Lichter, A. S., Fraass, B. A., and Yanke, B.: Treatment techniques in the conservative management of breast cancer. Semin. Radiat. Oncol., *2*:94, 1992a.

Lichter, A. S., Lippman, M. E., Danforth, D. N., et al.: Mastectomy versus breast-conserving therapy in the treatment of stage I and II carcinoma of the breast: A randomized trial at the National Cancer Institute. J. Clin. Oncol., *10(6)*:976, 1992b.

Lingos, T., Recht, A., Vicini, F., et al.: Radiation pneumonitis in breast cancer patients treated with conservative surgery and radiation therapy. Int. J. Radiat. Oncol. Biol. Phys., *21*:355, 1991.

Lippman, M. E., Lichter, A. S., Edwards, B. K., et al.: The impact of primary irradiation treatment of localized breast cancer on the ability to administer systemic adjuvant chemotherapy. J. Clin. Oncol., *2*:21, 1984.

Matory, W.E., Wetheimer, M., Fitzgerald, T.J., et al.: Aesthetic results following partial mastectomy and radiation therapy. Plast. Reconstr. Surg., *85(5)*:739, 1990.

McCormick, B.: Invasive breast carcinoma: Patient selection for conservative management. Semin. Radiat. Oncol., *2*:74, 1992.

McCormick, B., Yahalom, J., Cox, L., et al.: The patient's perception of her breast following radiation and limited surgery. Int. J. Radiat. Oncol. Biol. Phys., *17*:1299, 1989.

Montebello, J. F., and Hartson-Eaton, M. The palliation of osseous metastasis with 39P or 89Sr compared with external beam and hemibody irradiation: A historical perspective. Cancer Invest., 7:139, 1989.

National Institutes of Health Consensus Development Conference Statement, Treatment of Early-Stage Breast Cancer. J. Am. Med. Assoc., 265:391–395, 1991.

Nattinger A. B., Gottlieb M. S., Veum J., et al.: Geographic variation in the use of breast-conserving treatment for breast cancer. N. Engl. J. Med., 326:1102, 1992.

Olivotto, I. A., Rose, M. A., Osteen, R. T., et al.: Late cosmetic outcome after conservative surgery and radiotherapy: Analysis of causes of cosmetic failure. Int. J. Radiat. Oncol. Biol. Phys., 17:747, 1989.

Osteen, R. T., Steele, G. D., Menck, H. R., et al.: Regional differences in surgical management of breast cancer. CA Cancer J. Clin., 42:39, 1992.

Patanaphan, V., Salazar, O. M., and Poussin-Rosillo, H.: Prognosticators in recurrent breast cancer. Cancer, 54:228, 1984.

Paterson, R., and Russell, M.H.: Clinical trials in malignant disease. III. Breast cancer: Evaluation of post-operative radiotherapy. Clin. Radiol., 10:175, 1959.

Patterson, M. P., Pezner, R. D., Hill, L. R., et al.: Patient self-evaluation of cosmetic outcome of breast-preserving cancer treatment. Int. J. Radiat. Oncol. Biol. Phys., 11:1849, 1985.

Peters, M. V.: Cutting the "Gordian knot" in early breast cancer. Ann. R. Coll. Phys. Surg. (Can.), 8:186, 1976.

Pierce, L., and Glatstein, E.: Management of locally advanced breast cancer: The changing role of radiotherapy. Admin. Radiol., May 1992, pp. 43–47.

Pierquin, B., Huart J., Raynal, M., et al.: Conservative treatment for breast cancer: Long-term results (15 years). Radiother. Oncol., 20:16, 1991.

Poulter, C. A., Cosmatos, D. P, and Rubin, P.: A report of RTOG 8206: A phase III study of whether the addition of single dose hemibody irradiation to standard fractionated local field irradiation is more effective than local field irradiation alone in the treatment of symptomatic osseous metastases. Int. J. Radiat. Oncol. Biol. Phys., 23:207, 1992.

Ray, G. R., Fish, V. J., Marmor, J. B., et al.: Impact of adjuvant chemotherapy on cosmesis and complications in stages I and II carcinoma of the breast treated by biopsy and radiation therapy. Int. J. Radiat. Oncol. Biol. Phys., 10:837, 1983.

Recht, A., Come, S. E., Gelman, R. S., et al.: Integration of conservative surgery, radiotherapy, and chemotherapy for the treatment of early-stage, node-positive breast cancer: Sequencing, timing, and outcome. J. Clin. Oncol., 9:1662, 1991a.

Recht, A., Pierce, S. M., Abner, A., et al.: Regional nodal failure after conservative surgery and radiotherapy for early-stage breast carcinoma. J. Clin. Oncol., 9(6):988, 1991b.

Ribeiro, G.: Personal communication to Harris Hellman, 1987. Mentioned in Harris, J. R., and Hellman, S.: Put the "Hockey Stick" on ice. Int. J. Radiat. Oncol. Biol. Phys., 15:497–499, 1988.

Rissanen, P. M.: A comparison of conservative and radical surgery combined with radiotherapy in the treatment of stage I carcinoma of the breast. Eur. J. Radiol., 42:423, 1969.

Rivkin, S. E., Green S., Metch, B., et al.: Adjuvant CMFVP versus melphalan for operable breast cancer with positive axillary nodes: 10-year results of a Southwest Oncology Group study. J. Clin. Oncol., 7:1229, 1989.

Robertson, J., Clarke, D., Peyzner, M., et al.: Breast conservation therapy: Severe breast fibrosis after radiation in patients with collagen vascular disease. Cancer, 18:502, 1991.

Rodger, A., Montague, E., and Fletcher, G.: Preoperative or postoperative irradiation as adjunctive treatment with radical mastectomy in breast cancer. Cancer, 51:1388, 1983.

Rose, C. M., Botnick, L., Weinstein, M., et al.: Axillary sampling in the definitive treatment of breast cancer by radiation therapy and lumpectomy. Int. J. Radiat. Oncol. Biol. Phys., 9:339, 1983.

Rosner, D., Bedwani, R. N., Vana J., et al.: Noninvasive breast cancer. Ann. Surg., 192:139, 1980.

Rubin, P.: The Franz Buschke Lecture. Late effects of chemotherapy and radiation therapy. A new hypothesis. Int. J. Radiat. Oncol. Biol. Phys., 10:5, 1984.

Rutqvist, L. E., Cedermark, B., Glas, U., et al.: Radiotherapy, chemotherapy and tamoxifen as adjuncts to surgery in early breast cancer: A summary of three randomized trials. Int. J. Radiat. Oncol. Biol. Phys., 16:629, 1989.

Rutqvist, L. E., Lax, I., Fornander, T., et al.: Cardiovascular mortality in a randomized trial for adjuvant radiation therapy versus surgery alone

in primary breast cancer. Int. J. Radiat. Oncol. Biol. Phys., 22:887, 1992.

Salazar, O. M., Rubin, P., Hendrickson, F. R., et al.: Single dose half-body irradiation for palliation of multiple bone metastases from solid tumors. Cancer, 58:29, 1986.

Sarrazin, D., Le, M. G., Arriagada, R., et al.: Ten-year results of a randomized trial comparing a conservative treatment to mastectomy in early breast cancer. Radiother. Oncol., 14:177–184, 1989.

Schwaibold, F., Fowble, B. L., Slin, L. J., et al.: The results of radiation therapy for isolated local regional recurrence after mastectomy. Int. J. Radiat. Oncol. Biol. Phys., 21:299, 1991.

Silverstein, M. J., Rosser, R. J., and Gierson, E. D.: Axillary lymph node dissection for intraductal breast carcinoma—is it indicated? Cancer, 59:1819, 1987.

Silverstein, M. J., Waisman, J. R., and Gierson, E. D.: Radiation therapy for intraductal carcinoma. Is it an equal alternative? Arch. Surg., 126:424, 1991.

Solin, L. J.: Radiation treatment volumes and doses for patients with early-stage carcinoma of the breast treated with breast-conserving surgery and definitive irradiation. Semin. Radiat. Oncol., 2:82, 1992.

Solin, L., Fowble, B., and Goodman, R.: Response to "Is radiotherapy as curative as mastectomy for patients with ductal carcinoma in situ?" Int. J. Radiat. Oncol. Biol. Phys., 19:1103, 1990b.

Solin, L. J., Fowble, B., and Schultz: D. J.: Age as a prognostic factor for patients treated with definitive irradiation for early stage breast cancer. Int. J. Radiat. Oncol. Biol. Phys., 16:373, 1989.

Solin, L. J., Fowble, B. L., Schultz, D. J., et al.: Definitive irradiation for intraductal carcinoma of the breast. Int. J. Radiat. Oncol. Biol. Phys., 19:843, 1990a.

Solin, L. J., Fowble, B. L., Schultz, D. J., et al.: The significance of the pathology margins of the tumor excision on the outcome of patients treated with definitive irradiation for early stage breast cancer. Int. J. Radiat. Oncol. Biol. Phys., 21:279, 1991a.

Solin, L. J., Recht, A., Fourquet A., et al.: Ten-year results of breast-conserving surgery and definitive irradiation for intraductal carcinoma (ductal carcinoma in situ) of the breast. Cancer, 68:2337, 1991b.

Spanos, W. J., Montague, E. D., and Fletcher, G. H.: Late complications of radiation only for advanced breast cancer. Int. J. Radiat. Oncol. Biol. Phys., 6:1473, 1980.

Spitalier, J. M., Gambarelli, J., Brandone, H., et al.: Breast conserving surgery with radiation therapy for operable mammary carcinoma: A 25-year experience. World J. Surg., 10:1014, 1986.

Stadler, B., and Kogelnik, H. D.: Local control and outcome of patients irradiated for isolated chest wall recurrences of breast cancer. Radiother. Oncol., 8:105, 1987.

Stotter, A. T., McNeese, M. D., Ames, F. C., et al.: Predicting the rate and extent of local regional failure after breast conservation therapy for early breast cancer. Cancer, 64:2217, 1989.

Stotter, A. T., McNeese, M., Oswald, M. J., et al.: The role of limited surgery with irradiation in primary treatment of ductal in situ breast cancer. Int. J. Radiat. Oncol. Biol. Phys., 18:283, 1990.

Strom, E. A., McNeese, M. D., Fletcher, G. H., et al.: Results of mastectomy and postoperative irradiation in the management of locoregionally advanced carcinoma of the breast. Int. J. Radiat. Oncol. Biol. Phys., 21:319, 1991.

Sykes, H. F., Sim, D. A., Wong, C. J., et al.: Local-regional recurrence in breast cancer after mastectomy and adriamycin-based adjuvant chemotherapy: Evaluation of the role of postoperative radiotherapy. Int. J. Radiat. Oncol. Biol. Phys., 16:641, 1989.

Tang, G., Gillick, L., and Hendrickson, F. R.: The palliation of symptomatic osseous metastases. Final results of the study by the Radiation Therapy Oncology Group. Cancer, 50:893, 1982.

Thoms, W. W., McNeese, M. D. Fletcher, G. H., et al.: Multimodal treatment for inflammatory breast cancer. Int. J. Radiat. Oncol. Biol. Phys., 17:739–745, 1989.

Toonkel, L. M., Fix, I., Jacobson, L. H., et al.: Postoperative radiation therapy for carcinoma of the breast: Improved results with elective irradiation of the chest wall. Int. J. Radiat. Oncol. Biol. Phys., 8:977, 1982.

Toonkel, L. M., Fix, I., Jacobson, L. H., et al.: The significance of local recurrence of carcinoma of the breast. Int. J. Radiat. Oncol. Biol. Phys., 9:33, 1983.

Tubiana, M., Arriagada, R., and Sarrazin, D.: Human cancer natural history, radiation-induced immunodepression and post-operative radiation therapy. Int. J. Radiat. Oncol. Biol. Phys., 12:477, 1986.

Van Dongen, J. A., Bartelink, H., Aaronson, H., et al.: Randomized clinical trial to assess the value of breast-conserving therapy in Stage II breast cancer: EORTC Trial 10801. Proceedings of the NIH consensus Development Conference, June 18–21, 1990, pp. 25–27.

Van Limbergen, E., Rijnders, A., van der Schueren, E., et al.: Cosmetic evaluation of breast conserving treatment for mammary cancer. A quantitative analysis of the influence of radiation dose, fractionation schedules and surgical treatment techniques on cosmetic results. Radiother. Oncol., *16*:253, 1989.

Van Limbergen, E., Van der Bogaert, W., Van der Schueren, et al.: Tumor excision and radiotherapy as primary treatment of breast cancer analysis of patient and treatment parameters and local control. Radiother. Oncol., *8*:1, 1987.

Veronesi, U., Rilke, F., and Luini, A.: Distribution of axillary node metastases by level of invasion: An analysis of 539 cases. Cancer, *59*:682, 1987.

Wallgren, A., Arner, O., Bergstrom, J., et al.: Preoperative radiotherapy in operable breast cancer. Cancer, *42*:1120–1125, 1978.

Wilson, J. F., Destouet, J. M., Winchester, D. P., et al.: Current controversies in the management of ductal carcinoma in situ of the breast. Radiology, 185:77–81, 1992.

Winchester, D. P., and Cox, J. D.: Standards for breast-conservation treatment. CA Cancer J. Clin., *42*:134–162, 1992.

Zafrani, B., Vielh, P. Fourquet, A., et al.: Conservative treatment of early breast cancer: Prognostic value of the ductal *in situ* component and other pathological variables on local control and survival. Eur. J. Cancer Clin. Oncol., *25*:1645, 1989.

20 Chemotherapy of Breast Cancer

Janell Seeger
Thomas M. Woodcock

Systemic chemotherapy has an important role in the palliative treatment of breast cancer and as an adjuvant to local treatment for patients with and without node involvement.

ADVANCED DISEASE

Disseminated breast cancer currently is not curable, and patients at this stage of the disease will die from progressive tumor. Nevertheless, metastatic breast cancer is very treatable and is one of the solid tumors most responsive to cytotoxic chemotherapy. Patients whose disease responds survive longer and enjoy better quality of life. Typically, patients receive either hormonal or cytotoxic agents, and, if response occurs, months or years of palliation associated with prolonged survival can be expected, including a 10% to 20% chance of complete remission. With continued treatment, the disease becomes resistant, tumor progresses, and therapy must be changed. Continuing changes lead to increased toxicity of treatment, and decreases in rate and duration of response.

Since the initial use of cytotoxic drugs in humans in 1942, virtually every new drug developed has been tested for breast cancer. The classes of active antineoplastic agents are summarized in Table 20–1.

Single-Drug Chemotherapy

The most extensively studied and most active alkylating agent is cyclophosphamide; however, virtually all of the alkylating agents are active. Cyclophosphamide kills tumor cells by interacting chemically with deoxyribonucleic acid (DNA) and causing miscoding of base pairs. The many doses and schedules that are active against breast cancer range from low-dose oral regimens frequently used in combination with other drugs for adjuvant therapy to higher-dose therapy that requires bone marrow support. Toxicity varies with dose but effects include nausea, vomiting, alopecia, and, uniquely, hemorrhagic cystitis. Cystitis is common with high-dose therapy, when prolonged excretion of metabolites of cyclophosphamide causes local irritation of the bladder. Hydration, diuresis, and bladder irrigation can be protective.

Doxorubicin hydrochloride (Adriamycin), an anthracycline antibiotic, is the most active single agent against breast cancer. Its mechanisms of action are complex: doxorubicin may intercalate in the DNA helix and activate DNA cleavage by topoisomerase II, and it may generate free radicals that react with oxygen to produce toxic superoxides. Generation of free radicals is probably the mechanism of cardiotoxicity that is unique to anthracyclines. The major site of metabolism is the hepatoenteric circulation, which puts the patient at risk of hyperbilirubinemia or he-

Table 20–1. SINGLE-AGENT ACTIVITY IN BREAST CANCER

	No. of Responders	Total	Per Cent
Alkylating Agents			
Cyclophosphamide	182	529	34
L-Phenylalanine mustard	20	86	23
Nitrogen mustard	32	92	35
Chlorambucil	11	54	20
Thiotepa	48	162	30
Antimetabolites			
5-Fluorouracil	324	1263	26
Methotrexate	120	356	34
Arabinosyl cytosine	6	64	9
Hydroxyurea	2	16	12
Mitotic Inhibitors			
Vincristine	47	226	20
Vinblastine	19	95	20
Antitumor Antibiotics			
Adriamycin (doxorubicin hydrochloride)	67	193	35
Actinomycin D	5	44	11
Mitomycin C	23	60	38
Bleomycin	0	8	0
Mithramycin	5	32	16
Miscellaneous			
BCNU	16	76	21
CCNU	18	155	12
Methyl-CCNU (MeCCNU)	2	33	6
Hexamethylmelamine	11	39	28
Imidazole carboxamide	2	29	7
Procarbazine	1	21	5
6-Thioguanine	1	23	5

(Modified from Carter, S. K.: Integration of chemotherapy into combination modality treatment of solid tumors. Cancer Treat. Rev., 3:141, 1976.)
Abbreviations: BCNU = bischlorethylnitrosurea; CCNU = N-(2-chloroethyl)-N'-cyclohexyl-N-nitrosourea.

patic failure and may require dose reduction or discontinuation of treatment.

The standard dose of doxorubicin for adjuvant therapy or advanced disease is 60 to 75 mg/M^2 every 3 weeks intravenously, but doses and schedules can be varied. In some patients an infusion of 60 mg/M^2 over 24 to 96 hours may avoid nausea and vomiting without compromising therapeutic effect (Legha et al., 1982), and patients with a prohibitive cardiac history tolerated weekly doses of 10 mg/M^2 well (Chlebowski et al., 1979).

Response rates of up to 50% are reported in previously untreated patients (Ahmann et al., 1974). Its success as a single agent has fostered many regimens based on doxorubicin. Two popular combinations are doxorubicin and cyclophosphamide (AC) and 5-fluorouracil, doxorubicin, and cyclophosphamide (FAC).

Of the several anthracycline analogues evaluated to date, only mitoxantrone has found a role in the treatment of breast cancer. Mitoxantrone is an anthraquinone that causes DNA damage by stabilizing the DNA–topoisomerase II complex and kills both proliferating and resting cells. Several trials confirm its efficacy in advanced breast cancer (Coleman et al., 1984; Cornbleet et al., 1984). In a randomized crossover study of mitoxantrone versus doxorubicin, response rates, duration of response, and survival were equivalent. Quality of life assessment suggested less toxicity as manifested in alopecia, nausea, vomiting, and mucositis, as well as less cardiotoxicity (Henderson and Dukhart, 1984, Shenkenberg and Von Hoff, 1986). Mitoxantrone, in doses of 10 to 14 mg/M^2 every 3 weeks, is substituted for doxorubicin hydrochloride in many standard combinations.

Triethylenethiophosphoramide (thiotepa) is an alkylating agent first used in humans in the 1960s. It is active against breast cancer, the only common side effect being pancytopenia. In the 1990s this drug is being studied in combination with other active drugs in standard doses and in high doses with bone marrow or growth factor support (Lyding et al., 1992).

A pyrimidine analog modestly active against breast cancer is 5-fluorouracil (5-FU). It has several mechanisms of action: incorporation into ribonucleic acid (RNA), inhibition of thymidylate synthesis, and incorporation into DNA. Complex interaction among the administered dose, the schedule of and interaction with other drugs, (methotrexate or leucovorin) can direct the drug to favor a specific mechanism of action. In the body 5-FU is metabolized extensively, and some metabolites (fluonocatrate) may contribute to nonhematologic toxicities such as cerebellar dysfunction. Other common side effects include diarrhea, mucositis, and, occasionally, hyperpigmentation. It functions by inhibiting thymidylate synthase and synthesis of DNA. It is active in several combinations (Table 20–2). The biochemical modulation of 5-FU with leucovorin potentiates cell kill in vivo by selectively reducing thymidine biosynthesis (Rustum et al., 1987). In phase II trials response rates with the combination of 5-FU and leucovorin range from 17% to 48%, depending on the amount of previous therapy.

Cisplatin, a drug widely used for gynecologic and urologic malignancies, was initially thought to have limited activity against breast cancer. The bone marrow–sparing characteristics, however, make it an attractive drug for sal-

Table 20–2. COMMON CYCLOPHOSPHAMIDE- AND ADRIAMYCIN-BASED CHEMOTHERAPY REGIMENS

Cyclophosphamide-Based Regimens

CMFVP (Copper, 1969)

C	= Cyclophosphamide	2 mg/kg/d orally
M	= Methotrexate	0.7 mg/kg/wk intravenously × 8 wk
F	= 5-Fluorouracil	12 mg/kg/d × 4, then 500 mg/wk intravenously
V	= Vincristine	0.035 mg/kg/wk intravenously
P	= Prednisone	0.75 mg/kg/d orally

CMF (DeLena et al., 1975)

C	= Cyclophosphamide	100 mg/m^2/d orally on days 1–14
M	= Methotrexate	30–40 mg/m^2 intravenously on days 1 and 8 28 d
F	= 5-Fluorouracil	400–600 mg/m^2 intravenously on days 1 and 8 every 28 d

CFP (Broder and Tormey, 1974)

C	= cyclophosphamide	150 mg/m^2/d orally × 5
F	= 5-Fluorouracil	300 mg/m^2/d intravenously × 5 q 6 wk
P	= Prednisone	30 mg/d × 7

Adriamycin-Based Regimens

FAC (Blumenschein et al., 1974)

F	= 5-Fluorouracil	500 mg/m^2 intravenously on days 1 and 8
A	= Adriamycin (doxorubicin hydrochloride)	50 mg/m^2 intravenously on day 1
C	= Cyclophosphamide	500 mg/m^2 intravenously on day 1. Repeat cycle every 28 d

ACMF (Kennealey et al., 1978)

A	= Adriamycin	40 mg/m^2 on day 21
C	= Cyclophosphamide	1000 mg/m^2 on day 1
M	= Methotrexate	30 mg/m^2 on days 21, 28, and 35
F	= 5-Fluorouracil	400–600 mg/m^2 on days 21, 28, and 35. Repeat cycle q 6 wk

AC (Salmon and Jones, 1974)

A	= Adriamycin	40 mg/m^2
C	= Cyclophosphamide	200 mg/m^2 on days 3 to 6. Repeat cycle q 21 d

vage therapy. Several active combinations are reported (mitomycin C and cisplatin, 5-FU, leucovorin, and cisplatin, etoposide and cisplatin), but they remain third-line regimens.

Taxol (paclitaxel) is a new drug that has generated much interest. Taxol interferes with cell division by enhancing the stability of microtubules required for mitosis. Holmes and colleagues (1991) reported a 56% objective response rate for advanced breast cancer in a population largely pretreated with doxorubicin (Holmes et al., 1991). The dose-limiting toxic effect was brief granulocytopenia and chronic peripheral sensory neuropathy. Steroids, antihistamines, and histamine H2 blockers must be used to prevent acute hypersensitivity reactions. In phase II trials, Taxol as a single agent produced high response rates in patients with previously untreated metastatic breast cancer (56% to 62%) as well as respectable response rates in previously heavily treated patients (25%). Efficacy seems to be additive when it is given sequentially after adriamycin. Ongoing trials are investigating optimal infusion schedules (3-hour, 24-hour, and 72-hour) as well as a potential role in adjuvant therapy. Taxotere, a semisynthetic analogue of Taxol, is in phase I clinical trials (Pazdur, 1992).

Vinorelbine (Navelbine), a new semisynthetic vinca alkaloid not yet approved by the U.S. Food and Drug Administration (FDA), is also showing promise in advanced breast cancer. Izzo and coworkers (1992) reported high levels of activity in visceral disease in a dose-intensity study of continuous infusion.

Combination Chemotherapy

With such a variety of drugs that are active as single agents against advanced breast cancer, combinations of drugs can be created that have independent mechanisms of action and varying toxicity. The first investigator to apply this concept in advanced breast cancer was Greenspan, as early as 1963. He combined cytotoxic and hormonal agents in a five-drug regimen and reported a 50% response rate (Greenspan, 1966).

The five-drug combination reported by Cooper in 1969 was controversial and was investigated extensively. The drugs were cyclophosphamide, methotrexate, 5-FU, vincristine, and prednisone (CMFVP). Doses and schedules are listed in Table 20–2. The initial abstract reported a 90% rate of complete remission in 60 patients whose disease was refractory to hormone therapy (Cooper, 1969). Several cooperative groups adopted the CMFVP regimen with modifications of dose or schedule or both. Between 1972 and 1974, 11 different studies were reported; response rates were 20% to 70%. Although none was able to reproduce Cooper's results, combining drugs greatly improved results over those achieved with single agents. Cooper's program is still used today.

Randomized trials comparing single drugs to various combinations confirm the benefits of multidrug therapy (Table 20–3). Two cooperative groups compared giving CMFVP on continuous or on intermittent schedules, and results favored the continuous regimen (Smalley et al., 1973; Broder et al., 1974). The CMFVP regimen was then studied in clinical trials that removed drugs one at a time to see if response was affected. Of all the permutations studied, the combination of cyclophosphamide, methotrexate, and 5-FU (CMF) reproducibly achieved a 50% response rate, and this became the standard combination chemotherapy for advanced breast cancer (Fisher et al., 1975).

Because doxorubicin (represented with an "A" for "Adriamycin" when acronyms are used to designate drug combinations) is still the most active drug against breast cancer, doxorubicin-based programs are also prevalent (Blum and Carter, 1974). Table 20–4 shows that doxorubicin alone and CMFVP are equally efficacious. Patients treated with doxorubicin responded earlier but the responses were somewhat shorter lived. Many doxorubicin-based combinations, such as FAC (5-FU, doxorubicin, and cyclophosphamide), AC (Adriamycin and cyclophosphamide), and ACMF (doxorubicin plus CMF) have been used extensively (see Table 20–2). There appears to be no advantage in response rates to using a combination of more than three drugs because the associated more intense mye-

Table 20–3. SINGLE AGENTS VERSUS COMBINATION CHEMOTHERAPY

Drugs	No. of Patients	Response (%)	Median Response (Mo)	Reference
L-PAM (6 mg/m²/d × 5) versus	91	21	3.3	Canellos et al., 1976
CMF	93	53	6.3	
Cyclophosphamide versus	27	25	7.0	Mouridsen et al., 1977
CMFVP	28	63	13.0	
Cyclophosphamide versus	49	55	5.5	Rubens et al., 1975
CMF + Velban	50	62	7.0	

Abbreviations: L-PAM = L-phenylalanine mustard.

losuppression requires reducing the dose (Muss et al., 1977). It is generally accepted that, for standard community care in the absence of investigational protocols, CMF and FAC programs offer a 50 per cent chance of response and are used first for advanced breast cancer.

Several salvage regimens are available after first-line therapy fails. One combination that contains neither cyclophosphamide nor doxorubicin is 5-FU and methotrexate. Biochemical experiments suggest that the antitumor effects of these two drugs may be enhanced by giving them in sequence. Methotrexate is given in doses of 200 mg/m² intravenously followed in 1 hour by 5-FU, 600 mg/m² on days 1 and 8 every 28 days. Leucovorin rescue, 10 mg/m² by mouth every 6 hours for six doses, is instituted 24 hours after each methotrexate dose. Gewirtz and Cadman (1981) reported a response in 11 of 17 patients so treated. Other investigators saw similar responses with smaller doses of methotrexate (100 mg/m²) administered in the same sequence with 5-FU (Plotkin et al., 1985). This regimen can be used by patients who are no longer able to take Adriamycin and by those with little bone marrow reserve.

Using Adriamycin-based regimens as initial therapy for patients with metastatic breast cancer results in complete remissions in 10% to 25% of patients. Legha and coworkers (1979) were able to achieve complete remission with combined drug therapy in 116 patients with advanced breast cancer. The median duration of remission was 17 months, but tumors tended to recur in sites of prior involvement while the patients were taking maintenance therapy. It is obvious that, even with complete disappearance of all disease clinically, only a fraction of tumor cells were killed. Thus, studies that alternated drugs with different mechanisms of cell kill (sequential noncross-resistant combinations) evolved.

Exposing tumor cells to alternating combinations of drugs theoretically should delay the development of resistant populations of cells. Two major studies have alternated doxorubicin–based combinations with cyclophosphamide-based ones (Abeloff et al., 1977; Brambilla et al., 1978). Neither study showed improvement in survival with this approach.

Table 20-4. SINGLE AGENTS SEQUENTIALLY VERSUS COMBINATION CHEMOTHERAPY

	No. of Patients	Response (%)	Median Duration (Mo)	Reference
5-FU, Cyclophosphamide, Vincristine	30	53	—	Baker et al., 1974
versus				
CFV	46	43	6.0	
5-FU, Methotrexate, Cyclophosphamide Vincristine, Prednisone	34	18	4.0	Smalley et al., 1976
versus				
CMFVP continuous	35	46	7.0	
versus				
CMFVP intermittent	33	27	8.5	
Adriamycin		55	5.0	Hoogstraten and George, 1974
versus				
CMFVP continuous	200 total	65	13.5	
versus				
CMFVP intermittent		59	9.0	
Adriamycin	20	45	—	Ahmann et al., 1975
versus				
CFP	28	43	—	

Abbreviations: 5-FU = 5-Fluorouracil.

High-Dose Therapy

Although multiple chemotherapy regimens produce high response rates and can prolong survival, a woman with metastatic breast cancer will ultimately die of the disease. Even a complete clinical remission achieved with standard dose therapy represents only a small reduction in total tumor burden. For this to translate into cure, nearly total tumor cell kill must be achieved.

Several facts about dose-intensive therapy make its application to breast cancer appealing. Many drugs active against breast cancer have a steep dose-response curve in vivo, which means that doubling the dose may more than double tumor cell kill. Investigators have also shown that resistance to alkylating agents is difficult to induce in cell culture, and even when a low level of resistance was produced the cells did not exhibit cross-resistance to other alkylating agents. Phase I trials showed short-lived responses in previously refractory tumors induced by doses of alkylating agents escalated up to 30 times the usual dose. Further studies showed that multiple alkylating agents could be synergistic. The approach currently favored is aggressive combination chemotherapy using standard doses to induce the best remission, followed by dose intensification with autologous bone marrow or peripheral stem cell support.

The drugs selected for dose intensification have a steep dose-response curve and myelosuppression is the dose-limiting toxic effect. Autologous bone marrow reinfusion is a toxicity-limiting strategy that allows otherwise lethal doses of chemotherapy to be given with low rates of morbidity and mortality. Hematopoietic stem cells harvested in advance from peripheral blood may also be used to prevent fatal pancytopenia after high-dose chemotherapy.

Marrow harvest is done with the patient under general anesthesia using multiple pelvic marrow aspirations. For the highest yield the harvest is done after the patient has recovered from standard chemotherapy, when the bone marrow is rebounding. Subsequent high-dose chemotherapy is given using various protective maneuvers against acute toxicity. The marrow is then reinfused. A period of bone marrow aplasia results until the harvested marrow engrafts and matures, usually in 28 days. During the period of aplasia, intensive support is necessary to minimize or treat opportunistic infections and to provide blood product replacement.

Circulating peripheral stem cells can be harvested to supplement (or in the future perhaps supplant) bone marrow. With repeated leukophoresis, the number of stem cells recovered can be equal to that of bone marrow. Peripheral stem cells offer an advantage in the immediate aplastic period, as they are already committed progenitor cells and can shorten the number of days of absolute aplasia.

The commercial availability of colony-stimulating factors has helped reduce toxicity from high-dose therapy and from dose-intensified standard therapy. Granulocyte-macrophage colony–stimulating factor (GM-CSF) and granulocyte colony–stimulating factor (G-CSF) are natural cytokines that have an endogenous role in regulating granulocytes. Superphysiologic doses in normal patients causes a sustained, dose-dependent increase in circulating granulocytes. In patients receiving standard-dose chemotherapy, the degree and duration of neutropenia is diminished by these growth factors.

Intensification of standard chemotherapy is now possible for adjuvant treatment of breast cancer. With high-dose therapy growth factors enhance granulocyte recovery and reduce the risk of infections. After bone marrow transplantation these growth factors enhance granulocyte recovery and reduce infections. Growth factors are also used to stimulate the number of circulating peripheral stem cells to augment the harvest by leukophoresis. All of these uses are being investigated to better define the appropriate use of growth factors. New growth factors are being developed, such as macrophage CSF and interleukin-2 combined with

G-CSF to stimulate stem cells and to facilitate recovery of platelets.

Toxicity

Chemotherapy affects organs and tissues in the body to varying degrees. The drugs distinguish poorly between malignant and normal cells. Familiarity with side effects is necessary to maximize the therapeutic usefulness of treatment while minimizing toxicity.

Bone marrow is composed of rapidly dividing cells and is susceptible to damage by many chemotherapeutic drugs. Frequent blood counts are necessary to adjust the dose and schedule of drug administration. Granulocytes, which have a half-life of 6 hours, are usually affected first. If the absolute granulocyte count is suppressed to less than 1000 leukocytes per microliter, the patient is at risk for sepsis from endogenous organisms and should receive broad-spectrum antibiotics for any febrile episode. Recovery time is a function of agent, dose, rate of metabolism, and degree of myelosuppression. Platelets (half-life 5 to 7 days) are suppressed next, but thrombocytopenia is rarely the dose-limiting factor. Anemia usually is not dose limiting because of the long half-life of red blood cells (120 days) and the ease of replacement (Hoagland, 1982). Growth factors are changing the spectrum and severity of bone marrow toxicity.

Skin changes can range from minor hyperpigmentation with 5-FU and bleomycin to total alopecia with doxorubicin hydrochloride and high-dose cyclophosphamide, to severe extravasation reactions produced by vesicants such as vincristine, doxorubicin hydrochloride, and mitomycin C. The radiation recall phenomenon is an exacerbation of normal skin reaction to radiation in tissues previously or concurrently exposed to adriamycin or actinomycin D.

Cardiotoxicity, though not common, can be refractory, progressive, and fatal. Doxorubicin hydrochloride and daunorubicin are the major offenders. Acute electrocardiographic abnormalities can be demonstrated while these drugs are being administered and immediately afterward. Arrhythmias and ST-T wave changes are evident and usually resolve without symptoms or treatment. Doxorubicin hydrochloride and daunorubicin may also cause a cumulative, dose-dependent cardiomyopathy. The risk increases greatly after a total lifetime dose of 550 mg/m². Other factors such as age, underlying heart disease, cyclophosphamide therapy, and previous mediastinal irradiation also contribute to the overall risk. Attempts to avoid this devastating complication include monitoring cardiac function with MUGA (multiple gated acquisition) scans or endomyocardial biopsies, and development of less toxic analogues and cardioprotectors (Von Hoff et al., 1982).

Pulmonary signs of toxicity from chemotherapy can progress from dry cough and exertional dyspnea to fatal pulmonary insufficiency. Classic interstitial fibrosis is found on histologic examination. Bleomycin is the drug most often implicated. Risk factors include advanced age, previous thoracic irradiation, and cumulative drug doses of 500 units or more. No effective therapy is known. Pulmonary function tests, including diffusion capacity of the lung

with carbon monoxide, may be useful to document early damage. Bischlorethylnitrosourea (BCNU) can produce pulmonary toxicity when doses exceed 1400 mg/m² (Ginsberg et al., 1982).

Gastrointestinal side effects are the most clinically apparent to the patient. Nausea and vomiting, aside from being psychologically distressing, contribute to malnutrition and dehydration. Much effort has been spent to develop effective antiemetic regimens. Metoclopramide (Reglan), an effective antiemetic agent especially for cisplatin-induced nausea, improves patient tolerance. Ondansetron (Zofran) is a selective serotonin 5-HT3 receptor antagonist that much reduces the nausea and vomiting associated with chemotherapy of all types. Mucositis and diarrhea are often associated with chemotherapy because of the rapid turnover of the cells lining the gastrointestinal tract (Mitchell et al., 1982). Only symptomatic support is available at this time.

The list of new toxic effects of chemotherapy is growing as clinical use expands. Some that physicians consider minor inconveniences may be of more consequence to the patient. Cushing's syndrome or masculinization after steroid and sex hormone administration can be particularly distressing. Chemically induced menopause is often part of therapy. The most common complaints of women receiving adjuvant chemotherapy are weight gain and malaise, and both reduce compliance.

The risk of second malignancies after adjuvant chemotherapy remains a concern. Recent studies of patients who have received adjuvant chemotherapy for breast cancer have not suggested a significant long-term cancer risk. The physician who administers chemotherapy must be prepared to manage minor toxic effects as well as the life-threatening ones (Perry et al., 1984).

ADJUVANT CHEMOTHERAPY

Stage III and Inflammatory Breast Cancer

Stage III breast cancer is locally advanced. This means the patient has a large primary tumor or extensive node involvement but no demonstrable distant metastases. This group of patients' prognosis is poor. Inflammatory breast cancer is a unique clinicopathologic subset of Stage III breast cancer that is particularly aggressive. The clinical presentation is typical: inflammatory skin changes without a distinct mass. Findings of histologic examination are not diagnostic, though they often show involvement of dermal lymphatic vessels with cancer.

Radical surgery alone cannot cure locally advanced breast cancer. Of 122 patients treated with radical mastectomy, 49% had a local recurrence after 5 years and only 1% were alive and free of disease (Haagensen and Stout, 1943). Radiation therapy alone improved local control but not survival (Baclesse, 1949). Radiotherapy is more effective for achieving local control when bulky tumor is removed and doses greater than 6000 cGy are used (Balawajder et al., 1983). With megavoltage radiotherapy by external beam or interstitial implant, local control improved to 75% at 5 years (Bruckman et al., 1979).

Combination chemotherapy is necessary to improve survival of patients with Stage III disease. Preoperative administration is preferred, for several theoretical reasons. Subclinical metastasis, the harbinger of systemic disease, can be treated as well as the primary disease and may facilitate later resection. Drug delivery may be more consistent if tumor vasculature is unaltered by surgery or radiation. The physician can also observe tumor response to the chemotherapy and confirm sensitivity (Papaioannou, 1985).

Most regimens combine chemotherapy with radiation, surgery, or both. DeLena and colleagues (1975) performed a randomized trial to compare mastectomy and radiation for local-regional control; both groups received aggressive chemotherapy beforehand and afterward. There was no difference in treatment failure, duration of response, or survival after 3 years, but a 5-year update showed a significant survival advantage for the mastectomy group. Another report involved induction chemotherapy followed by local radiation. Mastectomy was performed if residual tumor was present, and was followed by resumption of chemotherapy. Hu and coworkers (1985) reported 100% local control and 87% relapse-free survival with this approach. Hortobagyi and colleagues (1983) advocate an Adriamycin-based regimen (FAC) followed by local therapy (simple mastectomy, radiotherapy, or both) followed by a cyclophosphamide-based regimen (CMF) to complete 2 years of treatment. At 5 years, 40% of patients remained free of disease. Many other combinations of drugs have improved overall survival.

Because the poor prognosis of Stage III breast cancer can be altered by chemotherapy, high-dose therapy with bone marrow support has promise. Studies include Stage II patients if more than 10 lymph nodes are involved because their prognosis is nearly as dismal as that for women with Stage III disease. The regimen often involves induction with standard-dose therapy followed by high-dose therapy with bone marrow or stem cell support. Most clinical trials have short follow-up periods, but initial results are encouraging enough to proceed to Phase III randomized trials.

Stage II (Node-Positive) Cancer

State II breast cancer has been extensively studied in the adjuvant setting, probably because a relatively small fraction of patients are cured by surgery alone. Prognosis is directly related to the number of nodes histologically involved with metastases: the prognosis is distinctly worse when that number is four or more. After radical mastectomy, surgical investigators report that patients with metastases in lymph nodes have a 10-year survival rate of 25% to 48% (DeVita et al., 1982). Survival for those with one to three involved nodes ranges from 34% to 63% and from 16% to 27% for those with at least four "positive" nodes. The goal of adjuvant chemotherapy is to kill any remaining breast cancer cells after definitive surgery; this should translate into an increased disease-free interval and cure.

Concepts about the biologic behavior of cancer have come full circle since the 2nd century A.D., when Galen considered cancer a systemic disease caused by excess black bile and thus not surgically curable. Laboratory data and clinical experience suggest that in most patients breast cancer is a systemic disease. In 1869, Ashworth observed circulating malignant cells in the blood. Hematogenous dissemination was markedly increased by manipulation of or trauma to the primary tumor. Theoretically, effective antitumor drugs administered postsurgically would kill these cells and prevent dissemination, a feat demonstrated in vitro with a mouse model by Martin (1959).

The rationale of adjuvant chemotherapy was to prevent implantation of hematogenously disseminated cells and eradicate subclinical metastases. By the early 1960s, several trials began using a single alkylating agent, triethylenethiophosphoramide (Thiotepa) in the immediate postoperative period. The cooperative group of the National Surgical Adjuvant Breast Project (NSABP) designed a prospective randomized trial of brief low-dose thiotepa versus placebo. At 10 years, a statistically significant survival benefit was seen in treated premenopausal women who had four or more involved nodes (Fisher, 1968). Another clinical trial initiated by Donegan and coworkers in 1963 extended surgical adjuvant thiotepa therapy postoperatively for 1 year. The most recent update after a median interval of more than 15 years' follow-up showed a significant survival benefit for patients with negative axillary nodes, but a neutral and a detrimental effect, respectively, for patients with one to three involved nodes and four or more (Donegan et al., 1985). The European experience with intensive postoperative chemotherapy given as a brief course compared with no therapy demonstrated benefit for the treated group. Nissen-Meyer and colleagues (1978) reported a multicenter randomized trial from Scandinavia in which women were treated with cyclophosphamide for 6 days after mastectomy. Although there was no stratification for node status, after 10 years' follow-up a small but significant reduction in recurrence and death was seen. One interesting piece of statistical data was that benefit from chemotherapy was lost if therapy was delayed more than 3 weeks after surgery. These early single-agent trials are summarized in Table 20–5. The results were encouraging, but skepticism remained because of lack of stratification and variations in other treatments of the study patients.

Laboratory studies continue to contribute new information about the biologic behavior of breast cancer. It has been shown that breast cancer cells are capable of metastasizing via the blood and lymphatics interchangeably even before cancers grow large enough to be clinically detectable. Instead of just killing breast cancer cells released by surgical manipulation, adjuvant therapy must also kill established but microscopic metastases. Micrometastases are known to have a high growth fraction, which should make them more sensitive to cytotoxic drugs. Much has been learned about cell cycle kinetics and growth regulation of malignant cells. Tumor cells replicate by four distinct phases of growth, and cytotoxic drugs are active in different phases. By combining multiple drugs that are tumorcidal at different stages of replication, cell kill should be maximized and drug resistance circumvented. Recent clinical trials apply this understanding of tumor biology. The first major trial of adjuvant chemotherapy conducted by the NSABP (Protocol B-05) entered patients with Stage II breast cancer after treatment with radical or modified radical mastectomy.

Table 20–5. EARLY SINGLE-AGENT TRIALS FOR SURGICAL ADJUVANT THERAPY

Study	Drug	Conclusion	Reference
NSAPB (1958)	Thiotepa versus placebo	Premenopausal women with 4+ nodes benefited	Fisher et al., 1975
Donegan (1966)	Thiotepa versus no therapy	Relapse-free survival advantage in node-negative patients	Donegan, 1974
NSABP (1972)	L-PAM versus placebo	Premenopausal women 1–3+ nodes benefited	Fisher et al., 1980
Nissen-Meyer (1965)	Cyclophosphamide versus no therapy	Longer overall survival in treated group at 12 y	Nissen-Meyer, 1978

Abbreviations: NSABP = National Surgical Adjuvant Breast Project; L-PAM = L-Phenylalanine mustard.

Patients were stratified by age and degree of node involvement. Patients received either L-phenylalanine mustard (L-PAM) orally for 5 days every 6 weeks for 2 years or placebo. Disease-free and overall survival rates were significantly improved in the treated group—by 8% and 5%, respectively. The greatest benefit was seen in premenopausal women, whose mortality rate was reduced by 37% (Fisher et al., 1986). Adjuvant therapy was most effective against anaplastic tumors among premenopausal and postmenopausal women. After this study, another clinical trial (B-07) was designed using two drugs with different actions. All parameters of eligibility and stratification were the same, but this study compared L-PAM alone to L-PAM plus 5-FU. At 5 years a slight benefit was evident for women treated with two drugs as compared with those treated with one, but the most significant improvement was in postmenopausal women who had four or more involved nodes. These two NSABP trials and subsequent B-08 and B-09 protocols are summarized in Table 20–6. In 1973, the Instituto Nationale Tumori, in Milan, Italy, began an adjuvant program for operable breast cancer. The first study tested combination chemotherapy with an active drug combination for advanced disease, CMF (Bonadonna et al., 1976). After radical mastectomy, patients received CMF on days 1 and 8 of a 28-day cycle for 12 cycles. Annual analysis of relapse-free survival showed significant benefit for the treated group—64% versus 48% for controls at 5 years (Rossi et al., 1980). Benefit was seen in premenopausal

women who had one to three involved nodes. Subsequent protocols comparing 12 cycles of therapy with six cycles showed equal efficacy (Tancini et al., 1979). Although a shorter treatment did not reduce the survival advantage, reducing the dose did. When patients received less than 75% of the optimal dose of drugs, relapse-free survival and overall survival were reduced (Bonadonna et al., 1979). Many older postmenopausal women required dose reduction because of hematologic toxicity, and this was thought to be a major factor in the failure of adjuvant CMF therapy in postmenopausal women.

Another cooperative group, the Southwest Oncology Group, compared CMFVP to L-PAM as an adjuvant. Not only was relapse-free survival improved in the group treated with combination chemotherapy, but postmenopausal women benefited as well as premenopausal women (Glucksberg et al., 1979).

The same concept of alternating therapy with drugs that do not induce cross-resistance developed for advanced breast cancer was applied to adjuvant therapy. Table 20–7 shows the results of a study with CMFP for six cycles followed by AV for four. This study could not demonstrate benefit from what has been termed *late-intensification, or reinduction, chemotherapy.* The NSABP incorporated this biologic question in protocols B-15 and B-16, with similar results. AC followed by CMF was not superior to AC alone. It was observed that 2 months of AC (four cycles) was as effective as 6 months of CMF (Fisher et al., 1990).

Table 20–6. NATIONAL SURGICAL ADJUVANT BREAST PROJECT: ADJUVANT CHEMOTHERAPY FOR OPERABLE BREAST CANCER

NSABP Protocol	Drugs	Relapse-Free Survival (%)	Conclusion	Reference
B-05	L-PAM	55	Benefit greatest in premenopausal women with 1–3+ nodes	Fisher et al., 1980
	versus			
	Placebo	44		
B-07	L-PAM	50	Benefit first seen in postmenopausal women with 4+ nodes	Fisher et al., 1977
	versus			
	L-PAM + 5 FU	54		
B-08	L-PAM + 5 FU	74	No increased benefit 2 versus 3 drugs	Fisher et al., 1980
	versus			
	L-PAM, 5-FU, MTX	70		
B-09	L-PAM + 5 FU	74.8	Superior relapse-free survival in women ≥ 50 y of age with any node + ER > 10 fmol/mg	Fisher et al., 1980
	versus			
	L-PAM + 5 FU + Tamoxifen	80.1		

Abbreviations: MTX = methotrexate; ER = estrogen receptor.

Table 20-7. CYCLOPHOSPHAMIDE-METHOTREXATE-5-FLUOROURACIL–BASED ADJUVANT CHEMOTHERAPY FOR OPERABLE BREAST CANCER

Drugs	Relapse-Free Survival (%)	Conclusion	Reference
CMF × 12 cycles versus	64	Benefit in women with 1–3+ nodes, premenopausal only	Bonadonna et al., 1976
no therapy	48		
CMF × 12 cycles versus	46	No significant difference in 6 versus 12 cycles	Tancini et al., 1979
CMF × 6 cycles	54.8		
CMFVP versus	47	Premenopausal and postmenopausal benefits regardless of nodal status	Glucksberg et al., 1979
L-PAM	26		
CMFP × 6 cycles + AV × 4 cycles versus	46.4	No significant benefit seen by late intensive chemotherapy	Bonadonna et al., 1985
CMF	55		

With the availability of growth factors for bone marrow support, Adriamycin-based regimens are being used extensively for Stage II breast cancer. The acute toxicity of CMF versus AC suggests that, despite total alopecia, AC is tolerated better. Perhaps this is due to the shorter duration of treatment for the AC regimen, which is considered more intensive and is completed in four 3-week cycles. This also keeps the total dose of Adriamycin well under the maximum tolerated lifetime dose. AC is now considered one of the standard regimens for node-positive breast cancer.

In response to evidence that high-dose therapy may make adjuvant therapy more effective (Hryniuk et al., 1986), the NSABP piloted a feasibility study of escalating doses of cyclophosphamide in the AC combination using growth factor support (Hryniuk et al., 1986). Designed for "poor-prognosis" Stage II and III patients or initial treatment for those with advanced breast cancer, these trials (BP-53 and BP-54) demonstrated that dose escalation was safe. The subsequent protocols for Stage II breast cancer used three arms of AC with increasing doses of cyclophosphamide up to 2400 mg/m² and (G-CSF) growth factor support.

Stage I (Node Negative) Cancer

Approximately 20% to 25% of women with Stage I breast cancer eventually develop disseminated disease. Before 1980, however, the surgical cure rate was considered too high to warrant adjuvant therapy. The first clinical trials of adjuvant therapy for Stage I disease were designed with minimally toxic drugs because the potential benefit was to a small number of patients.

Four studies were completed by various groups, and all showed improvement in disease-free survival. The first study published was the Milan IV trial conducted at the Milan Cancer Institute. It randomized node-negative, estrogen receptor–negative breast cancer patients to CMF for 9 months or to observation. The treated group had an overall survival rate of 84%, versus 58% for the untreated group. This trial was criticized for its small size (only 90 patients) and for the larger proportion of patients with large tumors in the untreated group.

Three other studies were completed and published by 1989. The NSABP B-13 trial randomized women to methotrexate and 5-FU for 12 months and had a no-treatment control arm. Again, a disease-free survival advantage was shown, 76% versus 67%, and survival benefit was greatest for women aged 50 years or older. The Intergroup 0011 trial (Mansour et al., 1989) and the Ludwig V trial (The Ludwig Breast Cancer Study Group, 1989) both showed significant improvement in disease-free survival as compared with no therapy.

A comprehensive meta-analysis of adjuvant therapy was reported by the Early Breast Cancer Trialists' Collaborative Group (1992). This report analyzed 133 randomized trials involving 75,000 women including both polychemotherapy and adjuvant hormonal manipulations. Although the types of chemotherapy varied (mostly CMF), the summary data indicated significant benefit, in both reduced recurrence and improved survival, for node-positive and node-negative patients (Fig. 20–1). The greatest benefit was seen with at least 6 months' polychemotherapy, and response was age related (best results in younger patients; Table 20–8).

A National Institutes of Health Consensus Statement summarized current recommendations for Stage I breast cancer. Patients should be made aware of the risks and benefits of adjuvant systemic therapy. This involves discussing with each patient, at her level of understanding, the individual prognostic factors, toxic effects of accepted reg-

Table 20-8. META-ANALYSIS OF 47 ADJUVANT CHEMOTHERAPY TRIALS: 10-YEAR RESULTS

Age (Yr)	Cases (No.)	Reduction in Recurrence (%)	Reduction in Deaths (%)
< 50 Premenopausal	3138	36	25
< 50 Postmenopausal	225	37	
50–59 Premenopausal	911	25	23
50–59 Postmenopausal	3128	29	13
60–69	3774	20	10

Data from Early Breast Cancer Trialists' Collaborative Group-1992

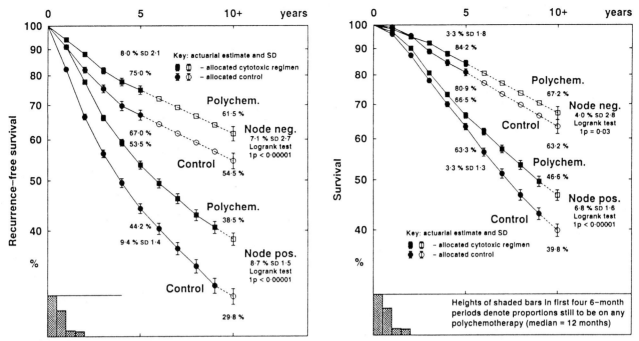

Figure 20-1. Ten-year outcome of adjuvant polychemotherapy trials according to node status. Meta-analysis of international randomized trials of adjuvant chemotherapy by the Early Breast Cancer Trialists' Collaborative Group. Significant improvement in disease free survival and survival is demonstrated for patients with and without axillary metastases. (From Early Breast Cancer Trialists' Collaborative Group: Systemic treatment of early breast cancer by hormonal, cytotoxic, or immune therapy. Lancet, *339*:71–84, 1992. © by *The Lancet Ltd.*, 1992.)

imens, and expected benefit. While all node-negative patients are at some risk for recurrence, patients with invasive tumors no larger than 1 cm diameter have an excellent prognosis and do not require adjuvant systemic therapy outside of clinical trials (NIH 1991).

SUMMARY

Chemotherapy offers palliation for patients with advanced breast cancer and an improved prognosis for some with local and regional disease. The trend for adjuvant therapy has been toward dose intensification and shorter duration of treatment. The availability of growth factors and autologous bone marrow support facilitates this approach. Adjuvant chemotherapy offers benefit for both node-positive and node-negative cases, but prognostic factors are needed to select more accurately the cases that will benefit.

References

Abeloff, M. D., and Ettinger, D. S.: Treatment of metastatic breast cancer with Adriamycin-cyclophosphamide induction followed by alternating combination therapy. Cancer Treat. Res., *61*:1685, 1977.

Ahmann, D. L., Bisel, H. F., Eagan, R. T., et al.: Controlled evaluation of Adriamycin (NSC-123127) in patients with disseminated breast cancer. Cancer Chemother. Rep., *58*:877, 1974.

Ahmann, D. L., Bisel, H. F., Edmonson, J. H., et al.: An analysis of a multiple-drug program in the treatment of patients with advanced breast cancer utilizing 5-fluorouracil, Cytoxan, prednisone with or without vincristine. Cancer *36*:1925, 1975.

Baclesse, R.: Roentgen therapy as the sole method of treatment of cancer of the breast. A.J.R. Am. J. Roentgenol., *62*:311, 1949.

Baker, L. H., Vaughn, C. B., Al-Sarref, M., et al.: Evaluation of combination vs. sequential cytotoxic chemotherapy in the treatment of advanced breast cancer. Cancer, *33*:513, 1974.

Balawajder, I., Antich, P. P., and Boland, J.: An analysis of the role of radiotherapy alone and in combination with chemotherapy and surgery in the management of advanced breast carcinoma. Cancer, *51*:574, 1983.

Blum, R. D., and Carter, S. K.: A new anticancer drug with significant clinical activity. Ann. Intern. Med., *80*:249, 1974.

Bonadonna, G., Brusamolino, E., Valagussa, P., et al.: Combination chemotherapy as an adjuvant treatment in operable breast cancer. N. Engl. J. Med., *294*:405, 1976.

Bonadonna, G., Valagussa, P., Rossi, A., et al.: CMF adjuvant chemotherapy in operable breast cancer. *In* Jones, S. E., and Salmon, S. E. (Eds.): Adjuvant Therapy of Cancer II. New York, Grune & Stratton, 1979, p. 227.

Bonadonna, G., Valagussa, P., Rossi, A., et al.: Ten-year experience with CMF-based adjuvant chemotherapy in resectable breast cancer. Breast Cancer Res. Treat., *5*:95, 1985.

Brambilla, C., Valagussa, P., and Bonadonna, G.: Sequential combination chemotherapy in advanced breast cancer. Cancer Chemother. Pharmacol., *1*:35, 1978.

Broder, L. E., and Tormey, D. C.: Combination chemotherapy of carcinoma of the breast. Cancer Treat. Res., *1*:183, 1974.

Bruckman, J. E., Harris, J. R., Levene, M. B., et al.: Results of treating stage III carcinoma of the breast by primary radiation therapy. Cancer, *43*:985, 1979.

Canellos, G. P., Pocock, S. J., Taylor, S. F. III, et al.: Combination chemotherapy for metastatic breast carcinoma: Prospective comparison of multiple drug therapy with L-phenylalanine mustard. Cancer, *38*:1882, 1976.

Chlebowski, R., Pugh, R., Paroly, W., et al.: Adriamycin on a weekly schedule: Clinically effective with low incidence of cardiotoxicity. Clin. Res., *27*:53A, 1979.

Coleman, R. E., Maisey, M. N., Knight, R. K., et al.: Mitoxantrone in advanced breast cancer: A phase II study with special attention to cardiotoxicity. Eur. J. Cancer Clin. Oncol., *20*:771–776, 1984.

Cooper, R.: Combination cytotoxic chemotherapy in hormone-resistant breast cancer (abstract). Proc. Am. Assoc. Cancer Res. Am. Soc. Clin. Oncol. *10*:15, 1969.

Cornbleet, M. A., Stuart-Harris, R. C., Smith, I. E., et al.: Mitoxantrone for the treatment of advanced breast cancer: Single-agent therapy in previously untreated patients. Eur. J. Cancer Clin. Oncol., *20*:1141, 1984.

DeLena, M., Brambilla, C., Morabito, A., et al.: Adriamycin plus vincristine compared to and combined with cyclophosphamide, methotrexate, and 5-fluorouracil for advanced breast cancer. Cancer, *35*:1108, 1975.

DeVita, V. T., Hellman, S., and Rosenberg, S. A.: Cancer.: Principles and Practice of Oncology. Philadelphia, J. B. Lippincott, 1982, p. 920.

Donegan, W. L.: Extended surgical adjuvant thiotepa for mammary carcinoma. Arch. Surg., *109*:187, 1974.

Donegan, W. L., and Kardinal, C. G.: Long-term results of extended adjuvant thiotepa for operable breast cancer (Abstract). Proc. A.S.C.O., *4*:75, 1985.

Early Breast Cancer Trialists' Collaborative Group: Systemic treatment of early breast cancer by hormonal, cytotoxic, or immune therapy. Lancet, *339*:71–84, 1992.

Fisher, B., Ravdin, R. G., Ausman, R. K., et al.: Surgical adjuvant chemotherapy in cancer of the breast. Results of a decade of cooperative investigation. Ann. Surg., *168*:337, 1968.

Fisher, B., Ravdin, R. G., Ausman, R. K., et al.: L-phenylalanine mustard (L-PAM) in the management of primary breast cancer: A report of early findings. N. Engl. J. Med., *292*:117, 1975.

Fisher B., Fisher E. R., Redmond, C., et al.: Ten-year results from the National Surgical Adjuvant Breast and Bowel Project (NSABP) clinical trial evaluating the use of L-phenylalanine mustard (L-PAM) in the management of primary breast cancer. J. Clin. Oncol., *4*:929–941, 1986.

Fisher, B., Brown, A. M., Dimitrov, N. V., et al.: Two months of doxorubicin-cyclophosphamide with and without interval reinduction therapy compared with 6 months of cyclophosphamide, methotrexate, and fluorouracil in positive-node breast cancer patients with tamoxifen-nonresponsive tumors: Results from the National Surgical Adjuvant Breast and Bowel Project B-15. J. Clin. Oncol., *8*:1483–1496, 1990.

Fisher, B., Ravdin, R. G., Ausman, R. K., et al.: Surgical adjuvant chemotherapy in cancer of the breast: Results of a decade of cooperative investigation. Ann. Surg., *168*:337, 1968.

Fisher, B., Ravdin, R. G., Ausman, R. K., et al.: L-Phenylalanine mustard (L-PAM) in the management of primary breast cancer: A report of early findings. N. Engl. J. Med., *292*:117, 1975.

Fisher, B., Redmond, C., Fisher, E. R., et al.: The contribution of recent NSABP clinical trials of primary breast cancer therapy to an understanding of tumor biology—an overview of findings. Cancer, *46*:1009, 1980.

Fisher, B., Slack, N., Katrych, D., et al.: Ten-year follow up results of patients with carcinoma of the breast in a cooperative clinical trial evaluating surgical adjuvant chemotherapy. Surg. Gynecol. Obstet., *140*:528, 1975.

Gewirtz, A. M., and Cadman, E.: Preliminary report on the efficacy of sequential methotrexate and 5-fluorouracil in advanced breast cancer. Cancer, *47*:2552, 1981.

Ginsberg, S., and Comis, R. L.: The pulmonary toxicity of antineoplastic agents. Semin. Oncol., *9*:34, 1982.

Glucksberg, H., Rivkin, S. E., and Rasmussen, S.: Adjuvant chemotherapy for stage II breast cancer: A comparison of CMFVP versus L-PAM. *In* Jones, S. E., and Salmon, S. E. (Eds.): Adjuvant Therapy of Cancer II. New York, Grune & Stratton, 1979, p. 261.

Greenspan, E. M.: Combination cytotoxic chemotherapy in advanced disseminated breast carcinoma. J. Mt. Sinai Hosp., *33*:1, 1966.

Haagensen, C. D., and Stout, A. P.: Carcinoma of the breast: Criteria of operability. Ann. Surg., *118*:859, 1943.

Halsted, W. S.: The results of radical operations for the cure of cancer of the breast. Ann. Surg., *4*:1, 1907.

Henderson, I. C., and Dukhart, G.: A randomized trial comparing mitoxantrone with doxorubicin in patients with metastatic breast cancer (Abstract). Proc. A.S.C.O., *3*:120, 1984.

Hoagland, H. C.: Hematologic complications of chemotherapy. Semin. Oncol., *9*:95, 1982.

Holmes, F. A., Walters, R. S., Theriault, R. L., et al.: Phase II trial of taxol, an active drug in the treatment of metastatic breast cancer. J. Nat. Cancer Insti. *83*:1797–1805, 1991.

Hoogstraten, B., and George, S.: Adriamycin and combination chemotherapy in breast cancer: A Southwest Oncology Group study. Proc. A.A.C.R., *15*:70, 1974.

Hortobagyi, G. N., Blumenschein, G. R., Spanos, W., et al.: Multimodal treatment of locoregionally advanced breast cancer. Cancer, *51*:763, 1983.

Hrynivk, W. M., Levine, M. N., and Levin, L: Analysis of dose intensity for chemotherapy in early (Stage II) and advanced breast cancer. NCI Monogr., *1*:87–94, 1986.

Hu, E., Stockdale, F. E., Carlson, R. W., et al.: Locally advanced breast cancer patients (T_3/T_4 or N_3) treated with a sandwich approach of chemotherapy, radiotherapy and chemotherapy. Proc. A.S.C.O., *4*:58, 1985.

Izzo, J., Toussiant, C., Chabot, G., et al.: High activity and dose intensity (DI) relationship in advanced breast cancer (ABC) with continuous infusion (CIV) of navelbine (NVB). Proc. A.S.C.O., *11*:71, 1992.

Legha, S. S., Benjamin, R. S., Macray, B., et al.: Adriamycin therapy of continuous intravenous infusion in patients with metastatic breast cancer. Cancer, *49*:1762, 1982.

Legha, S. S., Buzdar, A. U., Smith, T. L., et al.: Complete remissions in metastatic breast cancer treated with combination drug therapy. Ann. Intern. Med., *91*:847, 1979.

Logan, W. P. D.: Cancer of the breast: No decline in mortality. W.H.O. Chron., *29*:462, 1975.

The Ludwig Breast Cancer Study Group: Prolonged disease-free survival after one course of perioperative adjuvant chemotherapy for node-negative breast cancer. N. Engl. J. Med., *320*:491, 1989.

Lyding, J., Damon, L., Wolf, J., et al.: High-dose cyclophosphamide, thiotepa, and mitoxantrone with autologous bone marrow transplant for breast cancer. Proc. A.S.C.O., *11*:70, 1992.

Mansour, E. G., Gray, R., Shatila, A. H., et al.: Efficacy of adjuvant chemotherapy in high-risk node-negative breast cancer. N. Engl. J. Med., *320*:485, 1989.

Martin, D. S.: An appraisal of chemotherapy as an adjuvant to surgery for cancer. Am. J. Surg., *97*:685, 1959.

Mitchell, E. P., and Schein, P. S.: Gastrointestinal toxicity of chemotherapeutic agents. Semin. Oncol., *9*:52, 1982.

Mouridsen H. T., Brahm, T. P. M., and Rahbek, I.: Evaluation of single-drug versus multiple drug chemotherapy in the treatment of advanced breast cancer. Cancer Treat. Rep., *61*:47, 1977.

Muss, H. B., White, D. R., Cooper, M. R., et al.: Combination chemotherapy in advanced breast cancer: A randomized trial comparing a three- vs five-drug program. Arch. Intern. Med., *137*:1711, 1977.

National Institutes of Health Consensus Conference: Treatment of early stage breast cancer. J.A.M.A., *265*:391, 1991.

Nissen-Meyer, R., Kjellgren, K., Malmio, K., et al.: Surgical adjuvant chemotherapy: Results with one short course with cyclophosphamide after mastectomy for breast cancer. Cancer, *41*:2088, 1978.

Papaioannou, A. N.: Preoperative chemotherapy: Advantages and clinical application in Stage III breast cancer. Recent Results Cancer Res., *98*:67, 1985.

Pazdur, R., Newman, R. A., Newman, B. M., et al.: Phase I trial of taxotere (RP56976). Proc. A.S.C.O., *11*:111, 1992.

Perry, M. C., and Yarbro, J. W.: Toxicity of Chemotherapy. New York, Grune & Stratton, 1984.

Plotkin, D., Waugh, W., and Peng, J.: Sequential methotrexate–5-fluorouracil in advanced breast cancer (Abstract). Proc. A.S.C.O., *4*:62, 1985.

Rossi, A., Bonadonna, G., Valagussa, P., et al.: CMF adjuvant program for breast cancer: Five-year results. Proc. A.A.C.R., *21*:404, 1980.

Rubens, R. D., Knight, R. K., and Daywood, J. L.: Chemotherapy of advanced breast cancer: A controlled randomized trial of cyclophosphamide versus a 4 drug combination. Br. J. Cancer, *32*:730, 1975.

Rustum, Y. M., Trave, F., Zakrzewski, S. F., et al.: Biochemical and pharmacologic basis for potentiation of 5-fluorouracil action by leucovorin. Monogr. Natl. Cancer Inst., *5*:165–170, 1987.

Shenkenberg, T. D., and Von Hoff, D. D.: Mitoxantrone: A new anticancer drug with significant clinical activity. Ann. Intern. Med., *105*:67–81, 1986.

Smalley, R. V., Murphy, S., Chan, Y. K., et al.: Comparison of two five-drug regimes vs sequential chemotherapy in metastatic breast carcinoma. Cancer Chemother. Rep., *57*:110, 1973.

Tancini, G., Bajetta, E., Marchiini, S., et al.: Preliminary 3-year results of 12 versus 6 cycles of adjuvant CMF in premenopausal breast cancer. Cancer Clin. Trials, *2*:285, 1979.

Von Hoff, D. D., Rozencweig, M., and Piccart, M.: The cardiotoxicity of anticancer agents. Semin. Oncol., *9*:23, 1982.

21

Chemosensitivity of Cultured Human Breast Cancer

Ricky J. Ballou
Michael T. Tseng

The advent of cell-culturing technologies and highly defined cell lines has proved very beneficial in the study of breast cancer. The ability to observe cells and tissues in isolation became practical with the advancement of Harrison's "hanging drop" coverslip method in 1907. This led to the development of the culture flask with a unique side arm, enabling investigators to propagate and subculture their initial cell population (Carrel and Burrows, 1911). Carrel was one of the first investigators to recognize the value of cell culture as a means of investigating, and possibly combating, neoplastic diseases (Carrel and Burrows, 1911; and Carrel 1923). Wright and coworkers (1957) as well as DiPaolo and Dowd (1961) were pioneers in the use of a patient's own tumor tissue for in vitro prediction of drug sensitivity. The concept of customized treatment planning was promoted initially by favorable experience with advanced ovarian carcinomas (Limburg and Krahe, 1964). A plethora of in vitro methods has since been developed. These include the clonogenic assay, introduced in the early 1970s by Park and colleagues (1971); and the MTT assay developed by Mosmann (1983). All of these procedures have a common endpoint: predicting the clinical response of a patient to a specific treatment. The commercial availability of synthetic cell culture media since the 1950s has made it possible for many researchers to develop in vitro screening of anticancer drugs. These anticancer agents are often tested on cells grown in monolayer (anchorage-dependent) cultures, and the results are assessed according to (1)

morphologic criteria (Wright et al., 1957; Holmes and Little, 1974; and Lickiss et al., 1974); (2) the degree of metabolic inhibition (Laszlo et al., 1958; DiPaolo and Dowd, 1961; and Roper and Drewinko, 1976); (3) inhibited incorporation of radiolabeled precursors into deoxyribonucleic acid (DNA), ribonucleic acid, and proteins (Livingston et al., 1974, 1980; and Volm, 1981) and (4) colorimetric determination of mitochondrial viability (Mosmann, 1983). Although the anchorage-dependent culture technique permits growth of the heterogeneous cell population of a solid tumor, inability to distinguish cells that possess unlimited capacity for division from those that are terminally differentiated has increased interest in culturing clones of cells in soft agar (Agrez et al., 1982; and Alberts et al., 1982). In 1961, Till and McCulloch showed that a subpopulation comprising fewer than 1% of the spleen cells of normal mice can repopulate the hematopoietic tissues of lethally irradiated syngeneic recipients. Pike and Robinson (1970) reported the formation of cell colonies when cells were maintained in an anchorage-independent two-layer soft agar (clonogenic) system. This clonogenic cell growth technique (anchorage-independent) was subsequently introduced into the in vitro chemosensitivity test system by Salmon and colleagues in 1978. The principal difference between this chemosensitivity test and others is the method of cell maintenance (Fig. 21–1).

Although the clonogenic assay permits determination of the reproductive potential of selected cell subpopulations, it

Figure 21–1. A comparison of two major cell culture techniques used for chemosensitivity testing. Anchorage-dependent cultures form a monolayer on the bottom of the dish. Anchorage-independent cultures form spherical colonies at the interphase of a semisolid and a solid agar basal layer.

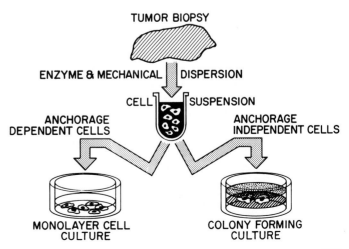

is a laborious technique, plagued by low plating efficiency and long incubation periods. In contrast, the anchorage-dependent cell cultures proliferate rapidly, preserve greater cell heterogeneity, and permit rapid and accurate quantification of results. Thus, in the authors' laboratory, the anchorage-dependent cell culture technique was chosen as the standard method, and the soft agar clonogenic assay was employed only when specimens permitted the maintenance of parallel cultures.

CHEMOSENSITIVITY OF BREAST TISSUE IN PRIMARY CULTURE

The ability to determine the sensitivity of bacteria to antibiotics by in vitro methods had a major impact on the selection of effective drug treatments for infectious diseases. A similar benefit might be realized in the treatment of advanced breast cancer by the use of chemosensitivity screening procedures; however, predicting clinical response with in vitro assays is complicated by multiple factors that cannot easily be reproduced in the laboratory. A solid tumor is a three-dimensional expanding structure that often outgrows its vascular supply. This dynamic tissue-microvascular interaction affects the cytotoxicity of various agents. Poor perfusion of the tumor mass results in lactic acid buildup, even in the presence of adequate tissue oxygenation. The localized acidosis that results can enhance or decrease the efficacy of cytotoxic agents. An acidic tissue environment has been exploited to therapeutic advantage for several years with thiotepa in the treatment of transitional cell carcinomas (Groos et al., 1986). Conversely, regional hypoxia and hyperosmolarity in large solid tumors can increase drug resistance. Hypoxia results in poor cellular proliferation and thus the accumulation of cells in the G_1-phase of the cell cycle. This can result in reduced efficacy of certain cytotoxic agents that specifically exert their effects during the S-phase of cell growth. In addition, hypoxia decreases free radicals of oxygen, which decreases the efficacy of several cytotoxic agents, as well as radiotherapy (Moulder and Rockwell, 1987). Hyperosmolar states result in a poor response to platinum compounds (Smith and Brock, 1989). Some cytotoxic agents exert their effects via active metabolites. The most obvious example is cyclophosphamide, which requires hepatic microsomal enzyme activation. The base compound is useless for testing in vitro (Connors, 1970). The influence of cell kinetics on the effectiveness of cytotoxic agents is well known and is fundamental to the evaluation of chemosensitivity assays (Drewinko et al., 1981). Until confluency is reached cells grown in culture typically are growing in an exponential fashion. A tumor mass has cells that are in a quiescent state, rendering the tumor less susceptible to cytotoxic agents that require incorporation into cellular DNA. These factors and others conspire to influence the outcome of chemotherapy.

RESISTANCE

Human neoplasms are heterogeneous. Some progress slowly with virtually no mortality, whereas others prove fatal in a matter of months. Tumors are heterogeneous cell populations not only in terms of histologic composition but also in terms of biochemical sensitivity. In human solid tumors as many as 15% to 30% of the cells may be resistant to a single agent such as cis-platinum, and as many as 10% may be resistant to a five-drug combination (Ahmann, 1983). On average, a tumor that is clinically detectable consists of approximately 10^9 cells (Speafica and Garattini, 1978); therefore, an average of 150 million to 300 million cells would be resistant, still a substantial tumor burden. In addition to this initial drug resistance, cyclic treatment with single or combination drugs frequently results in the selection of cells that are resistant to specific drugs. Nonresponsiveness is wide ranging and may extend to unrelated classes of drugs to which the patient has had no previous exposure. The appearance of chromosomes with expanded regions was reported by Biedler and Spengler (1976) in methotrexate-resistant Chinese hamster–lung cell lines. Chromosomal abnormality in the unstable amplified state is manifested in paired extrachromosomal elements called "double minute chromosomes" (Brown et al., 1983). The consequence of gene amplification is the overproduction of one or more proteins, which enable cells to effectively eliminate compounds such as antibiotics from cytoplasm (Wahl et al., 1979; Beach and Palmiter, 1981; Rossana et al., 1982; Young and Ringold, 1983; and McConlogue et al., 1984). Rath and coworkers (1984) examined methotrexate-resistant 3TG cells and found that dehydrofolate reductase (DHFR)–amplified genes are generated by selection instead of being a distinct, pre-existing subpopulation. Similar conclusions were reached when a transplantable murine breast tumor became resistant to melphalan, cisplatin, and cyclophosphamide after repeated treatments (McMillan et al., 1985). Chromosomal abnormalities indicative of gene amplification have been observed in human, Chinese hamster, and mouse cell lines with high levels of acquired resistance to vincristine. One specific protein, V-19, is overproduced in these resistant cells (Schimke, 1984; and Meyers et al., 1985). Regardless of whether resistant cells are pre-existing or selected for, increased copies of DHFR genes have been observed clinically in patients with leukemia (Cardman et al., 1984; and Horns et al, 1984), in oat cell carcinoma of the lung (Curt et al., 1983), and in patients with ovarian adenocarcinoma (Trent et al., 1984) following treatment with methotrexate. Fivefold DHFR gene amplification may be sufficient to convey resistance to the conventional dosage of methotrexate.

In addition to the perplexing problem of resistance is the phenomenon of "tumor evolution." From their inception, tumors are continually changing. As a tumor enlarges, alterations occur in the kinetics of the cell population. The most probable explanation is that, as a tumor mass grows, the cells in the central core receive progressively fewer nutrients, which slows their metabolic activity (Carter and Livingston, 1982). This concept is of clinical importance because most of the agents used to treat malignant neoplasms have as their mode of action the ability to interfere with normal DNA synthesis. Therefore, cells undergoing mitosis are more sensitive than resting cells. Smaller tumors have a greater proportion of their cells actively synthesizing DNA and consequently are more sensitive to chemotherapy than larger tumors (Griswold, 1975; Schabel, 1977; and Skipper, 1978). Reducing the tumor mass by surgery, even when it is known that the procedure will not be curative, has been shown to increase the rate of cell division in the cells that remain at the surgical margins. Consequently, these cells become more dangerous to the patient while at the same time they become more sensitive to adjuvant chemotherapy. It must be remembered that chemosensitivity testing by in vitro methods utilizes tissue that has been removed from the tumor bulk. In addition, the tumor tissue actually used may be from the primary tumor, whereas the chemotherapy may be directed toward metastatic growths that may have different kinetic properties.

From the oncologist's point of view, a tumor is a "moving target." In vitro testing must be viewed as a procedure for selecting the best antitumor agent for a particular patient at a specific time in the course of the disease.

CORRELATIONS BETWEEN LABORATORY TESTS AND CLINICAL RESPONSES

Sensitivity of a specific tumor to chemotherapy cannot be predicted from either clinical symptoms or histologic examination. It has also been recognized for many years that the experimental models previously used to study chemosensitivity (i.e., continuous cell lines and tumors chemically induced) in animals have limitations. As models for human cancer, they provide data on the possible effects of an agent on a given type of tumor, but they fail to give accurate data on the behavior of an individual tumor. Thus, a number of groups began to investigate the possibility of using the patient's own tumor tissue for in vitro drug screening (Wright et al., 1957; and DiPaolo and Dowd, 1961).

In 1964, Limburg and Krahe reported substantial improvement in the median survival time of patients with advanced ovarian carcinomas when treatment was based on results of in vitro testing. Over the next decade, disaggregated biopsy specimens containing either single cells, tissue explants, or tumor slices were used to establish suspension, monolayer, or organ cultures. During the past 30 years, various procedures have been used to test the sensitivity of tumor cells to antitumor drugs. A number of methods use fresh tumor material and can be carried out in a few hours (Bickis et al., 1966; Krummer et al., 1970; Wüst and Matthes, 1970; Volm et al., 1979; Volm, 1981; and Sondak et al., 1984). Others require culturing of the tumor cells for 1 to 3 days (Wright et al., 1957; Limburg and Krahe, 1964; Tanneberger and Bacigalupo, 1970; Holmes and Little, 1974; Ebeling and Spitzbart, 1977; and Dendy, 1980) or 2 to 4 weeks (Hamburger and Salmon, 1977; Salmon et al., 1978; Meyshens and Salmon, 1981; and Von Hoff et al., 1981), or even 2 to 3 months (Fujita et al., 1980; and Shorthouse et al., 1980). None of the methods has acquired widespread clinical use (Limburg and Krahe, 1964; Salmon et al., 1978; Volm et al., 1979; and Sondak et al., 1984).

The ideal chemosensitivity screening system must be simple, sensitive, specific, easily standardized, inexpensive, rapid, and flexible and must provide results that correlate with clinical data (Hamburger and Salmon, 1977). Therefore, a test of intermediate duration has attractive features.

The degree of cytoxicity can be measured by isotope uptake, cell counts, or colorimetric changes, all of which are easily automated. These techniques frequently use microtiter plates, which simplifies the handling of 60 to 96 replicate samples. With a large number of replicate cultures derived from a relatively small amount of tumor material, it is possible to produce dose-response curves over a large range of drug concentrations, to test a statistically acceptable number of samples within each drug concentration, and to test combinations of drugs.

In the United States, the National Cancer Institute developed an anticancer drug–screening program that adopted a colorimetric assay for quick analysis of a large number of compounds. The screening assay utilizes microtiter plates on which standardized amounts of cells are used to establish a monolayer culture. Then the cultures are incubated with various test compounds for 48 hours. At the end of the incubation period the cells are evaluated for growth inhibition and cell death by use of the protein stain sulforhodamine. This detects the ability of remaining living cells to reduce a tetrazolium-based compound (MTT) to a formazan compound, which imparts a color change in the supernatant of each microtiter well (Kerkvliet, 1990; and Mosmann, 1983). Both systems are rapid, sensitive, and inexpensive methods for measuring cellular protein content of adherent or suspension cultures in microtiter plates. These assays have recently been adapted from a screening technique for antineoplastic compounds to a chemosensitive assay with promising results. Furukawa and coworkers (1991) used a modification of the MTT technique to evaluate adjuvant chemotherapy treatment of patients having advanced gastrointestinal malignancies. Cytotoxic agents previously shown to be effective in vitro resulted in a significant increase ($P < .05$) in long-term survival rates when compared to agents that were not effective in vitro.

In vitro testing of malignant tumors has received much attention in the scientific literature over the past decade. A number of different assays have been developed, all of which take tissue directly from the patient and test the cultured cells against a panel of agents. The initial aim is to predict the response of an individual patient to a proposed treatment regimen. The predictive value of these assays varies; however, it has been clearly documented that most assays are more effective for predicting drug resistance than for predicting chemosensitivity (Phillips et al., 1990). Dendy (1980) and Shorthouse (1980) reported that drug sensitivity tests accurately predicted subsequent clinical results. When patient populations were comparable in age, clinical stage, and histologic grade, the patients treated according to results of in vitro drug screening survived longer than patients treated by empirical drug selection. Investigators have subsequently shown that drug resistance in vitro correlates positively with resistance to drug treatment in vivo, at or above the 90% confidence level. Additionally, sensitivity in vitro correlates with tumor response in vivo in about 60% to 70% of the cases (Holmes and Little, 1974; Salmon et al., 1980; Sondak et al, 1984; Furukawa et al., 1991; and Phillips et al., 1990). Thus, the predictive value of these assays is similar to those of other widely accepted tests such as the estrogen receptor assay or the bacterial sensitivity tests used in most clinical laboratories (Von Hoff, 1990).

SUMMARY

Assays capable of selecting a subset of patients who would benefit significantly from chemotherapy would be desirable. The ability to forecast resistance in vivo to cytotoxic agents commonly used to treat breast cancer would also be desirable, as it could spare patients harmful treatment with ineffective agents and avoid delay of alternative therapy.

References

Agrez, M. V., Kovach, J. S., and Vert, R. W.: Human colorectal carcinoma: Patterns of sensitivity to chemotherapeutic agents in human stem cell assay. J. Surg. Oncol., 20:187, 1982.

Ahmann, F. R.: Chemotherapy and hormonal therapy of advanced breast cancer. In Feig, S. A., and McLelland, R. (Eds.): Breast Cancer—Current Diagnosis and Treatment. New York: Masson, 1983, p. 533.

Alberts, D. S., Mackel, C., Pocelinko, R., and Salmon, S. E.: Phase I clinical investigation of 9,10-anthracenedicarboxaldehyde bis[(4,5-dihydro-1H-imidazol-2-yl)hydrazone] dihydrochloride with correlative in vitro human tumor clonogenic assay. Cancer Res., 42:1170, 1982.

Beach, L. R., and Palmiter, R. D.: Amplification of the methallothionein-I gene in cadmium-resistant mouse cells. Proc. Natl. Acad. Sci. U.S.A., 78:2110, 1981.

Bickis, I. J., Henderson, I. W., and Quastel, J. H.: Biochemical studies of human tumors. II. In vitro estimation of individual tumor sensitivity to anticancer agents. Cancer, 19:103, 1966.

Biedler, J. L., and Spengler, B. A.: Metaphase chromosomes anomaly: Association with drug resistance and cell-specific products. Science, 191:185, 1976.

Brown, P. C., Johnston, R. N., and Schimke, R. T.: Approaches to the study of mechanisms of selecting gene amplification in cultured mammalian cells. In Subtelny, S. (Ed.): Gene Structure and Regulation in Development. New York: Alan R. Liss, 1983, p. 197.

Cardman, M. D., Schornegal, J. H., Rivest, R. S., et al.: Resistance to methotrexate due to gene amplification in patients with acute leukemia. J. Clin. Oncol., 2:16, 1984.

Carrel, A.: A method for physiological studies of tissues in vitro. J. Exp. Med., 38:47, 1923.

Carrel, A., and Burrows, M. T.: Cultivation in vitro of malignant tumors. J. Exp. Med., 13:571, 1911.

Carter, S. K., and Livingston, R. B.: Principles of cancer chemotherapy. In Carter, S. K., Glatstein, E., and Livingston, R. B. (Eds.): Principles of Cancer Treatment. New York: McGraw-Hill, 1982, p. 95.

Connors, T. A., Grover, P. L., and McLaughlin, A. M.: Microsomal activation of cyclophosphamide in vivo. Biochem. Pharmacol., 19:1533, 1970.

Curt, G. A., Carney, D. M., and Cowen, K. H., et al.: Unstable methotrexate resistance in human small-cell carcinoma associated with double minute chromosomes. N. Engl. J. Med., 308:199, 1983.

Dendy, P. P.: The use of in vitro methods to predict tumor response to chemotherapy. Br. J. Cancer, 41(Suppl IV):195, 1980.

DiPaolo, J. A., and Dowd, J. E.: Evaluation of inhibition of human tumor tissue by cancer chemotherapeutic drugs with an in vitro test. J. Natl. Cancer Inst., 27:807, 1961.

Drewinko, B., Patchen, M., Yung, L., et al.: Differential killing efficacy of twenty antitumor drugs on proliferating and nonproliferating human tumor cells. Cancer Res., 41:2328, 1981.

Ebeling, K., and Spitzbart, H.: Zur Erfassung zytostatischer Effekte an Zellkulturen in vitro und deren gegenwartige Bedeutung für eine individualisierte Tumorchemotherapie der fortgeschrittenen Ovarialkarzinoma. Zentralbl. Gynaekol., 99:1041, 1977.

Fujita, M., Hayata, S., and Taguchi, T.: Relation of chemotherapy on human cancer xenographs in nude mice to clinical response in donor patients. J. Surg. Oncol., 15:211:1980.

Furukawa, T., Kubota, T., Suto, A., et al.: Clinical usefulness of chemosensitivity testing using the MTT assay. J. Surg. Oncol., 48:188, 1991.

Griswold, D. S.: The potential for murine tumor models in surgical adjuvant chemotherapy. Cancer Chemother. Rep., 5:187, 1975.

Groos, E., Walker, L., and Masters, J. W. R.: The influence of pH on drug cytoxicity in vivo. Br. J. Cancer, 54:180, 1986.

Hamburger, A. W., and Salmon, E.: Primary bioassay of human tumor stem cells. Science, 197:461, 1977.

Holmes, H. L., and Little, J. M.: Tissue culture microtest for predicting response of human cancer to chemotherapy. Lancet, 2:985, 1974.

Horns, R. C., Dower, W. J., and Schimke, R. T.: Gene amplification in a leukemic patient treated with methotrexate. J. Clin. Oncol., 2:1, 1984.

Kerkvliet, G. I.: Drug discovery screen adapts to changes. J. Natl. Cancer Inst., 82:1087, 1990.

Krummer, H., Muhlenen, A., and Laissue, J.: Survival of labelled and non-labelled platelets in the lethally irradiated dog: An evaluation of the 51-chromate method. Helv. Med. Acta, 35:226, 1970.

Laszlo, J., Stengle, J., Wright, K., et al.: Effects of chemotherapeutic agents on metabolism of human acute leukemia cells in vitro. Proc. Soc. Exp. Biol. Med., 97:127, 1958.

Lickiss, J. N., Cane, K. A., and Baikie, A. G.: In vitro drug selection in antineoplastic chemotherapy. Eur. J. Cancer 10:809, 1974.

Limburg, H., and Krahe, M.: Die Züchtung von menschlichem Krebsgewebe in der Gewebekultur und seine Sensibilitätstestung gegen neuere Zytostatika. Dtsch. Med. Wochenschr., 89:1938, 1964.

Livingston, R. B., Ambus, U., George, S. L., et al.: In vitro determination of thymidine-[³H] labeling index in human solid tumors. Cancer Res., 34:1376, 1974.

Livingston, R. B., Titus, G. A., and Heilbrum, L. H.: In vitro effects on DNA synthesis as a prediction of biologic effect from chemotherapy. Cancer Res., 40:2209, 1980.

McConlogue, L., Gupta, A., Wu, M., et al.: Molecular cloning and expression of the mouse ornithine decarboxylase gene. Proc. Natl. Acad. Sci. U.S.A., 81:540, 1984.

McMillan, T. J., Stephens, T. C., and Steel, G. G.: Development of drug resistance in murine mammary tumors. Br. J. Cancer, 52:823, 1985.

Meyers, M. B., Spengler, A., Chang, T. D., et al.: Gene amplification associated cytogenetic aberrations and protein changes in vincristine resistant chinese hamster, mouse, and human cells. J. Cell Biol., 100:588, 1985.

Meyshens, F. L., and Salmon, S. E.: Modulation of clonogenic human melanoma cells by follicle-stimulating hormone, melatonin, and nerve growth factor. Br. J. Cancer, 43:111, 1981.

Mosmann, T.: Rapid colometric assay for cellular growth and survival: Application assays. J. Immunol. Methods, 65:55, 1983.

Moulder, J. E., and Rockwell, S.: Tumor hypoxia: Its impact on cancer therapy. Cancer Metast. Rev., 5:313, 1987.

Park, C. H., Bergsagel, D. E., and McCulloch, E. A.: Mouse myeloma tumor stem cells: A primary culture assay. J. Natl. Cancer Inst., 46:411, 1971.

Phillips, R. M., Bibby, M. C., and Double, J. A.: A critical appraisal of the predictive value of in vitro chemosensitivity assays. J. Natl. Cancer Inst., 82:1457, 1990.

Pike, B. R., and Robinson, W. A.: Human bone marrow colony growth in agar-gel. J. Cell Physiol., 76:77, 1970.

Rath, H., Tisty, T., and Schimke, R. T.: Rapid emergence of methotrexate resistance in cultured mouse cells. Cancer Res., 44:3303, 1984.

Roper, P. R., and Drewinko, B.: Comparison on in vitro methods to determine drug induced cell lethality. Cancer Res., 36:2182, 1976.

Rossana, E., Rao, L. G., and Johnson, L. F.: Thymidine synthesis overproduction in 5-fluorodeoxyuridine-resistant mouse fibroblasts. Molec. Cell Biol., 2:1118, 1982.

Salmon, S. E., Alberts, D. S., Meyshens, F. L., et al.: Clinical correlations of in vitro drug sensitivity. In Salmon, S. E. (Ed.): Cloning of Human Tumor Stem Cells. New York: Alan R. Liss, 1980, p. 223.

Salmon, S. E., Hamburger, A. W., Soehnlen, B., et al.: Quantification of different sensitivity of human tumor stem cells to anticancer drugs. N. Engl. J. Med., 298:1321, 1978.

Schabel, F.: Surgical adjuvant chemotherapy of metastatic murine tumors. Cancer, 40:558, 1977.

Schimke, R. T.: Gene amplification, drug resistance and cancer. Cancer Res., 44:1735, 1984.

Shorthouse, A. J., Smyth, J. F., Steel, G. G., et al.: The human tumor xenograft: A valid model in experimental chemotherapy? Br. J. Surg., 67:715, 1980.

Skipper, H. E.: Adjuvant chemotherapy. Cancer, 41:936, 1978.

Smith, E., and Brock, A. P.: The effect of reduced osmolarity on platinum drug toxicity. Br. J. Cancer, 59:873, 1989.

Sondak, V. K., Berelsen, C. A., Tanigawa, N., et al.: Clinical correlation with chemosensitivities measured in a rapid thymidine incorporation assay. Cancer Res., *44*:1725, 1984.

Speafica, F., and Garattini, S.: Chemotherapy of experimental metastasis. *In* Baldwin, R. W. (Ed.): Secondary Spread of Cancer. London, Academic, 1978, p.101.

Tanneberger, S., and Bacigalupo, G.: Einige Erfahrungen mit individuellen zytostatischen Behandlung maligner Tumoren nach prätherapeutischer Zytostatika-Sensibilitätsprüfung in vitro. Arch. Geschwulstforsch. 35:44, 1970.

Till, J. E., and McCulloch, E. A.: A direct measurement of the radiation sensitivity of normal mouse bone marrow cells. Radiat. Res., *14*:213, 1961.

Trent, J. M., Buick, R. M., Olson, S., et al.: Cytologic support for gene amplification in methotrexate-resistant cells obtained from a patient with ovarian adenocarcinoma. J. Clin. Oncol., *2*:8, 1984.

Volm, M.: In vitro short-term test to determine the resistance of human tumors to chemotherapy. Cancer, *48*:2127, 1981.

Volm, M., Wayss, K., Kaufmann, M., et al.: Pretherapeutic detection of tumor resistance and the results of tumor chemotherapy. Eur. J. Cancer, *15*:983, 1979.

Von Hoff, D. D.: He's not going to talk about in vitro predictive assays again, is he? J. Natl. Cancer Inst., *82*:96, 1990.

Von Hoff, D. D., Casper, J., Bradley, E., et al.: Association between human tumor colony-forming assay results and response of an individual patient's tumor to chemotherapy. Am. J. Med., *70*:1027, 1981.

Wahl, G. M., Padgett, R. A., and Stark, G. R.: Gene amplification causes overproduction of the first three enzymes of UMP synthesis in *N*-(phosphoacetyl-1-aspartate)–resistant hamster cells. J. Biol. Chem., *254*:8679, 1979.

Wright, J. C., Cobb, J. P., Gumport, S. L., et al.: Investigation of the relation between clinical and tissue culture response to chemotherapeutic agents on human cancer. N. Engl. J. Med., *257*:1207, 1957.

Wüst, G. P., and Matthes, K. J.: In vitro–Messung des Einbes von ³H-Thymidin in Jensen Sarkom unter Cytostaticaeinwirkung mit Hilfe der Flüssigkeits-Szintillations-Spektrometrie. S. Krebsforsch., *73*:204, 1970.

Young, A. P., and Ringold, G. M.: Mouse 3GT cells that overproduce glutamine synthetase. J. Biol. Chem., *258*:1126, 1983.

22 Endocrine Therapy of Breast Cancer

Carl G. Kardinal

Almost 100 years have passed since Beatson empirically performed the first oophorectomy for the treatment of metastatic breast cancer. Only now are we beginning to understand the molecular biology that explains why Beatson was successful—and why other forms of hormone therapy are useful in the treatment of mammary carcinomas. In the 27 years since the first edition of this text, endocrine therapy of breast cancer has evolved from the palliative treatment of advanced disease predominantly through ablative procedures to adjuvant therapy to prevent recurrence of Stage I and II tumors, and to a possible method for the prevention in women at high risk for developing breast cancer.

Before the description of the estrogen receptor (ER) in the 1970s and its role in predicting response to both additive and ablative hormone therapy, the trend was shifting away from endocrine therapy for breast cancer toward combination chemotherapy. Endocrine therapy was unreliable, producing only a 20% to 30% objective response rate and requiring as long as 6, or even 12, weeks for the response to occur. Combination chemotherapy, on the other hand, induced objective response in 60% to 70% of unselected cases, and the response was reasonably rapid. It seemed during the 1980s that chemotherapy might even replace hormone therapy altogether, and, owing to better understanding of tumor cell kinetics and pharmacology, that the chemotherapeutic cure of advanced breast cancer was only months to a few years away. Needless to say, this did not happen; the results of combination chemotherapy have "plateaued," and there were few advances from the 1970s to the 1990s (Kardinal, 1992).

Endocrine therapy, however, has continued to advance in the 1990s with the development of new agents such as the pure antiestrogen toremifene, the antiprogestational agent mifepristone, the new aromatase inhibitor fadrozole, a variety of new luteinizing hormone–releasing hormone (LH-RH) analogues, and development of the somatostatin analogue octreotide. There is now better understanding of the development of hormonal resistance and of possible methods of overcoming it (Jiang and Jordan, 1992). This is, indeed, a promising era for hormone therapy.

THE ENDOCRINE BASIS OF THERAPY

The normal development and function of the mammary gland depend on the coordinated action of several hormones: prolactin, estrogen, progesterone, adrenal cortico-steroids, insulin, growth hormone, and thyroid hormone (Frantz and Wilson, 1985) (Fig. 22–1). Ductal growth is promoted by estrogen. Lobuloalveolar development is promoted by prolactin and progesterone; lactation is fostered by prolactin. By far the two most important hormones involved in mammary physiology, and presumably mammary pathology, are estrogen and prolactin (Calandra et al., 1984).

Estrogen

Estrogen is a highly potent mammary mitogen. Currently all forms of endocrine manipulation for the treatment of breast cancer are directed toward inhibiting, ablating, or otherwise interfering with estrogen activity (Lippman, 1985). However, in the stimulation of breast development, estrogen is ineffective in the absence of anterior pituitary hormones (Lyons et al., 1958). Estrogen increases growth hormone secretion, and together they promote ductal development (Frantz and Rabkin, 1965). Estrogen appears to inhibit prolactin and acts to regulate prolactin receptors in breast tissue (Frantz and Wilson, 1985).

Estrogen is the major stimulus for the growth of hormone-dependent breast cancer (Santen, 1982). The ovaries and the placenta are the principal sites of estrogen synthesis; however, estrogen is synthesized in multiple other areas, such as the adrenal gland, adipose tissue, and in mammary tumors themselves (Miller et al., 1982; and Siiteri, 1982). Estrogens are synthesized by the aromatization of androgens via the enzyme aromatase (Fig. 22–2). Aromatase is the rate-limiting step in estrogen production. Consequently, there has been a concentrated effort to synthesize pharmacologic aromatase inhibitors as potential therapeutic agents for hormonally sensitive breast cancer. As already indicated, aromatase is not restricted to classic endocrine tissues such as the ovary and the adrenal gland, but is also present in adipose tissue and the hypothalamus, and, in small amounts, in muscle, fibroblasts, and even cancer tissue (Lipton et al., 1987). Estradiol was believed to stimulate breast growth (mitogenesis) by binding to a receptor, which in the cell nucleus stimulates increase in ribonucleic acid polymerase activity (Jordan et al., 1980). Through immunohistochemical and cell enucleation techniques, it has been recognized that the estrogen receptor is located in the nucleus of the cell, not the cytoplasm (Jordan et al., 1992).

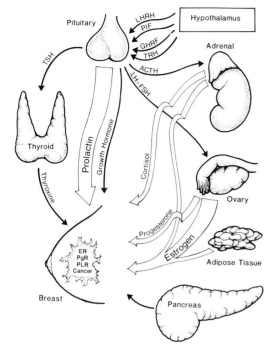

Figure 22-1. The endocrine basis of breast cancer therapy. Estrogen and prolactin are the dominant mitogens to normal breast tissue. However, the role of prolactin in human breast cancer is not yet established. Ductal growth is promoted by estrogen in the presence of growth hormone; lobular development is promoted by prolactin and progesterone. Estrogen is synthesized not only in the ovary but also in adrenal and adipose tissue. The roles of cortisol, thyroxine, and insulin are permissive rather than regulatory. LHRH = luteinizing hormone–releasing hormone; PIF = prolactin inhibitory factor; GHRF = growth hormone–releasing factor; ACTH = adrenocorticotropic hormone; LH = luteinizing hormone; FSH = follicle-stimulating hormone; TSH = thyroid-stimulating hormone; ER = estrogen receptor; PgR = progesterone receptor; PLR = prolactin receptor.

Estrogen Replacement Therapy in Patients with Breast Cancer

Estrogen is clearly implicated in the pathogenesis of breast cancer, and blocking the effects of estrogen by additive or ablative means is therapeutic in many patients with advanced metastatic disease. For years, investigators have debated whether or not menopausal estrogen replacement therapy increases a woman's risk of developing breast cancer (Colditz et al., 1990; and Dupont and Page, 1991). A recent meta-analysis indicated that the risk of breast cancer did increase after 5 years of estrogen use. Moreover, after 15 years of use, there was a 30% increase in the risk of breast cancer; that is, an increase in the relative risk from 1.0 to 1.3 (Steinberg et al., 1991).

The more difficult question is: Can a woman who has successfully been treated for breast cancer receive estrogen replacement therapy? The answer has always been no, but is this correct? There is a widely held general belief that hormone replacement therapy increases the risk of recurrence, but there are in fact no hard data to support this conclusion. There is indirect evidence of an adverse effect, in that obese women with breast cancer are at increased

risk of recurrence, and obesity is associated with increased circulating levels of estrogen (Spicer et al., 1990). However, two small prospective studies do not confirm increased risk. The first of these was by Stoll (1989, 1990) of St. Thomas' Hospital in London. Stoll selected patients with severe menopausal symptoms and treated them with a combination of conjugated equine estrogen and norgestrel for 3 months. Treatment was continued for 3 months longer if menopausal symptoms had not completely abated. At a minimum follow-up interval of 2 years there was no case of tumor reactivation. The second study is by Wile and colleagues (1991). They performed a case-control trial in 25 women with favorable-prognosis breast cancer. Of the 16 patients whose ER status was known, 13 were ER positive. Each of the 25 women who received hormone replacement therapy was matched with two women with similar stage breast cancer. With a median follow-up of 25.3 months, there was one breast cancer–related death in the treated group and two in the control group. It may not be justifiable to withhold hormone replacement from women with low-risk breast cancer, particularly in light of the known benefit of estrogen replacement with regard to cardiovascular disease and osteoporosis. This issue is unresolved. There appears to be a need for a large controlled clinical trial to evaluate estrogen replacement therapy in women treated for breast cancer (Bluming 1993; DiSaia 1993; and Marchant 1993).

Prolactin

Next to estrogen, prolactin is the most important hormone involved in breast development and function. Like estrogen, prolactin is a potent mitogen to breast tissue (Shiu and Friesen, 1980). In the absence of prolactin and growth hormone, estrogen alone is ineffective in inducing ductal development or other mammary growth. Conversely, prolactin requires estrogen as a stimulator of epithelial cell

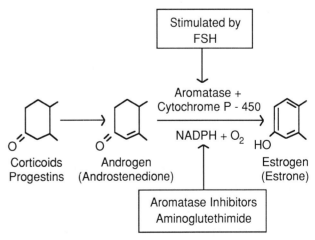

Figure 22-2. Synthesis of estrogen by the aromatization of androgens (adrostenedione) via the enzyme aromatase. This is the major source of estrogen production in postmenopausal women. Aromatization by aromatase is the rate-limiting step in estrogen synthesis and is the target of the drugs aminoglutethimide, fadrozole, and 4-hydroxyandrostenedione.

proliferation. Along with progesterone, prolactin fosters lobuloalveolar development. Prolactin receptors are present in human mammary tissue and increase in number during pregnancy and lactation (Dhadly and Walker, 1983). High-affinity receptors for prolactin have also been demonstrated in human breast cancer (Peyrat et al., 1984). Considering the known effect of prolactin on cell multiplication, this hormone could have a role in the development of breast cancers in humans. The prolactin analogues buserelin and pergolide have direct growth-inhibiting effects on human breast cancer cells in tissue culture (Wiznitzer and Benz, 1984). It has been shown that basal and perphenazine-stimulated levels of prolactin are significantly decreased after the first pregnancy, and that this decrease may persist for 12 to 13 years (Musey et al., 1987). It is interesting to speculate that this may be the mechanism through which early pregnancy protects against breast cancer development. It has also been shown that diets rich in saturated fats are associated with increased prolactin levels (Ingram et al., 1990), a possible explanation for another breast cancer risk factor.

Other Hormones

The other hormones involved in the physiology of normal breast development and function all interact with estrogen or prolactin, or both. *Progesterone* has no effect unless there is concomitant or preceding estrogen stimulation. Under these conditions, progesterone interacts with prolactin to promote lobuloalveolar development (Freeman and Topper, 1978). Growth hormone appears to synergize with prolactin to promote ductal development (Frantz and Wilson, 1985). Insulin and glucocorticoids are necessary for most phases of breast growth and secretion, but they probably exert a permissive rather than a regulatory role (Shyamala, 1973; and Topper and Oka, 1974).

Thyroid hormone is not essential for breast development or lactation, but both processes may be adversely affected in states of thyroid hormone excess or deficiency (Cowie et al., 1980). It has been reported, however, that among women undergoing screening mammography the prevalence of breast cancer was higher for those receiving thyroid hormone than for those who were not (Kapdi and Wolfe, 1976). This increased risk could not be confirmed in two subsequent carefully performed studies (Hoffman et al., 1984; and Shapiro et al., 1980). The final word seems to be that the use of thyroid supplements does not increase the risk of developing breast cancer.

MOLECULAR BIOLOGY OF BREAST CANCER

Most normal cells require the addition of specific peptides for growth in tissue culture, whereas malignant cells no longer require these same peptides and grow autonomously without an exogenous source. To explain this phenomenon, the autocrine hypothesis was proposed, which held that cells became malignant by the endogenous production of peptides that stimulate their own growth (Sporn and Rob-

erts, 1992). The demonstration of these growth factors and their role in the autonomous stimulation of tumor growth are the basis of our current understanding of tumor biology and tumor-hormone interactions.

It is important for the clinician to understand the molecular biology of breast cancer since cellular mechanisms are the basis of hormone activity and the foundation for novel therapeutic strategies (Fig. 22–3).

Estrogen plays a critical role in the pathogenesis and proliferation of breast cancer. Estrogen-dependent cells dominate the early proliferative phase of all breast cancers. Cellular proliferation is stimulated by a series of autocrine and paracrine growth factors whose biosynthesis is enhanced by estrogen. *Autocrine* growth factors are released by one cell type, such as a breast cancer epithelial cell, and act on the same cell type, through cell surface receptors. *Paracrine* growth factors are released by one cell type, such as a breast cancer stromal cell, and modulate the function of adjacent or neighboring epithelial cells (Lippman et al., 1986; Mori et al., 1991; and Dickson and Lippman, 1992).

Growth factors that act as the mediators or modulators of steroid hormone action are the transforming growth factors TGFα and TGFβ and epidermal growth factor (EGF). In hormonally responsive cells, both estrogen and progesterone enhance the production of the *growth-stimulating factors* TGFα and EGF, and suppress the production of the *growth-inhibiting factor* TGFβ. Tamoxifen, on the other hand, augments secretion of TGFβ (Thompson et al., 1991; and Dreicer and Wilding, 1992).

EGF and TGFα are closely related peptides that act through a single receptor, the EGF receptor (EGFR). A similar EGFR is the gene product of the oncogene *erb* B₂ (HER-2/neu). Amplification of the *erb* B₂ oncogene has

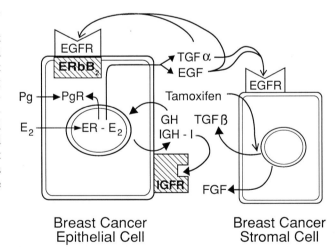

Breast Cancer Epithelial Cell   Breast Cancer Stromal Cell

Figure 22–3. Diagrammatic representation of autocrine and paracrine stimulation of breast cancer epithelial cells by the transforming growth factors (TGFα and TGFβ), epidermal growth factor (EGF), and fibroblast growth factor (FGF). The induction of insulin-like growth factor I (IGF-I) by growth hormone (GH) is shown, as is the induction of EGF and TGFα by estradiol (E₂) and progesterone (Pg) via their specific receptors (ER and PgR, respectively). The *erb* B₂ oncogene product EGFR (epidermal growth factor receptor) and its relationship to TGFα and EGF are noted. Finally, the inhibitory growth factor TGFβ is induced by tamoxifen.

been associated with more aggressive and hormonally un-responsive tumors. There is an inverse relationship between EGFR expression and the ER content of a tumor. This suggests that EGFR-expressing tumors may have arisen from hormonally responsive cells. However, EGFR expression is associated with hormone-independent tumor growth and poor prognosis (Ciardiello et al., 1989; Dotzlaw et al., 1990; and Toi et al., 1990).

Insulin-like growth factor-I (IGF-I) is a potent mitogen of breast cancer cells and is indirectly stimulated by estrogen. IGF-I is growth hormone (GH) dependent. GH secretion is stimulated by estrogen. *Tamoxifen* blocks IGF-I production by blocking estrogen receptors in the hypothalamic-pituitary axis. This function of tamoxifen is independent of the ER content of the primary breast cancer. Both the amplification of TGFβ and the suppression of IGF-I are mechanisms through which tamoxifen is inhibitory in ER-positive as well as ER-negative breast cancers (Baum et al., 1990; Jordan, 1990; Pollak et al., 1990; Jordan 1993; and Noguchi et al., 1993). *Somatostatin* (SMS) also inhibits GH and IGF-I production (Foekens et al., 1989). Therefore, an SMS-tamoxifen combination might have an additive, or even a synergistic, effect on metastatic breast cancer; this combination is being tested by the North Central Cancer Treatment Group.

Other growth factors produced by breast cancer epithelial or stromal cells do not as yet have clearly defined roles or hormonal relationships. These include IGF-II, platelet-derived growth factor (PDGF), and fibroblast-related growth factor. These growth factors may be involved in tumor angiogenesis and in the development of the stromal support of breast cancers.

In addition to *erb* B$_2$ (HER 2/neu), other oncogenes such as c-*myc, hst,* and *int-2* are frequently amplified in breast cancer (Le Roy et al., 1991). Of these, c-*myc* amplification appears to be an independent prognostic variable in node-positive and node-negative breast cancer and a much more sensitive prognostic indicator than HER-2/neu (Berns et al., 1992) (Fig. 22–4).

HORMONE RESISTANCE

Breast cancers inevitably progress from a hormone-responsive to a hormone-resistant state. Since most of the actions of estrogens and antiestrogens are mediated through the ER, resistance could result from a loss of steroid receptor protein or the formation of a variant ER with different functional capability (Raam et al., 1988; Katzellenbogen, 1991; and Fuqua, 1992). Tamoxifen may interact with cells with

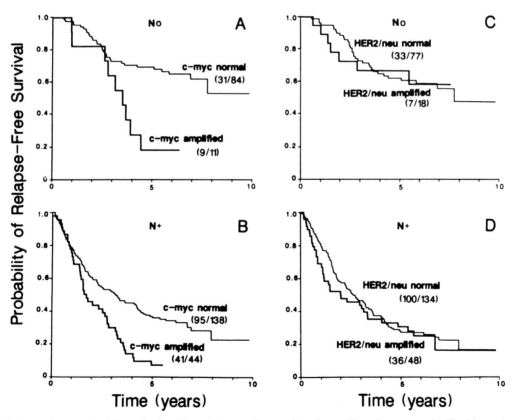

Figure 22–4. Relapse-free survival in patients with node-negative and node-positive disease as stratified by c-*myc* and *HER-2/neu* status. *A and B,* Survival for node-negative patients (NO) and node-positive patients (N+) as a function of c-*myc* amplification, respectively. *C and D,* Survival as a function of *HER-2/neu* amplification for node-negative and node-positive patients, respectively. Median follow-up was 74 months. Normal = two copy numbers of the respective gene; amplified = more than two copies of the gene. Numbers in parentheses reflect the number of failures of the total number of patients in each group. *Bold lines* signify the group of amplified genes. (From Berns, M. J. J., Klijn, J. G. M., van Putten, W. L. J., et al.: c-*myc* amplification is a better prognostic factor than *HER-2/neu* amplification in primary breast cancer. Cancer Res., *52*:1107–1113, 1992.)

variant ER and be ineffective, or a tamoxifen metabolite may exert a paradoxical effect. It is now well documented that, as resistance develops, increased production of estrogenic tamoxifen metabolites may stimulate tumor growth (Osborne et al., 1991, 1992; and Wiebe et al., 1992). With the development of hormonal autonomy production of EGF, TGFα, and IGF-I increases. As complete hormonal resistance develops, stromal cells fail to produce the inhibitory growth factor TGFβ in response to tamoxifen, and total tumor cell autonomy emerges.

HISTORICAL ASPECTS

In 1836, Sir Astley Cooper (Keynes, 1922) observed that advanced breast cancer waxed and waned during a patient's menstrual cycle. By the late 19th century, it was well recognized that the gonads influenced a variety of other tissues and that these influences could be altered by removal of the testes or ovaries. Hormones were not described as the chemical mediators of these responses until the 1920s (Rossof, 1980). Believing that younger women with advanced breast cancer had a poorer prognosis than older ones, Schinzinger in 1889 asked, "... whether it would be permissible to make the ladies old more quickly by removing their ovaries, which would cause the mammary gland to atrophy and give the tumor the opportunity to be encapsulated in the shrinking tissue of the gland." Schinzinger further suggested, "In women who are still menstruating, one should first perform a castration before operating for breast cancer in order to prevent it from spreading locally or to stop a too rapid growth." Evidently Schinzinger never actually performed oophorectomy for breast cancer, nor was he able to convince his German colleagues to do so.

It is unclear whether Beatson was aware of the writings of Schinzinger or whether he performed the first oophorectomy for breast cancer based purely on his own research. Beatson wrote his thesis for the doctor of medicine degree on the subject of lactation and was convinced that the ovary sent out influences "more subtle and more mysterious" than those from the nervous system. Regardless of the exact reason, Beatson performed the first therapeutic bilateral oophorectomy for the treatment of advanced breast cancer on June 15, 1895. The procedure was performed on a 33-year-old woman with a locally recurrent breast cancer that developed 5 to 6 months following mastectomy. Beatson initially treated the patient with thyroid tablets, but as there was no change in the local area after 1 month he proceeded with the oophorectomy. Following the oophorectomy, the thyroid tablets were resumed to function as "a powerful lymphatic stimulant." Eight months after the operation, "all vestiges of the previous cancerous disease had disappeared" (Beatson, 1896). The patient was thought to have been cured and, indeed, remained in remission 46 months before she suffered a relapsed of her disease and died. Interestingly, the use of thyroid hormone with oophorectomy continued until the 1970s, when the Cooperative Breast Cancer Group confirmed that the effects of surgical castration were not enhanced by the addition of thyroid hormone (O'Bryan et al., 1974).

Following Beatson's initial report, oophorectomy became widely practiced, but after only 10 years the procedure was largely abandoned, probably for the reasons that (1) the procedure was not truly curative, as had initially been hoped, and (2) castration by irradiation came into use and was safer.

In 1902, Thompson reported on 80 cases treated with oophorectomy and noted the duration of response to be 6 to 12 months. In 1905, Lett reviewed 99 cases and reported that the response rate in premenopausal women was 29.3%. Surgical oophorectomy fell into disrepute and was ignored for nearly half a century, yet this was the first demonstration of an effective systemic treatment for cancer of any type (Yarbro, 1985).

By the early 1940s, the structural framework was in place for the resurrection of endocrine therapy. The hormones testosterone and estrogen had been discovered, and their physiologic action was described. Interestingly, it was not an endocrinologist but a urologist, Charles Huggins, who sparked the revival (Kardinal, 1985). Huggins and associates (Huggins and Hodges, 1941; and Huggins and Bergenstal, 1952) reported on the relationship between prostate cancer, testosterone, and acid phosphatase and on the response of prostate cancer to surgical orchiectomy, estrogens, and later adrenalectomy. For this work Huggins was awarded the Nobel prize in 1966.

Huggins' success with prostate cancer stimulated interest in castration for the treatment of advanced breast cancer. In 1945, Adair and colleagues reviewed 304 women castrated radiotherapeutically and 31 women castrated surgically, noting equivalent results. Rossof (1980) also reported good results with six cases of male breast cancer treated with surgical orchiectomy.

By 1948, the value of additive hormone therapy using androgens or estrogens was recognized and was reported by Taylor and colleagues. Taylor also introduced the use of progestins in 1951 (Taylor and Morris, 1951). Thus, what might be considered the first golden age of hormone therapy had begun. The Cooperative Breast Cancer Group organized under the chairmanship of Albert Segaloff of the Ochsner Clinic, concerned itself with comparative evaluations of estrogens and androgens, the role of thyroid hormone with oophorectomy, and the role of megestrol acetate as an adjuvant. Perhaps the most important contribution of this group of investigators was the establishment of objective criteria for the evaluation of response to treatment in patients with advanced breast cancer (Segaloff, 1966). With slight modification, these criteria were adopted by the International Union Against Cancer (Hayward et al., 1977) and remain in use today.

It was established during the 1960s that the objective response rate to hormonal manipulation, whether additive or ablative, was no greater than 25% to 30%, and that the median duration of response was approximately 12 months. In 1969, Cooper reported to the American Association for Cancer Research an objective response rate of 80% for hormonally refractory breast cancers to the five-drug regimen cyclophosphamide, methotrexate, 5-fluorouracil, vincristine, and prednisone. Response rates of this magnitude were unknown with hormone therapy. The first golden age of hormone therapy came to an abrupt end. Recent advances in the understanding of hormonal mechanisms seem to be ushering in a second one.

PRINCIPLES OF HORMONE THERAPY

The clinical presentation of breast cancer has changed dramatically in the past decade. In the early 1980s, there were 130,000 new cases per year in the United States. Almost all of the tumors were found by women themselves. The median diameter was at least 3 cm, and more than half were associated with involvement of the axillary lymph nodes. Ultimately, 70% of these women developed recurrence and died of their disease (Baum, 1984). In fact, it was questioned whether or not breast cancer was a curable disease. Rutqvist and coworkers (1984) reviewed 14,731 cases from the Cancer Registry of Norway and found a continuing late mortality (Table 22–1). Stage I disease was associated with the longest median survival time, implying that patients with an initially small tumor burden are at risk of recurrence for considerably longer periods (Clark et al., 1987).

In the 1990s, on average, 180,000 new cases of breast cancer will be discovered every year, but the clinical spectrum of the disease is considerably different. The average tumor is no larger than 2 cm, 75% to 80% being clinical Stage I or II, and almost two-thirds without axillary node involvement (NIH Consensus Conference, 1990). It is now estimated that only 30% of newly diagnosed patients will develop recurrence and ultimately die of metastatic breast cancer. Dramatic improvements can be attributed to better breast cancer awareness, mammographic screening, and improved systemic adjuvant therapy for operable breast cancer.

Once a breast cancer has recurred as distant (even a local) metastasis, the disease is no longer curable by currently available methods. The goals of treatment change from cure to palliation of symptoms and prolongation of a useful, productive life. Advanced breast cancer clearly is a systemic disease and must be treated systemically. Currently the only effective systemic treatments available are endocrine therapy (additive and ablative) and cytotoxic chemotherapy. Perhaps in the near future biologic response modifiers and monoclonal antibodies may play a role in the management of advanced breast cancer (Schlom et al., 1984; and Kardinal, 1985).

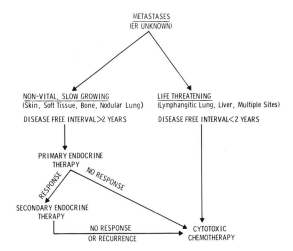

Figure 22–5. Clinical management of a patient with advanced breast cancer when the receptor status is unknown. This was the standard approach to the patient in the 1970s, the prereceptor era. It is still valid in the 1990s if a patient's receptor status is unknown.

The treatment of patients with advanced disease has undergone considerable change over the past three decades. In the 1960s, when chemotherapy was in its infancy, sequential hormone therapy was developed. During the 1970s, the selection of therapy for advanced breast cancer was based on clinical judgement (Segaloff, 1975). The use of hormonal receptors did not come into wide clinical use until the late 1970s and early 1980s. The clinical decision to use hormone therapy, as opposed to chemotherapy, was based on these major criteria: (1) the site of metastasis and the number of metastatic sites; and (2) the disease-free interval (Fig. 22–5; Tables 22–2, 22–3).

Cutler and associates (1969) recognized certain sites where metastasis could be considered "dire," such as the liver, lymphangitic pulmonary metastases, and central nervous system (see Table 22–2). Skin, soft tissue, bone, and nodular pulmonary metastases (unless multiple and bilateral) were associated with a better prognosis. From this it could be deduced that, if the patient had multiple sites of metastasis or a site of dire prognosis were involved, the clinician could not risk taking the necessary 6 to 8 weeks to determine whether the patient would be one of the 25%

Table 22–1. LONG-TERM FOLLOW-UP OF BREAST CANCER PATIENTS' DATA FROM THE CANCER REGISTRY OF NORWAY

Stage	Cured Fraction	Median Survival of Noncured Patients
I	54 ± 3(%)	7.6 (yr)
II	27 ± 1(%)	3.4 (yr)
III	19 ± 2(%)	2.1 (yr)
IV	2 ± 1(%)	0.7 (yr)

(Data from Rutqvist, L. E., et al.: Is breast cancer a curable disease? A study of 14,731 women with breast cancer from the Cancer Registry of Norway. Cancer, *53*:1793, 1984.)

Table 22–2. THE EFFECT OF THE NUMBER OF METASTATIC SITES ON SURVIVAL

Sites (N)	Cases (N)	Median Survival
1	249	19 (mo)
2*	200	13 (mo)
3*	114	10 (mo)
4*	51	6 (mo)
"Dire"†	111	6 (mo)

(Modified from Cutler, S. J., et al.: Classification of patients with disseminated cancer of the breast. Cancer, *24*:861, 1969.)
*Does not include a "dire" prognosis site.
†"Dire" = liver, peritoneum, brain, or spinal cord metastases.

Table 22–3. THE EFFECT OF DISEASE-FREE INTERVAL ON SURVIVAL AFTER DISSEMINATION

Disease-Free Interval	Cases (N)	Median Survival After Dissemination
<1 (yr)	135	7 (mo)
1–2 (yr)	142	7 (mo)
2–5 (yr)	208	15 (mo)
5+ (yr)	129	25 (mo)

(Modified from Cutler, S. J., et al.: Classification of patients with disseminated cancer of the breast. Cancer, 24:861, 1969.)

Table 22–4. RELATIONSHIP BETWEEN ESTROGEN RECEPTOR STATUS OF BREAST CANCER AND OBJECTIVE RESPONSE TO ENDOCRINE THERAPY

ER+ (Proportion/Rate)	ER− (Proportion/Rate)
522/977 (53%)	36/567 (6%)

(Data from the NIH Consensus Development Conference on Steroid Receptors in Breast Cancer. Modified from Wittliff, J. L.: Steroid-hormone receptors in breast cancer. Cancer 53:630, 1984.)

to 30% who would respond to hormones. Instead, the patient had to be treated directly with cytotoxic chemotherapy, which had a more rapid onset of action and a higher response rate.

The other important prognostic factor recognized during the 1960s and 1970s was the disease-free interval (Cutler et al., 1969; and Carter, 1972). Disease-free interval is defined as the time between primary therapy and recurrence. The greater the disease-free interval, the longer was survival time after development of metastases (see Table 22–3). There is a direct relationship between the disease-free interval and hormonal responsiveness. Tumors with prolonged disease-free intervals are slower growing, more highly differentiated, and more likely to remain hormone responsive (Rozencweig and Heuson, 1975). Disease-free interval, the site of the tumor, and the number of metastatic sites remain important, clinically relevant predictors of hormone responsiveness, especially in patients whose receptor status is unknown.

EVALUATING HORMONE DEPENDENCY: ESTROGEN AND PROGESTERONE RECEPTORS

The pioneering work of Jensen and colleagues (1971), McGuire (1973), Wittliff (1974), and DeSombre and coworkers (1976) established the relationship between the presence of ER in the cytosol of breast cancer tissue and response to hormone manipulation. By the use of the ER alone, and by restricting hormonal manipulation to patients who are ER positive ($\geq$ 10 fmol/mg protein), the response rate to hormone manipulation can be increased from between 25% and 30% in unselected cases to 55% in ER-positive cases (Wittliff, 1984). The ER data from the National Institutes of Health (NIH) Consensus Development Conference on Steroid Receptors in Breast Cancer are summarized in Table 22–4. The response rates to additive (56%) and ablative (55%) forms of hormone manipulation in ER-positive cases are equivalent (McGuire et al., 1975) (Table 22–5). This probably reflects the fact that both additive and ablative therapy are designed to block estrogen production or action.

In 1975, Horwitz and colleagues hypothesized that the presence of progesterone receptor (PgR) in human breast cancer would be a sensitive predictor of response to endocrine therapy. PgR was found in 56% of tumors with ER,

and in preliminary observation it was noted that only tumors with PgR regressed after endocrine therapy. Horwitz and coworkers further postulated that because the synthesis of PgR is estrogen dependent, the presence of PgR indicated that the tumor was capable of synthesizing at least one end product under estrogen regulation and remained endocrine responsive. This is basically true. The response rate of tumors that contain both ERs and PgRs is 78%. The Horwitz hypothesis was evaluated in a prospective trial by the Southwest Oncology Group (SWOG) (Ravdin et al., 1992), which evaluated the prognostic significance of PgR levels in ER-positive breast cancer patients treated with tamoxifen. This study demonstrated that ER-positive tumors with higher PgR values had a higher response rate to tamoxifen therapy than ER positive ones with low PgR values. No group of ER-positive tumors, however, had such a low response rate as to preclude consideration of the use of tamoxifen, even if they were PgR-negative. In contrast to the SWOG data, Bezwoda and colleagues (1991) reported that response to tamoxifen correlated with the ER level but not the PgR level. Patients with an ER level greater than 30.1 fmol/mg protein had an 80% rate of response to tamoxifen therapy. They concluded that a quantitative estimation of ER level is the best predictor of response to hormone therapy with tamoxifen in advanced breast cancer. From this it can be concluded, as Allegra (1984*a*) has done, that receptors are necessary for a tumor to be hormone dependent but that they are not, in themselves, sufficient. The data on hormone responsiveness and receptor status (ER-positive, PgR-positive; ER-positive, PgR-negative; ER-negative, PgR-negative) are summarized in Table 22–6 (Wittliff, 1984). The ER-negative, PgR-positive group, with its small numbers and relatively high hor-

Table 22–5. RELATIONSHIP BETWEEN ESTROGEN RECEPTOR STATUS AND RESPONSE TO ADDITIVE AND ABLATIVE ENDOCRINE THERAPY

	ER+ (Proportion/Rate)	ER− (Proportion/Rate)
Additive hormone treatment	59/105 (56%)	12/109 (11%)
Ablative endocrine therapy	59/107 (55%)	8/94 (8%)
Total	118/212 (56%)	20/203 (10%)

(Modified from McGuire, W. L., Carbone, P. O., and Vollmer, E. P. (Eds.): Estrogen Receptors in Human Breast Cancer. New York: Raven, 1975.)

Table 22–6. RELATIONSHIP BETWEEN ESTROGEN (ER) AND PROGESTERONE (PgR) RECEPTOR STATUS AND RESPONSE TO ENDOCRINE THERAPY

ER+, PgR+	ER+, PgR−	ER−, PgR−	ER−, PgR+
135/174	55/164	16/165	5/11
78%	34%	10%	45%

(Modified from Wittliff, J. L.: Steroid-hormone receptors in breast cancer. Cancer, *53*:630, 1984.)

mone response rate (45%), may well be an artifact that reflects a false-negative ER, possibly owing to improper specimen handling when the tissue is obtained (Bridges et al., 1983). Kiang and Kollander (1987) demonstrated that in nine of nine ER-negative, PgR-positive patients studied, ER could be demonstrated in the nucleus with the enzyme immunoassay or the immunocytochemical staining method using monoclonal antibodies to ER. They postulated that endogenous estrogen may be partly responsible for the false-negative ER by the conventional dextran charcoal assay.

As might be anticipated, there is a quantitative relationship between estrogen receptor concentration in breast cancer tissue and response to endocrine therapy (Osborne et al., 1980; and Allegra, 1983*a*) (Table 22–7). The higher the ER, the more likely a response. There is also a striking difference in response when PgR is evaluated as a function of ER concentration (Osborne et al., 1980) (Table 22–8).

The difference in response to endocrine manipulation in ER-positive tumors by metastatic site is not as great as might be anticipated (Allegra, 1983*b*) (Table 22–9). The old belief, which goes as far back as Beatson (1896), that visceral metastases respond poorly to endocrine manipulation, is not necessarily valid. What is true is that patients with a heavy tumor cell burden in visceral sites may not be able to afford to wait 6 to 8 weeks for the onset of an endocrine response. Patients with smaller metastatic tumor cell burdens in visceral sites, however, may have good objective responses to hormonal manipulation. For patients with high receptor-positive tumor burdens in visceral sites, consideration should be given to initial therapy with six to eight cycles of anthracycline-based chemotherapy followed by maintenance hormone therapy with tamoxifen or megestrol acetate (MA).

Receptor status varies as a function of age (Allegra,

Table 22–7. QUANTITATION OF ER AND RESPONSE TO ENDOCRINE THERAPY

ER (fmol/mg)	Primary Cancer (%)	Metastatic Biopsy (%)
0–10	9	8
10–50	50	40
100	83	61

(Data from Allegra, J. C.: Methotrexate and 5-fluorouracil following tamoxifen and Premarin in advanced breast cancer. Semin. Oncol., *10*(Suppl. 2):23, 1983*a*; and from Osborne, C. K., Yochmowitz, M. G., Knight, W. A., et al.: The value of estrogen and progesterone receptors in the treatment of breast cancer. Cancer, *46*:2884, 1980.)

Table 22–8. RESPONSE TO ENDOCRINE THERAPY BY QUANTITATIVE ER VERSUS QUALITATIVE PgR

Measure	Response Rate (%)
ER	
3–100 fmol/mg	34
>100 fmol/mg	63
PgR	
Negative (<5 fmol/mg)	31
Positive (≥5 fmol/mg)	80

(Modified from Osborne, C. K., et al.: The value of estrogen and progesterone receptors in the treatment of breast cancer. Cancer, *46*:2884, 1980.)

1984*b*) (Table 22–10) and thus with menopausal status (Wittliff, 1984) (Table 22–11). The younger the patient, the more likely she is to be receptor negative and hormonally unresponsive. Conversely, the older the patient, the more likely she is to be receptor positive and hormonally responsive. This difference in receptor content by age and menopausal status probably explains why premenopausal patients have a poorer prognosis than postmenopausal women. However, when receptor content and node status are comparable, response rates and survival are equivalent in premenopausal and postmenopausal women.

Changes in Receptors

ER- and PgR positivity diminish with progression of the malignancy (Nomura et al., 1985; and Kamby et al., 1989) (Table 22–12). Differences in the receptor content between the primary lesion and metastatic sites have been observed by several investigators (Brennan et al., 1979; Allegra et al., 1980; Hull et al., 1983; and Kamby et al., 1989). When changes in receptivity occur, they are almost always in the direction from positivity to negativity, implying tumor dedifferentiation. Changes in receptor status from negative to positive are, however, reported (Holdaway and Bowditch, 1983; Rosen et al., 1977; and Nomura et al., 1985).

The tumor dedifferentiation theory may not explain why receptor-positive tumors tend to become receptor negative. During the course of their disease, almost all patients with

Table 22–9. OBJECTIVE RESPONSES TO ENDOCRINE THERAPY IN ER-POSITIVE TUMORS BY DOMINANT SITE OF METASTATIC DISEASE

Site	Response (%)
Skin	52
Soft tissue	57
Nodes	61
Lung	62
Liver	55
Bone	50
Bone marrow	67
Central nervous system	0

(Modified from Allegra, J. C.: The use of steroid hormone receptors in breast cancer. *In* Margolese, R. (Ed.): Breast Cancer. New York, Churchill Livingstone, 1983, p. 187.)

Table 22–10. THE RELATIONSHIP BETWEEN RECEPTOR STATUS AND AGE

Age (yrs)	ER+ (%)	PgR+ (%)
40	44	31
40–49	48	36
50–59	53	42
60–69	58	36
70	69	29

(Modified from Allegra, J. C.: *In* The Management of Breast Cancer Through Endocrine Therapies. Amsterdam, Excerpta Medica, 1984, pp. 1–13.)

Table 22–12. CHANGES IN RECEPTOR CONTENT WITH PROGRESSION OF DISEASE

Disease Status	ER+ (%)	PgR+ (%)
Primary lesion	53.8	26.3
First relapse	56.5	24.5
Second relapse	39.0	19.1
Preterminal	20.0	3.4

(Data from Nomura, Y., et al.: Changes of steroid hormone receptor content by chemotherapy and/or endocrine therapy in advanced breast cancer. Cancer, *55*:546, 1985.)

advanced breast cancer receive multiple types of treatment, such as chemotherapy and hormone therapy. Some observed changes in receptor status may be induced by treatment (Table 22–13). It appears that hormone therapy has a greater tendency to induce changes from ER positive to ER negative status than does cytotoxic chemotherapy (Nomura et al., 1985; and Hawkins et al., 1990), which implies that chemotherapy kills cells indiscriminately, regardless of their receptor status, leaving the same proportion of ER-positive and ER-negative cells (Kardinal et al., 1986). However, hormone therapy selectively interferes with ER-positive cells. Allegra and coworkers (1980) suggested that the observed conversion of ER-positive tumors to ER-negative status after treatment with tamoxifen may occur because the drug occupies the ER sites, causing artificially low ER determinations. This suggests that ER-positive breast cancers that become ER negative after antiestrogen therapy may still respond to second-line endocrine therapy.

In addition to ER and PgR, a series of other receptors have been demonstrated on breast cancer cells. These include LH-RH receptors, somatostatin (SMS) receptors, and EGF receptors (Fekete et al., 1989; and Reubi and Torhorst, 1989). All tumors that contain SMS receptors are ER positive and tend to be EGFR negative. In contrast, EGFR-positive tumors tend to be ER negative. Perhaps it will become possible to correlate the levels of these receptors with clinical parameters to better identify endocrine-responsive neoplasms.

Receptors and Breast Cancer Biology

Over the past several years, it has become apparent that the ER and PgR status of a breast cancer is an important prog-

nostic indicator as well as an indicator of response to endocrine therapy (Gapinski and Donegan, 1980; Clark and McGuire, 1983; McGuire and Clark, 1983; Winstanley et al., 1991; and Nomura et al., 1992). It has also been demonstrated that receptors correlate with the cell turnover rates, nuclear grade, and degree of histologic differentiation (Fisher et al., 1987*a*). Meyer and colleagues (1977) demonstrated that tumors with low thymidine-labeling indices; i.e., low cellular replication rates, tended to be ER positive and, conversely, those with a high thymidine-labeling indices tended to be ER negative. Fisher and coworkers (1980) and Parl and colleagues (1984) demonstrated that ER-positive tumors tend to be well differentiated and ER-negative tumors tend to be poorly differentiated. It can be deduced from this that the more like normal breast tissue a breast cancer is (i.e., the better-differentiated the tumor), the more likely the tumor is to be ER positive and hormonally responsive, and the better the prognosis.

Allegra and colleagues (1979) and Knight and associates (1977) demonstrated that the ER status of a primary tumor is associated with the disease-free interval. ER positivity is associated with long disease-free intervals and ER negativity with shorter disease-free intervals (Fig. 22–6). This association is independent of age, menopausal status (Fig. 22–7), tumor size (Fig. 22–8), or nodal status (Fig. 22–9). Thus, it appears that receptor status is an independent prognostic variable. Also, the purely clinical observation that prolonged disease-free intervals tend to be associated with persistence of hormone responsiveness has been confirmed by scientific findings.

The role of progesterone receptors as a prognostic variable was critically evaluated by Clark and associates (1983),

Table 22–11. RELATIONSHIP OF RECEPTOR STATUS AND MENOPAUSAL STATUS

Receptor Status	Menopausal Status	
	Premenopausal (%)	Postmenopausal (%)
ER+, PgR+	45	63
ER+, PgR−	12	15
ER−, PgR−	28	17
ER−, PgR+	15	5

(Modified from Wittliff, J. L.: Steroid-hormone receptors in breast cancer. Cancer, *53*:630, 1984.)

Table 22–13. CHANGES IN ER CONTENT BY TREATMENT

Treatment	Pretreatment ER+ (%)	Posttreatment ER+ (%)
Antiestrogen	71	43
Adreno-oophorectomy	64	25
Chemotherapy	36	32
Chemoendocrine therapy	60	28
Between first and last treatment	63	16

(Modified from Nomura Y., et al.: Change of steroid hormone receptor content by chemotherapy and/or endocrine therapy in advanced breast cancer. Cancer, *55*:546, 1985.)

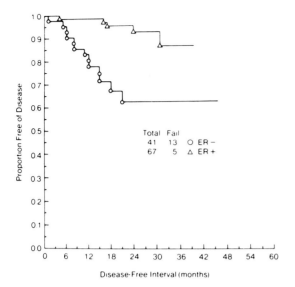

Figure 22-6. The relationship between disease-free interval and ER status in patients with breast cancer not receiving adjuvant therapy. (From Allegra, J. C.: Role of hormone receptors in determining treatment of breast cancer. *In* Allegra, J. C. (Ed.): The Management of Breast Cancer Through Endocrine Therapies. Amsterdam, Excerpta Medica, 1984, p. 8.)

who noted that, when analyzed separately, the presence and quantity of either ER or PgR was positively correlated with disease-free survival (Fig. 22–10). The presence of PgR was more significant than that of ER for predicting time to recurrence (Fig. 22–11). When patients were divided into tumor groups (ER-positive, PgR-positive; ER-positive, PgR-negative; ER-negative, PgR-negative [there were too few ER-negative, PgR-positive tumors to evaluate]), disease-free survival for the ER-positive, PgR-positive group was significantly longer than for either the ER-positive, PgR-negative or the ER-negative, PgR-negative group (Fig. 22–12). In addition, the disease-free survival of the ER-positive, PgR-negative group was only marginally longer than that of the ER-negative, PgR-negative group.

It has been assumed that all breast cancers are hormone dependent initially, and that in due course they dedifferentiate, losing endocrine responsiveness and becoming increasingly receptor negative. One would then anticipate that early, impalpable tumors would more often be ER positive, PgR positive than palpable operable tumors, which in turn would more frequently be ER positive, PgR positive than locally advanced or metastatic tumors. This is indeed the case. The confirmatory data of Tinnemans and colleagues (1990), are summarized in Table 22–14.

Axillary node metastases are a critical prognostic variable, and patients with negative axillary nodes do considerably better than patients with any degree of axillary node involvement (Bonadonna et al., 1976; and Fisher et al., 1968, 1975, 1983a) (Table 22–15). In addition, patients with one to three involved nodes have a better prognosis than those with more than four. Among those with more than four involved nodes, patients with four to six do better than those with 7 to 12, who in turn do better than those with more than 13 involved nodes (Fisher et al., 1983a) (Fig. 22–13).

Most investigators (Allegra et al., 1979; Hartviet et al.,

1980; Croton et al., 1981; Clark and McGuire, 1983; and McGuire et al., 1986) have confirmed that hormone receptors are an independent prognostic variable. However, it is now apparent that ER and PgR have their greatest prognostic significance for patients with Stage II breast cancer (Table 22–16). The presence of ER and PgR is highly predictive of recurrence and survival in node-positive patients. Receptor status alone is insufficient to identify the 20% to 30% of node-negative patients who will eventually suffer relapse and die of metastatic breast cancer (Butler et al., 1985; Henderson et al., 1989; and Tsangaris et al., 1992). Despite conflicting data, there appears to be no difference in disease-free survival time or overall survival for premenopausal or postmenopausal women with ER-positive or ER-negative, node-negative breast cancer.

Another important observation is that receptor-positive patients have a significantly longer survival from the date

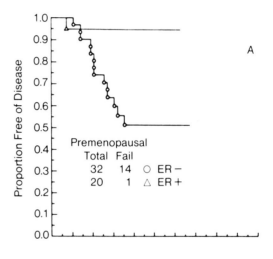
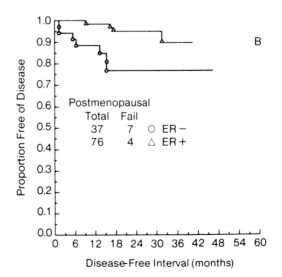

Figure 22-7. The relationship among disease-free interval, ER status, and menopausal state in patients with breast cancer. (From Allegra, J. C.: Role of hormone receptors in determining treatment of breast cancer. *In* Allegra, J. C. (Ed.): The Management of Breast Cancer Through Endocrine Therapies. Amsterdam, Excerpta Medica, 1984, p. 9.)

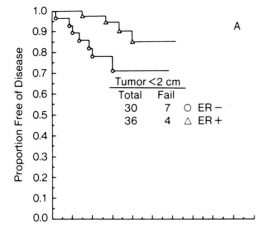

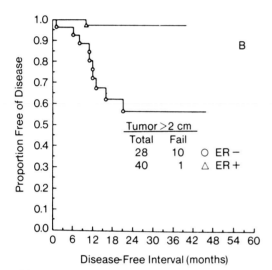

Figure 22–8. Relationship among disease-free interval, ER-status, and tumor size in patients with breast cancer. (From Allegra, J. C.: Role of hormone receptors in determining treatment of breast cancer. *In* Allegra, J. C. (Ed.): The Management of Breast Cancer Through Endocrine Therapies. Amsterdam, Excerpta Medica, 1984, p. 10.)

of first recurrence than receptor negative patients (Godolphin et al., 1981; and Kinne et al., 1981) (Fig. 22–14). In addition, within the receptor-positive group, those whose quantitative ER value is the highest (≥ 160 fmol/mg) do better than those with lower levels of positivity (10–159 fmol/mg). After recurrence, the poorer prognosis for the receptor-negative group may be due to the fact that ER-negative patients are more likely than ER-positive patients to develop visceral metastases, and ER-positive tumors are more often associated with the more indolent osseous metastases (Qazi et al., 1984; Sherry et al., 1986a; and Clark et al., 1987).

Carcinoembryonic Antigen, CA 15-3, and Other Serum Markers

The usefulness of the plasma level of carcinoembryonic antigen (CEA) for monitoring response to treatment, as a

predictor of early relapse, and as a prognostic factor in colorectal cancer—is well documented (Kardinal and Bush, 1985). In the past few years, it has become apparent that the cytosolic concentration of CEA may have similar use-

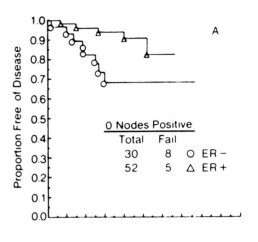

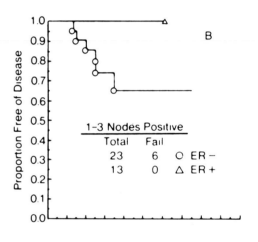

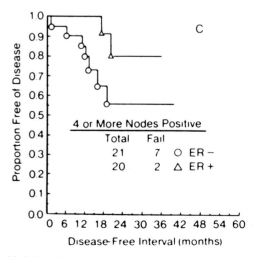

Figure 22–9. Relationship among disease-free survival, ER status, and the degree of axillary node involvement in patients with breast cancer. (From Allegra, J. C.: Role of hormone receptors in determining treatment of breast cancer. *In* Allegra, J. C. (Ed.): The Management of Breast Cancer Through Endocrine Therapies. Amsterdam, Excerpta Medica, 1984, p. 11.)

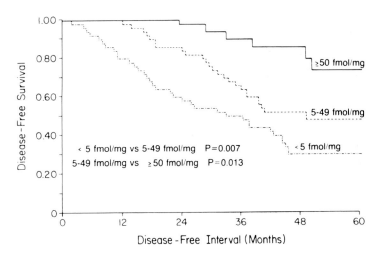

Figure 22–10. Relationship between disease-free survival and quantitative PgR levels. Patients with PgR levels of ≥ 50 fmol/mg of protein (N = 41) have a significantly longer disease-free survival than patients with a PgR level that is 5 to 49 fmol/mg (N = 68); patients in each of these groups have a longer disease-free period than patients with a PgR level <5 fmol/mg (N = 41). (From Clark, G. M., McGuire, W. L., Huybay, C. A., et al.: Progesterone receptors as a prognostic factor in stage II breast cancer. N. Engl. J. Med., *309*:1343, 1983.)

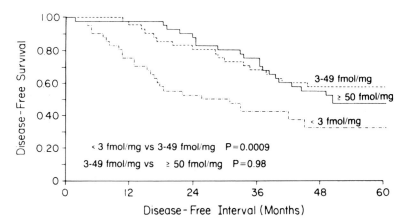

Figure 22–11. Relationship between disease-free survival and quantitative ER levels. Patients with ER levels <3 fmol/mg (N = 45) had significantly shorter disease-free survival than those with moderate or high levels. No difference was observed between patients with 3 to 49 fmol/mg (N = 82) and those with at least 50 fmol/mg (N = 62). (From Clark, G. M., McGuire, W. L., Huybay, C. A., et al.: Progesterone receptors as a prognostic factor in stage II breast cancer. N. Engl. J. Med., *309*:1343, 1983.)

Figure 22–12. Relationship between ER and PgR status and disease-free survival. Patients who are ER-positive, PgR-positive (N = 104) have a significantly longer disease-free survival than patients who are ER-positive, PgR-negative (N = 39) or patients who are ER-negative, PgR-negative (N = 40). (From Clark, G. M., McGuire, W. L., Huybay, C. A., et al.: Progesterone receptors as a prognostic factor in stage II breast cancer. N. Engl. J. Med., *309*:1343, 1983.)

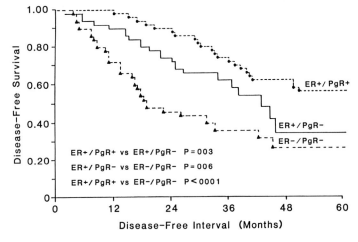

Table 22–14. RECEPTOR PHENOTYPE IN POSTMENOPAUSAL PATIENTS AT DIFFERENT STAGES OF BREAST CANCER

Disease Status	Patients (N)	ER+ PgR+ (%)*	ER+ PgR− (%)	ER− PgR+ (%)	ER− PgR− (%)
Nonpalpable	38	71	21	2	5
Primary operable	125	54	15	0	30
Locally advanced	42	50	24	3	19
First metastasis	42	40	29	0	31
Late metastasis	122	33	30	4	34

(From Tinnemans, J. G. M., Beex, L. V. A. M., Wobbes, T., et al.: Steroid-hormone receptors in nonpalpable and more advanced stages of breast cancer. Cancer, 66:1165–1167, 1990.)
Abbreviations: ER = estrogen receptor; PgR = progesterone receptor.
*χ^2 for ER+ PgR+ = 22.34, df = 4, P = 0002.

Table 22–15. TREATMENT FAILURE AFTER STANDARD RADICAL MASTECTOMY

Patient & Disease Status		Treatment Failures (%)			
	Number	18 mo	3 yr	5 yr	10 yr
All patients	370	19	—	39.7	49.5
Negative nodes	198	6	—	17.7	24.1
Positive nodes	172	35	—	71.0	76.1
Premenopausal					
Negative nodes	52	6	17	21.2	25.5
Positive nodes	60	50	61	70.0	76.3
1–3	24	13	—	45.8	56.6
≥4	36	64	82	86.1	88.9
Postmenopausal					
Negative nodes	146	8	15	16.4	23.6
Positive nodes	112	22	50	62.5	76.0
1–3	58	18	37	51.7	67.9
≥4	54	48	62	74.1	84.3

(Data from Fisher, B., Ravdin, R. G., Ausman, R. K., et al.: Surgical adjuvant chemotherapy in cancer of the breast. Results of a decade of cooperative investigation. Ann. Surg., 163:337, 1968; Fisher, B., Slack, N., Katrych, D., et al.: Ten year follow-up results of patients with carcinoma of the breast in a cooperative clinical trial evaluating surgical adjuvant chemotherapy. Surg. Gynecol. Obstet., 140:528, 1975; and Fisher, B., Bauer, M., Wickerham, D. L., et al.: Relation of number of positive axillary nodes to the prognosis of patients with primary breast cancer. An NSABP update. Cancer, 52:1551, 1983.)

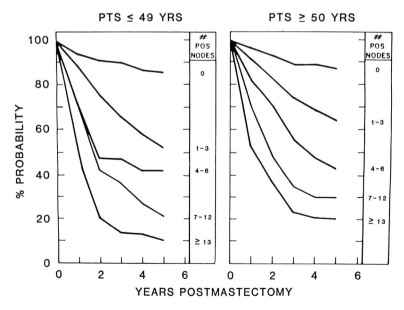

Figure 22–13. Disease-free survival relative to age and number of positive axillary nodes for patients (PTS) ≤49 years of age and those ≥50 years of age. (From Fisher, B., Bauer, M., Wickerham, D. L., et al.: Relation of number of positive axillary nodes to the prognosis of patients with primary breast cancer: An NSABP update. Cancer, 52:1551, 1983.)

Table 22–16. PROGNOSTIC VALUE OF RECEPTORS FOR DISEASE-FREE SURVIVAL AND OVERALL SURVIVAL IN PATIENTS WITH STAGE II BREAST CANCER (MULTIVARIATE ANALYSIS OF 1529 PATIENTS)

	P Value	
Factor	Disease-Free Survival	Overall Survival
Positive nodes	<.0001	<.0001
Tumor size	<.0001	.0001
Progesterone receptor status	.0001	.0001
Endocrine therapy	.0004	.0017
Chemotherapy	.0731	.0191
Estrogen receptor status	.1376	.0017
Age	.8990	.0622

(From McGuire, W. L., Clark, G. M., Dressler, L. G., et al.: Role of steroid hormone receptors as prognostic factors in primary breast cancer. Natl. Cancer Inst. Monogr., *1*:19–23, 1986.)

fulness in breast cancer (Duffy et al., 1983; and Mansour et al., 1983). Schwartz and colleagues (1985) demonstrated that the cytosolic CEA value is related to pathologic stage and is independent of ER status, histologic differentiation, and other pathologic variables. The CEA value may, therefore, provide information on some other biologic characteristic of breast cancer. Falkson and coworkers (1982) demonstrated that, in patients receiving postsurgical adjuvant chemotherapy, a rising CEA level is a more sensitive predictor of recurrence than is the lactic dehydrogenase or alkaline phosphatase level. Also, changes in the plasma CEA level during hormone therapy or chemotherapy reflect an increasing or decreasing tumor cell burden (Silva et al., 1982). The high cost of CEA assays and their relative

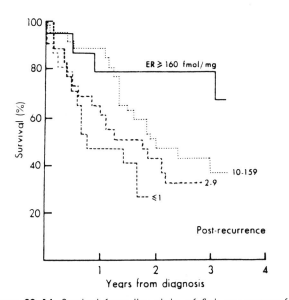

Figure 22–14. Survival from the date of first recurrence for breast cancer patients in four groups by ER concentration. (From Godolphin, W., Elwood, J. M., and Spinelli, J. J.: Estrogen receptor quantitation and staging as complementary prognostic indicators of breast cancer: A study of 583 patients. Int. J. Cancer, *28*:677, 1981. Reprinted by permission of Wiley-Liss, a division of John Wiley and Sons, Inc. Copyright © 1981.)

insensitivity prohibit their routine use in breast cancer patients (Loprinzi and Ahmann, 1986).

Other serum markers, particularly CA 15-3 and mucin-like carcinoma-associated antigen (MCA or BCM) are currently being evaluated as indicators of tumor activity and tumor burden (Colomer et al., 1989; Garcia et al., 1990; Bates, 1991; O'Dwyer et al., 1990; Miserez et al., 1991; Safi et al., 1991; and Daly et al., 1992). Elevated CA 15-3 levels are found in patients with breast cancer, but the specificity is low since such elevated levels are also associated with other malignancies (of ovary, endometrium, and occasionally lung), benign breast disease, and benign liver disease. Like CEA, CA 15-3 is elevated in only a small percentage of Stage I or II breast cancers, making it a poor diagnostic or screening tool. CA 15-3 is more sensitive than CEA for detecting recurrent or metastatic breast cancer, being increased in 75% to 80% of patients with progressive disease, but CA 15-3 is a poor barometer of response since it decreases in only 38% of patients who exhibit objective clinical improvement. MCA or BCM may be a more sensitive indicator of the clinical course of breast cancer than either CEA or CA 15-3, but further trials should be done. There appears to be considerable overlap among CEA-positive, CA 15-3–positive, and MCA-positive populations, which phenomenon limits the usefulness of marker combinations. Since therapy for recurrent or metastatic breast cancer is palliative rather than curative, it can be questioned whether the early detection (and thus early treatment) of metastasis is critical to long-term survival. Routine use of CEA, CA 15-5, or MCA cannot be recommended at this time.

ABLATIVE HORMONE THERAPY

Oophorectomy

Surgical castration remains an effective first- or second-line treatment for hormonally responsive breast cancer in premenopausal women (Veronesi et al., 1981; Wells and Santen, 1984; Conte et al., 1989). As reviewed by Haas (1981), the overall response rate in unselected cases is 31% (365 responders in 1163 patients), and the median response duration is 12 months, but responses lasting 25 years have been reported (Mecklenburg and Lipsett, 1973). The response rate can be increased to 55% by restricting oophorectomy to ER-positive patients and to 78% by restricting it to ER-positive, PgR-positive patients. Oophorectomy should not be performed in ER-negative women because the response rate is less than 10%. The contraindications to surgical castration are listed in Table 22–17.

The traditional role of oophorectomy as the primary mode of endocrine therapy in premenopausal women is currently being challenged by the antiestrogen tamoxifen (Haas, 1981; Buchanan et al., 1986; and Ingle et al., 1986). Response rates and response durations appear to be equivalent (Margreiter and Wiegele, 1984; and Planting et al., 1985). In fact, Pritchard and coworkers (1984) stated that response to tamoxifen is a good predictor of response to oophorectomy. This implies that tamoxifen should be used as primary therapy and that oophorectomy should be re-

Table 22–17. CONTRAINDICATIONS TO SURGICAL CASTRATION

Uncontrolled central nervous system metastases
Massive hepatic metastases
Pulmonary lymphangitic metastases or bloody pleural effusion
Uncontrolled hypercalcemia
Myelophthisic anemia
More than 1 year postmenopausal
ER-negative receptor status

stricted to patients who have previously responded to tamoxifen. That tamoxifen is a good predictor of response to oophorectomy could not be confirmed by the SWOG (Hoogstraten et al., 1982, 1984). In the SWOG trial, none of 14 premenopausal patients who responded to tamoxifen responded to oophorectomy, whereas 5 of 22 patients who failed to respond to tamoxifen responded to oophorectomy followed by continued tamoxifen therapy. Kalman and associates (1983) also reported response to oophorectomy after failure to respond to tamoxifen in a premenopausal patient. The use of tamoxifen in premenopausal patients is discussed in the section on *Additive Hormone Therapy*. High-dose medroxyprogesterone acetate versus oophorectomy has been evaluated as first-line therapy for advanced breast cancer. There was no difference in response rate, response duration, or survival, though two of four patients who failed to respond to oophorectomy responded to subsequent medroxyprogesterone acetate (Martoni et al., 1991).

Oophorectomy and Chemotherapy

Attempts have been made to improve the response to oophorectomy by adjunctive cytotoxic chemotherapy. Four prospective, randomized trials were done before assays of estrogen or progesterone receptors were available (van Dyk and Falkson, 1971; Ahmann et al., 1977; Falkson et al., 1979, 1987; and Rossof et al., 1982). In each of those trials, the response rate was higher in patients treated with oophorectomy plus chemotherapy than in those who underwent oophorectomy alone, but the response did not exceed that reported for chemotherapy alone. However, Falkson and coworkers (1994) have reported a median survival of 59 months for premenopausal women with ER-positive metastatic breast cancer treated with chemotherapy plus oophorectomy compared with 26 months for those treated with chemotherapy alone.

To add to the confusion, Forbes and coworkers (1992) reported that the complete and partial response rates for premenopausal women with advanced breast cancer who were treated with cytotoxic chemotherapy (Adriamycin and cyclophosphamide) were equivalent to those for women treated with oophorectomy. (A third group of women treated with chemotherapy and oophorectomy did significantly worse, suggesting a negative treatment interaction.) The results of these studies emphasize that there is no clear benefit from chemotherapy plus hormone therapy, and that since the goal is palliation, hormone therapy and chemo-

therapy should be used sequentially and not in combination (Glauber and Kiang, 1992). Less toxic hormone therapy should be used initially, followed, as the disease progresses, by the more toxic chemotherapeutic regimens.

Radiation Oophorectomy

The use of irradiation for castration of women with locally advanced and disseminated breast cancer began in the early 1920s, using a technique described by Halberstadter in 1905 (de Courmeller, 1922; and Wintz, 1926; Ahlbom, 1930). The procedure was safe, and the results were equivalent to those of surgical castration (Adair et al., 1945; and Diczfalusy et al., 1959). With radiotherapy the reduction of estrogen production is considerably slower than with surgery, and it may take 3 to 5 months to reach the basal level (Block et al., 1958). The argument that radiation oophorectomy still is indicated for patients who are too sick to undergo surgical oophorectomy is not valid; it is hardly acceptable to wait 3 to 5 months for a therapeutic response, and alternative modes of therapy should be instituted. So many alternative treatments are available, such as tamoxifen, aminoglutethimide, and even cytotoxic chemotherapy, that there are few if any indications for radiation oophorectomy.

Oophorectomy in the Adjuvant Setting

Schinzinger, in 1889, proposed oophorectomy as an adjuvant, and he repeated his plea in 1905, stating that his objective was to slow the growth rate of the cancer (cited by Nissen-Meyer, 1991). The first trial of prophylactic castration was instituted by Taylor in 1934. After 4 years, the results in 50 patients castrated therapeutically were sufficiently similar to those of 47 patients treated prophylactically that Taylor concluded that the production of artificial menopause was not advantageous (Taylor, 1939). Numerous other investigators reported conflicting results with prophylactic oophorectomy, and the procedure continued to be practiced widely until the 1970s. In 1961, the National Surgical Adjuvant Breast Project (NSABP) initiated a prospective, randomized trial of surgical oophorectomy as an adjunct to radical mastectomy for the treatment of operable breast cancer (Ravdin et al., 1970). In all, 699 patients were entered into the study. No significant differences were seen in recurrence or survival rates. When the data were interpreted in terms of the nodal status of the different treatment groups, still no differences were found. Nonetheless, two more recent studies show marginal improvement in late survival in the prophylactically oophorectomized group (Bryant and Weir, 1981; and Meakin et al., 1983). For neither of these studies were hormonal receptor data available, and in neither were the results impressive enough to recommend that the procedure be adopted. Finally, in 1985 and updated in 1990, the International (Ludwig) Breast Cancer Study Group (1990) reported the results of a study that randomized premenopausal women with Stage II breast cancer and four or more involved axillary nodes to (1) adjuvant chemotherapy with cyclophosphamide, methotrexate, 5-fluorouracil, and prednisone (CMFP) or (2) CMFP plus oophorectomy (Ludwig Breast Cancer Study Group, 1985). No difference was found in disease-free or absolute survival, even in receptor-positive cases. This study should have laid adjuvant oophorectomy to rest, but like the phoenix, the issue is again rising from the ashes.

The Early Breast Cancer Trialists' Collaborative Group more recently (1992) reported a meta-analysis of essentially every prospective, randomized trial of systemic adjuvant therapy for early breast cancer. It is estimated that 90% of patients who were ever "randomized" were included in this study. Twelve prospective, randomized trials of ovarian ablation had been initiated before 1985, and data were available for analysis from 10 of these trials involving 3000 women; 2000 were younger than age 50 at randomization and, so, were presumed to be premenopausal. Women older than 50 years had no benefit from prophylactic (adjuvant) oophorectomy, but for women younger than 50, despite the fact that none of the 10 trials individually confirmed benefit, after 10 years, 47% of the control group were alive, as compared to 57% of the oophorectomized group ($P < .01$) (Fig. 22–15). Benefit was noted in both node-positive and node-negative cases. Although the data may be valid, one can question the meta-analysis technique of pooling data from different times and different investigators worldwide. The oophorectomy studies, in general, were initially reported more than 15 to 20 years ago, before hormone receptors were generally available. The benefit of ovarian ablation for women selected for high receptor levels might be even more striking. Perhaps ovarian ablation deserves reexamination as an adjuvant for premenopausal women with receptor-positive tumors.

Adjuvant Chemotherapy–Induced Amenorrhea

The meta-analysis reported by the Early Breast Cancer Trialists' Collaborative Group (1992) seems to confirm, or at least raise the question of, benefit from adjuvant oophorectomy for premenopausal women. This raises a second question: How much of the benefit gained from adjuvant chemotherapy in premenopausal women is an endocrine effect? Many women receiving adjuvant chemotherapy become temporarily or permanently amenorrheic. Bianco and co-workers (1991) from the University of Naples evaluated the prognostic role of drug-induced amenorrhea (DIA) on 221

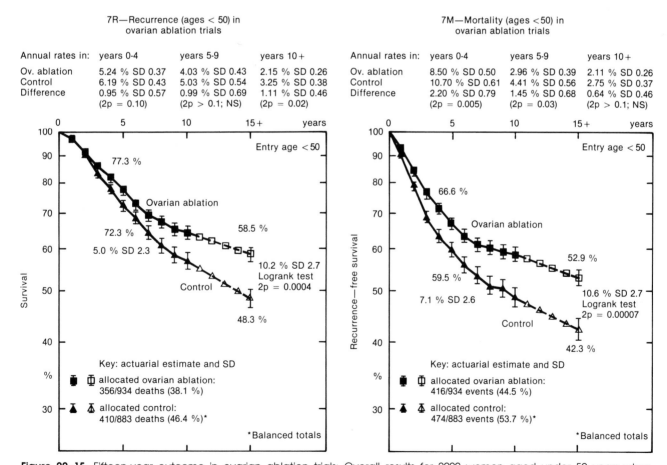

Figure 22–15. Fifteen-year outcome in ovarian ablation trials: Overall results for 2000 women aged under 50 years when randomized. 7R = recurrence (disease-free survival) curves; 7M = mortality curves. (From Early Breast Cancer Trialists' Collaborative Group: Systemic treatment of early breast cancer by hormonal, cytotoxic, or immune therapy: 133 randomised trials involving 31,000 recurrences and 24,000 deaths among 75,000 women. Lancet, *399*:1–15, 71–85, 1992. © by *The Lancet Ltd.,* 1992.)

premenopausal women treated with regimens containing adjuvant cyclophosphamide, methotrexate, and 5-fluorouracil (CMF). DIA, defined as drug-induced cessation of menses for at least 3 months, occurred in 166 of 221 patients (75.1 per cent). At a median follow-up interval of 69 months, patients who developed DIA had a significantly longer disease-free survival (Fig. 22–16) than those who did not. In this study, DIA as a prognostic variable was independent of age, number of involved nodes, or tumor size. Similar observations have been reported by Reyno and associates (1993).

The Danish Breast Cooperative Group evaluated the effects of DIA in a group of 1032 premenopausal and perimenopausal women randomized to observation alone, cyclophosphamide monotherapy, or CMF (Brincker et al., 1987). CMF improved relapse-free survival, regardless of whether DIA was induced; however, cyclophosphamide alone improved relapse-free survival only in patients who developed DIA and it had no effect in patients who retained normal menstrual function. In each of these studies an inverse relationship was evident between age and duration of treatment required to induce ovarian suppression (Dnistrian et al., 1983). Amenorrhea is generally induced within 2 to 4 months in women older than 40 years. Women aged 30 to 39 years require larger cumulative doses to induce ovarian dysfunction, and women younger than 30 years, as a rule, continue to menstruate and exhibit no major alterations in hormone levels despite adjuvant chemotherapy.

The NSABP reported no association between disease-free survival time and depressed ovarian function (Fisher et al., 1979). In the NSABP series, improvement in disease-free survival was better for younger groups of women with a lower incidence of DIA. Bonadonna (1989) reported that women treated with CMF adjuvant chemotherapy who developed DIA and subsequently relapsed had the same response to therapeutic castration as those who did not develop DIA. Collectively, these data imply that the effect of adjuvant cytotoxic chemotherapy in premenopausal women who develop DIA is mediated through two mechanisms, endocrine ablation and a direct cytotoxic effect.

Adrenalectomy and Hypophysectomy

Adrenalectomy and hypophysectomy are effective modes of therapy in hormonally responsive breast cancer, but they are seldom practiced today and currently are of historic interest only. Although the operative mortality rates associated with adrenalectomy and hypophysectomy are low, appreciable morbidity is associated with these procedures (Fracchia et al., 1967). These operations have been replaced by treatment with tamoxifen and the adrenal-blocking agent aminoglutethimide (Wells and Santen, 1984), two simpler, less expensive, and safer means of suppressing estrogen levels. Adrenalectomy became popular in the 1950s as a treatment for metastatic breast cancer in postmenopausal women or in premenopausal women who had previously responded to oophorectomy (Harris and Spratt, 1969). The procedure became possible in 1951 with the introduction of cortisone acetate for adrenal replacement. The first report on adrenalectomy for advanced breast cancer was by Huggins and Bergenstal in 1952.

Hypophysectomy was introduced by Luft and Olivecrona in 1953 as an alternative to adrenalectomy. Response rates of adrenalectomy and hypophysectomy proved to be equivalent, and the choice between the two procedures was one of available expertise (McDonald, 1962): because general surgeons were more readily available than neurosurgeons, adrenalectomy became the more popular procedure.

Santen and coworkers (1981) reported a prospective, randomized clinical trial of surgical versus medical adrenalectomy using aminoglutethimide plus hydrocortisone. Ninety-six postmenopausal women were stratified by disease-free interval, site of dominant disease, and ER status. Estrogen levels decreased similarly in response to either treatment. No significant differences were seen in response rate, response by dominant site of metastatic disease, or response duration (Fig. 22–17). Santen and colleagues concluded that medical adrenalectomy with aminoglutethimide plus hydrocortisone can be logically chosen in place of surgical adrenalectomy.

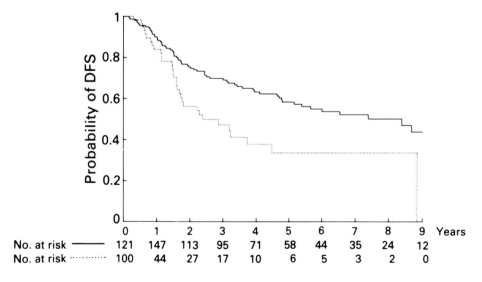

Figure 22–16. Disease-free survival (DFS) curves for premenopausal women with drug-induced amenorrhea (DIA) (solid line) versus women who did not develop amenorrhea (dotted line) after receiving adjuvant chemotherapy, $P < 0.001$. (From Bianco, A. R., Del Mastro, L., Gallo, C., et al.: Prognostic role of amenorrhea induced by adjuvant chemotherapy in premenopausal patients with early breast cancer. Br. J. Cancer, 63:799–803, 1991.)

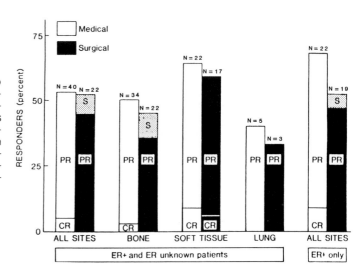

Figure 22–17. Percentage of patients with a response to treatment with medical adrenalectomy. *Open bars* represent patients treated with aminoglutethimide and hydrocortisone; *solid* or *shaded bars* represent patients treated with surgical adrenalectomy. CR = complete response; PR = partial response; S = stable disease. (From Santen, R. J., Worgul, T. J., Samojlik, E., et al.: A randomized trial comparing surgical adrenalectomy with aminoglutethimide plus hydrocortisone in women with advanced breast cancer. N. Engl. J. Med., *305*:545, 1981.)

Kiang and associates (1980) reported equivalent response rates and response duration in 26 patients randomized to hypophysectomy or tamoxifen. Nemoto and colleagues (1984) reported equivalent response rates in 51 patients randomized to tamoxifen or adrenalectomy.

ADDITIVE HORMONE THERAPY

The term "additive hormone therapy" is something of a misnomer. Before the introduction of tamoxifen, which is a competitive inhibitor of hormonal activity, medical hormonal therapy was truly "additive" and consisted of high-dose estrogen, androgens, progestins, and even corticosteroids. Now the armamentarium of additive hormone therapy is being expanded further to include a group of inhibitory compounds such as the aromatase inhibitors aminoglutethimide and fadrozole, the LH-RH agonists, and somatostatin analogues. However, the term "additive hormone therapy" remains in popular use. Perhaps it should be replaced by the term "medical hormone therapy," to distinguish it from the surgical ablative forms of treatment. Nonetheless, medical forms of hormone manipulation have largely replaced the surgical ablative procedures, not because they are more effective but because they are associated with lower morbidity and better patient acceptance.

In (1) patients likely to be hormonally responsive (that is, patients who are ER positive—or, even better, ER positive, PgR positive), (2) patients with a disease-free interval greater than 2 years, and (3) patients without immediately life-threatening visceral or central nervous system metastases, hormonal manipulation is appropriate first-line therapy.

Primary hormone therapy can be expected to produce an objective response in 50% of ER-positive and 70% of ER-positive, PgR-positive patients. For *premenopausal* patients, the primary therapy of choice is either tamoxifen or oophorectomy; though, newer approaches involving total estrogen suppression with tamoxifen plus an LH-RH analogue, or increased growth factor suppression with tamoxifen plus SMS analogues, are under investigation. For *postmenopausal* women, the primary hormone therapy of

choice is tamoxifen, but megestrol acetate—or even diethylstilbestrol (DES)—produces an essentially equivalent response.

Secondary hormone therapy is a more difficult problem. There are several agents to choose from, but it is unclear which factors predict response. Classically, it has been taught that the best predictor of response to a second form of hormone therapy is an initial response to a primary form of hormone therapy. In general this is true; however, response rates to second-line hormone therapy in prior responders are often low (from 14% to 40%), and responses as high as 30% have been reported in patients who fail to respond to initial therapy (Wilson, 1983). Wilson's data on secondary responses are summarized in Table 22–18. Seymour and coworkers (1990) from South Africa have tried further to define who will respond to second-line chemotherapy. They studied a group of 22 patients who had previously responded to first-line hormone therapy. Nine of 22 responded to second-line hormone treatment. Approximately 50 per cent of patients remained ER positive, but the responses were equivalent between ER-positive and ER-negative cases. However, 8 of 12 patients with diploid tumors responded, whereas only 1 of 10 patients with aneuploid tumors did.

Secondary responses to hormone therapy are, therefore, difficult to predict. Nevertheless, secondary, and even tertiary, responses to hormonal manipulation do occur and can be durable. Secondary hormone therapy is most appropriate for patients with indolent metastatic disease such as soft tissue– and bone-dominant metastases (Sherry et al., 1986a, 1986b; Hortobagyi, 1991; and Yamashita et al., 1991). Secondary hormone therapy is not appropriate for patients with visceral-dominant disease.

For patients with *metastatic disease to bone,* the bone scan and serum alkaline phosphatase may be unreliable parameters of response to hormone therapy or chemotherapy. Twelve of sixteen patients observed to have healing lytic lesions on x-ray exhibited paradoxical deterioration on bone scan after 3 months' treatment. This was characterized by increased activity of baseline lesions and even by the appearance of new foci of tracer uptake (Coleman et al., 1988). These changes are attributed to a "flare" of osteo-

Table 22–18. SECONDARY RESPONSE TO HORMONE THERAPY AFTER RESPONSE OR FAILURE TO INITIAL HORMONAL THERAPY

First Treatment	Second Treatment	Patients (N)	Response to First Treatment No. (%)	Response after First Response No. (%)	Response after First Failure No. (%)
Androgen	Tamoxifen	51	26 (51)	18 (69)	9 (36)
Tamoxifen	Androgen	26	11 (42)	4 (36)	3 (20)
Estrogen	Tamoxifen	25	12 (48)	12 (100)	8 (62)
Tamoxifen	Estrogen	5	2 (40)	2 (100)	1 (33)
Progestin	Tamoxifen	7	3 (58)	2 (67)	3 (75)
Tamoxifen	Progestin	12	7 (58)	1 (14)	1 (20)
Oophorectomy/ Adrenelectomy	Tamoxifen	18	8 (44)	2 (25)	0 (0)
Hypophysectomy	Tamoxifen	16	12 (75)	7 (58)	0 (0)
Tamoxifen	Hypophysectomy	58	26 (45)	15 (58)	8 (25)
Tamoxifen	Aiminoglutethimide	91	41 (45)	22 (54)	16 (32)
Aminoglutethimide	Tamoxifen	31	16 (52)	5 (31)	2 (13)
	TOTALS	330	164 (50)	90 (55)	51 (31)

(Modified from Wilson, A. J.: Response in breast cancer to a second hormonal therapy. Rev. Endocrine-Related Cancer, *14*:5, 1983.)

blast activity induced by successful treatment, as confirmed by a rise in serum osteocalcin and alkaline phosphatase bone isoenzyme. New lesions that appeared after 6 months indicated progressive disease. The flare response seems to be the rule rather than the exception after successful systemic therapy for bone metastases. The appearance of new lesions during the first 3 months of therapy is as likely to herald a clinical response as it is to indicate disease progression. These findings have been confirmed in a much larger study by Vogel and coworkers (1992). In the absence of corroborating evidence of disease progression, patients with early bone scan changes or x-ray changes of increasing osteoblastic activity should continue on therapy until more definitive evidence of response or progression is observed.

Tamoxifen

Tamoxifen (Nolvadex) entered clinical trials in Europe in 1971 (Jordan, 1992). It was approved in the United States by the U. S. Food and Drug Administration on December 30, 1977 for the treatment of metastatic breast cancer in postmenopausal women. Tamoxifen rapidly became the treatment of choice for this indication because of high response rate, safety, and few side effects (Ingle et al., 1981; Bloom and Fishman, 1983; Lippman, 1983; and Manni et al., 1979). Currently, tamoxifen is approved for the treatment of all stages of breast cancer in both pre- and postmenopausal women and it is being investigated in both Europe and the United States as a possible chemopreventive agent in women at high risk of developing breast cancer.

Tamoxifen is a nonsteroidal triphenylethylene compound that is structurally related to DES (Legha, 1988). Tamoxifen acts primarily by blocking the binding of estrogen to ER, but it also exerts ER-independent suppressive activity by enhancing production of inhibitory growth factor TGFβ and blocking production of the enhancing growth factor IGF-I. Breast cancer cells treated with tamoxifen accumulate in the G_0/G_1 stage of the cell cycle, with resultant inhibition of growth (Love, 1989). The drug is not cytocidal but is cytostatic in its antitumor action, and tamoxifen should be considered chemosuppressive rather than chemotoxic (Lerner and Jordan, 1990). It has long been recognized that the cytostatic effect of tamoxifen is potentially reversible (Lippman et al., 1976; and Manni et al., 1977), and cells can be "rescued" from the tamoxifen-induced cell cycle blockade by excess estrogen (Lippman and Bolan, 1975). It has also been demonstrated that once tamoxifen is cleared from a rat with mammary cancer, the malignant cells are reactivated, and palpable tumors develop (Jordan et al., 1980). In the *N*-nitrosourea–induced model of rat mammary carcinoma, continuous administration of tamoxifen completely suppresses the appearance of palpable tumors. Cessation of therapy, however, results in the appearance of mammary tumors in as many as 50% of animals (Jordan et al., 1991*a*). These data demonstrate that the effect of tamoxifen is reversible, and they provide the experimental basis for prolonged tamoxifen therapy. (Jordan, 1983; and Jordan et al., 1984). Tamoxifen therapy given early in disease is not curative but suppressive, and the favorable effect of tamoxifen may be in delaying recurrence, it is hoped indefinitely, with prolonged use of the drug (Love, 1989).

Tamoxifen Dose

After oral administration of the standard dose (10 mg twice daily) a steady-state serum concentration is not achieved until the fourth week of therapy. The parent compound has a half-life of 7 days; that of the active metabolite, *N*-desmethyltamoxifen, is 14 days. Tamoxifen can be detected in the serum for 4 weeks after treatment is discontinued (Legha, 1988; and Love, 1989). Because of the marked delay in achieving a steady-state serum concentration, one would not anticipate a therapeutic effect from tamoxifen in less than 4 weeks, and, indeed, it may take as long as 12 weeks to induce a favorable response. Although tamoxifen dosage is generally 10 mg twice daily, the same biologic effect can be achieved with a single daily dose of 20 mg because of its long half-life (Buzdar et al., 1994).

Tamoxifen does not have a significant dose-response

curve, and response rates are not enhanced by dose escalation to 40 mg, 90 mg, or even 120 mg per day (Manni and Pearson, 1980 and Ingle, 1984). Doses of 120 mg per day are more effective in suppressing menses in premenopausal patients; however, the response rate to 20 mg per day is equivalent to that of larger doses, despite the fact that estrogenic effects are incompletely blocked and most premenopausal women continue to menstruate.

Tamoxifen Flare

"Tamoxifen flare" was described in 1978 by Plotkin and coworkers. This curious phenomenon, characterized by increased bone or soft tissue pain, and occasionally by hypercalcemia, occurs in approximately 10% of cases. When a flare occurs, it develops in the first few weeks of therapy. Contrary to what may seem like progression, a flare generally heralds a response to treatment. Flares should be treated with analgesics or other symptomatic therapy, and full-dose tamoxifen should be continued. Brooks and Lippman (1985) proposed that the flare occurs because it takes several weeks for tamoxifen to reach therapeutic levels, and at lower concentrations the drug may be estrogenic and stimulatory, as has been noted in tissue culture. In the M. D. Anderson series, hypercalcemic flares were peculiar to patients who had osteolytic or mixed lytic and blastic bone metastases (Legha et al., 1981). Hypercalcemia can generally be managed with hydration and continuation of tamoxifen therapy; though, if the hypercalcemia is severe, tamoxifen should be discontinued temporarily and reinstituted cautiously at a reduced dose, with or without a short course of corticosteroids. Even though hypercalcemia is a potentially serious complication of tamoxifen therapy, it is generally short lived and can be controlled with supportive measures. A hypercalcemic flare in a breast cancer patient with bone metastases usually heralds a therapeutic response and should not be misinterpreted as disease progression (Legha, 1988).

Tamoxifen as Primary Therapy in Elderly Patients

Tamoxifen has been evaluated as primary therapy for breast cancer in elderly and frail women who are not believed to be candidates for surgery (Bradbeer and Kyngdon, 1983; and Auclerc et al., 1990). In women 70 years and older, intercurrent illness can prevent conventional treatment, and death from causes other than cancer occurs in 30% to 50% of patients. Horobin and coworkers (1990, 1991) reported on long-term follow-up of 113 patients, aged 70 to 93 years, with operable local-regional breast cancer who were treated with tamoxifen, 20 mg twice daily, as their sole primary therapy. There were 38 (34%) complete responses with a median duration of 50 months, 17 (15%) partial responses for 18 months, 34 (30%) cases of disease stabilization for 21 months, and 24 (21%) cases of disease progression. The median survival for the entire group was 5 years, but more than half of the responders had local relapse by that time. Similar findings were reported by Akhtar and

colleagues (1991) in a group of 100 elderly women with a median age of 76.3 years. It can be concluded from these data that, in the short term, tamoxifen is a valid alternative to conventional therapy for operable breast cancer in elderly women, provided they are followed closely. More than half the patients treated with tamoxifen alone will require a change in management to maintain local control (Bates et al., 1991). These patients may be even poorer operative candidates when their disease progresses.

Tamoxifen in Premenopausal Women

The traditional role of oophorectomy as the primary mode of hormonal therapy in receptor-positive, premenopausal women is being challenged successfully by tamoxifen. In randomized, controlled trials of more than 200 patients, the rate of response and the duration of response to tamoxifen were equivalent to those with oophorectomy; Buchanan et al., 1986; (Haas, 1981; Margreiter and Wiegele, 1984; Planting et al., 1985 and Ingle et al., 1986). Many of these investigators now feel that tamoxifen is the primary hormonal treatment of choice for premenopausal women as well as for postmenopausal women with hormonally responsive metastatic disease.

It is important to point out that, even though tamoxifen is an antiestrogen, it is not a contraceptive. In fact, tamoxifen has been used to induce ovulation in subfertile women (Jordan, 1992). In premenopausal women with breast cancer, tamoxifen therapy is associated with elevations in serum estradiol and progesterone (Jordan et al., 1991b). Initially, it was believed that the high circulating levels of estrogen induced by tamoxifen might prevent tamoxifen from binding to ER and nullify its therapeutic effect, or worse, result in tumor stimulation (Legha, 1988). This has not been observed clinically (Sunderland and Osborne, 1991).

Since tamoxifen is a competitive inhibitor of estrogen, one might anticipate an enhanced effect in a low-estrogen environment. There are no reports on the simultaneous impact of ovarian ablation and tamoxifen; however, there are now three reports of the combined use of the LH-RH agonist goserelin (Zoladex) and tamoxifen for advanced breast cancer in premenopausal women (Robertson et al., 1989; Nicholson et al., 1990; and Dixon et al., 1991). Goserelin reduces the release of pituitary gonadotropins, with a resultant reduction in ovarian steroidogenesis to postmenopausal levels, in essence producing medical oophorectomy (Jordan, 1992). Preliminary data from these trials show that there is no increase in the response rate for patients treated with goserelin plus tamoxifen, though the time to disease progression is extended.

Adjuvant Tamoxifen in Operable Breast Cancer

Risk Assessment. The most reliable risk factor for predicting the probability of recurrence in operable breast cancer is the status of axillary lymph nodes (Bonadonna et al., 1976; Fisher et al., 1975, 1983a, 1968) (see Table 22–15).

Essentially a quantitative relationship exists between the number of involved axillary lymph nodes and disease-free survival (see Fig. 22–15) as well as absolute survival. Steroid hormone receptors (ER, PgR) are reliable risk factors in Stage II breast cancer; "receptor-positive patients" have a significantly better prognosis than receptor-negative ones.

Determining the risk of recurrence of node-negative breast cancer has been considerably more difficult. Hormone receptor status has not been a consistently reliable prognostic indicator. A variety of other risk factors are being evaluated, e.g. *erb* B_2 (HER 2/neu) oncogene amplification (Tandon et al., 1989; Paik et al., 1990; and Wiltschke et al., 1994), cathepsin D (Tandon et al., 1990), nm 23 RNA (Bevilacqua et al., 1989), haptoglobin-related protein (Kuhajda et al., 1989), Ki 67 immunostaining (Sahin et al., 1991), occult bone marrow micrometastases (Cote et al., 1991), DNA ploidy and S-phase fraction (Joensuu et al., 1990; Keyhani-Rofagha et al., 1990; Clark et al., 1992). Elaborate schemata have been developed to integrate these so that appropriate therapeutic decisions can be made in node-negative cases (McGuire et al., 1990; and McGuire and Clark, 1992). This large series of potential prognostic factors has not produced reliable, reproducible data and should not yet be incorporated into the clinical decision-making process. Currently, the only consistently reliable prognostic indicator in node-negative breast cancer is *tumor size* (Rosen et al., 1989a, 1989b, 1991; and Tabár et al.,

1992). Persons with tumors smaller than 1 cm in maximum diameter have a disease-free survival rate at 10 years of 92%, whereas that for tumors 1.0 to 1.9 cm is 78%, and for those of at least 2 cm is 69%. Because of the good prognosis for patients with tumors smaller than 1 cm in diameter they probably are not candidates for adjuvant therapy with cytotoxic drugs. These persons, however, may still benefit from tamoxifen. Clearly, there is a need for more reliable markers in node-negative breast cancer, so that adjuvant therapy can be reserved for patients at high risk of recurrence (Gasparini et al., 1993).

Tamoxifen in Node-Negative Breast Cancer

In the Early Breast Cancer Trialists' Collaborative Group (1992) meta-analysis of 133 randomized trials of systemic adjuvant therapy for early breast cancer, 30,000 women were in tamoxifen trials. There were highly significant reductions in the annual rates of both recurrence (25%) and death (17%) for the tamoxifen-treated groups ($P < .00001$). There were no differences between different doses of tamoxifen (20, 30, or 40 mg per day); however, longer courses of tamoxifen therapy (2–5 years) were significantly more effective than shorter courses (< 2 years). Of the 30,000 women in tamoxifen trials, nearly 13,000 had "neg-

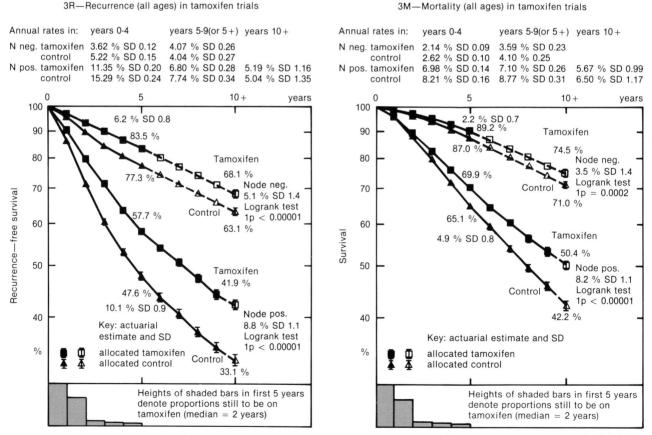

Figure 22–18. Ten-year outcome of tamoxifen trials, subdivided by nodal status. 3R = recurrence (disease-free survival); 3M = mortality. (Early Breast Cancer Trialists' Collaborative Group: Systemic treatment of early breast cancer by hormonal, cytotoxic, or immune therapy: 133 randomised trials involving 31,000 recurrences and 24,000 deaths among 75,000 women. Lancet, *339*: 1–15, 71–85, 1992. © by *The Lancet Ltd.*, 1992.)

Table 22-19. RANDOMIZED TRIALS OF ADJUVANT TAMOXIFEN ALONE (VERSUS CONTROL) IN NODE-NEGATIVE BREAST CANCER

Trial	Daily Dose	Duration of Therapy	Premenopausal	Postmenopausal	Disease-Free Survival	Survival
NSABP B-14*	20 mg	5 and 10 years	812	1832	p<0.0001	p≤0.05
NATO†	20 mg	2 years	0	604	p≤0.05	p≤0.05
Christie Hospital‡	20 mg	1 year	0	382	N.S.	N.S.
Stockholm§	40 mg	2 and 5 years	0	696	p<0.01 in ER +	N.S
CRC¶	20 mg	2 years	316	571	p≤.05	N.S.
Scottish#	20 mg	5 years	212	539	p<0.1>0.05	N.S.

(Adapted from Love, R. R.: Tamoxifen therapy in primary breast cancer: Biology, efficacy, and side effects. J. Clin. Oncol., 7:803, 1989.)
*National Surgical Adjuvant Breast and Bowel Project (Fisher et al., 1989a).
Abbreviation: N.S. = No significant difference.
†Nolvadex Adjuvant Trial Organization (Baum et al., 1983; 1985; 1988).
‡(Ribiero and Palmer, 1983; Ribiero and Swindell, 1985, 1988).
§(Rutqvist et al., 1989; Fornander et al., 1989).
¶(Bartlett et al., 1987; Stewart, 1992).
#Cancer Research Campaign (Abram et al., 1988).

ative'' axillary lymph nodes. Tamoxifen in node-negative patients was associated with a significant reduction in relapse-free survival and overall survival times for women of all ages. In fact, the odds of death from any cause were reduced for women treated with tamoxifen. Data from the Early Breast Cancer Trialists' Collaborative Group in both node-positive and node-negative patients are graphically displayed in Figure 22–18 (Allegra, 1984b). The data from several adjuvant tamoxifen trials in node-negative breast cancer are summarized in Table 22–19 (Love, 1989).

Data from NSABP trial B-14 is the only adjuvant trial designed specifically to evaluate the effects of tamoxifen on node-negative breast cancer. It is the largest trial ever performed for node-negative breast cancer, and the results from this trial are the basis for a tamoxifen chemoprevention trial in women at high risk (Fisher et al., 1989a, 1989b, 1992). The NSABP conducted a prospective, randomized, double-blind, placebo-controlled trial of adjuvant tamoxifen, 10 mg twice daily, in 2644 ER-positive (≥10 fmol/mg of protein) patients with breast cancer and histologically negative axillary lymph nodes. At the time of the initial publication of this trial, a highly significant prolongation of disease-free survival was observed in women treated with tamoxifen as compared to those receiving placebo (83%

disease free at 4 years, compared to 77% [*P* < .00001]). Although there was not as yet a survival advantage for tamoxifen-treated cases, with further maturation of the data, a survival advantage was observed. Improved disease-free survival was observed in all subsets analyzed in the group treated with tamoxifen, whether they were grouped by age (women ≤49 years vs. women ≥50 years); by tumor size (≤2 cm or >2 cm); or ER (10–49 fmol, 50–99 fmol, or ≥100 fmol). The disease-free survival rates for women aged 49 years and younger and 50 and older are graphically displayed in Figure 22–19. The sites of treatment failure are listed in Table 22–20. It is important to emphasize three things depicted in this table: (1) Local control was improved with tamoxifen; (2) survival free of distant metastases was improved with tamoxifen; and (3) women treated with tamoxifen had a significant reduction in the rate of development of cancer in the opposite breast.

The drug was tolerated amazingly well, and the side effects reported by patients enrolled in NSABP B-14 were essentially the same for those treated with tamoxifen and those who received placebo (Table 22–21). It should be pointed out that a larger proportion of women younger than 40 years reported hot flashes, vaginal discharge, and irregular menses than did women (aged 40 to 49 or >50). A

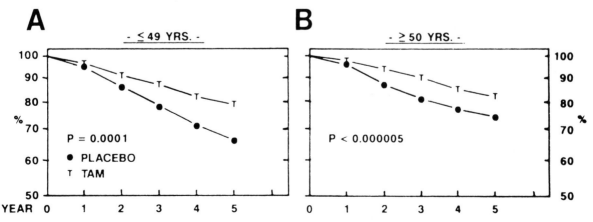

Figure 22–19. Effect of tamoxifen (T) on disease-free survival related to age. *A,* Placebo: 438 patients, 111 events; tamoxifen: 440 patients, 59 events (TAM = T = tamoxifen). *B,* Placebo: 988 patients, 207 events; tamoxifen: 977 patients; 130 events. (From Fisher, B., Wickerham, D. L., Redmond, C.: Recent developments in the systemic adjuvant therapy of breast cancer. Semin. Oncol., *19:*263–277, 1992.)

Table 22–20. SITE OF RECURRENCE AFTER TREATMENT FAILURE FOR 1318 PATIENTS TREATED WITH TAMOXIFEN AND 1326 WHO RECEIVED PLACEBO

| Site of Recurrence | Treatment Failures (No.) | | P Value† |
	Placebo*	Tamoxifen*	
Local	37	7	<.0001
Chest wall and surgical scar	26	7	.0006
Ipsilateral breast after lumpectomy‡	11	0	.0008
Regional	11	8	.4
Distant	117	73	.0005
Opposite breast§	29	13	.0089
Skeletal	46	28	.0221
Respiratory	23	13	.07
All other distant recurrences	19	29	.9
Second primary cancer¶	12	15	.6
Death without breast cancer	15	15	.9

(From Fisher, B., Costantino, J., Redmond, C., et al.: A randomized clinical trial in the treatment of patients with node-negative breast cancer who have estrogen receptor–positive tumors. N. Engl. J. Med., *320*:479–484, 1989. Reprinted with permission from *The New England Journal of Medicine*.)

*Site unknown in one patient.
†By comparison of the average hazard rates.
‡Lumpectomy was performed in 499 patients in the placebo group and 496 in the tamoxifen group.
§Includes second primary breast cancer.
¶Excludes cancers of the opposite breast.

very similar side effect profile was reported by Love and coworkers (1991). The treatment of tamoxifen-induced hot flashes has been difficult. Transdermal clonidine use has been found disappointing (Goldberg et al., 1994). Clonidine by mouth (0.1mg/d) may be more effective. Low-dose megestrol acetate (20 mg twice daily) has been reported to ameliorate tamoxifen-induced hot flashes in a placebo-controlled clinical trial (Loprinzi et al., 1994).

Tamoxifen in Stage II Breast Cancer

The data from several trials of adjuvant tamoxifen alone are summarized in Table 22–22. Data from the Early Breast Cancer Trialists' Collaborative Group on both node-positive and node-negative breast cancer are graphically displayed in Figure 22–18. The first of the major tamoxifen adjuvant trials to confirm a survival advantage of patients treated with tamoxifen as a single agent was the Nolvadex Adjuvant Trial Organization (NATO) trial, under the chairmanship of Prof. Michael Baum of King's College Hospital

Table 22–21. RATES OF SIDE EFFECTS IN NATIONAL SURGICAL ADJUVANT BREAST AND BOWEL PROJECT (NSABP) B-14 FOR 1422 PATIENTS TREATED WITH TAMOXIFEN AND 1439 WHO RECEIVED PLACEBO

Side Effects	Placebo (%)	Tamoxifen (%)
Hot flashes	46.2	62.4
Fluid retention	28.6	30.9
Vaginal discharge	14.2	28.4
Irregular menses	17.6	23.6
Skin rash	14.3	17.7
Diarrhea	12.9	9.8
Toxicity that forced withdrawal	6.2	9.4

(Data from Fisher, B., Costantino, J., Redmond, C., et al.: A randomized clinical trial in the treatment of patients with node-negative breast cancer who have estrogen receptor–positive tumors. N. Engl. J. Med., *320*:479–484, 1989.)

in London. The NATO trial studied 1285 patients 75 years of age or younger. The study included premenopausal node-positive patients as well as postmenopausal node-negative and node-positive patients (Baum et al., 1983, 1985, 1988). The patients were randomized to tamoxifen, 10 mg twice daily, for 2 years or to no further treatment. The results are displayed in Figure 22–20. The benefits of tamoxifen therapy in the NATO trial appear to be independent of menopausal, nodal, or ER status, though in other large series, benefit was restricted to ER-positive patients (Pritchard et al., 1984, Rutqvist et al., 1984; Rose et al., 1985a and 1985b; and Pritchard, 1987).

Adjuvant Tamoxifen Plus Chemotherapy in Stage II Breast Cancer

The early trials of combination adjuvant therapy were basically designed to determine whether the addition of tamoxifen to chemotherapy would enhance the effect of chemotherapy. The NSABP performed the largest such study (Fisher et al., 1981, 1983b, 1986). In this study, 1891 women with primary operable breast cancer and positive axillary nodes were randomized to receive melphalan (L-PAM) plus 5-fluorouracil, that is, PF or PF plus tamoxifen. Tamoxifen was administered as 10 mg twice daily for 2 years. The initial results of this trial are illustrated graphically in Figure 22–21. Women aged 50 years or older derived a clear benefit from the addition of tamoxifen to PF, and this benefit increased with the level of both the ER and PgR. For women aged 49 years or younger, the addition of tamoxifen provided no benefit, regardless of the ER or PgR level. Another important observation was that postmenopausal women treated with tamoxifen began to suffer relapses in the third year, that is, 1 year after tamoxifen was discontinued. This prompted the NSABP to test whether women who were disease free at 2 years would benefit from an

Table 22–22. RANDOMIZED TRIALS OF ADJUVANT TAMOXIFEN ALONE (VERSUS CONTROL) IN NODE-POSITIVE BREAST CANCER

Trial	Daily Dose (mg)	Duration of Therapy (yr)	Patients (N)		Survival (P Value)	
			Premenopausal	Postmenopausal	Disease-Free Survival	Total
NATO*	20	2 y	128	393	≤.05	p≤0.05
Christie Hospital†	20	1 y	0	206	<.1>.05	N.S.
Stockholm‡	40	2 y	0	1407	≤.05	N.S.
CRC§	20	2 y	140	232	<.01	N.S.
Scottish¶	20	5 y	0	456	≤.05	p≤0.05
Danish#	30	1 y	0	1650	≤.05	N.S.

(Adapted from Love, RR: Tamoxifen therapy in primary breast cancer: Biology, efficacy, and side effects. J. Clin. Oncol., 7:803–815, 1989.)
*Nolvadex Adjuvant Trial Organization (Baum et al., 1983; 1985; 1988).
†(Ribiero and Palmer, 1983; Ribiero and Swindell, 1985; 1988).
‡(Rutqvist et al., 1989; Fornander et al., 1989).
§Cancer Research Campaign (Abram, 1988).
¶(Bartlett et al., 1987; Stewart, 1992).
#(Rose et al., 1985).

additional year of tamoxifen, and, indeed, they did (Fisher et al., 1987*b*) (Fig. 22–22). This is the first clinical trial to confirm Jordan's laboratory data that tamoxifen is cytostatic rather than cytocidal, that discontinuation of tamoxifen allows reactivation of latent tumor cells, and that more prolonged tamoxifen therapy yields more benefit than shorter courses. Several other clinical trials have confirmed that short courses of tamoxifen (1 year) fail to enhance the effect of chemotherapy in both premenopausal and postmenopausal women (Ingle et al., 1988*a*, 1989; Taylor et al., 1989; Tormey et al., 1990; Dombernowsky et al., 1992). The value of adding long-term (5 years') tamoxifen therapy to chemotherapy for treating postmenopausal, node-positive women has been confirmed by the Eastern Cooperative Oncology Group (Falkson et al., 1990).

The trials of chemotherapy with or without tamoxifen do not separate out the effect of tamoxifen alone. Given the beneficial effects of tamoxifen alone (particularly in postmenopausal women) reported in the European literature, one cannot help but wonder what, if any, additional effect is contributed by the chemotherapy. Again, the definitive trial was performed by the NSABP (Fisher et al., 1990, 1992), which randomized 1124 eligible postmenopausal, receptor-positive, node-positive women to one of three treatment arms: (1) tamoxifen (T) alone for 5 years; (2) tamoxifen for 5 years plus four cycles of Adriamycin plus cyclophosphamide (AC); or (3) tamoxifen for 5 years plus a prolonged course of L-PAM (P) plus 5-fluorouracil (F), with or without Adriamycin (PF or PAF). The data from this trial confirm that the addition of chemotherapy (AC,

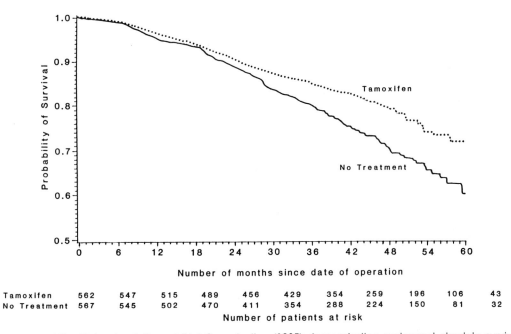

Figure 22–20. Results of the Nolvadex Adjuvant Trial Organization (1985) demonstrating prolonged absolute survival in breast cancer patients treated with adjuvant tamoxifen. (Modified from Baum, M., Brinkley, D. M., Dosset, J. A., et al.: Controlled trial of tamoxifen as single adjuvant agent in the management of early breast cancer: Analysis at six years by Nolvadex Adjuvant Trial Organization. Lancet, i:836, 1985.)

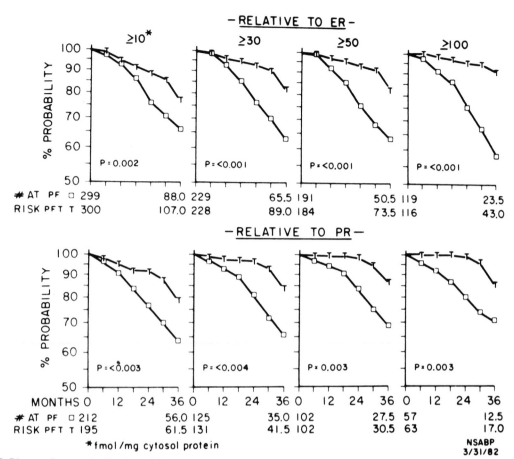

Figure 22-21. Disease-free survival in stage II breast cancer patients age 50 years or older treated with PF (L-PAM + 5-fluorouracil) versus those treated with PFT (PF + tamoxifen) relative to ER and PgR (PR) concentration. (From Fisher, B., Redmond, C., Brown, A., et al.: Influence of tumor estrogen and progesterone receptor levels on the response to tamoxifen and chemotherapy in primary breast cancer. J. Clin. Oncol., *1*:227, 1983.)

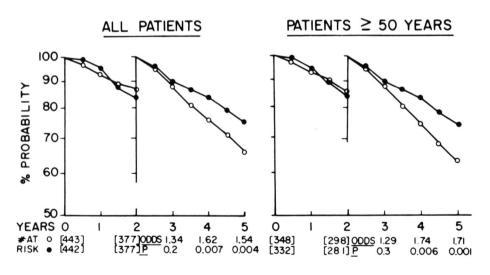

Figure 22-22. Effect of an additional year of tamoxifen on the disease-free survival of patients who were free of disease 2 years after surgery. *Open circles* indicate women who received melphalan, fluorouracil, and tamoxifen alone, and *closed circles* indicate women who received this treatment plus an additional year of tamoxifen. (Reproduced with permission from Fisher, B., Brown, A., Wolmark, N., et al.: Prolonging tamoxifen therapy for primary breast cancer. Ann. Intern. Med., *106*:649–654, 1987.)

PF, or PAF) clearly enhances the disease-free survival and overall survival for postmenopausal women treated long-term with tamoxifen. They also confirm that a short course of four cycles of AC is equivalent in effect to longer-term chemotherapy with PF or PAF. The data for AC plus tamoxifen versus tamoxifen alone are shown in Figure 22–23.

An Italian study has been reported that did not show an advantage from the addition of chemotherapy to long-term tamoxifen (Boccardo et al., 1990*a*). However, the benefit of adding chemotherapy to tamoxifen in postmenopausal, node-positive women has been confirmed by Pearson and coworkers (1989) as well as by the large meta-analysis performed by the Early Breast Cancer Trialists' Collaborative Group (1992).

Tamoxifen for Breast Cancer Prevention

In May, 1992, the NSABP initiated a major clinical trial to evaluate the role of tamoxifen in the prevention of breast cancer in women at high risk. The rationale is based on the efficacy of tamoxifen in the treatment of advanced breast cancer, its relatively low toxicity profile, and the observation that women treated long term with adjuvant tamoxifen are at significantly lower risk of developing carcinoma of the opposite breast (Fornander et al., 1989; Fisher and Redmond, 1991; and Rutqvist et al., 1991); (Fisher, 1992). The Early Breast Cancer Trialists' Collaborative Group (1992) confirmed a 39% odds reduction in the risk of carcinoma of the opposite breast for women treated with adjuvant tamoxifen (122 cases in 9128 women) compared to controls (184 in 9135 women) ($P < .00001$).

The NSABP Breast Cancer Prevention Trial (BCPT) will involve 16,000 women in the United States and Canada who are at increased risk for the development of breast cancer. These women will be randomized to tamoxifen, 20 mg daily as a single dose for 5 years, or to placebo for 5 years. All women aged 60 and older will be eligible for the BCPT, as well as women aged 35 to 59 who have additional risk factors that increase their risk to at least that of a woman aged 60 or older. A woman of 60 years has a risk of developing breast cancer of 335 per 100,000 females per year, whereas a woman aged 35 who has no other risk factors has a risk of developing breast cancer of 66 per 100,000 females per year. In other words, a woman of 60 is five times more likely to develop breast cancer based on age alone. Other risk factors to be considered in women aged 35 to 59 are the number of first-degree relatives (mother, sister, daughter) with breast cancer, a history of lobular carcinoma in situ, a history of atypical hyperplasia, previous breast biopsy for benign disease, nulliparity, age at first live birth (≥age 29), and menarche before age 12 years. The estimates of risk are then calculated according to the Gail risk model (Gail et al., 1989; and Jordan, 1992) (Fig. 22–24). Two studies have validated the Gail model for predicting individual breast cancer risk (Bondy et al., 1994; and Spiegelman et al., 1994).

The primary objective of the BCPT is to determine whether tamoxifen can reduce the incidence of breast cancer in women who are at increased risk. However, tamoxi-

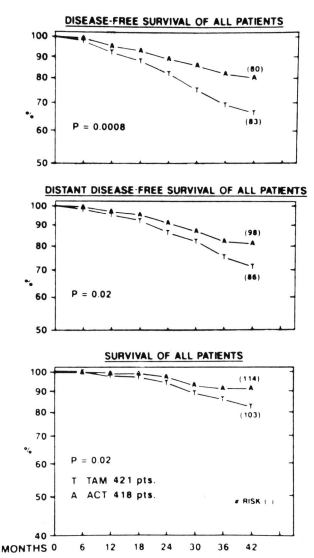

Figure 22–23. Disease-free survival, distant disease-free survival, and survival of patients treated postoperatively with ACT (Adriamycin, cytoxan, and tamoxifen) versus those treated with TAM (tamoxifen) alone. A = Adriamycin; T = tamoxifen. (From Fisher, B., Wickerham, D. L., Redmond, C.: Recent developments in the systemic adjuvant therapy of breast cancer. Semin. Oncol., *19*:263–277, 1992.)

fen has selective estrogen-agonist effects on bone and lipid metabolism. Tamoxifen may therefore reduce the risk of osteoporotic fractures as well as that of coronary artery disease (Nayfield et al., 1991). In the meta-analysis performed by the Early Breast Cancer Trialists' Collaborative Group (1992), women treated with tamoxifen had a significant reduction in breast cancer–unrelated deaths as well as in breast cancer–related deaths. The reduction in breast cancer–unrelated deaths was due predominantly to a reduction in vascular mortality.

Potential Breast Cancer–Unrelated Benefits of the Breast Cancer Prevention Trial

Cardiovascular Risk Factors. Cardiovascular disease is a major cause of morbidity and mortality in postmenopausal

To Determine the Worth of Tamoxifen
For Preventing Breast Cancer

**POTENTIAL
PARTICIPANTS:**

> 60 years old -   with / without risk factors
35-59 years old -   with risk factors:
    • LCIS
    • relative with BC
    • breast biopsy
    • atypical hyperplasia
    • > 25 1st child
    • no children
    • menarche < 12

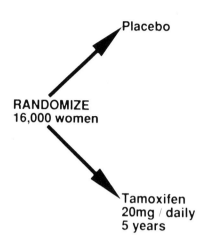

Placebo

**RANDOMIZE
16,000 women**

Tamoxifen
20mg / daily
5 years

Figure 22–24. Schema for the National Surgical Adjuvant Breast and Bowel Project (NSABP) Breast Cancer Prevention Trial. Entry requirements are shown on the left of the diagram. Women between the ages of 39 and 59 years must have an accumulation of risk factors that are the same or in excess of the risks of a 60-year-old woman. LCIS = lobular carcinoma in situ; BC = breast cancer. (From Jordan, V. C.: The role of tamoxifen in the treatment and prevention of breast cancer. Curr. Probl. Cancer, *16*:131–176, 1992.)

(but not premenopausal) women, presumably, owing to the favorable effects of estrogen on lipid metabolism. There had been concern that tamoxifen, an antiestrogen, might accelerate the development of atherosclerosis, but it appears that tamoxifen exerts an estrogen agonist effect rather than an antiestrogen effect on the blood lipid profile (Love et al., 1990; Schapira et al., 1990; Rutqvist et al., 1993; and Thangaraju et al., 1994). The mean cholesterol level declines 34.6 ± 3.6 mg/dL in women taking tamoxifen. Serum cholesterol fell by more than 10 mg/dL in 73% of women taking tamoxifen, and by more than 40 mg/dL in 40%. The decrease is due predominantly to a decrease in low-density lipoprotein cholesterol; only minor changes are observed in high-density lipoprotein cholesterol. This has translated into

a significant decrease in fatal myocardial infarctions in the tamoxifen-treated group in the Scottish Adjuvant Tamoxifen Trial (McDonald and Stewart, 1991). Tamoxifen given for 5 years as an adjuvant for early-stage breast cancer seems to have a cardioprotective, estrogen-like effect in postmenopausal women. One would expect to see this same cardioprotective effect in participants in the BCPT who do not have breast cancer.

Effects on Bone Mineral Density. The concern that tamoxifen would have an antiestrogen effect in bone and accelerate the development of osteoporosis appears unfounded (Turken et al., 1989; and Fornander et al., 1990). In a study from the University of Wisconsin, the lumbar spine bone mineral density of postmenopausal women

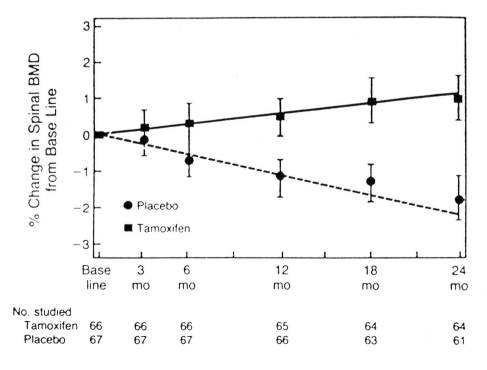

Figure 22–25. Change in mean (± SE) lumbar-spinal bone mineral density (BMD) in women with breast cancer given either tamoxifen or a placebo for 2 years. The *solid* and *dashed lines* represent the mean regression lines for the tamoxifen and placebo groups, respectively, as determined from the individual regression lines for each woman (only women with ≥3 data points were included in this analysis). (From Love, R. R., Mazess, R. B., Barden, H. S., et al.: Effects of tamoxifen on bone mineral density in postmenopausal women with breast cancer. N. Engl. J. Med., *326*:852–856, 1992. Reprinted with permission from *The New England Journal of Medicine*.)

No. studied

	Base line	3 mo	6 mo	12 mo	18 mo	24 mo
Tamoxifen	66	66	66	65	64	64
Placebo	67	67	67	66	63	61

treated with tamoxifen increased 0.61% per year, whereas in those given placebo it *decreased* 1.00% per year (Love et al., 1992*a*) (Fig. 22–25).

Potential Risks

Since the NSABP BCPT is the largest trial of long-term tamoxifen in women who do not have a malignancy, there is great concern about potential side effects and the long-term risks of this medication. In general the side effect profile of tamoxifen is quite favorable: most reported side effects are distributed equally between the tamoxifen-treated and the placebo control groups. There are, however, three major areas of potential risk from long-term tamoxifen: thromboembolic events, ocular toxicity, and the induction of new primary tumors.

Thromboembolic Events. Several reports indicate a possible association between long-term tamoxifen treatment and thromboembolic disease (Lipton et al., 1984; Levine et al., 1988; and Saphner et al., 1991). The thromboembolic events range from arterial thrombi, to superficial thrombophlebitis, to deep vein thromboses, and even to fatal pulmonary emboli. The exact incidence is unknown, but it has been estimated to be one per 800 treatment years greater than the rate for placebo treatment (Love et al., 1992*b*). It has also been estimated that the incidence of thromboembolic complications is greater in patients treated with chemotherapy plus tamoxifen than in those treated with tamoxifen alone (Levine et al., 1988; Saphner et al., 1991). Several investigators have evaluated coagulation in patients receiving tamoxifen (Enck and Rios, 1984; Auger and Mackie, 1988; and Love et al., 1992*b*). Antithrombin III levels decreased but not to clinically significant levels, fibrinogen levels decreased by 15%, and platelet counts decreased by 7% to 9% after 6 months of tamoxifen therapy. These changes do not explain the increased risk of thromboembolic disease associated with tamoxifen. The thromboembolic events that occurred in patients treated on NSABP protocol B-14 (tamoxifen versus placebo in node-negative, receptor-positive breast cancer) are listed in Table 22–23.

Life-threatening drug interactions between tamoxifen and warfarin have been reported (Tenni et al., 1989). One patient developed a subdural hematoma and another, severe hematuria. Patients receiving tamoxifen may require only 2 to 3 mg of warfarin per day to maintain appropriate prothrombin times.

Ocular Toxicity. There is some direct and indirect evidence that tamoxifen may cause ocular toxicity in humans. The long-term use of triphenylethylenes causes cataracts in rats, and doses of tamoxifen in excess of 200 mg per day cause retinal changes in humans (Jordan, 1992). A series of case reports document retinopathy, keratopathy, and optic neuritis in patients receiving treatment with tamoxifen. In general, these changes are reversible with discontinuation of the drug (Pugesgaard and Von Eyben, 1986; Ashford et al., 1988; Gerner, 1989; and Costa et al., 1990). Prospective evaluation of larger series of patients has yielded conflicting results. Longstaff and coworkers (1989) were not able to demonstrate changes in tear production, corneal sensitivity, or central visual field red thresholds in women taking tamoxifen; however, Pavlidis and coworkers (1992) found that 4 of 63 tamoxifen-treated patients developed retinopathy or keratopathy, or both. The ophthalmic findings consisted of decreased visual acuity, macular edema, and paramacular exudates. Again, these findings were largely reversible upon tamoxifen withdrawal. Potential ocular toxicity will be monitored during the BCPT.

Induction of New Primary Tumors

Endometrial Cancer. Although an association between endometrial cancer and tamoxifen was first reported in 1985, it was not until the report from Stockholm by Fornander and colleagues (1989) that a generalized concern arose (Killacke et al., 1985; and Gusberg, 1990). The Stockholm group noted 13 cases of endometrial cancer in 931 tamoxifen-treated patients (40 mg/day for 2 to 5 years), and 2 cases in 915 untreated controls ($P < .01$). Subsequently, other investigators reported elevated risk of endometrial cancer in patients treated long term with tamoxifen (Table 22–24).

As a whole, the endometrial cancers associated with tamoxifen therapy have been low-grade and early-stage tumors with good ''curability potential.'' In fact, the Early Breast Cancer Trialists' Collaborative Group documented only two deaths from endometrial cancer in more than 15,000 women treated with tamoxifen. However, four deaths from uterine cancer have been reported in tamoxifen-treated women participating in the NSABP B-14 trial (Fisher et al., 1994). Tamoxifen does appear to have an estrogenic stimulatory effect on the human uterus, as it does on rat and mouse uteri (Jordan, 1992). This is further verified by an increased incidence of endometrial hyperplasia and endometrial polyps in postmenopausal women treated with tamoxifen (Neven et al., 1990; De Muylder et al., 1991; and Gal et al., 1991).

Hepatocellular Carcinoma. Estrogens are promoters of liver carcinogenesis in rats. Tamoxifen is sufficiently estrogenic when given in large doses (20 to 100 times the human dose) to cause hepatic tumors in rats (Jordan, 1992). Tamoxifen induces liver tumors in rats only when given in large doses and for extended periods. Not a single case of hepatocellular carcinoma developed in the several thousand patients treated in NSABP adjuvant tamoxifen studies, nor has any case of hepatocellular carcinoma been reported in

Table 22–23. RATES OF THOMBOEMBOLIC EVENTS IN THE NATIONAL SURGICAL ADJUVANT BREAST AND BOWEL PROJECT (NSABP) B-14 FOR 1422 PATIENTS TREATED WITH TAMOXIFEN AND 1440 WHO RECEIVED PLACEBO

Thromboembolic Event	Placebo No. (%)	Tamoxifen No. (%)
Superficial phlebitis (mild)	0 (0.0)	3 (0.2)
Vein thrombosis (moderate)	0 (0.0)	4 (0.3)
Deep vein thrombosis (requiring hospitalization)	2 (0.1)	6 (0.4)
Pulmonary emboli	1 (0.1)	6 (0.4)
Death	0 (0.0)	2 (0.1)
Total	3 (0.2)	21 (1.5)

Table 22–24. INCIDENCE OF ENDOMETRIAL CANCER IN PATIENTS TREATED LONG-TERM WITH TAMOXIFEN

	Tamoxifen Treated Patients			Controls	
	Daily Dose (mg)	Endometrial Cancers	Total Treated	Endometrial Cancers	Total Controls
Stockholm Trial*	40	13	931	2	915
Danish Trial†	30	7	864	2	846
Scottish Trial‡	20	0	539	2	531
Christie Hospital Trial§	20	1	282	1	306
NSABP B-14¶	20	23	1422	2	1439
Totals		44	4038	9	4037

(Data from Fornander et al., 1989*; Andersson et al., 1991†; Stewart, 1992‡; Ribiero and Swindell, 1988§; NSABP [Fisher et al., 1989a]; Fisher et al., 1994.)

any adjuvant trial using tamoxifen at a dose of 20 mg per day. Fornander and colleagues (1989) from Stockholm observed two cases of hepatocellular carcinoma in 931 women treated with 40 mg of tamoxifen per day. It seems exceedingly unlikely that there will be an increased incidence of hepatocellular carcinoma among women receiving tamoxifen during the NSABP BCPT.

Other Breast Cancer Prevention Trials

The group at the Royal Marsden Hospital in England has completed a pilot feasibility study in 200 women with a family history of breast cancer (Powles et al., 1989). The design of this trial is essentially the same as that of the NSABP BCPT, with women randomized between placebo and tamoxifen, 20 mg per day. Compliance was high, and the frequency of side effects, except for hot flashes, was similar in both groups. Bone mass and clotting factors were not adversely affected by tamoxifen, though there was a significant reduction in serum cholesterol (principally low-density lipoprotein) in the tamoxifen-treated group. The study has been expanded to as many as 1000 women; however, in order to detect a 25% reduction in the incidence of breast cancer, at least 300 cancers would have to develop. This would require 10,000 women and 10 years' follow-up (Powles et al., 1990), a figure similar to the projected accrual (16,000 women) for the NSABP BCPT.

Another agent, fenretinide [*N*-(4-hydroxyphenyl) retinamide] or 4-HPR, is of considerable interest as a possible chemopreventive agent for breast cancer (Atiba and Meyskens, 1992). Fenretinide is an effective inhibitor of *N*-nitroso *N*-methylurea–induced breast cancer in rats. Unlike other synthetic retinoids, 4-HPR has few side effects and doses of 200 mg per day can be tolerated for prolonged periods (Rotmensz et al., 1991). This prompted the group at the Milan Cancer Institute to evaluate 4-HPR in preventing contralateral primary tumors in women already treated for breast cancer (Veronesi and Costa, 1988). In the *N*-methyl *N*-nitrosourea rat mammary carcinoma model, the combination of 4-HPR and tamoxifen is more effective than either drug alone for prevention of rat mammary carcinomas (Ratko et al., 1989).

Pure Antiestrogens

A series of new compounds with pure antiestrogenic properties are now entering clinical trials. These include ICI 164,384 and ICI 182,780, which are 17α-alkylsulfinyl derivatives of 17β-estradiol, droloxifene (3-OH tamoxifen), and toremifene, which is a triphenylethylene derivative structurally related to tamoxifen (Valavaara et al., 1990; Deschenes, 1991; Hamm et al., 1991; Pritchard et al., 1991; Wakeling et al., 1991; and DeFriend et al., 1994). As a group, these compounds inhibit estrogen- or tamoxifen-induced uterine growth in immature rats and mice and reduce mature uterine weight (Jordan, 1992). Preliminary findings indicate that the pure antiestrogens do not induce hepatic neoplasms in rodents (Love, 1989). This reflects their low degree of estrogenicity.

The pure antiestrogens may offer advantages and disadvantages when compared to tamoxifen. The pure antiestrogens do not induce a tumor flare in patients with bone metastases and would not be expected to induce or stimulate occult endometrial cancers. However, in the absence of any estrogenic activity, the pure antiestrogens would be expected to accelerate the development of osteoporosis and induce atherosclerosis. These drugs would therefore be poor choices for long-term adjuvant therapy or chemoprevention.

It is anticipated that the main clinical role for the pure antiestrogens will be in the treatment of metastatic breast cancer in patients in whom tamoxifen has failed. One of the mechanisms of tamoxifen failure is the induction of estrogenic metabolites that may actually stimulate tumor growth, but these patients may remain responsive to therapy with a pure antiestrogen. However, major cross-resistance between tamoxifen and toremifine has been reported (Vogel et al., 1993)

Progestins

When used as first-line agents, the progestins, megestrol acetate (MA; Megace) and medroxyprogesterone acetate (Provera), are very active against receptor-positive metastatic breast cancer in postmenopausal women (Johnson et al., 1988; Sedlacek, 1988; Becher et al., 1989; and Etienne et al., 1992). The side effects of the progestins are minimal and consist primarily of mild glucocorticoid activity and weight gain (Ingle, 1984; Gregory et al., 1985; and Cruz et al., 1990). Four prospective, randomized trials have compared MA to tamoxifen as first-line hormone therapy for metastatic breast cancer (Morgan, 1985; Ettinger et al., 1986; Muss et al., 1985, 1987, 1988; and Paterson et al., 1990). In each of the trials, the response rates are equivalent, but response duration and survival were greater for tamoxifen-treated patients in one of them (Fig. 22–26).

Since tamoxifen has been widely accepted as the drug of choice for first-line hormone therapy for metastatic breast cancer, MA is relegated to a second-line position. However, the rate of response to MA after tamoxifen failure averages only 20% (range 0–31%) (Ross et al., 1982; Muss et al., 1988; Paterson et al., 1990; and Schacter et al., 1990). Rates of response to tamoxifen after MA failure are equally poor (14–25%). Clearly, better second-line hormone therapy is needed.

Progestins have a direct cytotoxic effect on human breast cancer cells in long-term tissue culture, but their dominant activity is antiestrogenic and is mediated through the progesterone receptor (Rochefort, 1984; and Allegra and Kiefer, 1985). Progestins are clearly more active against recep-

tor-positive disease, and not surprisingly, PgR is the single best predictor of response (Blumenschein, 1983; and Johnson et al., 1983).

MA is currently the progestational agent of choice because of its ease of administration, safety, and efficacy. The standard dose is 40 mg four times daily, but 160 mg once daily has comparable therapeutic efficacy (Carpenter and Peterson, 1985; and Pronzato et al., 1990). Hypercalcemia and pain *flares* have also been reported with MA; like a tamoxifen flare, an MA flare may herald a response to treatment (Greenwald, 1983; and Otteman and Long, 1984).

It has been proposed for many years that progestational agents, unlike tamoxifen, have a steep dose-response curve and that larger doses are associated with increased bioavailability and therapeutic responsiveness (Pannuti et al., 1979; Cavilli et al., 1984; and Roberts et al., 1990). A series of reports of small trials comparing large and small doses of medoxyprogesterone acetate and of MA had conflicting results and tended to support larger doses (Aisner et al., 1987; Lundgren et al., 1989; Muss et al., 1990; and Parnes et al., 1991). In the definitive dose-response trial of MA in metastatic breast cancer, performed by the Cancer and Leukemia Group B (Aisner et al., 1992), a group of 368 women with metastatic breast cancer were randomized to receive 160 mg, 800 mg, or 1600 mg per day. Response rates were virtually identical at the three dose levels (24, 24, and 28%, respectively); however, the duration of response at the highest dose level was significantly shorter than that at the two lower dose levels (7.8 versus 13.9 and 14.2 months, respectively). The incidence of serious vascular complications, arterial thrombi, and pulmonary emboli was higher at the higher dose level. It can safely be concluded that there is no advantage to the large dose over the standard dose of MA.

Megestrol Acetate in Cachexia

Since patients with metastatic breast cancer who are treated with MA frequently gain weight, a series of studies have been performed that evaluate MA in cancer anorexia and cachexia as well as acquired immunodeficiency syndrome (AIDS) (Aisner et al., 1988, 1990; Loprinzi et al., 1990 and 1993; Schmoll et al., 1991; and Tchekmedyian et al., 1991). The dose of MA in these studies ranged from 320 to 1600 mg per day. MA consistently improved appetite and food intake in patients with AIDS or cancer. This resulted in nonfluid weight gain in many patients as well as a decrease in disease-associated nausea. At this time, a specific dose of MA for the treatment of cancer-related anorexia and cachexia cannot be recommended based on available data, but more than 160 mg per day probably is necessary.

Antiprogestins

The success of the antiestrogens in the treatment of breast cancer led to a search for antiprogestational agents for possible use as anticancer drugs (Jordan et al., 1992). Currently, two compounds, onapristone (ZK 112,993 from

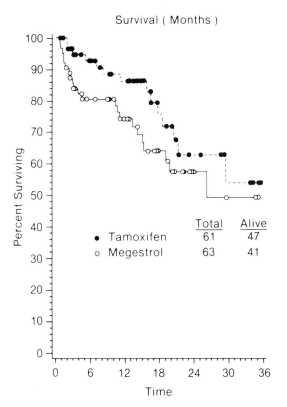

Figure 22–26. Even though there is a trend in favor of the use of tamoxifen, as yet there is no definite survival advantage (*P* = 0.16). (From Muss, H. B., Paschold, E. H., Black, W. R., et al.: Megestrol acetate versus tamoxifen in advanced breast cancer: A phase III trial of the Piedmont Oncology Association. Semin. Oncol., *12*(Suppl. 1):55, 1985.) Recent data (Muss et al., 1987) have demonstrated a significantly greater disease-free survival for patients treated initially with tamoxifen (*P* = 0.009).

Shering Laboratories) and mifespristone (RU 486 from Roussel-Uclaf Laboratories), are in preclinical and early clinical trials (Klijn et al., 1989; Michna et al., 1989; Bakker et al., 1990; and Spitz and Bardin, 1993). These drugs have an affinity for progesterone receptor that is five times greater than that of progesterone itself; they block progesterone- and estradiol-mediated proliferative effects in rat mammary tumor models. The antitumor activity of the antiprogestins is enhanced when they are used in combination with an antiestrogen or an LH-RH agonist. The side effects are due mainly to the antiglucocorticoid properties of the drugs. Mifespristone binds to glucocorticoid receptors with an affinity that is two to three times greater than that of dexamethasone. Attempts are ongoing to synthesize an antiprogestin with fewer antiglucocorticoid properties.

The antiprogestins are controversial in the United States because of their effects on the endometrium and decidua. The antiprogestational properties not only have anticancer effects but also contraceptive and abortofacient ones. All of the preclinical and clinical studies are being conducted in Europe.

Aromatase Inhibitors

In postmenopausal and oophorectomized premenopausal women, the main source of estrogen production is the aromatase system (see Fig. 22–2). Estrogen production in adrenal tissue, adipose tissue, and even breast cancer tissue is mediated by the enzyme aromatase, which stimulates the conversion of androstenedione to estrone (Miller et al., 1982; and Siiteri, 1982). Inhibitors of the aromatase system have been under intensive investigation since the 1960s (Cash et al., 1967).

Currently, the only commercially available aromatase inhibitor is aminoglutethimide (AG). Postmenopausal women treated with AG exhibit a 72% decline in plasma estrone levels and an 85% decrease in urinary estrone excretion over a 12-week period (Samojlik et al., 1982). It is well established that AG is an active agent in postmenopausal women and in oophorectomized premenopausal women with metastatic breast cancer (Santen et al., 1981; and Nemoto et al., 1989), and it is equivalent to surgical adrenalectomy for treatment of advanced breast cancer (see Fig. 22–7).

Since AG blocks adrenal steroidogenesis, hydrocortisone replacement is required with standard-dose AG therapy. AG also has a series of other undesirable side effects, such as lethargy in 48% of patients, skin rash in 33%, orthostatic hypotension in 20%, ataxia in 10%, and drug fever in 2.5%. In addition, leukopenia, thrombocytopenia, and even pancytopenia occur in as many as 5% of patients (Ingle, 1984). For these reasons, AG has not become a popular drug.

The standard dose schedule for AG is 250 mg twice daily for 14 days, increasing to four times a day thereafter, plus hydrocortisone, 20 to 30 mg daily, in a single morning dose. Low-dose AG (250 mg twice daily), with or without hydrocortisone replacement, is reported to be equivalent to standard-dose AG and has fewer side effects (Crivellari et al., 1989; and Cocconi et al., 1992).

Two new aromatase inhibitors, 4-hydroxyandrostene-dione (4-OHA) and fadrozole (CGS 16949A), are currently entering clinical trials (Höffken et al., 1990; Lipton et al., 1990; Stein et al., 1990; Lnning et al., 1991; Santen et al., 1991; and Raats et al., 1992). These drugs have the advantage that they are selective aromatase inhibitors that do not block adrenal steroidogenesis. Therefore, concurrent cortisol replacement is not required. The other undesirable side effects of AG are also greatly reduced. The main side effects of these new drugs are hot flashes in 28%, nausea and vomiting in 13%, and anorexia in 5%. No hematologic toxicity has been observed. Fadrozole and 4-OHA appear to be as active as AG in preliminary studies. Fadrozole is administered orally in doses of 1 to 4 mg daily; 4-OHA is given intramuscularly in doses of 250 to 500 mg every 1 to 2 weeks.

Estrogens

Before the introduction of tamoxifen, DES, a synthetic estrogen, was the hormone of choice for treatment of postmenopausal women with advanced breast cancer (Ingle et al., 1981). Large doses of estrogens produced the highest response rate and the most prolonged remissions (Kennedy, 1974). In postmenopausal women, the overall response rate to estrogens is 36%, but response increases with age and the number of years following menopause (Council on Drugs, 1960). The overall rate of response to DES in ER-positive tumors is 63%. In general, the median duration of response to estrogen is 12 to 18 months, but responses of longer than 5 years have been documented. It is important to point out that tamoxifen has never been superior to DES in terms of response rate or response duration. It only has fewer side effects than DES. Given the poor response to MA in tamoxifen failures, DES should be reevaluated as second-line hormone therapy in postmenopausal women (Boyer and Tattersall, 1990).

The mechanism by which estrogens act on metastatic breast cancer is unknown. Tumor cells that contain ERs bind estrogens with great affinity and specificity. Large doses of estrogen may flood the system and, by mass action, may actually be antiestrogenic. Hall (1974) proposed that tumor cells that respond to large doses of estrogen may be more like normal cells, and that massive doses of a normal differentiation-promoting substance might cause the tumor to mature, differentiate, and stop proliferating. It was recently shown that large doses of estrogen reduce the fluidity of the cell membrane of human breast cancer cells. This cytotoxicity appears not to be ER mediated (Clarke et al., 1990).

The most commonly used estrogen remains DES, in doses of 5 mg three times daily. Other estrogen preparations used are ethinyl estradiol, 3 mg daily, and conjugated equine estrogens, 30 mg daily. Nausea, the most common early side effect of DES, may be avoided by increasing the dose incrementally; that is, starting with 5 mg daily for 7 to 10 days, increasing to 5 mg twice a day for the next 7 to 10 days, and then giving 5 mg three times daily. Vomiting, anorexia, and even diarrhea may occur, but the gastrointestinal side effects of DES usually subside within 2 weeks. Increased nipple, areolar, and axillary pigmentation is frequent. Fluid retention occurs in about a third of cases and it may aggravate or even precipitate congestive heart failure. The use of large doses of estrogens may be associated with thromboembolic phenomena.

Breakthrough or withdrawal uterine bleeding occurs in 40% of postmenopausal women receiving estrogen therapy. It usually has little clinical significance and responds to cessation of treatment or abates spontaneously with continued therapy, but if the problem is persistent, dilation and curettage may be necessary. Persistent uterine bleeding associated with estrogen therapy may signal the presence of an endometrial carcinoma.

Hypercalcemic flares occur in 10% to 25% of women treated with DES (Kennedy et al., 1953). In breast cancer patients, spontaneous or induced hypercalcemia occurs only in association with osseous metastases. Induced hypercalcemia from any additive form of hormone therapy seems to indicate that the tumor has retained its endocrine responsiveness and often heralds a response to continued hormonal treatment (Hall et al., 1963; and Muggia and Heinemann, 1970).

Estrogen Rebound Regression

Patients who respond to estrogen therapy and who later cease to respond and exhibit progression of metastatic disease may respond to the sudden withdrawal of estrogens with another period of tumor regression. Rebound regression, originally described by Escher (1949), occurs in as many as 32% of estrogen responders (Kaufman and Escher, 1961; and Baker and Vaitkevicius, 1972). Patients who show a rebound response have a significantly longer disease-free interval before estrogen therapy was instituted than those who do not. The duration of rebound regression is usually 3 to 10 months, but Nesto and colleagues (1976) reported that the median duration was in excess of 18 months.

■

Case History (No. 63-31885, EFSCH)

In September 1963, a 66-year-old black woman complained of a mass in the right breast of 1 month's duration. The entire right breast was found to be occupied by a mass that was hard and fixed to the skin. Axillary adenopathy was present on the side of the lesion, and the largest lymph node measured 1.5 by 2.0 cm. Needle biopsy of the breast mass revealed poorly differentiated adenocarcinoma. Because of the locally advanced stage of the lesion, the patient was not considered a candidate for mastectomy and was treated with DES, 5 mg orally three times a day. She continued to take this medication for almost 2 years and showed symptomatic improvement and almost total regression of the primary neoplasm. In September 1965, the breast mass measured only 2.0 by 2.5 cm; though progression was evident in the form of newly developing subcutaneous nodules in the involved breast, a 1-cm right supraclavicular lymph node, and a 1.5-cm hard lesion in the opposite breast. DES was discontinued, and after 1 month all palpable lesions had diminished in size. Three months after therapy was suspended, all masses, including the original one

in the right breast, were absent, and the only evidence of residual disease was a 1.5-cm lymph node in the right axilla. In November 1973 the patient was still free of disease. She died in March 1974 at age 77 years, almost 11 years after her initial treatment.

Androgens

Androgens were the first additive agents to prove useful for hormone therapy of mammary cancer. Through the animal research of Lacassagne and Raynaud (1939), it became evident that testosterone could inhibit certain implantable and spontaneously occurring neoplasms. In London in the same year, Loeser (1939) reported two cases in which postoperative recurrence of mammary cancer had not reappeared for one and a half years after incidental androgen treatment directed toward menstrual problems. Ulrich (1939) in Paris noted marked shrinkage of breast tumors in two women who were receiving androgens. Fels (1944) in Argentina also noted favorable results in three women aged 34, 48, and 54 years who were treated with testosterone. Farrow and Woodward (1942) treated 33 patients with testosterone and first reported the rise of serum calcium level, which often is induced by androgens when bony metastases are present. Further experience with androgens established their palliative value in both premenopausal and postmenopausal women with disseminated disease.

The Cooperative Breast Cancer Group amassed considerable experience with androgenic agents. In 1964, this group reported the results of therapy in 564 postmenopausal women with metastatic mammary cancer treated with testosterone proprionate (Cooperative Breast Cancer Group, 1964). An overall objective regression rate of 21% was observed. Based on pre-ER data, the response of osseous metastases to androgens is equivalent to that for estrogens, 25% to 30%, but the response rate of soft tissue metastases (breast, skin, nodes) to androgens (20–25%) is significantly less than the 35% to 45% reported for estrogens (Kennedy, 1974). Fewer than 18% of visceral metastases respond to androgens (Kennedy, 1965). Because of the inferior response rate of visceral and soft tissue lesions, metastatic bone disease should be considered the primary indication for the use of androgens (Fig. 22–27).

Androgens display their antitumor effect in receptor-positive patients by two mechanisms of action: (1) blocking of pituitary gonadotropin release and subsequent ovarian secretion of estrogen; and (2) an antiestrogenic effect (Rochefort, 1984). Androgens exert their antiestrogenic effect by complex interactions with three receptors: ER, PgR, and androgen receptor. In large doses androgens stimulate human breast cancer cells in tissue culture, and this effect is mediated via the ER (Zava and McGuire, 1978). In smaller doses, androgens compete with estradiol for ER and are antiestrogenic. Androgens can also bind to PgR and may have progestin-like actions. Because the dose of androgen required to give an antiestrogenic effect saturates the androgen receptors but is too low to saturate the ERs, it postulated that the therapeutic effect is mediated via androgen receptors. This is verified to some degree by the observation

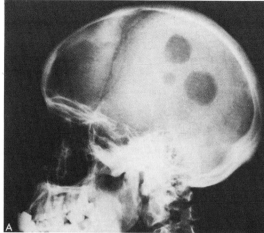
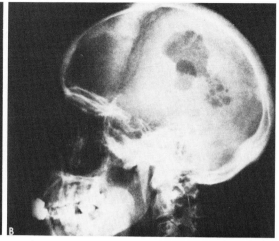
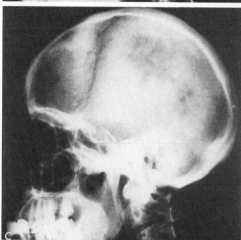

Figure 22–27. This 65-year-old black woman had a right modified mastectomy in June 1975 for an invasive carcinoma of the right breast with axillary metastases, and she received postoperative irradiation. *A,* Sixteen months after her operation, lytic metastases became evident in the skull and pelvis. She was placed on diethylstilbestrol, 5 mg orally 3 times daily, and after 6.5 months, x-rays showed a mixed response *(B)*. The two most prominent lesions had enlarged, and small new ones had appeared peripheral to them. The posterior defect had recalcified, but within it lytic areas suggested the growth of estrogen-resistant clones of cells. Estrogen use was discontinued, and, after a 1-month delay, fluoxymesterone therapy was begun at a dose of 10 mg twice daily. *C,* Three months later, all lesions were recalcifying and eventually healed. This patient's tumor appeared to represent a mixed population of cells, some of which were sensitive to estrogens and some of which were sensitive to androgens.

that, in tissue culture of rat mammary carcinomas and human breast cancer, antiandrogens such as cyproterone inhibit the antiestrogenic effect of androgens (Rochefort, 1984).

The subjective, hematopoietic, and anabolic effects of androgens are notable. Androgens stimulate erythropoiesis, probably via erythropoietin (Kennedy, 1962). Patients treated with androgens may experience an increased sense of well-being, pain relief, increased appetite, and weight gain. According to Kennedy (1974), however, it is not unusual to observe continued progression of disease despite excellent symptomatic improvement.

The side effects of androgens are predominantly those associated with the physiologic effects of male hormones, that is, virilization with frontal baldness, plethora, acne, hirsutism, fluid retention, and, less commonly, increased libido and clitoral hypertrophy. The virilizing effects vary with the androgenic preparation used. They occur in more than 50% of patients treated with testosterone propionate, in 35% to 40% of patients treated with fluoxymesterone, and in none treated with testolactone. Unfortunately, the virilizing and therapeutic effects of androgens may not be totally separable; the objective response rate to testolactone is only 14% (Volk et al., 1974). Androgens with a 17α-methyl substitution, such as fluoxymesterone and methyltestosterone, may cause reversible cholestatic jaundice and,

rarely, a multifocal hepatocellular necrosis termed peliosis hepatis (Naeim et al., 1973; and Bagheri and Boyer, 1974). The large areas of cystic hemorrhagic necrosis of peliosis hepatis may cause an abnormal liver scan that can be confused with metastases.

Fluoxymesterone (Halotestin) has emerged as the androgen of choice because it is at least as potent as testosterone propionate, is less virilizing, and can be taken orally. The daily dose of fluoxymesterone is 20 to 30 mg by mouth. Stanozol, an anabolic steroid with fewer androgenic properties, is entering clinical trials. It has activity in metastatic breast cancer, but its role relative to other androgens is not yet defined (Daniel et al., 1991).

Adrenal Corticosteroids

There are only limited indications for the use of corticosteroids as single agents for metastatic breast cancer. Responses to corticosteroids are generally nonspecific, but temporary objective regression of tumor occurs in approximately 18% of cases (Kelley, 1971). Specific tumor responses appear to be limited to premenopausal patients with a history of response to castration and to postmenopausal women with a history of response to other forms of additive therapy (Kennedy, 1965). Unlike aminoglutethimide, the use of corticosteroids does not constitute medical adrenal-ectomy.

Corticosteroids may be helpful in the treatment of jaundice due to hepatic metastases and restricted lung function due to lymphangitic pulmonary metastases, but data are sparse. Corticosteroids are often used in combination with cytotoxic agents, but the contribution of corticosteroids to combination chemotherapy remains questionable.

Adrenal corticosteroids are particularly helpful in the medical management of brain or spinal cord metastases. For the acute management of increased intracranial pressure, a loading dose of dexamethasone, 8 mg intravenously, can be given, followed by 4 mg intravenously or orally every 6 hours. Long-term use of large daily doses of dexamethasone can precipitate fluid and electrolyte imbalances and steroid myopathies. Hyperosmolar states can also develop in patients with a tendency toward diabetes mellitus. The dose of dexamethasone during radiation therapy for brain or spinal cord metastases should be 4 mg every 6 to 8 hours. Following completion of radiation therapy, the dexamethasone dose should be tapered over 2 to 3 weeks (Kornblith et al., 1985).

Corticosteroids may be a useful adjunct in the management of patients with far advanced or preterminal disease because they frequently cause euphoria, stimulate appetite, and decrease pain (Schell, 1972). Schell demonstrated that the narcotic requirement was often decreased. Subjective improvement occurs in as many as 75% of patients. Bruera and coworkers (1985) reported a randomized, double-blind study of methylprednisolone versus placebo in terminally ill cancer patients and confirmed Schell's observations. Such patients treated with 32 mg of methylprednisolone daily had less intense pain, increased appetite, and an increased sense of well-being, as compared with placebo-treated controls.

It is difficult to make dose recommendations because no dose-response data are available for breast cancer. Objective tumor regression has followed cortisone acetate, 100 to 400 mg daily, and prednisone, 30 to 250 mg daily. The smaller doses may be as effective as large ones (Gardner et al., 1962; and Stoll, 1963). Euphoria can be produced by a dose of 20 to 40 mg of oral prednisone daily.

The well-known side effects of long-term corticosteroid administration are sodium and fluid retention, aggravation or precipitation of diabetes mellitus, hypertension, hypokalemia, muscle weakness, peptic ulcer, defects of cell-mediated immunity, and overt Cushing's syndrome.

NEWER AGENTS FOR HORMONE MANIPULATION

Luteinizing Hormone–Releasing Hormone Agonists

In animals, long-term treatment with supraphysiologic doses of LH-RH agonists causes (1) decreased gonadotropin (follicle-stimulating hormone and LH) secretion, (2) decreased prolactin secretion, (3) decreased plasma concentration of sex steroid, (4) reduction in weight of secondary sex organs, and (5) inhibition of the actions of the sex

steroids at their target organs (Klijn et al., 1984). LH-RH analogues, therefore, act directly or indirectly on the pituitary, the gonads, and the target organs of the sex steroids. Schally and coworkers (1984) demonstrated significantly decreased tumor weight and volume in mouse and rat mammary cancers treated with D-Trp^6-LH-RH (decapeptyl). After administration of an LH-RH agonist, serum concentrations of estradiol, LH, and follicle-stimulating hormone are significantly depressed. Mean serum estradiol levels fall to castrate or postmenopausal levels after 2 to 3 weeks of therapy (Kaufmann et al., 1989). In essence, the LH-RH agonists produce medical oophorectomy that is reversible with discontinuation of therapy.

The LH-RH analogues goserelin (Zoladex), leuprolide (Lupron), buserelin (Suprefact), and decapeptyl are in clinical trials for metastatic breast cancer (Klijn and de Jong, 1982; Klijn et al., 1984; Harvey et al., 1985; Dixon et al., 1990; and Dowsett et al., 1990). As would be anticipated by the mechanism of action, responses are seen predominantly in premenopausal women, but responses in postmenopausal women have been reported (Mathé et al., 1987; and Schwartz et al., 1988; and Saphner et al., 1993). In the largest series so far reported, of 134 premenopausal and perimenopausal women with metastatic breast cancer treated with the LH-RH agonist goserelin, the overall objective response rate was 44.9% (10.2% complete response and 34.7% partial) (Kaufmann et al., 1989). The median time to response was 4 months, and the median duration was 8+ months. Responses were more common in ER-positive tumors (49.3%), but responses were also observed in ER-negative ones (33.3%). All patients developed amenorrhea in the first month of treatment, and 63% (84 of 134) developed hot flashes. Other side effects were minimal.

The LH-RH agonists are not approved in the United States for the treatment of breast cancer, but leuprolide and goserelin are approved for the treatment of metastatic prostate cancer.

Trials of total estrogen blockade using an LH-RH agonist plus tamoxifen are being conducted (Robertson et al., 1989; Nicholson et al., 1990; and Dixon et al., 1991). Preliminary data imply that the combination of LH-RH agonists plus tamoxifen may induce a greater response rate than tamoxifen alone, and the duration of response may be prolonged (Buzzoni et al., 1994; and Jonat et al., 1994).

Danazol

Danazol (2,3-isoxazol-17α-ethinyl testosterone) has four important mechanisms of action: (1) inhibition of pituitary gonadotropin secretion, probably by inhibition of gonadotropin-releasing hormone; (2) inhibition of adrenal and gonadal steroidogenesis; (3) binding to androgen and progesterone receptors; and (4) binding to sex hormone–binding globulin and corticosteroid-binding globulin (Barbieri and Ryan, 1981). Danazol is relatively nontoxic and has been released by the FDA for the treatment of endometriosis and relief of the pain and nodularity associated with chronic cystic mastopathy (Ingle, 1984).

Peters and coworkers (1977) reported a 66% objective rate of response to danazol in the treatment of dimethylbenzanthracene-induced mammary cancers in rats. In doses of 100 to 200 mg three times daily (the same dosage range used to treat chronic cystic mastopathy), objective responses in 7 of 37 postmenopausal patients treated with danazol were reported by Coombes and associates (1980).

Somatostatin

Somatostatin (SMS) inhibits growth hormone release, prolactin secretion, insulin and glucagon release, and pentagastrin-induced gastric secretion (Schally et al., 1986; and Karashima and Schally, 1987). SMS inhibits autocrine growth factors, particularly IGF-I and EGF. SMS receptors have been demonstrated on breast cancer cells, which may facilitate a direct inhibitory effect on cell growth (Fekete et al., 1989). SMS analogues possess significant antitumor activity in experimental tumor systems, including rat mammary carcinomas (Schally et al., 1987). Naturally occurring SMS is a tetradecapeptide with an exceedingly brief circulatory half-life (3 minutes). The only available SMS analogue is octreotide (Sandostatin), which, has a relatively prolonged half-life (still, only 113 minutes). The peptide nature of the compound and the short half-life necessitate that octreotide be administered subcutaneously every 8 to 12 hours. The frequency of injections has greatly limited the appeal of SMS for the treatment of advanced breast cancer. Longer-acting preparations, such as RC 160 (half-life 2 weeks) are being evaluated in rat mammary carcinomas and, it is hoped, will soon be available for clinical trials (Schally, 1988). Despite the short half-life and the need for frequent injections, clinical trials of the SMS analogue octreotide are being explored for advanced breast cancer by Pollak and collaborators (1992) and by the North Central Cancer Treatment Group.

Combination Hormone Therapy

Numerous combinations of hormonal agents have been evaluated for treatment of metastatic breast cancer: fluoxymesterone with ethinyl estradiol, DES with testosterone propionate, tamoxifen with MA, tamoxifen with medoxyprogesterone acetate, tamoxifen with DES, tamoxifen with prednisone, tamoxifen with AG, and ethinyl estradiol with medoxyprogesterone acetate. In general, the results of these trials have shown only marginal improvement in small subsets of patients, or no improvement in response rates or survival over single-agent therapy (Ingle et al., 1988b, 1991). This is what would be anticipated since the mechanism of action of each of these agents is basically the same, that is, inhibition of the synthesis or action of estrogen. The toxicity of combination endocrine therapy is almost always additive, and the concurrent use of a combination of additive hormonal agents may result in a loss of sequential endocrine responses (Henderson et al., 1987). Combinations of the traditional hormonal agents (tamoxifen, MA, fluoxymesterone, DES, AG, or prednisone) cannot be recommended.

A series of new combination hormonal trials is now in progress. These include the use of hormonal agents with biologic response modifiers such as tamoxifen plus interferon-α (Macheledt et al., 1991; and Vandenberg and Skillings, 1992), hormonal agents plus retinoids (Boccardo et al., 1990b; and Rechia et al., 1991), LH-RH agonists plus tamoxifen (Dixon et al., 1991), LH-RH agonists plus SMS (Schally, 1988), and tamoxifen plus SMS. These new combinations may be expected to have additive, or even synergistic, effects beyond estrogen blockade alone.

Combination Chemohormonal Therapy

The rationale for the use of combination therapy with cytotoxic drugs and hormone manipulation is based on three assumptions: (1) tumors are heterogeneous (i.e., breast cancers are composed of various proportions of receptor-positive and receptor-negative cells); (2) receptor-positive and receptor-negative cells have different responses to cytotoxic chemotherapy and hormone therapy; and (3) neither chemotherapy nor hormone therapy interferes with the action of the other form of treatment, so response rates for combined therapy are additive and not antagonistic. Unfortunately, these three assumptions may not be totally valid.

One limitation of the methods currently available for assaying ER and PgR in tissue cytosol is the inability to assess heterogeneity within the breast cancer itself (DeSombre et al., 1984). Various histologic methods of staining for ER have been attempted, but though they seem to confirm tissue heterogeneity with regard to ER, the results have been inconsistent with those of cytosolic ER assays (DeSombre, 1982). King and colleagues (1982) described the use of a specific monoclonal antibody to human breast cancer ER in lightly fixed and frozen sections of tissue. Using this technique in ER-rich breast cancer, all of the staining is restricted to the cell nuclei. This implies that ER is a nuclear receptor rather than a cytoplasmic receptor, and there is a difference between what is cytosolic and what is truly cytoplasmic. Using a similar technique, Nenci (1984) was able to demonstrate that breast tumors rarely display homogeneous cell types (i.e., they are rarely composed of only ER-positive or only ER-negative cells); almost all breast tumors prove to be composed of mixed receptor-positive and receptor-negative cell populations in varying proportions. Nenci (1984) also noted that positivity of 20% of the cell population was sufficient to produce evidence of a positive ER by cytosolic assay. These observations of cell heterogeneity in breast cancer seem clinically relevant and may explain why the probability of tumor regression after endocrine therapy correlates better with a quantitative than with a simply qualitative receptor assay.

Salmon (1984) asked, "Is the estrogen receptor expressed clonally in the human tumor clonogenic assay with some colonies positive and others negative, or is it expressed over time in all colonies that grow in the assay (the latter being more consistent with ER as a differentiation antigen)?" (p. 18). Using the MCF-7 human breast cancer cell line, he was able to demonstrate that at the small cluster stage of growth the proportion of ER-positive cells was small and variable, and some ER-negative clusters were present. ER positivity increased progressively with time, the greatest positivity occurring at the colony stage of growth. Once the colony stage was reached, ER was expressed in 70% of the cells in colonies, and none of the colonies was ER negative. These findings support the concept that ER is proliferation-differentiation dependent and that cells are not clonally ER positive or ER negative. Salmon (1984) went on to postulate that ER is expressed increasingly in transitional cells and end cells rather than in tumor stem cells. Therefore, endocrine therapy acts beyond the level of the tumor stem cell and will suppress but not eradicate breast cancer clones. In contrast, cytotoxic agents appear to kill cells in both stem cell and transitional cell compartments.

Salmon's observations demonstrate that breast cancers may not be heterogeneous with reference to ER but rather may be at different phases of cellular differentiation.

Receptor-positive cells have a well-documented differential response to hormone therapy. An important question is whether receptor-positive and receptor-negative cells respond differently to cytotoxic chemotherapy, or whether chemotherapy kills ER-positive and ER-negative cells indiscriminately, as Salmon's (1984) human tumor clonogenic assay tissue culture data seem to imply.

In 1978, Lippman and colleagues reported a retrospective study of 70 patients with metastatic breast cancer treated with cytotoxic chemotherapy. Objective responses were seen in 34 of 45 (75%) ER-negative (<10 fmol/mg) patients, but only 3 of 25 (12%) ER-positive (≥ 10 fmol/mg) patients responded ($P = .0001$). These data were so striking that they seemed to establish a differential response to chemotherapy for ER-positive and ER-negative cells, but 6 months later, in another retrospective study, Kiang and associates (1978) reported the opposite finding. In women treated with chemotherapy, 24 of 28 (86%) ER-positive patients responded, compared to 13 of 36 (36%) ER-negative patients ($P < .0001$). Clearly, there was a problem. Since then, a variety of retrospective studies have been reported, some confirming that ER-positive tumors respond better to chemotherapy (Mortimer et al., 1981; and Paone et al., 1981), some confirming that those tumors respond poorly to chemotherapy (Lippman and Allegra, 1980), and some reporting no difference in response to chemotherapy (Pouillart et al., 1982; Corle et al., 1984; Falkson et al., 1985). To establish firmly whether or not ER-positive and ER-negative cells respond differently to cytotoxic chemotherapy, the Cancer and Leukemia Group B performed a prospective, randomized study from January 1980 to August 1982 (Kardinal et al., 1983; and Perry et al., 1984). All of the patients were postmenopausal and were stratified by ER status (< 7 or ≥ 7 fmol/mg) and site of dominant metastatic disease. Objective responses were observed in 26 of 37 (70%) ER-negative patients and in 20 of 40 (50%) ER-positive patients ($P = .07$). A differential response to cytotoxic chemotherapy between ER-positive and ER-negative cells cannot be confirmed; chemotherapy kills both types indiscriminately. It can be concluded that, at least with reference to ER-positive cells, chemotherapy and hormone therapy are competing for the same cell population (Kardinal et al., 1986).

The third assumption necessary to propose an additive effect between chemotherapy and hormone therapy is that there is no interference between the two types of treatment. The experimental data of Sutherland and coworkers (1983) and Osborne and colleagues (1983) have demonstrated that tamoxifen acts as a cell cycle inhibitor, arresting cells in the G_0–G_1 phase of the cell cycle. Drugs that are cell cycle specific, such as methotrexate and 5-fluorouracil, require for a cytotoxic effect that the target cells be actively dividing. Even the cell cycle–nonspecific drugs, such as the alkylating agents and the antitumor antibiotics, are most effective against actively dividing cells. At least theoretically, tamoxifen potentially interferes with cytotoxic drugs by slowing cell replication. This has not been confirmed in clinical chemohormonal trials.

To date, there are no convincing data to indicate that the addition of a hormonal agent such as tamoxifen to a standard chemotherapeutic regimen, such as CMF or cyclophosphamide, Adriamycin, and 5-fluorouracil (CAF) has increased the rate or duration of response over that of either regimen alone. Perry and associates (1987) reported a prospective, randomized study of 246 postmenopausal patients with advanced cancer of the breast, stratified by ER-receptor status and dominant site of metastatic disease, who were treated with CAF versus CAF plus tamoxifen. No difference in response rate or response duration to CAF or CAF plus tamoxifen was seen with respect to ER status or dominant site of metastatic disease. Two other studies evaluated tamoxifen alone versus tamoxifen plus CMF (Glick et al., 1980; and Bezwoda et al., 1982). In neither of these studies was the addition of CMF advantageous. Krook and associates (1985) also demonstrated no advantage in time to disease progression or survival by the addition of tamoxifen to cyclophosphamide, 5-fluorouracil, and prednisone over the use of the last three drugs alone.

The failure to demonstrate an advantage from the addition of hormonal agents to cytotoxic chemotherapy does not rule out the possibility that the kinetic effects of tamoxifen might be used to increase chemotherapeutic effectiveness. Preliminary data of Allegra (1983*a*) demonstrated that tumor cell synchronization by tamoxifen, followed with recruitment by equine estrogens (Premarin priming), enhanced the response to cytotoxic chemotherapy.

Conte and coworkers (1985) have been able to confirm in vivo estrogen-induced expansion of the growth fraction in human breast cancer. They evaluated 16 previously untreated women with locally advanced breast cancer who received DES, 1 mg daily for 3 days, followed by 5-fluorouracil, Adriamycin, and cyclophosphamide chemotherapy. DES induced a significant increase in labeling index in 8 of 16 patients. Following this preliminary observation, Conte and coworkers (1987, 1990) expanded their clinical trials to include 117 patients with metastatic breast cancer and 86 patients with locally advanced breast cancer. There was no difference in response rate, progression-free survival time, or total survival time between women treated with estrogen priming prior to chemotherapy and women treated with chemotherapy alone. These investigators confirmed that patients were not harmed by estrogen recruitment. The failure of estrogenic recruitment to enhance chemotherapeutic responsiveness has been reported by other investigators (Paridaens et al., 1993; and Ingle et al., 1994).

It therefore seems clear that combination hormonal ther-

APPROACH TO THE PATIENT
WITH METASTATIC BREAST CANCER
(Receptors Known)

Premenopausal	Premenopausal & Postmenopausal	Postmenopausal
(ER+ PgR+)	(ER- PgR-)	(ER+ PgR+)

Primary   Life Threatening Metastases   Life Threatening Metastases   *Primary*

TAM or OOPHX   TAM or Megestrol

Secondary   No Response →   ← No Response   *Secondary*

OOPHX or TAM   Combination Cytotoxic Chemotherapy   Megestrol or DES

Tertiary   No Response →   ← No Response   *Tertiary*

AG or Megestrol   DES or AG

Quarternary   No Response   No Response   *Quarternary*

Fluoxymesterone   Fluoxymesterone

Patients with ER-positive, PgR-negative and ER-negative, PgR-positive metastases should be managed in the same manner.
TAM = tamoxifen; OOPHX = oophorectomy; AG = aminoglutethimide; DES = diethylstilbestrol.

Figure 22–28. Diagram depicting a series of *clinical judgment* issues in the treatment of premenopausal and postmenopausal women with metastatic breast cancer. All ER-negative, PgR-negative patients should be treated with chemotherapy. Women with receptor-positive but immediately life-threatening metastases should be treated initially with chemotherapy but can be maintained on hormonal therapy. Receptor-positive patients with non–life-threatening metastases should be treated with a primary form of hormonal manipulation. If a response occurs, other forms of hormonal treatment may be useful for progression. Secondary, tertiary, and even quarternary hormonal responses may occur, but they are not common. A judgment must be made at each sequential step.

apy and chemotherapy offers no advantage to women with locally advanced or metastatic breast cancer, nor does estrogen recruitment before chemotherapy. These data further emphasize the importance of a sequential, rather than a combined, approach to advanced breast cancer. As outlined in the next section the initial therapeutic consideration should be whether or not the patient with advanced breast cancer is a candidate for hormonal manipulation. If she is, primary hormone therapy should be initiated. At treatment failure, secondary hormone therapy should be considered before initiation of the more toxic chemotherapeutic regimens.

PATIENT MANAGEMENT

The approach to the patient with metastatic breast cancer depends on three major factors: (1) the tumor's ER and PgR status, (2) the patient's menopausal status, and (3) the distribution of disease (Fig. 22–28). Clinical judgment involves determining how potentially life-threatening the disease is when therapy is initiated. If the disease is immediately life threatening, the patient should be treated directly with cytotoxic chemotherapy because of its more rapid onset of action, regardless of tumor receptor status. Potentially life-threatening are lymphangitic pulmonary metastases and

EFFICACY

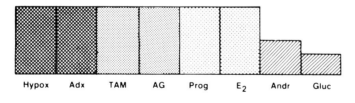

Hypox   Adx   TAM   AG   Prog   E₂   Andr   Gluc

PROBLEMS WITH THERAPY

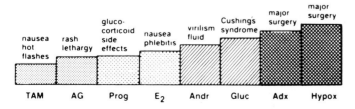

TAM   AG   Prog   E₂   Andr   Gluc   Adx   Hypox

Figure 22–29. Considerations in choosing endocrine therapy. Hypox = hypophysectomy; Adx = adrenalectomy; TAM = tamoxifen; AG = aminoglutethimide; Prog = progestins; E_2 = estrogen; Andr = androgens; Gluc = glucocorticoids. (From Santen, R. J.: Basic principles in choosing endocrine therapy. *In* Allegra, J. C. (Ed.): Management of Breast Cancer Through Endocrine Therapies. Amsterdam, Excerpta Medica, 1984, p. 19.)

massive hepatic metastases. Central nervous system metastases, although life threatening, respond to neither chemotherapy nor hormone therapy. If the clinical situation is not life threatening (i.e., if the patient can safely wait 6 to 8 weeks for the onset of action) and the tumor is ER positive, it is very desirable to treat the patient with some form of hormone manipulation. Hormone therapy is preferred in the appropriate clinical setting because the response rates are high in ER-positive, PgR-positive patients and hormone therapy is relatively free of side effects, in contrast to cytotoxic chemotherapy.

After the judgment is made that the patient is a candidate for hormone manipulation, how does the clinician decide which form of therapy is most appropriate and in what sequence, since the patient may respond not only to the primary form of hormone manipulation but to secondary, and even tertiary, endocrine therapy?

Most hormone manipulations, additive or ablative, induce approximately the same overall rate and duration of response. Selection is based primarily on side effects or other morbidity associated with the therapy (Allegra, 1984*b*) (Fig. 22–29). Sequential approaches to hormone manipulation in premenopausal and postmenopausal patients with advanced breast cancer are illustrated in Figure 22–28.

The therapist can be more liberal with hormonal manipulation for ER-positive, PgR-positive tumors because the response rate is very high (78%) (see Table 22–6). That is, the physician may be more willing to take greater risks and to treat sicker patients. When patients are ER positive, PgR negative or ER negative, PgR positive, whose response rates are only 30% to 40%, more caution in patient selection must be used. In these cases, hormone therapy should be reserved for patients with indolent disease, such as bone metastases, soft tissue metastases, and possibly nodular lung metastases. ER-negative, PgR-negative patients should not be treated with hormone therapy because response rates are consistently lower than 10%. Management of the patient with metastatic breast cancer whose receptor status is unknown is illustrated in Figure 22–5.

References

Abram, W. P., Baum, M., Berstock, D. A., et al.: Cyclophosphamide and tamoxifen as adjuvant therapies in the management of breast cancer: Preliminary analysis by the CRC Adjuvant Breast Trial Working Party. Br. J. Cancer, *57*:604, 1988.

Adair, F. E., Treves, N., Farrow, J. H., et al.: Clinical effects of surgical and x-ray castration in mammary cancer. J.A.M.A., *128*:161, 1945.

Ahlbom, H.: Castration by roentgen rays as auxiliary treatment in the radiotherapy of cancer mammae at Radiumhemmet, Stockholm. Acta Radiol., *11*:614, 1930.

Ahmann, D. L., O'Connell, M. J., Hahn, R. G., et al.: An evaluation of early or delayed adjuvant chemotherapy in premenopausal patients with advanced breast cancer undergoing oophorectomy. N. Engl. J. Med., *297*:356, 1977.

Aisner, J., Berry, D., Henderson, I. C., et al.: A phase III dose-response trial of megestrol acetate (MA) in metastatic breast cancer (MBC) (Abstract). Proc. Am. Soc. Clin. Oncol., *11*:56, 1992.

Aisner, J., Parnes, H., Tait, N., et al.: Appetite stimulation and weight gain with megestrol acetate. Semin. Oncol., *17*(Suppl. 9):2, 1990.

Aisner, J., Tchekmedyian, N. S., Moody M., et al.: High-dose megestrol acetate for the treatment of advanced breast cancer: Dose and toxicities. Semin. Hematol., *24*(Suppl. 1):48, 1987.

Aisner, J., Tchekmedyian, N. S., Tait, N., et al.: Studies of high-dose megestrol acetate: Potential applications in cachexia. Semin. Oncol., *15*(Suppl. 1):68, 1988.

Akhtar, S. S., Allan, S. G., Rodger, A., et al.: A 10-year experience of tamoxifen as primary treatment of breast cancer in 100 elderly and frail patients. Eur. J. Surg. Oncol., *17*:30, 1991.

Allegra, J. C.: Methotrexate and 5-fluorouracil following tamoxifen and premarin in advanced breast cancer. Semin. Oncol., *10*(2 Suppl. 2):23, 1983*a*.

Allegra, J. C.: Mechanism of hormone response and resistance: Clinical studies. Rev. Endocrine-Related Cancer, *14*(Suppl.):53, 1984*a*.

Allegra, J. C.: The use of steroid hormone receptors in breast cancer. *In* Margolese, R. (Ed.): Breast Cancer. New York, Churchill Livingstone, 1983*b*, p. 187.

Allegra, J. C.: Role of hormone receptors in determining treatment of breast cancer. *In* The Management of Breast Cancer Through Endocrine Therapies. Amsterdam, Excerpta Medica, 1984*b*, pp. 1–13.

Allegra, J. C., Barlock, A., Huff, K. K., et al.: Changes in multiple or sequential estrogen receptor determinations in breast cancer. Cancer, *45*:792, 1980.

Allegra, J. C., and Kiefer, S. M.: Mechanisms of action of progestational agents. Semin. Oncol., *12*(1 Suppl. 1):3, 1985.

Allegra, J. C., Lippman, N. E., Simon, R., et al.: Association between steroid hormone receptor status and disease-free interval in breast cancer. Cancer Treat. Rep., *63*:1271, 1979.

Andersson, M., Storm, H. H., and Mouridsen, H. T.: Incidence of new primary cancers after adjuvant tamoxifen therapy and radiotherapy for early breast cancer. J. Natl. Cancer Inst., *83*:1013, 1991.

Ashford, A. R., Donev, I., Tiwari, R. P., et al.: Reversible ocular toxicity related to tamoxifen therapy. Cancer, *61*:33, 1988.

Atiba, J. O., and Meyskens, F. L., Jr.: Chemoprevention of breast cancer. Semin. Oncol., *19*:220, 1992.

Auclerc, G., Khayat, D., Borel, C., et al.: Tamoxifen as sole treatment in patients (PTS) aged 65 years and over with primary breast cancer. A multicenter study with 78 PTS (Meeting abstract). Proc. Am. Soc. Clin. Oncol., *9*:A173, 1990.

Auger, M. J., and Mackie, M. J.: Effects of tamoxifen on blood coagulation. Cancer, *61*:1316, 1988.

Bagheri, S. A., and Boyer, J. L.: Peliosis hepatis associated with androgenic–anabolic steroid therapy. Ann. Intern. Med., *81*:610, 1974.

Baker, L. H., and Vaitkevicius, V. K.: Reevaluation of rebound regression in disseminated carcinoma of the breast. Cancer, *29*:1268, 1972.

Bakker, G. H., Setyono-Han, B., Portengen, H., et al.: Treatment of breast cancer with different antiprogestins: Preclinical and clinical studies. J. Steroid Biochem. Molec. Biol., *37*:789, 1990.

Barbieri, R. L., and Ryan, K. J.: Danazol: Endocrine pharmacology and therapeutic applications. Am. J. Obstet. Gynecol., *141*:453, 1981.

Bartlett, K., Eremin, O., Hutcheon, A., et al.: Adjuvant tamoxifen in the management of operable breast cancer: The Scottish trial. Report from the Breast Cancer Trials Committee, Scottish Cancer Trials Office (MRC), Edinburgh. Lancet, *2*:171, 1987.

Bates, S. E.: Clinical applications of serum tumor markers. Ann. Intern. Med., *115*:623, 1991.

Bates, T., Riley, D. L., Houghton, J., et al.: Breast cancer in elderly women: A cancer research campaign trial comparing treatment with tamoxifen and optimal surgery with tamoxifen alone. The Elderly Breast Cancer Working Party. Br. J. Surg., *78*:591, 1991.

Baum, M.: Does treatment influence the natural history of breast cancer? Rev. Endocrine-Related Cancer, *14*(Suppl.):193, 1984.

Baum, M., Brinkley, D. M., Dossett, J. A., et al.: Controlled trial of tamoxifen as adjuvant agent in management of early breast cancer: Interim analysis at four years by Nolvadex Adjuvant Trial Organisation. Lancet, *1*:257, 1983.

Baum, M., Brinkley, D. M., Dossett, J. A., et al.: Controlled trial of tamoxifen as single adjuvant agent in management of early breast cancer: Analysis at six years by Nolvadex Adjuvant Trial Organisation. Lancet, *1*:836, 1985.

Baum, M., Brinkley, D. M., Dossett, J. A., et al.: Controlled trial of tamoxifen as a single adjuvant agent in the management of early breast cancer: Analysis at eight years by Nolvadex Adjuvant Trial Organisation. Br. J. Cancer, *57*:608, 1988.

Baum, M., Ebbs, S., Brooks, M., et al.: Biological fallout from the trials of adjuvant tamoxifen in early breast cancer. *In* Salmon, S. (Ed.): Adjuvant Therapy of Cancer VI. Philadelphia, W. B. Saunders, 1990, pp. 269–274.

Beatson, G. T.: On the treatment of inoperable cases of carcinoma of the mamma: Suggestions for a new method of treatment with illustrative cases. Lancet, 2:104, 162, 1896.

Becher, R., Miller, A. A., Höffken, K., et al.: High-dose medroxyprogesterone acetate in advanced breast cancer: Clinical and pharmacokinetic study with a combined oral and intramuscular regimen. Cancer, 63:1938, 1989.

Berns, E. M. J. J., Klijn, J. G. M., van Putten, W. L. J., et al.: C-*myc* amplification is a better prognostic facter than *HER2/neu* amplification in primary breast cancer. Cancer Res., 52:1107, 1992.

Bevilacqua, G., Sobel, M. E., Liotta, L. A., et al.: Association of low *nm23* RNA levels in human primary infiltrating ductal breast carcinomas with lymph node involvement and other histopathological indicators of high metastatic potential. Cancer Res., 49:5185, 1989.

Bezwoda, W. R., Derman, D., De Moor, N. G., et al.: Treatment of metastatic breast cancer in estrogen receptor positive patients. A randomized trial comparing tamoxifen alone versus tamoxifen plus CMF. Cancer, 50:2747, 1982.

Bezwoda, W. R., Esser, J. D., Dansey, R., et al.: The value of estrogen and progesterone receptor determinations in advanced breast cancer: Estrogen receptor level but not progesterone receptor level correlates with response to tamoxifen. Cancer, 68:867, 1991.

Bianco, A. R., Del Mastro, L., Gallo, C., et al.: Prognostic role of amenorrhea induced by adjuvant chemotherapy in premenopausal patients with early breast cancer. Br. J. Cancer, 63:799, 1991.

Block, G. E., Vial, A. B., and Pullen, F. W.: Estrogen excretion following operative and irradiation castration in cases of mammary cancer. Surgery, 43:415, 1958.

Bloom, N. D., and Fishman, J. H.: Tamoxifen treatment failures in hormonally responsive breast cancers. Correlation with steroid receptors. Cancer, 51:1190, 1983.

Blumenschein, G. R.: The role of progestins in the treatment of breast cancer. Semin. Oncol., 10(Suppl. 4):7, 1983.

Bluming, A. Z.: Hormone replacement therapy: Benefits and risks for the general postmenopausal female population and for women with a history of previously treated breast cancer. Semin. Oncol., 20:662–674, 1993.

Boccardo, F., Rubagotti, A., Bruzzi, P., et al.: Chemotherapy versus tamoxifen versus chemotherapy plus tamoxifen in node-positive, estrogen receptor–positive breast cancer patients: Results of a multicentric Italian study. J. Clin. Oncol. 8:1310, 1990*a.*

Boccardo, F., Canobbio, L., Resasco, M., et al.: Phase II study of tamoxifen and high-dose retinyl acetate in patients with advanced breast cancer. J. Cancer Res. Clin. Oncol., *116*:503, 1990*b.*

Bonadonna, G.: Conceptual and practical advances in the management of breast cancer. J. Clin. Oncol., 7:1380, 1989.

Bonadonna, G., Rossi, A., Valaguassa, P., et al.: Adjuvant chemotherapy trial with CMF (Meeting abstract). *In* Breast Cancer: A Report to the Profession 1976. Bethesda, MD, National Cancer Institute, 1976, p. 52.

Bondy, M. L., Lustbader, E. D., Halabi, S., et al.: Validation of a breast cancer risk assessment model in women with a postive family history. J.N.C.I. J. Natl. Cancer Inst., 86:620–625, 1994.

Boyer, M. J., and Tattersall, M. H.: Diethylstilbestrol revisited in advanced breast cancer management. Med. Pediatr. Oncol., *18*:317, 1990.

Bradbeer, J. W., and Kyngdon, J.: Primary treatment of breast cancer in elderly women with tamoxifen. Clin. Oncol., 9:31, 1983.

Brennan, M. J., Donegan, W. L., and Appleby, D. E.: The variability of estrogen receptors in metastatic breast cancer. Am. J. Surg., *137*:260, 1979.

Bridges, K. G., Keshgegian, A. A., Kumar, H. A., et al.: Influences of surgical technique on estrogen and progesterone receptor determinations in breast cancer. Cancer, *51*:2317, 1983.

Brincker, H., Rose, C., Rank, F., et al.: Evidence of a castration-mediated effect of adjuvant cytotoxic chemotherapy in premenopausal breast cancer. J. Clin. Oncol., 5:1771, 1987.

Brooks, B. J., Jr., and Lippmann, M. E.: Tamoxifen flare in advanced endometrial carcinoma. J. Clin. Oncol., 3:222, 1985.

Bruera, E., Roca, E., Cedaro, L., et al.: Action of oral methylprednisolone in terminal cancer patients: A prospective randomized double-blind study. Cancer Treat. Rep., 69:751, 1985.

Bryant, A. J., and Weir, J. A.: Prophylactic oophorectomy in operable instances of carcinoma of the breast. Surg. Gynecol. Obstet., 153:660, 1981.

Buchanan, R. B., Blamey, R. W., Durrant, K. R., et al.: A randomized comparison of tamoxifen with surgical oophorectomy in premenopausal patients with advanced breast cancer. J. Clin. Oncol., 4:1326, 1986.

Butler, J. A., Bretsky, S., Menendez-Botet, C., et al.: Estrogen receptor protein of breast cancer as a predictor of recurrence. Cancer, 55:1178, 1985.

Buzdar, A. U., Hortobagyi, G. N., Frye, D., et al.: Bioequivalence of 20-mg once-daily tamoxifen relative to 10-mg twice-daily regimens for breast cancer. J. Clin. Oncol., *12*:50–54, 1994.

Calandra, R. S., Chaneau, E. H., Giaroli, A. R., et al.: Incidence of estrogen, progesterone, and prolactin receptors in human breast cancer. *In* Gurpide, E., Colandra, R., Levy, C., et al. (Eds.): Hormones and Cancer. New York, Alan R. Liss, 1984, pp. 97–108.

Carpenter, J. T., Jr., and Peterson, L.: Use of megestrol acetate in advanced breast cancer on a single-daily-dose schedule. Semin. Oncol., *12*(Suppl 1):40, 1985.

Carter, S. K: Single and combination nonhormonal chemotherapy in breast cancer. Cancer, 30:1543, 1972.

Cash, R., Brough, A. J., Cohen, M. N., et al.: Aminoglutethimide (Elipten-Ciba) as an inhibitor of adrenal steroidogenesis: Mechanism of action and therapeutic trial. J. Clin. Endocrinol. Metab., 27:1239, 1967.

Cavilli, F., Goldhirsch, A., Jungi, F., et al.: Randomized trial of low-versus high-dose medroxyprogesterone acetate in the induction treatment of postmenopausal patients with advanced breast cancer. J. Clin. Oncol., 2:414, 1984.

Ciardiello, F., Kim, N., Liscia, D. S., et al.: mRNA expression of transforming growth factor-alpha in human breast carcinomas and its activity in effusions of breast cancer patients. J. Natl. Cancer Inst., 81:1165, 1989.

Clark, G. M., and McGuire, W. L.: Prognostic factors in primary breast cancer. Breast Cancer Res. Treat., 3(Suppl.):S69, 1983.

Clark, G. M., Mathieu, M.-C., Owens, M. A., et al.: Prognostic significance of S-phase fraction in good-risk, node-negative breast cancer patients. J. Clin. Oncol., 10:428, 1992.

Clark, G. M., McGuire, W. L., Hubay, C. A., et al.: Progesterone receptors as a prognostic factor in stage II breast cancer. N. Engl. J. Med., 309:1343, 1983.

Clark, G. M., Sledge, G. W. Jr., Osborne, C. K., et al.: Survival from first recurrence: Relative importance of prognostic factors in 1015 breast cancer patients. J. Clin. Oncol., 5:55, 1987.

Clarke, R., van den Berg, H. W., Murphy, R. F.: Reduction of the membrane fluidity of human breast cancer cells by tamoxifen and 17β-estradiol. J. Natl. Cancer Inst., 82:1702, 1990.

Cocconi, G., Bisagni, G., Ceci, G., et al.: Low-dose aminoglutethimide with and without hydrocortisone replacement as a first-line endocrine treatment in advanced breast cancer: A prospective randomized trial of the Italian Oncology Group for Clinical Research. J. Clin. Oncol., 10:984, 1992.

Colditz, G. A., Stampfer, M. J., Willett, W. C., et al.: Prospective study of estrogen replacement therapy and risk of breast cancer in postmenopausal women. J.A.M.A., 264:2648, 1990.

Coleman, R. E., Mashiter, G., Whitaker, K. B., et al.: Bone scan flare predicts successful systemic therapy for bone metastases. J. Nucl. Med., 29:1354, 1988.

Colomer, R., Ruibal, A., and Salvador, L.: Circulating tumor marker levels in advanced breast carcinoma correlate with the extent of metastatic disease. Cancer, 64:1674, 1989.

Conte, P. F., Fraschini, G., Alama, A., et al.: Chemotherapy following estrogen-induced expansion of the growth fraction of human breast cancer. Cancer Res., 45:5926, 1985.

Conte, P. F., Pronzato, P., Rubagotti, A., et al.: Conventional versus cytokinetic polychemotherapy with estrogenic recruitment in metastatic breast cancer: Results of a randomized cooperative trial. J. Clin. Oncol., 5:339, 1987.

Conte, C. C., Nemoto, T., Rosner, D., et al.: Therapeutic oophorectomy in metastatic breast cancer. Cancer, 64:150, 1989.

Conte, P. F., Gardin, G., Miglietta, L., et al.: Chemotherapy with estrogenic recruitment in locally advanced (LABC) and metastatic breast cancer (MBC): Results of two randomized trials (Meeting abstract). Proc. Am. Soc. Clin. Oncol., 9:A162, 1990.

Coombes, R. C., Dearnaley, D., Humphreys, J., et al.: Danazol treatment of advanced breast cancer. Cancer Treat. Rep., 64:1073, 1980.

Cooperative Breast Cancer Group: Testosterone propionate therapy in breast cancer. J.A.M.A., *188*:1069, 1964.

Cooper, R.: Combination chemotherapy in hormone resistant breast cancer (Abstract). Proc. Am. Assoc. Cancer Res., *10*:15, 1969.

Corle, D. K., Sears, M. E., and Olson, K. B.: Relationship of quantitative estrogen-receptor level and clinical response to cytotoxic chemotherapy in advanced breast cancer: An extramural analysis. Cancer, *54*:1554, 1984.

Costa, R. H., Dhooge, M. R., Van Wing, F., et al.: Tamoxifen retinopathy. A case report. Bull. Soc. Belge. Opthalmol., *238*:161, 1990.

Cote, R. J., Rosen, P. P., Lesser, M. L., et al.: Prediction of early relapse in patients with operable breast cancer by detection of occult bone marrow micrometastases. J. Clin. Oncol., *9*:1749, 1991.

Council on Drugs: Report to the Council. Androgens and estrogens in the treatment of disseminated mammary carcinoma. Retrospective study of nine hundred forty-four patients. J.A.M.A., *172*:1271, 1960.

Cowie, A. T., Forsyth, I. A., and Hart, I. C.: Hormonal Control of Lactation. Berlin, Springer-Verlag, 1980.

Crivellari, D., Galligioni, E., Frustaci, S., et al.: Low-dose aminoglutethimide plus steroid replacement in advanced breast cancer patients resistant to conventional therapies. Cancer Invest., *7*:113, 1989.

Croton, R., Cooke, T., Holt, S., et al.: Oestrogen receptors and survival in early breast cancer. Br. Med. J., *283*:1289, 1981.

Cruz, J. M., Muss, H. B., Brockschmidt, J. K., et al.: Weight changes in women with metastatic breast cancer treated with megestrol acetate: A comparison of standard versus high-dose therapy. Semin. Oncol., *17*(Suppl. 9):63, 1990.

Cutler, S. J., Asire, A. J., and Taylor, S. G., III: Classification of patients with disseminated cancer of the breast. Cancer, *24*:861, 1969.

Daly, L., Ferguson, J., Cram, G. P. Jr., et al.: Comparison of a novel assay for breast cancer mucin to CA15-3 and carcinoembryonic antigen. J. Clin. Oncol., *10*:1057, 1992.

Daniel, F., Rao, D. G., and Tyrrell, C. J.: A pilot study of stanozolol for advanced breast carcinoma. Cancer, *67*:2966, 1991.

deCourmeller, F. V.: La radiotherapie indirecte, ou dirigée par les correlations organiques. Arch. Elect. Med., *32*:264, 1922.

DeFriend, D. J., Howell, A., Nicholson, R. I., et al.: Investigation of a new pure antiestrogen (ICI 182780) in women with primary breast cancer. Cancer Res., *54*:408–414, 1994.

De Muylder, X., Neven, P., De Somer, M., et al.: Endometrial lesions in patients undergoing tamoxifen therapy. Int. J. Gynaecol. Obstet., *36*:127, 1991.

Deschenes, L.: Droloxifene, a new antiestrogen, in advanced breast cancer. A double-blind dose-finding study. The Droloxifene 002 International Study Group. Am. J. Clin. Oncol., *14*(Suppl. 2):S52, 1991.

DeSombre, E. R.: Breast cancer: Hormone receptors, prognosis and therapy. Clin. Oncol., *1*:191, 1982.

DeSombre, E. R., Kledzik, G., Marshall, S., et al.: Estrogen and prolactin receptor concentrations in rat mammary tumors and response to endocrine ablation. Cancer Res., *36*:354, 1976.

DeSombre, E. R., Greene, G. L., King, W. J., et al.: Estrogen receptors, antibodies and hormone dependent cancer. *In* Gurpide, E., Calandra, R., Levy, C., et al. (Eds.): Hormones and Cancer. New York, Alan R. Liss, 1984, pp. 1–22.

Dhadly, M. S., and Walker, R. A.: The localization of prolactin binding sites in human breast tissue. Int. J. Cancer, *31*:433, 1983.

Dickson, R. B., and Lippman, M. E.: Molecular determinants of growth, angiogenesis, and metastases in breast cancer. Semin. Oncol., *19*:286, 1992.

Diczfalusy, E., Notter, G., Edsmyr, F., et al.: Estrogen excretion in breast cancer patients before and after ovarian irradiation and oophorectomy. J. Clin. Endocrinol. Metab., *19*:1230, 1959.

DiSaia, P. J.: Hormone-replacement therapy in patients with breast cancer. Cancer, *71*:1490–1500, 1993.

Dixon, A. R., Robertson, J. F. R., Jackson, L., et al.: Goserelin (Zoladex) in premenopausal advanced breast cancer: Duration of response and survival. Br. J. Cancer, *62*:868, 1990.

Dixon, A. R., Robertson, J. F., Jackson, L., et al.: Zoladex and tamoxifen in premenopausal advanced breast cancer (Meeting abstract). Br. J. Cancer, *64*(Suppl 15):8, 1991.

Dnistrian, A. M., Schwartz, M. K., Fracchia, A. A., et al.: Endocrine consequences of CMF adjuvant therapy in premenopausal and postmenopausal breast cancer patients. Cancer, *51*:803, 1983.

Dombernowsky, P., Zedeler, K., Hansen, M., et al.: Randomized trial of adjuvant CMF + radiotherapy (RT) vs CMF alone vs CMF + tamoxifen (TAM) in pre- and menopausal stage II breast cancer (Abstract). Proc. Am. Soc. Clin. Oncol., *11*:54, 1992.

Dotzlaw, H., Miller, T., Karvelas, J., et al.: Epidermal growth factor gene expression in human breast cancer biopsy samples: Relationship to estrogen and progesterone receptor gene expression. Cancer Res., *50*:4204, 1990.

Dowsett, M., Mehta, A., Mansi, J., et al.: A dose-comparative endocrine-clinical study of leuprolide in premenopausal breast cancer patients. Br. J. Cancer, *62*:854, 1990.

Dreicer, R., and Wilding, G.: Steroid hormone agonists and antagonists in the treatment of cancer. Cancer Invest., *10*:27, 1992.

Duffy, M. J., O'Connell, M., O'Sullivan, F., et al.: CEA-like material in cytosols from human breast carcinomas. Correlation with biochemical and pathologic parameters. Cancer, *51*:121, 1983.

Dupont, W. D., and Page, D. L.: Menopausal estrogen replacement therapy and breast cancer. Arch. Intern. Med., *151*:67, 1991.

Early Breast Cancer Trialists' Collaborative Group: Systemic treatment of early breast cancer by hormonal, cytotoxic, or immune therapy: 133 randomised trials involving 31,000 recurrences and 24,000 deaths among 75,000 women. Lancet, *339*:1–15, 71–85, 1992.

Enck, R. E., and Rios, C. N.: Tamoxifen treatment of metastatic breast cancer and antithrombin III levels. Cancer, *53*:2607, 1984.

Escher, G. C.: Clinical improvement in inoperable breast carcinoma under steroid treatment. *In* Council of Pharmacy and Chemistry, American Medical Association: Proceedings of the First Conference on Steroid Hormone and Mammary Carcinoma. Chicago, American Medical Association, 1949, p. 92.

Etienne, M. C., Milano, G., Frenay, M., et al.: Pharmacokinetics and pharmacodynamics of medroxyprogesterone acetate in advanced breast cancer patients. J. Clin. Oncol., *10*:1176, 1992.

Ettinger, D. S., Allegra, J., Bertino, J. R., et al.: Megestrol acetate *v* tamoxifen in advanced breast cancer: Correlation of hormone receptors and response. Semin. Oncol., *13*(Suppl. 4):9, 1986.

Falkson, G., Falkson, H. C., Glidewell, O., et al.: Improved remission rates and remission duration in young women with metastatic breast cancer following combined oophorectomy and chemotherapy: A study of Cancer and Leukemia Groupe B. Cancer, *43*:2215, 1979.

Falkson, H. C., Falkson, G., Portugal, M. A., et al.: Carcinoembryonic antigen as a marker in patients with breast cancer receiving postsurgical adjuvant chemotherapy. Cancer, *49*:1859, 1982.

Falkson, G., Gelman, R. S., Tormey, D. C., et al.: The Eastern Cooperative Oncology Group experience with cyclophosphamide, Adriamycin, and 5-fluorouracil (CAF) in patients with metastatic breast cancer. Cancer, *56*:219, 1985.

Falkson, G., Gelman, R. S., Tormey, D. C., et al.: Treatment of metastatic breast cancer in premenopausal women using CAF with or without oophorectomy: An Eastern Cooperative Oncology Group study. J. Clin. Oncol., *5*:881, 1987.

Falkson, G., Gelman, R. S., Tormey, D. C., et al.: Median survival of 59 months for premenopausal women with ER-positive metastatic breast cancer: An ECOG study (Abstract 31). Proc. Am. Soc. Clin. Oncol., *13*:57, 1994.

Falkson, H. C., Gray, R., Wolberg, W. H., et al.: Adjuvant trial of 12 cycles of CMFPT followed by observation or continuous tamoxifen versus four cycles of CMFPT in postmenopausal women with breast cancer: An Eastern Cooperative Oncology Group phase III study. J. Clin. Oncol., *8*:599, 1990.

Farrow, J. H., and Woodward, H. Q.: The influence of androgenic and estrogenic substances on the serum calcium. In cases of skeletal metastases from mammary cancer. J.A.M.A., *118*:339, 1942.

Fekete, M., Wittliff, J. L., and Schally, A. V.: Characteristics and distribution of receptors for [D-TRP⁶]-luteinizing hormone–releasing hormone, somatostatin, epidermal growth factor, and sex steroids in 500 biopsy samples of human breast cancer. J. Clin. Lab. Anal., *3*:137, 1989.

Fels, E.: Treatment of breast cancer with testosterone propionate: A preliminary report. J. Clin. Endocrinol., *4*:121, 1944.

Fisher, B.: Experimental and clinical justification for the use of tamoxifen in a breast cancer prevention trial: A description of the NSABP effort (Abstract). Proc. Am. Assoc. Cancer Res., *33*:567, 1992.

Fisher, B., and Redmond, C.: New perspective on cancer of the contralateral breast: A marker for assessing tamoxifen as a preventive agent (Editorial). J. Natl. Cancer Inst., *83*:1278, 1991.

Fisher, B., Ravdin, R. G., Ausman, R. K., et al.: Surgical adjuvant chemotherapy in cancer of the breast: Results of a decade of cooperative investigation. Ann. Surg., *163*:337, 1968.

Fisher, B., Slack, N., Katrych, D., et al.: Ten-year follow-up results of patients with carcinoma of the breast in a cooperative clinical trial evaluating surgical adjuvant chemotherapy. Surg. Gynecol. Obstet., *140*:528, 1975.

Fisher, B., Sherman, B., Rockette, H., et al.: L-Phenylalanine mustard (L-PAM) in the management of premenopausal patients with primary breast cancer. Lack of association of disease-free survival with depression of ovarian function (Abstract). Cancer, *44*:847, 1979.

Fisher, B., Constantino, J. P., Redmond, C. K., et al.: Endometrial cancer in tamoxifen-treated breast cancer patients: Findings from the National Surgical Adjuvant Breast and Bowel Project (NSABP) B-14. J.N.C.I. J. Natl. Cancer Inst., *86*:527–537, 1994.

Fisher, E. R., Redmond, C. K., Liu, H., et al.: Correlation of estrogen receptor and pathologic characteristics of invasive breast cancer. Cancer, *45*:349, 1980.

Fisher, B., Redmond, C., Brown, A., et al.: Treatment of primary breast cancer with chemotherapy and tamoxifen. N. Engl. J. Med., *305*:1, 1981.

Fisher, B., Bauer, M., Wickerham, D. L., et al.: Relation of number of positive axillary nodes to the prognosis of patients with primary breast cancer: An NSABP update. Cancer, *52*:1551, 1983*a*.

Fisher, B., Redmond, C., Brown, A., et al.: Influence of tumor estrogen and progesterone receptor levels on the response to tamoxifen and chemotherapy in primary breast cancer. J. Clin. Oncol., *1*:227, 1983*b*.

Fisher, B., Redmond, C., Brown, A., et al.: Adjuvant chemotherapy with and without tamoxifen in the treatment of primary breast cancer: 5-year results from the National Surgical Adjuvant Breast and Bowel Project Trial. J. Clin. Oncol., *4*:459, 1986.

Fisher, B., Brown, A., Wolmark, N., et al.: Prolonging tamoxifen therapy for primary breast cancer: Findings from the National Surgical Adjuvant Breast and Bowel Project Clinical Trial. Ann. Intern. Med., *106*:649, 1987*b*.

Fisher, E. R., Sass, R., and Fisher, B.: Pathologic findings from the national surgical adjuvant breast project: Correlations with concordant and discordant estrogen and progesterone receptors. Cancer, *59*:1554, 1987*a*.

Fisher, B., Constantino, J., Redmond, C., et al.: A randomized clinical trial evaluating tamoxifen in the treatment of patients with node-negative breast cancer who have estrogen-receptor–positive tumors. N. Engl. J. Med., *320*:479, 1989*a*.

Fisher, B., Redmond, C., Wickerham, D. L., et al.: Systemic therapy in patients with node-negative breast cancer: A commentary based on two National Surgical Adjuvant Breast and Bowel Project (NSABP) clinical trials. Ann. Intern. Med., *111*:703, 1989*b*.

Fisher, B., Redmond, C., Legault-Poisson, S., et al.: Postoperative chemotherapy and tamoxifen compared with tamoxifen alone in the treatment of positive-node breast cancer patients aged 50 years and older with tumors responsive to tamoxifen: Results from the National Surgical Adjuvant Breast and Bowel Project B-16. J. Clin. Oncol., *8*:1005, 1990.

Fisher, B., Wickerham, D. L., and Redmond, C.: Recent developments in the use of systemic adjuvant therapy for the treatment of breast cancer. Semin. Oncol., *19*:263, 1992.

Foekens, J. A., Portengen, H., Janssen, M., et al.: Insulin-like growth factor-1 receptors and insulin-like growth factor-1–like activity in human primary breast cancer. Cancer, *63*:2139, 1989.

Forbes, J. F., Byrne, M., Snyder, R., et al.: Oophorectomy (OOX) versus cytotoxic chemotherapy (AC) versus concurrent modality therapy (OOX + AC). A randomised trial in premenopausal women with advanced breast cancer (Abstract). Proc. Am. Soc. Clin. Oncol., *11*:80, 1992.

Fornander, T., Cedermark, B., Mattsson, A., et al.: Adjuvant tamoxifen in early breast cancer: Occurrence of new primary cancers. Lancet, *1*:117, 1989.

Fornander, T., Rutqvist, L. E., Sjöberg, H. E., et al.: Long-term adjuvant tamoxifen in early breast cancer: Effect on bone mineral density in postmenopausal women. J. Clin. Oncol., *8*:1019, 1990.

Fracchia, A. A., Randall, H. T., and Farrow, J. H.: The results of adrenalectomy in advanced breast cancer in 500 consecutive patients. Surg. Gynecol. Obstet., *125*:747, 1967.

Frantz, A. G., and Rabkin, K. J.: Effects of estrogen and sex difference on

secretion of human growth hormone. J. Clin. Endocrinol. Metab., *25*:1470, 1965.

Frantz, A. G., and Wilson, J. D.: Endocrine disorders of the breast. *In* Wilson, J. D., and Foster, D. W. (Eds.): Williams Textbook of Endocrinology. 7th Ed. Philadelphia, W.B. Saunders, 1985, pp. 402–421.

Freeman, C. S., and Topper, Y. J.: Progesterone is not essential to the differentiative potential of mammary epithelium in the male mouse. Endocrinology, *103*:186, 1978.

Fuqua, S. A.: Where is the lesion in hormone-independent breast cancer? (Editorial). J. Natl. Cancer Inst., *84*:554, 1992.

Gail, M. H., Brinton, L. A., Byar, D. P., et al.: Projecting individualized probabilities of developing breast cancer for white females who are being examined annually. J. Natl. Cancer Inst., *81*:1879, 1989.

Gal, D., Kopel, S., Bashevkin, M., et al.: Oncogenic potential of tamoxifen on endometria of postmenopausal women with breast cancer—preliminary report. Gynecol. Oncol., *42*:120, 1991.

Gapinski, P. V., and Donegan, W. L.: Estrogen receptors and breast cancer: Prognostic and therapeutic implications. Surgery, *88*:386, 1980.

Garcia, M. B., Blankenstein, M. A., van der Wall, E., et al.: Comparison of breast cancer mucin (BCM) and CA 15-3 in human breast cancer. Breast Cancer Res. Treat., *17*:69, 1990.

Gardner, B., Thomas, A. N., and Gordan G. S.: Antitumor efficacy of prednisone and sodium liothyronine in advanced breast cancer. Cancer, *15*:334, 1962.

Gasparini, G., Pozza, F., Harris, A. L.: Evaluating the potential usefulness of new prognostic predictive indicators in node-negative breast cancer patients. J.N.C.I. J. Natl. Cancer Inst., *85*:1206–1219, 1993.

Gerner, E. W.: Ocular toxicity of tamoxifen. Ann. Ophthalmol., *21*:420, 1989.

Glauber, J. G., and Kiang, D. T.: The changing role of hormonal therapy in advanced breast cancer. Semin. Oncol., *19*:308, 1992.

Glick, J. H., Creech, R. H., Torri, S., et al.: Tamoxifen plus sequential CMF chemotherapy versus tamoxifen alone in postmenopausal patients with advanced breast cancer: A randomized trial. Cancer, *45*:735, 1980.

Godolphin, W., Elwood, J. M., and Spinelli, J. J.: Estrogen receptor quantitation and staging as complementary prognostic indicators in breast cancer: A study of 583 patients. Int. J. Cancer, *28*:677, 1981.

Goldberg, R. M., Loprinzi, C. L., O'Fallon, J. R., et al.: Transdermal clonidine for ameliorating tamoxifen-induced hot flashes. J. Clin Oncol., *12*:155–158, 1994.

Greenwald, E. S.: Megestrol acetate flare (Letter). Cancer Treat. Rep., *67*:405, 1983.

Gregory, E. J., Cohen, S. C., Oines, D. W., et al.: Megestrol acetate therapy for breast cancer. J. Clin. Oncol., *3*:155, 1985.

Gusberg, S. B.: Tamoxifen for breast cancer: Associated endometrial cancer (Editorial). Cancer, *65*:1463, 1990.

Haas, H. A. D.: A trial of oophorectomy against Nolvadex (tamoxifen). Rev. Endocrine-Related Cancer, *10*(Suppl.):27, 1981.

Hall, T. C.: Predictive tests in cancer. Br. J. Cancer, *30*:191, 1974.

Hall, T. C., Dederick, M. M., and Nevinny, H. B.: Prognostic value of hormonally induced hypercalcemia in breast cancer. Cancer Chemother. Rep., *30*:21, 1963.

Hamm, J. T., Tormey, D. C., Kohler, P. C., et al.: Phase I study of toremifene in patients with advanced cancer. J. Clin. Oncol., *9*:2036, 1991.

Harris, H. S. Jr., and Spratt, J. S. Jr.: Bilateral adrenalectomy in metastatic mammary cancer. An analysis of sixty-four cases. Cancer, *23*:145, 1969.

Hartviet, F., Maartmann-Moe, H., Sta, K. F., et al.: Early recurrence of oestrogen receptor–negative breast carcinomas. A preliminary report. Acta Chir. Scand., *146*:93, 1980.

Harvey, H. A., Lipton, A., Max, D. T., et al.: Medical castration produced by the GnRH analogue leuprolide to treat metastatic breast cancer. J. Clin. Oncol., *3*:1068, 1985.

Hawkins, R. A., Tesdale, A. L., Anderson, E. D. C., et al.: Does the oestrogen receptor concentration of a breast cancer change during systemic therapy? Br. J. Cancer, *61*:877, 1990.

Hayward, J. L., Carbone, P. P., Heuson, J. C., et al.: Assessment of response to therapy in advanced breast cancer: A project of the programme on Clinical Oncology of the International Union Against Cancer, Geneva, Switzerland. Cancer, *39*:1289, 1977.

Henderson, I. C., Hayes, D. F., Come, S., et al.: New agents and new medical treatments for advanced breast cancer. Semin. Oncol., *14*:34, 1987.

Henderson, I. C., Harris, J. R., Kinne, D. W., et al.: Cancer of the breast. *In* DeVita, V., Hellman, S., and Rosenberg, S. A. (Eds.): Cancer: Principles and Practice of Oncology. 3rd ed. Philadelphia, J. B. Lippincott, 1989, pp. 1197–1268.

Höffken, K., Jonat, W., Possinger, K., et al.: Aromatase inhibition with 4-hydroxyandrostenedione in the treatment of postmenopausal patients with advanced breast cancer: A phase II study. J. Clin. Oncol., *8*:875, 1990.

Hoffman, D. A., McConabey, W. M., Brinton, L. A., et al.: Breast cancer in hypothyroid women using thyroid supplements. J. A. M. A., *251*:616, 1984.

Holdaway, I. M., and Bowditch, J. V.: Variation in receptor status between primary and metastatic breast cancer. Cancer, *52*:479, 1983.

Hoogstraten, B., Fletcher, W. S., Gad-el-Mawla, N., et al.: Tamoxifen and oophorectomy in the treatment of recurrent breast cancer: A Southwest Oncology Group study. Cancer Res., *42*:4788, 1982.

Hoogstraten, B., Gad-el-Mawla, N., Maloney, T. R., et al.: Combined modality therapy for first recurrence of breast cancer: A Southwest Oncology Group Study. Cancer, *54*:2248, 1984.

Horobin, J. M., Preece, P. E., Dewar, J. A., et al.: 5-12-Year follow-up of 113 elderly patients with localized breast cancer whose sole primary treatment was tamoxifen (Meeting abstract). Br. J. Cancer, *62*(Suppl. 12):12, 1990.

Horobin, J. M., Preece, P. E., Dewar, J. A., et al.: Long-term follow-up of elderly patients with locoregional breast cancer treated with tamoxifen only. Br. J. Surg., *78*:213, 1991.

Hortobagyi, G: Bone metastases in breast cancer patients. Semin. Oncol., *18*(Suppl. 5):11, 1991.

Horwitz, K. B., McGuire, W. L., Pearson, O. H., et al.: Predicting response to endocrine therapy in human breast cancer: A hypothesis. Science, *189*:726, 1975.

Huggins, C., and Bergenstal, D. M.: Inhibition of human mammary and prostatic cancer by adrenalectomy. Cancer Res., *12*:134, 1952.

Huggins, C., and Hodges, C. V.: Studies on prostatic cancer. Effect of castration, of estrogen and of androgen injection on serum phosphatases in metastatic carcinoma of the prostate. Cancer Res., *1*:293, 1941.

Hull, D. F. 3rd., Clark, G. M., Osborne, C. K., et al.: Multiple estrogen receptor assays in human breast cancer. Cancer Res., *43*:413, 1983.

Ingle, J. N.: Additive hormonal therapy in women with advanced breast cancer. Cancer, *53*:766, 1984.

Ingle, J. N., Ahmann, D. L., Green, S. J., et al.: Randomized clinical trial of diethylstilbestrol versus tamoxifen in postmenopausal women with advanced breast cancer. N. Engl. J. Med., *304*:16, 1981.

Ingle, J. N., Krook, J. E., Green, S. J., et al.: Randomized trial of bilateral oophorectomy versus tamoxifen in premenopausal women with metastatic breast cancer. J. Clin. Oncol., *4*:178, 1986.

Ingle, J. N., Everson, L. K., Wieand, H. S., et al.: Randomized trial of observation versus adjuvant therapy with cyclophosphamide, fluorouracil, prednisone with or without tamoxifen following mastectomy in postmenopausal women with node-positive breast cancer. J. Clin. Oncol., *6*:1388, 1988*a*.

Ingle, J. N., Twito, D. I., Schaid, D. J., et al.: Randomized clinical trial of tamoxifen alone or combined with fluoxymesterone in postmenopausal women with metastatic breast cancer. J. Clin. Oncol., *6*:825, 1988*b*.

Ingle, J. N., Everson, L. K., Wieand, H. S., et al.: Randomized trial to evaluate the addition of tamoxifen to cyclophosphamide, 5-fluorouracil, prednisone adjuvant therapy in premenopausal women with node-positive breast cancer. Cancer, *63*:1257, 1989.

Ingle, J. N., Twito, D. I., Schaid, D. J., et al.: Combination hormonal therapy with tamoxifen plus fluoxymesterone versus tamoxifen alone in postmenopausal women with metastatic breast cancer: An updated analysis. Cancer, *67*:886, 1991.

Ingle, J. N., Foley, J. F., Mailliard, J. A., et al.: Randomized trial of cyclophosphamide, methotrexate, and 5-fluorouracil with or without estrogenic recruitment in women with metastatic breast cancer. Cancer, *73*:2337–2343, 1994.

Ingram, D. M., Nottage, E. M., Roberts, A. N., et al.: Prolactin and breast cancer risk. Med. J. Aust., *153*:469, 1990.

International Breast Cancer Study Group: Late effects of adjuvant oophorectomy and chemotherapy upon premenopausal breast cancer patients. Ann. Oncol., *1*:30, 1990.

Jensen, E. V., Block, G. E., Smith, S., et al.: Estrogen receptors and breast cancer response to adrenalectomy. Natl. Cancer Inst. Monogr., *34*:55, 1971.

Jiang, S.-Y., and Jordan, V. C.: Growth regulation of estrogen receptor–negative breast cancer cells transfected with complementary DNAs for estrogen receptor. J. Natl. Cancer Inst., *84*:580, 1992.

Joensuu, H., Toikkanen, S., and Klemi, P. J.: DNA index and S-phase fraction and their combination as prognostic factors in operable ductal breast carcinoma. Cancer, *66*:331, 1990.

Johnson, P. A., Bonomi, P. D., Anderson, K. M., et al.: Progesterone receptor level as a predictor of response to megestrol acetate in advanced breast cancer: A retrospective study. Cancer Treat. Rep., *67*:717, 1983.

Johnson, P. A., Muss, H., Bonomi, P., et al.: Megestrol acetate as primary hormonal therapy for advanced breast cancer. Semin. Oncol., *15*(Suppl 1):34, 1988.

Jonat, W., Kaufmann, M., Blamey, R. W., et al.: A randomized trial comparing "Zoladex" (Goserelin) with "Zoladex" Plus "Novaldex" (tamoxifen) as first-line treatment for pre-menopausal advanced breast cancer (Abstract 33). Proc. Am. Soc. Clin. Oncol., *13*:58, 1994.

Jordan, V. C.: Laboratory studies to develop general principles for the adjuvant treatment of breast cancer with antiestrogens: Problems and potential for future clinical applications. Breast Cancer Res. Treat., *3*(Suppl.):73, 1983.

Jordan, V. C.: Estrogen receptor–mediated direct and indirect antitumor effects of tamoxifen (Editorial). J. Natl. Cancer Inst., *82*:1662, 1990.

Jordan, V. C.: The role of tamoxifen in the treatment and prevention of breast cancer. Curr. Probl. Cancer, *16*:129, 1992.

Jordan, V. C.: Growth factor regulation by tamoxifen is demonstrated in patients with breast cancer. Cancer, *72*:1–2, 1993.

Jordan, V. C., Allen, K. E., and Dix, C. J.: Pharmacology of tamoxifen in laboratory animals. Cancer Treat. Rep., *64*:745, 1980.

Jordan, V. C., Mirecki, D. M., and Gottardis, M. M.: Continuous tamoxifen treatment prevents the appearance of mammary tumors in a model system. *In* Jones, S. E., and Salmon, S. E. (Eds.): Adjuvant Therapy of Cancer IV. New York, Grune & Stratton, 1984, pp. 27–34.

Jordan, V. C., Lababidi, M. K., and Langan-Fahey, S.: Suppression of mouse mammary tumorigenesis by long-term tamoxifen therapy. J. Natl. Cancer Inst., *83*:492, 1991*a*.

Jordan, V. C., Fritz, N. F., Langan-Fahey, S., et al.: Alteration of endocrine parameters in premenopausal women with breast cancer during long-term adjuvant therapy with tamoxifen as the single agent. J. Natl. Cancer Inst., *83*:1488, 1991*b*.

Jordan, V. C., Jeng, M.-H., Jiang, S.-Y., et al.: Hormonal strategies for breast cancer: A new focus on the estrogen receptor as a therapeutic target. Semin. Oncol., *19*:299, 1992.

Kaiser-Kupfer, M. L., and Lippman, M. E.: Tamoxifen retinopathy. Cancer Treat. Rep., *62*:315, 1978.

Kalman, A. M., Thompson, T., and Vogel C. L.: Response to oophorectomy after tamoxifen failure in a premenopausal patient. Cancer Treat. Rep., *66*:1867, 1983.

Kamby, C. Rasmussen, B. B., and Krinstensen, B.: Oestrogen receptor status of primary breast carcinomas and their metastases. Relation to pattern of spread and survival after recurrence. Br. J. Cancer, *60*:252, 1989.

Kapdi, C. C., and Wolfe, J. N.: Breast cancer. Relationship to thyroid supplements for hypothyroidism. J. A. M. A., *236*:1124, 1976.

Karashima, T., and Schally, A. V.: Inhibitory effects of somatostatin analogs on prolactin secretion in rats pretreated with estrogen or haloperidol (42518). Proc. Soc. Exp. Biol. Med., *185*:69, 1987.

Kardinal, C. G.: Cancer chemotherapy. Historical aspects and future considerations. Postgrad. Med., *77*:165, 1985.

Kardinal, C. G.: Chemotherapy of breast cancer. *In* Perry, M. C. (Ed.): The Chemotherapy Source Book. Baltimore, Williams & Wilkins, 1992, pp. 948–988.

Kardinal, C. G., and Bush, D. J.: Complications of treatment for advanced colorectal cancer. *In* Ferrari, B. T., Ray, J. E., and Gathright, J. B. (Eds.): Complications of Colon and Rectal Surgery: Prevention and Management. Philadelphia, W.B. Saunders, 1985, pp. 267–300.

Kardinal, C. G., Perry, M. C., Weinberg, V., et al.: Chemoendocrine therapy vs. chemotherapy alone for advanced breast cancer in postmenopausal women: Preliminary report of a randomized study. Breast Cancer Res. Treat., *3*:365, 1983.

Kardinal, C. G., Perry, M. C., Korzun, A. H., et al.: Lack of differential response of estrogen receptor–positive (ER+) vs. ER negative (ER−) breast cancer to Cytoxan and Adriamycin and 5-fluorouracil (CAF) chemotherapy (Abstract). Proc. Am. Soc. Clin. Oncol., *5*:74, 1986.

Katzellenbogen, B. S.: Antiestrogen resistance: Mechanisms by which breast cancer cells undermine the effectiveness of endocrine therapy (Editorial). J. Natl. Cancer Inst., *83:*1434, 1991.

Kaufman, R. J., and Escher, G. C.: Rebound regression in advanced mammary carcinoma. Surg. Gynecol. Obstet., *113:*635, 1961.

Kaufmann, M., Jonat, W., Kleeberg, U., et al.: Goserelin, a depot gonadotrophin-releasing hormone agonist in the treatment of premenopausal patients wtih metastatic breast cancer. J. Clin. Oncol., *17:*1113, 1989.

Kelley, R. M.: Hormones and chemotherapy in breast cancer. Cancer, *28:*1686, 1971.

Kennedy, B. J.: Stimulation of erythropoiesis by androgenic hormones. Ann. Intern. Med., *57:*917, 1962.

Kennedy, B. J.: Hormonal therapy for advanced breast cancer. Cancer, *18:*1551, 1965.

Kennedy, B. J.: Hormonal therapies in breast cancer. Semin. Oncol., *1:*119, 1974.

Kennedy, B. J., Tibbetts, D. M., Nathanson, I. T., et al.: Hypercalcemia, a complication of hormone therapy of advanced breast cancer. Cancer Res., *13:*445, 1953.

Keyhani-Rofagha, S., O'Toole, R. V., Farrar, W. B., et al.: Is DNA ploidy an independent prognostic indicator in infiltrative node-negative breast adenocarcinoma? Cancer, *65:*1577, 1990.

Keynes, G.: The life and works of Sir Astley Cooper. St. Bartholomew's Hosp. Rep., *15:*9, 1922.

Kiang, D. T., and Kollander, R.: Breast cancers negative for estrogen receptor but positive for progesterone receptor, a true entity? J. Clin. Oncol., *5:*662, 1987.

Kiang, D. T., Frenning, D. H., Goldman, A. I., et al.: Estrogen receptors and responses to chemotherapy and hormonal therapy in advanced breast cancer. N. Engl. J. Med., *299:*1330, 1978.

Kiang, D. T., Frenning, D. H., Vosika, G. J., et al.: Comparison of tamoxifen and hypophysectomy in breast cancer treatment. Cancer, *45:*1322, 1980.

Killacke, M. A., Hakes, T. B., and Pierce, V. K.: Endometrial adenocarcinoma in breast cancer patients receiving antiestrogens. Cancer Treat. Rep., *69:*237, 1985.

King, W. J., Jensen, E. V., Miller, L., et al.: Immunocytochemical detection of estrogen receptor in frozen sections of human breast tumors with monoclonal antireceptor antibodies. Abstr. Endocrine Soc., 1982, p. 258.

Kinne, D. W., Ashikari, R., Butler, A., et al.: Estrogen receptor protein in breast cancer as a predictor of recurrence. Cancer, *47:*2364, 1981.

Klijn, J. G., and de Jong, F. H.: Treatment with a luteinising-hormone–releasing hormone analogue (buserelin) in premenopausal patients with metastatic breast cancer. Lancet, *1:*1213, 1982.

Klijn, J. G., de Jong, F. H., Blankenstein, M. A., et al.: Anti-tumor and endocrine effects of chronic LHRH agonist treatment (buserelin) with or without tamoxifen in premenopausal metastatic breast cancer. Breast Cancer Res. Treat., *4:*209, 1984.

Klijn, J. G. M., de Jong, F. H., Bakker, G. H., et al.: Antiprogestins, a new form of endocrine therapy for human breast cancer. Cancer Res., *49:*2851, 1989.

Knight, W. A., Livingston, R. B., Gregory, E. J., et al.: Estrogen receptor as an independent prognostic factor for early recurrence in breast cancer. Cancer Res., *37:*4669, 1977.

Kornblith, P. L., Walker, N. D., and Cassady, J. R.: Treatment of metastatic cancer. *In* DeVita, V. T., Hellman, S., and Rosenberg, S. A. (Eds.): Cancer: Principles and Practice of Oncology. 2nd ed. Philadelphia, J. B. Lippincott, 1985, p. 2101.

Krook, J. E., Ingle, J. N., Green, S. J., et al.: Randomized clinical trial of cyclophosphamide, 5-FU, and prednisone with or without tamoxifen in postmenopausal women with advanced breast cancer. Cancer Treat. Rep., *69:*355, 1985.

Kuhajda, F. P., Piantadosi, S., Pasternack, G. R.: Haptoglobin-related protein (Hpr) epitopes in breast cancer as a predictor of recurrence of the disease. N. Engl. J. Med., *321:*636, 1989.

Lacassagne, A., and Raynaud, A.: Sur le mechanisme d'une action preventive de la testosterone sur le carcinome mammaire de la souris. Compt. Rend. Soc. Biol., *131:*586, 1939.

Le Roy, V., Escot, C., Brouillet, J. P., et al.: Decrease of c-*erb*B-2 and c-*myc* RNA levels in tamoxifen-treated breast cancer. Oncogene, *6:*431, 1991.

Legha, S. S.: Tamoxifen in the treatment of breast cancer. Ann. Intern. Med., *109:*219, 1988.

Legha, S. S., Powell, K., Buzdar, A. U., et al.: Tamoxifen-induced hypercalcemia in breast cancer. Cancer, *47:*2803, 1981.

Lerner, L. J., and Jordan, V. C.: Development of antiestrogens and their use in breast cancer: Eighth Cain Memorial Award Lecture. Cancer Res., *50:*4177, 1990.

Lett, H.: An analysis of 99 cases of inoperable breast cancer treated by oophorectomy. Lancet, *1:*227, 1905.

Levine, M. N., Gent, M., Hirsh, J., et al.: The thrombogenic effect of anticancer drug therapy in women with stage II breast cancer. N. Engl. J. Med., *318:*404, 1988.

Lippman, M. E.: Antiestrogen therapy of breast cancer. Semin. Oncol., *10*(4 Suppl. 4):11, 1983.

Lippman, M. E.: Endocrine responsive cancers of man. *In* Wilson, J. D., and Foster, D. W. (Eds.): Williams Textbook of Endocrinology. 7th Ed. Philadelphia, W. B. Saunders, 1985, pp. 1309–1326.

Lippman, M. E., and Allegra, J. C.: Quantitative estrogen receptor analyses: The response to endocrine and cytotoxic chemotherapy in human breast cancer and the disease-free interval. Cancer, *46:*2829, 1980.

Lippman, M. E., and Bolan, G.: Oestrogen-responsive human breast cancer in long-term tissue culture. Nature (Lond), *256:*592, 1975.

Lippman, M., Bolan, G., and Huff, K.: Interactions of antiestrogens with human breast cancer in long-term tissue culture. Cancer Treat. Rep., *60:*1421, 1976.

Lippman, M. E., Allegra, J. C., Thompson, E. B., et al.: The relation between estrogen receptors and response rate to cytotoxic chemotherapy in metastatic breast cancer. N. Engl. J. Med., *298:*1223, 1978.

Lippman, M. E., Dickson, R. B., Bates, S., et al.: Autocrine and paracine growth regulation of human breast cancer. Breast Cancer Res. Treat., *7:*59, 1986.

Lipton, A., Harvey, H. A., and Hamilton, R. W.: Venous thrombosis as a side effect of tamoxifen treatment. Cancer Treat. Rep., *68:*887, 1984.

Lipton, A., Santner, S. J., Santen, R. J., et al.: Aromatase activity in primary and metastatic human breast cancer. Cancer, *59:*779, 1987.

Lipton, A., Harvey, H. A., Demers, L. M., et al.: A phase I trial of CGS 16949A. A new aromatase inhibitor. Cancer, *65:*1279, 1990.

Lnning, P. E., Jacobs, S., Jones, A., et al.: The influence of CGS 16949A on peripheral aromatisation in breast cancer patients. Br. J. Cancer, *63:*789, 1991.

Loeser, A. A.: Male hormone in treatment of cancer of the breast. Acta Un. Int. Contre Cancer, *4:*375, 1939.

Longstaff, S., Sigurdsson, H., O'Keefe, M., et al.: A controlled study of the ocular effects of tamoxifen in conventional dosage in the treatment of breast carcinoma. Eur J. Cancer Clin. Oncol., *25:*1805, 1989.

Loprinzi, C. L., and Ahmann, D. L.: Carcinoembryonic antigen. A routine test in patients with breast carcinoma? (Editorial). Arch. Intern. Med., *146:*2125, 1986.

Loprinzi, C. L., Ellison, N. M., Goldberg, R. M., et al.: Alleviation of cancer anorexia and cachexia: Studies of the Mayo Clinic and the North Central Cancer Treatment Group. Semin. Oncol., *17*(Suppl. 9):8, 1990.

Loprinzi, C. L., Michalak, J. C., Schaid, D. J., et al: Phase III evaluation of four doses of megestrol acetate as therapy for patients with cancer, anorexia, and/or cachexia. J. Clin. Oncol., *11:*762–767, 1993.

Loprinzi, C. L., Michalak, J. C., Quella, S. K., et al.: Placebo-controlled clinical trial of megestrol acetate (MA) for ameliorating hot flashes in both men and women: A North Central Cancer Treatment Group Study (Abstract 1482). Proc. Am. Soc. Clin. Oncol., *13:*432, 1994.

Love, R. R.: Tamoxifen therapy in primary breast cancer: Biology, efficacy, and side effects. J. Clin. Oncol., *7:*803, 1989.

Love, R. R., Newcomb, P. A., Wiebe, D. A., et al.: Effects of tamoxifen therapy on lipid and lipoprotein levels in postmenopausal patients with node-negative breast cancer. J. Natl. Cancer Inst., *82:*1327, 1990.

Love, R. R., Cameron, L., Connell, B. L., et al.: Symptoms associated with tamoxifen treatment in postmenopausal women. Arch. Intern. Med., *151:*1842, 1991.

Love, R. R., Mazess, R. B., Barden, H. S., et al.: Effects of tamoxifen on bone mineral density in postmenopausal women with breast cancer. N. Engl. J. Med., *326:*852, 1992*a*.

Love, R. R., Surawicz, T. S., Williams, E. C.: Antithrombin III level, fibrinogen level, and platelet count changes with adjuvant tamoxifen therapy. Arch. Intern. Med., *152:*317, 1992*b*.

Ludwig Breast Cancer Study Group: Chemotherapy with or without oophorectomy in high-risk premenopausal patients with operable breast cancer. J. Clin. Oncol., *3:*1059, 1985.

Luft, R., and Olivecrona, H.: Experiences with hypophysectomy in man. J. Neurosurg., *10:*301, 1953.

Lundgren, S., Kvinnsland, S., and Utaaker, E.: Oral high-dose progestins as treatment for advanced breast cancer. Acta Oncol., *28:*811, 1989.

Lyons, W. R., Li, C. H., and Johnson, R. E.: The hormonal control of mammary growth and lactation. Recent Prog. Horm. Res., *14:*219, 1958.

Macheledt, J. E., Buzdar, A. U., Hortobagyi, G. N., et al.: Phase II evaluation of interferon added to tamoxifen in the treatment of metastatic breast cancer. Breast Cancer Res. Treat., *18:*165, 1991.

Manni, A., and Pearson, O. H.: Antiestrogen-induced remissions in premenopausal women with stage IV breast cancer: Effects on ovarian function. Cancer Treat. Rep., *64:*779, 1980.

Manni, A., Trujillo, J. E., and Pearson, O. H.: Predominant role of prolactin in stimulating the growth of 7, 12-dimethylbenz(a)-anthracene–induced rat mammary tumor. Cancer Res., *37:*1216, 1977.

Manni, A., Trujillo, J. E., Marshall, J. S., et al.: Antihormone treatment of stage IV breast cancer. Cancer, *43:*444, 1979.

Mansour, E. G., Hastert, M., Park, C. H., et al.: Tissue and plasma carcinoembryonic antigen in early breast cancer. A prognostic factor. Cancer, *51:*1243, 1983.

Marchant, D. J.: Estrogen-replacement therapy after breast cancer: Risks versus benefits. Cancer, *71:*2169–2176, 1993.

Margreiter, R., and Wiegele, J.: Tamoxifen (Nolvadex) for premenopausal patients with advanced breast cancer. Breast Cancer Res. Treat., *4:*45, 1984.

Martoni, A., Longhi, A., Canova, N., et al.: High-dose medroxyprogesterone acetate versus oophorectomy as first-line therapy of advanced breast cancer in premenopausal patients. Oncology, *48:*1–6, 1991.

Mathé, G., Keiling, R., Prévot, G., et al.: LH-RH agonist: Breast and prostate cancer. *In* Klijn, J. G. M., et al. (Eds.): Hormonal Manipulation of Cancer: Peptides, Growth Factors, and New Anti-Steroidal Agents. New York, Raven, 1987, pp. 315–319.

McDonald, C. C., and Stewart, H. J.: Fatal myocardial infarction in the Scottish Adjuvant Tamoxifen Trial. The Scottish Breast Cancer Committee. Br. Med. J., *303:*435, 1991.

McDonald, I.: Endocrine ablation in disseminated mammary carcinoma. Surg. Gynecol. Obstet., *115:*215, 1962.

McGuire, W. L.: Estrogen receptors in human breast cancer. J. Clin. Invest., *52:*73, 1973.

McGuire, W. L., and Clark, G. M.: The prognostic role of progesterone receptors in human breast cancer. Semin. Oncol., *10*(Suppl. 4):2, 1983.

McGuire, W. L., and Clark, G. M.: Prognostic factors and treatment decisions in axillary node–negative breast cancer. N. Engl. J. Med., *326:*1756, 1992.

McGuire, W. L., Carbone, P. O., and Vollmer, E. P.: Estrogen Receptors in Human Breast Cancer. New York, Raven, 1975.

McGuire, W. L., Clark, G. M., Dressler, L. G., et al.: Role of steroid hormone receptors as prognostic factors in primary breast cancer. Natl. Cancer Inst. Monogr., *1:*19, 1986.

McGuire, W. L., Tandon, A. K., Allred, D. C., et al.: How to use prognostic factors in axillary node–negative breast cancer patients. J. Natl. Cancer Inst., *82:*1006, 1990.

Meakin, J. W., Allt, W. E. C., Beale, F. A., et al.: Ovarian irradiation and prednisone following surgery and radiotherapy for carcinoma of the breast. Breast Cancer Res. Treat., *3*(Suppl. 1):S45, 1983.

Mecklenburg, R. S., and Lipsett, M. B.: Disappearance of metastatic breast cancer after oophorectomy. N. Engl. J. Med., *289:*845, 1973.

Meyer, J. S., Rao, B. R., Stevens, S. C., et al.: Low incidence of estrogen receptor in breast carcinomas with rapid rates of cellular replication. Cancer, *40:*2290, 1977.

Michna, H., Schneider, M. R., Nishino, Y., et al.: The antitumor mechanism of progesterone antagonists is a receptor-mediated antiproliferative effect by induction of terminal cell death. J. Steroid Biochem., *34:*447, 1989.

Miller, W. R., Hawkins, R. A., and Forrest, A. P.: Significance of aromatase activity in human breast cancer. Cancer Res., *42*(Suppl.):3365s, 1982.

Miserez, A. R., Gunes, I., Muller-Brand, J., et al.: Clinical value of a mucin-like carcinoma-associated antigen in monitoring breast cancer patients in comparison with CA 15-3. Eur. J. Cancer, *27:*126, 1991.

Morgan, L. R.: Megestrol acetate vs tamoxifen in advanced breast cancer in postmenopausal patients. Semin. Oncol., *12*(1 Suppl. 1):43, 1985.

Mori, T., Morimoto, T., Komaki, K., et al.: Comparison of estrogen recep-

tor and epidermal growth factor receptor content of primary and involved nodes in human breast cancer. Cancer, *68:*532, 1991.

Mortimer, J., Reimer, R., Greenstreet, R., et al.: Influence of estrogen receptor status on response to combination chemotherapy for recurrent breast cancer. Cancer Treat. Rep., *65:*763, 1981.

Muggia, F. M., and Heinemann, H. O.: Hypercalcemia associated with neoplastic disease. Ann. Intern. Med., *73:*281, 1970.

Musey, V. C., Collins, D. C., Musey, P. I., et al.: Long-term effect of a first pregnancy on the secretion of prolactin. N. Engl. J. Med., *316:*229, 1987.

Muss, H. B., Paschold, E. H., Black, W. R., et al.: Megestrol acetate v tamoxifen in advanced breast cancer: A phase III trial of the Piedmont Oncology Association (POA). Semin. Oncol., *12*(Suppl. 1):55, 1985.

Muss, H., Paschold, E., Black, W., et al.: Megestrol acetate (M) vs. tamoxifen (T) in advanced breast cancer (ABC): A five-year report (Abstract). Proc. Am. Soc. Clin. Oncol., *5:*55, 1987.

Muss, H. B., Wells, H. B., Paschold, E. H., et al.: Megestrol acetate versus tamoxifen in advanced breast cancer: 5-year analysis—a phase III trial of the Piedmont Oncology Association. J. Clin. Oncol., *6:*1098, 1988.

Muss, H. B., Case, L. D., Capizzi, R. L., et al.: High- versus standard-dose megestrol acetate in women with advanced breast cancer: A phase III trial of the Piedmont Oncology Association. J. Clin. Oncol., *8:*1797, 1990.

Naeim, F., Copper, P. H., and Semion, A. A.: Peliosis hepatis. Possible etiologic role of anabolic steroids. Arch. Pathol., *95:*284, 1973.

National Institutes of Health: National Institutes of Health Consensus Development Conference Statement. Treatment of Early Stage Breast Cancer, June 18–21, 1990.

Nayfield, S. G., Karp, J. E., Ford, L. G., et al.: Potential role of tamoxifen in prevention of breast cancer. J. Natl. Cancer Inst., *83:*1450, 1991.

Nemoto, T., Patel, J., Rosner, D., et al.: Tamoxifen (Nolvadex) versus adrenalectomy in metastatic breast cancer. Cancer, *53:*1333, 1984.

Nemoto, T., Rosner, D., Patel, J. K., et al.: Aminoglutethimide in patients with metastatic breast cancer. Cancer, *63:*1673, 1989.

Nenci, I.: Charting steroid-cell interactions in normal and neoplastic tissues. *In* Gurpide, E., Calandra, R., Levy, C., et al. (Eds.): Hormones and Cancer. New York, Alan R. Liss, 1984, pp. 23–26.

Nesto, R. W., Cady B., Oberfield, R. A., et al.: Rebound response after estrogen therapy for metastatic breast cancer. Cancer, *38:*1834, 1976.

Neven, P., De Muylder, X., Van Belle, Y., et al.: Hysteroscopic follow-up during tamoxifen treatment. Eur. J. Obstet. Gynecol. Reprod. Biol., *35:*235, 1990.

Nicholson, R. I., Walker, K. J., McClelland, R. A., et al.: Zoladex plus tamoxifen versus Zoladex alone in pre- and peri-menopausal metastatic breast cancer. J. Steroid Biochem. Molec. Biol., *37:*989, 1990.

Nissen-Meyer, R.: Primary breast cancer: The effect of primary ovarian irradiation. Ann. Oncol., *2:*343, 1991.

Noguchi, S., Motomura, K., Inaji, H., et al.: Down-regulation of transforming growth factor-α by tamoxifen in human breast cancer. Cancer, *72:*131–136, 1993.

Nomura, Y., Tashiro, H., and Shinozuka, K.: Changes of steroid hormone receptor content by chemotherapy and/or endocrine therapy in advanced breast cancer. Cancer, *55:*546, 1985.

Nomura, Y., Miura, S., Koyama, H., et al.: Relative effect of steroid hormone receptors on the prognosis of patients with operable breast cancer. A univariate and multivariate analysis of 3089 Japanese patients with breast cancer from the study group for the Japanese Breast Cancer Society on Hormone Receptors and Prognosis in Breast Cancer. Cancer, *69:*153, 1992.

O'Bryan, R. M., Gordon, G. S., Kelley, R. M., et al.: Does thyroid substance improve response of breast cancer to surgical castration? Cancer, *33:*1082, 1974.

O'Dwyer, P. J., Duffy, M. J., O'Sullivan, F., et al.: CEA and CA 15-3 in primary and recurrent breast cancer. World J. Surg., *14:*562, 1990.

Osborne, C. K., Yochmowitz, M. G., Knight, W. A. III, et al.: The value of estrogen and progesterone receptors in the treatment of breast cancer. Cancer, *46:*2884, 1980.

Osborne, C. K., Boldt, D. H., Clark, G. M., et al.: Effects of tamoxifen on human breast cancer cell cycle kinetics: Accumulation of cells in early G1-phase. Cancer Res., *43:*3583, 1983.

Osborne, C. K., Coronado, E., Allred, D. C., et al.: Acquired tamoxifen resistance: Correlation with reduced breast tumor levels of tamoxifen and isomerization of *trans*-4-hydroxytamoxifen. J. Natl. Cancer Inst., *83:*1477, 1991.

Osborne, C. K., Wiebe, V. J., McGuire, W. L., et al.: Tamoxifen and the isomers of 4-hydroxytamoxifen in tamoxifen-resistant tumors from breast cancer patients. J. Clin. Oncol., *10:*304, 1992.

Otteman, L. A., and Long, H. J.: Hypercalcemic flare with megestrol acetate. Cancer Treat. Rep., *68:*1420, 1984.

Paik, S., Hazan, R., Fisher, E. R., et al.: Pathologic findings from the National Surgical Adjuvant Breast and Bowel Project: Prognostic significance of erbB$_2$ protein overexpression in primary breast cancer. J. Clin. Oncol., *8:*103, 1990.

Pannuti, F., Martoni, A., Di Marco, A. R., et al.: Prospective, randomized clinical trial of two different high dosages of medroxyprogesterone acetate (MAP) in the treatment of metastatic breast cancer. Eur. J. Cancer, *15:*593, 1979.

Paone, J. F., Abeloff, M. D., Ettinger, D. S., et al.: The correlation of estrogen and progesterone receptor levels with response to chemotherapy for advanced carcinoma of the breast. Surg. Gynecol. Obstet., *152:*70, 1981.

Paridaens, R., Heuson, J. C., Julien, J. P., et al.: Assessment of estrogenic recruitment before chemotherapy in advanced breast cancer: A double-blind randomized study. J. Clin. Oncol., *11:*1723–1728, 1993.

Parl, F. F., Schmidt, B. P., Dupont, W. D., et al.: Prognostic significance of estrogen receptor status in breast cancer in relation to tumor stage, axillary node metastasis and histopathologic grading. Cancer, *54:*2237, 1984.

Parnes, H. L., Abrams, J. S., Tchekmedyian, N. S., et al.: A phase I/II study of high-dose megestrol acetate in the treatment of metastatic breast cancer. Breast Cancer Res. Treat., *18:*171, 1991.

Paterson, A. H. G., Hanson, J., Pritchard, K. I., et al.: Comparison of antiestrogen and progestogen therapy for initial treatment and consequences of their combination for second-line treatment of recurrent breast cancer. Semin. Oncol., *17*(Suppl. 9):52, 1990.

Pavlidis, N. A., Petris, C., Briassoulis, E., et al.: Clear evidence that long-term, low-dose tamoxifen treatment can induce ocular toxicity: A prospective study of 63 patients. Cancer, *69:*2961, 1992.

Pearson, O. H., Hubay, C. A., Gordon, N. H., et al.: Endocrine versus endocrine plus five-drug chemotherapy in postmenopausal women with stage II estrogen receptor–positive breast cancer. Cancer, *64:*1819, 1989.

Perry, M. C., Kardinal, C. G., Weinberg, V., et al.: Chemotherapy compared to chemotherapy plus hormone therapy in the treatment of postmenopausal women with advanced breast cancer: An interim report. *In* Amers, F. C., Blumenschein, G. R., and Montague, E. D. (Eds.): Current Controversies in Breast Cancer. Austin, University of Texas Press, 1984, p. 477.

Perry, M. C., Kardinal, C. G., Korzun, A. H., et al.: Chemohormonal therapy in advanced carcinoma of the breast: Cancer and Leukemia Group B Protocol 8081. J. Clin. Oncol., *5:*1534, 1987.

Peters, T. G., Lewis, J. D., Wilkinson, E. J., et al.: Danazol therapy in hormone-sensitive mammary carcinoma. Cancer, *40:*2797, 1977.

Peyrat, J. P., Djiane, J., Kelly, P. A., et al.: Characterization of prolactin receptors in human breast cancer. Breast Cancer Res. Treat., *4:*275, 1984.

Planting, A. S., Alexieva-Figusch, J., Blonk-v. d. Wijst, J., et al.: Tamoxifen therapy in premenopausal women with metastatic breast cancer. Cancer Treat. Rep., *69:*363, 1985.

Plotkin, D., Lechner, J. J., Jung, W. E., et al.: Tamoxifen flare in advanced breast cancer. J.A.M.A., *240:*2644, 1978.

Pollak, M., Costantino, J., Polychronakos, C., et al.: Effect of tamoxifen on serum insulinlike growth factor I levels in stage I breast cancer patients. J. Natl. Cancer Inst., *82:*1693, 1990.

Pollak, M., Poisson, R., Major, D., et al.: Octreotide with or without a prolactin suppressive agent for patients with breast cancer refractory to antiestrogens (Abstract). Proc. Am. Soc. Clin. Oncol., *11:*87, 1992.

Pouillart, P., Madgelenat, H., Jouve, M., et al.: Metastatic breast cancer: Prognostic significance and sensitivity to cytotoxic chemotherapy according to the results of the estradiol and progesterone receptor assay. Bull. Cancer (Paris), *69:*461, 1982.

Powles, T. J., Hardy, J. R., Ashley, S. E., et al.: Chemoprevention of breast cancer. Breast Cancer Res. Treat., *14:*23, 1989.

Powles, T. J., Tillyer, C. R., Jones, A. L., et al.: Prevention of breast cancer with tamoxifen—an update on the Royal Marsden Hospital Pilot Programme. Eur. J. Cancer, *26:*680, 1990.

Pritchard, K. I.: Current status of adjuvant endocrine therapy for resectable breast cancer. Semin. Oncol., *14:*23, 1987.

Pritchard, K. I., Meakin, J. W., Boyd, N. F., et al.: A randomized trial of adjuvant tamoxifen in postmenopausal women with axillary node–positive breast cancer. *In* Jones, S. E., and Salmon, S. E. (Eds.): Adjuvant Therapy of Cancer IV. New York, Grune & Stratton, 1984, pp. 339–348.

Pritchard, K. I., Paterson, A. H., Deschenes, L., et al.: A randomized double-blind trial of the antiestrogen droloxifene (3-OH tamoxifen) in previously untreated postmenopausal women with estrogen (ER)- or progesterone receptor (PGR)–positive or unknown metastatic or locally unresectable breast cancer (Meeting abstract). Proc. Am. Soc. Clin. Oncol., *10:*A52, 1991.

Pronzato, P., Brema, F., Amoroso, D., et al.: Megestrol acetate: Phase II study of a single daily administration in advanced breast cancer. Breast Cancer Res. Treat., *17:*51, 1990.

Pugesgaard, T., and Von Eyben, F. E.: Bilateral optic neuritis evolved during tamoxifen treatment. Cancer, *58:*383, 1986.

Qazi, R., Chuang, J. L., and Drobyski, W.: Estrogen receptors and the pattern of relapse in breast cancer. Arch. Intern. Med., *144:*2365, 1984.

Raam, S., Robert, N., Pappas, C. A., et al.: Defective estrogen receptors in human mammary cancers: Their significance in defining hormone dependence. J. Natl. Cancer Inst., *80:*756, 1988.

Raats, J. I., Falkson, G., and Falkson, H. C.: A study of fadrozole, a new aromatase inhibitor, in postmenopausal women with advanced metastatic breast cancer. J. Clin. Oncol., *10:*111, 1992.

Ratko, T. A., Detrisac, C. J., Dinger, N. M., et al.: Chemopreventive efficacy of combined retinoid and tamoxifen treatment following surgical excision of a primary mammary cancer in female rats. Cancer Res., *49:*4472, 1989.

Ravdin, P. M., Tandon, A. K., Allred, D. C., et al.: Cathepsin D by western blotting and immunohistochemistry: Failure to confirm correlations with prognosis in node-negative breast cancer. J. Clin. Oncol., *12:*467–474, 1994.

Ravdin, R. G., Lewison, E. F., Slack, N. H., et al.: Results of a clinical trial concerning the worth of prophylactic oophorectomy for breast cancer. Surg. Gynecol. Obstet., *131:*1055, 1970.

Ravdin, P. M., Green, S., Dorr, T. M., et al.: Prognostic significance of progesterone receptor levels in estrogen receptor–positive patients with metastatic breast cancer treated with tamoxifen: Results of a prospective Southwest Oncology Group study. J. Clin. Oncol., *10:*1284, 1992.

Rechia, F., Marchionni, F., and Rabitti, G.: Phase II trial of tamoxifen (TAM), beta-interferon (BIFN) and retinoids (R) in metastatic breast cancer (MBC) (Meeting abstract). Proc. Am. Soc. Clin. Oncol., *10:*A88, 1991.

Reubi, J.-C., and Torhorst, J.: The relationship between somatostatin, epidermal growth factor, and steroid hormone receptors in breast cancer. Cancer, *64:*1254, 1989.

Reyno, L. M., Levine, M. N., Skingley, P., et al.: Chemotherapy-induced amenorrhoea in a randomised trial of adjuvant chemotherapy duration in breast cancer. Eur. J. Cancer, *29A:*21–23, 1993.

Ribeiro, G., and Palmer, M. K.: Adjuvant tamoxifen for operable carcinoma of the breast: Report of clinical trial by the Christie Hospital and Holt Radium Institute. Br. Med. J., *286:*827, 1983.

Ribeiro, G., and Swindell, R.: The Christie Hospital tamoxifen (Nolvadex) Adjuvant Trial for Operable Breast Carcinoma—7-yr results. Eur. J. Cancer Clin. Oncol., *21:*897, 1985.

Ribeiro, G., and Swindell, R.: The Christie hospital adjuvant tamoxifen trial—status at 10 years. Br. J. Cancer, *57:*601, 1988.

Roberts, J. T., Bates, T., Bozzino, J. M., et al.: Treatment of carcinoma of the breast with high dose oral medroxyprogesterone acetate: Does increased bioavailability improve the therapeutic ratio? Clin. Oncol. (R. Coll. Radiol.), *2:*324, 1990.

Robertson, J. F., Walker, K. J., Nicholson, R. I., et al.: Combined endocrine effects of LHRH agonist (Zoladex) and tamoxifen (Nolvadex) therapy in premenopausal women with breast cancer. Br. J. Surg., *76:*1262, 1989.

Rochefort, H.: Biochemical basis of breast cancer treatment by androgens and progestins. *In* Gurpide, E., Calandra, R., Levy, C., et al. (Eds.): Hormones and Cancer. New York, Alan R. Liss, 1984, pp. 79–96.

Rose, C., Mouridsen, H. T., Thorpe, S. M., et al.: Antiestrogen treatment of postmenopausal breast cancer patients with high risk of recurrence: 72 months of life table analysis and steroid hormone receptor status. World J. Surg., *9:*765, 1985*a*.

Rose, C., Thorpe, S. M., Anderson, K. W., et al.: Beneficial effect of adjuvant tamoxifen therapy in primary breast cancer in patients with high oestrogen receptor values. Lancet, *1:*16, 1985*b*.

Rosen, P. P., Menendez-Botet, C. J., Urban, J. A., et al.: Estrogen receptor protein (ERP) in multiple tumor specimens from individual patients with breast cancer. Cancer, *39:*2194, 1977.

Rosen, P. P., Groshen, S., Saigo, P. E., et al.: A long-term follow-up study of survival in stage I (T1N0M0) and stage II (T1N1M0) breast carcinoma. J. Clin. Oncol., *7:*355, 1989*a*.

Rosen, P. P., Groshen, S., Saigo, P. E., et al.: Pathological prognostic factors in stage I (T1N0M0) and stage II (T1N1M0) breast carcinoma: A study of 644 patients with median follow-up of 18 years. J. Clin. Oncol., *7:*1239, 1989*b*.

Rosen, P. P., Groshen, S., and Kinne, D. W.: Prognosis in T2N0M0 stage I breast carcinoma: A 20-year follow-up study. J. Clin. Oncol., *9:*1650, 1991.

Ross, M. B., Buzdar, A. U., and Blumenschein, G. R.: Treatment of advanced breast cancer with megestrol acetate after therapy with tamoxifen. Cancer, *49:*413, 1982.

Rossof, A. H.: The early history of hormone manipulation in human cancer—an appreciation of Sir George Thomas Beatson. Rev. Endocrine-Related Cancer, *6*(Suppl.):7, 1980.

Rossof, A. H., Gelman, R., and Creech, R. H.: Randomized evaluation of combination chemotherapy vs. observation alone following response or stabilization after oophorectomy for metastatic breast cancer in premenopausal women. Am. J. Clin. Oncol., *5:*253, 1982.

Rotmensz, N., De Palo, G., Formelli, F., et al.: Long-term tolerability on fenretinide (4-HPR) in breast cancer patients (Abstract). Eur. J. Cancer, *27:*1127, 1991.

Rozencwieg, M., and Heuson, J. C.: Breast cancer: Prognostic factors and clinical evaluation. *In* Staquet, M. S. (Ed.): Cancer Therapy: Prognostic Factors and Criteria of Response. New York, Raven Press, 1975, pp. 139–147.

Rutqvist, L. E., and Mattsson, A.: Cardiac and thomboembolic morbidity among postmenopausal women with early-stage breast cancer in a randomized trial of adjuvant tamoxifen. J.N.C.I. J. Natl. Cancer Inst., *85:*1398–1406, 1993.

Rutqvist, L. E., Wallgren, A., and Nilsson, B.: Is breast cancer a curable disease? A study of 14,731 women with breast cancer from the Cancer Registry of Norway. Cancer, *53:*1793, 1984.

Rutqvist, L. E., Cedermark, B., Fornander, T., et al.: The relationship between hormone receptor content and the effect of adjuvant tamoxifen in operable breast cancer. J. Clin. Oncol., *7:*1474, 1989.

Rutqvist, L. E., Cedermark, B., Glas, U., et al.: Contralateral primary tumors in breast cancer patients in a randomized trial of adjuvant tamoxifen therapy. J. Natl. Cancer Inst., *83:*1299, 1991.

Safi, F., Kohler, I., Röttinger, E., et al.: The value of the tumor marker CA 15-3 in diagnosing and monitoring breast cancer: A comparative study with carcinoembryonic antigen. Cancer, *68:*574, 1991.

Sahin, A. A., Ro, J., Ro, J. Y., et al.: Ki-67 immunostaining in node-negative stage I/II breast carcinoma: Significant correlation with prognosis. Cancer, *68:*549, 1991.

Salmon, S. E.: In vitro observations in clonogenic assay and potential extrapolations to adjuvant therapy of cancer. *In* Jones, S. E., and Salmon, S. E. (Eds.): Adjuvant Therapy of Cancer IV. New York, Grune & Stratton, 1984, pp. 17–26.

Samojlik, E., Santen, R. J., Kirschner, M. A., et al.: Steroid hormone profiles in women treated with aminoglutethimide for metastatic carcinoma of the breast. Cancer Res., *42:*3349s, 1982.

Santen, R. J.: Introduction to the conference, Aromatase: New perspectives for breast cancer. Cancer Res., *42*(Suppl.):3268s, 1982.

Santen, R. J.: Basic principles in choosing endocrine therapy. *In* Allegra, J. C. (Ed.): The Management of Breast Cancer Through Endocrine Therapies. Amsterdam, Excerpta Medica, 1984, pp. 14–28.

Santen, R. J., Worgul, T. J., Samojlik, E., et al.: A randomized trial comparing surgical adrenalectomy with aminoglutethimide plus hydrocortisone in women with advanced breast cancer. N. Engl. J. Med., *305:*545, 1981.

Santen, R. J., Demers, L. M., Lynch, J., et al.: Specificity of low dose fadrozole hydrochloride (CGS 16949A) as an aromatase inhibitor. J. Clin. Endocrinol. Metab., *73:*99, 1991.

Saphner, T., Tormey, D. C., and Gray, R.: Venous and arterial thrombosis in patients who received adjuvant therapy for breast cancer. J. Clin. Oncol., *9:*286, 1991.

Saphner, T., Troxel, A. B., Tormey, D. C., et al.: Phase II study of Goserelin for patients with postmenopausal metastatic breast cancer. J. Clin Oncol., *11:*1529–1535, 1993.

Schacter, L. P., Rozencweig, M., Canetta, R., et al.: Overview of hormonal therapy in advanced breast cancer. Semin. Oncol., *17*(Suppl. 9):38, 1990.

Schally, A. V.: Oncological applications of somatostatin analogues. Cancer Res., *48:*6977, 1988.

Schally, A. V., Redding, T. W., and Comaru-Schally, A. M.: Inhibition of the growth of some hormone dependent tumors by D-Trp6-LH-RH. Med. Oncol. Tumor Pharmacother., *1:*109, 1984.

Schally, A. V., Cai, R.-Z., Torres-Aleman, 1., et al.: Endocrine, gastrointestinal and antitumor activity of somatostatin analogues. *In* Moody, T. W. (Ed.): Neural and Endocrine Peptides and Receptors. New York, Plenum, 1986.

Schally, A. V., Redding, T. W., Cai, R.-Z., et al.: Somatostatin analogs in the treatment of various experimental tumors. *In* Klijn, J. G. M. (Ed.): Hormonal Manipulation of Cancer: Peptides, Growth Factors, and New (Anti-)Steroidal Agents. New York, Raven, 1987, pp. 431–440.

Schapira, D. V., Kumar, N. B., and Lyman, G. H.: Serum cholesterol reduction with tamoxifen. Breast Cancer Res. Treat., *17:*3, 1990.

Schell, H. W.: Adrenal corticosteroid therapy in far-advanced cancer. Geriatrics, *27:*131, 1972.

Schinzinger, A. S.: Über carcinoma mammae. Beilage zum Centralblatt fur Chirurgie *16:*55, 1889.

Schlom, J., Greiner, J., Hand, P. H., et al.: Monoclonal antibodies to breast cancer–associated antigens as potential reagents in the management of breast cancer. Cancer, *54:*2777, 1984.

Schmoll, E., Wilke, H., Thole, R., et al.: Megestrol acetate in cancer cachexia. Semin. Oncol., *18*(Suppl 2):32, 1991.

Schwartz, L., Guiochet, N., and Keiling, R.: Two partial remissions induced by an LHRH analogue in two postmenopausal women with metastatic breast cancer. Cancer, *62:*2498, 1988.

Schwartz, M. R., Randolph, R. L., and Panko, W. B.: Carcinoembryonic antigen and steroid receptors in the cytosol of carcinoma of the breast. Relationship to pathologic and clinical features. Cancer, *55:*2464, 1985.

Sedlacek, S. M.: An overview of megestrol acetate for the treatment of advanced breast cancer. Semin. Oncol., *15*(Suppl. 1):3, 1988.

Segaloff, A.: Assessment of response to treatment by the Cooperative Breast Cancer Group. *In* Hayward, J. L., and Bulbrook, R. D. (Eds.): Clinical Evaluation in Breast Cancer. London, Academic Press, 1966, p. 125.

Segaloff, A.: Hormone treatment of breast cancer. J. A. M. A., *234:*1175, 1975.

Seymour, L., Bezwoda, W. R., Meyer, K.: Response to second-line hormone treatment for advanced breast cancer: Predictive value of ploidy determination. Cancer, *65:*2720, 1990.

Shapiro, S., Slone, D., Kaufman, D. W., et al.: Use of thyroid supplements in relation to the risk of breast cancer. J. A. M. A., *244:*1685, 1980.

Sherry, M. M., Greco, F. A., Johnson, D. H., et al.: Breast cancer with skeletal metastases at initial diagnosis: Distinctive clinical characteristics and favorable prognosis. Cancer, *58:*178, 1986*b*.

Sherry, M. M., Greco, F. A., Johnson, D. H., et al.: Metastatic breast cancer confined to the skeletal system. An indolent disease. Am. J. Med., *81:*381, 1986*a*.

Shiu, R. P., and Friesen, H. G.: Mechanism of action of prolactin in the control of mammary gland function. Ann. Rev. Physiol., *42:*83, 1980.

Shyamala, G.: Specific cytoplasmic glucocorticoid hormone receptors in lactating mammary glands. Biochemistry, *12:*3085, 1973.

Siiteri, P. K.: Review on studies of estrogen biosynthesis in the human. Cancer Res., *42*(Suppl.):3269s, 1982.

Silva, J. S., Leight, G. S., Haagensen, D. E. Jr., et al.: Quantitation of response to therapy in patients with metastatic breast carcinoma by serial analysis of plasma gross cystic disease fluid protein and carcinoembryonic antigen. Cancer, *49:*1236, 1982.

Spicer, D., Pike, M. C., and Henderson, B. E.: The question of estrogen replacement therapy in patients with a prior diagnosis of breast cancer. Oncology (Williston Park), *4:*49, 1990.

Spiegelman, D., Colditz, G. A., Hunter, D., et al.: Validation for the Gail et al. model for predicting individual breast cancer risk. J.N.C.I. J. Natl. Cancer Inst., *86:*600–607, 1994.

Spitz, I. M., and Bardin, C. W.: Mifepristone (RU 486): A modulator of progestin and glucocorticoid action. N. Engl. J. Med., *329:*404–412, 1993.

Sporn, M. B., and Roberts, A. B.: Autocrine secretion—10 years later. Ann. Intern. Med., *117:*408, 1992.

Stein, R. C., Dowsett, M., Hedley, A., et al.: The clinical and endocrine effects of 4-hydroxyandrostenedione alone and in combination with goserelin in premenopausal women with advanced breast cancer. Br. J. Cancer, *62:*679, 1990.

Steinberg, K. K., Thacker, S. B., Smith, S. J., et al.: A meta-analysis of the effect of estrogen replacement therapy on the risk of breast cancer. J.A.M.A., *265:*1985, 1991.

Stewart HJ: The Scottish trial of adjuvant tamoxifen in node-negative breast cancer. Natl. Cancer Inst. Monogr., *11:*117, 1992.

Stoll, B. A.: Corticosteroids in therapy of advanced mammary cancer. Br. Med. J., *2:*210, 1963.

Stoll, B. A.: Hormone replacement therapy in women treated for breast cancer. Eur. J. Cancer Clin. Oncol., *25:*1909, 1989.

Stoll, B. A.: Hormone replacement therapy for women with a past history of breast cancer (Editorial). Clin. Oncol., *2:*309, 1990.

Sunderland, M. C., and Osborne, C. K.: Tamoxifen in premenopausal patients with metastatic breast cancer: A review. J. Clin. Oncol., *9:*1283, 1991.

Sutherland, R. L., Green, M. D., Hall, R. E., et al.: Tamoxifen induces accumulation of MCF 7 human mammary carcinoma cells in the G0/G1 phase of the cell cycle. Eur. J. Cancer Oncol., *19:*615, 1983.

Tabár, L., Fagerberg, G., Day, N. E., et al.: Breast cancer treatment and natural history: New insights from results of screening. Lancet, *339:*412, 1992.

Tandon, A. K., Clark, G. M., Chamness, G. C., et al.: HER-2/*neu* oncogene protein and prognosis in breast cancer. J. Clin. Oncol., *7:*1120, 1989.

Tandon, A. K., Clark, G. M., Chamness, G. C., et al.: Cathepsin D and prognosis in breast cancer. N. Engl. J. Med., *322:*297, 1990.

Taylor, G. W.: Evaluation of ovarian sterilization for breast cancer. Surg. Gynecol. Obstet., *68:*452, 1939.

Taylor, G. W.: Artificial menopause in carcinoma of the breast. N. Engl. J. Med., *211:*1138, 1934.

Taylor, S. G. III, and Morris, R. S. Jr.: Hormones in breast metastasis therapy. Med. Clin. North Am., *35:*51, 1951.

Taylor, S. G. III, Slaughter, D. P., Smejkal, W., et al.: The effect of sex hormones on advanced carcinoma of the breast. Cancer, *1:*604, 1948.

Taylor, S. G. IV, Knuiman, M. W., Sleeper, L. A., et al.: Six-year results of the Eastern Cooperative Oncology Group trial of observation versus CMFP versus CMFPT in postmenopausal patients with node-positive breast cancer. J. Clin. Oncol., *7:*879, 1989.

Tchekmedyian, N. S., Hickman, M., and Heber, D: Treatment of anorexia and weight loss with megestrol acetate in patients with cancer or acquired immunodeficiency syndrome. Semin. Oncol., *18*(Suppl. 2):35, 1991.

Tenni, P., Lalich, D. L., Byrne, M. J., et al.: Life threatening interaction between tamoxifen and warfarin (Abstract). Br. Med. J., *298:*93, 1989.

Thangaraju, M., Kamar, K., Gandhirajan, R., et al.: Effect of tamoxifen on plasma lipids and lipoproteins in postmenopausal women with breast cancer. Cancer, *73:*659–663, 1994.

Thompson, A.: Analysis of cases in which oophorectomy was performed for inoperable carcinoma of the breast. Br. Med. J., *4:*1538, 1902.

Thompson, A. M., Kerr, D. J., and Steel, C. M.: Transforming growth factor-beta₁ is implicated in the failure of tamoxifen therapy in human breast cancer. Br. J. Cancer, *63:*609, 1991.

Tinnemans, J. G. M., Beex, L. V. A. M., Wobbes, Th., et al.: Steroid-hormone receptors in nonpalpable and more advanced stages of breast cancer. A contribution to the biology and natural history of carcinoma of the female breast. Cancer, *66:*1165, 1990.

Toi, M., Nakamura, T., Mukaida, H., et al.: Relationship between epidermal growth factor receptor status and various prognostic factors in human breast cancer. Cancer, *65:*1980, 1990.

Topper, Y. J., and Oka, T.: Some aspects of mammary gland development in the mature mouse. *In* Larson, B. L., and Smith, V. R. (Eds.): Lactation: A Comprehensive Treatise. New York, Academic, 1974, pp. 327–348.

Tormey, D. C., Gray, R., Gilchrist, K., et al.: Adjuvant chemohormonal therapy with cyclophosphamide, methotrexate, 5-fluorouracil, and predisone (CMFP) or CMFP plus tamoxifen compared with CMF for premenopausal breast cancer patients: An Eastern Cooperative Oncology Group trial. Cancer, *65:*200, 1990.

Tsangaris, T. N., Knox, S. M., and Cheek, J. H.: Tumor hormone receptor status and recurrences in premenopausal patients with node-negative breast carcinoma. Cancer, *69:*984, 1992.

Turken, S., Siris, E., Seldin, D., et al.: Effects of tamoxifen on spinal bone density in women with breast cancer. J. Natl. Cancer Inst., *81:*1086, 1989.

Ulrich, P.: Testosterone (hormone male) et son role possible dans le trâitement de certains cancers du sein. Acta Un. Int. Cancre, *4:*377, 1939.

Valavaara, R., Tuominen, J., Johansson, R.: Predictive value of tumor estrogen and progesterone receptor levels in postmenopausal women with advanced breast cancer treated with toremifene. Cancer, *66:*2264, 1990.

Vandenberg, T., and Skillings, J.: Phase II study of interferon-alpha and tamoxifen in patients with metastatic breast cancer previously unresponsive to tamoxifen (Meeting abstract). Proc. Am. Assoc. Cancer Res., *33:*213, 1992.

van Dyk, J. J., and Falkson, G.: Extended survival and remission rates in metastatic breast cancer. Cancer, *27:*300, 1971.

Veronesi, U., and Costa, A.: Chemoprevention of contralateral breast cancer with the synthetic fetinoid fenretinide (Abstract). Cancer Invest., *6:*55, 1988.

Veronesi, U., Cascinelli, N., Greco, M., et al.: A reappraisal of oophorectomy in carcinoma of the breast. Ann. Surg., *205:*18, 1981.

Vogel, C. L., Shemano, I., Reynolds, R., et al.: The ''worsening'' bone scan in breast cancer clinical trials: A potentially significant source of error in response evaluation (Abstract). Proc. Am. Soc. Clin. Oncol., *11:*50, 1992.

Vogel, C. L., Shemano, I., Schoenfelder, J., et al.: Multicenter phase II efficacy trial of toremifene in tamoxifen-refractory patients with advanced breast cancer. J. Clin. Oncol., *11:*345–350, 1993.

Volk, H., Deupree, R. H., Goldenberg, I. S., et al.: A dose response evaluation of delta-1-testololactone in advanced breast cancer. Cancer, *33:*9, 1974.

Wakeling, A. E., Dukes, M., and Bowler, J.: A potent specific pure antiestrogen with clinical potential. Cancer Res., *51:*3867, 1991.

Wells S. A. Jr., and Santen, R. J.: Ablative procedures in patients with metastatic breast carcinoma. Cancer, *53:*762, 1984.

Wiebe, V. J., Osborne, C. K., McGuire, W. L., et al.: Identification of estrogenic tamoxifen metabolite(s) in tamoxifen-resistant human breast tumors. J. Clin. Oncol., *10:*990, 1992.

Wile, A. G., Opfell, R. W., Margileth, D. A., et al.: Hormone replacement therapy does not affect breast cancer outcome (Meeting abstract). Proc. Am. Soc. Clin. Oncol., *10:*A106, 1991.

Wilson, A. J.: Response in breast cancer to a second hormonal therapy. Rev. Endocrine-Related Cancer, *14:*5, 1983.

Wiltschke, C., Tyl, E., Speiser, P., et al.: Increased natural killer cell activity correlates with low or negative expression of the HER-2/neu oncogence in patients with breast cancer. Cancer, *73:*135–139, 1994.

Winstanley, J., Cooke, T., George, W. D., et al.: The long-term prognostic significance of oestrogen receptor analysis in early carcinoma of the breast. Br. J. Cancer, *64:*99, 1991.

Wintz, H.: Experience in irradiation of breast cancer. Br. J. Radiol., *31:*100, 1926.

Wittliff, J. L.: Specific receptors of the steroid hormones in breast cancer. Semin. Oncol., *1:*109, 1974.

Wittliff, J. L.: Steroid-hormone receptors in breast cancer. Cancer, *53:*630, 1984.

Wiznitzer, I., and Benz, C.: Direct growth-inhibiting effects of the prolactin antagonists burserelin and pergolide on human breast cancer (Abstract). Proc. Am. Assoc. Cancer. Res., *25:*208, 1984.

Yamashita, K., Ueda, T., Komatsubara, Y., et al.: Breast cancer with bone-only metastases: Visceral metastases-free rate in relation to anatomic distribution of bone metastases. Cancer, *68:*634, 1991.

Yarbro, J. W.: Cancer research and the development of cancer centers. *In* Gross, S. C., and Garb, S. (Eds.): Cancer Treatment and Research in Humanistic Perspective. New York, Springer, 1985, pp. 3–15.

Zava, D. T., and McGuire, W. L.: Human breast cancer: Androgen action mediated via estrogen receptor. Science, *199:*787, 1978.

23

Immunology, Serum Markers, and Immunotherapy of Mammary Tumors

Muthukumaran Sivanandham
Marc K. Wallack

Although immunotherapy is often regarded as a new approach to cancer treatment, both theoretical tumor immunology and clinical immunotherapy originated independently near the turn of the present century (Coley, 1891; Ehrlich, 1909). The history of tumor immunology has been linked to that of specific immunotherapy by association with the dramatic success that immunization against microbes has had in prevention of infectious disease. Unfortunately, a comparison of tumor-specific antigens and microbial antigens reveals an inherent problem; tumor antigens are generally weakly immunogenic and often are identical to normal tissue components expressed during differentiation (Lennox, 1985). The original concept of immune surveillance (Ehrlich, 1909; Thomas, 1959; Burnet, 1970), which was based on the inherent ability of the immune system to recognize and eliminate tumor cells, has been difficult to confirm experimentally. On the other hand, the relationship of an intact immune system to prevention of malignancy is being demonstrated dramatically in the current epidemic of Kaposi's sarcoma associated with acquired immunodeficiency syndrome (Fahey et al., 1986).

An important factor in mammary tumorigenesis, as in all tumorigenesis, is the escape of tumor cells from host immune surveillance, which can be related to several mechanisms: (1) inability to induce immune responses owing to similarity of tumor cells and normal cells; (2) induction of tumor-induced immunosuppression; (3) insufficient amount of tumor rejection antigens to induce immune responses; (4) defective host immune system; and (5) insufficient antitumor activity to fight against the growing tumor. Recent studies have shown that immunogenic tumors such as melanoma, renal carcinoma and colon carcinoma are promising candidates for immunotherapeutic approaches. Mammary tumor cells express a variety of tumor-associated antigens (TAAs) identified by monoclonal antibodies. This characteristic of the mammary tumor makes it a candidate for specific immunotherapy. Moreover, in experimental animal models breast cancer offers one of the best examples of malignancy with immunologic implications. There are animal models in which tumor-associated antigens have been demonstrated and against which successful immunotherapeutic regimens have been developed. The human disease itself has a course of histopathologic development that strongly suggests participation of the host immune response. The availability of surgical specimens from lymph node dissection has provided opportunities for relating reactive changes in these nodes to prognosis. For these reasons, breast cancer has been cited as a model for cancer immunology (Black et al., 1984).

Until recently, therapy of breast cancer emphasized the three standard treatment methods—surgery, radiotherapy, and chemotherapy. In a wide variety of combinations, these methods of treatment have had variable success against other malignancies and some success in the treatment of breast cancer. The use of hormone therapy in conjunction with adjuvant chemotherapy has generated much interest. Despite the encouraging results with this approach, however, there is little evidence for substantial improvement in the long-term survival of breast cancer patients (Urban, 1986).

It is therefore clear that different approaches are needed. Although immunotherapy is a very old concept with a long history of promise and disappointment, in recent years it has developed into a legitimate fourth method of treatment that has been included under the classification of biologic response modifiers (Oldham, 1984). Advances in basic biologic and genetic research and technical achievements in immunobiology during the last decade have revolutionized this approach.

This chapter briefly reviews the history of immunologic studies of mammary cancer. The immunology and immunotherapy of breast cancer have been reviewed comprehensively (Nathanson, 1977; Nauts, 1984; Black & Zachrau, 1987). This chapter, therefore, emphasizes the most recent contributions.

TAAs are expressed in breast cancer tissue, owing to the activation of genes in some cases and to their amplification in others. The expression of mammary TAAs also occurs because of the loss in the regulation of normal biochemical processes. Changes in biochemical and gene regulation cause overexpression of some biochemicals, which are often immunogenic and serve as markers for diagnosis and prognosis. In the case of mammary cancer, these biochemicals are demonstrated in sera of breast cancer patients and in breast cancer tissues.

IMMUNOBIOLOGY OF TUMORS

Breast Tumor–Associated Antigens

The existence of organ-specific neoantigens in breast cancer is based on the serologic specificity of circulating antibodies such as the complement-dependent antibodies (Hindsley et al., 1979) or the ability of crude tumor extracts to elicit delayed skin responses (Austin et al., 1982).

The search for tumor-specific antigens that in the past preoccupied tumor immunologists has recently been supplanted by the recognition that, although many antigens exist in higher concentration on tumor cells than on normal cells, it is questionable whether truly tumor-specific antigens exist (Lennox, 1985). The term "tumor-associated antigens" has become increasingly useful in diagnosis, staging, monitoring, and therapy. The identification and characterization of TAAs was revolutionized by the advent of hybridoma technology and the resultant proliferation of monoclonal antibodies. Some important breast TAAs and the monoclonal antibodies against them are listed in Table 23–1. They can generally be classified as follows: (1) antigens related to mouse mammary tumor virus; (2) antigens expressed only in breast cancer (i.e., not shared with other tumors or normal cells); (3) antigens of normal breast tissue (present in increased amounts in breast tumors); and (4) antigens common to adenocarcinomas. The most extensive body of research with experimental mammary tumors has been with the mouse mammary tumor virus (MMTV). Certain strains of mice have a predictably high incidence of mammary tumors arising from immunologically related endogenous viruses (Gross, 1947).

The MMTV model has recently been used to study the ability of active immunization with vaccines prepared from spontaneous mammary tumors to prevent the occurrence of spontaneous or virus-induced tumors in other mice. Vaccines prepared from cells of primary spontaneous mammary tumors of RIII/IMr, GR/Imr, C3H/IMr, A/Imr, and C3HfC57BL/Imr mice were used to immunize MMTV-free BALB/c/Imr and C57BL/Imr mice before challenge with MMTV from the respective strains. Mammary tumor vaccines from C3H-strain tumor cells protected BALB/c and C57BL mice from developing tumors from all four mammary tumor viruses and significantly enhanced development of A-MMTV–induced tumors. The need for viral antigens, acting alone or in concert with cellular antigens, was indicated by the failure of vaccines prepared from C3HfC57BL tumor cells free of C3H-MMTV to induce protection. Moreover, a second set of experiments was conducted in which the same vaccines were used to immunize mice from the homologous strains that have a high incidence of spontaneous tumors that result from natural infection with MMTV. These experiments showed that tumorigenesis was not prevented in any of these strains, though delayed appearance of tumor was observed in RIII and GR mice (Girardi et al., 1985).

This MMTV system has been useful as a model for studying tumor virus–host interaction, although a human equivalent to MMTV has yet to be demonstrated. Nonetheless, there is an abundance of immunologic evidence associating MMTV-related antigens and human mammary tumors. First, it was observed that leukocytes of patients with breast cancer react with MMTV in leukocyte migration assays (Black et al., 1974). There have been several reports of antibodies to MMTV-related antigens in sera of patients with breast carcinoma (Day et al., 1981; Tomana et al.,

Table 23–1. COMMONLY EXPRESSED BREAST CANCER–ASSOCIATED ANTIGENS AND MONOCLONAL ANTIBODIES THAT REACT TO EPITOPES OF THE ANTIGENS

Antigen/Antibody	Characteristics	Use	Reference
Epithelial membrane antigen (DF3)	High–molecular weight glycoprotein, 300 kd	Prognosis Diagnosis?	Hayes et al., 1991
CA15.3	High–molecular weight glycoprotein	Prognosis	Gion et al., 1991; Nicolini et al., 1991
B72.3	Glycoprotein >10^6 kd mucin	Diagnosis of primary and metastatic breast cancer	Lamki et al., 1991; Mottolese et al., 1991
83D4 (BCAA)	Mucin epitope of B72.3, 300–1000 kd	Diagnosis	Pancino et al., 1991
Breast epithelial antigen	Epitope of mucin	Diagnosis	Ceriani and Rosenbaum, 1991
Milk fat globule membrane antigen	150 kd (CA549), 70 kd, 40 kd, 46 kd	Diagnosis	Larocca et al., 1991
1BE12	Epitope of milk fat globule membrane antigen, 900 kd	Diagnosis	Pancino et al., 1990
Anti–epidermal growth factor receptor (*HER-2* or c-*erb* B$_2$)	Glycoprotein 185–190 kd	Prognosis for ER+ tumor, and possible therapy	Borg et al, 1990
Antibody BCA-200	Resembles c-*erb* B$_2$	Prognosis	Ring et al., 1991
Antibody Ki-67	Proliferating cell nuclear antigen	Prognosis by cell cycle analysis	Bacus et al., 1989
Anti–hepatoglobulin related protein	Hepatoglobulin-related protein	Prognosis	Kuhajda et al., 1989; Shurbaji et al., 1991
Laminin receptor	Glycoprotein, 62–75 kd	Prognosis	Marques et al., 1990; Castronovo et al., 1990
Insulin-like growth factor-I receptor	130 kd	Prognosis	Foeken et al., 1990

1981). The antigen is related to the major envelope glyco-protein of MMTV (Mesa-Tejada et al., 1978; Dion et al., 1980). Further study of this antigen has revealed its presence in metastases of human mammary cancers as well as in human breast carcinoma cell lines. Clonal derivatives of cell lines have been shown to contain retrovirus particles that have antigenic cross-reactivity with gp52, the major external protein of MMTV (Keydar et al., 1978). These cross-reactive antigens are further characterized as two gly-cosylated polypeptides with molecular weights of 68 and 60 kd, the larger of which is present in the viral particles shed by human breast carcinoma lines (Segev et al., 1985). Further evidence for a human mammary tumor virus includes the demonstration of retrovirus-like particles with reverse transcriptase activity in human milk samples (Key-dar, et al., 1978) and the detection of sequences related to the MMTV genome in the deoxyribonucleic acid of human mammary tumors (Callahan et al., 1982; May et al., 1983). MMTV gp52–related antigens have been detected on the surface of normal human lymphocytes (Lopez, 1986). By analogy with the mouse system in which MMTV ribonu-cleic acid is expressed on a subset of B lymphocytes (Lopez et al., 1985), the deoxyribonucleic acid sequences that code for this molecule may function as a proto-oncogene that has an important role in the growth or differentiation (or both) of cells of bone marrow–derived lymphoid cells.

The classic example of an antigen that is present in normal cells in a naked form but is detected in serum and tumor tissue of breast cancer patients is the Thomsen-Frie-denreich antigen (Springer et al., 1980). This antigen, known as the T antigen, is a precursor of the human blood group system MN and, therefore, is readily demonstrable in red blood cells. The T antigen has also been used to elicit a specific delayed hypersensitivity skin reaction in breast cancer patients. It is important to note that the majority of healthy subjects and patients with benign breast disease lacked the antigen (Springer, et al., 1980). A sensitive immunofluorescence method for detecting single metastatic adenocarcinoma cells of the breast is based on the specific binding of peanut agglutinin to the terminal disaccharide sequence of asialoglycophorin A, the MN precursor substance that identified the Thomsen-Friedenreich antigen (Seitz et al., 1984).

A 43 kd membrane glycoprotein present in breast cancer cells but not in normal cells has been characterized by immunoprecipitation with a monoclonal antibody (Edwards et al., 1986). This antigen was, however, found in tumors of other origin.

The antigen recognized by the monoclonal antibody B72.3 is a tumor-associated glycoprotein complex termed TAG-72. This is detectable in small amounts on normal secretory cells and is modulated by the spatial configuration of cells in culture (Horan-Hand et al., 1985). This antibody reacts with the tumor-associated glycoprotein complex of primary breast cancers and also with 85% of colon carcinomas. Carcinoembryonic antigen (CEA), although associated with colon carcinoma, serves as a useful indicator of breast cancer (Colcher et al., 1984).

Monoclonal antibodies useful for diagnosis and monitoring of breast cancer are not limited to those that identify breast cancer–specific antigens or even restricted TAAs.

Monoclonal antibodies that are directed against estrogen-regulated proteins may be very useful in diagnosis of breast cancer (Brabon et al., 1984; Garcia et al., 1985).

Monoclonal antibodies that identify components of the delipidated human milk fat globule membrane (Hilkens et al., 1981; Taylor-Papadimitrious, 1981), although not specific for a tumor antigen, have proved valuable (Wilkinson et al., 1984). On the other hand, some, such as 10-302 (Soule et al., 1983), bind to all breast carcinomas but not to normal mammary epithelium or other normal tissues. Several (Colcher et al., 1984) recognize carcinoma antigens shared by several tumors in addition to breast cancer but are nonreactive with normal cells. Although murine monoclonal antibodies with selective reactivity to human breast cancer cells have been described (Papsidero et al., 1983; White et al., 1985), the antigens recognized by these reagents have not been characterized.

A new monoclonal antibody, 3E1-2, stains breast carcinomsa, but also has weaker reactivity with some other tumors and with normal tissues (Stacker et al., 1985). Two monoclonal antibodies produced against milk fat globule membranes have proved highly discriminatory in detecting breast cancer (Feller, et al., 1985).

Even HLA antigens, which are broadly shared with normal tissue, may under controlled conditions serve as suitable tumor markers on the basis of relative depression (Natali et al., 1983; Bernard et al., 1985). At an international workshop on breast cancer research and treatment, a wide variety of normal gene products detectable by monoclonal antibodies were shown to be potentially useful markers for diagnosis. These included cytokeratins, glycosphingolipids, and human oncogene products (Peterson and Ceriani, 1985).

Some of the most promising monoclonal antibodies for breast cancer prognosis are the anti–estrogen receptor antibodies D547Sp-gamma and D75Sp-gamma. Enzyme-linked immunosorbent assay procedures employing these antibodies on breast cancer tissue and the estrogen receptor (ER) immunocytochemical assay using these antibodies compare very favorably to the estrogen-binding procedure previously employed (Pertschuk, 1985).

Although mouse monoclonal antibodies are useful if they achieve recognition of TAAs or normal antigens that are expressed in high concentration on breast cancer cells, a major goal of immunodiagnosis and therapy is to characterize breast TAA responses. The most promising means of achieving this is through production of human monoclonal antibodies by fusion of lymphocytes from human lymphoblastoid lines. Fusion with a nonsecretory variant of murine myeloma cells results in the production of human monoclonal antibodies. Preliminary screening of the resultant clones showed that 15 of 81 clones produced human monoclonal antibody that preferentially bound to breast carcinoma cells (Iman et al., 1985). These results have important implications for both active and passive immunotherapy.

SERUM MARKERS

Tumorigenesis involves several genetic and biochemical alterations—activation of oncogenes, inactivation of tumor suppressor genes, increased secretion of hormones and growth factors, elevated expression of hormone and growth factor receptors and gene products associated with invasion and metastasis, and, finally, increased organ-specific products. These changes lead to alterations in the expression of several antigens in the host system. Upward and downward regulation of these markers provide useful means by which to evaluate the potential efficacy of therapy.

The role of MMTV in human carcinogenesis is unproved, but MMTV cross-reactive antigens provide potentially useful markers. Antibodies against MMTV have been detected by several investigators in the sera of American women with breast cancer, and more often than in healthy women or patients with benign breast disease (Day et al., 1981; Tomana et al., 1981). Fewer than 5.0% of women from mainland China who have breast cancer were MMTV reactive. The MMTV-associated marker may define a subset of patients whose prognosis is poor. For example, the MMTV-related antigen that is expressed in metastases is more prevalent in Tunisian patients suffering from a rapidly progressive form of breast cancer known as *pousée evolutive* (Levine et al., 1984).

CEA, human beta-chorionic gonadotrophin, ceruloplasmin, and casein hydroxyproline have been evaluated as serum markers in breast cancer patients. Of these markers, CEA is associated with increased risk of disease progression and increased tumor burden and is elevated in at least 71% of patients, though CEA is also elevated in patients with colorectal cancer, benign liver disease, and inflammatory bowel disease. Therefore, CEA alone has limited specificity.

Several mucin-glycoprotein and high–molecular weight proteoglycan antigens are expressed on breast cancer cells. Two antibodies, B72.3 (reacting to high–molecular weight glycoprotein antigen) and CA15.3 (reacting to an epitope of the mucin antigen), are found in sera of breast cancer patients. CA15.3 antibody levels are correlated with stage of the disease. The CA15.3 antigen is present in the sera of 73% of breast cancer patients. However, a significant elevation was also seen in 71% of those who had nonmalignant lesions and in 44% with benign hepatic lesions. Based on multivariate analysis, a combination of CEA and CA15.3 was more sensitive than the CA15.3 alone for determining the presence of breast cancer (Colomer et al., 1989).

Monoclonal antibodies to epitopes of milk fat globule membrane antigen (HMFG1 and HMFG2) have been explored for the immunohistochemical detection of mammary cancer. The monoclonal antibody DF3, which recognizes an epitope of mucinlike breast carcinoma–associated antigen, is correlated with longer disease-free survival (Bacus et al., 1989).

A more sensitive and specific assay is the CA549 assay, which uses antibodies to both breast epithelial antigen and milk fat globule membrane antigen. Compared with the CEA assay it is superior for monitoring tumor progression, and stability (Beveridge et al., 1988). Another technical modification is the use of recombinant antigens. Recombinant antigen NP5, which binds to monoclonal antibody MC5, in a radioimmunoassay system had higher sensitivity and specificity than CEA (Ceriani et al., 1991).

In a multivariate analysis two recently developed anti-mucin monoclonal antibodies CAM26 and CAM29 were useful in measuring respective epitopes of the antigen in cancer patients' sera. Results were compared with those obtained from an assay system that employed carcinoma-specific antibodies such as CA125 and CA15.3. Although the reactivity of the CAM26 was similar to CAM29, CAM26 was a specific marker for squamous cell carcinoma; CAM29 was useful for ovarian carcinoma (Yemada et al., 1991). Such epitope-specific antibodies will serve as better markers for breast cancer.

Antigens on breast tumor cells can serve as markers for diagnosis and prognosis. Expression of mucinous carcinoma–associated antigen was analyzed by immunohistochemistry and correlated with disease progression. Disease-free survival was significantly correlated. This antigen can be identified in paraffin sections (Eskelien, 1990). Epitopes of hepatoglobulin-related protein antigen were analyzed in paraffin-embedded breast cancer tissues by immunohistochemical methods and were found to be associated with early recurrence. Furthermore, in combination with progesterone receptor (PR) status hepatoglobulin-related protein antigen expression was strongly related to prognosis (Kuhajda, 1989). A monoclonal antibody Ki-67, which reacts with a nuclear antigen expressed in cycling cells but not in resting cells, has been used in the immunohistochemical measure of deoxyribonucleic acid ploidy. This analysis, combined with PR and estrogen receptor (ER) status, was prognostically useful in patients with small breast cancers (Bacus et al., 1989).

Some nonimmunogenic biochemicals can serve as useful markers, either alone or in combination with breast cancer–associated antigens. Expression of sex hormone receptors divides breast cancers into two categories. The following is a brief summary of the use of hormones and receptors, and hormone-regulated biochemicals.

Plasma prolactin levels are sometimes elevated in breast cancer patients, and they change with disease progression (Bhatavdekar et al., 1990). Dehydroepiandrosterone is a secretory product of the adrenal gland that is metabolized to estrogen. The serum level of the dehydroepiandrosterone derivative in persons at high risk of developing breast cancer was reduced 10% compared with that of matched controls. Furthermore, estrogen-regulated protein pS2 identifies a subclass of ER-expressing tumors (Kida et al., 1989). Patients lacking the pS2 protein often exhibit a poor response to hormone therapy and early disease recurrence. While aromatase activity (an enzyme complex that converts androgen to estrogen) in primary cancers is correlated with early relapse, there is no correlation between aromatase activity and overall survival, histologic tumor grade, menopausal status, or ER. Estrogen-regulated lysosomal protease cathepsin-D levels can be elevated in breast cancer tissues, a finding that predicts reduced disease-free survival (Tandon et al., 1990). Cathepsin-D enzyme activity has also been elevated in ER-negative tumor tissues and may have prognostic importance in breast cancer (Zara et al., 1991). Immunoreactive estrogen-regulated protein pS2 and cathepsin-D are being evaluated as prognostic markers in preliminary pilot studies.

Biochemicals involved in tumor cell metastases are increased in breast cancer tissues and can be used as markers to predict metastases. Hyaluronic acid activity is associated with cell motility, and possibly with tumor cell metastases. Sera from breast cancer patients with measurable tumor contained increased hyaluronic acid–stimulating activity not observed in sera from volunteers or in breast cancer patients with no evidence of disease. Conclusive evidence for its role in metastasis needs further study. Considerable evidence suggests that the plasmin-plasminogen system plays a role in tumorigenesis and metastasis. Tissue plasminogen activator was higher in association with breast cancer than with benign disease (O'Grady et al., 1985) and could serve as a useful marker to differentiate benign from malignant tissue.

Enhanced tyrosine kinase activity is associated with cellular proliferation and in breast cancer tissue has been correlated with early systemic relapse (Hennipman et al., 1989). However, tyrosine kinase activity is not restricted to breast cancer and can be associated with all biologically aggressive tumors.

Activated oncogenes in tumor cells are involved in neoplastic transformation. Oncogenes products are expressed on tumor cells and often are immunogenic. Although dysregulation of the c-*myc*, c-Ha-*ras*, and c-*erb* B_2 oncogenes have been established in breast cancer, the c-*erb* B_2 is significantly correlated with progression. (Benz et al., 1989; Danovan-Peluso et al., 1991). The *ras* oncogene mutation is rarely involved in either initiation or progression of breast cancer (Rochlitz et al., 1989). Amplification of c-*erb* B_2 indicates a poor prognosis (Salomon et al., 1987). The c-*erb* B_2 gene amplification was tested in node-negative patients and node-positive patients. Amplification of c-*erb* B_2 predicted a high percentage of metastases in node-negative patients (Ro et al., 1989) and was correlated with poor survival in node-positive patients (Borg et al., 1990). The c-*erb* B_2 oncogene protein and epithelial mucin antigen are measurable in the serum of breast cancer patients and in tumor cytosol. It is too early to decide whether these markers can be used as diagnostic and prognostic tools.

Summary

Several immunogenic antigens are useful as markers for breast cancer. CEA, epithelial mucin antigen, MMTV antigen, and c-*erb* B_2 are the best. These antigens are also the best candidates for active specific immunotherapy.

IMMUNOCOMPETENCE AND IMMUNOTHERAPY

Clinical evidence for the protective role of a competent immune system in breast cancer includes reports of higher incidence, and more severe disease, in immunocompromised patients. Reports cite a better prognosis for patients who have been able to mount an immune response. Lymphocytes from breast cancer patients have depressed proliferative responses, possibly mediated by a serum component (Whittiker and Clark, 1971). It has been suggested that the failure of postmastectomy radiation therapy to improve sur-

vival may be due to the depression of absolute lymphocyte counts, which persists for years (Meyer et al., 1970).

A variety of clinical conditions related to compromised immunity are associated with an increased incidence or severity of breast cancer. Immunodeficiency associated with autoimmune processes, such as myasthenia gravis, in which thymomas are common, are associated with a high incidence of breast cancer and a high frequency of bilateral disease. The protective effect of thymectomy in these cases is similar to that achieved in experimental animals, although the endocrine and immune factors involved remain to be clarified (Papatestas et al., 1977).

The largest group of patients in which immunodeficiency may be associated with enhanced disease is the elderly. Immunosenescence may contribute to the poor prognosis for breast cancer in patients of advanced age (Mueller and Amers, 1978). A comprehensive study of immune function related to breast cancer stage indicated that two different phases of immunosuppression can be discriminated. The first, associated with early breast cancer, is primary and patient related. The second is a tumor-induced depression of the immune response and characterizes advanced metastatic breast cancer (Adler et al., 1980). Modulation of Class I and Class II major histocompatibility complex antigens are observed in these two phases. These antigens are important for antitumor cytolytic and helper T-cell recognition. The major histocompatibility complex Class I antigens are "down-regulated" on micrometastatic breast cancer cells and are associated with a higher frequency of bone marrow metastases (Pantel et al., 1991).

Immunosuppression in breast cancer patients is perhaps due to defects in tumor antigen processing and presentation to T cells. Evidence for this suppression is a decreased number of Langerhans cells, which are efficient antigen-presenting cells, in the epidermis of breast cancer patients who have metastases as compared with the number of these cells found in patients with benign breast disease or localized breast cancer. This suggests a link between decreased antigen presentation and decreased cellular immune response as measured by skin hypersensitivity responses.

Perhaps the most controversial issue related to immune function and prognosis after surgery concerns the removal of uninvolved lymph nodes. It is clear that a negative correlation exists between lymph node activity and stage of breast cancer (Reiss et al., 1983), but the cause-and-effect relationship remains unclear. A dilemma related to the role of lymph node immune responsiveness and surgery involves concern for residual disease, on the one hand, and lowering of regional immunity by lymph node dissection, on the other hand (Fisher and Fisher, 1972).

Autologous immune responsiveness to breast cancers is evident in serologic and cellular assays and in histopathologic observations. The first suggestion of a relationship between immune recognition of breast cancer–associated antigen and prolonged survival was based on the histologic appearance of a proliferative reaction in the axillary lymph nodes (Halsted, 1898). Since this original observation, much additional evidence has accumulated that suggests that morphologic manifestations, including lymphoid infiltrates (MacCarty, 1922) and sinus histiocytosis (Black et al., 1953), are associated with survival and cure and represent cell-mediated immune responses. Cell-mediated immune response, assessed with skin window reactivity to autologous breast cancer, has proved a useful test for prognosis. Positive skin window reactivity is associated with significantly reduced risk of metastases (Black et al., 1988).

A phenomenon that suggests that immune modification influences the occurrence of breast cancer is an apparent protective effect of early first pregnancy on the risk of developing breast cancer. One hypothesis is that exposure to fetal antigens (shared with tumors) during pregnancy provides a natural vaccination against tumorigenesis. Evidence to support this theory has been based largely on observations that women with low immunoglobulin levels are at high risk, and breast cancer patients with low levels of immunoglobulin are likely to have a poor prognosis (Papatestas et al., 1979; Lamoureux et al., 1982). Production of circulating antibodies against breast tumor antigens correlate well with fewer lymph node metastases and better prognosis (Hudson et al., 1974). Circumstantial evidence for the importance of cell-mediated immunity to the occurrence and progression of human breast cancer is based on observations relating development of cell-mediated immunity to in situ cancers and to the stage and time of diagnosis of second breast cancers (Black et al., 1984). These observations are consistent with the immunogenicity of breast cancer and the protective effect of cell-mediated responses. Other evidence supporting the role of cell-mediated immunity is the significant inverse correlation between peripheral lymphocyte count and chance of recurrence (Papatestas and Kark, 1974; Lee, 1984). This point is supported by evidence that the depleted lymphocytes include a T-cell subpopulation responsible for cell-mediated reactions against breast cancer cells (Felix et al., 1981).

Another approach to demonstrate autologous immune responses to breast TAAs is to elicit skin responses with tumor extracts (Oldham and Herberman, 1979). This method is used to monitor the development of cell-mediated immunity. Extracts of autologous tumors have been used with some success to skin test patients undergoing active immunotherapy (Humphrey et al., 1984). In another approach, crude membrane (CM) extracts prepared from cultured human breast tumor lines were infected with vesicular stomatitis virus (VSV) to augment antigenicity. These were then injected intradermally into breast cancer patients. One of these extracts, VSB-MCF-7, elicited positive skin test responses in 78.9% of patients, as compared with 13.3% and 15.4% of patients with lung carcinoma and melanoma, respectively (Austin et al., 1982). Although the tumor antigens involved in eliciting these responses remain to be characterized further biochemically, the demonstration of antigenic cross-reactivity with a large number of breast cancer patients is a finding of great importance for potential immunotherapy.

The frequency of surface immunoglobulin (sIg) isotypes in axillary lymph nodes was significantly increased in sIgM positive lymphocytes in those patients with lymph node metastases (Richters and Paller, 1979). This confirms a significant increase in IgM production locally in certain breast tumors (Roberts et al., 1973). Half the antiestrogen-treated breast cancer patients have shown increased numbers of immunoglobulin-secreting cells, suggesting an im-

munoregulatory effect of the antiestrogen (Paavonen et al., 1991), which could lead to increased survival.

The early suggestions of a cellular response to carcinoma in situ prompted many attempts to demonstrate cellular immune responses. Those techniques that measure general immune responsiveness, such as blastogenic response to nonspecific mitogens in vitro and skin test response to common recall antigens and the synthetic antigen dinitrochlorobenzene, appeared useful for determining prognosis. Other techniques that detect reactivity to TAAs include leukocyte migration inhibition, macrophage arming, lymphocytotoxicity, and blastogenesis with specific antigen preparations.

In vitro evidence has been obtained for reactivity of axillary node lymphocytes against breast carcinoma. In one study the response of lymphocytes from lymph nodes was significantly greater in patients who had no metastatic involvement as compared with patients who had extensive metastases. Moreover, in six patients from whom peripheral lymphocytes as well as lymph node lymphocytes were available, a greater response to tumor cells was manifested by lymph node lymphocytes (Crile, 1969). Other studies with in vitro cell-mediated responses have implicated MMTV-associated antigens (discussed earlier). In these studies women with metastatic breast cancer have diminished responsiveness to mitogens, but their T lymphocytes exhibit heightened reactivity to MMTV. These results suggest an altered proportion of T-cell subsets in the peripheral blood of patients with metastatic breast cancer (Lopez, 1986). Other investigators have demonstrated changes in peripheral lymphocyte subsets related to breast cancer. Substantial differences in lymphocyte subsets between Stages I and Stage II breast carcinoma have been demonstrated using a panel of monoclonal antibodies and two-color flow cytometric analysis. For instance, a markedly increased number of helper T cells was seen in regional lymph nodes of patients with Stage II disease. These results suggest that change in subsets may be related to metastasis of breast cancer to regional nodes (Morton et al., 1986).

More direct evidence associating regional lymphoid changes and immune response to carcinoma in situ has been obtained from immunohistochemical studies. The cells infiltrating human breast carcinomas have been characterized using anti–mononuclear cell monoclonal immunoperoxidase stains of frozen sections. Although both lymphoid and myelomonocyte lineage cells were demonstrated in the infiltrated tumors, there was a predominance of T4 cells associated with HLA-DR-positive phenotype (Gottlinger et al., 1985). Functional studies of lymphocytes recovered from infiltrated human mammary carcinomas also support the predominance of T4-bearing effector cells that display cytolytic activity (Whiteside et al., 1986). Furthermore, an in vitro lymphocyte proliferation assay against autologous tumor cells predicted the course of the disease. Absence of a cell-mediated response correlated directly with aggressive systemic breast cancer (Cannon et al., 1988, 1989).

Tumor-infiltrating lymphocytes (TILs) express specific immune responses to melanoma and renal cell carcinoma. In breast cancer patients TILs showed larger numbers of CD4-positive T cells when compared with peripheral blood lymphocytes and lymph node lymphocytes. The mitogenic proliferation index was greater for lymphocytes from PBLs and lymph nodes than for lymphocytes from the tumor. On stimulation with mitogen, TILs secreted immunomodulating cytokines such as interleukin 2 (IL-2), interferon-gamma (IFN-γ), and tumor necrosis factor (TNF). Lymph node lymphocytes produce low levels of IFN-γ but high levels of IL-2 and TNF. Mitogen-mediated TNF secretion increased after addition of autologous mammary tumor cells to the TIL and lymph node lymphocyte cultures (Rubbert et al., 1991), suggesting that antigens on the autologous mammary tumor cells were involved in stimulating the lymphocytes. In another study, the majority of TILs from breast cancers were CD8 (cytolytic/suppressor)-bearing phenotypes rather than CD4 (helper). No relationship between the degree of lymphocytic infiltration and tumor stage could be established, but an inverse correlation with estrogen receptor level in the tumor was demonstrated. In the TIL population, activated T lymphocytes (a marker for the existence of immune responses) were present along with markers such as high-affinity IL-2 receptor and HLA-DR antigen. The activated TILs had more CD8-positive cells than CD4-positive cells (Whitford, 1990). These studies suggest the presence of T-cell immune activation.

Because lymphocytes isolated from regional lymph nodes of breast cancer patients are exposed to tumor antigens it is worth studying the lymphocytes' immune responses to autologous tumor cells, in order to understand host cellular immunity. Lymphocytes from draining lymph nodes of 12 patients with primary breast cancer were analyzed, and it was found that 31% of lymphocytes proliferated when stimulated with autologous tumor cells and IL-2. No conclusive evidence was obtained from the phenotypic and functional properties of T lymphocytes stimulated by autologous tumor antigen (Hoover et al., 1991); however, PBL isolated from a breast cancer patient released cytokines (i.e. granulocyte-macrophage colony–stimulating factor, TNF, and IFN-γ) when stimulated with autologous tumor cells (Schwartzentruber et al., 1991), suggesting stimulation of T cells.

A unique technique to demonstrate T-cell immune response against breast cancer is to identify functionally specific T-cell clones. T-lymphocyte clones from breast tumor biopsy specimens were studied by Whiteside and coworkers (1986) for phenotypic and functional properties. Most of the T-cell clones expressed CD4 phenotype. Although this study demonstrated that T-cell clones can be expanded from the TILs of the breast cancer tissues, helper and cytolytic specificity for tumor cells could not be demonstrated (Whiteside et al., 1986). In an another study, cytolytic T-lymphocyte (CTL) clones derived from breast cancer were reported. These clones specifically lysed autologous tumor cells, suggesting that functionally specific CTL clonal responses exist in breast cancer patients.

Although specific immunity by CTL is an important function of the immune system, nonspecific effector function by natural killer (NK) cells is also important and has been demonstrated in breast cancer patients. Stage I breast cancer patients with no evidence of disease have greater NK activity than patients with recurrence (Brenner et al., 1991). High NK activity predicts longer survival of breast cancer patients during disease progression (Levy, 1991).

Furthermore, NK cell sensitivity of ER-positive breast cancer cells was enhanced when the cells were treated with estradiol, but no response was found with ER-negative tumor cells, suggesting that a hormone-mediated signaling system helps in the NK cell–tumor interaction (Screpanti et al., 1991). These results are derived from experiments in vitro using allogenic tumor cells, and the role of estradiol in the enhancement of NK activity needs to be demonstrated with patient's lymphocytes against autologous tumor cells.

A combination of cytolytic T-cell activity and NK activity could enhance antitumor response. This was investigated using fresh lymphocytes isolated from tumor, lymph nodes, and peripheral blood of breast cancer patients. Although fresh lymphocytes from each of the sources did not show NK or CTL activity, potent (and sometimes tumor-specific) cytolytic activity was observed after expansion of the lymphocytes in vitro with IL-2 (Rubbert et al., 1991). This study suggests that breast cancer patients could have autologous tumor-specific cytolytic activity and are suitable candidates for adoptive immunotherapy with lymphocytes stimulated and expanded in vitro.

Immunomodulatory drugs enhance immunity against tumor cells. Levamisole has many different effects on immunity. One is to restore NK activity through the inhibition of soluble suppressor factors. Levamisole with chemotherapy resulted in an increased survival rate in patients treated in one study (Klefstrom and Nuortio, 1991). Further studies are necessary to clarify levamisole's role.

An important step in further development of immunotherapy for breast cancer is to identify specific antigens that induce either cellular or humoral immune responses. Although various studies demonstrate the existence of both arms of the immune response in breast cancer patients, antigens in these patients that induce an immune response have not been studied. The recent finding that an epitope of the breast cancer–associated mucin antigen binds with major histocompatibility complex–unrestricted cytotoxic T cells suggests participation of the antigen in T-cell immunity. Further evidence for participation of the mucin antigen in T-cell immunity is the observation that a soluble purified mucin induced proliferation of breast tumor–restricted T cells (Brand et al., 1989). These findings suggest that breast cancer–associated antigens are involved in T-cell immune responses (Jerome et al., 1991). These antigens need to be further delineated.

Summary

A great deal of evidence in the literature supports a relationship between immune responsiveness and breast cancer occurrence and progression. Much of this evidence has been drawn from correlations between lymph node reactivity and progression of systemic disease. Other evidence is from skin tests and assays in vitro. These findings support the rationale for immunotherapy.

CLINICAL IMMUNOTHERAPY
Nonspecific Active Immunotherapy

The first form of biologic therapy for cancer can legitimately be attributed to nature and is based on reports of tumor regression in association with concurrent acute bacterial infection. A total of 449 such cases of so-called spontaneous regression have been recorded, of which 93 were breast cancers (Nauts, 1984).

The first attempt to induce bacterial infection as a therapeutic measure for breast cancer was made more than 200 years ago. The pioneer of this approach in the United States was Coley, who developed a vaccine from a mixture of bacteria (MBV), also known as Coley's mixed toxin, which was prepared from *Streptococcus pyogenes* and *Bacillus prodigiosus* (now *Serratia marcescens*). A total of 896 microscopically proved cases of cancer were treated with mixed bacteria vaccine, of which 78 involved the breast. This study did not include a large number, and was without concurrent controls (Nauts, 1980).

The most important result of mixed bacteria–vaccine research was the stimulation of interest in other bacterial vaccines, such as *bacille Calmette-Guérin* (BCG). Though BCG, an attenuated form of the tubercle bacillus, was first used as a vaccine against tuberculosis, it was found to be a potent stimulator of the reticuloendothelial system. Such stimulation was associated with prevention of tumor growth in mice (Old et al., 1959), an observation that stimulated interest in clinical trials, which ushered in the era of nonspecific immunotherapy (Nauts, 1984). BCG was first used to treat disseminated breast cancer in combination with chemotherapy which included 5-fluorouracil (5-FU), doxorubicin hydrochloride (Adriamycin), and cyclophosphamide in combination, (FAC). Compared with FAC alone, rates of remission were similar but remission lasted longer when BCG was included (Gutterman et al., 1976). Many clinical studies using immunotherapy have since reported prolonged disease-free intervals, especially when it is used in combination with chemotherapy (Buzdar et al., 1979). Some protocols have included radiotherapy with this combination and have had success in treating patients with inflammatory breast carcinoma (Krutchik et al., 1979). However in a randomized prospective trial of patients with Stage II breast cancer with 9-year follow-up, BCG in conjunction with chemotherapy and tamoxifen failed to produce a better overall disease-free survival rate than chemotherapy in combination with tamoxifen (Fisher et al., 1990).

Another organism able to stimulate the reticuloendothelial system is *Corynebacterium parvum.* In a killed vaccine, it was able to inhibit tumor growth (Halpern et al., 1966). Large numbers of patients with disseminated disease were treated with *C. parvum,* including many with metastatic breast cancer. These trials showed significant increases in survival for certain patients and complete remission in isolated cases (Nathanson, 1977), but 8-year follow-up of a trial of chemotherapy in combination with *C. parvum* failed to show a better disease-free survival rate or overall survival for patients with Stage II breast cancer (Fisher et al., 1990).

These studies failed to support the use of nonspecific immunotherapy using BCG or *C. parvum,* alone or in combination with chemotherapy, for breast cancer patients.

Nonspecific Passive Immunotherapy

Although the term "passive immunotherapy" suggests a lack of participation of the host, several substances that have direct nonspecific antitumor properties, and therefore are considered to confer resistance passively, may actually exert an indirect antitumor effect based on modulation of the immune response. A great many biologic mediators produced by cells of the immune system (lymphokines, monokines, or cytokines) enhance antitumor immune response and have direct cytotoxic or antiproliferative effects (Oldham, 1984; Torrence, 1986).

Interferon is the classic example of a biologic response modifier that has multiple biologic effects (Hooks and Detrick, 1986). Growth inhibition and immunostimulation were shown to be responsible for the antitumor effects of interferon in vitro and in animal models, but clinical trials were limited by the small amount of material that could be prepared from human buffy coat cells stimulated with virus or mitogen. Successful cloning of the gene(s) for cytokines, which allowed mass production of recombinant molecules, ushered in the modern era of biologic immunotherapy and a new wave of optimism.

Relatively few clinical trials have evaluated IFN-α against breast cancer per se. In the trials that were performed, a minority of patients showed major objective tumor regression, but considerable toxicity was reported (Gutterman et al., 1980; Borden et al., 1984). Similar trials with recombinant (leukocyte) IFN-α, either alone or in combination with one or more cytokines, are currently under way.

It should be emphasized that the majority of clinical trials have been performed with clone A IFN-α. Several other clonotypes of recombinant α-interferon have only recently been cloned, but its immunoregulatory properties have already been characterized, and the recombinant molecule is in use in a number of clinical trials. It should be noted that doses and schedules of interferon treatment have been derived empirically.

Another cytokine of great interest was first described as a possible mediator of the antitumor activity of bacterial endotoxin (Carswell et al., 1975). TNF is so named because it is believed to mediate endotoxin-induced tumor necrosis. The gene for TNF is cloned and expressed in a vector. Recombinant TNF has been extensively characterized for its functional properties. A similar molecule produced by lymphocytes, named lymphotoxin, has also recently been obtained as a cloned gene product and is closely related to the original TNF (Old, 1985). Clinical trials with TNF are currently under way (Flick and Gifford, 1986). In these trials, TNF has shown toxicity such as fever, rigors, noncardiac pulmonary edema due to vascular leakage, and dose-limiting hypotension (Schiller et al., 1991). Modification of TNF to reduce side effects is being pursued.

Perhaps the lymphokine of greatest interest for immunotherapy at present is IL-2. IL-2 exerts antitumor effects in mouse models, especially in conjunction with adoptive immunotherapy. The clinical experience with IL-2 is similar to that in the mouse (i.e., limited effectiveness alone, synergism with adoptively transferred cells that have been activated with IL-2 in vitro, and significant toxicity in large doses) (Rosenberg et al., 1985). Only one in five breast cancer patients showed a partial response (West, 1989) on adoptive immunotherapy with continuous infusion of IL-2. Studies from larger populations are needed to evaluate the effect of the IL-2 therapy, alone or in combination with adoptive transfer of immune cells.

Certain synthetic drugs are also potentially useful as immune response modifiers. A number of synthetic immunomodifiers exert their biologic effects through induction of IFN. Most notable of these are the polynucleotides polyriboinosinic acid: polyribocytidylic acid (poly I:C) and polyadenylate:polyuridylate (poly A:U). Both are good inducers of IFN, but poly A:U is preferred because of its more rapid rate of depolymerization in vivo and its lesser toxicity. Poly A:U treatment as an adjunct to simple mastectomy and radiation was evaluated in a large randomized trial in France and was found to result in a 4-year relapse-free survival rate of 77% versus 57% in controls (Lacour et al., 1982).

A synthetic immune modifier of uncertain action is levamisole, a drug originally used in veterinary medicine as an anthelminthic. The immunopotentiating properties of levamisole demonstrated in vitro and in animal models prompted clinical evaluation. Promising results with the use of levamisole in treating advanced breast cancer were correlated with an increase in lymphocyte counts and delayed hypersensitivity skin reactions (Rojas et al., 1976). Other studies, however, reported no differences in survival compared with chemotherapy (Hirshaut et al., 1978) and an actual increase in recurrences compared with postoperative radiation (Anthony, 1980). The high frequency of side effects resulted in suspension of other trials (Retsas et al., 1978).

A nonspecific immunotherapeutic approach that could be considered either active or passive, depending on the interpretation of the mechanism of action, is extracorporeal immunoadsorption on bacterial cell wall component chambers. The mode of action of this procedure is believed to involve complexes, although some investigators postulate that cellular activation is also involved (Bertram, 1985). Protein A immunoadsorption treatment was performed in seven breast cancer patients in a Phase I study (Anisworth et al., 1988). Although a 50% regression of measurable tumor volume occurred in four of seven patients, mild to moderate side effects resulted. A randomized study with more patients may determine the effectiveness of this treatment.

The other major approach in this category is adoptive immunity, in which the effectors of antitumor immunity are whole cells rather than soluble cell products. Until very recently, this approach was directed entirely toward the transfer of lymphocytes from patients who had experienced tumor regression. The problems of this approach were similar to those encountered with soluble products from single patient sources (e.g., poor quality control and limited quantities). The major breakthrough in adoptive immunotherapy came with the discovery of T-cell growth factors, which enable us to prepare large quantities of homogeneous cell populations. Such expanded T-cell lines and clones were initially shown to be antigen specific, but after further culture they exhibited nonspecific killing activity. In mice these nonspecific cells were activated by IL-2 in vitro and were capable of lysing fresh tumor cells nonspecifically. These lymphokine-activated killer (LAK) cells caused dramatic regression of various murine tumors when adminis-

tered along with IL-2 (Mule et al., 1986). This approach was used to treat advanced cancer in trials that included IL-2 alone, LAK cells alone, or LAK cells in combination with IL-2. The results confirmed the effectiveness of the LAK–IL-2 combination in advanced cancers of all histologic types (Rosenberg et al., 1985). The major drawbacks remain the cumbersome nature of the procedure, the small number of patients who can be treated, and the toxicity associated with large doses of IL-2. Overcoming these problems will undoubtedly result in a treatment method that will impact favorably on breast cancer in the near future.

In a recent study, newly characterized TILs expressing high specificity for autologous tumor cells have been investigated. These TILs also possess tumor-targeting potential (Fisher et al., 1989). Breast cancers contain infiltrating lymphocytes and so afford an opportunity to use TIL in adoptive immunotherapy.

One of the latest advances in immunotherapy is the use of gene-transfected TIL therapy. The idea is to use the tumor-targeting potential of the TILs. Gene-transfected TILs have been studied in patients with advanced melanoma. In this study the TNF gene was transfected into autologous TILs and injected back into patients. A preliminary study evaluated the toxicity and side effects of this approach (Rosenberg et al., 1990). This can be attempted in breast cancer patients who have infiltrating lymphocytes in their tumor.

Specific Active Immunotherapy

Specific active immunotherapy is based on the assumption that tumor-associated antigens exist that can elicit an autologous antitumor response. Although chemically and virally induced experimental tumors possess sufficient immunogenicity to confer resistance to rechallenge, it has been more difficult to demonstrate this with spontaneous tumors of low antigenicity (Kreider and Bartlett, 1985).

The most appropriate setting for active specific immunotherapy is in the presence of minimal tumor burden. Thus, this approach is best evaluated as an adjuvant to surgery. Of the several immunotherapy adjuvant studies that have been performed in breast cancer, most have involved combination chemotherapy or radiotherapy, or both, and relatively few have included adjuvant immunotherapy alone. Humphrey and coworkers (1980) reported promising preliminary data from treatment of breast cancer patients with a breast tumor–derived antigen preparation after radical mastectomy. The survival rates in this study with Stage I patients compared favorably with those that used radiation therapy as the principal treatment (Humphrey et al., 1980).

Since the major drawback to the development of a tumor vaccine is the relatively weak immunogenicity of autologous breast cancer antigens, attempts to augment the immunogenicity of these tumors have been many and varied. These approaches include several physical, chemical, and biologic modifications of tumor cells to xenogenize them (i.e., to render them ''foreign'') (Kobayashi, 1982). One of the more promising is to use viral infection to augment tumor cell antigenicity. Several different viruses have been used to infect tumors (or tumor cell lines), and the resulting whole cells or membrane preparations, called oncolysates, have increased resistance to rechallenge in mouse models. Similar preparations have been used to treat a variety of tumors in the adjuvant setting (Austin & Boone, 1979). Although breast cancer has not been treated with oncolysates, vesicular stomatitis virus–infected breast tumor line extracts have elicited positive skin test results in a greater proportion of breast cancer patients than extracts prepared from uninfected cells (Austin et al., 1982). Promising results have been obtained with gynecologic malignancies treated with an influenza oncolysate. Patients with ovarian carcinoma show a clinical response and augmentation of NK cell activity (Lotzova et al., 1984). Extended disease-free survival of vulvar carcinoma patients was achieved coincident with development of humoral and cellular immune responses (Freedman et al., 1983).

A major problem with specific active immunotherapy is the identification and purification of relevant antigens. By observation of patients' responses to their own tumors and to crude vaccines, and with identification of breast-associated tumor antigens with monoclonal antibodies, the relevant antigens should ultimately be identified. These molecules' genes might then be cloned and recombinant vaccines be obtained for active specific immunotherapy.

Recently, the epithelial tumor antigen, an antigen commonly expressed on breast cancer cells, was cloned in vaccinia virus vector. This tumor antigen–encoded vaccinia virus vaccination showed protective immunity in a study with an experimental animal model (Hareuveni et al., 1990).

Oncogene products are expressed on tumor cells and, provided they are immunogenic, could stimulate immune responses. The *neu* oncogene expressed in rat systems is homologous to c-*erb* B_2 oncogene expressed in human breast cancer cells. The c-*erb* B_2 gene product stimulated an antibody response in immunized rats and showed protective immunity to *neu* gene–transfected NIH 3T3 cells. This experiment suggests a possible therapeutic application for the oncogne product in human breast cancer. Numerous oncogne products can be tested.

Specific Passive Immunotherapy

The concept of passive immunotherapy for cancer by administration of preformed antibodies is a direct extension of the classic approach to antimicrobial and antitoxic serotherapy, which, though now largely replaced by antibiotic therapy, is still used to rescue victims of acute intoxication (as with snake venoms). Although the concept of transfer of specific immunity to cancer is theoretically sound if a strong immune response to tumor-associated antigens has been generated, little success has been achieved, either in animal models or in clinical attempts to passively transfer whole serum from persons who have successfully rejected tumors to patients with established cancers. The reasons for this failure may include both the predominance of cellular rather than serologic antitumor immunity and the inability to achieve high enough concentrations of specific antibodies when using polyvalent serum.

The advent of hybridoma technology generated renewed interest in serotherapy. With serotherapy, unlimited quantities of homogeneous antibody with restricted specificity for TAAs can be generated. The wide variety of monoclonal antibodies potentially useful in diagnosis and prognosis of breast cancer was reviewed earlier. Although many of these antibodies have potential, either alone or conjugated to drugs, toxins, or radionuclides, few clinical trials have actually been performed. One monoclonal antibody directed against HMFG-2 has been radiolabeled and administered intraperitoneally to deliver radiation to ovarian tumors (Burchell and Taylor-Papadimitrious, 1985). A toxin conjugated with monoclonal antibody to breast-associated antigen was internalized specifically by breast cancer cells (Yu et al., 1990). A paracarcinoma monoclonal antibody (NR-LU-10) conjugated to endotoxin A was used to eliminate breast cancer cells from bone marrow (Bjorn et al., 1985, 1990).

The other major approach to specific passive immunotherapy, the adoptive transfer of lymphocytes that can recognize and kill tumor targets, has been developed. This technique was used widely in animal models in which the availability of inbred strains allows pooling of lymphocytes from several donors to achieve sufficient numbers but has held few possibilities for human immunotherapy because of the inability to collect sufficient numbers of cells (Rosenberg and Terry, 1977). Renewed interest in this approach resulted from the discovery of T-cell growth factor (Morgan et al., 1976), now designated IL-2, and the development of T cell–cloning technology (Fathman and Frelinger, 1983), which allows the production of monoclonal effector cells. It has been demonstrated that specific T-cell clones expanded in IL-2 can mediate regression of established solid tumor metastases in a mouse model (Shu et al., 1986). This approach continues to have limited applicability in the clinical setting, however, because of the need for autologous cells and the technical complexity and time required to select and clone the appropriate effector cells and grow them in large numbers. Moreover, the additional cloning required for this approach seems unnecessary in light of the success achieved with nonspecific LAK cells (Rosenberg, 1986).

SUMMARY

Until recently immunotherapy of breast cancer has been limited to nonspecific immunopotentiation with a variety of bacterial products and lymphokines of variable potency. These attempts, which have largely been limited to Phase I trials with patients with advanced disease, have been only marginally successful. The prospects for successful immunotherapy of breast cancer in the near future are, however, improved. This new-found optimism is, in large part, based on the dramatic breakthroughs in basic science, which have redefined immunobiology in molecular terms. The development of hybridoma technology has far-reaching effects on both active and passive approaches to immunotherapy, because monoclonal antibodies allow the purification and characterization of TAAs. The monoclonal antibodies themselves, or as conjugates with drugs, toxins, or radionuclides, are potentially ideal reagents for seeking out residual tumor cells. Recombinant deoxyribonucleic acid technology allowed the cloning and synthesis of a number of molecules that are now available in unlimited quantities in pure form. The first of these molecules, IFN, was not the magic bullet hoped for, but it is showing promise and has yet to be thoroughly evaluated. Other lymphokines, such as IL-2, which act through activation of killer cells, show promise. The new biotechnology promises to provide significant advances in immunotherapy of breast cancer.

References

Adler, A., Stein, J. A., et al.: Active specific immunotherapy of stage III breast cancer: Results of an exploratory study. Cancer Immunol. Immunother., *10*:45, 1980.

Anisworth, S. K., Pilia, P. A., Pepkowitz, S. K., et al.: Toxicity following protein A treatment of metastatic breast adenocarcinoma. Cancer, *61*:1495, 1988.

Anthony, H. M.: Adjuvant levamisole in breast cancer. Lancet, 2:1123, 1980.

Austin, F. C., and Boone, C. W.: Virus augmentation of the antigenicity of tumor cell extracts. Adv. Cancer Res., *30*:301, 1979.

Austin, F. C., Boone, C. W., Levin, D. L., et al.: Breast cancer skin test antigens of increased sensitivity prepared from vesicular stomatitis virus–infected tumor cells. Cancer, *49*:2034, 1982.

Bacus, S. S., Goldschmidt, R., Chin, D., et al.: Biological grading of breast cancer using antibodies to proliferating cells and other markers. Am. J. Pathol., *135*:1152, 1989.

Bernard, D. J., Maurizis, J. C., Chassagne, J., et al.: Comparison of class II HLA antigen expression in normal and carcinomatous human breast cells. Cancer Res., *45*:1152, 1985.

Benz, C. C., Scott, G. K., Santos, G. F., et al.: Expression of c-*myc*, c-Ha-*ras*1, and c-*erb* B₂ protooncogenes in normal and malignant human breast epithelial cells. J Natl. Cancer Inst., *81*:1704, 1989.

Bertram, J. H.: Staphylococcus protein A column: Its mechanism of action. *In* Reif, R., and Mitchell, M. S. (Eds.): Immunity to Cancer. Orlando, FL, Academic Press, 1985, p. 499.

Beveridge, R. A., Chan, D. W., Damron, D., et al.,: A new biomarker in monitoring breast cancer: CA 549. J. Clin. Oncol., *6*:1815, 1988.

Bhatavdekar, J. M., Shah, N. G., Balar, D. B., et al.: Plasma prolactin as an indicator of disease progression in advanced breast cancer. Cancer, *65*:2028, 1990.

Bjorn, M. J., Manger, R., Sivam, G., et al.: Selective elimination of breast cancer cells from human bone marrow using an antibody–*Pseudomonas* exotoxin A conjugate. Cancer Res., *50*:5992, 1990.

Bjorn, M. J., Ring, D., and Frankel, A.: Evaluation of monoclonal antibodies for the development of breast cancer immunotoxins. Cancer Res., *45*:1214, 1985.

Black, M. M., Kerpe, S., and Speer, F. D.: Lymph node structure in patients with cancer of the breast. Am. J. Pathol., *29*:505, 1953.

Black, M. M., and Zachrau, R. E.: Immune mechanisms: Prognostic, therapeutic and preventive significance. *In* Ariel, I. M., and Cleary, J. B. (Eds.): Breast Cancer: Diagnosis and Treatment. New York, McGraw-Hill, 1987, p. 128.

Black, M. M., Hankey, B. F., Aron, J. L., et al.: Possible immunological implications of an association between the first stages of first and second independent breast cancer. Breast Cancer Res. Treat., *4*:95, 1984.

Black, M. M., Moore, D. H., Shore, B., et al.: Effect of murine milk samples and human breast tissues on human leukocyte migration indices. Cancer Res., *34*:1054, 1974.

Black, M. M., Zachrau, R. E., Hankey, B. F., et al.: Skin window reactivity to autologous breast cancer: An index of prognostically significant cell-mediated immunity. Cancer, *62*:72, 1988.

Borden, E. C., and Balkwill, F. R.: Preclinical and clinical studies of interferons and interferon inducers in breast cancer. Cancer, *53*:783, 1984.

Borg, A., Tandon, A. K., Sigurdsson, H., et al.: *HER-2/neu* amplification predicts poor survival in node positive breast cancer. Cancer Res., *50*:4332–4337.

Brabon, A. C., Williams, J. F., and Cardiff, R. D.: A monoclonal antibody

to a human breast tumor protein released in response to estrogen. Cancer Res., *44*:2704, 1984.

Brand, D. L., Lan, M., Metzgar, R., et al.: Specific MHC unrestricted recognition of tumor associated mucin by human cytotoxic T-cells. Proc. Natl. Acad. Sci. USA., *86*:7159, 1989.

Brenner, B. G., Gryllis, C., Gornitsky, M., et al.: Differential effects of chemotherapy-induced and HIV-1–induced immunocompromise on NK and LAK activities using breast cancer and HIV-1 seropositive patient populations. Anticancer Res., *11*:969, 1991.

Buessow, S. C., Paul, R. D., and Lopez, D. M.: Influence of mammary tumor progression on phenotype and function of spleen and in situ lymphocytes in mice. J Natl. Cancer Inst., *73*:249, 1984.

Burchell, J. M., and Taylor-Papadimitriou, J.: Monoclonal antibodies to breast cancer and their application. *In* Baldwin, R. W., and Byers, V. S. (Eds.): Monoclonal Antibodies for Cancer Detection and Therapy. New York, Academic Press, 1985, p. 1.

Burnet, F. M.: The concept of immunological surveillance. Progr. Exp. Tumor Res., *13*:1, 1970.

Buzdar, A. U., Blumenschein, G. R., Smith, T. L., et al.: Adjuvant chemoimmunotherapy following regional therapy for isolated recurrences of breast cancer (Stage IV NED). J. Surg. Oncol., *12*:27, 1979.

Callahan, R., Drohan, W., Tronick, S., et al.: Detection and cloning of human DNA sequences related to the mouse mammary tumors by immunoperoxidase staining of paraffin sections. Proc. Natl. Acad. Sci., *79*:5503, 1982.

Cannon, G. B., and Pomerantz R.: Cell-mediated immune responses—prognostic indicators of survival from breast cancer. Int. J. Cancer, *44*:995, 1989.

Cannon, G. B., McCoy, J., Promerantz, R., et al.: 10-Year survival in breast cancer patients predicted by clinical and immunological parameters (Abstract). Proc. Am. Assoc. Cancer Res., *29*:382, 1988.

Carswell, E. A., Old, L. J., Kassel, R. L., et al.: An endotoxin-induced serum factor that causes necrosis of tumors. Proc. Natl. Acad. Sci., *72*:3666–3670, 1975.

Castronovo, V., Colins, C., Claysmith, A. P., et al.: Immunodetection of metastases-associated laminin receptor in human breast cancer cells obtained by fine needle aspiration biopsy. Am. J. Pathol., *137*:1373, 1990.

Ceriani, R. L., and Rosenbum, E. H.: Breast epithelial antigens in the circulation of breast cancer patients. Immunol. Ser., *53*:223, 1991.

Colcher, D., Horan-Hand, P., Wunderlich, D., et al.: Potential diagnostic and prognostic applications of monoclonal antibodies to human mammary carcinomas. *In* Wright, G. L. (Ed.): Monoclonal Antibodies and Cancer. New York, Marcel Dekker, 1984, p. 121.

Coley, W. B.: Contributions to the knowledge of sarcoma. Ann. Surg., *14*:199, 1891.

Colomer, R., Ruibal, A., and Salvador, L.: Circulating tumor marker levels in advanced breast carcinoma correlated with the extent of metastatic disease. Cancer, *64*:1674, 1989.

Crile, G. Jr.: Possible role of uninvolved nodes in preventing metastasis from breast cancer. Cancer, *24*:1283, 1969.

Danovan-Peluso, M., Contento, A. M., Tobon, H., et al.: Oncogene amplification in breast cancer. Am. J. Pathol., *138*:835, 1991.

Day, N. K., Wilkin, S. S., Sarkar, N. H., et al.: Antibodies reactive with murine mammary tumor virus in sera of patients with breast cancer: Geographic and family studies. Proc. Nat. Acad. Sci. USA, *78*:2483, 1981.

Edwards, D. P., Grzyb, K. T., Dressler, L. G., et al.: Monoclonal antibody identification and characterization of a M 43,000 membrane glycoprotein associated with human breast cancer. Cancer Res., *46*:1306, 1986.

Ehrlich, P. (1909): Uber den jetzgen Stand der Karzinom-forschung. *In* Himmelweit, F. (Ed.): The Collected Papers of Paul Ehrlich. Vol. II. Immunology and Cancer Research. London, Pergamon Press, 1957, p. 559.

Eskelinen, M., Lipponen, P. and Collan, Y.: Immunohistochemical staining of human breast cancer with new tumor marker MCA: Relating to axillary lymph node involvement, metastases, and survival. Anticancer Res., *10*:519, 1990.

Fahey, J. L., Taylor, J. M., Korns, E., et al.: Diagnostic and prognostic factors in AIDS. Mt. Sinai J. Med., *53*:567, 1986.

Fathman, C. G., and Frelinger, J. G.: T-lymphocyte clones. Annu. Rev. Immunol., *1*:633, 1983.

Felix, E., Katz, S., Teodorescu, A., et al.: Enumeration of lymphocytes and their subpopulation identified by bacterial adherence in blood smears of patients with breast tumors. J. Surg. Oncol., *18*:323, 1981.

Feller, W., Kantor, J., Hilkens, J., et al.: Monoclonal antibody defined antigens in plasma of breast cancer patients (Abstract 589). Proc. Am. Assoc. Cancer Res., 26:149, 1985.

Fisher, B., and Fisher, E. R.: Studies concerning the regional lymph nodes in cancer. II. Maintenance of immunity. Cancer, 29:1496, 1972.

Fisher, B., Brown, A., Wolmark, N., et al.: Evaluation of the worth of *Corynebacterium parvum* in conjunction with chemotherapy as adjuvant treatment for primary cancer. Cancer, 66:220, 1990.

Fisher, B., Packard, B. S., Read, E. J., et al.: Tumor localization of adoptively transferred Indium-111–labeled tumor infiltrating lymphocytes in patients with metastatic melanoma. J. Clin. Oncol., 7:250, 1989.

Flick, D. A., and Gifford, G. E.: Tumor necrosis factor. *In* Torrence, P. F. (Ed.): Biological Response Modifiers: New Approaches to Disease Intervention. Orlando, FL, Academic Press, 1986, p. 171.

Foeken, J. A., Portengen, H., van Puttern, W. L. J., et al.: Prognostic value of receptors for insulin-like growth factor 1, somatostatin, and epidermal growth factor in human breast cancer. Cancer Res., 49:7002, 1990.

Freedman, R. S., Bowen, J. M., Herson, J. H., et al.: Immunotherapy for vulvar carcinoma with virus-modified homologous extracts. Obstet. Gynecol., 62:707, 1983.

Garcia, M., Capony, F., Derocq, D., et al.: Characterization of monoclonal antibodies to the estrogen-regulated Mr 52,000 glycoprotein and their use in MCF7 cells. Cancer Res., 45:709, 1985.

Gion, M., Mione, R., Nascimben, O., et al.: Tumor-associated antigen CA15.3 in primary breast cancer evaluation of 667 cases. Br. J. Cancer, 63:809, 1991.

Girardi, A. J., Dion, A. S., and Holben, J. A.: Immunologic studies with mouse mammary tumor viruses: Comparative studies with spontaneous mammary tumor call vaccines from five inbred mouse strains. J. Natl. Cancer Inst., 74:105, 1985.

Gottlinger, H. G., Gokel, J. M., Lohe, K. J., et al.: Infiltrating mononuclear cells in human breast carcinoma: Predominance of T4+ monocytic cells in the tumor stroma. Int. J. Cancer, 35:199, 1985.

Gross, L.: Immunological relationship of mammary carcinomas developing spontaneously in female mice of a high-tumor line. J. Immunol., 55:297, 1947.

Gutterman, J., Blumenschein, G. R., Hortobagyi, G., et al.: Immunotherapy for breast cancer. Breast, 2:29, 1976.

Gutterman, J. U., Blumenschein, G. R., Alexanian, R., et al.: Leukocyte interferon-induced tumor regression in human metastatic breast cancer, multiple myeloma, and malignant lymphoma. Ann. Intern. Med., 93:399, 1980.

Halpern, B. N., Biozzi, G., Stiffel, C., et al.: Inhibition of tumor growth by administration of killed *Corynebacterium parvum*. Nature, 212:853, 1966.

Halsted, W. S.: A clinical and histological study of certain adenocarcinomata of the breast. J.A.M.A., 14:114, 1898.

Hareuveni, M., Gautier, C., Kieny, M. P., et al. Vaccination against tumor cells expressing breast epithelial tumor antigen. Proc. Natl. Acad. Sci. USA, 87:9498, 1990.

Hayes, D. F., Mesa-Tesa-Tejada, R., Papsidero, L. W., et al.: Prediction of prognosis in primary cancer by detection of high molecular weight mucin-like antigen using monoclonal antibodies DF3, F36/22, and CU18: A cancer and leukemia group study. J. Clin. Oncol., 9:1113, 1991.

Hennipman, A., van Orischot, B. A., Smits, J., et al.: Tyrosine kinase activity in breast cancer, benign breast disease, and normal breast tissue. Cancer Res., 49:516, 1989.

Hilkens, J., Tager, J. M., Bujis, F., et al.: Monoclonal antibodies against human acid alpha-glycosidase. Biochim. Biophys. Acta, 678:7, 1981.

Hindsley, J. P., Avis, I., Newsome, J. F., et al.: Certain aspects of analysis of complement dependent antibody in breast cancer patients. J. Surg. Oncol., 11:107, 1979.

Hirshaut, Y., Kesselheim, H., Pinsky, C. M., et al.: Levamisole as an immunoadjuvant: Phase I study and application in breast cancer. Cancer Treat. Res., 62:1693, 1978.

Hooks, J. J., and Detrick, B.: Immunoregulatory functions of interferon. *In* Torrence, P. F. (Ed.): Biological Response Modifiers: New Approaches to Disease Intervention. Orlando, Academic Press, 1986, p. 57.

Hoover, S. K., Frank, J. L., McCrady, C., et al.: Activation and in vitro expansion of tumor reactive T lymphocytes from nodes draining human primary breast cancers. J. Surg. Oncol., 46:117, 1991.

Horan-Hand, P., Colcher, D., Salmon, D., et al.: Influence of spatial configuration of carcinoma cell population on the expansion of tumor associated glycoprotein. Cancer Res., 45:833, 1985.

Hudson, M. J. K., Humphrey, L. J., Mantz, F. A., et al.: Correlation of circulating serum antibody to the histologic findings in breast cancer. Am. J. Surg., 128:756, 1974.

Humphrey, L. J., Singla, O., and Volenec, F. J.: Immunologic responsiveness of the breast cancer patient. Cancer, 46:893, 1980.

Humphrey, L. J., Taschler-Collins, S., and Volenec, F. J.: Treatment of primary breast cancer with immunotherapy. Am J. Surg., 148:649, 1984.

Iman, A., Drushella, M. M., Taylor, C. R., et al.: Generation and immunohistological characterization of human monoclonal antibodies to mammary carcinoma cells. Cancer Res., 45:263, 1985.

Jerome, K. R., Barnd, D. L., Bendt, K. M., et al.: Cytotoxic T lymphocytes derived from patients with breast adenocarcinoma recognize an epitope present on the protein core of mucin molecule preferentially expressed by malignant cells. Cancer Res., 11:2908, 1991.

Keydar, I., Mesa-Tejada, R., Ramanarayanan, M., et al.: Detection of viral proteins in mouse mammary tumors by immunoperoxidase staining of paraffin sections. Proc. Natl. Acad. Sci., 75:1524, 1978.

Kida, N., Yoshimura, T., Mori, K., et al.: Hormonal regulation of synthesis and secretion of protein relevant to growth of human breast cancer cells (MCF-7). Cancer Res., 49:3494, 1989.

Klefstrom, P., and Nuortio, L.: Levamisole in the treatment of advanced breast cancer. A ten-year follow-up of a randomized study. Acta. Oncol., 30:340, 1991.

Kobayashi, H.: Modification of tumor antigenicity in therapeutics: Increase in immunologic foreignness of tumor cells in experimental model systems. *In* Mihich, E. (Ed.): Immunological Approaches to Cancer Therapeutics. New York, John Wiley & Sons, 1982, p. 405.

Kreider, J. W., and Bartlett, G. L.: Increased immunogenicity of a spontaneous variant clone of the 13762A rat mammary adenocarcinoma. J. Natl. Cancer Inst., 75:141, 1985.

Krutchik, A. N., Buzdar, A. U., Blumenschein, G. R., et al.: Combined chemoimmunotherapy and irradiation therapy of inflammatory breast carcinoma. J. Surg. Oncol., 11:325, 1979.

Kuhajda, F. P., Piantadosi, S., and Pasternack, G. R.: Hepatoglobulin-related protein (Hpr) epitopes in breast cancer as a predictor of recurrence of the disease. N. Engl. J. Med., 321:636, 1989.

Lacour, F., Lacour, J., Spiras, A., et al.: A new adjuvant treatment with polyadenylic-polyuridylic acid in operable breast cancer. Recent Results Cancer Res., 80:200, 1982.

Lamki, L. M., Buzdar, A. U., Singletary, S. E., et al.: Indium labeled B72.3 monoclonal antibody in the detection and staging of breast cancer phase I study. J. Nucl. Med., 32:1326, 1991.

Lamoureux, G., Mandeville, R., Poisson, R., et al.: Biologic markers and breast cancer: A multiparametric study. I. Increased serum protein levels. Cancer, 49:502, 1982.

Larocca, D., Peterson, J. A., Urrea, R., et al.: A Mr 46,000 human milk fat globule protein that is highly expressed in human breast tumors contains factor VIII–like domains. Cancer Res., 51:4994, 1991.

Lee, Y.-T.: Delayed cutaneous hypersensitivity, lymphocyte count, and blood tests in patients with breast carcinoma. J. Surg. Oncol., 27:135, 1984.

Lennox, E. S.: What are tumor antigens? *In* Reif, A. E., and Mitchell, M. S. (Eds.): Immunity to Cancer. Orlando, Academic Press, 1985, p. 17.

Levine, P. H., Mesa-Tejada, R., Keydar, I., et al.: Increased incidence of mouse mammary tumor virus–related antigen in Tunisian patients with breast cancer. Int. J. Cancer, 33:305, 1984.

Levy, S. M., Herberman, R. B., Lippman, M., et al.: Immunological and psychological predictors of disease recurrence in patients with early stage breast cancer. Bhev. Med., 17:67, 1991.

Lopez, D. M.: New developments in breast cancer immunology. *In* Rich, M. A., Hager, J. C., and Taylor-Papadimitrious, J.: Breast Cancer: Origins, Detection and Treatment. Boston, Martinus Nijhoff, 1986, p. 112.

Lopez, D. M., Charyulu, V., and Paul, R. D.: B cell subsets in spleens of Balb/c mice: Identification and isolation of MMTV-expressing and MMTV-responding subpopulations. J. Immunol., 134:603, 1985.

Lotzova, E., Savary, C. A., Freedman, R. S., et al.: Natural killer cell cytotoxic potential of patients with ovarian carcinoma and its modulation with virus-modified tumor cell extract. Cancer Immunol. Immunother., 16:124, 1984.

MacCarty, W. C.: Factors which influence longevity in cancer. Ann. Surg., 76:9, 1922.

Marques, L. A., Franco, E. L. F., Torloni, H., et al.: Independent prognostic value of laminin receptor expression in breast cancer survival. Cancer Res. 50:1479, 1990.

May, F. E., Westley, B. R., Rockefort, H., et al.: Mouse mammary tumor virus–related sequences are present in human DNA. Nucleic Acid Res., *11*:4127, 1983.

Mesa-Tejada, R., Keydar, I., Ramanarayanan, M., et al.: Immunohistochemical detection of cross-reacting virus antigen in mouse mammary tumors and human breast carcinomas. J. Histochem. Cytochem., *26*:532, 1978.

Meyer, K. K., Boselli, B. D., Weaver, D. R., et al.: Cellular immune response to mastectomy and radiation. Guthrie Clin. Bull., *40*:48, 1970.

Morgan, D. A., Ruscetti, F. W., and Gallo, R. C.: Selective in vitro growth of T-lymphocytes from normal human bone marrows. Science, *193*:1007, 1976.

Morton, B. A., Ramey, W. G., Paderon, H., et al.: Monoclonal antibody–defined phenotypes of regional lymph node and peripheral blood lymphocyte subpopulations in early breast cancer. Cancer Res., *46*:2121, 1986.

Mottolese, M., Bigotti, G., Coli, A., et al.: Potential use of monoclonal antibodies in the diagnostic distinction of gynecomastia from breast carcinoma in men. Am. J. Clin. Pathol., *96*:233, 1991.

Mueller, C. B., and Amers, F.: Bilateral carcinoma of the breast: Frequency and mortality. Can. J. Surg., *21*:459, 1978.

Mule, J. J., Shu, S., Schwartz, S. L., et al.: Adoptive immunotherapy of established pulmonary metastases with LAK cells and recombinant interleukin-2. Science, *225*:1487, 1986.

Natali, P. G., Giacomini, P., Bigotti, A., et al.: Heterogeneity in the expression of HLA and tumor-associated antigens by surgically removed and cultured breast carcinoma cells. Cancer Res., *43*:660, 1983.

Nathanson, L.: Immunology and immunotherapy of human breast cancer. Cancer Immunol. Immunother., *2*:209, 1977.

Nauts, H. C.: The Beneficial Effects of Bacterial Infections on Host Resistance to Cancer. End Results in 449 Cases. A Study and Abstracts of Reports in the World Medical Literature (1775–1980) and Personal Communications. Monograph 8. 2nd ed. New York, Cancer Research Institute, 1980.

Nauts, H. C.: Breast Cancer: Immunological Factors Affecting Incidence, Prognosis and Survival. Monograph 18. New York, Cancer Research Institute, 1984.

Nicolini, A., Colombini, C., Luciani, L., et al.: Evaluation of serum CA15-3 determination with CEA and TPA in the post-operative follow-up of breast cancer patients. Br. J. Cancer, *64*:599, 1991.

O'Grady, P., Lijnen, H. R., and Duffy, M. J.: Multiple form of plasminogen activator in human breast tumors. Cancer Res., *45*:6216, 1985.

Old, L. J.: Tumor necrosis factor (TNF). Science, *230*:630, 1985.

Old, L. J., Clarke, D. A., and Benacerraf, B.: Effect of bacillus Calmette-Guerin infection on transplanted tumors in the mouse. Nature, *184*:291, 1959.

Oldham, R. K.: Biologicals and biological response modifiers: Fourth modality of cancer treatment. Cancer Treat. Rep., *68*:221, 1984.

Oldham, R. K., and Herberman, R. B.: Delayed hypersensitivity skin tests with tumor extracts. *In* Herberman, R. B., and McIntire, K. R. (Eds.): Immunodiagnosis of Cancer. New York, Marcel Dekker, 1979, p. 940.

Paavonen, T., Aronen, H., Pyrhonen, S., et al.: The effect of toremifene therapy on serum immunoglobulin levels in breast cancer. APMIS, *99*:849, 1991.

Pancino, G., Charpin, C., Osinaga, E., et al.: Characterization and distribution in human tissues of a glycoprotein antigen defined by monoclonal antibody 1BE12 raised against the human breast cancer cell line T47D. Cancer Res., *50*:7333, 1990.

Pancino, G., Osnaga, E., Carpin, C., et al.: Purification and characterization of breast cancer–associated glycoprotein not expressed in normal breast and identified by monoclonal antibody 83D4. Br. J. Cancer, *63*:390, 1991.

Pantel, K., Schlimok, G., Kutter, D., et al.: Frequent down-regulation of major histocompatibility class I antigen expression on individual micrometastatic carcinoma cells. Cancer Res., *51*:4712, 1991.

Papatestas, A., and Kark, A. E.: Peripheral lymphocyte counts in breast carcinoma. Cancer, *34*:2014, 1974.

Papatestas, A. E., Bramis, J., and Aufses, A. H.: Serum immunoglobulins in women with breast cancer. J. Surg. Oncol., *12*:155, 1979.

Papatestas, A. E., Mulvhill, M., Genkins, G., et al.: Thymus and breast cancer-plasma androgens, thymic pathology and peripheral lymphocytes in myasthenia gravis. J. Natl. Cancer Inst., *59*:1583, 1977.

Papsidero, L. D., Croghan, G. A., O'Connell, M. J., et al.: Monoclonal antibodies (F36/22 and M7/105) to human breast carcinoma. Cancer Res., *43*:1741, 1983.

Pertschuk, L. P.: Monoclonal antibodies to localized breast cancer receptors. Organ Systems Newslett. *2*:8, 1985.

Peterson, J. A., and Ceriani, R. L.: International workshop on monoclonal antibodies and breast cancer. Breast Cancer Res. Treat., *5*:207, 1985.

Reiss, C. K., Humphrey, M., Singla, O., et al.: The role of the regional lymph node and systemic reactivity. J. Surg. Oncol., *22*:249, 1983.

Retsas, S., Phillips, R. H., Hanham, I. W. F., et al.: Agranulocytosis in breast cancer patients treated with levamisole. Lancet, *2*:324, 1978.

Richters, A., and Paller, M.: The relationship between sIgM-positive lymph-node lymphocytes and breast cancer metastasis. J. Surg. Oncol., *11*:79, 1979.

Ring, D. B., Clark, R. and Saxena, A.: Identity of BCA200 and c-*erb* B₂ indicated by reactivity of monoclonal antibodies with recombinant c-*erb* B₂. Molec. Immunol., *28*:915, 1991.

Ro, J., El-Naggar, A., Ro, J. Y., et al.: *cerb* B₂ Amplification in node-negative human breast cancer. Cancer Res., *49*:6941, 1989.

Roberts, M. M., Bass, E. M., Wallack, I. W. J., et al.: Local immunoglobulin production in breast cancer. Br. J. Cancer, *27*:269, 1973.

Rochlitz, C. F., Scott, G. K., Dodson, J. M., et al.: Incidence of activating *ras* oncogene mutation associated with primary and metastatic human breast cancer. Cancer Res., *49*:357, 1989.

Rojas, A. F., Feierstein, J. N., Mickiewicz, E., et al.: Levamisole in advanced human breast cancer. Lancet, *1*:211, 1976.

Rosenberg, S. A.: Adoptive immunotherapy of cancer using lymphokine activated killer cells and recombinant IL-2. *In* DeVita, V. T. Jr., Hellman, S., and Rosenberg, S. A. (Eds.): Important Advances in Oncology, 1986. Bethesda, MD, National Cancer Institute, 1986, p. 55.

Rosenberg, S. A., and Terry, W.: Passive immunotherapy of cancer in animals and man. Adv. Cancer Res., *24*:323, 1977.

Rosenberg, S. A., Aebersold, P., Cornetta, K., et al.: Gene transfer into immunotherapy of patients with advanced melanoma, using tumor infiltrating lymphocytes modified by retroviral gene transduction. N. Engl. J. Med., *323*:570, 1990.

Rosenberg, S. A., Lotze, M. T., Mull, L. M., et al.: Observation of the systemic administration of autologous lymphokine-activated killer cells and recombinant interleukin-2 to patients with metastatic cancer. N. Engl. J. Med., *313*:1485, 1985.

Rubbert, A., Manger, B., Lang, N., et al.: Functional characterization of tumor-infiltrating lymphocytes, lymph-node lymphocytes and peripheral blood lymphocytes from patients with breast cancer. Int. J. Cancer, *49*:25, 1991.

Salomon, D. J., Clark, G. M., Wong, S. G., et al.: Human breast cancer correlation of relapse and survival with amplification of the *HER-2/neu* oncogene. Science (Wash. DC), *235*:177, 1987.

Schiller, J. H., Storer, B. E., Witt, P. L., et al.: Biological and clinical effects of intravenous tumor necrosis factor–alpha administered three times weekly. Cancer Res., *51*:1651, 1991.

Schwartzentruber, D. J., Topalian, S. L., Mancini, M. et al.: Specific release of granulocyte-macrophage colony–stimulating factor, tumor necrosis factor–alpha, and IFN-gamma by human tumor-infiltrating lymphocytes after autologous tumor stimulation. J. Immunol., *146*:3674, 1991.

Screpanti, I., Felli, M. P., Toniato, E., et al.: The enhancement of natural killer cell susceptibility of human breast cancer cells by estradiol and v-Ha-*ras* oncogene. Int. J. Cancer, *47*:445, 1991.

Seitz, R. C., Fischer, K., Stegner, H. E., et al.: Detection of metastatic breast carcinoma cells by immunofluorescent demonstration of Thomsen-Friedenreich antigen. Cancer, *54*:830, 1984.

Segev, N., Hizi, A., Kirenberg, F., et al.: Characterization of a protein released by the T47d cell line, immunologically related to the major envelope protein of mouse mammary tumor virus. Proc. Natl. Acad. Sci., *82*:1531, 1985.

Seto, M., Takahashi, T., Nakamura, S., et al.: Effector mechanism in antitumor activity of monoclonal antibodies produced against an ascitic mouse mammary tumor. Cancer Res., *46*:2056, 1986.

Shu, S., Chou, T., and Rosenberg, S. A.: In vitro sensitization and expansion with viable tumor cells and interleukin-2 in the generation of specific therapeutic effector cells. J. Immunol., *136*:3891, 1986.

Shurbaji, M. S., Pastenack, G. R., and Kuhada, F. P.: Expansion of hepatoglobulin-related protein in primary and metastatic breast cancers. A longitudinal study of 48 fetal tumors. Am. J. Clin. Pathol., *96*:238, 1991.

Soule, H. R., Linden, E., and Edgington, T. S.: Membrane 126-kilodalton phosphoglycoprotein associated with human carcinomas identified by a hybridoma antibody to mammary carcinoma cells. Proc. Nat. Acad. Sci. USA, *80*:1332, 1983.

Springer, G. F., Murthy, M. S., Desai, P. R., et al.: Breast cancer patient's cell-mediated immune response to Thomsen-Friedenreich (T) antigen. Cancer, *45*:2949, 1980.

Stacker, S. A., Thompson, C., Riglar, C., et al.: A new breast carcinoma antigen defined by a monoclonal antibody, J Natl. Cancer Inst., *75*:801, 1985.

Tandon, A. K., Clark, G. M., Chamness, G. C., et al.: Cathepsin D and prognosis in breast cancer. N. Engl. J. Med., *322*:297, 1990.

Taylor-Papademitrious, J., Peterson, J. A., Arklie, J., et al.: Monoclonal antibodies to epithelium-specific components of the human milk fat globule membrane: Production and reaction with cells in culture. Int. J. Cancer, *28*:7, 1981.

Thomas, L.: Discussion: Reactions to homologous tissue antigens. *In* Lawrence, H. S. (Ed.): Cellular and Humoral Aspects of the Hypersensitivity States. New York, Hoeber-Harper, 1959, p. 529.

Tomana, M., Kajados, A. H., Niedermeier, W., et al.: Antibodies to mouse mammary tumor virus–related antigen in sera of patients with breast carcinoma. Cancer, *47*:2696, 1981.

Torrence, P. F. (Ed.): Biological Response Modifiers: New Approaches to Disease Intervention. Orlando, FL, Academic Press, 1986.

Urban, J. A.: Breast cancer 1985: What have we learned? Cancer, *57*:636, 1986.

West, W. H.: Continuous infusion of recombinant interleukin-2 (rIL-2) in adoptive cellular therapy of renal carcinoma and other malignancies. Cancer Treat. Rev., *16*:83, 1989.

White, C. A., Dulbecco, R., Allen, R., et al.: Two monoclonal antibodies selective for human mammary carcinoma. Cancer Res., *45*:1337, 1985.

Whitford, P., Mallon, E. A., George, W. D., et al.: Flow cytometric analysis of tumor infiltrating lymphocytes in breast cancer. Br. J. Cancer, *62*:971, 1990.

Whiteside, T. L., Miescher, S., Hurlimann, L., et al.: Clonal analysis and in situ characterization (Abstract). Fed. Proc., *45*:849, 1986.

Whittiker, M. G., and Clark, C. G.: Depressed lymphocyte function in carcinoma of the breast. Br. J. Surg., *58*:717, 1971.

Wilkinson, M. J., Homell, A., Harris, M., et al.: The prognostic significance of two epithelial membrane antigens expressed by human mammary carcinomas. Int. J. Cancer, *33*:299, 1984.

Yemada, K. A., Kenemans, P., Wobbes, T., et al.: Carcinoma associated mucin serum markers CA M26 and CA M29: Efficacy in detecting and monitoring patients with cancer of the breast, colon, ovary, endometrium and cervix. Int. J. Cancer, *47*:170, 1991.

Yu, Y. H., Cooper, C. K., Ramakrishnan, S., et al.: Use of immunotoxin in combination to inhibit clonogenic of human breast carcinoma cells. Cancer Res., *50*:3231, 1990.

Zara, D. T., Dollbaum, C. M., Farsi, N., et al.: Cathepsin D in human breast cancer. Proc. Am. Assoc. Cancer Res., *32*:165, 1991.

24 Screening and Follow-Up

John S. Spratt
William L. Donegan

"Screening" is the routine examination of asymptomatic populations for disease. The principal purpose of screening for breast cancer is to reduce mortality from the disease through early diagnosis and treatment. The high incidence of breast cancer in the female population, mortality rates that remain undiminished, and the knowledge that small asymptomatic breast cancers are very curable all provide the rationale for screening. Treatment might also be associated with less morbidity if cancers were detected earlier.

The rationale for screening patients after treatment, otherwise known as follow-up, is similar. Recurrence is a frequent sequela to treatment; and, if it is discovered early morbidity and mortality might be reduced by re-treatment. Additional objectives of follow-up include management of treatment-related complications, evaluation of alternative treatments, and early diagnosis of new primary lesions in the opposite breast. Psychosocial support for the patient is also among the benefits of follow-up.

Either type of screening is simpler in concept than in application. The presumption is that the morbidity and mortality associated with the disease can be altered favorably by earlier treatment and that the morbidity and mortality of the techniques used for earlier detection and treatment do not reduce survival or increase morbidity. The issues that must be addressed include who should be screened, with what, and how often, and, considering the effort and expense involved, to what extent are the objectives attained?

Mammography provides a means of detecting breast cancer while it is clinically occult and is integral to most screening efforts. Breast self-examination (BSE) and clinical breast examination (CBE) play complementary roles (Hurley and Kaldor, 1992). Screening would be uncontroversial were it not for several real and potential liabilities: expense, discomfort, unnecessary additional procedures prompted by false positive results, overtreatment of some abnormalities, possible radiation-induced cancers, and, in some cases, false reassurance. While controlled trials demonstrate that screening for breast cancer can save lives, the balance between benefits and liabilities continues to receive critical attention. Among the questions that remain unresolved are these: (1) How effective is the combination of mammography and physical examination in reducing mortality in women 40 to 49 years old? (2) What is the contribution of mammography to the reduction in mortality for women aged 50 to 59 years? (Bailar, 1976; Shapiro, 1977) (3) Can better assessment of risk factors for the selection of populations to be screened increase screening efficacy? (4) What is the natural history of "minimal breast cancer" identified by mammography alone? Such knowledge is important for measuring the value of its discovery and planning how frequently to rescreen. (5) What is the cost-benefit ratio? This information is essential for setting public policy on health expenditures, particularly government subsidized ones (Eddy, 1989). For example, the Kentucky General Assembly in 1989 mandated a health benefit requiring third-party carriers to fund one screening mammogram for every woman between the ages 35 and 39 years, a mammogram every 2 years between the ages 40 and 59 years, and an annual mammogram after age 50 years. When the experience and costs for the year 1991 were reviewed, it was found that 65% of all mammograms were done on women younger than 50 years. Mammograms were actually performed on children as young as 8 years. Eight cancers were diagnosed in women under age 50, but seven had physical findings at the time the mammograms were performed. Numerous states mandate mammography as a health benefit. The value of all legislatively mandated health benefits should be monitored for value and cost (Spratt and Pope, 1992).

Cadman and associates (1984) summarized the conditions that must be met to justify a screening program. The effectiveness of the program must be confirmed by a randomized trial. Efficacious treatment for the disease must exist. The mortality and morbidity produced by the disease must warrant screening. An effective and acceptable screening test must exist. The screening program must reach those in need of screening. The health care system must have the professionals and resources that the program requires. Persons with positive findings on screening must comply with advice and accept effective treatment. All the conditions listed are applicable to screening for breast cancer.

Table 24–1 contains terms intrinsic to various concepts as they affect the design, description, and evaluation of screening. On the first screen of a population prevalent disease that has accumulated over time is discovered. Repeated annually, screening discovers the disease that has accumulated during the preceding year. When cases discovered by annual screening are added to cases that appear in the interval between screens (interval cancers), the annual incidence rate (cases per 1000 screened) for the screened population may be determined. The duration of disease before discovery by screening can be estimated by dividing the prevalence rate at first screen by the annual incidence rate when the annual incidence rate is constant. The interval cancer rate can be calculated as the number of interval cancers divided by the sum of these interval cancers and screening-detected cancers; that figure is then multiplied by 100. The proportional incidence of interval cancers, that is, the per cent of symptomatic cancers that screening failed to

Table 24–1. GLOSSARY OF TERMS ESSENTIAL FOR EPIDEMIOLOGIC DESCRIPTION OF ANY SCREENING PROGRAM

True positive = Those testing positive who *do have* the disease.
False positive = Those testing positive who *do not have* the disease.
False negative = Those testing negative who *do have* the disease.
True negative = Those testing negative who *do not have* the disease.

$$\text{Sensitivity} = \frac{\text{True positives}}{\text{True positives and false negatives}} = \frac{\text{True positives}}{\text{All of those with the disease}}$$

$$\text{Specificity} = \frac{\text{True negatives}}{\text{True negatives and false positives}} = \frac{\text{True negatives}}{\text{All of those without the disease}}$$

Terminal = The disease is no longer curable, either before detection or after. Terminal state may be reached before a cancer is clinically detectable.

Lethal = Time of host death.

Failures = Undetectable disease that has already reached a terminal point.

e = Effectiveness.

$$e = \frac{\text{failures (no screen)} - \text{failures (screen)}}{\text{failures (no screen)}}$$

Time of onset = Requires concise definition for the disease in question.

Onset of symptoms = Requires concise definition of symptoms in question.

Threshold of measurement = That minimum size or level below which the method of measurement has a sensitivity which approaches zero (i.e., unable to detect).

Variability in interpretation:

(1) Interindividual: representing inconsistency of interpretation among different readers of x-ray films or other clinical and laboratory measurements.

(2) Intraindividual: reflecting the failure of a reader to be consistent with himself or herself in independent interpretations of the same set of films or other clinical or laboratory evaluations.

$$\text{Incidence rate per 1000} = \frac{\text{Number of new cases of a disease occurring in a population during a specific period (as annual)}}{\text{Number of persons exposed to risk of developing the disease during that period}} \times 1000$$

$$\text{Prevalence rate per 1000} = \frac{\text{Number of cases of disease present in the population at a specified time}}{\text{Number of persons in the population at that specified time}} \times 1000$$

Prevalence rate = incidence rate × duration of the disease in a stable population

  or

$$\text{Incidence rate} = \frac{\text{Prevalence rate}}{\text{Duration of the disease}}$$

Cancer control window = Time in the life history of a cancer elapsing between the threshold of measurement and the time a cancer becomes terminal.

Lead time bias = The bias introduced into the evaluation of the end results of cancer treatment in which the improved end results are incorrectly attributed to earlier diagnosis. If the earlier diagnosis is made *after* the cancer has become *terminal* but earlier in the terminal period, the patient lives longer from the time of treatment but *not* from the terminal point. The lead time bias is the time interval at which discovery is made earlier in the life history of the cancer but after the terminal point.

Length bias = The bias introduced into the interpretation of screening programs when the fact is not recognized that slower growing, often more biologically favorable cancers are present for great *lengths* of time thereby enhancing the possibility that slower growing more indolent cancers are the ones discovered by periodic screening. Once again, end results from treatment will look better as cancers discovered by screening are more biologically favorable in the first place.

Interval surfacing cancers = These are cancers that become evident by any means of discovery and are confirmed by histologic examination within a specified time interval after an examination from which no recommendation for biopsy resulted but before the next scheduled rescreen at the end of a constant time, as annual.

prevent, is determined using the following formula: interval cancer rate × 100/control group incidence. The sensitivity of screening is therefore equal to 100 minus the proportional incidence of interval cancers (Roberts et al., 1990).

MODELS OF SCREENING

Planning a screening strategy for the discovery of asymptomatic cancer is facilitated by a model of the screening problem and a model of breast cancer itself. The complex behavior of breast cancer is modeled in Table 24–2 according to Spratt and Spratt (1985) as adapted from Walter and Day (1983) and the complicated nature of the screening problem in Figure 24–1. Conflicting conclusions are frequently drawn about the value of different approaches toward screening for new or recurrent cancers. To construct a model of breast cancer screening and to test its solutions, data of consistent quality and sufficient amount are needed. The conclusions drawn from models vary with the definition of the optimal endpoints. What is *optimal* is often determined by concensus rather than by any scientific mode (Spratt, 1991).

A major consideration of any model is the minimum size of detectable cancers. The threshold size is determined by the Weber-Fechner law (Spratt, 1969), which states that an organism's response to a stimulus is proportional to the logarithm of the magnitude of the stimulus. Paraphrased for cancer, the ability of the examiner or examining method to detect a cancer is such that the distribution of the sizes of cancers at diagnosis would be lognormal. Size at diagnosis is, therefore, stochastic and not deterministic. The frequency distribution of the sizes of newly detected cancers is, in fact, lognormal, as predicted by the Weber-Fechner law. This is a major factor in the wide variation in size at discovery, so there is always the risk that a portion of

cancers will have exceeded the size at which the cancer metastasizes. Growth rate may affect size at discovery but not the threshold of discoverable size. Basically, a large cancer with a short history probably has a more rapid growth rate than a small cancer with a long history. This phenomenon is the cause of length bias in screening. Acute or rapidly progressing cancers have many characteristics that are different from those of slower-growing cancers discovered by screening (Spratt et al., 1983).

Eddy (1978) synthesized screening programs for breast cancer into a simulation model. With his model, many runs could be made on the computer to predict the characteristics of a screening program with different data. Eddy's model has the capacity for coping with the various financial costs, intangible costs, and discount rates on the input side and the total expected value on the output side (Table 24–3). Using recent data on screening from controlled clinical trials Eddy (1989) concluded that screening annually for 10 years with physical examination alone might decrease the probability of death from breast cancer by 25 per 10,000 women. The average increase in life expectancy would be 20 days. The addition of annual mammography might decrease the probability of dying from breast cancer by an additional 25 per 10,000 women and would increase the life expectancy an additional 20 days. When discounted at 5% the numbers are lower, ranging from 2 to 10 days only. Eddy observed that the average benefit from controlled clinical trials was slightly less than these predictions. During 10 years of screening 2500 false positive diagnoses could be expected per 10,000 women. With a program that targeted only 25% of American women between ages 40 and 75, the number of deaths from breast cancer might be reduced by 4000 per year by the year 2000, at a net *annual cost* of $1.3 billion. The evidence to support screening for women under age 50 was inconsistent. Assuming that 175,000 women per year are diagnosed as having breast

Table 24–2. MODEL OF BREAST CANCER PROGRESSION

Asymptomatic Disease Below Threshold Size for Detection—Local, Local-Regional, Distant Normal	Asymptomatic Disease Above Threshold Size for Detection	Symptomatic	Endpoints	
T_v Biologic onset	T_w Disease now detectable if screen done Screening takes place, can be true positive or also negative	T_x Disease becomes symptomatic Patient comes for diagnosis of symptomatic disease	T_y Death without treatment	T_z Death with treatment
$T_a = T_w - T_v$: $T_b = T_x - T_w$: $T_c = T_a + T_b$: $T_y - T_v$: $T_z - T_v$:	Undetectable sojourn Detectable asymptomatic sojourn (same as maximum lead time) Delay time Natural sojourn of undiagnosed, untreated disease Natural sojourn of diagnosed disease, treated without treatment mortality		T_v: Onset T_w: Detectable but asymptomatic T_x: Symptomatic T_z: Time of death with treatment T_y, T_z: Determined by lifelong follow-up to avoid truncation of results	
Cancer Control Window (CCW): Time that cancer disseminates and is no longer local-regional less T_w. The CCW can be negative if dissemination occurs before T_w.				

(From Spratt, J. S., and Spratt, J. A.: What is breast cancer doing before we can detect it? J. Surg. Oncol., *30*:156, 1985. Reprinted with permission.)

The sojourn times in various intervals are dependent on cancer growth rates, biologic properties of cancers, and the sensitivity and specificity of diagnostic methods.

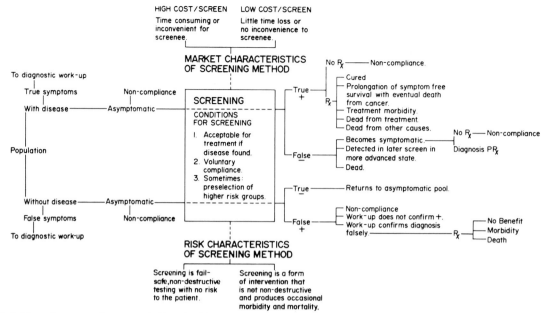

Figure 24–1. Flow diagram of representative decisions and outcomes in any screening program. Quality control at many points is essential to the reduction of errors. The existence of effective treatment determines the ultimate benefit of screening. A controlled clinical trial is generally essential to test hypotheses on the benefit of screening. (From Spratt, J. S.: Epidemiology of screening for cancer. Curr. Probl. Cancer, 6:1–58, 1982. Reprinted with permission.)

cancer and that 48% (84,000) die of the cancers, he concluded that deaths from breast cancer annually would be reduced by 7%; 93% of deaths would remain unaffected. Clearly, this reflects a limited impact on breast cancer mortality.

Although several workable mathematical models now exist to assist in the selection of optimal screening strategies, the quality of the models often exceeds the quality of available data. Any screening model ultimately must be extended to complete cancer management strategies, permitting the sequential selection of decisions that give optimal benefit to large numbers of people. Screening has value only if functional longevity is enhanced. The general hypothesis to be tested by any model might be stated as follows: A population screened and managed by a particular strategy has greater functional longevity than an unscreened population or a population screened and managed by a different strategy. Evaluation of a screening program in isolation from the total clinical management process is impossible. Furthermore, on studying the flow diagram in Figure 24–1, the benefit of an acceptable screening program could vary from laboratory to laboratory, radiology department to radiology department, and clinic to clinic, depending on the ability of the local system to minimize false negative and false positive results, comparability of treatment, and other deviations. Studies from one program could not be accepted as equivalent for another program unless the entire screening, quality control, and management strategy of the first system were mirrored by the second. An optimal strategy gives the highest probability of providing the maximum number of functional person-days with the least amount of nonfunctional time and at a tolerable cost (Spratt 1975a, 1975b). In any cancer screening and management system some end point must be defined whose

value is to be maximized or minimized. Wagner (1974) emphasized that most decision makers cannot make consistent judgments about the relative desirability of different strategies. The impact of actions on outcome can take unexpected turns, and data rather than intuition are necessary for design and evaluation.

CANCER CONTROL WINDOW

The ability to discover cancer while it is still localized is addressed by the cancer control window (CCW) concept. The CCW is that segment in the natural history of a cancer between the moment the cancer is large enough to be detected and the moment it disseminates (i.e., is no longer curable; Fig. 24–2). The CCW cannot exceed the time required for a cancer to double its volume (DT_{act}) 14-fold—and probably cannot exceed the time required to double its volume 9-fold (Spratt, 1981). Those cancers that disseminate before they attain a threshold size that permits detection have a negative CCW and are never discoverable in a curable state. The variable lengths of positive CCWs are shown in Tables 24–4 and 24–5. Those cancers below the line in Table 24–4 could all traverse the CCW in periods of less than a year and so might escape an annual screening effort. There is strong evidence that many breast cancers have a (DT_{act}) of less than 20 days in their predetectable phase; all of these would become evident in less than 1 year, leading to probable self-detection. The studies by Osborne and coworkers (1991), which report the prevalence of breast cancer cells in the bone marrow associated with early-stage breast cancers, provide an example of cancers with negative cancer control windows. Aron and Prorok

Table 24–3. SIMULATION MODEL FOR SCREENING PROGRAMS FOR BREAST CANCER

Data that must be put into the simulation model (input)
  Patient age
  Relative risk category
  Age-specific incidence rates
  Age-specific mortality rates
  Complication rates of diagnostic and therapeutic
    procedures (e.g., the operative mortality rates of a breast
    biopsy done under general anesthesia)
  The effectiveness of mammography
  The effectiveness of patient behavior
  The effectiveness of therapy
  Radiation effect
  Previous history of physical examinations of the breast
  Schedule for future physical examinations of the breast
  Schedule for future mammographic examinations
Data that can be derived from the simulation model (output)
  The probability that the patient will be diagnosed as having
    breast cancer in any given year in the future
  The probability that the patient will be a surviving breast
    cancer patient during any year in the future
  The probability that the patient will die of breast cancer in
    any year
  The probability that the patient will die of other cancers in
    any year
  Five, 10, 15 year survival and patient life expectancy
  The probability that the patient will have a malignant lesion
    detected by a physical examination, a mammogram, or
    the patient herself in any given interval of time in the
    future
  The survival rates of patients according to method of
    detection
  The probability that the patient will have a biopsy in any
    year
  A comparison of the mortality rate of a lesion detected at
    a screening session, with the mortality rate of that lesion if
    the patient postponed the screening appointment or
    waited until the lesion became apparent on self-
    examination

(From Eddy, D. M.: Screening for Breast Cancer: Theory, Analysis, and Design. © 1980, pp. 172, 173. Reprinted with permission of Prentice-Hall, Inc., Englewood Cliffs, NJ.)

(1986) concluded that some but not all breast cancer cases detected early through screening have a reduced mortality rate. The authors concluded that future research should relate reductions in breast cancer mortality to mathematical models of disease progression and screening.

LENGTH BIAS AND LEAD TIME

Whenever a disease is discovered by periodic screening, and the preclinical sojourn of that disease is of variable

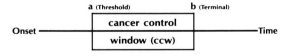

c = number of net doublings between a and b

d = $DT_{(act)}$ between a and b

c.c.w. = c × d

c.c.w. is negative when b < a

Figure 24–2. Diagram of the cancer control window.

Table 24–4. DURATION OF THE CANCER CONTROL WINDOW IN DAYS*

$DT_{(act)}$ (d)	Number of Doublings of the Volume of a Cancer						
	2	4	6	8	10	12	14
1000	2000	4000	6000	8000	10000	12000	14000
500	1000	2000	3000	4000	5000	6000	7000
100	200	400	600	800	1000	1200	1400
50	100	200	300	400	500	600	700
20	40	80	120	160	200	240	280†
10	20	40	60	80	100	120	140
5	10	20	30	40	50	60	70

(From Spratt, J. S.: The relationship between the rates of growth of cancer and the intervals between screening examinations necessary for effective discovery. Cancer Detect. Prevent., *4*:301, 1981. Reprinted with permission.)
*Duration of cancer control window (CCW) = DT_{act} times number of net doublings of cells occurring between threshold size and terminal size.
†CCWs below this line all have durations of less than 1 year.

duration, the cases of longest sojourn stand a greater probability of being discovered by screening. This introduces *length bias* into the screening process, ensuring that less aggressive, and presumably more favorable, cancers will be the ones discovered by screening. A circumscribed cancer margin and papillary intraductal growth are associated with more slowly growing cancers, a feature that permits them more frequently to be discovered by annual mammography (length bias). The cancers discovered by screening also have a longer lead time (the length of time before they would otherwise have been discovered) and hence appear to have a more favorable prognosis than cancers not discovered by screening. In uncontrolled screening projects these biases appear to favor screening, and population-based controlled clinical trials are necessary to avoid them.

An estimation of lead time may be obtained by multiplying the number of doublings required for cancer to grow from a lesion detectable by mammography to one detectable by BSE by the DT_{act}. In the Louisville Breast Cancer Detection Demonstration Project (BCDDP), no breast cancer smaller than 2.1 mm was diagnosed on mammograms, even on retrospective review. A study on the value of BSE by Foster and coworkers (1978) showed the mean maximum tumor diameter discovered by monthly BSE to be 20.4 mm. Some nine or 10 doublings of the tumor volume

Table 24–5. VARIABLES DETERMINING THE DURATION OF THE CANCER CONTROL WINDOW (CCW)

a = Threshold of detectable size
b = Terminal size (size at which cancer has disseminated and is no longer local-regional)
c = Number of net doublings of the cancer cells present at threshold size (a) that must occur to produce a cancer of terminal size (b)
d = Net tumor volume doubling time
CCW = Cancer control window duration
CCW = c × d

When b < a, the cancer control window has a negative value and the detection of local-regional cancer is not possible.

would be required for a cancer to grow from 2.1 mm to 20.4 mm in diameter. Using the DT_{act} for grossly measurable breast cancers, which varies from 944 to 109 days, the lead time bias for these cases could vary from 8496 days (9 × 944) to 981 days (9 × 109) (median 2943 days [9 × 327]). These estimates would be shorter or longer, depending on growth rates. For interval cancers, lead time would be shorter and length bias negligible. Unfortunately, fast-growing breast cancers probably are not the ones detected by mammographic screening; instead, they are self-detected in the intervals between annual mammography.

Moskowitz and Fox's data (1979) were useful for estimating the lead time gained by vigorous mammographic screening. Before age 50 years the lead time was estimated to be 2.2 years (± 0.4), and after age 50 years it was 3.2 years (± 0.4). In the Louisville BCDDP prevalence rate at the first screen divided by the incidence rate in subsequent years of screening gave a lead time estimated at 1.8 to 6.9 years, but this varied with age (Heuser et al., 1979a; Spratt et al., 1986).

Groups At High Risk

Screening is more efficient when it is targeted at persons at high risk for breast cancer. Thus, identification of those at high risk is important in the design of screening strategies. Risk may be defined as a probability, rate, or ratio at which an adverse event occurs (Spratt et al., 1989). Of all risk factors for breast cancer, age is the most significant. Once pediatric cancers are set aside, the vast majority of cancers increase in incidence with age.

Breast cancer can strike any woman at any age and any man about 1% as frequently. Breast cancer even occurs in children, though infrequently (McDivitt et al., 1966). Collectively, fewer than 2% of all breast cancers are diagnosed before age 30 years (Noyes et al., 1982). The infrequency of cancer in younger women, and the density of their breasts, make screening less effective in the younger age group. Moreover, when mammography is used to screen the breasts of younger women, the theoretical risk of radiation exposure is greater.

About 25% of breast cancers occur in women aged 30 to 50 years, and the remainder develop after age 50. Although some risk factors for breast cancer are known, the fact remains that more than two thirds of all breast cancers occur in women who have no recognized risk factors (Seidman et al., 1982). In summarizing the significance of risk factor data, Berg (1984) pointed out that no adult American woman is at such a low risk as to merit exclusion from an effective breast cancer control program. Even among Native American women in New Mexico, who have the lowest incidence of breast cancer in the United States, the risk before age 75 years is 1 in 40 (2.5%). At the time of Berg's assessment, American women in general had 1 chance in 12 (8.2% cumulative prevalence) of developing breast cancer before age 75 years. Among women with no recognized risk factors, this dropped to only 5.9% (1 in 17). The rate of 1:40 far exceeds those for other common cancers, except the risk of lung cancer for heavy smokers. By targeting women who have risk factors for screening one may create

unnecessary anxiety in women at risk and a false sense of security in those who are not.

TRIALS OF SCREENING

Studies of population screening are of three general types: (1) randomized trials, (2) screening projects, and (3) case-control studies. In *randomized trials*, women are assigned randomly to be screened or to a control group in which they usually follow their customary health practices. Prospective randomized trials avoid lead time and length bias. In *screening projects*, the results obtained in a screened population are compared with the findings in the general population or a selected segment of that population. In *case-control studies* the prevalence of screening in women who die of breast cancer is compared with the prevalence of screening in age-matched women who die of other causes. The relative risks of dying from breast cancer after screening or no screening are then determined.

These interventions demonstrate that women are receptive to screening, that cancers are detected at earlier stages by screening, and that, when mammography is included, mortality from breast cancer can be reduced as much as 30% in a screened population. Improvement in prognosis is also enduring—still demonstrable at least 18 years later. Screening trials also demonstrate that some cancers grow so fast that they become symptomatic in the interval between annual examinations, and the problem increases with longer intervals between examinations. Younger women are predisposed to these faster-growing "interval" cancers, but whether more frequent examinations will serve them better is unclear. The most appropriate interval for examinations remains in doubt, as does whether they should be age-specific. The relative contributions of mammography and physical examination to detection are unresolved, though it is clear that each makes an independent contribution. An improvement in survival for women younger than 50 years through screening is inconclusive: Some seems evident, but it is less than that for older women, is expressed later, and to date has not been demonstrated consistently (Fig. 24–3). Experience is also scant with screening of elderly women, who are not included in many projects and who do not respond as readily to invitations. No more than 3% of breast cancers in women 70 years or older seen at cancer centers in the United States are detected by screening (Singletary et al., 1993).

Health Insurance Plan of Greater New York Trial

The first randomized trial of screening, and the only one performed to date in the United States, was the Health Insurance Plan of Greater New York (HIP) trial (Shapiro, 1989). In 1963, 62,000 women aged 40 to 64 years and enrolled in a health insurance program were randomized to screening or to routine care, the latter serving as the control group. Screening consisted of a two-view mammogram and a physical examination. Members of the study group were offered an initial examination and three additional exami-

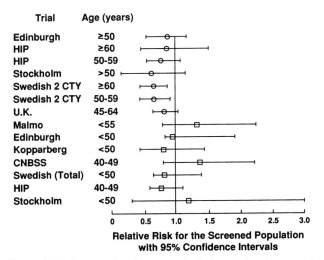

Trial	Age (years)
Edinburgh	≥50
HIP	≥60
HIP	50-59
Stockholm	>50
Swedish 2 CTY	≥60
Swedish 2 CTY	50-59
U.K.	45-64
Malmo	<55
Edinburgh	<50
Kopparberg	<50
CNBSS	40-49
Swedish (Total)	<50
HIP	40-49
Stockholm	<50

**Relative Risk for the Screened Population
with 95% Confidence Intervals**

Figure 24–3. The relative risk of mortality from breast cancer is shown for screened women in randomized trials by age group. A relative risk of less than 1.0 indicates benefit, but a 95% confidence interval that includes 1.0 means it may not be significant. Reduced risk is more consistent and reliable for women older than 50 years of age. (Data from Hurley and Kaldor, 1992; Tabar et al., 1993; Nystron et al., 1993.)

nations at yearly intervals. About 67% responded and had an initial examination. The number attending subsequent examinations gradually decreased, but 59% of the responders attended all four examinations. Follow-up has continued 18 years. The incidence of axillary node involvement in the screened group was lower (46%) than in the controls (57%), despite the fact that 32% of cancers were diagnosed in the intervals between screening examinations. In this early study, 33% of cancers were found solely by mammography and 44% only by physical examination, illustrating the contribution of both to detection (Strax et al., 1973). Within 7 years after entry, 425 cases of breast cancer were diagnosed in the study group and 443 cases in the control group, from which 165 and 212 deaths resulted, respectively. At 10 years, mortality in the study group from breast cancer diagnosed within 5 to 7 years of the start of the study was reduced by 30% compared with controls, and at 18 years the decrease was 23 to 24%. The reduction was statistically significant overall and for women aged 50 and older (Fig. 24–4). Reviews by Habbema and coworkers (1986) and by Chu and colleagues (1988) indicated reduced mortality for women 40 to 49 years of age at entry as well as for those aged 50 to 64 years, but improvement in the younger women became evident later (after they had reached age fifty), and was not as great as for the women over fifty. Improved survival for the younger group with cancers did not become statistically significant until 9 years after entry, whereas it was evident within 4 years in the older group.

The Breast Cancer Detection Demonstration Project

The encouraging results of the HIP study led in 1973 to a national screening project, the Breast Cancer Detection

Demonstration Project (BCDDP) sponsored by the American Cancer Society and the National Cancer Institute. The purpose was to demonstrate that widespread screening for breast cancer was feasible. Women 35 to 74 years of age were offered five annual screenings with physical examination, two-view mammography, and thermography, and 280,222 women were screened at 29 centers. In 1975, thermography was discontinued and mammography was limited to women aged 50 and older, unless they were at high risk, because of doubt about its efficacy in younger women and concern about carcinogenic risk. The population that responded was largely well-educated white women with a family history of breast cancer, and more than half were younger than 50 years of age. A total of 39,019 breast biopsies were recommended as a result of the examinations and 29,390 were performed to diagnose 4275 breast cancers, a ratio of almost seven biopsies per cancer found (Smart et al., 1993). Improvement in mammography was evident in the fact that 42% of cancers were detected by mammography alone (compared with 33% in the HIP study). It detected 89% of all cancers found in women aged 40 to 49 years and 95% in those aged 60 to 69 years. Noninvasive and small invasive cancers (< 1 cm in diameter) constituted 33% of all cancers found, and the frequency of interval cancers (25%) was less than the 32% in the HIP study. On pathologic review, some errors were found: 31 of the lesions diagnosed as cancer were considered benign, and 147 women with cancer were found to have lymph node involvement that had not previously been appreciated.

The fact that the BCDDP involved no control group has continued to complicate evaluation. Comparison of the results with data relating to breast cancer mortality in the national Surveillance Epidemiology and End Results registry, assuming a 1-year lead time in the screened population, suggested a 20% reduction in deaths from breast cancer at a point 9 years after the project began (Morrison et al., 1988). In an analysis at 14 years, the similarity of death rates and relative survival rates for screenees aged 40 to 49, 50 to 59, and 60 to 69 years suggested that screening benefited women in all three groups (Smart et al., 1993).

During the first 4 years of the BCDDP at Louisville, 115 cancers were found among 10,128 women. Serial measurements were possible by xeromammography in 32 cases. Twenty-three of these tumors exhibited doubling times that ranged from 109 to 944 days. The log mean of the actual doubling times was 327 days. The predominant geometric shape of small primary breast cancers observed on mammography was spheroidal with a long axis following the direction of the ducts. The frequency distribution of the doubling times of the spheroids was lognormal, confirming a highly skewed distribution of growth rates (Heuser et al., 1979a,b). Forty-three percent of these cases (49 of 115) were cancers diagnosed in the intervals between annual mammograms. Of these, 7.8% (9 of 115), or 28% of the cases observed by two or more mammograms (9 of 32), consisted of cancers that grew too slowly to permit measurement of growth over periods of 1 to 4 years. The annual prevalence of cancers increased from 0.064% to 0.239% over the first 3 years of the project and dropped to 0.144% in the fourth year, when women younger than 50 years

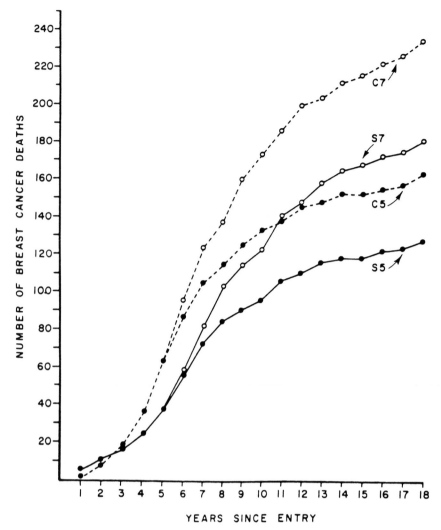

Figure 24-4. Cumulative deaths from breast cancer over the course of 18 years in the HIP study of screening women with cancers diagnosed within 5 to 7 years of entry had a significant benefit from screening with physical examination and mammography. (S, screened group; C, control group; 5, cancers diagnosed within 5 years; 7, cancers diagnosed within 7 years.) (From Shapiro, S.: Determining the efficacy of breast cancer screening. Cancer, *63*:1873–1880, 1989.)

were excluded from mammographic screening. The conclusions of the Louisville study were that a very large percentage of all breast cancers exhibited exceedingly rapid growth and that annual screening was primarily subdividing breast cancers into three subsets determined by growth rates (i.e., rapidly growing interval cancers, indolent prevalent cancers, and nongrowing cancers) (Heuser et al., 1979*a,b*). The faster-growing cancers were more likely to metastasize.

Numerous studies of screening followed the HIP trial and BCDDP project in other parts of the world. These have employed various intervals, age groups, and methods. Seven additional prospective randomized controlled trials have utilized mammography (Hurley et al., 1992).

Swedish Two-Counties Study

A trial begun in 1977 involved communities in the counties of Kopparberg and Ostergotland, in Sweden. Women 40 years of age and older were cluster randomized for a single-view mammogram or their usual care. Screening examinations were conducted at 2-year intervals for those aged 40 to 49 and at 33-month intervals for those aged 50 to 74. Study and control groups numbered 78,085 and 56,782, respectively. About 13% of controls had mammography as part of their usual care. Interval cancers increased during the early years of the trial, reaching 45% of the value in controls by the third interval in women over 50 years of age and 68% in younger women, despite the shorter interval of screening (Tabar et al., 1987). The high frequency of interval cancers, particularly in young women, suggested that annual screening would be more appropriate for the 40- to 49-year-old group, and every 2 years for older women. A 31% reduction in mortality from breast cancer was found among women 40 to 74 years old after 8 years of follow-up. Although no significant reduction in mortality was found specifically for women 40 to 49 years old, no difference in effect was apparent between age groups. Reduction in mortality for the 40- to 49-year-old group in the Kopparberg part of the trial was 26%. Results with single-view and two-view mammograms were similar (Tabar et al., 1993).

Malmö Trial

Begun in 1976, this trial individually randomized 42,284 women 45 to 69 years old to a two-view mammogram every 18 to 24 months for five rounds or to usual care (which for 24% of the control group involved at least one mammogram). Seventeen per cent of cancers were interval cancers. Initially more women in the study group died of breast cancer, but after 7 years the reverse was true. A nonsignificant 4% reduction in breast cancer mortality in favor of screening was found after a mean period of 8.8 years. For women 55 years or older the reduction was far greater, that is, 20% (Andersson et al., 1988). The relative risk of death from breast cancer in the study group was reduced to 0.9 at 11 years.

Stockholm Trial

In this study, which began in 1981, women 40 to 64 years old were randomized individually to have a single-view mammogram on two occasions 28 months apart or to have no screening. The screened group numbered 40,318 and the controls 20,000. After 5 years the controls were also invited for screening. After 7 years of follow-up a nonsignificant 29% reduction in mortality was observed in the screened group.

Gothenborg Trial and Combined Swedish Studies

The Gothenborg study dates from 1982 and involved individual randomization of 52,000 women 40 to 59 years of age to screening with two-view mammograms at 18-month intervals. It was included in an overview of the five trials conducted in Sweden since 1976, and the relative risk (RR) of death from breast cancer in the screened population, compared with that of the control group, was 0.84 (Nystrom et al., 1993, Chamberlain, 1993).

The overview of Swedish trials involved 2.5 million woman-years of follow-up of women 40 to 74 years of age. In the combined studies, a highly significant risk reduction of 24% was found for women invited for screening. (RR of death from breast cancer 0.76 with 95% confidence intervals of 0.66 to 0.87.) For women aged 50 to 69 years the reduction was 29%, but for those 40 to 49 years old it was 13% and not significant. The reduction in mortality appeared earlier (at 4 to 5 years) in the older women than in those younger than 50, in whom it did not become evident until 8 years after screening began.

Edinburgh Trial

In this trial 84 general practices in Edinburgh were randomized to offer or not to offer women 45 to 64 years old seven screening examinations. Screening consisted of a yearly physical examination and a biennial mammogram. Participants were recruited from 1979 to 1981, and 61% of the study population reported for an initial examination. A disproportionate number of the 23,226 women screened were socioeconomically advantaged, as compared with the 21,904 controls. Ninety-six per cent of 88 prevalent cancers were detected with mammography and 74% with physical examination. Only 3% were detected solely by physical examination. In years when both examinations were performed, they detected 90% of incident cancers. Seven years after the trial began a 17% reduction in breast cancer mortality was found in the screened population, but this reduction was not statistically significant (Roberts et al., 1990).

Anderson and colleagues (1986) reviewed the histologic characteristics of 210 cancers discovered in the Edinburgh screening project and confirmed that prevalent cancers have more favorable pathologic characteristics than cancers discovered by incidence screening, as predicted by the epidemiologic theory of screening.

United Kingdom Trial

The United Kingdom Trial included the Edinburgh trial as part of a larger effort in which breast cancer mortality was compared between health districts that offered (1) screening with annual physical examination and biennial mammography, (2) training in BSE, or (3) neither (UK Trial, 1988). After 7 years and some adjustments for different inherent breast cancer mortality rates, an overall comparison of districts detected a 20% reduction in breast cancer mortality associated with screening, which was not a significant difference. The difference was observed only after the first 5 years of the trial, and no reduction was detected for women offered only instruction in BSE.

Canadian National Breast Screening Study (NBSS)

A trial designed specifically to test the value of screening women 40 to 49 years of age was conducted at 15 urban centers in Canada between 1980 and 1985. The 50,430 women in this age group were individually randomized to have annual physical examination and two-view mammography or to have only an initial physical examination (Miller et al., 1992a). All were taught BSE. Unexpectedly, at the initial examination more node-positive cancers were found in the screened group than in the control group. Seven years after initiation of the study 38 breast cancer deaths had occurred in the screened group and 28 in the control group. As in the early results of the Malmö trial, the proportion of deaths in the screened population, as compared to the controls (1.36), reflected a higher risk associated with screening. Survival rates were similar in the two groups. So far this study fails to show a benefit from screening women younger than 50 years of age, but it has been criticized on several points, including randomization and quality control of mammograms (Moskowitz, 1992; Mettlin et al., 1993).

A parallel study in the NBSS that pertained to women aged 50 to 59 years was designed to determine whether mammography added significantly to clinical breast examination (CBE) for screening. All participants received an annual CBE and were taught BSE, but half were randomized to receive an annual mammogram as well. Evaluation at 7 years indicated that mammography doubled the number of cancers discovered, particularly cancers in situ and node-negative cancers, but overall survival and death rates from breast cancers in the two groups were not significantly different (Miller et al., 1992*b*).

Union of Soviet Socialist Republic/World Health Organization Controlled Trial of Breast Self-Examination

The first randomized trial of BSE alone as a screening measure was begun in Leningrad and Moscow in 1985, to determine whether this simple and inexpensive technique can lower mortality from breast cancer. Six district polyclinics and ten enterprise polyclinics were randomly assigned to teach BSE or to serve as a control (not to teach BSE), and the target population numbered approximately 150,000 women aged 40 to 64 years. In Leningrad, 31,186 were recruited into the BSE group and 31,066 into the control group in the first 15 months (Semiglazov et al., 1987). More than a quarter (27.8%) of instructed women practiced BSE 12 times or more per year, and 55% maintained this frequency for at least 12 months. BSE resulted in a fivefold increase in the number of women who sought consultation for breast complaints in this initial period (i.e., 4.8% of the BSE population). For those subsequently diagnosed as having breast cancer, delay before consultation was shorter in the BSE group than in the control group (91 versus 125 days). Consultation led to a diagnosis of breast cancer in 36 (1.15 per 1000) BSE-exposed women and 16 controls (0.51 per 1000). The average size of breast cancers was 1.3 cm smaller in the BSE group. Two patients have died from breast cancer, one in each group. This study demonstrates the *feasibility* of BSE as a screening measure, but its *effectiveness* remains uncertain.

CASE-CONTROL STUDIES OF SCREENING

Three population-based screening projects have been evaluated using case-control methods, two in the Netherlands and one in Italy.

The Nijmegen Project, begun in 1975, consisted of a single-view mammogram every 2 years for women 35 to 65 years of age. More than 23,000 women were invited for examinations. Eighty per cent responded, and after four screenings 46 women who died of breast cancer diagnosed after the screening began were compared with randomly selected controls who died of other causes. The relative risk of death from breast cancer among women who had been screened was less than half (0.48) that of controls. A later analysis indicated a significant 19% reduction in breast cancer deaths for screened women, but a significant reduction could not be confirmed in women younger than 50 years or older than 64 years (Verbeek et al., 1985).

The DOM Project was conducted in Utrecht, The Netherlands, beginning in 1974. Women between ages 50 and 64 were offered screening with physical examination and xeromammography, initially and again after 12, 18, and 24

months. Slightly fewer than three quarters (14,796) of 20,555 invited women responded. A less sensitive method of analysis was used in which all cases of death from breast cancer following the onset of the project were compared with those for controls. Thus, some may have been diagnosed before the project and so did not have an opportunity for screening. An analysis through 1981 found that 20% of 46 women who died of breast cancer after the project began had been screened, versus 43% of 138 controls. This resulted in a 70% lower relative risk of death from breast cancer for screened women, and the reduction was most evident in women 60 to 64 years of age (Collette et al., 1984).

The Florence, Italy, Project, an uncontrolled screening program, was initiated in 1970 and continued 11 years. An analysis based on 57 breast cancer deaths and 285 deaths from other causes (controls) produced an adjusted relative risk of breast cancer death in women who had been screened of 0.53 compared with controls. This risk reduction persisted and became statistically significant for women aged 50 years and older, but not for younger women (Palli et al., 1989).

INTERVAL CANCERS

Interval cancers are a constant feature of screening efforts. Panousspoulos and coworkers (1977) first called attention to the self-detected cancers that appear in the intervals between annual mammograms. Any breast cancer whose DT_{act} is less than 17 days could be an interval cancer. Cancers with a DT_{act} of 9 days or less could arise after an annual mammogram and lead to the host's death in less than 1 year. Interval cancers are associated more frequently with an anaplastic nuclear grade, absence of mammographic and microscopic calcification, patients younger than 50 years, no family history of breast cancer, and presence of a mammographic pattern classified as dysplastic. The prognosis is worse for interval cancers. DeGroote and coworkers (1983) provided further confirmation of the greater lethality of interval cancers. Dividing 120 newly diagnosed breast cancers into three subsets, they reported that cancers diagnosed in the intervals between screens had significantly higher percentages of positive axillary lymph nodes, higher overall mortality rates, and a lower 6-year survival rate than prevalent cancers detected at the first screen or than cancers detected at scheduled screens.

The nature of cancers does vary with the manner of discovery. Cancers discovered by mammographic examination are smaller and of lower grade than those discovered by palpation and are more likely to be noninvasive. In one screening program (Feig et al., 1981), Grade I cancers were discovered nearly 90% of the time by mammography but only 25% of the time by physical examinations. Grade I cancers were all smaller than 3.0 cm. Tubular cancers were less frequently apparent on physical examination.

BREAST SELF-EXAMINATION

BSE requires no physician and costs nothing, but it will not find cancers as small as those found by mammography (Fig. 24–5). Whether BSE can improve survival remains

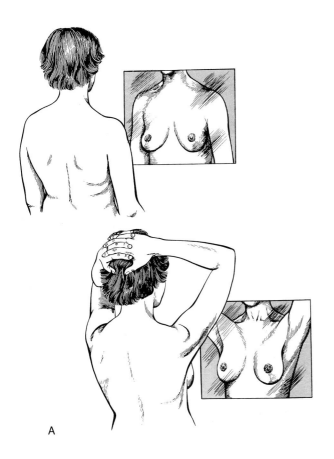

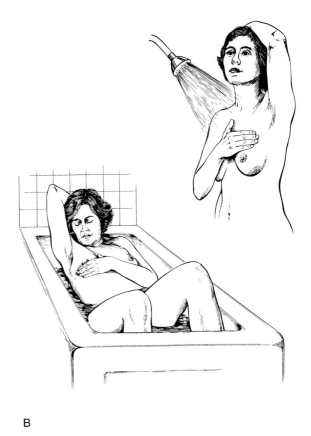

A

B

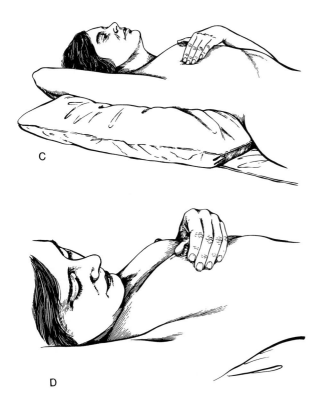

C

D

Figure 24–5. A technique of BSE. Self-examination can result in earlier diagnosis of clinically detectable breast cancers. Monthly self-examination is recommended by the American Cancer Society for all women older than 20 years. BSE consists of inspection *A*, palpation often when bathing, *B*, examination of the breast and axilla, *C*, and compression of the nipple, *D*. (From Danforth, D. N., and Scott, J. R. (Eds.): Diseases of the Breast in Obstetrics and Gynecology. Philadelphia, J. B. Lippincott, 1986, p. 1170.)

unproven, but it is the most cost-effective approach to detecting smaller breast cancers. Foster (1978) reported a retrospective survey of 335 women with breast cancer that correlated their BSE practices with clinical stage at the time of diagnosis. The maximum tumor diameter for women who practiced monthly BSE was 19.7 ± 2.2 mm (mean ± standard error of the mean), compared with 24.7 ± 2.0 mm for lesions of women who practiced BSE less often than monthly. The tumor diameter for women who never practiced BSE was 35.9 ≤ 1.5 mm. The relationship between the frequency of BSE and axillary lymph node metastases did not reach statistical significance. This series was expanded to 1004 women, with follow-up to correlate survivorship with BSE practices (Foster et al., 1984). These investigators observed that more frequent BSE was associated with a greater chance that a woman would find the cancer and that there would be less delay between discovery and histologic diagnosis. The cancers were found at an earlier clinical stage and were smaller, and fewer had involved axillary lymph nodes. At the median follow-up interval (52 months), 14% of the women who performed monthly BSE and 26% of those who did not had died of breast cancer. The 5-year survival rate was 75% for women who performed BSE and 57% for the others. They estimated that a lead time of 3 years would have to exist to negate the apparent beneficial effects of BSE on survivorship. In making this estimate, they used a tumor volume DT of 100 days and estimated that the diameter would double every 300 days at this rate. Actually, the DT_{act} of tumors is extremely variable and in the predetectable phase is much faster than 100 days. The size of tumors at discovery was 19.7 ± 2.2 mm with monthly BSE and 24.7 ± 2 mm with BSE at intervals of more than a month. The volume of a sphere, using these dimensions, averaged 4003 mm^3 for tumors discovered with monthly BSE and 7890 mm^3 for the others. The cell replication between these two points is trivial in comparison to the total number of cells in the tumors. This increase in volume would require less than one doubling. Thus, on average, less than one additional doubling occurred without monthly BSE. Prolonged follow-up is required on this study population to strengthen or refute the argument that BSE contributes to a reduction in mortality.

Saltzstein (1984) conducted a pathologic review of breast cancers diagnosed before and after an intense public education program on BSE. He found that neither the size of newly diagnosed cancers—before the education (average, 2.77 ± 2.06 cm, median, 2.0 cm) or after the education (average = 2.68 ± 1.72 cm median, 2.3 cm)—nor the prevalence of involved axillary lymph nodes had changed significantly as a result of the public education program.

The preliminary results of the trial of BSE in Moscow and Leningrad confirm that smaller cancers are found by practitioners of BSE and that the delay between discovery and contact with a physician is shorter. Whether mortality from breast cancer will be reduced has yet to be determined (Semiglazov et al., 1987). Training, paradoxically, increases the rate of false positive findings among trainees. Hall and coworkers (1980) concluded that a "more complex training model for breast lesions" than that provided by silicone models would be needed to reduce false positive

results. Because of the considerable individual variation among breasts, the best training model is a woman's own breasts. After instruction in the location and extent of breast tissue, each woman needs to become familiar with the consistency and shape of her own breasts. With monthly BSE, she then looks for changes.

COST-BENEFIT AND HARM-BENEFIT VARIABLES OF SCREENING

Screening programs are expensive and must be evaluated with respect to cost and benefit. Determining the cost per case of cancer found becomes complex. With any first screen, the prevalence rate is high and the cost per case of cancer found looks promisingly low. In subsequent years, discovery rates drop to age-specific annual incidence rates and the cost per case of cancer rises. The cost of treating earlier cancers may be less than that of treating more advanced cases, but the magnitude of this saving has not been well studied. Conceivably, it could more than counterbalance the high cost per case of cancer found in a low-yield screening program. Evens (1986) estimated that charges for mammography would generate an annual cost of $2.6 billion if used as recommended for all American women at risk. The cost per cancer found would be $14,000. This did not include the cost of biopsies done for benign changes and falsely positive mammograms.

The impact of breast cancer screening on a population may be viewed from the perspective of harm versus benefit. Wright (1987) analyzed biopsy rates, detection of benign disease, and mortality rates. He concluded that 2041 women would have to be screened for one to benefit. If women undergoing biopsy for benign disease were considered harmed, the harm-benefit ratio ranges up to 62:1. The harm-benefit ratio might be lower for the screening of high-risk groups. In the BCDDP at Louisville, 9.9 biopsies were performed for each cancer diagnosed.

PUBLIC EDUCATION

A byproduct of a screening program should be patient education (Monaco et al., 1972). The screener's role can be made more effective by educating and motivating people to participate in their own health maintenance. Public education reduces anxiety and facilitates compliance. Reinforcement by education of family and peers further enhances compliance. Education also minimizes dependence on others in the self-surveillance process.

Participation of knowledgeable women in self-care is effective and low in cost. Vickery and colleagues (1983) reported decreases in total medical visits and minor illness visits in three separately educated experimental groups as compared with a control group. They estimated savings of $2.50 to $3.50 for each dollar spent on education. Standard curriculum materials save time by reducing iterative teaching and errors of omission.

Education of women in screening programs should include the understanding that participants are exposed to risks as well as benefits. These risks include negative biopsies and false-negative examination findings. They should also realize that participation does not ensure curability if cancer is found. Cancers may already have spread by the time they are detected by mammography, so that detection does not lead to cure.

The majority of positive mammograms are false-positive, but they require biopsy of the breast. Moskowitz and Fox (1979) remain proponents of frequent mammographic screening and earlier biopsy. This approach accepts a high false-positive rate in the interest of achieving earlier diagnosis. The net effect is that more biopsies are done on disease-free women.

Mammography can provide a false sense of security if the mammogram is used to exclude the presence of cancer when physical findings are suspicious. That mammograms may be falsely negative in the presence of cancer has been documented repeatedly (Martin et al., 1979; Holland et al., 1983; Mann et al., 1983). The reasons for this range from radiographic technique and interpretation to characteristics of the cancers themselves. Histologic characteristics that make them occult to mammographic discovery include diffuse invasive pattern, poor desmoplastic reaction, and lack of microcalcifications. Dense breasts conceal cancers. Mammographically occult cancers may grow large. For example, a mean diameter of 50 mm has been reported for invasive lobular cancers that are occult on mammograms (Holland et al., 1983). The conclusion is obvious: a normal finding on mammographic examination does not rule out cancer. As a result, even if a recent mammogram is negative, a lump in the breast, a discharge, bloody or otherwise, from the nipple, or other breast symptoms, warrants medical evaluation. Women must remain vigilant between negative screening examinations, because a number of cancers in patients undergoing screening are found between examinations. Monthly BSE is an essential complement to any screening effort.

GUIDELINES FOR SCREENING

Guidelines for screening were first recommended by the American Cancer Society (ACS) in 1977, and continue under review. In 1987 a consensus was reached by 12 organizations on the following essentials for screening asymptomatic women: First, CBE and mammography are the basic methods of detection, and both are necessary for optimal screening since physical examination detects some cancers missed with mammography. Second, the screening process should begin by age 40 and should consist of annual CBE and a mammogram every 1 to 2 years. The ACS and others recommend that screening with mammography begin at age 40, despite controversy about its survival value, because 25% of cancers occur in the population aged 40 to 49 years and many can be diagnosed in an early, potentially more curable stage. Third, beginning at age 50 women should have clinical examinations of the breasts and mammograms annually (Dodd, 1992). For women 40 to 49 years old breast cancer in a close relative is generally the indication for mammography every year rather than at 2-year intervals. The ACS no longer recommends a baseline mammogram for women at 35 to 40 years of age, but

it places no upper age limit on screening. As long as life expectancy is sufficient to realize benefits, screening of elderly women is desirable. Although BSE has no proven survival benefit, cancers are detected at a smaller size by women who practice it. As the technique is harmless and inexpensive, and potentially useful, it is included in the current ACS guidelines for screening shown in Table 24–6.

FOLLOW-UP AFTER TREATMENT

Follow-up after treatment of cancer is a well-established clinical practice. In fact, it represents screening of a special high-risk population. Follow-up can be justified on the basis of providing emotional support, determining success of treatment, monitoring the natural history of cancers, and achieving timely identification of treatable recurrences. For years follow-up was linked to cancer registries that generated information for end-results studies. Schedules were adopted without proof that they contributed to decreased morbidity and mortality (Eiseman et al., 1982). Recommendations represent the consensus of experienced clinicians from multiple disciplines. These recommendations are not supported by models or controlled studies. They do not emphasize patient and family education or self-surveillance. As the role of mammography in follow-up has not received controlled study, periodic mammographic examinations do not have proven value.

The demands of follow-up can add to economic costs of care without improving outcome. When in the 1960s the thousands of patients who came from all parts of Missouri to the Ellis Fischel State Cancer Hospital (EFSCH) for follow-up exceeded the capacity of the staff and the facilities to accommodate them, a series of studies on optimal schedules for follow-up were performed. The entire scope of issues for determining the value of follow-up to the patient was reconsidered: What patients benefit from follow-up and how often must they be evaluated? What examinations are of value for enhanced survivorship? When does the timely discovery of recurrences, metastases, and new primary tumors benefit the patient? If discovery is beneficial, how can the greatest benefit be achieved for the least cost? When is follow-up no longer necessary? The

Table 24–6. SCREENING RECOMMENDATIONS OF THE AMERICAN CANCER SOCIETY*

Age (Yr)	Recommendation
>20	BSE every month
20–40	BSE every month, CBE every 3 years
40–49	BSE every month, CBE every year, mammography every 1 to 2 years, depending on personal risk
50+	BSE every month, CBE every year, mammography every year

(From Dodd, G. D.: American Cancer Society guidelines on screening for breast cancer. Cancer, *60(Suppl.)*:1885–1887, 1992.)
*At the time of this writing, these recommendations for mammography for patients between the ages of 40 and 49 are not supported by The National Cancer Institute because there is insufficient evidence for a reduction in the risk of death from breast cancer (Spratt, 1994).

economic problem was immediate, as the hospital had a legislatively fixed appropriation. The budget could not be increased by charging for visits or for laboratory and radiographic studies. Without a plan that had value to the patients, fiscal resources could have been expended with little measurable benefit. The question was, How many person-years of productive life and how much comfort and function are added as a result of follow-up? To study the existing system, a simple device was used. The interval rate of recurrence was determined for different cancers. This was done by dividing the number of persons alive and free of recurrence at the beginning of successive monthly intervals into the number of persons who developed recurrences during the succeeding month. These interval rates were then matched to the existing follow-up system. Gross disparities in the existing schedule were evident. Patients had been seen too seldom during the first 2 post-treatment years, when the interval recurrence rate was highest, and too frequently after the third year. For breast cancer the schedule of follow-up examinations was changed to 1, 6, 12, 18, 24, 36, 48, and 60 months. After 5 years the patients were contacted annually but were seen only every 2 years through the 10th year. They were seen at any time if they were concerned or developed a sign or symptom. This system reduced visits, but there was no evidence that patient survival was any better or worse than it would have been with trained self-surveillance.

Duration of follow-up was also an issue, since recurrence of breast cancer continues for decades (Fig. 24–6). Several studies question whether survivorship ever returns to normal after treatment for breast cancer (Mueller, 1978; Pocock et al., 1982; Haybittle, 1990). A statistical cure is said to exist when, after long follow-up, a proportion of patients shows an annual rate of dying from all causes that is similar to that in the ''normal'' population of the same age (Haybittle 1990). No long-term study has shown a statistical

cure for breast cancer. A clinical cure requires that long-term survivors have no greater risk of dying from breast cancer than do women of similar age in the general population. A personal cure occurs when a person treated for breast cancer has no further evidence of breast cancer during the remaining life span. Haybittle concluded from data derived from England and Wales that no more than 26% of the afflicted enjoy a personal cure.

TESTS FOR RECURRENT CANCER

Whenever diagnostic tests are used, certain principles should govern. First, the test should offer a high probability that the results are accurate. Diagnostic tests should be obtained only when the results will lead to altered management. If the change in management cannot lead to an improved clinical outcome, the test generally has no value (Sox, 1986). Many tests for recurrence are used without the research necessary to establish either the optimal schedule or the contribution to patient care.

Osseous Metastases

Pauwels and coworkers (1982) concluded that routine bone scans, done in follow-up, did not justify the cost. Bone pain and an elevated alkaline phosphatase level were associated with positive scans. When bony metastases did occur, they generally did so in the first 2 years postmastectomy. Early protocols of the National Surgical Adjuvant Breast Project (NSABP), required radionuclide bone scans every 6 months for the first 3 years postoperatively, and yearly thereafter (Wickerham et al., 1984). In the evaluation of 7984 bone scans performed to document first treatment failure in 2697 persons with involved lymph nodes, 779 patients had failed treatment, with 163 (20.9%) limited to bone. Only 52 (0.6%) of the total scans detected metastases in asymptomatic patients. As a result, NSABP protocols were changed to require follow-up bone scans only to evaluate symptoms. Bone scans have also been used to assay response to chemotherapy, but they have proved to be very crude monitors of response (Bitran et al., 1980). The association between bone pain and positive bone scans is not as strong as was once thought. Front and colleagues (1979) evaluated the association of bone pain and the findings of technetium 99m methylene diphosphonate bone scintigraphy. Of the 66 patients with positive scans, 21 (32%) did not complain of bone pain. Among 155 skeletal sites of metastatic disease suggested by scans, only 50 sites were associated with pain. There was no correlation between the involvement of weight-bearing bones and pain. Other studies similarly have questioned the frequency and rationale for bone scans (Forrest, 1979).

Hepatic Metastases

Hepatic metastases from breast cancer are a frequent problem and they carry a poor prognosis. Tempero and coworkers (1982) evaluated the comparative sensitivity of different

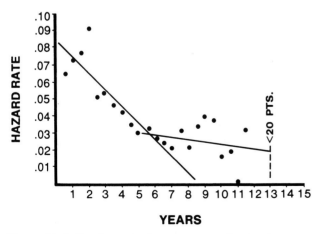

**HAZARD RATES FOR RECURRENT BREAST CA
961 PATIENTS MCW 1967-79**

Figure 24–6. The hazard of recurrence after treatment of breast cancer persists. The pattern suggests bimodal risk, probably reflecting early recurrence of rapidly growing tumors followed by a continued lower rate from more indolent ones. (MCW = Medical College of Wisconsin.)

Figure 24–7. Circulating tumor markers are unreliable for staging and not sensitive enough for routine follow-up, but they do provide a means for evaluating the success or failure of treatment for advanced disease. This graph shows the response of two tumor markers, carcinoembryonic antigen (CEA) and CA 15–3, to treatment of disseminated breast cancer with hormones. Tamoxifen produced a reduction in CA 15–3 as well as a rebound reduction when it was discontinued. Treatment with the progestational agent Megace produced a temporary reduction in both serum markers before the disease eventually progressed (Case of WLD).

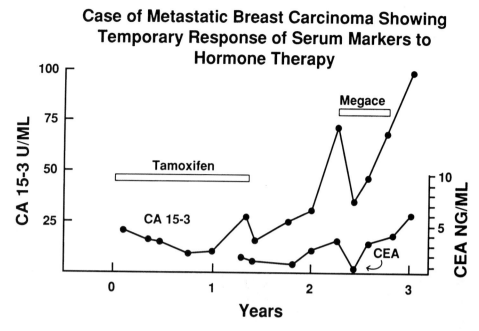

Case of Metastatic Breast Carcinoma Showing Temporary Response of Serum Markers to Hormone Therapy

testing methods. They found biochemical testing to be the most sensitive and least expensive approach and concluded that liver scans should be reserved for patients with elevated biochemical values. The biochemical tests used were alkaline phosphatase, aspartate aminotransferase, lactic dehydrogenase, and total bilirubin levels. Any test result value more than 10% above normal was considered abnormal. The liver scans were done with technetium 99m sulfur colloid. The rate of false positive scans (focal defects in the absence of metastatic liver disease) reached 35%. DeRivas and colleagues (1980) correlated serum alkaline phosphatase, hepatic ultrasonography, and hepatic scintigraphy, with the hepatic findings at autopsy for 282 patients with breast cancer. At the time of primary treatment, only 1.5% of patients had evidence of metastases on scintiscan, and only 1.2% had such evidence on hepatic ultrasonography. Alkaline phosphatase was elevated in only 6.4%. On diagnosis of first metastasis the serum alkaline phosphatase value was elevated in 35.3% of the patients. In a majority of the 51 patients with hepatic metastasis at autopsy there had been a progressive rise in alkaline phosphatase over the preceding year. However, within the 3 months before death, the liver scintiscans and ultrasonograms were positive in fewer than 30% of the examinations.

Pulmonary Metastases

Thoracic radiographs in search of asymptomatic pulmonary metastases are seldom revealing. Whenever a single tumor shadow is discovered on a chest film, particularly in a woman who smokes, a new primary lung cancer must be suspected.

Cerebral Metastases

Methods exist for the discovery of cerebral metastases, but no support for using these tests on persons free of central

nervous systems symptoms can be found in the literature. These tests, therefore, are not part of routine follow-up evaluation for asymptomatic metastatic disease in breast cancer patients. The appearance of neurologic symptoms in a patient under follow-up should be evaluated according to the symptoms.

Tumor Markers

A variety of circulating tumor markers for breast cancer are reported. Carcinoembryonic antigen (CEA), apparently the strongest of these, is present in 5% to 80% of breast tumor cell populations, but it is not associated with a particular cytologic type or degree of differentiation. The tumor and plasma concentrations of CEA are not strongly correlated. Thus, when CEA is present in breast cancer it is not always released in measurable amounts. The serum level of CEA correlates with the pretreatment size of the primary cancer; however, the values are still too low to be of any value for screening. A lowered CEA level is often seen in patients who have undergone curative treatment. The CEA level rises postoperatively in some patients with metastatic disease progression, but convincing evidence that CEA is useful in routine postoperative follow-up is elusive. Unless any lead time offered by CEA elevation can be put to therapeutic benefit, it would be of little value.

The identification and evaluation of a variety of serum markers continues to be an active area of research. To date, none are suitable for routine use in screening or follow-up. Serum markers are most useful for evaluating treatment of metastatic disease when increasing and decreasing levels predict progression and regression of residual disease, respectively (Fig. 24–7).

STUDIES OF FOLLOW-UP

Detecting disseminated cancer when it is asymptomatic rather than symptomatic offers no opportunity for salvage as in either instance it is incurable. Detection of asymptomatic local recurrence or a second primary in the remaining breast may be another story. Using an intensive follow-up schedule Marrazzo and associates (1986) found 28.1% of recurrences while asymptomatic, but they pointed out that no study had yet demonstrated benefit from detecting asymptomatic recurrences. Zwaveling's group (1987) found a similar proportion of recurrences while asymptomatic (27%) but could detect no survival difference from the time of mastectomy between patients with symptomatic recurrences and those with asymptomatic ones. They suggested visits whenever symptoms appeared, otherwise only an annual follow-up for physical examination and a mammogram and to maintain contact. In evaluating 192 relapses, Dewar and Kerr (1985) concurred that follow-up visits could be reduced. Survival was superior when local recurrences were found while asymptomatic rather than when they were found by the patient, but potentially curable relapses (local or in the opposite breast) were found at only 1% of follow-up visits. Wagmen and coworkers (1991) also suggested that physical examination and mammograms might be the only useful examinations. In a review of 64 patients with a recurrence or a new breast primary, total survival time from initial treatment was better for the patients whose disease was detected at routine visits only when new primary tumors in the second breast were included.

Tomin and Donegan (1987) conducted a review of the impact on the ultimate prognosis of different diagnostic procedures used in follow-up for the detection of recurrent breast cancer. The study population consisted of 1230 patients treated for cure of invasive breast cancer. Diagnostic interventions included history, physical examination, radiography, scanning, blood tests, and various clinical procedures, all used according to a predetermined follow-up schedule. The categories of recurrences used were local (mastectomy scar, skin flaps, or tissues underlying skin flaps), regional (supraclavicular, internal mammary, or axillary lymph nodes), pulmonary (parenchymal or pleural, with or without effusions), skeletal, visceral (brain, liver intestines, bladder, or ovaries), and multiple sites. Physician-discovered recurrences were considered asymptomatic; patient-discovered recurrences were considered symptomatic recurrences.

Among 248 patients who developed recurrences during the study, 64.1% were symptomatic and only 35.9% asymptomatic. Symptoms included bone pain, skin nodules, enlarging lymph nodes, cough, malaise, fatigue, and weakness. Shortness of breath, nausea, jaundice, and weight loss were less frequent. Symptoms varied with sites of metastases. From the time of recurrence, the median survival time was 22 months. Two thirds of patients survived 12 months. The 5-year survival rate was 15.6%; the 7-year rate was 4.6%. Survival for patients with asymptomatic recurrences was significantly longer than for women with interval recurrences ($P = 0.0017$), with the respective median survival times being 29 and 17 months. The respective 5-year survival rates were 25% and 11%. Survival also varied according to the site of recurrence (Fig. 24–8). Disease-free intervals between treatment and recurrence were not significantly related to prognosis. Estrogen receptor–positive cancers had a better prognosis, regardless of category (Fig. 24–9).

Relevant to the pattern of follow-up was the comparison of survivorship of two groups: (1) patients with recurrences who complied with a specified schedule of laboratory, x-ray, and scanning studies and (2) patients whose tests were irregular or who were not compliant. The difference in survivorship was not significant (Fig. 24–10). The percentage of patients with interval recurrence was no different in the two groups. The overvigorous use of many costly laboratory, radiographic, and nuclear medicine studies seemed only to add a lead time bias to survival data. As is true of all screening efforts performed at fixed intervals, the more indolent problems are present longer, which increases the probability of discovery and introduces length bias to the sample. The more rapidly progressive neoplasms become manifest as recurrences between scheduled examinations.

Cowan and Kies (1981) confirmed that history and physical examination lead to the discovery of two thirds of recurrences. They identified 115 sites of metastatic breast cancer in 55 patients; bone, lung, liver, and skin were the most frequent sites. Of 36 patients with bony metastases, only 15 were identified by bone scan while they were asymptomatic. Among 31 patients with pulmonary metastases, 12 were asymptomatic when these were discovered by radiographs. For metastases to liver, skin, lymphatic sites, central nervous system, and eye, initial discovery was purely clinical. Cowan and Kies observed low yields for liver function tests and radionuclide examinations of the brain and liver when findings of clinical evaluations were normal. Whether survivorship was improved when asymptomatic metastases were discovered by laboratory or radiographic studies remained unanswered. Rutgers and coworkers (1989) also concluded that history and physical examination alone provided adequate follow-up. They reported experience with different diagnostic procedures used in following 416 patients who had undergone treatment of primary breast cancers intended for cure. The follow-up period ranged from 2.5 to 13.5 years and included 4533 routine outpatient visits. Among 8005 radiographs only 24 (0.3%) revealed asymptomatic metastases. Seventeen thousand laboratory tests led to the discovery of only six asymptomatic bony and four asymptomatic hepatic recurrences. Screening for metastases did not lead to a reduction in lead time, as the disease-free interval was equal in symptomatic and asymptomatic patients. Forty-two of forty-six locoregional recurrences were found by physical examination alone, and in thirty-seven instances the patients noted the recurrences first. Periodic mammographic examination of the remaining breast was endorsed. They discounted the argument that a smaller tumor burden would be discovered by more aggressive follow-up testing by pointing out that, for both symptomatic and asymptomatic metastases the existing tumor burden would exceed 10^{10} cells.

Schapira and Urban (1991) provided an analysis of follow-up costs with a review of the literature and strongly endorsed a minimalist follow-up surveillance strategy. They estimated that the cost of routine surveillance testing could easily reach "$1 billion in 1990 dollars by the year 2000." If the surveillance testing in follow-up is based on the proposition that survivorship is enhanced, this is unproven. Most recurrences are perceived first by the patient and are predominantly pathognomonic of disseminated disease.

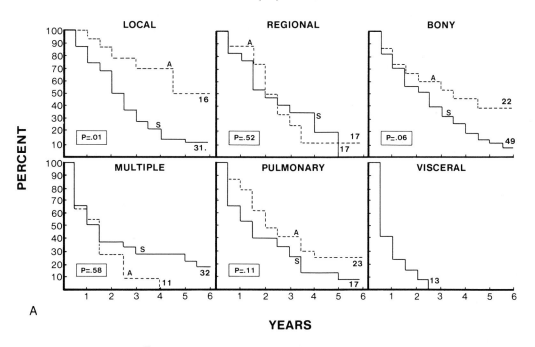

SURVIVAL AFTER SYMPTOMATIC (S)
VS
ASYMPTOMATIC (A) RECURRENCE BY SITE

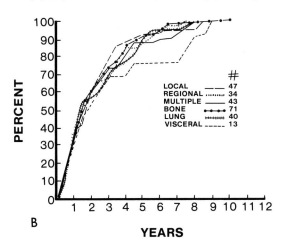

CUMULATIVE RECURRENCE BY SITE

Figure 24–8. A, Only patients with local recurrence derive significant survival benefit from detection of recurrence when it is asymptomatic. B, Rate of recurrence is similar for all sites. (From Tomin, R., and Donegan, W. L.: Screening for recurrent breast cancer—its effectiveness and prognostic value. J. Clin. Oncol., 5:62, 1987. Reproduced with permission.)

If the question for follow-up is, What tests do we do and how often? no final answer is available. For guidelines, a test should have a dependable level of accuracy, be economically feasible, and place the patient at negligible risk. The information gained should have a logical link to a plan of action that benefits the patient.

MULTIPLE BREAST CANCERS

Early detection of second primary breast cancers is an important function of follow-up. Women with cancer in one

breast are likely to develop another in the second breast. The earlier in life a woman develops a breast cancer, the greater is the risk of a synchronous or subsequent additional breast cancer. As Egan (1982) reported, women with multiple synchronous breast cancers constitute a unique group. Their annual mortality rate is higher than that for women with a single breast cancer. Women with bilateral synchronous cancers have a higher mortality rate than women with metachronous bilateral cancers. Since the risk for developing a new breast cancer in the contralateral breast is constant and is increased, particularly if the first breast cancer

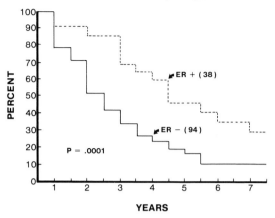

SURVIVAL AFTER RECURRENCE BY TUMOR ESTROGEN RECEPTOR

Figure 24–9. The survival after recurrence of patients with ER-positive tumors is significantly better than that of patients with ER-negative tumors. (From Tomin, R., and Donegan, W. L.: Screening for recurrent breast cancer—Its effectiveness and prognostic value. J. Clin. Oncol., 5:62, 1987. Reproduced with permission.)

occurs before age 50 years, a strategy for observation of the contralateral breast is useful. Mellink and colleagues (1991) reported that asynchronous cancers of the contralateral breast were more likely to be discovered when they are smaller in size with annual mammograms than with physical examination alone; however, the study did not document a survival benefit from this practice.

FOLLOW-UP OF THE IRRADIATED BREAST

Follow-up of patients who have been managed with breast conservation presents a number of unique problems. The response of breast tissue to irradiation can obscure recurrence (Welch, 1986). Changes, both early and late, include redness, edema, and fibrosis. The portion of the underlying lung included in the field undergoes fibrosis, and in some cases there may be symptoms of radiation pneumonitis. Fibrosis added to surgical defects may produce a distorted breast. Fibrosis and fat necrosis are more extensive in obese women and in women with fatty breasts. Tanning and atrophy of the skin tends to be greater at sites treated with radiation boosts. Changes produced by radiation tend to progress, and results that initially were acceptable from the cosmetic standpoint may become less acceptable with the passage of time. A longitudinal study by Clarke and associates (1983) found significant fibrosis in 20%, myositis in 5%, and arm edema in 1%. Chemotherapy can add to the effects of radiotherapy. It can enhance desquamation, myositis, rib fractures, edema, pericarditis, and pneumonitis. Breast retraction may also increase. Masses in irradiated breasts pose a particularly vexing problem. The clinical manifestations of benign and malignant disease in the irradiated breast are often indistinguishable, and reoperation is fraught with the risks of delayed wound healing, infection, and necrosis.

Denshaw and associates (1992) reported a series of 43 breast recurrences in 42 women. Recurrences were detected by mammography in 18, physical examination alone in 14, and by both modalities in 11. Recurrences were more frequent in women younger than 50 years and occurred earliest at the site of the original cancer. When cancer appeared in the breast away from the primary site the mean interval was longer—69 months versus 34 months. They concluded that the efficacy of mammography was diminished in the treated breast. Among 1030 women who underwent excisional biopsy for Stage I or II breast cancer with axillary dissection and irradiation between 1978 and 1986, 65 had developed recurrences in the treated breast, nine of which were associated with distant metastases. Detection of recurrence was accomplished by mammography in 29%, physical examination in 50%, and by both modalities in 21%. The median interval to recurrence was 34 months. The majority (65%) were in the vicinity of the original cancer, and the balance in other quadrants of the breast. Fifty-two underwent "salvage" mastectomy.

Boyages and colleagues (1990) reported on the relationships between various clinical, pathologic, and treatment characteristics and the risk of local recurrences in a series of 783 patients with Stage I or II breast cancer managed by excisional biopsy, axillary dissection, and radiotherapy. By 80 months' follow-up, 91 patients had developed breast recurrences. Recurrences were more frequent in patients whose tumors exhibited an extensive intraductal component (EIC) and in young patients. Similar conclusions were reported by Peterse and coworkers (1988) regarding the association of an EIC and breast recurrences.

Biopsy of the irradiated breast for suspected recurrence may be necessary during follow-up, and some concern is justified about the capacity of irradiated tissues to heal (Spratt and Sala, 1962). Pezner and coworkers (1992) reviewed their experience with breast biopsies after breast conservation and reported that 14% of patients subsequently had biopsies with benign outcomes. Twenty-seven open biopsies of irradiated breasts were followed by infection in 8 cases (30%) and by a seroma in one. They noted that cosmetic advantages may be lost from contractures

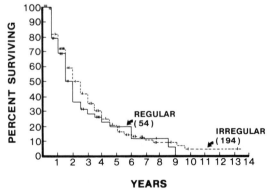

SURVIVAL AFTER RECURRENCE OF BREAST CARCINOMA ACCORDING TO REGULAR OR IRREGULAR FOLLOW-UP EXAMINATIONS

Figure 24–10. Survival after recurrence is similar whether or not patients adhere to a predetermined schedule of followup examinations after their primary treatment. (From Tomin, R., and Donegan, W. L.: Screening for recurrent breast cancer—Its effectiveness and prognostic value. J. Clin. Oncol., 5:62, 1987. Reproduced with permission.)

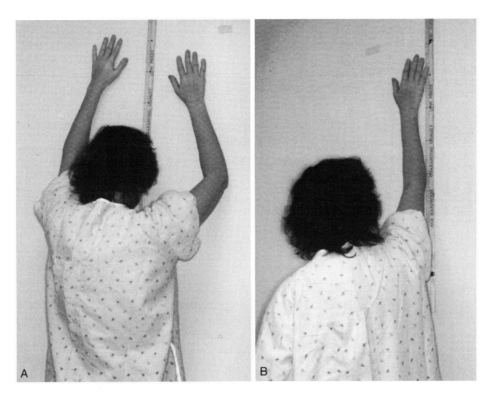

Figure 24–11. After drains are removed, patients perform prescribed shoulder exercises. Upward reach in the forward A and lateral B position is measured and compared at each visit until the range of shoulder motion is restored to normal. This can be expected within a month. A yardstick on the wall is used to measure the patient's progress.

associated with any delays in wound healing. No problems were noted when needle biopsies were performed.

REHABILITATION

Functional rehabilitation is an important objective in follow-up. Whenever axillary dissection is performed or the axilla is irradiated, reduced shoulder function and changes in the lymph physiology are risks that require attention. Active shoulder exercises are instituted after treatment. Passive or isometric exercises increase lymph formation but do not provide the lymph-pumping action of active exercises. A program of exercises is instituted after drains are removed, and the patient's upward reach is measured on the

wall in the forward and lateral positions at each visit to monitor progress and to compare with the opposite arm (Fig. 24–11). If full motion is not achieved by the fourth postoperative week, referral is made for physical therapy. Progress is more rapid after breast conservation than after mastectomy. Failure to restore full range of motion is rare.

Both axillary dissection and irradiation of the axilla permanently decrease lymph flow. The capacity for lymph flow never returns to normal, and the patient is predisposed to lymphedema. Patients must be educated to practice preventive measures, avoid minor trauma, avoid venipuncture, treat even minor trauma and infections as emergencies, and not to allow incipient levels of soft lymphedema to persist. Soft lymphedema is rapidly converted to permanent fibrokeratotic lymphedema by the ingrowth of fibroblasts into

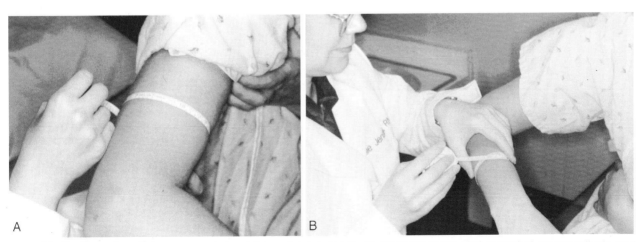

Figure 24–12. Circumferential measurements of the arms are made at standard levels and recorded preoperatively and postoperatively. These are used to evaluate any future problem with lymphedema. The arm is measured 15 cm proximal and distal to the olecranar with the elbow bent in a right angle.

Table 24–7. KARNOFSKY PERFORMANCE STATUS SCALE

General Category	Index	Specific Criteria
Able to carry on normal activity	100	Normal, no complaints, no evidence of disease
	90	Able to carry on normal activity, minor signs or symptoms of disease
	80	Normal activity with effort, some signs of symptoms of disease
Unable to work, able to live at home and care for most personal needs, varying amount of assistance needed	70	Cares for self, unable to carry on normal activity or to do work
	60	Requires occasional assistance from others but able to care for most needs
	50	Requires considerable assistance from others and frequent medical care
Unable to care for self, requires institutional or hospital care or equivalent, disease may be rapidly progressing	40	Disabled, requires special care and assistance
	30	Severely disabled, hospitalization indicated, death not imminent
	20	Very sick, hospitalization necessary, active supportive treatment necessary
	10	Moribund
	00	Dead

(From Mor, V., Laliberte, L., Morris, J. N., et al.: The Karnofsky performance status scale—an examination of its reliability in a research setting. Cancer, *53*:2002, 1984. Reprinted with permission.)

the protein-rich lymph. A useful practice early in the postoperative period is to measure the circumference of both upper extremities at standard levels (i.e., 15 cm above and below the olecranon process) and to record these measurements for future reference (Fig. 24–12).

An economic and societal problem still encountered by persons who have survived an episode with cancer is job discrimination. Hoffman (1991) estimates that a quarter of the six million persons in the United States with a history of cancer suffer from this discrimination, which persists even though it is illegal. Persons subjected to such discrimination need appropriate legal counseling and advocacy on their behalf by treating physicians.

RADIATION-INDUCED SARCOMAS

A late effect of irradiation is the induction of sarcomas of the chest wall. Souba and coworkers (1986) provided a review of 16 such cases, 10 of which developed after irradiation for breast cancer. The mean dose for 14 patients

Table 24–8. ANALYSIS OF VARIANCE RELATING PATIENTS' KARNOFSKY PERFORMANCE STATUS SCORE TO LONGEVITY

Karnofsky Score	Mean Longevity	Standard Deviation	Median Longevity	Number
10	17.6	20.5	9.5	13
20	27.1	29.4	17.8	84
30	45.7	43.4	31.9	239
40	64.1	52.4	46.7	244
50	72.0	52.8	59.7	105
Overall	53.5	48.9	36.6	685

(From Mor, V., Laliberte, L., Morris, J. N., et al.: The Karnofsky performance status scale—an examination of its reliability in a research setting. Cancer, *53*:2002, 1984. Reprinted with permission.)
F-ratio: 19.2
$p < 0.001$.
"Eta squared": 0.09

whose radiation dose was known was 4900 rad (range, 4200 to 5500 rad). The latent period between irradiation and the appearance of the sarcoma ranged from 5 to 28 years (mean, 13 years). The presenting symptom included pain in 10 patients (63%) and swelling or mass in 13 (75%). The mean age at diagnosis was 47 years (range, 18 to 77 years). These sarcomas proved to be difficult to treat effectively, and 13 of the 16 patients died of the sarcomas. Only one was a long-term survivor. Wang and colleagues (1992) reported four cases of periclavicular postirradiation sarcoma and two of clavicular osteoradionecrosis occurring within 10 years after radiotherapy for breast cancer. The patients had generally been treated with hypofractionation or large doses per fraction.

In an analysis of nationwide cancer registry material from Finland, Wiklund and colleagues (1991) report six postirradiation sarcomas of the breast occurring 7.5 to 15.8 years (average, 12.65 years) after irradiation for breast cancer. The sarcomas were predominantly fibrosarcomas and osteogenic sarcomas. Edeiken's group (1991) reported two cases of angiosarcoma of the breast following tylectomy and radiation therapy for carcinoma of the breast and reviewed the literature. The average interval between treatment and the appearance of this relatively infrequent cancer was 8.6 years. Souba and colleagues reviewed the current literature to confirm that radiation-induced sarcomas are being reported with increasing frequency. Their prevalence, and the resultant morbidity and mortality, must ultimately be considered when evaluating the outcome of treatment.

PERFORMANCE STATUS IN FOLLOW-UP

An important consideration in follow-up is evaluation of a treated individual's performance. Because of the chronic nature of breast cancer and the potential morbidity of treatment, quantifying the functional capacity of the patient is important. The Karnofsky Performance Status Scale (KPSS) (Karnofsky, 1948; Karnofsky et al., Burchenal,

Table 24–9. KARNOFSKY PERFORMANCE STATUS BY RANGE OF LONGEVITY

Patient Longevity	KPS Level (Per Cent)					
	10	**20**	**30**	**40**	**50**	**Total**
1–18 d	71.4	52.2	29.1	13.9	8.7	24.2
19–36 d	21.4	25.0	27.6	26.6	20.9	25.8
37 d or more	7.1	22.6	43.3	59.6	70.4	50.0
Total	1.9	12.3	34.8	35.6	15.4	100.0

(From Mor, V., Laliberte, L., Morris, J. N., et al.: The Karnofsky performance status scale—an examination of its reliability in a research setting. Cancer 53:2202, 1984. Reprinted with permission.)
 Number = 685.
 KPS; Karnofsky Performance Status.

1949) is standard for this purpose (Table 24–7). Mor and coworkers (1984) reported on the statistical evaluation and prognostic utility of the KPSS in the National Hospice Study (Table 24–8). After training, and only 4 months' field experience, raters were highly reliable at categorizing patients. As a predictor of survival, an increase in one KPSS level yielded an increase of approximately 15 days' survival (Table 24–9).

SCREENING AND FOLLOW-UP OF AGED PATIENTS

In Figure 24–13 the data for the 1990 census have been translated into person-days of residual life by age and sex. An appreciation for the limits of potential gain (i.e., the average number of days of useful life remaining according to age, sex, and ethnicity) is worthwhile. At the level of public health, arguments deal with the allocation of all health dollars and the ranking of competitive priorities in terms of the potential gain from screening. Just finding a cancer or a precancerous condition does not confirm that screening per se leads to enhanced cure. When this cannot be shown, screening programs may still be justifiable if reduced morbidity and treatment costs and enhanced survivorship can be attributed to the screening strategy and to subsequent treatment.

Mortality and morbidity from complicated diagnostic studies and therapy are greater in elderly, fragile patients. They need care that will ensure comfort and dignity without requiring unnecessary trips to medical centers. These facts have a bearing on screening and follow-up of elderly persons. Eventually, family, family physician, and community medical resources are more helpful than long trips to a screening or follow-up clinic. With the passage of time the probability of recurrence decreases, as does the justification for follow-up examinations. The patient needs only prompt access to a physician or hospital should signs or symptoms develop. For the purpose of end-results studies, names of previously treated patients can be sent to the Vital Statistics Service in most states annually to be matched against death certificates. For special studies the patient or family could be contacted (Hoag, 1963).

Mueller (1978) provided a longitudinal study of 3558 women diagnosed with breast cancer and performed an analysis through 15 years. He reaffirmed that the use of fixed–end point survival rates, such as 5-year survival rates, were meaningless. It is the force of mortality (the time-dependent death rate) that is most important in understanding the natural history of breast cancer and the impact of interventions. Mueller's data indicated two rates of dying—one for those who die quickly, within 3 years of diagnosis, and one for those who live longer than 3 years. Of all women who developed breast cancer, 80% to 85% ultimately died of their cancer, and the likelihood was even greater for those who were young at the time of diagnosis. The annual death rate averaged 8% through the 12th year after diagnosis, significantly in excess of the expected rate of dying. For elderly women who develop breast cancer, the death rate from accumulating conditions of aging is great enough to conceal the more rapid rate of dying during the first 3 years, if it exists at all for the elderly. Mueller concluded that the quality of life attained by treating the manifestations of cancer as they occur might be a more meaningful way to assess benefit. This observation on the elderly was supported by Stoll (1976), who reported that the survival rates for women past age 70 years were nearly the same regardless of whether the disease was limited or extensive at presentation. Survivorship was also independent of the treatment. Stoll concluded that survivorship in the over-70 age group was principally a function of the general medical condition at the time of diagnosis. At some point, diminishing returns of screening become evident, increasing the risk of more harm than good or of cost in excess of value to the screened population. This is a limitation imposed by function, however, rather than chronologic age.

AUTOPSY AS THE END POINT OF FOLLOW-UP

The autopsy for final assessment of both treatment and follow-up remains valuable but underutilized. Viadana and colleagues (1973) reported on the autopsies of 647 women with primary carcinoma of the breast. The frequency with which a particular anatomic site contained metastatic cancer is given in Table 24–10. Autopsies showed the diffuseness of terminal breast cancer. The authors were unable to confirm a time sequence for the appearance of metastases in different organs. Hagemeister and coworkers (1980) reported on 166 patients who died of breast cancer between 1973 and 1977. The autopsies consistently disclosed more tumor involvement than had been suspected on clinical evaluation. The unsuspected areas were most often endocrine organs (40%), lungs (28%), cardiovascular system (21%), genitourinary system (21%), bones (10%), and central nervous system (14%). The causes of death included pulmonary insufficiency (26%), infection (24%), cardiac disease (15%), hepatic insufficiency (14%), hemorrhage (9%), central nervous system dysfunction (9%), and hypercalcemia (3%). Forty-two per cent of all deaths were related directly to uncontrolled metastatic cancer. Although infection was the second leading cause of death, only 27% of the deaths were associated with neutropenia. Similarly, only 9% of the patients who died of hemorrhage had thrombocytopenia. The authors concluded that deaths related to chemotherapy were infrequent and that deaths from terminal infections had not increased with the availability of chemotherapy.

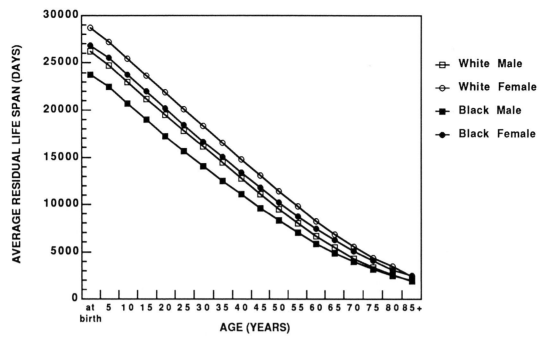

Figure 24–13. Person days of average residual survivorship by age, race, and sex calculated from the U.S. Bureau of the Census Statistical Abstract of the United States, 112th ed. Washington, D.C., U.S. Bureau of the Census, 1992.

Autopsy is essential to determining the lethality of any disease. A tendency in collecting vital statistics is to attribute the cause of death of anyone diagnosed as having had cancer to the cancer. As autopsy sometimes reveals a totally unsuspected cause of death, the results serve to assess the diagnostic accuracy of clinical, laboratory, and radiographic procedures used in follow-up (Goldman et al., 1983). In a review and commentary on the value of the autopsy in oncology, Hill and Anderson (1991) compared antemortem assessments of the extent of cancer with autopsy findings. They reported that the rate of false positive test results for clinical cancer ranged from 0% to 9% and that of false negative diagnoses from 5% to 56%. The review documents the importance of autopsies on cancer patients for quality assurance, improved therapy, enhancing the value of controlled clinical trials and other protocol studies, more accurate vital statistics, medical education, assistance in the grieving process, and assistance to families in obtaining insurance benefits, occupational benefits, and genetic assessments. Clear discussions of autopsy findings and their implications can be of benefit to families. Clearly, autopsy must be regarded as an essential component of follow-up.

Table 24–10. NUMBER AND PERCENTAGE OF CASES WITH METASTASES FROM CARCINOMA OF THE BREAST CONFIRMED AT AUTOPSY (647 CASES)

Site	Number	Per Cent
Stomach	62	10
Pancreas	70	12
Liver	397	61
Lungs	401	66
Bones	450	70
Uterus	86	13
Peritoneum	156	20
Kidney	86	13
Central nervous system	161	25
Lymph nodes: Neck	233	36
Thorax	359	56
Abdomen	250	38.5
Pelvis	107	16.6
Pituitary or parathyroid, or both	130	20
Adrenals	176	38
Thyroid	132	20
Ovaries	61	15

(Adapted from Viadana, E., Cotter, R., Pickren, J. W., et al.: An autopsy study of some routes of dissemination of cancer of the breast. Br. J. Cancer, *27*:336, 1973.)

RECOMMENDATIONS FOR FOLLOW-UP

We recommend that patients be taught self-surveillance for the signs and symptoms of recurrence. The treating physician must be rapidly responsive to patients who develop these signs and symptoms. Patients need to be seen promptly when recurrence is suspected, either to confirm and manage or to reassure. After treatment patients need to be seen periodically for examination and to have a mammogram of the remaining breast. The same rule applies to the conserved breast. Visits should be concentrated in the period of greatest risk for recurrence, usually the first 24 to 36 months. Patients at appreciable risk for recurrence should be encouraged to follow research protocols that offer promise for improving prognosis. These protocols generally have specific follow-up plans (Table 24–11).

In designing follow-up examinations a reasonable plan should reflect the pattern of recurrence. The pattern of recurrent breast cancer provides no rationale for changing the type of examination over time, as the relative risk for recurrence at various sites does not change. For example, local recurrences do not appear earlier than distant ones. As Fig-

Table 24–11. SAMPLE FOLLOW-UP SCHEDULE FOR PATIENTS WITH INVASIVE CARCINOMA ON NATIONAL SURGICAL ADJUVANT BREAST AND BOWEL PROJECT ADJUVANT CHEMOTHERAPY AND HORMONE THERAPY CLINICAL RESEARCH PROTOCOL

	Schedule			
	Year 1	*Years 2 and 3*	*Years 4 and 5*	*Years 5+*
History and physical examination	q 3 mo	q 3 mo	q 6 mo	q 12 mo
Complete blood count, platelet count	q 3 mo	q 3 mo	q 6 mo*	q 6 mo*
Blood chemistry: BUN, creatinine, bilirubin, alkaline phosphatase, SGOT, SGPT, calcium	q 3 mo	q 3 mo	q 6 mo*	q 6 mo*
Chest radiography	q 12 mo	q 12 mo	q 12 mo	prn
Bone scan†	prn	prn	prn	prn
Mammogram of remaining breast(s)	q 12 mo	q 12 mo	q 12 mo	q 12 mo

*For duration of tamoxifen therapy.
†Only as needed for symptoms after baseline bone scan before treatment.
Key: prn, as indicated for symptoms.

ure 24–8*B* shows, cumulative recurrences at all sites of dissemination have the same temporal pattern. Only the overall frequency of recurrence varies, and, thus, the need for examinations. As risk for recurrence decreases with time, schedules of routine follow-up should be designed so that examinations are most frequent early during the period of greatest risk and become less frequent as the risk declines. A schedule such as that presently used by one of the

Table 24–12. SUGGESTED INTERVALS FOR TESTING AFTER PRIMARY TREATMENT IN NONPROTOCOL FOLLOW-UP

	Months After Initiation of Treatment		
	0–24	*25–60*	*>60*
Invasive Carcinoma			
Physical examination	q 3 mo	q 6 mo	q 12 mo
Chest radiography	q 6 mo	q 12 mo	q 12 mo
Liver functions†	q 6 mo	q 6 mo	q 12 mo
Complete blood count*			
Mammogram (ipsilateral)†	q 6 mo	q 12 mo	q 12 mo
Mammogram (contralateral)	q 12 mo	q 12 mo	q 12 mo
Bone scan (for symptoms)			
Ductal Carcinoma in Situ			
Physical examination	q 6 mo	q 6 mo	q 12 mo
Chest radiography	q 12 mo	q 12 mo	q 12 mo
Liver functions†	q 12 mo	q 12 mo	q 12 mo
Complete blood count*			
Mammogram (ipsilateral)†	q 6 mo	q 12 mo	q 12 mo
Mammogram (contralateral)	q 12 mo	q 12 mo	q 12 mo
Bone scan (for symptoms)			
Lobular Carcinoma in Situ			
Physical examination	q 6 mo	q 6 mo	q 6 mo
Mammogram (ipsilateral)	q 12 mo	q 12 mo	q 12 mo
Mammogram (contralateral)	q 12 mo	q 12 mo	q 12 mo

*One time only, 3 months after surgical treatment: otherwise as indicated by adjuvant treatment.
†For patients treated with breast conservation.
‡Or as indicated by adjuvant treatment.
Note: No proof exists that this schedule of follow-up leads to longer survival when compared with other schedules or with self-surveillance and prompt evaluation of symptoms. Despite follow-up programs such as this, the majority of recurrent cancers are discovered by patients.

authors (WLD) provides a starting point to compare with other variations, and perhaps with trials of self-surveillance (Table 24–12).

CONCLUSIONS

Much work has been done to define the value of both screening and follow-up examinations, but much more is needed. Any program of routine testing needs to be used in combination with an effective treatment strategy or research protocol. A natural question for both endeavors is, What tests should be done? A test should have a dependable level of accuracy, a tolerable cost, and be of negligible risk to the patient. The information gained from the test should have a logical link to a plan of action based on the results that will lead to a beneficial outcome for the patient. Furthermore, the tests and the test schedules should be known to provide a better outcome than less complicated plans such as patient self-surveillance and evaluation of symptoms when they arise. Information from the literature and from this review should serve only as guidelines and as points of departure for evaluating screening and follow-up as an integrated system of cancer care. Screening is not an activity done in isolation from the total system.

References

Anderson, D. E., and Badzioch, M. D. Survival in familial breast cancer patients. Cancer *58*:360–365, 1986.

Anderson, T. J., Lamb, J., Alexander, F., et al.: Comparative pathology of prevalent and incident cancers detected by breast screening. Lancet, *i*:519–522, 1986.

Andersson, I., Aspegren, K., Janzon, L., et al.: Mammographic screening and mortality from breast cancer: The Malmö mammographic screening trial. Br. Med. J., *297*:943–948, 1988.

Aron, J. L., and Prorok, P. C.: An analysis of the mortality effect in a breast cancer screening study. Int. J. Epidemiol., *15*:36, 1986.

Bailar, J. III: Mammography: A contrary review. Ann. Intern. Med., *84*:77, 1976.

Basinski, A. S. H. The Canadian national breast screening study: Opportunity for a rethink. Can. Med. Assoc. J., *147*:1431–1487, 1992.

Berg, J. W.: Clinical implications of risk factors for breast cancer. Cancer, *53*:589, 1984.

Bitran, J. D., Bekerman, C., and Desser, R. K.: The predictive value of serial bone scans in assessing response to chemotherapy in advanced breast cancer. Cancer, *45*:1562, 1980.

Boyages, J., Recht, A., Connolly, J. L., et al.: Early breast cancer: Predictors of breast recurrence for patients treated with conservative surgery and radiation therapy. Radiother. Oncol., *19*:29–41, 1990.

Cadman, D., Chambers, L., Feldman, W., et al.: Assessing the effectiveness of community screening programs. J.A.M.A., *251*:1580, 1984.

Chamberlain, J.: Firmer evidence on the value of breast screening—the Swedish Overview. Eur. J. Cancer, *29A*(13):1804–1805, 1993.

Chu, K. C., Smart, C. R., and Tarone, R. E.: Analysis of breast cancer mortality and stage distribution by age for the Health Insurance Plan clinical trial. J. Natl. Cancer Inst., *80*:1125–1131, 1988.

Clarke, D., Martinez, A., and Cox, R. S.: Analysis of cosmetic results and complications in patients with Stage I and II breast cancer treated by irradiation. Int. J. Radiat. Oncol. Biol. Phys., *9*:1807, 1983.

Collette, H. J. A., Rombach, J. J., Day, N. E., et al.: Evaluation of screening for breast cancer in a non-randomised study (The DOM Project) by means of a case-control study. Lancet, *1*:1224–1226, 1984.

Corn, B. H., Trock, B. J., and Goodman, R. L.: Irradiation related ischemic heart disease. J. Clin. Oncol., *8*:741–750, 1990.

Cowan, J. D., and Kies, M. S.: Detection of recurrent breast cancer. South Med. J., *74*:910, 1981.

DeGroote, R., Rush, B. F., and Milazzo, J.: Interval breast cancer: A more aggressive subset of breast neoplasias. Surgery, *94*:543, 1983.

Denshaw, D. D., McCormick, B., and Osborne, M. P.: Detection of local recurrence after conservative therapy for breast cancer. Cancer *70*:493–496, 1992.

DeRivas, L., Coombes, R. C., McReady, V. R., et al.: Tests for liver metastases in breast cancer. Evaluation of liver scan and liver ultrasound. Clin. Oncol., *6*:225, 1980.

Dewar, J. A., and Kerr, G. R.: Value of routine follow up of women treated for early carcinoma of the breast. Br. Med. J., *291*:1465–1467, 1985.

Dodd, G. D.: American Cancer Society guidelines on screening for breast cancer. Cancer, *60*(Suppl.):1885–1887, 1992.

Danforth, D. N., and Scott, J. R. (Eds.): Diseases of the Breast in Obstetrics and Gynecology. Philadelphia, J. B. Lippincott, 1986, p. 1170.

Edeiken, S., Russo, D. P., Knecht, J., et al.: Angiosarcoma after tylectomy and radiation therapy for carcinoma of the breast. Cancer, *70*:644–647, 1991.

Eddy, D.: Screening for Cancer: Theory, Analysis and Design. Stanford, CA, Stanford University Press, 1978.

Eddy, D. M.: Screening for breast cancer. Ann. Intern. Med., *111*:389–399, 1989.

Egan, R. L.: Multicentric breast carcinomas: Clinical-radiographic-pathologic whole organ studies and 10 year survival. Cancer, *49*:1123, 1982.

Eiseman, B., Robinson, W. A., and Steele, G.: Follow-up of the Cancer Patient. New York, Thieme-Stratton, 1982.

Evens, R. G.: Screening mammography (Letter to the editor). N. Engl. J. Med., *314*:1451, 1986.

Feig, S. A., and Schwartz, G. F.: Pathologic discriminants of breast cancer detected on screening mammography and physical examination. Cancer Detect. Prevent., *4*:579, 1981.

Forrest, A. P., Cant, E. L. M., Roberts, M. M., et al.: Is the investigation of patients with breast cancer for occult metastatic disease worthwhile? Br. J. Surg., *66*:749, 1979.

Foster, R. S., Lang, S. P., Constanza, M. C., et al.: Breast self-examination practices and breast cancer stages. N. Engl. J. Med., *299*:265, 1978.

Foster, R. S., and Constanza, M. C.: Breast self-examination practices and breast cancer survival. Cancer, *53*:167, 1984.

Front, D., Schneck, S. O., Frankel, A., et al.: Bone metastases and bone pain in breast cancer—are they closely associated? J.A.M.A., *242*:1747, 1979.

Goldman, L., Sayson, R., Robbins, S., et al.: The value of the autopsy in three medical eras. N. Engl. J. Med., *308*:1000–1005, 1983.

Habbema, J. D. F., van Oortmerssen, G. J., van Putten, D. J., et al.: Age-specific reduction in breast cancer mortality by screening: An analysis of the results of the Health Insurance Plan of Greater New York study. J. Natl. Cancer Inst., *77*:317–320, 1986.

Hagemeister, F. B. Jr., Buzdar, A. U., Luna, M. A., et al.: Causes of death in breast cancer: A clinical pathologic study. Cancer, *46*:162, 1980.

Hall, D. C., Adams, C. K., Stein, G. H., et al.: Improved detection of human breast lesions following experimental training. Cancer, *45*:408, 1980.

Haybittle J. L.: Curability of breast cancer. Br. Med. Bull., *47*:319–323, 1990.

Heuser, L., Spratt, J. S., Polk, H. C. Jr., et al.: Growth rates of primary breast cancer. Cancer, *43*:1888, 1979a.

Heuser, L., Spratt, J. S., Polk, H. C. Jr., et al.: Relation between mammary cancer growth kinetics and the intervals between screenings. Cancer, *43*:857, 1979b.

Hill, R. B., and Anderson, R. E.: The autopsy in oncology. CA, *42*:47–56, 1991.

Hoag, M. G.: The follow-up of patients at the Ellis Fischel State Cancer Hospital, conducted by the Social Service Department. Missouri Med., *60*:1128, 1963.

Hoffman, B.: Employment discrimination: Another hurdle for cancer survivors. Cancer Invest., *9*:589–595, 1991.

Holland, R. T., Hendricks, J. H., and Mravunac, M.: Mammographically occult breast cancer. A pathologic and radiologic study. Cancer, *52*:1810, 1983.

Hurley, S. F., and Kaldor, J. M.: The benefits and risks of mammographic screening for breast cancer. Epidemiol. Rev., *14*:101–130, 1992.

Karnofsky, D. A., Abelmann, W. H., Craver, L. F., et al.: The use of nitrogen mustards in the palliative treatment of cancer. Cancer, *1*:634, 1948.

Karnofsky, D. A., and Burchenal, J. H.: The clinical evaluation of chemotherapeutic agents in cancer. *In* MacLeod, C. M. (Ed.): Evaluation of Chemotherapeutic Agents. New York, Columbia University Press, 1949, p. 191.

Mann, B. D., Giuliano, A. E., Bassett, L. W., et al.: Delayed diagnosis of breast cancer as a result of normal mammograms. Arch. Surg., *118*:23, 1983.

Marrazzo, A., Solina, G., Puccia, V., et al.: Evaluation of routine follow-up after surgery for breast carcinoma. J. Surg. Oncol., *32*:179–181, 1986.

Martin, J. E., Moskowitz, M., and Milbrath, J. R.: Breast cancer missed by mammography. Am. J. Roentgenol., *132*:737, 1979.

McDivitt, R. W., and Stewart, F. W.: Breast carcinoma in children. J.A.M.A., *195*:388, 1966.

Mellink, W. A. M., Holland, R., Hendricks, J. H. C. L., et al.: The contribution of routine follow-up mammography to an early detection of asynchronous contralateral breast cancer. Cancer, *67*:1844–1848, 1991.

Mettlin, C. J., and Smart, C. R. The Canadian national breast screening study. Cancer, *72*:1461–1465, 1993.

Miller, A. B., Baines, C. J., To, T., et al.: Canadian national breast screening study: Breast cancer detection and death rates among women aged 40 to 49 years. Can. Med. Assoc. J., *147*:1459–1476, 1992a.

Miller, A. B., Baines, C. J., To, T., et al.: Canadian national breast screening study: 2. Breast cancer detection and death rates among women aged 50 to 59 years. Can. Med. Assoc. J., *147*:1477–1488, 1992b.

Monaco, R., Salfen, L., and Spratt, J. S.: The patient as an education participant in health care. Missouri Med., *69*:932, 1972.

Mor, V., Laliberte, L., Morris, J. N., et al.: The Karnofsky performance status scale—an examination of its reliability in a research setting. Cancer, *53*:2002, 1984.

Morrison, A. S., Brisson, J., and Khalid, N.: Breast cancer incidence and mortality in the Breast Cancer Detection Demonstration Project. J. Natl. Cancer Inst., *80*:1540–1547, 1988.

Moskowitz, M., and Fox, S. H.: Cost analysis of aggressive breast screening. Radiology, *130*:253, 1979.

Moskowitz, M.: Response. J. Natl. Cancer Inst., *84*:1368–1371, 1992.

Mueller, C. B.: Breast cancer in 3558 women: Age as a significant determinant in the rate of dying and causes of death. Surgery, *83*:123, 1978.

Noyes, R. D., Spanos, W. J., and Montague, E. D.: Breast cancer in women age 30 and under. Cancer, *49*:1302, 1982.

Nystrom, L., Rutqvist, L. E., Wall, S., et al.: Breast cancer screening with mammography: Overview of Swedish randomised trials. Lancet, *341*:973–978, 1993.

Osborne, M. P., Wong, G. Y., Asina, S., et al.: Sensitivity of immunocytochemical detection of breast cancer cells in human bone marrow. Cancer Res. *57*:2706–2709, 1991.

Palli, D., Rosselli Del Turco, M., Buiatti, E., et al.: Time interval since last test in a breast cancer screening programme: A case-control study in Italy. J. Epidemiol. Commun. Health, *43*:241–248, 1989.

Panoussopoulos, D., Chang, J., and Humphrey, L. J.: Screening for breast cancer. Ann. Surg., *186*:356, 1977.

Pauwels, E. K. J., Heslinga, J. M., and Zwaveling, A.: Value of pretreatment and follow-up skeletal scintigraphy in operable breast cancer. Clin. Oncol., *8*:25, 1982.

Peterse, J. L., van Dongen, J. A., and Bartelink, H.: Recurrence of breast carcinoma after breast conserving treatment. Eur. J. Surg. Oncol., *14*:123–126, 1988.

Pezner, R. D., Lorant, J. A., Terz, J., et al.: Wound healing complications following biopsy of the irradiated breast. Arch. Surg., *127*:321–324, 1992.

Pocock, S. J., Gore, S. M., and Kerr, G. R.: Long-term survival analysis: The curability of breast cancer. Statistics Med., *1*:93, 1982.

Roberts, M. M., Alexander, F. E., Anderson, T. J., et al.: Edinburgh Trial of screening for breast cancer: mortality at seven years. Lancet, *335*:241–246, 1990.

Rutgers, E. J. Th., Van Slooten, E. A., and Kluck, H. M.: Follow-up after treatment of primary breast cancer. Br. J. Surg., *75*:187–190, 1989.

Saltzstein, S. L.: Potential limits of physical examination and breast self-examination in detecting small cancer of the breast—an unselected population based study of 1302 cases. Cancer, *54*:1443, 1984.

Schapira, D. V., and Urban, N.: A minimalist policy for breast cancer surveillance. J.A.M.A., *265*:380–382, 1991.

Seidman, H., Stellman, S. D., and Mushinski, M. H.: A different perspective on breast cancer risk factors: Some implications on non-attributable risk. CA, *32*:301, 1982.

Semiglazov, V. F., and Moiseenko, V. M.: Breast self-examination for the early detection of breast cancer: A USSR/WHO controlled trial in Leningrad. Bull. World Health Org., *65*:391–396, 1987.

Shapiro, S.: Evidence on screening for breast cancer from a randomized trial. Cancer, *39*:2772, 1977.

Shapiro, S.: Determining the efficacy of breast cancer screening. Cancer, *63*:1873–1880, 1989.

Singletary, S. E., Shallenberger, R., and Guinee, V. F.: Breast cancer in the elderly. Ann. Surg., *218*:667–671, 1993.

Smart, C. R., Hartmann, W. H., and Beahrs, O. H.: Insights into breast cancer screening of younger women. Cancer, *72*(Suppl.):1449–1456, 1993.

Souba, W. W., McKenna, R. J. Jr., Meis, J., et al.: Radiation-induced sarcomas of the chest wall. Cancer, *57*:610, 1986.

Sox, H. C. Jr.: Probability theory in the use of diagnostic tests—an introduction to critical study of the literature. Ann. Intern. Med., *104*:60, 1986.

Spratt, J. S.: The lognormal frequency distribution and human cancer. J. Surg. Res., *9*:151, 1969.

Spratt, J. S.: The relation of ''human capital'' preservation to health costs. Am. J. Econ. Soc., *34*:295, 1975a.

Spratt, J. S.: The physician's role in minimizing the economic morbidity of cancer. Semin. Oncol., *2*:411, 1975b.

Spratt, J. S.: The relationship between the rates of growth of cancers and the intervals between screening examinations necessary for effective discovery. Cancer Detect. Prevent., *4*:301, 1981.

Spratt, J. S.: Epidemiology of screening for cancer. Curr. Probl. Cancer, *6*:1, 1982.

Spratt, J. S.: The risky shift—fallacies of consensus decisions. J. Surg. Oncol., *48*:1–3, 1991.

Spratt, J. S., Chang, A. F. C., and Heuser, L. S., et al.: Acute carcinoma of the breast. Surg. Gynecol. Obstet., *157*:220, 1983.

Spratt, J. S., Greenberg, R. A., and Heuser, L. S.: Geometry, growth rates and duration of cancer and carcinoma-in-situ of the breast before detection by screening. Cancer Res., *46*:970, 1986.

Spratt, J. S., Greenberg, R. A., Kuhns, J. G., et al.: Breast cancer risk: A review of definitions and assessment of risk. J. Surg. Oncol., *41*:42–46, 1989.

Spratt, J. S., and Pope, R.: Legislatively mandated health benefits—mammography in Kentucky. Poster session, American Association for Cancer Education, Buffalo, NY, 1992.

Spratt, J. S., and Spratt, J. A.: What is breast cancer before we can detect it? J. Surg. Oncol., *30*:156, 1985.

Spratt, J. S.: Realities of breast cancer control, public expectations and the law. Surg. Oncol. Clin. North Am., *3*:25–33, 1994.

Spratt, J. S., and Sala, J. M.: The healing of wounds in irradiated tissue. Mo. Med., *59*:409–411, 1962.

Stoll, B. A.: Does the malignancy of breast cancer vary with age? Clin. Oncol., *2*:73, 1976.

Strax, P., Venet, L., and Shapiro, S.: Value of mammography in reduction of mortality from breast cancer in mass screening. Am. J. Roentgenol., *117*:686–689, 1973.

Tabar, L., Duffy, S. W., and Burhenne, L. W.: New Swedish breast cancer detection results for women aged 40–49. Cancer, *72*(Suppl.):1437–1448, 1993.

Tabar, L., Faberberg, G., Day, N. E., et al.: What is the optimum interval between mammographic screening examinations? An analysis based on the latest results of the Swedish two-county breast cancer screening trial. Br. J. Cancer, *55*:547–555, 1987.

Tempero, M. A., Peterson, R. J., Zetterman, R. K., et al.: Detection of metastatic liver disease. Use of liver scans and biochemical liver tests. J.A.M.A., *248*:1329, 1982.

Tomin, R., and Donegan, W. L.: Screening for recurrent breast cancer—its effectiveness and prognostic value. J. Clin. Oncol., *5*:62, 1987.

UK Trial of Early Detection of Breast Cancer Group: First results on mortality reduction in the UK trial of early detection of breast cancer. Lancet, 2:411–416, 1988.

Verbeek, A. L. M., Hendriks, J. H. C. L., Holland, R., et al.: Mammographic screening and breast cancer mortality: Age-specific effects in Nijmegen project, 1975–82. Lancet, *1*:865–866, 1985.

Viadana, E., Cotter, R., Pickren, J. W., et al.: An autopsy study of metastatic sites of breast cancer. Cancer Res., *33*:179, 1973.

Vickery, D. M., Kalmer, H., Lowry, D., et al.: Effect of a self-care education program on medical visits. J.A.M.A., *250*:2952, 1983.

Wagmen, L. D., Sanders, R. D., Terz, J. J., et al.: The value of symptom directed evaluation in the surveillance for recurrence of carcinoma of the breast. Surg. Gynecol. Obstet.: *172*:191–196, 1991.

Wagner, H. M.: Principles of Operations Research with Applications to Managerial Decisions. Englewood Cliffs, N. J., Prentice-Hall, 1974, p 364.

Walter, S. D., and Day, N. E.: Estimation of the duration of the preclinical disease state using screening data. Am. J. Epidemiol., *118*:865, 1983.

Wang, E. H. M., Sekyi-Otu, A., O'Sullivan, B., et al.: Management of long-term postirradiation periclavicular complications. J. Surg. Oncol., *51*:259–265, 1992.

Welch, J. S.: The postirradiated breast. Mayo Clin. Proc., *61*:392, 1986.

Wickerham, L., Fisher, B., Cronin, W., et al.: The efficacy of bone scanning in the follow-up of patients with operable breast cancer. Breast Cancer Res. Treat., *4*:303, 1984.

Wiklund, T. A., Bloomqvist, C. P., Raty, J., et al.: Postirradiation sarcoma. Analysis of nationwide cancer registry material. Cancer, *68*:524–531, 1991.

Wright, C. J.: Breast Cancer screening—a different look at the evidence. Surgery, *100*:594, 1986. [Letters to the editor on this paper: Surgery, *102*:106–114, 1987.]

Zwaveling, A., Albers, G. H. R., Felthuis, W., et al.: An evaluation of routine follow-up for detection of breast cancer recurrences. J. Surg. Oncol., *34*:194–197, 1987.

25 *Nursing Care*

Sharon L. Krumm
Patti M. Wilcox
Constance R. Ziegfeld
Jean M. Wainstock
Barbara W. Ashley
Catherine E. Mahaffy
Jennifer Dunn Bucholtz
Joy L. Fincannon

Nursing care for women with breast cancer is challenging and complex. Increasingly it is provided in multiple sites—hospitals, offices, clinics, hospices, and homes—in conjunction with specialists as well as generalists. Changes in reimbursement for medical care have resulted in shorter inpatient stays and more emphasis on ambulatory and home care settings. The case manager has become important in deciding how much care is provided and where. Nurses are challenged to deliver care with financial and clinical outcomes in mind. Careful systematic collection and recording of data is increasingly important for documenting clinical outcomes. Standards of practice developed by the Oncology Nursing Society, protocols, and clinical pathways are all useful tools for nurses caring for women with breast cancer and their families. Nurses are instrumental in ensuring that patients receive the care they need in multiple settings with multiple providers. Nursing practice includes prevention, screening and detection, acute care, rehabilitation, and support.

PREVENTION, SCREENING, AND DETECTION

Prevention of breast cancer remains controversial, but trials of chemoprevention (tamoxifen) and dietary intervention are under way. Discoveries in genetics have identified women at high risk who can consider prophylactic mastectomy. Genetic markers hold promise for early detection. Oncology nurses are active in clinical trials of prevention. They provide care and support to women in these trials while following the rigorous demands of the protocol. A great deal of education and psychosocial support is required to ensure the effective conduct of research.

Nurses should be familiar with the scientific basis for research related to prevention. As discussions about breast cancer prevention and risk often evoke a great deal of emotion, information must be provided in a manner that is sensitive and appropriate. Nurses should be familiar with principles of adult learning and with National Cancer Institute and American Cancer Society recommendations for screening.

Self-screening requires knowledge and skill in breast self-examination (BSE) and an orientation to self-care. Although 96% of women have heard of BSE (Lauver, 1987), Champion (1988) indicated that only some 18% to 36% actually practice it. Socioeconomically disadvantaged populations have increased rates of cancer morbidity and mortality (Nickens, 1990), but Esparza (1987) stated that low-income African Americans and Hispanics are less likely to know about and practice health screening. Older adults must compensate for visual and physical changes to successfully perform BSE (Ludwick, 1988). These are populations that require culturally appropriate health education. Innovative programs, such as the Maryland Health Services Cost Review Commission's breast cancer screening for low-income women and East Baltimore's African American church–based Heart, Body, and Soul, address these issues. In these programs nurses work with volunteers and neighborhood health workers to recruit women for free or low-cost mammography and clinical breast examinations. They are contacted through door-to-door campaigns, health fairs, community events, at food stamp distribution centers, senior citizen centers, and beauty shops. These programs provide a focused view of health care for high-risk populations and the homeless. Nurses and other providers coordinate transportation services, community workers, health care institutions, and community organizations to ensure the success of these programs. Nurses support screening and detection by teaching BSE, ensuring access to screening, and explaining procedures and options. Nurses should: (1) question patients about BSE, family history, and other risk factors for breast cancer; (2) encourage appropriate screening; and (3) demonstrate BSE. Education includes assessment of baseline knowledge about BSE, motivation for BSE, barriers to performing BSE, and BSE technique. Printed and video materials can be used to reinforce information. Teaching aids and printed materials are available form the American Cancer Society and the National Cancer Institute. The first step, however, is for each nurse to be proficient in

BSE and to serve as a role model by practicing it. Future research should address the cultural and learning needs of diverse populations and older adults. The impact of BSE on breast cancer detection and treatment also need to be determined.

In today's litigious environment nurses need to take measures to minimize legal risks. A recent survey (Heland, 1991) identified an increase in litigation related to failure to diagnose breast cancer. The following risk management measures are integral to good patient care and should be routine:

- Follow established standards for screening.
- Take patients' complaints seriously.
- Teach and stress BSE.
- Pursue diagnosis of *any* dominant mass.
- Be skeptical of a negative mammogram in a symptomatic woman.
- Ensure age-appropriate follow-up.
- Teach women about risks.
- Follow up on patient compliance.
- Don't overlook symptoms in younger women.
- Communicate with other health care providers about patient management (Heland, 1991).

Accurate, complete, and timely documentation relevant to each of these points is essential.

In addition to a history and physical examination, evaluation of symptoms often requires additional tests. Women need to be active participants in this process and to understand the nature, purpose, and expected outcome of diagnostic tests. Imaging techniques may not be clearly differentiated in the mind of the woman. Although women know that these tests contribute to the diagnosis of problems, they frequently lack knowledge about the process, limitations, and risks. For example, women who have had ultrasonography for prenatal care are knowledgeable about the procedure but frequently have unrealistic expectations. Many women ask appropriate questions about mammography equipment and staff, but most women do not appreciate the limitations of the procedure. Discomfort is a common complaint, but is more tolerable to women who understand the need for adequate compression. It is important for women to know the purpose of mammography and to understand the necessity for follow-up.

Surgical biopsy is the first step for a woman with breast cancer. Her concerns regarding pain associated with the breast biopsy, her ability to return to full activities, and risk of complications should be addressed in advance. It is important that the anticipated outcome of the biopsy be communicated. Women need information about preadmission testing, anesthesia, biopsy, and discharge.

Women undergoing diagnostic testing for a breast complaint are anxious about the outcome. Studies indicate that this is the most stressful time for women with breast cancer (Northouse, 1990). Careful explanations about procedures help women to cope with the process and the outcome.

SURGICAL THERAPY

Treatment for women with primary breast cancer usually involves either a mastectomy or lumpectomy followed by radiation therapy. Patients need reassurance that it is appropriate to take time to make decisions about treatment options and that survival is not affected by doing so. Information about treatments and opportunities to discuss options with physicians and nurses are essential (Lazovich et al., 1991). Referring women to other patients in the same age group and with similar symptoms who have recovered well may be helpful, as may referral to Reach to Recovery and local support groups. Furthermore, women should be reassured that decisions that are informed and consistent with their values will be affirmed by their physicians and nurses (Fetting, 1994).

Recent studies regarding the timing of mastectomy in relation to the woman's menstrual cycle have received a great deal of public attention but are controversial (Senie et al., 1991). Nurses should be aware of these issues and alert to their resolution. They must be prepared to answer questions about this and other relevant issues with as much factual information as possible.

Before undergoing an operation, the woman should understand the nature of the surgical procedure and what is expected of her postoperatively. Information should be given in the appropriate amount and in a manner that can be understood by the patient. Visual aids, such as simple line drawings or photographs, enhance learning. Because of the trend toward performing procedures in short-stay or ambulatory facilities, teaching must be effectively structured and planned. An example of a preoperative teaching plan is shown in Table 25–1. The plan is altered to meet individual circumstances, such as preparation for immediate reconstruction. Including family members or friends during teaching sessions, if acceptable to the woman, is desirable. The general aspects of surgery may be discussed, including the type and anticipated duration of anesthesia, what to bring to the hospital, and the expected recovery process.

In the operating room, the nurse is responsible for establishing a safe, therapeutic environment. This includes identifying the patient properly, positioning her safely and correctly, maintaining and monitoring the sterile technique of the operating room team, identifying and handling the surgical specimen correctly, and transporting the patient safely from the operating room suite. Attention is given to safety of the anesthetized patient. Extremities are positioned and padded to avoid pressure on nerves that can cause pareses.

The objectives of postoperative care are to promote wound healing and restore function to the extremity. Emphasis is placed on wound and drain care, comfort measures, precautions, and emotional support. Psychological adjustment of the patient and her family are also objectives. Complications that may attend mastectomy are hematoma, seroma, hemorrhage, wound infection, and pulmonary problems. Differences of opinion exist among surgeons about immobilization of the involved extremity. The physician's preference should be included in pre- and postoperative teaching. Following mastectomy, the woman is usually more comfortable using a pillow to support the involved arm. If the arm is not immobilized, the woman should know how to position it in a way that enhances gravitational flow of lymph and does not allow it to be dependent for long. Suction catheters placed under the skin flaps to remove exudate are kept free of obstructions and

Table 25–1. SAMPLE PREOPERATIVE TEACHING PLAN

Content Area Evaluation	Method of Presentation	Method of Evaluation
1. Turn, cough, deep breaths Use of incentive spirometer	a. Demonstration of procedure or activity	a. Return demonstration

2. Extremity exercises—
  a. isometric
  b. passive
  c. active
	a. Demonstration
	b. Patient practice
		a. Return demonstration
		b. Patient can state reasons for exercises

3. Immobilization of extremity (surgeon's preference)	a. Discussion b. Demonstration of methods of immobilization	a. Patient can state reasons for immobilization b. Patient maintains immobilization postoperatively
4. Dietary restrictions (diet progression, intravenous infusion)	a. Discussion b. Questioning about specific cultural or medical problems	a. Patient can state reasons for restrictions b. Patient complies with restrictions
5. Operative procedure, location and extent of incision, including axillary lymph node dissection	a. Discussion of operative procedure and function of axillary lymph nodes b. Visual aids	a. Patient can describe procedure and anticipated wound b. Patient can state function of axillary lymph nodes and describe how surgery may alter this c. Patient can discuss relationship of axillary node dissection to lymphedema and postoperative arm care d. Patient can describe relationship between axillary node dissection and diagnosis of extent of disease
6. Wound drainage system and dressings	a. Demonstration and explanation of equipment	a. Patient can state reason for use of equipment; return demonstration
7. Pain control and sensory changes	a. Demonstration of relaxation techniques b. Discussion of positions to decrease pain c. Discussion of potential sensory changes	a. Return demonstration b. Patient can express expectations of pain control c. Patient can state possible sensation in the chest wall and arm resulting from surgery
8. Body image changes	a. Discussion of concept b. Discussion of common reactions c. Discussion of influence on sexuality d. Include sex partner if appropriate	a. Patient can express feelings about her body b. Patient can identify potential concerns c. Patient can state problem-solving approaches
9. Coping strategies	a. Discussion of common responses and sources	a. Patient can express concerns b. Patient can identify sources of support c. Patient can state plans for coping
10. Rehabilitation	a. Brief discussion of Reach to Recovery, prostheses, reconstruction and postoperative exercise program	a. Patient can identify appropriate options

kinks, and sterility should be maintained. Instructing the woman to empty and care for these catheters is an important component of nursing care that requires demonstration and return demonstration. The woman should be taught to report to her physician or nurse any signs of infection (i.e., fever, redness, unusual pain). After the operation, blood pressure monitoring, venipuncture, or injections are *not* performed in the extremity ipsilateral to the operation. The best precaution is an informed patient who reinforces these restrictions.

The first dressing change may be traumatic, and the patient should know what to expect. She may choose not to see the wound at this point. The nurse respects the woman's privacy, listens, and offers information on request.

If exercises are not started immediately, the woman is given a date on which to begin them. When shoulder exercises are initiated, a mirror permits a self-check on posture and body alignment. The patient is encouraged to use the arm to care for her hair, brush her teeth, and perform other aspects of her usual daily routine. She should expect that her arm motion will be normal in approximately 1 month; if it is not, physical therapy should be initiated. Restoration of normal rotation and abduction of the shoulder joint is begun with gentle range of motion and stretching exercises. Unnecessary exercise of the elbow and wrist joints, which are not impaired, may result in accumulation of tissue fluid. Finger walking up the wall and overhead reaching are particularly beneficial. Tapes on the wall on which to mark progress provide a visible incentive to better previous efforts.

Each woman should understand the important aspects of skin and hand care on the side of the body from which axillary nodes were removed. A written list of *do's* and *don'ts* for her includes these:

- *Do not* cut cuticles.
- *Do* wear canvas gloves when gardening and rubber gloves when using steel wool. Avoid injury or infection.
- *Do* avoid burns; wear padded gloves when reaching into an oven.
- *Do* keep watchbands and jewelry loose on the involved arm.
- *Do* keep garment sleeves loose. Avoid pressure and tight bands.
- *Do not* use the affected arm to carry heavy purses or packages.
- *Do* use the **unaffected** arm for blood pressure monitoring, injections, and drawing blood samples.
- *Do* wear a thimble when sewing.
- *Do* wash the smallest break in the skin immediately with soap and water and cover with a bandage.
- *Do* use an electric razor for shaving underarm and avoid nicks and scrapes.
- *Do* use a good lanolin-based hand cream several times a day.
- *Do* give up smoking. If you insist on smoking hold cigarettes in the unaffected hand.
- *Do not* get sunburned. Use a sunscreen when out of doors.
- *Do* contact your physician or nurse if the arm feels hot or is red or swollen.
- *Do* continue normal activities.
- *Do* check with your doctor or nurse before using beauty creams or medications containing hormones.
- *Do* examine the remaining breast(s) monthly and report any changes to your doctor or nurse.

The patient should not wear a weighted prosthesis or a tight-fitting brassiere until the incision is healed. A loose-fitting cotton camisole or man's cotton undershirt is more comfortable; nylon and other synthetics may be uncomfortable. Once healing is complete, daily massage of the skin around the incision with cocoa butter can prevent dryness and promote skin mobility.

To promote continued recovery, the patient should be instructed to alter certain daily activities. For example, kitchen cabinets may be rearranged to force her to reach upward for articles used most frequently. Fatigue can be expected, and rest periods may be necessary. The fatigue will gradually decrease. Help from a home care nurse initially may be necessary for drain care or dressing changes. Small children or other adults in the home may require care. The patient should be encouraged to sit down while holding an infant or child. It is better to let small children climb up onto the lap than to pick them up.

Advice is useful regarding grooming and dressing. For example, it is best to insert the affected arm into sleeves first; brassiere extenders and prosthesis weights can be helpful. Feather and Lanigan (1985) suggest ways of altering swimsuits, sundresses, and nightgowns to overcome problems of style. Some women benefit from American Cancer Society (ACS)–sponsored programs, such as Reach to Recovery and Look Good, Feel Better. Information about these programs is available from the patient's local unit of the ACS. Nurses can help patients consider what they will say about their surgery to children, other family members, and friends.

Hypesthesia in the area of the incision may be permanent. Some women experience phantom breast sensations; others describe discomfort long after the incision has healed. Nurses can explain that this is not unusual.

A well-fitted breast prosthesis is an important part of many women's physical and psychological recovery. The patient should be encouraged to be fitted for such a prosthesis when healing is adequate, usually 3 to 4 weeks after the surgical procedure. Various types are available, including custom-made ones, and they range in price from $40 to $900. They are usually made of silicone and attempt to replicate the feel and weight of a normal breast. A well-fitting brassiere is important for holding the prosthesis in place, and special ones may be purchased or a pocket can be sewn inside a regular one to hold the prosthesis (McFadden, 1985). Most insurance plans cover all or part of the cost of the prosthesis and brassieres. A physician's prescription ensures reimbursement. Some women choose not to wear a prosthesis, and this decision is respected. However, problems with posture or neck, shoulder, and back soreness sometimes result from weight imbalance.

The role of reconstructive surgery is usually discussed by the surgeon. Nurses should respond to inquiries about the nature of the procedures and the relative advantages and risks. The timing ranges from the time of mastectomy to several months later. Concern about the use of silicone implants should be met with up-to-date information, including relevant U.S. Food and Drug Administration regulations. Various techniques are used to reconstruct the breast. Nurses promote recovery by reinforcing the surgeon's plan for immediate and long-range rehabilitation.

SYSTEMIC THERAPY

Women today have many options for treatment. Clinical research continues to broaden them and basic science research to investigate their foundations. Oncology nurses must keep abreast of this research so they can provide accurate information to women facing treatment. Nurses must respond as well to an increasingly knowledgeable public.

Treatment of breast cancer is planned in the context of a woman's menopausal, node, and hormone receptor status. Prognostic factors are important for nurses to know and understand. Their implications for women with breast cancer are profound. They include tumor size and node status. Estrogen receptor status and proliferative rates indicate hormone-dependency and metastatic potential. Tumor markers, Her-2/neu oncogene, and epidermal growth factors (EGF) indicate growth advantage and resistance to therapy (Davidson et al., 1992).

Systemic adjuvant therapy for breast cancer means treatment with cytotoxic agents or hormones. The goal of adjuvant therapy is to completely stop breast cancer's micrometastasis. Adjuvant therapy alters the course of breast cancer in most women (Bonadonna et al., 1985). Nurses play an important role in helping patients achieve the goals of therapy.

To treat women with distant metastases, hormone and cytotoxic therapy are the only options since the use of radiation and surgery are limited. The choice of drugs depends on prognostic factors, but also on what drugs the woman received as adjuvants. Antimicrotubular agents, such as navelbine and taxol, provide patients with new alternatives to cyclophosphamide (Cytoxan), doxorubicin (Adriamycin), 5F-fluorouracil, and methotrexate.

Toxicities from systemic therapy have changed in the last 15 years (Table 25–2). In the past most patients and families would voice concerns about nausea and vomiting, hair loss, and anorexia; today these symptoms have decreased. New antiemetics minimize the extent of nausea and vomiting from chemotherapy. Hair loss depends on what drugs are used, so patients may not need to wear wigs. It is interesting to note that fatigue, insomnia, and nausea are the most distressing side effects for women (Knobf, 1986; and Ehlke, 1988). When fatigue is severe, the nurse should advise moderation of activity and naps. Another side effect is weight gain, which can be distressing. Patients taking systemic adjuvant chemotherapy can expect an average weight gain of 4 kg (Knobf, 1986). The reason for this has not been determined, but counseling about nutrition and exercise can be successful.

Probably the most time-consuming toxicity for both the patient and nurse is hematologic toxicity. Blood counts need to be monitored and patients instructed to take appropriate precautions when counts are low. Although neutropenia is not distressing, it can be life threatening. The use of hematopoietic growth factors avoids most of the severe side effects from bone marrow depression.

Initiation of systemic therapy involves planning and patient education by both physicians and nurses. This requirement is heightened for clinical trials, which are often complex and time consuming and have less predictable outcomes. Watson (1982) suggested that the woman's learning style be determined by asking her how she would usually go about learning something new. The method and content are matched with the type of learning required—cognitive, psychomotor, or attitudinal. Initially the focus is on treatment options and on enhancing strategies for coping with physical and psychosocial changes. The primary objectives during this time are to have women acquire sufficient understanding to give informed consent, participate cooperatively in the treatment, and alleviate anxiety. Patients tend to forget or repress much of what is learned. Information should be given simply, concisely, and with frequent repetition.

Teaching then focuses on responsibility for self-care and coping. It is directed toward self-care and toward transferring these to home, work, or other settings. During this phase, women accept responsibility for their own care (Watson, 1982). Transfer of information is important. Nurses in physicians' offices, outpatient therapy centers, and home care practices must be informed about what is to be evaluated or reinforced. Women should be able to identify the care provider and how to contact him or her for additional information.

Treatment affects many of the body's systems. An underlying principle of oncology nursing is that nurses know and understand the anticipated effects of chemotherapy and hormone therapy. With such an understanding, nurses can intervene appropriately and be effective teachers, mentors, coaches, cheerleaders, and role models. Nursing interventions include the administration of pharmaceuticals, controlling the environment during treatment, and providing encouragement. Precise monitoring of response to treatment improves the probability of success. For example, the administration of antiemetics can be individualized and timed to obviate the onset of symptoms.

Nurses should anticipate physical and psychosocial reactions and prepare women to cope effectively with them.

Table 25–2. COMMONLY USED CHEMOTHERAPY AGENTS

Agent (Drug Class)	Dosage and Administration	Nadir (Days)	Side Effects or Toxic Effects
Cyclophosphamide (Cytoxan) (alkylating agent)	100 mg/m² orally days 1–14 every 28 day cycle	7–14	Bone marrow suppression; nausea and vomiting; mucositis-stomatitis; hemorrhagic cystitis (avoid by increased fluid intake prior to and during therapy); alopecia; ovarian damage
Methotrexate (antimetabolite)	30–40 mg/m² intravenously days 1 and 8 of each 28 day cycle	7–14	Bone marrow suppression; ulceration of mouth and digestive tract
5-Fluorouracil (5-FU) (antimetabolite)	500 mg/m² intravenously days 1 and 8 of each 28 day cycle	7–14	Bone marrow suppression; nausea and vomiting; gastrointestinal tract injury, resulting in stomatitis, mucositis, and diarrhea
Doxorubicin hydrochloride (Adriamycin) (antibiotic)	50–75 mg/m² intravenously every 3 weeks or 25–30 mg/m² intravenously days 1 and 8 of 28 day cycle Avoid extravasation	10–14	Bone marrow suppression; nausea and vomiting; severe alopecia; mucositis and stomatitis; diarrhea; urine will be red up to 7 days after administration; irreversible cardiotoxicity (dose related)
Vincristine (Oncovin) (vinca alkaloid)	0.5–1.5 mg/m² intravenously not to exceed 2 mg/dose	Not marrow suppressive	Areflexia; weakness; peripheral neuritis; nausea and vomiting; alopecia; paralytic ileus

(From Krakoff, I. H.: Cancer Chemotherapy Agents. New York, American Cancer Society Professional Education Publication, 1973.)

Her functional status or her role in the family may change. Ongoing assessment of these issues is enhanced by the use of standardized measures. Information that is rigorously recorded permits analysis of outcomes.

Nurses must adhere to guidelines for handling antineoplastic agents and patients' excreta. Evidence of mutagenic or teratogenic changes in the urine of nurses handling these agents is still contradictory, and the implications are unknown. Nurses should avoid taking unnecessary risks.

AUTOLOGOUS BONE MARROW TRANSPLANTATION

High-dose chemotherapy with alkylating agents followed by reinfusion of autologous bone marrow has a role in the treatment of metastatic breast cancer (Antman et al., 1992). The goal of therapy is to reduce or eliminate areas of metastasis. Autologous bone marrow transplantation (ABMT) significantly reduces the mortality and morbidity associated with prolonged aplasias and the organ toxicity seen with high-dose therapies (Kennedy et al., 1991). ABMT is employed primarily in Stage III and IV breast cancer, but clinical trials are under way for Stage II disease. At present, there is little justification for ABMT unless the patient is enrolled in a well-controlled clinical research program. ABMT is expensive, and reimbursement remains a controversial issue.

ABMT is aimed at producing a long-term remission. Women who responded to alkylating agents in conventional doses are likely to respond to dose intensification. Selected combinations of large doses of alkylating agents can produce high tumor cell kill without subsequent drug cross-resistance. Thus, steep dose-response curves are achieved in this population. Although not considered a curative therapy, ABMT achieves complete response rates of 28% 18 to 36 months after transplant, compared with 10% to 20% after standard therapy (Sledge et al, 1992).

The eligibility criteria for ABMT are listed in Table 25–3. The woman should understand that it is the stage of her disease that qualifies her as a candidate. Women with renal, hepatic, pulmonary, or cardiac insufficiency are considered too much at risk, as are patients with active central nervous system involvement. Unstable mental illness could interfere with the woman's ability to comply with the treatment and is a reason for exclusion. Table 25–4 lists what tests are required for evaluation. During the workup, most women try to deal with the reality of their disease and understand what transplant can offer them. Feelings of anxiety and fear may be apparent. Denial is seen. As the oncology nurse helps the woman prepare for the tests, she should seek to identify impaired coping skills. A multidisciplinary assessment during this phase should include a social worker in addition to the physician and the oncology nurse. Patient assessments are made at appropriate intervals throughout treatment.

Obtaining informed consent is an important step. The goal of therapy, expected effects and toxicity of drugs, potential risks, and potential complications are discussed. The woman should be informed about advanced directives.

Bone marrow harvest typically occurs under general an-

Table 25–3. ELIGIBILITY CRITERIA FOR AUTOLOGOUS BONE MARROW TRANSPLANTATION—STAGE IV BREAST CANCER

Age 18 to 60
Eastern Co-operative Oncology Group performance status < 2
Histologically proven adenocarcinoma of breast tissue which is metastatic, inoperable, or locally recurrent
Reported hormonal status
Achievement of clinically complete or stable partial response to therapy prior to study
Adequate organ function:

Creatinine ≤ 2.0	WBC > 3000; platelets > 100 K
Bilirubin ≤ 1.5	
Serum glutamic oxaloacetic transaminase ≤2× normal	Forced expiratory volume, functional vital capacity, ≥ 65–75%
	Left ventricular ejection fraction ≥ 45%

Absence of another major medical illness, CNS involvement, or any debilitating psychiatric illness that would preclude informed consent
Bone marrow aspirate and biopsy core morphologically negative for tumor and reserves adequate for harvest
Absence of excessive bone disease
No history of other malignant neoplasms (except cured basal cell or squamous cell carcinoma of skin, or ``cured'' cervical carcinoma in situ)
Negative pregnancy test and absence of major infection (HIV, hepatitis)
Signed informed consent

esthesia on the day of admission. Placement of a venous access device (VAD) is always necessary. A double-lumen or triple-lumen central line may be inserted at the time of harvest. Printed information is provided to enforce verbal teaching. It is important to remember that a great deal of information is shared with the woman by a number of health care providers. The woman's readiness and willingness to learn are just as important as the teaching. Following bone marrow harvest and VAD placement, pain is managed with analgesics—anything from acetaminophen to oxycodone or small IV doses of morphine, depending on the level of discomfort. General anesthesia may cause nausea and vomiting. Administering an antiemetic and preventing aspiration, especially if the woman is not totally alert, are key nursing responsibilities. Women are instructed to call for a nurse's assistance when getting out of bed for the first time, as they are prone to weakness and syncope.

ABMT can be divided into three distinct phases: (1) chemotherapy administration; (2) bone marrow reinfusion

Table 25–4. STANDARD ELIGIBILITY TESTS FOR ABMT

Bone scan
Radiographs of suspicious lesions on bone scan
CT of chest and abdomen
Radionuclide angiography
Pulmonary function test
Chest radiograph
Electrocardiogram
Bone marrow aspirate and biopsy
Blood work: blood counts, chemistries, liver function tests, herpes simplex virus and cytomegalovirus serology, HIV and hepatitis studies, and other studies as indicated

and myelosuppressive period; and (3) bone marrow engraftment. Nurses are responsible for the majority of teaching during these phases. Creative strategies must be employed to help the woman through the process. Hospitalization separates the woman from her family and friends. Identity roles and financial burdens are common concerns. Uncertainty about the future is expressed, often tearfully. Emotional support and an understanding manner help women through particularly difficult periods.

High-dose chemotherapy is given, as continuous infusion or as bolus injections, depending on the specific protocol, and toxicity should be anticipated (Table 25–5). Vigorous hydration before chemotherapy dilutes the urine and prevents bladder irritation. This helps to prevent nephrotoxicity and hemorrhagic cystitis, a side effect of large doses of cyclophosphamide. Drug metabolites adhere to the bladder wall and crystalize, causing tissue necrosis and bleeding (Ballard, 1991). Continuous bladder irrigation during administration of chemotherapy and vigorous hydration are both ways of preventing hemorrhagic cystitis.

Persistent nausea and vomiting are expected with high-dose chemotherapy. Ondansetron, given as a continuous infusion concurrently with the chemotherapy, is effective in controlling these side effects; however, most women also require additional antiemetics, such as prochlorperazine (Compazine) and lorazepam.

Mucositis is another gastrointestinal toxicity observed with high-dose thiotepa. Oral and esophageal effects range from mild erythema with plaque development to ulceration of the esophagus. Managing mucositis centers on pain control and prevention of infection. Table 25–5 lists toxicities and nursing interventions for them.

Hepatic toxicity occurs as veno-occlusive disease and can cause significant morbidity and mortality. Resting the liver as much as possible and monitoring for signs of hepatic insufficiency are two main objectives. Nurses are responsible for tracking the woman's weight, monitoring liver enzymes, measuring abdominal girth, and minimizing sodium solutions, as fluid retention is a key symptom.

Pulmonary fibrosis and development of adult respiratory distress syndrome (ARDS) may result from carmustine and cyclophosphamide in large doses. Carmustine typically produces dyspnea and fever. ARDS is most likely to develop within 1 to 2 weeks following chemotherapy. It is characterized by increasing dyspnea, wet lungs, pulmonary consolidation, and refractory hypoxia. Nursing management focuses on respiratory support, control of fluids, and monitoring for signs of infection.

The day of bone marrow reinfusion, Day 0, occurs after the chemotherapy has cleared the woman's system. Previous teaching about side effects should be reinforced on this day. Her vital signs will be taken during the reinfusion and for several hours afterward. The preservative dimethylsulfoxide, used to store bone marrow, can cause bradycardia, hypotension, arrhythmias, and allergic reactions. Pink urine may be seen initially secondary to red blood cell lysis.

White blood cell nadir occurs 1 to 7 days after the last doses of chemotherapy. The myelosuppressive period lasts roughly 21 days before bone marrow engraftment is adequate. Patients are at greatest risk for infection during this time. Infections account for 40% of the deaths associated with ABMT (Affronti, 1990). The majority of neutropenic fevers are due to bacterial contamination from the host's system. Fungal colonization also occurs early in the neutropenic period.

Nurses are responsible for meticulous daily hygiene and other strategies to prevent infection. For example, a routine is established for mouth care after meals, at bedtime, and following bouts of emesis. The woman should be prepared for periodic cultures of the throat, urine, and stool to help identify potential sources of infection (Table 25–6).

Women start receiving prophylactic antibiotics before myelosuppression. Antibiotic Profile Sheets developed by the transplant team reflect current research findings and clinical observations. Drugs include (1) oral norfloxacin, to prevent colonization of the gastrointestinal tract with resistant aerobic gram-negative organisms; (2) IV acyclovir, to provide protection against reactivation of herpes simplex if the titer is positive; (3) IV vancomycin, to prevent gram-positive infections associated with indwelling catheters; and, (4) oral fluconazole, to protect against fungal organisms (*Candida, Histoplasma, Cryptococcus* species) and to delay the use of amphotericin B. Table 25–6 lists infection prevention guidelines that were developed for immunocompromised patients.

In addition to leukopenia, patients develop anemia and thrombocytopenia. The duration and depth of aplasia determines how long women are dependent on blood product support. The woman should realize that she will receive red blood cell (RBC) transfusions to maintain her hematocrit level above 30% and that a low RBC count contributes to fatigue and dyspnea on exertion. Platelet transfusions are needed more frequently than RBCs, owing to the prolonged period required for engraftment and their short life span. Women are considered at risk for bleeding at counts below 50,000, but the rule of thumb is to transfuse with a count of 20,000 or less or when there are signs of bleeding. Nurses test urine, stool, and emesis for presence of blood. Bleeding precautions are especially important. These include wearing protective footwear, not cutting fingernails and toenails, and not using excessive force to blow the nose. Guidelines used at The Johns Hopkins Oncology Center are listed in Table 25–6.

Nutrition and activity are concerns during the period of myelosuppression. Owing to mucositis, anorexia, and malaise, eating becomes difficult. Severe throat pain and persistent nausea contribute. Eating becomes a task rather than a pleasure. Women are encouraged to eat and drink whenever possible but are not forced to do so. When a woman is unable to meet her caloric needs, hyperalimentation is used. A nutritionist evaluates each woman daily to determine when hyperalimentation should begin.

Activity is an integral part of recovery. A physical therapist can help motivate women to take regular walks and engage in other mild forms of activity. Patients are encouraged to stay out of bed as much as possible during the daytime, to promote a sense of well-being (Table 25–7).

Engraftment of the bone marrow starts around day 14. When the white cell count reaches 1000 or greater with an absolute neutrophil count greater than 50%, the patient is weaned from antibiotics. If amphotericin is being used for

Table 25–5. ORGAN TOXICITY ASSOCIATED WTIH HIGH-DOSE ALKYLATING AGENTS

Major Organ	Toxicity	Nursing Interventions
Heart	Hemorrhagic myocarditis	Assess for signs and symptoms: dyspnea, hypotension, fluid retention, tachycardia, and ↓ ECG voltage Manage and maintain monitoring equipment: pulmonary arterial catheters, intra-aortic balloon pump, arterial lines Administer and titrate inotropics, antiarrhythmics Monitor fluid status during diuresis: strict intake and outputs, continuous blood pressure, electrolyte balances, central venous pressure/mean arterial pressure/carbon monoxide readings Support respiratory effort: oxygen saturation monitoring
Lung	ARDS	Assess for signs and symptoms: increasing dyspnea, development of wet cough, fluid retention, labile blood pressure, refractory hypoxemia, and respiratory acidosis Assess for presence of ARDS exclusions: left ventricular heart failure, underlying lung disease Respiratory support and management: oxygen administration, ventilator support, arterial blood gases, frequent suctioning, oxygen saturation monitoring, chest radiographs Monitor and treat cardiac changes Fluid management: diuretics, strict intake and outputs, maintain intravascular circulation, weight (tid), electrolyte balances, renal function Monitor for development of infection: maintain sterile procedures, sputum cultures, chest radiographs Control symptoms of pulmonary bleeding Provide adequate sedation, analgesic relief, and emotional support
Urinary system	Hemorrhagic cystitis	Assess for signs and symptoms: hematuria, dysuria, continuous bladder irrigation to remove blood clots Administer blood products: platelets for clotting factors, pRBCs and plasma as volume expanders and to support the hematocrit Pain control for bleeding and cramping Monitor for infection
	Nephrotoxicity	Assess for signs and symptoms: serum creatinine > 1.8 mg/dL, oliguria, and fluid retention Administer IV fluids while maintaining strict intake and outputs Monitor renal status: serum creatinine, creatinine clearance, blood urea nitrogen and other electrolytes Monitor drug toxicity levels: aminoglycosides, amphotericin Assist with dialysis as needed for renal failure
Liver	Veno-occlusive disease	Assess for signs and symptoms: hyperbilirubinemia (> 5.0 mg/dL), ascites, and hepatomegaly Minimize drugs metabolized by the liver as much as possible Fluid management: sodium and free water restrictions, antibiotics and other drugs in minimal fluid, strict intake and outputs, diuresis, and abdominal girth and weight measurements Manage pain symptoms Monitor bilirubin levels
Gastrointestinal tract	Mucositis/esophagitis	Assess for severity of mucosal breakdown: Grade I–IV Administer medicines to help prevent or treat infection as ordered Culture all open lesions for surveillance Manage pain symptoms: topical anesthetics, iced saline rinses, and oral/intravenous narcotics Consider hyperalimentation for nutritional support Frequent mouth care especially after bouts of emesis
	Persistent nausea and vomiting/diarrhea	Help develop an antiemetic schedule that provides acceptable relief Monitor for development of dehydration and administer IV fluids to control volume Monitor electrolyte balances Culture stool per routine and as ordered; administer antidiarrheals as acceptable Encourage sitz baths after each loose stool Consider hyperalimentaiton for nutritional support
Skin	Skin rash	Assess for severity of involvement: percentage of body area affected, macular/papular presentation and level of patient discomfort Skin biopsy care to prevent infection Manage patient discomfort: antipruritics, menthol lotions, cool baths and antiinfective creams/powder as ordered

Hematopoietic system	Myelosuppression	Monitor daily blood counts:
		1. Anemia
		  • Transfuse pRBCs to maintain hematocrit above 28%
		  • Assess for symptoms of weakness, malaise, and shortness of breath
		2. Leukopenia
		  • Support aplastic period through infection prevention guidelines
		  • Trend absolute neutrophil count as bone marrow engrafts
		3. Thrombocytopenia
		  • Transfuse platelets to maintain count above 20 K or to control active bleeding
		  • Educate patients about bleeding precautions

Table 25–6. MANAGEMENT OF THE IMMUNOCOMPROMISED PATIENT

Indications
 When WBC count is below 1000 or neutrophil count below 500
 Receiving steroids at ≥ 1.5 mg/kg/day, antithymocyte globulin, Xomazyme, or cyclosporin A
  equivalent to 5 mg/IV/kg/day

Responsibility
 Physician will order complete blood count and differential as indicated.
 No fresh flowers, plants or plant material in patients' rooms.
 Visitors check with nurse if they have been exposed to any illnesses recently.
 Patients wear mask when leaving room.
 Physician will order cultures, including surveillance cultures, on solid tumor units.
 All staff and visitors wash hands upon entering and leaving patient's room.

Assessment
 WBCs and differential.
 Temperature q 4 hours.
 Potential areas for infection, qd
  Bone marrow aspirate and biopsy sites
  Mucous membranes
  Rectal area
  Genital area
  Groin
  Axilla
  Venipuncture sites/central venous line sites
  Skin integrity

Interventions
 Change all dressings at least qd unless otherwise noted by physician.
  Tegaderm dressings on Hickmans to be changed q4d.
 Surveillance cultures per routine.
  Tuesday and Friday or Monday and Thursday
 Culture any new or suspected infected lesion for bacteria and fungi.
 Any new onset or discolored secretions should be sent to bacteriology and mycology
  laboratories.
 Post "Immunocompromised Patient" card in front of room.
 Ensure daily hygiene.

Reportable Conditions
 Any new lesions or areas that appear reddened
 Discharge from any area
 Fever
 Hypotension
 Rigors, chills
 Cough, productive or dry

Documentation
See Also
 Standards of care for:
 • Altered body temperature
 • Altered mucous membranes
 • Impaired skin integrity
 • Impaired tissue integrity
 • Potentially impaired skin integrity
 • Potential for infection

resistant forms of *Candida* organisms, it is continued until the full course is completed. As treatment-related side effects resolve, women begin to eat and drink normally and are able to meet nutritional requirements without hyperalimentation. Daily platelet transfusions for thrombocytopenia are commonly required. Women are taught how to perform daily VAD dressing changes and how to flush the catheter with heparin solution. Return demonstrations and written instructions are used to reinforce instructions. The woman or a designated family member must be competent to do these things. Nutrition, activity, infection control measures, and what to expect during future visits are addressed. Family members are included as much as possible.

Follow-up lasts until care can be provided by the patient's own oncologist. At outpatient visits, blood specimens are obtained to monitor counts, electrolytes, and chemistry values. Chest radiography or scintigraphy may be needed. A physical examination is done to assess continued recovery. The woman may need blood product transfusions and electrolyte supplements. Coordination of care among inpatient and ambulatory nurses is critical for a smooth recovery.

Chemomodulators and growth factors are changing how ABMT patients respond to intensified chemotherapy. Novobiocin may enhance the effects of chemotherapy, so that intensification can be decreased, thus lessening organ toxicity. These drugs are not without their own side effects, however, and they may potentiate organ toxicity already induced by chemotherapy.

The use of peripheral blood progenitor cells (PBPCs) offers certain advantages in the transplant process. Many women with metastases have invasion of bone marrow. As

Table 25–7. ACTIVITY/EXERCISE GUIDELINES FOR ABMT PATIENTS

1. The following restrictions are based on varying levels of thrombocytopenia typically seen in transplant patients.
   - Platelet count ≤ 10 K: patient must have doctor's order for activity level
   - Platelet count 11–20 K: patient may ambulate (do "laps") in the hallways on her nursing floor or may leave the unit to go to a specified area accompanied by a staff person; no active PT, unless otherwise ordered by physician
   - Platelet count 21–30 K: patient may perform active ROM exercises and ambulate (do "laps"), unless otherwise ordered by physician
   - Platelet count 30–50 K: patient may do active ROM exercises, low-resistance stationary biking, aerobic bench steps; no resistive exercises, unless otherwise ordered by physician
   - Platelet count ≥ 50 K: patient may do restrictive activities (i.e., therabands, isotonic exercises, hand weights) and stationary biking with more resistance, unless otherwise ordered by physician

2. There may be other times when activity/exercise level may be restricted because of medications or treatments.

PBPCs do not contain marrow, the risk of transplanting tumor is minimal. Grafting is faster than with the use of bone marrow and is equally effective (Elias et al., 1991).

Nurses are continually challenged to provide comprehensive care for women undergoing ABMT. Management of symptoms, restoration of wellness, enhancement of quality of life, and education of patients and their families continue to be nurses' primary concerns. The focus continues to be on improving care, minimizing treatment-related side effects, and optimizing the benefit of ABMT.

RADIATION THERAPY

Radiation therapy may be the primary treatment for early or for advanced, inoperable breast cancer. It is also used to control chest wall recurrence. It must be emphasized that the choice between mastectomy and lumpectomy with radiation therapy for early-stage breast cancer is a personal choice for each woman after she learns the advantages and disadvantages of each. In the decision-making process the woman confronts her personal values (Valanis and Rumpler, 1985). She should not be rushed into making this decision. Furthermore, she should receive whatever support is required, including antianxiety medications if needed, to enable her decision.

Radiation therapy is essential to breast conservation, but the course can be long and tedious. As the primary treatment, radiation therapy is usually given five times a week for 5 weeks (5000 cGy) with a radioactive implant or electron boost of 2000 cGy (Wilson and Strohl, 1982). Nursing interventions are designed to (1) minimize the side effects of radiotherapy, (2) contribute to the patient's safety, (3) maintain an adequate nutritional status, (4) promote comfort, and (5) provide patient and family with emotional support. The most common side effects of radiation therapy are skin changes and fatigue. Less frequent ones are pneumonitis, pleural effusion, rib fracture, and lymphedema.

Information about treatment, side-effects, and self-care measures afford women a greater sense of control over what is happening to them (Dodd, 1988) (Table 25–8). The National Institutes of Health publication *Radiation Therapy: A Treatment for Early-Stage Breast Cancer* (NIH Publication No. 84–659, March, 1984) is an excellent resource, as is the ACS publication *Reach to Recovery, Breast Pres-*

Table 25–8. PATIENT'S SELF-CARE GUIDE FOR RADIATION THERAPY

Skin Care

We expect your skin to react to radiation in one of two ways. You will have either:
1. A "dry" reaction, characterized by red, dry skin with some flaking or cracking, *or*
2. A "wet" reaction, characterized by red, tender skin with areas that look like broken blisters.
   Skin reactions are *not* burns. They are the normal effects of radiation. Let your doctor or nurse know when you begin to notice a skin reaction. We will want to watch it. Look carefully for reactions in folds of skin, such as on the neck or under the breasts. *Skin reactions are temporary* and should clear within 6 to 8 weeks after your treatment.

If you have a dry skin reaction, you should take the following steps:
1. Keep the area clean.
2. Wash the area at least once daily with water and a mild oil-based soap such as Caress or Dove. Avoid strong deodorant soaps such as Dial. Be sure to rinse off the soap well.
3. Apply hydrolyzed lanolin or Aquaphor to dry skin several times a day to provide moisture and prevent cracking. Do *not* apply any lotion 30 minutes before your treatments.
4. Report flaking or cracking of the skin to the doctor or nurse. If the skin is cracked or becomes raw, do not apply lotions as this will irritate the area.

If you have a wet skin reaction, you should take the following steps:
1. Keep the area clean.
2. Wash the area at least three times a day with hydrogen peroxide that has been diluted with an equal amount of water.
3. Use a soft cloth for washing the skin. *Do not* use dry cotton balls on "weeping" areas, as they stick to skin. *Do not* rub or scrub. *Do not* pat or blot skin.
4. To dry the skin, leave the area open to the air as much as possible.
5. Wear only clean, soft cotton clothing over the affected area. Avoid synthetic fabrics as they trap moisture and increase irritation. Men's loose-fitting cotton tee shirts are especially comfortable.

Remember

Continue proper skin care after you have completed your treatment. For some people, skin reactions are greatest the first week or two following the *completion* of treatments. Do not be alarmed if this happens to you. Be sure to let your doctor or nurse know if you have questions or problems.

ervation/Radiation Therapy, A Patient Guide. As they are likely to be unfamiliar with radiation therapy equipment, women should be prepared for what they will see, hear, and feel during the treatment. They are told that the arm on the treated side will be raised during simulation and treatment and that this position may be uncomfortable. They must be assured that they are constantly observed and that assistance is available as needed.

Misconceptions about radiation burns and ''personal radioactivity'' must be dispelled (Fig. 25–1). General information may be provided in a group session and individual teaching for aspects peculiar to each patient's treatment. The use of printed and audiovisual materials enhances learning. The video *Radiation Therapy: An Option for Early Breast Cancer,* by Lange Productions is recommended (7661 Curson Terrace, Hollywood, CA 90046, telephone 213-874-0132).

Proper skin care is important. Skin integrity may be maintained by gently washing it with mild soap and applying a thin layer of hydrolyzed lanolin or an aloe-based product. Viscous lotions or creams, including deodorants, are not applied to the irradiated area. Constricting clothing, such as a tight bra strap, should not be worn. Patients are instructed not to expose irradiated areas to direct sunlight or sun lamps and to avoid tanning salons. They are not to apply ice, a heating pad, or an electric blanket, lest they injure the skin. Each patient should be provided printed instructions for skin care (Strohl, 1988).

Although radiation therapy frequently causes fatigue, most women are able to work and perform daily activities during the course of treatment. Some patients may require assistance in planning their work schedule and other activities to diminish the negative impact of fatigue on their lives. The treatment process is time consuming, though for each daily treatment the beam is actually on less than 3 minutes.

Irradiation of the lungs may cause pneumonitis with acute inflammatory changes, congestion, exudate, and infiltration. Dry, persistent cough and exertional dyspnea last for 4 to 6 weeks (Wilson et al., 1982). Fibrotic changes are permanent. Good pulmonary hygiene, adequate hydration, and humidification are valuable in controlling these side effects. Nurses should be alert for symptoms and should notify a physician if a patient develops dyspnea, restlessness, or cough.

A larger dose of radiation is often given to the lumpectomy area with an electron boost or interstitial implant. Boosts with electron beams from a linear accelerator are used to deliver approximately 1600 rad, usually over a period of 8 days. Interstitial implants of iridium ribbons are used to boost the radiation dose to a larger volume of breast tissue or when a larger dose is required to the tumor bed. Women usually experience only minor discomfort during this procedure. Potential side effects are arm edema (for 4% to 7% of patients) and rib fracture (for 1% to 5%) (Hassey, 1985; and McCarthy, 1987).

Women should be informed that it is possible to become pregnant and have normal, healthy children after receiving radiation therapy. Although it is recommended that a woman wait 2 years after primary breast radiation before becoming pregnant, a pregnancy before that does not generally require termination. Breast feeding is also possible following radiation therapy. If lactation occurs in the treated breast, and often it does not, the woman is usually instructed to nurse only with the nonirradiated breast. This precaution is taken to reduce the risk of mastitis in the irradiated breast, which is difficult to treat (Hassey, 1988).

Radiation therapy is often the treatment for oncologic emergencies caused by breast cancer, among them spinal cord compression, brain metastases, and bony metastases. It is important for the patient and family to know that it may take several radiation treatments to relieve the pain and that complete relief may not come until as long as 2 weeks following treatment. Patients with skeletal metastases are susceptible to pathologic fracture of involved bones. Nurses should be aware of this susceptibility and take precautions when moving the patient and when providing routine patient care. When a pathologic fracture is sus-

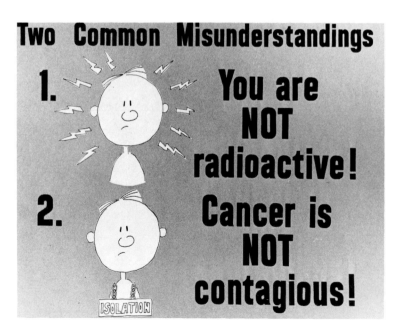

Figure 25–1. Selected page from a radiation therapy flip chart used in group teaching sessions.

pected, the patient's physician is notified at once and the suspected fracture is splinted. When the fractures involve long bones they frequently require prompt internal fixation. When weight-bearing bones are threatened, appropriately placed supports, braces, and bedboards may be indicated. Patients may be confined to bed or a wheelchair or need to use a cane or walker to decrease the possibility of fracture. Nurses can help patients understand the need for these measures. Active and passive exercises can be performed within limits. The patient is instructed not to lift heavy objects or to climb onto ladders or chairs. Carrying heavy grocery sacks or pushing a heavy vacuum cleaner are likewise avoided.

Multiple bony metastases from breast cancer can be treated with IV strontium 89. This pure beta radioisotope is given to the woman on an outpatient basis and requires very few radiation safety precautions. Patients may experience a great deal of pain from osseous metastases. Analgesics should be administered regularly and without hesitation. Nonsteroidal anti-inflammatory agents are often effective in relieving pain and discomfort. As the radiation begins to take effect, pain will decrease, as will the need for medication.

Metastases in the brain are treated with radiation therapy. The patient and her family need consistent support and reassurance during this time. Benefits may not be appreciable until several weeks after completion of treatment; however, dexamethasone (Decadron) at the outset can relieve symptoms quickly. Temporary alopecia is expected, usually in 2 weeks, and the patient and her family should be prepared for this. Information about wigs, turbans, and scarves should be provided. If the woman's memory is impaired, nurses should repeat instructions and formulate questions so that they can be answered easily. Patients with visual disturbances require a structured environment that provides a sense of security. The patient and her family need reassurance to help them deal effectively with behavioral and physical changes.

PSYCHOLOGIC ISSUES

The majority of women cope effectively with breast cancer and its sequelae. There are, however, unique aspects of adjustment related to each stage. The results of psychosocial research are a valuable guide for timely and appropriate nursing interventions.

Premorbid Factors

Premorbid factors that influence the response to breast cancer include age, personality, coping history, psychiatric history, experience with breast cancer, and social support. For example, the older woman with breast cancer may recognize cancer as a threat to life yet cope effectively. The younger woman is distressed by the threat to her body image and sexuality (Sinsheimer and Holland, 1987). The nurse's role is to determine a woman's reaction to her illness and provide a favorable influence.

Diagnosis

The time of diagnosis is one of anxiety and uncertainty. Anxiety and a deluge of information may compromise the ability of women to make decisions (Scott, 1983). Repeating information that cannot be assimilated immediately and helping to clarify choices all reduce anxiety.

Treatment Choice

Most studies that address the choice of mastectomy or lumpectomy with radiation therapy indicate no major differences between the two treatment options in terms of psychological morbidity (Kemeny et al., 1988; Maunsell et al., 1988; Holmberg et al., 1989; Wellisch et al., 1989; Fallowfield et al., 1990; and Ganz et al., 1992). This includes measures of anxiety, depression, sexual dysfunction, quality of life, mood disturbance, and social adjustment; however, women who choose lumpectomy enjoy a more intact and positive body image (Kemeny et al., 1988; Wellisch et al., 1989; and Ganz et al., 1992). Nurses who work with patients grappling with this decision can support whatever decision patients make, knowing that, psychologically, the outcomes are similar. Effective educational tools, such as the Breast Cancer Information Test-Revised (BCIT-R; Ward and Griffin, 1990), are important guides on this issue (Wainstock, 1991). After the treatment decision is made the nurse can focus on the anxiety related to a potentially life-threatening illness and address these fears collaboratively with the physician.

Mastectomy

The most obvious alteration of body image occurs in women who undergo mastectomy. This treatment may also affect psychological, sexual, and social adjustment for a limited time (Jones and Reznikoff, 1989). The nurse must quickly establish a therapeutic relationship and emphasize strengths and abilities that are not changed by the surgery. The spouse or partner is an important part of these discussions and should be encouraged to see the scar. Sexual activity may be resumed as soon as both are comfortable with it (Carroll, 1981). Referral to Reach to Recovery, an ACS volunteer organization for peer support, is often initiated at this time.

A decision about breast reconstruction is made at some point after mastectomy (Schain, 1985). Patient satisfaction is generally high after reconstruction (Stevens et al., 1984; Daniels, 1985; and Schain et al., 1985), which is viewed as an adaptive coping strategy. Issues such as timing of reconstruction and its impact on self-image are appropriate for discussion.

Radiation Therapy and Lumpectomy

A sensitive nursing approach makes bearable a long course of radiation therapy (some weeks) and its side effects

(Hughson et al., 1987). Being available as a consistent resource and not underestimating the emotional distress of treatment are paramount. Relaxation and imagery exercises can ease some of the anxiety and depression associated with radiation therapy (Bridge et al., 1982).

Adjuvant Chemotherapy

Adjuvant chemotherapy has its own psychological repercussions. The side effects, which include nausea and vomiting, alopecia, and weight gain, interfere with body image and well-being. Relaxation therapy, imagery, and hypnosis can be suggested as means of improving a sense of control over nausea. Nutritional counseling is another option for patients for whom weight gain is distressing (Knobf et al., 1983).

Schover (1991) proposes that chemotherapy-induced menopause is an under-recognized problem. Specific sexual concerns include vaginal dryness and reduced libido. The P-LI-SS-IT counseling model (Annon, 1974) may be used to initiate discussion of sexual issues. First, *P*ermission is given to the patient to broach the topic of sexual concerns. *L*imited *I*nformation, the next step, involves providing generalized, pertinent information. *S*pecific *S*uggestions, such as hugging, oral stimulation, fondling, caressing, and *I*ntensive *T*herapy may be offered as higher level interventions that maintain sexual intimacy. Discussions should include the partner, and the nurse must not assume that older women with breast cancer are not interested in resuming sexual intimacy.

Recurrence

Though few studies specifically address patients with recurrence, recurrence may be even more stressful than the initial cancer (Cella et al., 1990; and Mahon et al., 1990). The anxiety and depression, if accompanied by social withdrawal, loss of pleasure, hopelessness, or suicidal ideation, may require referral to a mental health professional (Jenkins et al., 1991).

Advanced Disease

The patient with advanced breast cancer is necessarily consumed with management of symptoms, but her concern about significant others contributes to her distress. Helping patients plan beyond death is a crucial role of nurses. Meaning and a sense of purpose are also important. Patients with advanced cancer may be less anxious and have higher self-esteem when they derive some meaning and purpose from their lives (Lewis, 1989). Support groups are one way of achieving a sense of purpose. Participants not only obtain support and validation of feelings but can help others in similar circumstances.

Coping

Adjustment is enhanced by a working knowledge of coping strategies. Keeping patients well-informed about resources and changes in their status increases their sense of control. Recent research suggests that emotional control, fatalism, helplessness, and psychological morbidity are linked (Watson et al., 1991). Cognitive strategies that address pain or stress, such as relaxation therapy and diversion, help cope with illness (Spiegel, 1990). Denial, when it does not interfere with function, and positive attitudes foster adaptation to uncertain circumstances (Greer et al., 1990).

Support groups expand social support and improve the ability to cope. Referral by a nurse provides an entry point for many patients. Information about support groups may be found through local chapters of the ACS or through regional cancer centers.

Social Support: Family

Sources of social support for the woman with breast cancer are her partner, her family, and her friends. Roles and family relationships change as a woman is diagnosed and treated. Northouse (1990) found that husbands of women with breast cancer were as emotionally distressed as their wives, underscoring the necessity for family-focused care. Children of mothers with breast cancer cope differently according to their age; younger children primarily fear the mother's death. One of the most telling questions to pose to families is whether children are pursuing routine activities (Issel et al., 1990). Daughters of breast cancer patients are understandably fearful about developing the disease (Kash et al., 1992). The nurse who has previously discussed risk factors may well address these concerns.

Nursing Staff Concerns

While nurses have many opportunities to influence psychological adaptation to breast cancer and its treatment, working with breast cancer patients also affects nurses. Often, the circumstances of the typical patient are similar to the nurse's (i.e., age, children, sexual concerns, femininity issues). This identification can produce reactions ranging from overinvolvement to deliberate distancing. Being aware of these personal feelings and of the need to manage them promotes a healthy, caring relationship between nurse and patient.

References

Affronti, M., Vanacek, K., and Peters, W. Autologous bone marrow transplant for the treatment of advanced breast cancer. Innov. Oncol. Nurs., 6:2–6, 19–21, 1990.

Annon, J. S.: The Behavioral Treatment of Sexual Problems. Honolulu, Mercantile Printing, 1974.

Antman, K., Ayash, L., Elias, A., et al.: A phase II study of high dose cyclophosphamide, thiotepa and carboplatin with autologous marrow support in women with measurable advanced breast cancer responding to standard-dose therapy. J. Clin. Oncol., 10:102–110, 1992.

Ballard, B.: (1991) Renal and hepatic compilations. *In* Whedon, M. (Ed.): *Bone Marrow Transplantation; Principles, Practice and Nursing Insights.* Boston, Jones and Bartlett, 1991, p. 252.

Bonadonna, G., and Vulagussa, P.: Adjuvant systemic therapy for resectable breast cancer. J. Clin. Oncol., 3:259–272, 1985.

Bosserman, G., McGuire, D., McGuire, W., et al.: Multidisciplinary management of vascular access devices. Oncol. Nurs. Forum, *17*:879–886, 1990.

Brandt, B.: Informational needs and selected variables in patients receiving brachytherapy. Oncol. Nurs. Forum, *18*:1221–1238, 1991.

Bridge, L., Benson, P., Pietroni, P., et al.: Relaxation and imagery in the treatment of breast cancer. Br. Med. J., *297*:1169–1172, 1982.

Bucholtz, J.: Radiation Therapy. *In* Ziegfeld, C. (Ed.): Core Curriculum for Oncology Nursing. Philadelphia, W. B. Saunders, 1987, p. 207–225.

Bucholtz, J. Implications of radiation therapy for nursing. *In* Clark, J., and McGee, R. (Eds.): Core Curriculum in Oncology Nursing. Philadelphia, W. B. Saunders, 1992, p. 319–328.

Carroll, R.: The impact of mastectomy on body image. Oncol. Nurs. Forum, *8*:29–32, 1981.

Cella, D. F., Mahon, S., and Donovan, M.: Cancer recurrence as a traumatic event. Behav. Med., *16*:15–22, 1990.

Champion, V.: Attitudinal variables related to intention, frequency, and proficiency of breast self-examination. Res. Nurs. Health, *11*:583–591, 1988.

Cloak, M., Connor, T., Stevens, K. et al.: Occupational exposure of nursing personnel to antineoplastic agents. Oncology Nursing Forum. *12*:33, 1985.

Daniels, E.: Breast reconstruction postmastectomy: A psychosocial study. Dissertation Abstracts International, *46*:1741B, 1985.

Davidson, N., and Abeloff, M.: Adjuvant systemic therapy in women with early stage breast cancer at high risk for relapse. J. Natl. Cancer Inst., *84*:301–304, 1992.

Dodd, M.: Patterns of self care in patients with breast cancer. West. J. Nurs. *10*:7–24, 1988.

Dow, K., and Hiderley, L. (Eds.): Nursing Care in Radiation Oncology. Philadelphia, W. B. Saunders, 1992.

Ehlke, G.: Symptom distress in breast cancer patients receiving chemotherapy in the outpatient setting. Oncol. Nurs. Forum, *15*:343–346, 1988.

Elias, A., Mazanet, R., Wheeler, C., et al.: Peripheral blood progenitor cells (PBPC): Two protocols using GM-CSF potentiated progenitor cell collection. *In* Dicke, K. A., and Armitage, I. (Eds.): Autologous Bone Marrow Transplantation–Proceedings of the International Symposium, 1991. Omaha, NE, University of Nebraska Medical Center, 1991.

Esparza, D.: Cancer prevention: implications for ethnic and racial minorities. Family Community Health, *11*:62–66, 1987.

Fallowfield, L., Hall, A., Maguire, G., et al.: Psychological outcomes of different treatment policies in women with early breast cancer outside a clinical trial. Br. Med. J., *301*:575–580, 1990.

Feather, B., and Lanigan, C.: The mastectome, her clothing and self-image. Unpublished Manuscript. The University of Missouri, 1985.

Fetting, J.: The Johns Hopkins Oncology Center. Personal Communication, 1994.

Fisher, F., Constantino, J., Redmond, C., et al.: Lumpectomy compared with lumpectomy and radiation therapy. N. Engl. J. Med., *328*:1581–1586, 1993.

Frei, E. III, Antman, K., Teicher, B., et al.: Bone marrow autotransplantation for solid tumors—prospects. J. Clin. Oncol., *7*:515–526, 1989.

Ganz, P., Schag, A., Lee, J., et al.: Breast conservation versus mastectomy: Is there a difference in psychological adjustment or quality of life in the year after surgery? Cancer, *69*:1729–1738, 1992.

Goodman, M.: Adjuvant systemic therapy of stage I and II breast cancer. Semin. Oncol. Nurs., *7*:175–186, 1991.

Grandt, N.: Hepatic veno-occlusive disease following bone marrow transplantation. Oncol. Nurs. Forum, *16*:813–817, 1989.

Greer, S., Morris, T., Pettingale, K., et al.: Psychological response to breast cancer and 15-year outcome. Lancet, *335*:49, 1990.

Hassey-Dow, K.: Breast cancer and fertility. NAACOG, Clinical Issues in Perinatal and Women's Health Nursing. *1*:444–452, 1990.

Hassey, K.: Demystifying care of patients with radioactive implants. Am. J. Nurs., *85*:788–792, 1985.

Hassey, K.: Pregnancy and parenthood after treatment for breast cancer. Oncol. Nurs. Forum, *15*:439–447, 1988.

Hassey, K.: Principles of radiation safety and protection. Semin. Oncol. Nurs., *3*:23–29, 1987.

Heland, K.: Breast cancer claims: The coming storm. OBG Management, *12*:19–33, 1991.

Hilderley, L.: Radiotherapy. *In* Groenwald, S., Frogge, M., Yarbro, C., et al. (Eds.): Cancer Nursing: Principles and Practice. Boston, Jones and Barlett, 1990, pp. 199–230.

Hillner, B., Smith, T., and Desch, C.: Efficacy and cost effectiveness of autologous bone marrow transplantation in metastatic breast cancer. J.A.M.A., *267*:2055–2061, 1992.

Holmberg, L., Omne-Ponten, M., Burns, T., et al.: Psychosocial adjustment after mastectomy and breast-conserving treatment. Cancer, *64*:969–974, 1989.

Hughson, A., Cooper, A., McArdle, C., et al.: Psychosocial effects of radiotherapy after mastectomy. Br. Med. J., *294*:1515–1518, 1987.

Issel, L., Ersek, M., and Lewis, F.: How children cope with mother's breast cancer. Oncol. Nurs. Forum, (Suppl.) *17*:5–13, 1990.

Iwamoto, R.: Radiation therapy. *In* Baird, S. (Ed.): A Cancer Source Book for Nurses. Atlanta, The American Cancer Society, 1991, pp. 63–72.

Jenkins, P., May, V., and Hughes, L.: Psychological morbidity associated with local recurrence of breast cancer. Int. J. Psychosoc. Med., *21*:149–159, 1991.

Jones, D., and Reznikoff, M.: Psychosocial adjustment to a mastectomy. J. Nervous Mental Dis., *177*:624–631, 1989.

Jones, R., Lee, K., Beschorner, W., et al.: Venooclusive disease of the liver following bone marrow transplantation. Transplantation, *44*:778–783, 1987.

Jordan, L., and Mantravandi, R.: Nursing care of the patient receiving high dose rate brachytherapy. Oncol. Nurs. Forum, *18*:1167–1174, 1235–1238, 1991.

Kash, K., Holland, J., Halper, M., et al.: Psychological distress and surveillance behaviors of women with a family history of breast cancer. J. Natl. Cancer Inst., *84*:24–30, 1992.

Kemeny, M., Wellisch, D., and Schain, W.: Psychosocial outcome in a randomized surgical trial for treatment of primary breast cancer. Cancer, *62*:1231–1237, 1988.

Kennedy, M., Beveridge, R., Rowley, S., et al.: High-dose chemotherapy with reinfusion of purged autologous bone marrow following dose-intense inductions as initial therapy for metastatic breast cancer. J. Natl. Cancer Inst., *83*:920–926, 1991.

Knobf, M.: Physical and psychologic distress associated with adjuvant chemotherapy in women with breast cancer. J. Clin. Oncol., *4*:678–684, 1986.

Knobf, M.: Primary breast cancer: Physical consequences and rehabilitation. Semin. Oncol. Nurs., *1*:214, 1985.

Knobf, M., Mullen, J., Xistris, D., et al.: Weight gain in women with breast cancer receiving adjuvant chemotherapy. Oncol. Nurs. Forum, *10*:28–33, 1983.

Lauver, D.: Theoretical perspectives relevant to breast self-examination. Advanced Nurs. Sci., *9*:16–24, 1987.

Lazovich, D., White, E., Thomas, D., et al.: Underutilization of breast conserving surgery and radiation therapy among women with stage I or II breast cancer. J.A.M.A., *266*:3433–3438, 1991.

Lewis, F. M.: Attributions of control, experienced meaning, and psychosocial well-being in patients with advanced cancer. J. Psychosoc. Oncol. *7*:105, 1989.

Ludwick, R.: Breast examination in the older adult. Cancer Nurs., *11*:99–102, 1988.

Mahon, S., Cella, D., and Donovan, M.: Psychosocial adjustment to recurrent cancer. Oncol. Nurs. Forum, *17*(Suppl.):47–54, 1990.

Maunsell, E., Brisson, J., and Deschenes, L.: Psychological distress after initial treatment for breast cancer: A comparison of partial and total mastectomy. J. Clin. Epidemiol., *42*:765–771, 1989.

McCarthy, C.: The role of interstitial implantation in the treatment of primary breast cancer. Semin. Oncol. Nurs., *3*:47–53, 1987.

McFadden, J.: Breast prostheses lessen trauma of mastectomies. Proc. Ellis Fischel Cancer Center, *3*:3, 1985.

Nickens, H.: Health promotion and disease prevention among minorities. Health Affairs, *3*:133–143, 1990.

Northouse, L.: A longitudinal study of the adjustment of patients and husbands to breast cancer. Oncol. Nurs. Forum, *17*(Suppl.):39–45, 1990.

Schain, W.: Breast reconstruction: Update of psychosocial and pragmatic concerns. Cancer, *68*(Suppl):1170–1175, 1990.

Schain, W., Wellisch, D., Pasnau, R., et al.: The sooner, the better: A study of psychological factors in women undergoing immediate versus delayed breast reconstruction. Am. J. Psychiatry, *142*:40–46, 1985.

Schover, L.: The impact of breast cancer on sexuality, body image, and intimate relationships. CA, *41*:112–120, 1991.

Scott, D.: Anxiety, critical thinking and information processing during and after breast biopsy. Nurs. Res., *32*:24–28, 1983.

Senie, R., Rosen, P., Rhodes, P., et al.: Timing of breast cancer excision during the menstrual cycle influences duration of disease-free survival. Ann. Intern. Med., *115*:337–342, 1991.

Sinsheimer, L., and Holland, J.: Psychological issues in breast cancer. Semin. Oncol., *14*:75–82, 1987.

Sitton, E.: Early and late radiation-induced skin alterations. Part II: Nursing care of irradiated skin. Oncol. Nurs. Forum, *19*:907–912, 1992.

Sledge, G. W. Jr., and Antman, K. H.: Progress in chemotherapy for metastatic breast cancer. Semin. Oncol., *19*:327, 1992.

Spiegel, D.: Facilitating emotional coping during treatment. Cancer, *66*:1422–1446, 1990.

Spiegel, D., Bloom, J., Kraemer, H., et al.: Effect of psychosocial treatment on survival of patients with metastatic breast cancer. Lancet, *ii*:888–891, 1989.

Stevens, L., McGrath, M., Druss, R., et al.: The psychological impact of immediate breast reconstruction for women with early breast cancer. Plastic Reconstruct. Surg., *73*:619–628, 1984.

Strohl, R.: The nursing role in radiation oncology: symptom management of acute and chronic reactions. Oncol. Nurs. Forum, *15*:429–434, 1988.

Valanis, B., and Rumpler, C.: Helping women to choose breast cancer treatment alternatives. Cancer Nurs., *8*:167, 1985.

Wainstock, J.: Breast cancer: Psychosocial consequences for the patient. Semin. Oncol. Nurs., *7*:207–215, 1991.

Ward, S., and Griffin, J.: Developing a test of knowledge of surgical options for breast cancer. Cancer Nurs., *13*:191, 1990.

Watkins-Bruner, D. (Ed.): Manual for Radiation Oncology Nursing Practice and Education. Pittsburgh, The Oncology Nursing Society, 1990.

Watson, M., Greer, S., Rowden, L., et al.: Relationships between emotional control, adjustment to cancer and depression and anxiety in breast cancer patients. Psychol. Med., *211*:51, 1991.

Watson, P.: Patient education: The adult with cancer. Nursing Clin. North Am., *17*:739, 1982.

Wellisch, D., DeMatteo, R., Silverstein, M., et al.: Psychosocial outcomes of breast cancer therapies: Lumpectomy versus mastectomy. Psychosomatics, *30*:165, 1989.

Wilson, C. A., and Strohl, R. A.: Radiation therapy as primary treament for breast cancer. Oncol. Nurs. Forum, *9*:12–15, 1982.

Yasko, J.: Care of the Client Receiving External Radiation Therapy. Reston, Va.: Reston Publishing Company, 1982.

26 Breast Reconstruction

Christian Paletta
Maurice J. Jurkiewicz

Reconstruction of the female breast, delayed or immediate, after surgical ablation of the organ for cancer has become an increasingly compelling consideration for the patient and her surgeon. Breast reconstruction following mastectomy has undergone tremendous growth in the past 15 years (Goldwyn, 1987). According to data collected by the American Society of Plastic and Reconstructive Surgeons, 42,888 patients underwent postmastectomy breast reconstruction in 1990, an increase of 114% since 1981. Four factors have contributed to this remarkable departure from traditional surgical thinking: (1) departure from traditional radical mastectomy; (2) development of better reconstructive techniques; (3) use of musculocutaneous flaps; and (4) development of tissue expansion techniques. First and most obvious was the switch from the Halsted radical mastectomy to some form of conservative operation. Preservation of the pectoralis major muscle was the first modification; increased flap thickness, the second. Other recent modifications include subtotal surgical mastectomy or tylectomy. Second, and occurring in parallel to the first, has been the development of reconstructive techniques that are reliable and give results that are aesthetically superior to those of previous reconstructive methods.

In the mid-1970s it was learned that skin was nourished, for the most part, by perforating vessels from underlying muscle. This resulted in the third improvement, the development of more modern techniques for myocutaneous flaps, especially the latissimus dorsi myocutaneous flap for breast reconstruction. In 1977, Schneider, Hill, and Brown introduced use of the latissimus dorsi myocutaneous flap as a one-stage procedure for breast reconstruction. This provided a significant advance over previous techniques, which involved either multiple stages with tubed abdominal flaps or inadequate breast mound formation with simple implants. In 1979, Bostwick and colleagues reported their experience with 60 latissimus dorsi flaps, thereby establishing this flap as a reliable and easily performed method for breast reconstruction.

The introduction of the latissimus dorsi flap provided the reconstructive surgeon with an abundance of well-vascularized tissue with which to build and shape a new breast. Experience with the latissimus dorsi flap generated a far superior reconstructive result than was hitherto possible. Publications on new and improved techniques flooded the literature, both lay and professional. At the same time, aesthetic refinements in breast surgery were being developed that became incorporated into breast reconstruction techniques. Advances such as the improvement in design and contour of implantable breast prostheses added signifi-

cantly to the aesthetic reconstructive result. First introduced by Cronin and Gerow in 1963, the ''natural-feel'' silicone (polydimethylsiloxane) prosthesis was a remarkable improvement over previous materials, which included paraffin injections, fat grafts, Ivalon polymer sponges, and silicone injections (Cronin et al., 1977).

In 1991, the silicone breast implant came under increased scrutiny by the Food and Drug Administration (FDA) (Kessler, 1992). It has been estimated that, since their introduction in 1963, between one and two million women have had silicone breast prostheses implanted, 80% for breast augmentation and 20% for breast reconstruction. Concern arose in the late 1980s regarding the safety of silicone breast implants. The primary controversial issues include these: (1) the possibility that the silicone gel implant could interfere with detection of breast disease on mammography and cause a delay in the diagnosis of breast cancer; (2) the possible link between a breast implant and the subsequent development of breast carcinoma or other soft tissue tumors such as sarcomas; (3) the longevity of the implant device; (4) the exact prevalence of silicone gel leakage and its local and systemic effects; and (5) a possible link between silicone and autoimmune disease. Unfortunately, many of the scientific concerns about the safety of silicone breast implants remain unanswered. While there have been many anecdotal reports of untoward reactions to silicone breast implants, retrospective series do not support a significant relationship (Fisher, 1992). A large retrospective review of 11,676 patients who underwent silicone implant breast augmentation failed to find any correlation between silicone implants and the subsequent development of breast cancer (Berkel, et al., 1992). And while the American College of Rheumatology has stated that there is no identifiable link between silicone and autoimmune disease, an antisilicone antibody has recently been identified in two patients with silicone shunts that were implanted for treatment of hydrocephalus (Goldblum et al., 1992).

Following a probing FDA hearing in February 1992, the use of silicone gel implants was restricted, and can be implanted only in patients taking part in an adjunctive study approved by the FDA. Silicone gel implants can no longer be used for breast augmentation, except in a very small number of patients entering into a study group. In order to be a participant in the Adjunct Study for silicone gel implants, a patient must meet certain criteria outlined by the FDA and the two remaining implant manufacturers. In addition, a retrospective breast implant registry has been mandated by the FDA.

The use of saline-filled breast implants has not been

affected by the recent controversy surrounding silicone gel implants. While interference with mammography remains a problem with saline implants, there is less concern about the systemic effect of saline leaked from an implant. There has been an increased use of saline breast implants since restrictions were placed on silicone implants. Though saline implants can provide an adequate alternative to silicone, problems—including the rippled contour of the overlying skin and the long-term deflation rate—need further investigation. Research into local and systemic effects of silicone and saline implants is under way. Several new implant products that use materials such as peanut oil are also being investigated. Whether any of these new products will be approved under the 1976 Medical Device Amendments remains to be seen.

A further milestone was reached in 1980, when Hartrampf performed the first successful reconstruction using the transverse rectus abdominis musculocutaneous (TRAM) flap (Hartrampf et al., 1982). The TRAM flap was an outgrowth of both experimental and clinical research on musculocutaneous flaps. The blood supply of the abdominal wall skin, as well as skin territories throughout the body, were redefined on the basis of a new understanding of perforating vessels from the underlying muscles and fascia. Using this new information, the TRAM flap created a whole new horizon for breast reconstruction. It not only eliminated the need for a foreign silicone prosthesis, but it also provided an abundance of fatty tissue from the lower abdomen for breast reconstruction while recontouring the abdomen with an abdominoplasty (Hartrampf, 1984).

With the development of microsurgery in the 1970s, breast reconstruction can now be performed using the free tissue transfer technique (Grotting et al., 1991). This represents the most complex method of breast reconstruction, but it can be highly successful in experienced hands. This technique can make available breast reconstruction for a patient who otherwise would not be a candidate, owing to implant failure, abdominal scarring, or severe radiation damage to the skin of the chest wall. Flaps used for this type of microsurgical breast reconstruction include (1) the free (TRAM) flap based on the inferior epigastric vessels, (2) the superior or inferior gluteal flap, and (3) the lateral transverse thigh flap based on the lateral femoral circumflex vessels. While this is a more complicated and costly approach, it can provide an excellent breast reconstruction for a patient when other methods have failed or would not yield a satisfactory result.

Finally, the development of tissue expansion techniques has led to yet another dimension in the field of breast reconstruction. First introduced by Radovan in 1976, tissue expanders have become increasingly popular, not only in breast reconstruction but also in many areas that require local tissue transfer (Radovan, 1982, 1984). They have been particularly useful in scalp reconstruction for burns or traumatic alopecia and in the reconstruction of various types of scar deformities. Tissue expansion is remarkable because of both its simplicity and its contribution to an acceptable cosmetic result (Bayet et al., 1991). Recent technological improvements in expanders have led to the development of textured surfaces that can diminish the development of firm capsules. Advances in valve design have also made available permanent expander-implants, which obviate the second surgical procedure to remove the expander and replace it with a permanent implant.

All of these techniques have a role in breast reconstruction. The reconstructive breast surgeon must be familiar and competent with each technique rather than relying solely on one technique for reconstruction of all breasts. This will result in more appropriate matching of a specific technique to a specific defect on each patient desiring reconstruction. For example, the tissue requirements for reconstruction following a Halsted radical mastectomy differ markedly from those following a simple mastectomy or subcutaneous mastectomy. In addition, certain techniques either will not be available or will be contraindicated in selected patients because of prior surgical procedures or preexisting medical illness.

Contributing to the growth in breast reconstruction has been the demand of the public for reconstructive surgery. Arguably as an outgrowth of the feminist movement in the 1960s and 1970s, women have become increasingly outspoken about—and opposed to—operations that involve removing part or all of the breast.

The number of women who develop breast cancer each year is large. The American Cancer Society estimates that, in 1993 182,000 women in the United States were diagnosed with breast cancer. Although the majority of women follow the traditional mode of therapy (i.e., modified radical mastectomy), more women, especially young women, are demanding alternative, more conservative treatment. There are essentially three reasons that women with breast cancer are choosing breast-conserving treatment. First, more breast cancers are being detected at an earlier stage, making the tumor amenable to less aggressive management. Second, randomized control studies have revealed that breast-conserving surgery followed by radiation can be as efficacious as modified radical mastectomy in terms of survival and local control of the disease. Last, the social structure of American society has changed, and the majority of women are in the workplace and would prefer a less disfiguring alternative to mastectomy.

An increasing number of women who have undergone mastectomy are seeking reconstruction. Though it is not requested by the majority of patients who undergo mastectomy, breast reconstruction (either immediate or delayed) meets a psychological need of many patients. In 1991, the American Society of Plastic and Reconstructive Surgeons constructed a demographic profile of women who have had breast reconstruction (Table 26–1). It is estimated that some 10% to 15% of women who have had a mastectomy seek reconstruction. Most centers have incorporated breast reconstruction into their comprehensive oncology program. For many women faced with the prospect of losing a breast, this has relieved some of the psychological trauma with the knowledge that the breast can be recreated if the patient so desires, either immediately or later.

Finally, the attitude of the general surgeon toward breast reconstruction has been changing. The Halstedian philosophy opposing breast reconstruction prevailed for more than a half century. Because of both the improved techniques and the finding that reconstruction does not interfere with survival or early detection of cancer recurrence, the attitude of the general surgical community toward breast reconstruction has become more favorable. As a result, the recon-

Table 26-1. PROFILE: WOMEN WHO HAVE BREAST RECONSTRUCTION (1991)

Demographics

Year Implants Inserted

Prior to 1975:	9%
1975–1984:	46%
1985–1990:	45%

Age at Time of Surgery

13–30 y:	11%
31–40 y:	26%
41 y up:	63%

How Soon After Mastectomy Implants Were Inserted

At same time:	49%	At 1–5 y:	16%
At 1 or less:	26%	At more than 5 y:	9%

Degree of Influence Other People Had on Decision

	Relatives	Husband/Lover	Friends
Great deal or some	25%	45%	22%
Little or none	75%	55%	78%

Degree of Support Shown By Others

	Relatives	Husband/Lover	Friends
Supportive/agreed to surgery	53%	64%	40%
Supportive/but believed surgery unnecessary	11%	14%	10%
Opposed	3%	2%	—
Not part of decision	33%	20%	50%

Marital Status at Time of Surgery

Married:	76%	Divorced or Separated:	13%
Widowed:	6%	Never Married:	5%

Overall Satisfaction

Satisfaction with Results of Reconstruction

Very satisfied:	47%
More satisfied than dissatisfied:	42%
More dissatisfied than satisfied:	7%
Very dissatisfied:	4%

Problems

Capsular Contracture (Tightening of Scar Tissue Around Implant)

How Breasts Feel Now

Soft and natural:	52%
Slightly firm*:	22%
Moderately firm*:	20%
Hard*:	6%

If Slightly Firm to Hard, Degree of Concern Felt

Not at all bothersome:	36%	Somewhat bothersome:	34%
Not very bothersome:	26%	Very bothersome:	4%

Scars

Almost invisible:	29%
Somewhat visible:	37%
Very visible:	34%

Other Problems Experienced?

No:	60%
Yes:	40% (includes appearance-related problems (14% of total), complaints such as pain and numbness (12%), and complications such as infection and implant leaks (10%).)

(Courtesy of the American Society of Plastic and Reconstructive Surgeons, Inc., Arlington Heights, IL.)
*Applies to one or both breasts.

structive surgeon in many instances is consulted even before the mastectomy.

Premastectomy consultation with the reconstructive surgeon achieves several goals. First, it provides the patient information on what can and what cannot be accomplished through reconstruction in her particular situation. It may help identify patients with unrealistic expectations, who generally are poor candidates for immediate reconstruction.

Second, premastectomy consultation can make it easier for the patient to choose mastectomy over a breast-conserving therapy that might not be appropriate in her particular case. Third, it permits improved communication between general and reconstructive surgeon. While taking steps to allow for adequate oncologic treatment, the surgeon may plan the position of the incision to anticipate a certain type of reconstruction. In conjunction with the patient's preference and stage of disease on presentation, the choice of immediate or delayed reconstruction can be considered.

PRINCIPLES AND TIMING OF RECONSTRUCTION

Several general principles should be followed when considering postmastectomy reconstruction. First and foremost is that reconstruction should not interfere with the early detection of recurrence or reduce the chances for survival from the disease. These two concerns were the primary reasons why postmastectomy reconstruction had not been generally accepted. The prevailing belief was that surgery to restore the breast was unnecessary and might even cause recurrence. As a result, early pioneers in breast reconstruction established strict guidelines and criteria for the selection of patients for reconstruction and its timing.

Early guidelines regarding selection and timing of reconstruction included these general principles: First, only patients with favorable lesions (e.g., Stage A in the Columbia Clinical Classification or Stage I in the International Classification) were considered candidates for reconstruction. Additionally, the presence of more than three involved lymph nodes was considered a contraindication to breast reconstruction. Pers (1981) found a local recurrence rate of less than 5% in patients with fewer than three involved axillary nodes. Second, many investigators found that approximately 75% of recurrences were manifested within the first 2 years after mastectomy.

The purpose of these early guidelines was to avoid performing reconstruction on a patient who was liable to develop local recurrence of disease. It was believed that if a patient succumbed to her disease within 1 to 5 years, reconstruction was unnecessary and wasteful. This negative approach has, for the most part, been abandoned over the past 15 years. Within reason, it is no longer necessary to deny a patient who desires it the satisfaction of a breast reconstruction by going through a waiting period to see if her tumor will recur. In fact, recently there has been a trend toward immediate reconstruction for selected patients (Marshall, 1982; Gilliland, 1983; Webster et al., 1984; Frazier et al., 1985; Noone et al., 1985). Immediate reconstruction, usually performed when patients have a favorable prognosis, offers several advantages. First, it reduces the psychological impact of the loss of a breast. Second, it reduces the cost of postmastectomy reconstruction. The second factor will become increasingly important in years to come. While immediate breast reconstruction is indicated for the majority of women desiring reconstruction, most plastic surgeons have reservations about performing it if postoperative radiation is planned or if the patient has a poor prognosis. Postoperative radiation after immediate breast reconstruction tends to increase wound complications and leads to more fibrosis around the breast implant. This yields a firmer breast and, overall, a less satisfactory aesthetic result.

As of 1992, approximately 50% of postmastectomy breast reconstructions were performed at the time of mastectomy; and 26%, within a year after mastectomy. In the majority of cases, immediate breast reconstruction is performed using a subpectoral tissue expander or subpectoral breast implant. In experienced hands, immediate breast reconstruction following mastectomy has not been associated with an increased rate of complications when compared with mastectomy alone (Vinton, 1990).

Immediate flap breast reconstruction (either latissimus dorsi flap or TRAM flap) is preferred by some surgeons for selected patients. While the total operative time and hospital stay are increased in this group of patients, many reconstructive surgeons feel that they can obtain a superior aesthetic result (Rosen, 1990; Beasley, 1991). Operative time can be reduced by flap elevations at the time of mastectomy.

The majority of reconstructions are performed as a delayed procedure, after the patient has recovered from her mastectomy and after adjuvant therapy (radiation or chemotherapy) has been completed. This is usually from 3 to 9 months after mastectomy, but reconstruction may be done many years after mastectomy.

Delayed reconstruction has several advantages. The patient and surgeon have a better idea of the stage and prognosis of her cancer. Generally a complicated flap procedure would not be recommended for a patient with a poor prognosis. In addition, some patients find that the deformity is acceptable and decide not to have reconstruction. Delaying the procedure also allows the patient additional time to assess her particular needs and discuss them with other women in similar situations. Although most patients rely on the reconstructive surgeon's advice as to the type of reconstruction, more and more are educating themselves through Reach to Recovery programs and similar sources of educational material (Bostwick & Berger, 1984). Some investigate the different types of reconstruction and decide which is the most suitable for them. Finally, whereas more than 90% of women are satisfied with their reconstructive result, a few expect an exact duplicate of their original breast. Delayed reconstruction demonstrates to these particular women what an improvement the reconstruction is over the postmastectomy deformity.

There was, and still remains, concern about a potential delay in early detection of breast cancer recurrence owing to deformities and scarring from breast reconstruction. Many authors who have addressed this fear find that the overwhelming majority of local recurrences occur at the site of the mastectomy scar (Zimmerman et al., 1966). The detection of recurrence in this site should not be influenced by either subpectoral implant or flap breast reconstruction. Furthermore, the prognosis for the patient, once a recurrence has occurred, generally is poor because local recurrence is usually associated with metastatic disease. Though it is too early to judge the influence of breast reconstruction on breast cancer survival, it appears doubtful that postmastectomy reconstruction will alter the natural history of the disease for the individual patient. A multicenter, long-term follow-up study will be necessary to answer this question.

TYPES OF RECONSTRUCTION

At the present time five different methods of breast reconstruction are available: (1) breast implant; (2) tissue expander followed by an implant; (3) latissimus dorsi flap with an implant or as a fleur-de-lis design without an implant; (4) TRAM; and (5) microvascular tissue transfer. Each

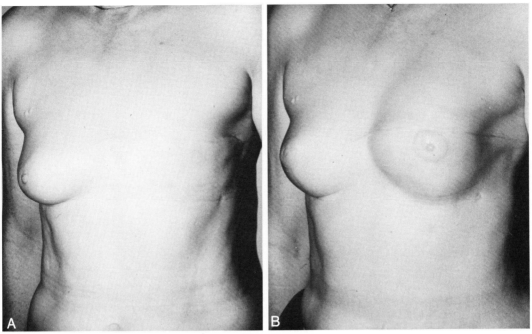

Figure 26-1. *A,* Patient following left modified radical mastectomy. *B,* Left breast reconstruction with a submuscular implant, nipple-areolar reconstruction, and right mastopexy. (Reproduced by permission from Bostwick, J.: Aesthetic and Reconstructive Breast Surgery. St. Louis, 1983, The C. V. Mosby Co.)

technique offers its own advantages and disadvantages. In addition, there are specific indications and contraindications for each technique (Bostwick, 1990).

Breast Implants Only

The simplest form of breast reconstruction following mastectomy involves replacing the breast with a silicone gel implant or a saline-filled implant (Fig. 26–1). This implant is most commonly placed beneath the pectoralis major muscle in the so-called submusculofascial space. This can be done as an immediate or as a delayed procedure. Most cases of immediate breast reconstruction involve either this technique or the placement of a tissue expander. The technique involves an incision through the lateral portion of the previous mastectomy scar. The scar is excised and sent to the pathology laboratory for examination. The pectoralis major muscle is split in the direction of its fibers over a course of 6 to 8 cm. Blunt dissection is then used to create a submuscular pocket beneath the pectoralis major muscle, the anterior portion of the serratus muscle, and the superior portion of the rectus abdominis and external oblique fasciae. The pocket is made larger than the implant, and extends 2 to 4 cm more inferior than the opposite inframammary crease. The implant is then inserted into this space, and the muscle is closed in an interrupted fashion with 3–0 or 4–0 Vicryl suture.

Reconstruction with an implant only is indicated when there is adequate skin coverage and adequate soft tissue in the infraclavicular space (Fig. 26–2). It is ideal for a patient after a modified radical mastectomy who has soft, well-healed skin flaps and an opposite breast dimension of 300 cm^2 or less (A or B cup). It is difficult to insert, as a primary procedure, an implant exceeding 300 cm^2 and maintain

adequate muscle coverage to prevent extrusion of the implant if there is necrosis of a portion of the mastectomy skin flaps. If this technique is used and the opposite breast is significantly larger, a reduction mammoplasty can be performed or progressively larger implants can be inserted as separate procedures to enlarge the reconstructed breast. In such cases, however, the use of a tissue expander is more appropriate. Complications include bleeding from the subpectoral dissection (usually blunt dissection), infection around the implant, extrusion of the implant as a result of either infection or inadequate muscle coverage, and scar contracture (capsule) around the implant, resulting in a firm, painful mound and poor aesthetic result. Placement of an implant is contraindicated when the patient has had a radical mastectomy, not only because of the impoverished blood supply to the attenuated skin and scar but also because an implant cannot replace the defect left by a radical mastectomy. Any patient with a skin deficiency or tight skin from the mastectomy should have reconstruction with the transfer of additional tissue (i.e, latissimus dorsi or TRAM). If an implant alone is used in such a case, the result, most surely, will be a disappointing compromise compared with the opposite breast.

Tissue Expander Technique

Tissue expanders (Fig. 26–3) added a new dimension to breast reconstruction (Argenta, 1984). Whereas the larger flap techniques are more appropriate for reconstruction following a radical mastectomy, the number of radical mastectomies being performed has decreased dramatically. The modified radical mastectomy or simple mastectomy with axillary dissection has replaced the Halstedian mastectomy, and surgeons have been leaving thicker skin flaps. As a

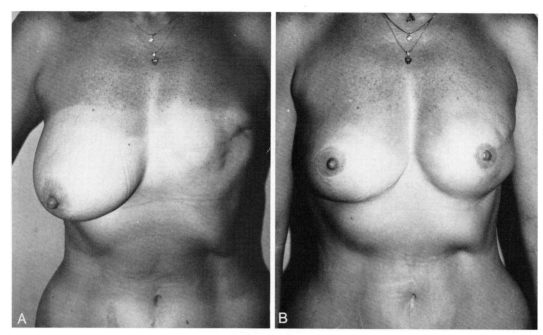

Figure 26-2. *A,* A 40-year-old patient following a left modified radical mastectomy. *B,* The left breast has been reconstructed with a submuscular implant. A right breast reduction has been performed for symmetry. (Reproduced by permission from Bostwick, J.: Aesthetic and Reconstructive Breast Surgery. St. Louis, 1983, The C. V. Mosby Co.)

result, the defect has qualitatively normal but quantitatively deficient skin. Tissue expansion provides a technique to enlarge the skin and pocket for the implant without requiring local or distant flaps. It provides gradual stretching of the skin in much the same way as the abdominal skin and abdominal wall musculature stretch during pregnancy (Slavin, 1990).

The technique is similar to that of reconstruction with an implant (Fig. 26–4). The mastectomy scar is excised, and the submusculofascial pocket is dissected bluntly. This can be performed either at the time of mastectomy or later. The expander is placed within this space. Some breast tissue expanders have self-contained reservoirs and do not require an additional dissection in the subcutaneous space laterally in the mid-axillary line for placement of a port. Other expanders have remote reservoirs connected to the expander with Silastic tubing. The remote reservoir is placed in a lateral position adjacent to the chest wall. At the time of insertion, the expander is inflated with 150 to 300 mL of saline solution, depending on the size and tightness of the pocket. After 2 to 3 weeks, 50 to 100 mL of saline solution is added to the expander weekly.

Most reconstructive breast surgeons prefer to overexpand the chest skin, with a total of anywhere from 400 to 1200 ml of saline in the expander depending on the size of the opposite breast. The expander is inflated over a period of 6 to 8 weeks. The overfilled expander is then left in place for several weeks to several months, depending on the pliability of the skin and the desires of the patient. The expander is then removed and replaced with the appropriate silicone gel or saline-filled implant. Postoperative planning and discussion with the patient determine whether the opposite breast should be reduced, changed in shape (mastopexy), or left alone.

Tissue expansion for breast reconstruction is a simple

technique. It provides additional skin coverage without the use of flaps. Matching of the opposite breast is made easier. The incidence of fibrous contracture after insertion of the implant may also be less than after insertion of an implant primarily. Complications of tissue expanders are essentially the same as those of implants. Placement of a tissue expander at the time of mastectomy is generally contraindicated if immediate postoperative radiation is planned, due to the likelihood of radiation fibrosis in the soft tissue.

Latissimus Dorsi Flap

The latissimus dorsi flap is ideally suited for breast reconstruction when there is a skin deficiency (e.g., a tight mastectomy scar, skin graft on the chest wall, or following radiation) or when there is a large defect, such as after radical mastectomy. A radical mastectomy defect may also be created if there has been damage to the lateral or medial pectoral nerves during a modified radical mastectomy. This will lead to atrophy of the pectoralis major muscle.

The latissimus dorsi muscle is a large, fan-shaped muscle situated in the lower part of the back. It has a very large site of origin that includes the spinous processes of the seventh through the twelfth thoracic vertebrae, the thoracolumbar fascia, and the posterior one-third of the iliac crest. As it ascends superiorly, it has an attachment to the inferior angle of the scapula. It then becomes a tendinous structure and inserts into the humerus.

On the basis of its vascular anatomy as defined by Mathes and Nahai (1981, 1982), the latissimus dorsi muscle is a Type V muscle. This means that it has one dominant pedicle and secondary segmental vascular pedicles. This allows the surgeon to rotate the muscle or skin island anteriorly using the thoracodorsal artery and vein or to cover

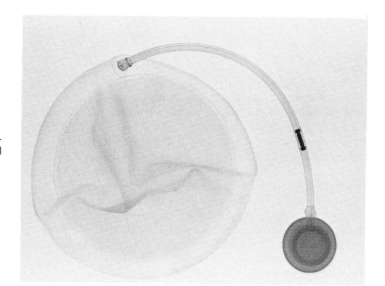

Figure 26-3. Tissue expander prior to insertion and inflation. The reservoir port through which the expander will be inflated is shown attached on the right.

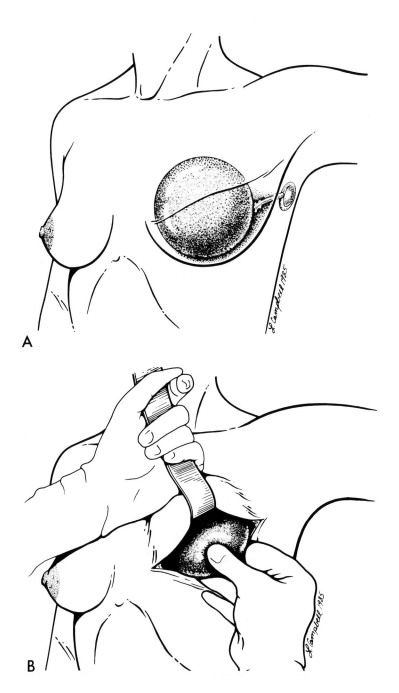

A

B

Figure 26-4. *A,* The tissue expander has been inserted through the previous mastectomy incision into a submuscular space. The reservoir is placed into a subcutaneous pocket beneath the axilla. *B,* After the expander has been fully inflated over 4 to 8 weeks, it is removed, and a permanent silicone implant is inserted into the submuscular pocket.

spinal defects using its medial thoracic and lumbar perforators.

The technique of latissimus dorsi breast reconstruction (Figs. 26–5 and 26–6) is well-described. Preoperatively, the surgeon must define not only the patient's anatomic deficiency but also the tissue requirements, to reestablish anatomic form. For example, if there is a deficiency or lack of an axillary fold, a portion of the bulk of the latissimus dorsi muscle may be used instead. Therefore, in the preoperative evaluation, careful examination of the latissimus dorsi muscle is mandatory. Although the thoracodorsal nerve is usually preserved during mastectomy, it may be injured. A helpful maneuver is to have the patient place her hand on her hip and push firmly while the surgeon tests for contraction of the latissimus dorsi muscle. It is necessary to feel for the contraction below the tip of the scapula. Contraction of the teres major muscle (innervated by a branch of the lower subscapular nerve) may be misinterpreted as contraction of the latissimus dorsi muscle. If the thoracodorsal nerve has been injured, leaving the muscle atrophic, the thin layer of muscle and its skin island may still be used for implant coverage when there is a large skin deficiency, but it cannot be used when muscle bulk is necessary to fill the defect created by a radical mastectomy.

During latissimus dorsi breast reconstruction, the patient is placed in the contralateral decubitus position. The skin island is usually designed transversely. A typical skin paddle measures 8 by 16 cm. The muscle is then detached from its wide origin, beginning inferiorly. Dissection continues beneath the muscle in a relatively avascular plane between the latissimus dorsi and chest wall. Care must be taken to exclude muscle fibers of the external oblique muscle inferiorly, the serratus anterior muscle superolaterally, and the teres major muscle superomedially, as these muscles are usually closely attached to the latissimus dorsi muscle in their respective locations. As the muscle is dissected toward the axilla, its vascular pedicle is identified. It is easily seen on the undersurface of the muscle in a slightly lateral position. Approximately 10 to 12 cm below the axillary vein, the thoracodorsal vessels communicate with a large serratus anterior collateral vessel. It is important not to divide this collateral, as the thoracodorsal vessels may have been ligated superiorly during the previous mastectomy. If the thoracodorsal complex has been ligated previously, the serratus collateral vessel can adequately nourish the latissimus dorsi flap (Fisher et al., 1983). Some surgeons prefer to transect the thoracodorsal nerve, in order to both decrease muscle bulk and prevent persistent muscle contraction. Other surgeons preserve the thoracodorsal nerve, feeling that the added muscle bulk can be advantageous and that persistent muscle contractions may help prevent periprosthetic capsule contracture.

Once the latissimus dorsi flap has been raised and its vascular pedicle isolated, its tendinous insertion may be divided to allow more complete rotation of the flap. This may be done, if necessary, through a separate transverse axillary incision. Detachment of the insertion of the latissimus dorsi muscle is helpful, when needed, to recreate the anterior axillary fold. Care must be taken to create a superior tunnel for the latissimus dorsi flap. If the tunnel is made too large or too far inferior, there is a risk that the implant will slide posterolaterad, underneath the arm.

When the flap has been raised and the tunnel dissected, the doner site on the back is closed after carefully ensuring hemostasis. A suction drain is placed into the latissimus dorsi donor site. A dressing is then placed over the wound and the patient is repositioned supine.

The previous mastectomy scar is removed and sent to the pathology laboratory. Superior and inferior skin flaps are then raised to create a pocket for the implant. The latissimus dorsi skin island is planned and placed as far inferior as possible, both to provide ptosis for the reconstructed breast and to keep the scars as far inferior as possible. The latissimus dorsi muscle is sutured inferiorly to the pectoralis muscle and rectus fascia at the level of the inframammary crease. It is sutured superiorly beneath the clavicle. If the patient has a large infraclavicular defect, the latissimus dorsi skin island can be "de-epithelialized" and used to fill this area.

After the muscle has been sutured into position and the appropriate aesthetic tailoring is completed, an appropriate-sized implant is placed beneath the muscle into its pocket. An implant can range in volume from 120 to 300 ml. If a larger implant is required to match the opposite breast and the pocket beneath the latissimus flap is not large enough to accommodate such an implant, a Becker expander-implant can be inserted. Approximately 3 to 4 weeks postoperatively, saline can be added to enlarge the breast mound. At the same time as the latissimus dorsi breast reconstruction, the opposite breast can be either reduced, enlarged, or changed in shape to provide a close match between the two (Fig. 26–7). The hospital stay can be as short as 2 days or as long as a week. Most patients are hospitalized 3 to 4 days and can return to work in 2 to 3 weeks.

McCraw recently introduced the fleur-de-lis latissimus dorsi flap for breast reconstruction (Fig. 26–8). This design utilizes the subcutaneous fat overlying the latissimus dorsi muscle. The subcutaneous fat is dissected with the latissimus muscle and much of the overlying skin is de-epithelialized. This flap is then transferred to the anterior chest wall and folded into a breast contour. In appropriate patients, it avoids the use of a breast implant. A patient must have an adequate amount of fatty tissue overlying the latissimus muscle in order for this design to be accomplished.

The latissimus dorsi flap is a very versatile and reliable one. The cutaneous blood supply is more direct and not as likely to be affected adversely by smoking as is the cutaneous blood supply of the TRAM flap. Complications relating to partial or total flap necrosis are seen in fewer than 5% of patients. Because an implant is used, capsular contracture resulting in a firm breast can still occur. A seroma develops in the donor site in 10% to 20% of patients. This is usually a minor problem and resolves with aspiration.

The latissimus dorsi flap is a very useful procedure for breast reconstruction, as there are many instances in which a TRAM flap is contraindicated. For heavy smokers with poor cutaneous circulation the latissimus dorsi flap is more reliable than a TRAM flap. If a patient has had multiple abdominal incisions, especially ones that divide the upper rectus abdominis muscle, a TRAM breast reconstruction may not be possible. Moderate to severe low back pain can be worsened by a TRAM flap, making the latissimus dorsi flap the procedure of choice. Finally, for patients with a paucity of lower abdominal fat a TRAM flap would not

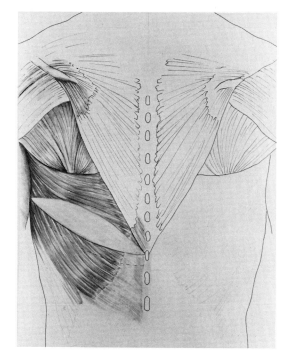

Figure 26–5. The latissimus dorsi muscle with an overlying skin island (shown here in a transverse direction).

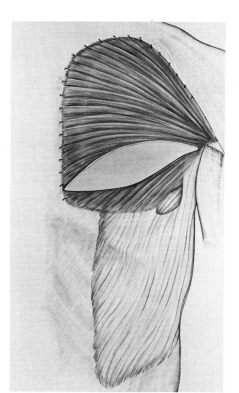

Figure 26–6. The latissimus dorsi musculocutaneous flap has been transferred to the chest wall. An implant is then placed beneath this flap.

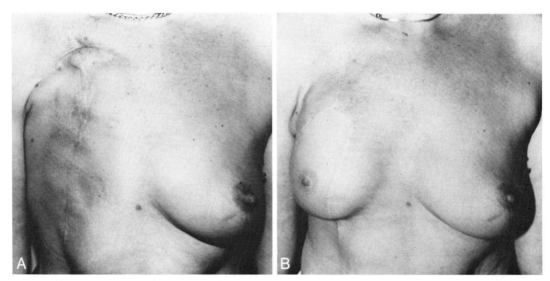

Figure 26–7. *A,* A 64-year-old patient after a right radical mastectomy. *B,* The right breast was reconstructed using a latissimus dorsi flap and implant. (Reproduced by permission from Bostwick, J.: Aesthetic and Reconstructive Breast Surgery. St. Louis, 1983, The C. V. Mosby Co.)

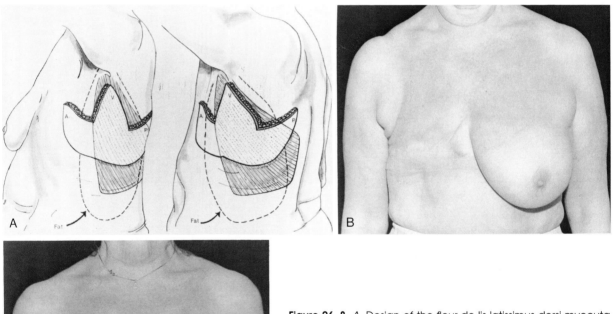

Figure 26–8. *A,* Design of the fleur-de-lis latissimus dorsi myocutaneous flap. *B,* Patient following right modified radical mastectomy. *C,* Right breast reconstruction with the fleur-de-lis latissimus dorsi flap. The muscle and subcutaneous tissue provide the breast mound bulk; thus, the use of a breast implant is avoided. (Reproduced by permission from Hartrampf, C. R.: Hartrampf's Breast Reconstruction with Living Tissue. New York, Raven Press, 1991.)

provide adequate fatty tissue for breast replacement without an implant. In such patients, a latissimus dorsi flap or free tissue transfer may be the best form of reconstruction.

Transverse Rectus Abdominis Myocutaneous Flap

The latest major addition to flap breast reconstruction, the TRAM flap, developed as an outgrowth of research with myocutaneous flaps. It offers many advantages over the latissimus dorsi flap. Because of the amount of fatty tissue transferred with the TRAM flap, the addition of an implant usually is not necessary. This avoids the possible development of a capsular contracture in the reconstructed breast. There is usually an abundance of subcutaneous tissue available with the TRAM flap, so that even very large defects can be reconstructed. In cases of bilateral reconstruction, each rectus muscle can be transferred with its corresponding skin and subcutaneous tissue at the same time. A second advantage of the TRAM flap is that, in addition to providing ample tissue for breast reconstruction, the abdominal wall reconstruction (i.e., abdominoplasty) results in an improved body contour. Finally, the contour and consistency of the transferred abdominal fat in the TRAM flap are very similar to those of the normal breast.

Development of the TRAM flap contributed to our understanding of the blood supply to the anterior abdominal wall. The rectus abdominis muscle is supplied primarily by the superior and inferior epigastric vessels but receives additional blood from lateral intercostal vessels. The superior and inferior epigastric vessels arborize within the muscle belly. There are anterior perforationg vessels that traverse the anterior rectus sheath and provide blood supply to a large island of anterior abdominal skin. The majority of these perforating vessels are located in the periumbilical area (Fig. 26–9). A large transverse elliptical island of middle to lower abdominal skin can be raised with one or both rectus abdominis muscles and a portion of the anterior rectus sheath. This can be mobilized up to the costal margin, taking care to include the medial and lateral rectus perforators. The lateral intercostal collateral vessels and intercostal nerves are divided in the process of raising the flap.

There are four separate methods of performing a TRAM breast reconstruction: (1) a single-pedicle TRAM (one rectus abdominis muscle); (2) a double-pedicle TRAM (both rectus abdominis muscles); (3) a ''supercharged'' single pedicle TRAM (augmenting the blood flow to the flap by anastomosing the inferior epigastric vessels to recipient vessels in the axilla); and (4) a free microvascular TRAM flap. The double-pedicle TRAM and free TRAM provide better vascularity to the cutaneous component of the flap (Fig. 26–10).

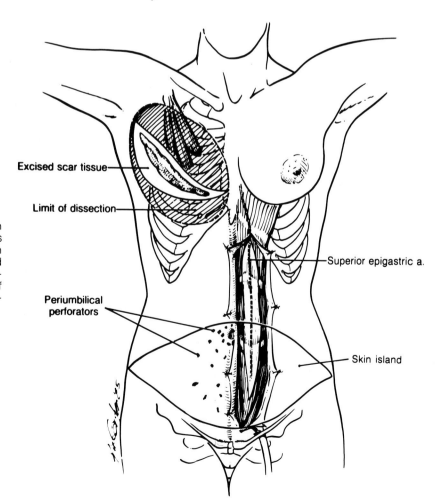

Figure 26–9. The TRAM flap consists of an elliptical island of skin and subcutaneous tissue from the lower abdomen based on the rectus abdominis muscle. (Reprinted with permission from Sando, W., and Jurkiewicz, M. J.: An approach to repair of radiation necrosis of chest wall and mammary gland. World J. Surg., *10*:206, 1986.)

Excised scar tissue

Limit of dissection

Periumbilical perforators

Superior epigastric a.

Skin island

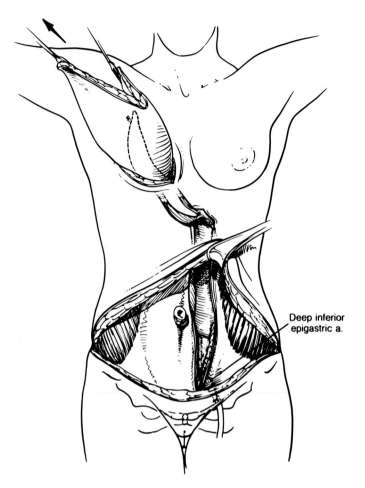

Figure 26-10. The TRAM flap has been elevated from its anatomic position, rotated in a clockwise fashion, and transferred to the chest wall. The deep inferior epigastric artery and vein are ligated. (Reprinted with permission from Sando, W., and Jurkiewicz, M. J.: An approach to repair of radiation necrosis of chest wall and mammary gland. World J. Surg., *10:*206, 1986.)

Deep inferior
epigastric a.

In the case of unilateral breast reconstruction with a single rectus pedicle, the contralateral rectus muscle is usually used, as this provides for a better arc of rotation of the vascular bundle. A tunnel is then made that communicates with the dissection used to raise the mastectomy skin flaps. The TRAM flap is placed gently through this tunnel. The appropriate trimming and contouring of the new breast is then accomplished (Figs. 26–11 and 26–12). The results obtained with the TRAM flap have been very satisfactory (Figs. 26–13 and 26–14).

Much attention is given to closure of the abdominal wall when a TRAM flap is used. Hartrampf (1985) performed more than 475 TRAM breast reconstructions and finds that abdominal wall closure can be accomplished with the existing anterior rectus sheath in the majority of cases. While Hartrampf reports an abdominal wall hernia rate of 1.3% in 475 patients, other surgeons report a rate between 5% and 15%. Bostwick (1985), on the other hand, perfers to strengthen the abdominal wall closure with Prolene mesh. He believes that adding Prolene mesh to the closure decreases the hernia rate. This also results in a tighter closure, and a more aesthetic abdominal contour. While Prolene mesh may not be necessary to reinforce the abdominal wall closure when a single rectus abdominis muscle is used, most surgeons feel that it gives a more secure abdominal fascial repair when both rectus muscles are elevated.

The TRAM flap is a technically demanding procedure for the surgeon and a physically demanding procedure for

the patient. Many fine details must be attended to to obtain a healthy, viable flap. Patient selection is critical. Most patients receive 2 units of blood during and immediately following the procedure. The hospital stay ranges between 5 and 7 days.

The TRAM flap is contraindicated for patients with a history of heavy smoking and should not be performed in any patient who has compromised cutaneous circulation (e.g., lupus erythematosus). A frequent complaint following a TRAM breast reconstruction is low back pain for several weeks. If the patient has had back difficulty before breast reconstruction, a TRAM flap can exacerbate it. A previous Kocher incision results in ligation of the right superior epigastric vessels. A TRAM based on the right rectus abdominis is therefore not possible in such cases, but the left TRAM can be used to reconstruct either breast. If both rectus abdominis muscles are necessary to the breast or chest wall reconstruction and one of the pedicles has been ligated, the corresponding deep inferior epigastric artery (DIEA) can be dissected with the muscle and anastomosed to the axillary vessels using microvascular technique. This principle of enhancement of the blood supply to the distal portion of a flap was first described by Longmire in 1945, in a modification of Roux's operation for esophageal reconstruction using jejunum (Longmire, 1947).

The complications of the TRAM flap are generally related to the skill and experience of the surgeon. Because of the large amount of dissection, postoperative hematomas

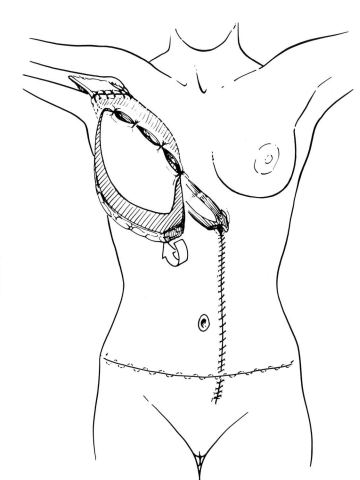

Figure 26–11. The left anterior rectus sheath and abdominal incision have been closed, the new umbilicus created, and the TRAM flap contoured and trimmed to reconstruct an aesthetic unit. (Reprinted with permission from Sando, W., and Jurkiewicz, M. J.: An approach to repair of radiation necrosis of chest wall and mammary gland. World J. Surg., *10*:206, 1986.)

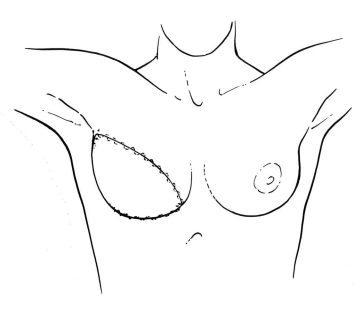

Figure 26–12. The completed breast reconstruction. (Reprinted with permission from Sando, W., and Jurkiewicz, M. J.: An approach to repair of radiation necrosis of chest wall and mammary gland. World J. Surg., *10*:206, 1986.)

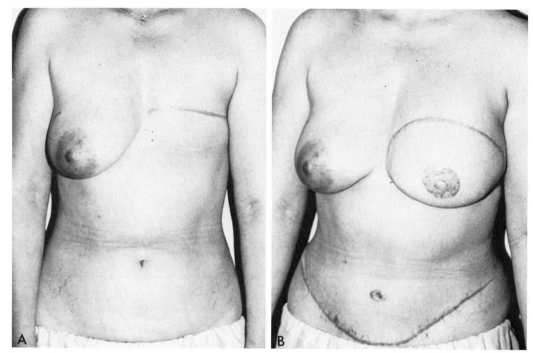

Figure 26-13. *A,* A 38-year-old patient following a left modified radical mastectomy. *B,* The patient is shown following a single pedicle TRAM reconstruction and nipple-areolar reconstruction. (From Hartrampf, C. R.: Transverse Abdominal Island Flap Technique. Rockville, MD, Aspen Systems Corporation, 1984, p. 41. Reprinted with permission.)

and seromas are a well-recognized complication. Partial or total flap loss can be kept to a minimum through careful patient selection and dissection. Abdominal wall hernias following TRAM flaps are infrequent, but they do occur. An as yet unanswered question regarding the TRAM flap is the long-term effect on the stability and strength of the abdominal wall. In the first 5 years of follow-up, this does not appear to be a major problem; however, long-term follow-up is necessary.

Microvascular Tissue Transfer in Breast Reconstruction

The advent of microsurgery in the past 10 years has had far-reaching effects on almost all areas of reconstruction. For breast reconstruction it can be used in very carefully selected patients (Serafin et al., 1982). Some patients do not have local flaps available to reconstruct their breast defect. These patients usually require replacement with a large amount of skin and soft tissue. The patient's largest source of local tissue (the TRAM flaps) may be either unavailable owing to prior surgery or deficient in very thin patients. In such patients, microsurgical tissue transfer (i.e., a free flap) can provide aesthetic breast reconstruction with an acceptable donor defect. Although many different free flaps have been described for breast reconstruction, the most promising appears to be the free TRAM flap, as reported by Grotting and coworkers (1989). This flap has proved to be reliable and offers a superior blood supply when compared with the conventional TRAM. Another source of free tissue transfer is the superior gluteal flap, as described by Shaw, and the inferior gluteal flap (Le-Quang, 1979; Shaw, 1983;

Nahai et al., 1993). In developing each flap, a large transverse island of skin with its underlying fat and a small segment of gluteal muscle is dissected with its corresponding gluteal vessel (Figs. 26–15 and 26–16). This composite flap is then transferred to the chest wall. The donor site on the abdomen or buttock is closed primarily. Microvascular transfer is performed using either the internal mammary vessels or the axillary vessels. Early reports on this technique have been promising. When used as an alternative to the TRAM flap, its primary disadvantage is that the microvascular technique is technically demanding.

NIPPLE-AREOLA RECONSTRUCTION

Nipple-areola reconstruction represents the final stage of breast reconstruction. The nipple and areola are usually reconstructed between 6 and 12 weeks after the initial breast reconstruction procedure. At this time, any additional scar revisions or fine adjustments of the original reconstruction may be accomplished.

The position of the nipple-areolar complex is determined with the patient standing or sitting. The area of the areola is then de-epithelialized over a circle measuring between 38 and 42 mm in diameter. A full-thickness skin graft is harvested from the upper, inner medial aspect of the thigh. The donor site is closed primarily using 3–0 or 4–0 chromic suture. The nipple is reconstructed either with a full-thickness skin graft from the thigh crease or, if the opposite nipple is sufficiently large, by excision of half the opposite nipple in a nipple-sharing technique.

The areolar and nipple grafts are sutured in place using a 3–0 silk stent dressing. This is left intact for 3 to 5 days,

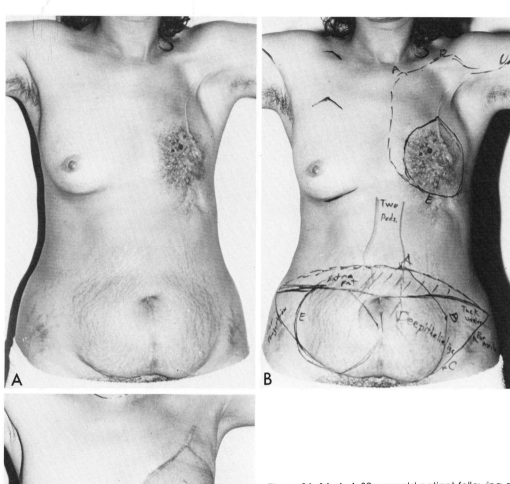

Figure 26–14. *A*, A 39-year-old patient following a left radical mastectomy and postoperative radiation. Radiation changes and necrosis are evident. *B*, Preoperative planning and design. A double-pedicle TRAM flap is required to adequately replace the absent skin and soft tissue. *C*, The patient following the double-pedicle TRAM and nipple-areolar reconstruction. (From Hartrampf, C. R.: Transverse Abdominal Island Flap Technique. Rockville, MD, Aspen Systems Corporation, 1984, p. 85. Reprinted with permission.)

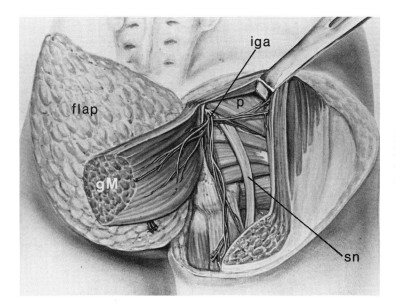

Figure 26–15. The anatomy and dissection of the inferior gluteal flap for microvascular free tissue transfer. gM = gluteus maximus; iga = inferior gluteal artery; sn = sciatic nerve; p = piriformis muscle.

Figure 26–16. The inferior gluteal flap has been transferred to the chest. The inferior gluteal vessels are anastomosed to the internal mammary vessels. If the internal mammary vein is not suitable for anastomosis, the cephalic vein or external jugular vein can be used. ej = external jugular vein; c = cephalic vein; im = internal mammary vessels.

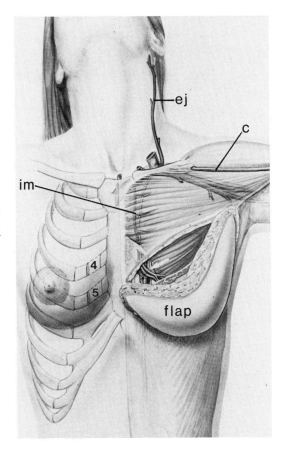

after which the stent is removed and the grafts are covered with Steristrips.

There have been many different techniques of nipple-areola reconstruction (Gruber, 1979). These include the use of small local flaps, ear cartilage, and other plastic techniques. Some early work is now being done using a permanent tattoo-type material similar to that used for the permanent eyeliner. Regardless of the type of technique used, the challenge is to provide nipple projection and permanent pigmentation of the areola.

SUMMARY

The current state of the art in breast reconstruction involves application of new and developing plastic surgery techniques (Bostwick, 1990). The results are far superior to those of the past. Although the results are good, it should not be forgotten that breast reconstruction is not an end unto itself. It has been developed to provide substantial psychological support, permitting patients to deal better with breast cancer and with the change in body image. Continual refinement and simplification of techniques should help to bring both cost and availability into equilibrium with need, demand, and societal resources (Kiser, 1985).

References

Argenta, L.: Reconstruction of the breast by tissue expansion. Clin. Plast. Surg., *11:*257, 1984.

Bayet, B., Mathieu, G., Lavand Homme, P., et al.: Primary and secondary breast reconstruction with a permanent expander. Eur. J. Plast. Surg., *14:*73, 1991.

Beasley, M.: Immediate breast reconstruction with a pedicled TRAM flap. Hartrampf's breast reconstruction with living tissue. New York, Raven Press, 1991.

Berkel, H., Birdsell, D. C., and Jenkins, H.: Breast augmentation: A risk factor for breast cancer? N. Engl. J. Med., *326:*1649, 1992.

Bostwick, J. III: Breast reconstruction following mastectomy. Contemp. Surg., *27:*15, 1985.

Bostwick, J. III: Plastic and Reconstructive Breast Surgery. St. Louis, Quality Medical Publishing, 1990.

Bostwick, J., and Berger, K: A Woman's Choice. St. Louis, C.V. Mosby, 1984.

Bostwick, J., Nahai, E., Wallace, J. G., et al.: Sixty latissimus dorsi flaps. Plast. Reconstr. Surg., *63:*31, 1979.

Cronin, T. D., Upton, J., and McDonough, J. M.: Reconstruction of the breast afer mastectomy. Plast. Reconstr. Surg., *59:*1, 1977.

Drever, J. M.: Immediate breast reconstruction after mastectomy using a rectus abdominis myodermal flap without an implant. Can. J. Surg., *25:*429, 1982.

Elliot, F.: The lateral transverse thigh flap. Breast reconstruction with living tissue. New York, Raven Press, 1991.

Fisher, J.: The silicone controversy—when will science prevail? N. Engl. J. Med., *326:*1696, 1992.

Fisher, J., Bostwick, J. III, and Powell, R. W.: Latissimus dorsi blood supply after thoracodorsal vessel division: The serratus collateral. Plast. Reconstr. Surg., *72:*502, 1983.

Frazier, T. G., and Noone, R. B.: An objective analysis of immediate simultaneous reconstruction in the treatment of primary carcinoma of the breast. Cancer, *55:*1202, 1985.

Gilliland, M.D.: Appropriate timing for breast reconstruction. Plast. Reconstr. Surg., *72:*335, 1983.

Goldblum, R. M., Pelley, R. P., O'Donell, A. A., et al.: Antibodies to silicone elastomers and reactions to ventriculoperitoneal shunts. Lancet, *340:*510, 1992.

Goldwyn, R.: Breast reconstruction after mastectomy. N. Engl. J. Med., *317:*1711, 1987.

Grotting, J.: The TRAM flap. Hartrampf's breast reconstruction with living tissue. New York, Raven Press, 1991.

Grotting, J., Urist, M. Maddox, W., et al.: Conventional TRAM flap versus free microsurgical TRAM flap for immediate breast reconstruction. Plast. Reconstr. Surg., *83:*828, 1989.

Gruber, R. P.: Nipple-areola reconstruction: A review of techniques. Clin. Plast. Surg., *6:*71, 1979.

Hartrampf, C. R.: Transverse abdominal island flap technique for breast reconstruction after mastectomy. Baltimore, University Park Press, 1984.

Hartrampf, C. R.: Closure of the donor defect for breast reconstruction with rectus abdominis myocutaneous flap (Discussion). Plast. Reconstr. Surg., *76:*563, 1985.

Hartrampf, C. R.: Hartrampf's Breast Reconstruction with Living Tissue. New York, Raven Press, 1991.

Hartrampf, C. R., and Bennett, G. K.: Autogenous tissue reconstruction in the mastectomy patient: A critical review of 300 patients. Ann. Surg., *205:*508, 1987.

Hartrampf, C. R., et al.: Breast reconstruction with a transverse abdominal island flap. Plast. Reconstr. Surg., *69:*216, 1982.

Kessler: Special report: The basis of the FDA's decision on breast implants. N. Engl. J. Med., *326:*1713, 1992.

Kiser, W. S.: Buying and selling health care: A battle for the medical marketplace. Bull. Am. Coll. Surg., *70:*2, 1985.

Le-Quang, C.: Two new free flaps proceeding from aesthetic surgery: The lateral mammary flap and the inferior gluteal flap. Transactions of the 7th International Congress of Plastic and Reconstructive Surgery, Rio De Janeiro, 1979.

Longmire, W. P. Jr.,: A modification of the Roux technique for antethoracic esophageal reconstruction. Surgery, *22:*94, 1947.

Marshall, D. R.: Immediate reconstruction of the breast following modified radical mastectomy for carcinoma. Br. J. Plast. Surg., *35:*438, 1982.

Mathes, S. J., and Nahai, F.: Classification of the vascular anatomy of muscles: Experimental and clinical correlation. Plast. Reconstr. Surg., *67:*177, 1981.

Mathes, S. J., and Nahai, F.: Clinical Applications for Muscle and Myocutaneous Flaps. St. Louis, C. V. Mosby, 1982.

McCraw, J., and Papp, C.: Latissimus Dorsi Myocutaneous Flap: ''Fleur-de-Lis'' Reconstruction. Hartrampf's Breast Reconstruction with Living Tissue. New York, Raven Press, 1991.

Nahai, F., Bostwick, J. III, and Paletta, C.: The inferior gluteal free flap in breast reconstruction (Abstract). Plast. Reconstr. Surg., *84:*875, 1989.

Noone, R. B., Murphy, J. B., Spear, S. L., et al.: A 6-year experience with immediate reconstruction after mastectomy for cancer. Plast. Reconstr. Surg., *76:*258, 1985.

Pers, M.: The selection of patients for reconstruction following mastectomy for carcinoma of the breast. Br. J. Plast. Surg., *34:*58, 1981.

Radovan, C.: Breast reconstruction after mastectomy using the temporary expander. Plast. Reconstr. Surg., *69:*195, 1982.

Radovan, C.: Tissue expansion is soft-tissue reconstruction. Plast. Recontr. Surg., *74:*482, 1984.

Rosen, P., Jabs, A., Kister, S., et al.: Clinical experience with immediate breast reconstruction using tissue expansion or transverse rectus abdominis musculocutaneous flaps. Ann. Plast. Surg., *25:*249, 1990.

Schneider, W. J., Hill, H. L., and Brown, R. G.: Latissimus dorsi myocutaneous flap for breast reconstruction. Br. J. Plast. Surg., *30:*277, 1977.

Serafin, D. Voci, V. E., and Georgiade, N. G.: Microsurgical composite tissue transplantation: Indications and technical considerations in breast reconstruction following mastectomy. Plast. Reconstr. Surg., *70:*24, 1982.

Shaw, W. W.: Breast reconstruction by superior gluteal microvascular free flaps without silicone implants. Plast. Reconstr. Surg., *72:*490, 1983.

Shaw, W.: The Gluteal Flap. Hartrampf's Breast Reconstruction with Living Tissue. New York, Raven Press, 1991.

Slavin, S. A., and Colen, S. R.: Sixty consecutive breast reconstructions with the inflatable expander: A critical appraisal. Plast. Reconstr. Surg., *86:*910, 1990.

Vinton, A., Traverso, W., and Zehring, D.: Immediate breast reconstruction following mastectomy is as safe as mastectomy alone. Arch. Surg., *125:*1303, 1990.

Webster, D., Mansel, R. E., and Hughes, L. E.: Immediate reconstruction of the breast after mastectomy: Is it safe? Cancer, *53:*1416, 1984.

Webster, J. P., and Gnudi, M. T.: The Life and Times of Gaspare Tagliacozzi, Surgeon of Bologna, 1545–1599. New York, Herbert Reichner, 1950.

Zimmerman, K. W., Montague, E. D., and Fletcher, G. H.: Frequency, anatomic distribution, and management of local recurrences after definitive therapy for breast cancer. Cancer, *19:*67, 1966.

Multiple Primary Cancers in Mammary and Extramammary Sites, and Cancers Metastatic to the Breast

William L. Donegan

John S. Spratt

The occurrence of multiple neoplasms in the same individual is not unusual. Their presence raises questions of predisposing causes and appropriate management. Clearly, any breast tissue that remains after treatment for an initial breast cancer remains at risk for a second primary tumor, and patients with breast cancer are not exempt from developing cancers of other organs. Primary cancers of remote sites may become evident by metastasizing to the breast.

In a review of 139,932 cases of breast cancer reported to the Surveillance, Epidemiology, and End Results (SEER) Program of the National Cancer Institute between 1972 and 1986, Robinson and coworkers (1993) found that 4.2% of patients had bilateral breast primary carcinomas; of these tumors, 41.7% (1.8% of patients) were simultaneous, and the remainder metachronous. Furthermore, after only a short follow-up, 3.6% of the patients had developed one or more extramammary cancers.

BREAST CANCER AND EXTRAMAMMARY CANCERS

If breast cancer did not predispose other organs to malignancy, one might expect women with breast cancer to develop additional cancers with a frequency comparable to that of the general population and, with continuing longevity, to display an accumulation of cancers. This appears to be the case. The three leading carcinomas among the general female population, in descending magnitude, are breast cancer, colorectal cancer, and lung cancer (Boring et al., 1993). Skin cancer of all types occurs with such great frequency that if it were included it would rank first. Thus, the predicted frequency of new cancers in a population treated for cancer of the breast would then be of the skin, breast, colorectum, and lung. Lee (1986) compared the frequency of nonmammary cancers in a population of 665 breast cancer patients studied during follow-up and found the data to be generally in accord with those from the SEER Program. The colorectum and the lung were the two most common sites of subsequent cancers. Rosen and associates

(1989*a*) also documented nonmammary malignancies. Of 644 breast cancer patients with a median follow-up duration of 18.2 years, 13% developed nonmammary cancers, a frequency approximately equal to that for the occurrence of second mammary primary cancers; however, these nonmammary cancers accounted for a death rate that was sevenfold greater than that associated with second primary tumors of the breast. Of the fatalities due to nonmammary primary cancers, most were caused by carcinomas of the ovaries, stomach, pancreas, and lung. Nonmammary cancers evidently constitute a substantial risk, and their detection should be among the goals of any follow-up program for breast cancer patients. Some of these "future" cancers are potentially preventable. Jouin and colleagues (1989) found that 20.5% of 161 patients diagnosed with breast cancer for the first time had adenomatous polyps on proctosigmoidoscopic examination, the removal of which could prevent colorectal cancer; this frequency of polyps is in the expected range (Vitale and Spratt, 1987).

The association between meningiomas and breast cancer, at least 43 cases of which have been reported through 1989, is noteworthy (Miller, 1986; and Rubinstein et al., 1989). Schoenberg and coworkers (1975) indicated that the coincidence of these two cancers exceeded expectations. Both tumors are more frequent in women than in men, appear to be stimulated by pregnancy, and contain estrogen and progesterone receptors (Donnell et al., 1979; and Rubenstein et al., 1989). Since breast cancer is the most frequent cause of intracranial metastases after cancer of the lung, there exists the hazard that curable symptomatic meningiomas will be mistaken for cerebral metastases from a previously treated breast cancer. As a result, a patient will erroneously be deemed incurable, will receive inappropriate treatment, and will die of a benign lesion. This tragic mistake is fostered by the fact that meningiomas are one of the most frequent intracranial tumors and can mimic metastases by being multiple. Meningioma should be suspected in the absence of systemic metastases when the location is typical and when the results of appropriate imaging procedures support the diagnosis.

Among 718 women with breast cancer seen at Ellis Fischel State Cancer Hospital (EFSCH) in Columbia, Missouri, and observed for a total of 3643 woman-years, 52 second cancers were diagnosed. Twenty-two of these (3.89%) were diagnosed synchronously with the diagnosis of breast cancer; in addition, within 20 years of diagnosis, the cumulative frequency of second cancers reached 24.5%. However, these rates were not significantly greater than the expected rates for a population of the same age or for those observed in a control population of women from the same hospital. The distribution of second cancers is shown in Table 27–1. The dominant sites for second cancers were the skin and any remaining breast tissue; cancers of the colorectum ranked a distant third. If the breast is classified as a skin appendage, 42 of 52 of the multiple primary cancers (81%) can be said to be of integumental origin (Spratt and Hoag, 1966; and Spratt, 1977). Considering the slow rate of neoplastic growth in humans, any population can be expected to accumulate ''simultaneous'' cancers before any of them are large enough to produce symptoms (Spratt and Spratt, 1964). The accumulated cancers are discovered simultaneously, but the chance of their having originated simultaneously is exceedingly small.

Statistical methods for the analysis of data relating to multiple cancers are complex and require large numbers of well-documented cases. Use of the actuarial method and further refinements have been valuable tools for determining that associations between cancers are not the result of chance alone (Spratt and Hoag, 1966; Schoenberg, 1977; and Drinkwater and Klotz, 1981). Cook (1966) reviewed the literature on multiple cancers paired at different anatomic sites and found only 12 sites that were associated significantly more often than by chance: breast cancer paired only with cancer of the endometrium. The association of breast and salivary gland cancer has been reported in several studies (Berg et al., 1968; Moertel and Elvebeck, 1969; and Dunn et al., 1972). However, Berg and associates and Moertel and Elvebeck were unable to confirm this association on analysis of the data from the California Tumor Registry. An Israeli experience with multiple primary cancers in breast cancer patients was reported for an 18-year period and for 12,302 cases (Schenker et al., 1984). During the period of observation, 984 patients (8%) had

more than 1 cancer, and 47 patients (0.4%) developed at least 2 cancers in addition to the breast cancer. The investigators concluded that the additional cancers occurred with an incidence greater than that expected for five other sites (the opposite breast, salivary glands, corpus uteri, ovaries, and thyroid gland). Cancers of the stomach and gallbladder occurred less frequently than was expected. Whenever breast cancer was treated with irradiation, the risk for developing carcinomas of the lung and hematopoietic system exceeded expectations.

It should be kept in mind that if persons cured of one cancer live to extremely old age, an estimated one-third of them can expect to develop an additional cancer of some other organ (Einhorn and Jakobsson, 1964; and Spratt and Hoag, 1966). Since these second cancers are the source of considerable morbidity and mortality, the detection of cancers at all sites while they are still in early stages should be the objective of a comprehensive follow-up program.

CANCERS OF THE SECOND BREAST

The breast is a paired organ, and because cancer of the breast is frequently a multifocal process, it is not unusual for women to develop independent cancers in both breasts. In fact, women with cancer in one breast are highly disposed to develop cancer in the second breast. The average annual rate of cancers in the second breast is reported to be between 0.53% and 0.8% in various studies (Rosen et al., 1989b). For the year 1979, the rate of breast cancer in the general female population in the United States was 85 per 100,000. This corresponds to a rate of 108 per 100,000 in the adult female population (which accounts for 78.5% of the total female population), or to an incidence of 0.108%. By dividing this into the annual rate of second breast cancers, one can estimate that women with one breast cancer are 4.9 to 7.4 times more likely to develop a second breast cancer than women in the general population are to develop an initial breast cancer. The annual rate of second breast cancers does not vary significantly. Rosen and colleagues (1989b) were able to demonstrate this during 20 years of follow-up. Hence, the cumulative percentage of patients who develop bilateral breast cancer is a function of time.

Second breast cancers found only with mammography tend to be localized, and a large proportion of these are noninvasive (Sterns and Fletcher, 1991). Unfortunately, not all second breast cancers are detected in this way. Rosen and colleagues (1989b) found that the stages of metachronous primary breast carcinomas tended to be similar. Since more than 80% of breast cancers are invasive ductal carcinomas, the histologic type of first and second primary cancers are usually similar as well; however, only a minority of these cancers are similar with respect to both histologic type and degree of differentiation (Sterns and Fletcher, 1991).

Criteria for Diagnosis

New primary tumors that occur in the opposite breast are potentially curable, whereas metastases to the opposite

Table 27–1. TYPES OF SECOND CANCERS DIAGNOSED AMONG 710 WOMEN WITH BREAST CANCER THROUGH 20 YEARS OF FOLLOW-UP (SIMULTANEOUS AND NONSIMULTANEOUS)

Site	Simultaneous or Within 1 Year of Diagnosis	Nonsimultaneous Diagnosed From 1 to 20 Years After First Diagnosis	Total
Skin	12	10	22
Cervix	1		1
Breast	8	12	20
Endometrium	1		1
Colorectum		4	4
Vulva		2	2
Hodgkin's disease		1	1
Esophagus		1	1
Total	22	30	52

breast are not. Hence, it is important to distinguish between the two. Billroth's original criteria for the diagnosis of independent cancers were stringent, requiring that the tumors have different histologic features, be located in different organs, and be responsible for separate metastases (Pennell, 1958; and Kapsinow, 1962). The more liberal criteria developed by Warren and Gates (1932)—which required only that the tumors be malignant and separate and that neither represent a metastasis—found greater general acceptance.

Except for a small group of special histologic types, the majority of breast cancers have similar features microscopically. Robbins and Berg (1964) appreciated this reality, and in defining a series of 94 patients with bilateral breast cancers, emphasized the following points for diagnosing second primary tumors:

1. Primary tumors can be expected to develop within breast tissue, most frequently in the upper outer quadrant, but not in the fatty tail of the breast: metastases appear in the fat at the periphery of the breast parenchyma, usually near the midline or in the fatty tail.

2. Metastases tend to be multiple and to show expansile growth rather than the infiltrative, stellate pattern characteristic of primary tumors.

3. Most importantly, primary tumors are often associated with contiguous in situ carcinoma, whereas metastases lack this feature. Medullary carcinoma, around which in situ cancer is not expected, is an exception to this observation.

In addition to these criteria, Leis (1971) accepted the diagnosis of a second primary tumor if the degree of nuclear differentiation was definitely greater than that of the first cancer or if the second lesion occurred more than 5 years after the first and in the absence of evidence of metastasis elsewhere.

Liberal criteria have been accepted in our own studies. If carcinoma was found in the parenchyma of the second breast at the time of or at any time subsequent to the treatment of the first primary tumor, and if thorough clinical, radiographic, and laboratory evaluations revealed no evidence of tumor elsewhere, then the lesion was considered an independent primary tumor rather than a metastasis. This gives a patient the benefit of the most optimistic interpretation of a lesion in the second breast. Any cancer in the second breast is more likely to be a new primary tumor than a metastasis, particularly if the interval after treatment of the first tumor is great (Shellito and Bartlett, 1967; and Egan, 1976). Over a comparable period of observation, only 1.5% of mastectomy patients at EFSCH developed metastases to the opposite breast, whereas 3% of them developed new primary tumors (Donegan, 1970).

Incidence of Cancers of the Second Breast

Bilateral cancers are categorized as simultaneous or nonsimultaneous (metachronous), depending on whether they are diagnosed at the same time or at different times (i.e., the second is diagnosed after the first cancer is treated or after some arbitrary interval, such as 6 months). Because neo-

plastic growth is variable, it is not always possible to determine whether and for how long two neoplasms have coexisted. According to 22 reports prior to 1965 collected from the literature by Leis and associates (1965), bilateral simultaneous mammary cancers were diagnosed in from 0.1% to 2% of cases. Nonsimultaneous second cancers developed in from 1% to 12% of cases during varying periods of observation, with a median rate of 3.2%. Most authors estimate that 7% to 10% of patients ultimately develop an independent cancer in the remaining breast (Kilgore, 1921; Harrington, 1946; Trevor, 1954; Fitts and Patterson, 1955; and Robbins and Berg, 1964).

The experience at EFSCH with simultaneous breast cancers was consistent with that of reports from other medical institutions. Fifty-two of 2620 women (2%) with cancer of the breast seen during the period from 1940 to 1965 initially had bilateral mammary cancers. The frequency of metachronous cancers varied somewhat in surgical series at EFSCH. In a 1967 review of the disease histories of 704 women with no previous cancers and treated with mastectomy who were observed for 5 to 18 years, it was found that 14 of them (2%) developed a second primary tumor of the breast within 7 years (Table 27–2). Later, 167 patients with clinically early unilateral cancers were treated with mastectomy between 1963 and 1972 and were closely observed for an average period of 63 months, during which 55.7% of the patients died. Five of these patients (3%) developed cancers in the remaining breast from 4 to 30 months after the original treatment. In two additional cases, occult cancers were diagnosed with elective biopsies of normal breasts, bringing the total rate of metachronous bilaterality to 4.2%.

Because detection of clinically apparent second primary cancers is a function of the duration of follow-up observation, the longer a group of patients is followed, the greater will be the morbidity from additional cancers. As illustrated in Table 27–3, the frequency of second mammary cancers ranged from 0% to 0.8% annually for the first 7 years after treatment, with no clear trend toward either increase or decrease.

In addition to total observation time, the detection of multiple cancers is distinctly a function of the age of a patient population. Data on incidence are recorded as the number of new cases per 100,000 people per year, but since the incidence varies at different ages, the rate is further defined for specific age ranges. The age-specific incidence of most cancers increases with time. When a patient has had one cancer, the pertinent question regarding additional cancers is whether the age-specific incidence is equal to, the same as, or less than the age-specific incidence of cancers among persons who have not had a previous cancer. A detailed analysis of EFSCH data was performed for 704 women who were at risk for developing a second mammary cancer after mastectomy for unilateral mammary cancer. The period of risk totaled 4663 woman-years, and during this time, 15 breast cancers appeared, corresponding to a frequency of 0.00321 cancers per woman-year of observation. This is equivalent to a frequency of 321 cancers per 100,000 people per year. The female control population with no mammary cancer was observed for 4244 woman-years, and 8 mammary cancers were diagnosed; this corre-

Table 27-2. SIMULTANEOUS AND NONSIMULTANEOUS SECOND PRIMARY BREAST CRCINOMAS AT EFSCH, 1940 TO JUNE 1958

	First Primary Treated				Simultaneous	Second Primary Treated				Survival After Treatment	
Age	Duration of Symptoms (mo)	Stage (CCC*)	Axillary Lymph Nodes	Diameter (cm)	Duration of Symptoms (mo)	Stage (CCC*)	Axillary Lymph Nodes	Diameter (cm)		First Primary (mo)	Second Primary (mo)
82	9	A	+	3.0	0	A	Unk†	2.5		21	20
68	24	A	−	2.0	28	B	−	2.4		126	122
56	12	A	+	5.0	25	B	+	5.0		182	181
68	25	A	−	1.0	2	A	−	2.5		93	92
63	1	B	+	Unk	3	A	+	3.3		42	40
49	12	B	−	8.5	6	B	+	7.0		19	19
78	9	C	Unk†	1.5	6	A	−	6.0		14	13

	First Primary				Nonsimultaneous Duration of Interval: Treatment of First to Symptoms of Second (mo)	Second Primary				Survival After Treatment	
Age	Duration of Symptoms (mo)	Stage (CCC*)	Axillary Lymph Nodes	Diameter (cm)		Duration of Symptoms (mo)	Stage (CCC*)	Axillary Lymph Nodes	Diameter (cm)	First Primary (mo)	Second Primary (mo)
68	21	A	−	3.0	79	4	A	−	4.0	120	40
38	3	A	+	6.0	48	7	B	+	8.0	61	6
61	4	A	−	<4.0	10	4	D	+	1.5	30	17
55	24	B	+	3.8	26	2	B	−	2.3	101	73
43	1	B	−	2.0	37	2	B	+	1.5	67	28
43	2	B	+	1.0	43	1	C	+	1.5	112	69
51	3	B	+	2.0	6	0	B	+	2.5	251	244
40	54	B	+	4.0	70	2	B	+	3.0	235	162
39	12	B	+	4.5	17	9	B	+	3.5	39	13
67	12	B	+	3.5	123	2	A	Unk†	2.0	177	53
74	18	B	+	4.0	45	7	B	−	3.0	159	107
76	48	B	−	9.0	79	1	D	+	2.0	97	19
72	6	B	−	2.0	27	8	B	+	4.5	166	131
75	24	C	+	5.0	14	1	A	−	1.0	91	77
51	6	C	+	7.5	13	3	A	+	5.0	24	8

*Columbia Clinical Classification.
†Unk = Unknown (simple mastectomy).
‡Local excision.

sponds to a frequency of 0.00188 cancers per women-year, which is equivalent to 188 cancers per 100,000 people per year. A 2 × 2 contengency table demonstrated no difference in the frequency of mammary cancers between the two populations (chi square test = 1.06; $P > .3$). The observed incidence of mammary cancer in Connecticut for adult females of equivalent ages ranged from 0.00123 to 0.00352 per woman-year (Griswold, 1955). However, the incidence of nonsimultaneous second mammary cancers did vary significantly above and below the age of 54 years (chi square

test = 6.21; $P = .01$) (Fig. 27–1). When these EFSCH data were compared with the ranges of the age-specific incidence of first cancers in New York State, there was a disproportionately large number of women younger than 50 years of age who were afflicted a second time (Fig. 27–2).

Concepts concerning the frequency of multiple primary breast cancers have changed as a result of information from detailed studies of mastectomy specimens, the widespread use of mammography, and biopsies of clinically normal breasts. Qualheim and Gall (1957) studied multiple sections

Table 27-3. RATE OF OCCURRENCE OF SECOND PRIMARY BREAST CARCINOMAS IN 704 PATIENTS FOLLOWING SURGERY FOR A PREVIOUS MAMMARY CANCER (EFSCH, 1940 TO JUNE 1958)

Years	Number at Risk	Number Dying	Number Withdrawn Alive	Annual Number Developing Second Primary	Annual Percentage Developing Second Primary	Cumulative Percentage with Second Primary
1	704	60	0	2	0.3	0.3
2	644	88	0	3	0.5	0.7
3	556	81	0	2	0.4	1.0
4	475	56	0	4	0.8	1.6
5	419	39	0	0	0.0	1.6
6	381	37	2	1	0.3	1.7
7	341	32	16	2	0.6	2.0

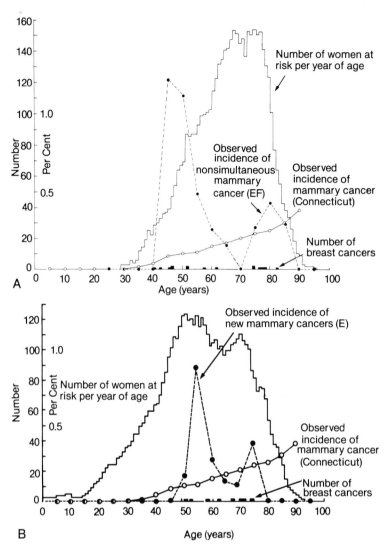

Figure 27-1. The age-specific percentage of new mammary cancers has been determined by averaging 5-year increments of observation. The number of woman-years of observation in each 5-year period was divided into the number of mammary cancers developing during the same period. Multiplying the dividend by 100 gives the age-specific percentage afflicted in 5-year averages. The 5-year average age-specific incidence rate for Connecticut (Griswold et al.) is plotted for comparison. The data in *A* are from a population of women who had had one mammary cancer resected. The data in *B* are from a population of women who had had one negative physical examination and were followed to determine the incidence of cancers developing subsequent to the examination. (From Spratt, J. S., and Hoag, T. L.: Incidence of multiple primary cancers per man-year of follow-up. Ann. Surg., *164:*775, 1966.)

of 157 breasts removed for cancer and found multiple independent sites of cancer in 54% of them, with involvement of multiple quadrants in 37%. These results were confirmed when Gallager and Martin (1969) found two or more (usually many) independent foci of cancer in 47% of subserial whole-organ histologic preparations of 47 breasts. Using only single histologic samples, Fisher and coworkers (1975*b*) found independent foci of cancer in quadrants other than those in which the clinical cancer arose in 13% of 904 mastectomy specimens. Multiplicity tends to be high even when the primary tumor is too small to palpate (Schwartz et al., 1988) and increases with tumor size (Ro-

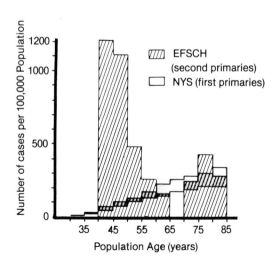

Figure 27-2. New mammary cancers in the breast remaining after mastectomy at EFSCH compared with the age-specific frequency of initial cancers in New York State. An excess is most notably evident in women younger than 55 years of age.

sen et al., 1975). Tinnemans and associates (1986) studied nonpalpable cancers treated with mastectomy using multiple 5-mm tissue sections. They took sections from any grossly or radiographically suspicious areas and defined multicentricity as additional sites of cancer in a quadrant different from the primary site or at least 5 cm away from the primary site if the latter was located beneath the nipple. These investigators found multifocal involvement in 33% of 57 cases of invasive cancer and in 48% of 25 cases of ductal carcinoma in situ. The data of these reports are clear evidence that carcinogenesis in the human breast is a diffuse phenomenon and is characterized by a more widespread tissue response than is appreciated clinically. Nielsen and associates (1986) reported an extensive histologic assessment of the contralateral breast in 84 consecutive autopsies of women with the clinical diagnosis of invasive breast cancer. Sixty-eight per cent of these women were found to have primary breast cancers in the contralateral breast (33% of these being invasive and 36% in situ cancers). Their study failed to identify any clinical or histopathologic characteristics that could have significantly predicted the occurrence of the contralateral cancers. Fibrocystic changes (type unspecified) were frequently associated with bilaterality.

The increased use of mammography increases the rate of detection of otherwise occult cancers. Mammography has contributed to earlier recognition of primary cancers and perhaps to their differentiation from metastatic cancers (Egan, 1976). Using mammography, Egan reported finding new contralateral cancers in 6% of 1112 women examined at Emory University between 1963 and 1973. Second mammary cancers were diagnosed in 26 (6.3%) of 414 women who underwent a previous mastectomy. Although the discovery rate in the total group was not unusually high, the proportion of cancers diagnosed simultaneously (27%) was higher and the proportion diagnosed subsequently lower (particularly during the first 6 months after mastectomy) than in series reported earlier in which routine mammography was not used. Second cancers were discovered more often while not palpable and at a smaller size than were the first cancers, although reduction in the frequency of axillary metastasis was not substantial. Thus, the effect of routine mammography was earlier detection, which resulted in the transfer of more second cancers into the simultaneous category.

The true significance of multicentric primary breast cancers remains incompletely resolved. Even the prevalence of the problem remains incompletely defined and varies with pathologic interpretation and with the inclusion or exclusion of in situ cancers. Necropsy data, for example, indicate carcinoma in situ to be 19 times as prevalent as invasive cancer (Kramer and Rush, 1973). The occurrence of two dominant cancers simultaneously is infrequent (~0.1%, according to Fisher and coworkers [1975*b*]), but new or progressive cancer in a treated breast is not infrequent if the breast is not removed. Hermann and associates (1984) reported the appearance of new primary cancers in the treated breast of 7% of women within 5 years of treatment with partial mastectomy. Thirty-seven per cent of Tagart's patients (1978) treated with local excision alone subsequently developed cancer in the same breast. Forty per cent of Fisher and coworkers' patients with operable cancers in the

National Surgical Adjuvant Breast Project Protocol B-06 who were treated with wide local excision alone developed progressive cancer in the treated breast within 8 years (Fisher et al., 1989). Whether or not breast irradiation is used, the most frequent site at which cancer reappears after partial mastectomy is the surgical area; suggesting that incomplete excision of the first cancer is the cause rather than the independent development of new cancers (Harris et al., 1981; and Fisher et al., 1989).

In Protocol B-04 of the National Surgical Adjuvant Breast Project, the appearance of cancers in the contralateral breast reached 3.7% for invasive cancers and 0.5% for noninvasive forms (Fisher et al., 1985*c*). Such longitudinal follow-up is essential to assay the importance of this problem.

An increase in the detection rate of simultaneous bilateral cancers can also be attributed to liberal indications for biopsy of the second breast. Urban (1967, 1969*b*) was the first to advocate routine contralateral biopsy as a method of detection. It was Urban's experience that breast biopsies performed in the presence of minimal physical signs yielded evidence of cancers in 11% of cases; many of the cancers detected in this way were also not suspected on mammography. Soon, Urban began to biopsy the second breast routinely. In the presence of a physically and mammographically normal breast, the "random" biopsies included 20% of the mammary parenchyma from the upper outer quadrant as well as from the location representing the "mirror image" of the area where the first primary tumor was located. Almost 1 in 10 of these biopsies (9.5%) revealed the presence of occult cancer (Urban, 1969*a*). Overall, 15% of 281 private patients proved to have contralateral cancers, 10% of which were simultaneous. The frequency of previous or simultaneous bilaterality rose to 20.4% among 337 private and clinic patients, and the total rate was 13% for 505 patients with and without contralateral biopsies who were seen between 1966 and 1968. The highest frequency of bilaterality was found in patients with in situ lobular carcinoma (54%), medullary carcinoma (25%), and noninfiltrating ductal carcinomas (19%). Sixty-three per cent of the simultaneous second cancers were found at a noninvasive stage, and only 6.2% of the invasive cancers had produced axillary metastases; both of these situations promised excellent chances of cure. Using elective biopsies, Pressman (1985) found that 10% of 250 consecutive women under the age of 65 years with Stage I or II cancers had cancers in the opposite breast. Some authors believe that the yield would probably be equally great if elective biopsies were limited to the upper outer quadrant of the breast rather than limited to the mirror image location (Fenig et al., 1975). Elective contralateral biopsy was adopted by some surgeons primarily for patients at a higher-than-average risk for the development of second cancers (Lewison, 1970; Wilson, 1973; Fenig et al., 1975; and Kessler et al., 1976).

The frequency of bilaterality detected with elective biopsies rivals that reported by Leis (1971) among carefully selected patients who had contralateral prophylactic mastectomies (17%) and is higher than that reported by Egan (1976) for physical examination and mammography. The fact that the frequency of bilateral cancers detected in this manner exceeds the 10% observed during follow-up suggests that some second primary cancers grow so slowly that they fail to evolve into clinical cancers during a patient's lifetime.

A major problem with elective biopsy is that failure to find cancer neither excludes its presence nor its future development. Fenig and colleagues (1975) reported on 314 "mirror image" biopsies, 23 of which (7.3%) confirmed the presence of cancer. Notably, 6 of 291 patients (2%) with negative results on biopsy subsequently developed cancer in the breast; in 3 of these, the cancers arose in the vicinity of the biopsy. Among 80 patients treated for lobular carcinoma in situ and observed for an average of 15 years, Rosen and associates (1981) found that the proportion of patients who developed cancers in the second breast after a negative contralateral biopsy (17.2%) was no smaller than that of patients who had no such biopsy (17.6%). One of the authors of this chapter (WLD) also found no obvious reduction in the occurrence of future cancers in patients with negative results on elective biopsy and thus abandoned this practice in favor of close follow-up. The natural history and malignant potential of many cancers diagnosed entirely on a microscopic basis (when they are both asymptomatic and clinically undetectable) remain undetermined.

Patients at High Risk for Cancer of the Second Breast

Several factors identify patients at high risk for bilateral cancers. These include youth, ability to survive the first cancer, a diffuse tissue response, and, possibly, a genetic predisposition.

Women Younger Than 50 Years of Age

The susceptibility of young women to bilateral primary tumors is clear. The risk for such patients is 10 to 14 times greater than expected for initial cancers in the general population (Robbins and Berg, 1964; Berndt et al., 1970; and Robinson et al., 1993). A partial explanation is the fact that young women who are cured of a first cancer have an extended period of risk for the development of a second.

Family History of Breast Cancer

The case control studies of Anderson (1973) indicated that patients with first-degree relatives who have breast cancer are two to five times more likely than average to develop bilateral cancers, with the highest risk among those who are 20 to 44 years old. Although this was not confirmed in a large population based study, the existence of a genetic predisposition to the disease that results in both an early onset and diffuse parenchymal involvement is likely (Adami et al., 1981).

Grossly Multifocal Cancer

Women who initially have two or more grossly evident, independent primary tumors in the same breast constitute less than 2% of all cases, but they have four times the average risk of developing additional cancers in the second breast (Robbins and Berg, 1964). Although a far greater number of women are found to have two or more occult cancers on detailed examination of the breast, the evidence for clinically relevant, diffuse carcinogenesis is most evident in patients with multiple gross cancers.

Lobular Carcinoma In Situ

Lobular carcinoma in situ (LCIS) accounts for less than 10% of mammary cancers, but much has been written about it, primarily because of its high bilaterality and controversial potential for malignancy. Haagensen (1971) minimized its potential and preferred to speak of lobular "neoplasia" rather than lobular carcinoma, but tumors demonstrating anaplasia (Type B) were considered more dangerous than well-differentiated tumors (Type A). At the other extreme, McDivitt and associates (1967) reported that 35% of women observed for up to 20 years developed invasive cancers in breasts known to harbor LCIS. One fact is uncontested: LCIS is unsurpassed for its occurrence bilaterally, which is detected in 25% to 40% of women with LCIS (Newman, 1963; Benfield et al., 1965; McDivitt et al., 1967; Urban, 1969b, Andersen, 1977; Fisher and Fisher, 1977; and Peters et al., 1977).

At EFSCH, random biopsies of the second breast of patients known to have LCIS or invasive lobular carcinoma of one breast revealed bilateral involvement in 11 of 36 cases (Donegan and Perez-Mesa, 1972). Seven were detected with elective biopsies in 20 patients, an incidence of 35% in clinically normal breasts. Bilaterality was diagnosed in 36% of 28 patients with LCIS. Although the cases were few, invasive lobular cancer seemed to carry the same implications as LCIS: one of five women from whom tissue was available had an invasive cancer in the opposite breast. Lobular cancer was multifocal in 76% of mastectomy specimens and often occurred in the presence of other histologic types of cancer. As cancers found in the second breast were not regularly lobular in type, LCIS appeared to be a marker for multiple cancers and not necessarily of their genesis. Baker and Kuhajda (1989) reviewed a series of patients treated for unilateral invasive lobular carcinoma and found no higher frequency of subsequent primary tumors in the second breast than in patients with invasive ductal cancers; however, the comparison was not controlled for the duration of the follow-up.

Ductal Carcinoma In Situ

Ductal carcinoma in situ (DCIS) tends to be multicentric or to extensively involve ducts by growth in continuity (Holland et al., 1990). Pomerantz and colleagues (1988) reviewed multiple factors associated with an increase in bilateral breast cancer in a series of 187 cases and concluded that the presence of multicentric in situ changes was the most significant predictor of metachronous cancer. The prognosis was favorable for patients who underwent definitive surgical treatment for each cancer. In a review of cases of noninvasive cancers at the Medical College of Wisconsin, 25% of women with DCIS in one breast had cancer in both breasts (Peters et al., 1977). This already had exceeded three times the general incidence of bilaterality. The high frequency of bilateral cancer in women with DCIS was also noted by Robbins and Berg (1964), by Robinson and coworkers (1993), and by Urban (1969*b*). Many patients with DCIS at the Medical College of Wisconsin had previously been treated for an invasive cancer. Twenty per cent of those whose initial cancer was DCIS developed bilateral cancers within 10 years. Webber and coworkers found no increase in bilaterality (1983).

Histologically Favorable Invasive Cancers

Mucinous carcinoma, erroneously called "colloid" carcinoma, is a relatively benign and rare type of cancer. Robbins and Berg (1964) found it to be associated with a mild excess of second primary cancers—that is, the second breast was affected at 1.23 times the expected rate. When in a pure form, tumors of this type are highly curable, thus leaving the patient at a prolonged risk for the development of cancer in the remaining breast. Among 44 pure mucinous carcinomas collected from three institutions (EFSCH, Milwaukee County Medical Complex, and Columbia Hospital in Milwaukee) over a period of 25 years, the authors observed that 2 patients (4.5%) had multifocal lesions in the first breast and that 4 patients (9%) had an independent primary tumor in the second breast. Sixteen of the patients with unilateral disease remained alive and at risk for second primary cancers.

Possibly at higher-than-average risk are patients with tumors of other benign histologic types, including tubular and medullary carcinomas. Slack and associates (1973) included patients with large cancers (those 6 cm or greater in diameter) in the high-risk category, but Robbins and Berg (1964) found no evidence for high risk.

Prognosis

Despite the fact that second primary mammary cancers are an acknowledged hazard, they are not always detected in their early stages. This was particularly true prior to the widespread use of mammography. At Memorial Sloan Kettering Cancer Center in New York City, second primary cancers generally were smaller than the first cancers, but only one-third of them were in early clinical stages (Robbins and Berg, 1964). The metachronous second cancers of 79 patients reported by Leis and coworkers in 1965 were not detected at stages earlier than were these patients' first primary tumors. During the same period, a conscientious follow-up program at EFSCH resulted in the discovery of second primary cancers at an average diameter (3.0 cm),

smaller than that of first ones (4.1 cm). However, no greater percentage of these cancers were found in early stages.

Since 1969, widespread use of mammography has improved detection. More recent series reflect that cancers in the second breast are smaller in size and that the frequency of nodal involvement is reduced when they are detected with mammography (Khafagy et al., 1975; Egan, 1976; Kessler et al., 1976; and Sterns et al., 1991).

The prognosis of patients with bilateral cancers is commensurate with the stages of the cancers (Huff, 1969; Slack et al., 1973; Wilson and Alberty, 1973; and Khafagy et al., 1975). Fourteen patients with bilateral simultaneous mammary cancers in operable stages treated at EFSCH prior to 1958 had an actuarial survival rate of 57% at 5 years. All except one patient underwent mastectomy. Fifteen cases of nonsimultaneous bilateral cancers were treated with mastectomy, with 5-year survival rates of 80% after treatment of the first cancer and of 47% after treatment of the second cancer. The capacity of a patient to live long enough to develop a second primary cancer in most instances reflects a prognostically favorable initial cancer. For comparison, 52.4% of 781 patients who developed no second breast cancers during this period survived for 5 years, and 34.3% survived for 10 years.

The favorable course of women after removal of a second mammary cancer has suggested to some investigators the possibility of a benefit from immunologic stimulation by the first cancer, particularly by in situ cancer (Black et al., 1972; Wilson and Alberty 1973; and Black, 1975). If it can be presumed that mammary cancers share common antigens, sequential cancers constitute, in effect, a natural experiment in immunotherapy. To support this thesis, Black and associates (1972) reported that cancers occurring subsequent to in situ cancers or to atypical hyperplasias were of a favorable type more often and had a better prognosis than those not preceded by these lesions.

It is clear that second breast cancers constitute an independent risk for treatment failure. Rosen and colleagues (1989*b*) estimated that they accounted for 5.1% of recurrences and for 2.6% of deaths from breast cancer. With matched controls, Robbins and Berg (1964) showed that a second mammary cancer reduced the expected survival in the group at risk. Robinson and coworkers (1993) reported a less favorable rate of survival for patients after treatment for a second breast cancer than after treatment for a single breast cancer; however, the difference was greater if both tumors were regional in extent than if they were both localized. Investigators have also found that the prognosis following a second breast cancer is better if it follows the first by a long interval, presumably because the competing risk of recurrence from the first cancer is diminished and less likely to be superimposed on that of the second (Michowitz et al., 1985; and Robinson et al., 1993). Simply stated, it would appear that the prognosis for surviving a second breast cancer is dependent on both the cancer's stage and its temporal occurrence. When breast cancers are simultaneous, the risk is additive, but the added risk of the second cancer is less likely to be appreciated if it is less extensive than the dominant cancer and if the prospects for cure of the dominant cancer are poor. When the second breast cancer is metachronous, its curability is diminished by the extent to which recurrence of the first cancer is a continuing risk.

Treatment

Operable primary cancers in one or both breasts should be treated optimistically with intent to cure. Treatment should not be compromised simply because both breasts contain cancer rather than only one breast. Each should be treated optimally. Except in unusual circumstances, both cancers can be treated simultaneously. Ratzer and associates (1966) described a two-team technique for performing simultaneous bilateral mastectomies, but a single team can perform this operation safely within a reasonable period of time and usually without the need for blood transfusion. When bilateral mastectomies are performed, the authors do not join the incisions across the midline because scars over the sternum and costal cartilage are prone to keloid formation. The central part of a continuous scar also tends to "bowstring" between the two breasts after breast reconstruction. Bilateral breast conservation, when the situation permits, is also feasible; however, experience in this area is still limited. The irradiation required for bilateral conservation is more extensive and more technically demanding than that for unilateral conservation. If the cancer on one side requires a mastectomy but that on the second side does not, the cancer on the second side can be treated with breast conservation if the patient prefers; however, the symmetry of breast reconstruction is usually improved if the second side also is treated with mastectomy.

PROPHYLACTIC MASTECTOMY

The threat imposed by second mammary cancers raises the issue of contralateral mastectomy as a preventive measure. It is not a new idea. Bloodgood suggested removing the uninvolved breast with simple mastectomy for this reason in 1921, as did Pack in 1951. Leis (1968) argued the case, emphasizing that a high-risk group for second cancers can be defined, that removal of the breast can be performed with negligible risk, that the procedure is acceptable to many women, and that for some women it is both a mental and physical benefit. Leis recommended the operation to women with small Stage I lesions; favorable histologic types of cancers, including in situ, medullary, and colloid cancers; a family history of breast cancer; and multiple primary tumors as well as to those younger than 50 years of age. Unsuspected cancers were found in 16 (17%) of 91 such mastectomy specimens, the majority of which (11) were not invasive (Leis, 1971). The 96.5% 5-year survival rate of Leis's cases suggests that selection was confined to women with a good prognosis and that occult second cancers were managed effectively.

The case for prophylactic mastectomy has been explored by others and been found wanting. The arguments against it are the following:

1. The anticipated benefits are small compared with the surgical morbidity.

2. With vigilance, second cancers can be detected early and treated effectively when they occur.

3. A large proportion of the mastectomies would be done needlessly for the possible benefit of relatively few women.

If mastectomy were adopted as a routine prophylactic measure, the magnitude of the undertaking would dwarf the anticipated rewards. Robbins and Berg (1964) estimated that only 1 in 20 such operations would be lifesaving. This is a conservative estimate. Using data on 2734 patients treated with mastectomies by members of the National Surgical Adjuvant Breast Project, Slack and associates (1973) found that within the first 5 years of follow-up, 3% of patients developed second mammary cancers. Assuming that one-third of the 3% ultimately would die of metastases from their first cancers and not be benefitted and that only 40% of the remaining 2% would have been saved by a prophylactic mastectomy (60% could still have been cured by treatment at the time of diagnosis), a maximum of 0.8% of all women (0.02 multipled by 0.40) would be saved from dying of a second breast cancer that had developed during the first 5 years. This salvage would require 98 nonbeneficial mastectomies for the potential benefit of 2 women. If the operation were confined to women who have five times the expected risk, the advantages would be increased, but not greatly. The same line of reasoning would lead to the conclusion that 90 useless mastectomies would have to be performed to save four patients' lives from new cancers diagnosed within 5 years of mastectomy. Although the rate of second cancers remains constant after this time, their absolute number is small because the number of surviving patients is greatly diminished. Breast tissue is so extensive in its anatomic spread and so intimate in its relation to the skin as to preclude its removal by any means of dissection short of a total mastectomy with thin skin flaps. Even after seemingly complete operations, both animal and human studies have shown that additional primary cancers still appear in any residual breast tissue (Klamer et al., 1983; and Jackson et al., 1984).

The usual "simple" mastectomy often fails to remove all breast tissue. Many examples of women who have had cancer develop in residual breast tissue at the site of simple mastectomies performed for nonmalignant conditions can be produced. This operation is thus an incomplete and, at best, an unproved guarantee against the occurrence of future mammary cancers (Hicken, 1940; and Holleb and Farrow, 1967). Considering the wide distribution of mammary parenchyma on the chest and in the axillae, a truly prophylactic operation is not the simple matter that it is often assumed to be.

The fact that second primary cancers are being discovered earlier with mammography, and often simultaneously with first primary cancers, makes prophylactic removal of breasts less attractive than when it was originally proposed. With current methods of diagnosis, it is likely that even fewer lives would be jeopardized if physicians were to maintain a policy of conscientious observation until therapeutic intervention is necessary. This conclusion was also reached by Al-Jurf and coworkers (1981) in a clinical study of 104 women with bilateral breast cancers. Based on the analysis of survivorship data, these authors believed that the problem of asynchronous second primary cancers was best addressed with detection through careful follow-up.

The problem of predicting who will develop a cancer in the second breast has been addressed by researchers in a search for effective clinical strategies. Some of these strategies are based on microscopic features of the first cancer (Fisher et al., 1975a; Schwartz et al., 1980; Lesser et al., 1982; Lewis et al., 1982; Martin et al., 1982; Haagensen et al., 1983; and Davis and Baird, 1984). An aggressive approach that included routine biopsies of the second breast was reported by Wanebo and coworkers (1985), who studied a series of 62 cases and used the morphologic findings to argue for this procedure. Without longitudinal studies to confirm the rate and frequency with which multicentric foci of in situ and invasive cancers become clinically significant, the ultimate outcomes of these approaches remain uncertain. When an initial cancer is unlikely to be cured, the threat of a future cancer in the second breast becomes of little consequence. When cure is likely, a patient's longevity may permit microscopic cancer and precancerous lesions in the second breast to develop into clinical disease.

The authors agree with those clinicians who believe that the indications for prophylactic mastectomy are few (Moffat et al., 1988; and Rosen et al., 1989b). After receiving a diagnosis of cancer in one breast, some patients insist on having bilateral mastectomies because of their overwhelming anxiety about the possible occurrence of subsequent second primary cancers; their overall well-being seems to require that such an operation be performed. Physicians encounter patients with combinations of circumstances (e.g., an exceptionally strong family history of breast cancer, biopsy evidence of extensive atypical hyperplasia, and a breast that defies reliable examination) for whom the request for bilateral mastectomy seems reasonable. The point can be added that bilateral mastectomy may simplify breast reconstruction. Although appealing in concept, the role of prophylactic mastectomy is not well established, even in circumstances of high risk for a second cancer.

METASTASES TO THE BREAST FROM NONMAMMARY CANCERS

Recognition of metastatic cancer to the breast is important not only for diagnosis of the second cancer but also to avoid unnecessary treatment of a patient's breast. Metastases to the breast may simulate all presentations of primary breast cancer, including those of inflammatory cancer (Hébert et al., 1991), and present a differential diagnostic challenge. In most cases, the cancer that produced the metastasis has been previously diagnosed. Multiple tumors, involvement principally of skin or subcutaneous tissues, or the presence of unusual histopathologic features suggests metastatic cancer. The results of histologic analysis also often suggest the site of the primary tumor, such as clear-cell carcinoma from the kidney or mucin-producing adenocarcinoma from the stomach or intestine. Undifferentiated carcinomas are less revealing but are consistent with melanoma. Vergier and coworkers (1991) found that immuno-histochemical studies often are helpful in identifying the source of metastases. Metastatic cancers tend to engulf or

displace mammary ducts and lobules, and the mammary epithelium does not participate in the neoplastic process (Silverman and Oberman, 1974). Metastases to the breast are indicative of a rapidly progressive disseminated cancer with a poor attendant prognosis. Only 1 of the 11 patients studied by Silverman and Oberman survived longer than 1 year.

Metastases to the breast originate from a wide variety of sites. Involvement by lymphoma and leukemia does occur but is usually excluded from consideration in reviews of this problem. Nance and coworkers (1966) reviewed cases reported between 1966 and 1936 and found fewer than 60. In their cases, metastases from a gastric cancer mimicked inflammatory cancer of the breast. Nielsen and associates (1981) found melanoma to be the most frequent source of metastases to the breast, followed in order of frequency by carcinomas of the lung, prostate gland, ovaries, and stomach. In 1991, Vergier and coworkers also found melanoma to be the most frequent source, followed by lung carcinoma and carcinoids. The English literature contained five definite cases of malignant carcinoid tumors that were metastatic to the breast, according to the research of Harrist and Kalisher (1977); to this set, these researchers added a sixth case. In their review, they noted that the most common secondary tumor of the female breast was metastatic cancer from the opposite breast. For the male breast, the most common secondary neoplasm was metastatic carcinoma from the prostate gland. The breast is also the occasional target for metastases from cancers originating in other organs, including the nasopharynx, uterus, kidney, pancreas, and liver (Nunez et al., 1989; Amichetti et al., 1990; Masters, 1990; and DiBonito et al., 1991). The authors have personal knowledge of patients with metastases to the breast from cancers of the lung (male breast), thyroid gland, cervix uteri, and stomach as well as from rhabdomyosarcoma (Figs. 27–3 and 27–4).

The tendency of melanomas to metastasize to the breast has been reported on a number of occasions. The presence of any breast mass in a patient with a past history of melanoma requires that melanoma be considered in the differential diagnosis and histologic evaluation. The absence of signs of systemic spread and a long disease-free

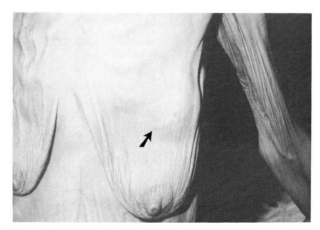

Figure 27–3. Metastasis to the breast from carcinoma of the thyroid.

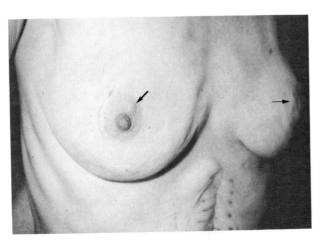

Figure 27–4. Multiple metastases to both breasts from an advanced adenocarcinoma of the stomach.

interval do not rule out the possibility of melanoma (Lanzafame et al., 1984). Nevertheless, metastasis of melanoma to the breast is still uncommon, and its frequency is eclipsed by melanoma's tendency to metastasize to other organs.

Peculiarly, the breast is a frequent site for metastases in children with rhabdomyosarcomas. Howarth and coworkers (1980) reported 7 cases of metastases to the breast in a series of 108 children and youths with rhabdomyosarcoma who ranged in age from 5 months to 20 years (median = 11.5 years).

Diagnosis of the occasional case of metastasis to the breast requires alert clinical and pathologic correlation. Management depends on the type of neoplasm and its extent. Mammography is useful to evaluate the extent of metastases within the breast. The objective of treatment is palliation. When an operation is necessary, wide local excision is usually adequate. Rarely, mastectomy may be necessary to control local progression. Occasionally, there is a palliative advantage to performing regional lymph node dissections when lymph nodes are enlarged from melanoma, even when they represent disseminated cancer.

TREATMENT-RELATED SECOND MALIGNANCIES

Increasing use of treatment methods that are themselves carcinogenic poses a risk of inducing additional cancers that is incompletely quantified (Boivin, 1990). This risk is evident after treatment of childhood cancers. Among 910 survivors of childhood cancer, Li and colleagues (1983) found four breast cancers in women aged 20, 25, and 38 years and in a man aged 38 years. Considering the ages of the patients and the duration of the period of follow-up, this number significantly exceeded that which would be expected. Dorr and Coltman (1985) reviewed cases of second cancers following antineoplastic therapy and found them to be infrequent. In the case of the breast, this involved induction of leukemia by chemotherapy and fibrosarcomas in fields of irradiation. The risk of radiation-induced sarcomas

of the chest wall may approximate 0.02%. Biopsy confirmation and wide local excision constitute the appropriate management of fibrosarcomas for most patients (Kardinal and Donegan, 1980).

Alkylating agents have the capacity to produce myelodysplastic syndromes and acute leukemia. Geller and coworkers (1989) reported two cases of acute myelocytic leukemia that developed 3 years after the initiation of adjuvant chemotherapy for early stage breast cancer. These authors stressed the importance of specifically identifying potential responders to adjuvant chemotherapy so that others may avoid exposure. The risk of leukemia after treatment of breast cancer was reported by the SEER program for 59,115 breast cancer patients treated between 1973 and 1980 (Curtis et al., 1984). A significant elevation was observed for patients who underwent chemotherapy in their first course of therapy (an occurred-to-expected ratio of 6:1.58). The excess risk peaked in the 3rd year after treatment, and the pattern of latency suggested a cause-and-effect relationship between chemotherapy and leukemia. In a review of 8483 patients treated for breast cancer in adjuvant protocols, Fisher and coworkers (1985a) found an increased relative risk of acute myelogenous leukemia in patients following postoperative regional irradiation and adjuvant chemotherapy. A two- to threefold increase in the occurrence of endometrial carcinoma has been observed in patients following adjuvant therapy with tamoxifen (Andersson et al., 1991).

Some have found an increase in the risk of developing leukemia following irradiation for breast cancer (Andersson et al., 1991); others have not (Curtis et al., 1984). Whether irradiation increases the risk of developing a second primary breast cancer is controversial (Moffat et al., 1988; and Rosen et al., 1989). Incidental radiation to the second breast as a consequence of adjuvant chest wall irradiation or of breast-conserving therapy with lumpectomy and breast irradiation can total between 50 and 200 cGy (Fraas et al., 1985). Parker and associates (1989) reviewed information on 1630 cases of breast cancer at the University of California at Los Angeles and found no difference in the incidence of subsequent contralateral primary cancers whether or not irradiation was a component of the initial treatment. The same was true in a study of 1985 cases performed by Holdener and colleagues (1982). In a review of 644 patients observed for a median duration of 18.2 years, Rosen and colleagues (1989b) found subsequent second breast primary tumors in 10.9% of previously irradiated patients compared with in 9.4% of unirradiated patients, but they concluded that the difference was not significant. Epidemiologic data, however, strongly suggest that the risk from irradiation may be increased for young women; furthermore, using data from the Connecticut Tumor Registry, Boice and coworkers (1992) found an elevated risk of a second breast primary tumor to be associated with irradiation among women who were younger than 45 years of age at the time of treatment (relative risk = 1.59). Radiation exposure after the age of 45 years entailed little if any risk (relative risk = 1.01). Any influence of irradiation is of considerable importance in view of the growing use of breast conserving therapy, particularly for the treatment of young women.

A PLAN OF MANAGEMENT

Constant suspicion must be maintained when considering the second breast of women with mammary carcinoma. To accomplish earlier diagnosis of a possible second primary cancer, the following plan, in conjunction with treatment of the first cancer, is recommended:

1. Perform a careful visual and palpatory examination of the second breast, the axillae, and the supraclavicular areas.
2. Order mammograms of both breasts.
3. Biopsy even minimally suspicious abnormalities found on palpatory examination or mammography.

Despite reassurance from these measures, the remaining breast continues to be at risk throughout a patient's life. Consequently, a component of the periodic examination after treatment for breast cancer should be a careful palpatory examination of the breast at each visit. In the authors' clinics, follow-up intervals are based primarily on the interval risk of recurrence of the first cancer. To supplement the physical examinations, mammography is performed annually. (Patients treated with breast conservation undergo ipsilateral mammography every 6 months for the first 2 years and every year thereafter.) As a final precaution, patients are instructed how to perform breast self-examination and are encouraged to do so at least once per month.

Circumstances may exist in which a prophylactic mastectomy is indicated for the physical and mental well-being of a patient. In the authors' opinion, situations in which adequate follow-up is neither possible nor practical or in which psychologic or cosmetic considerations are of overriding concern are infrequent, and patients for whom this procedure is to be performed must be carefully selected. A second, supporting opinion in these cases is helpful and prudent. To achieve its purpose, the operation must be a thorough, total mastectomy that includes removal of the nipple and meticulous removal of all breast tissue from the chest and axilla.

References

Adami, H. O., Hansen, J., Jung, B., et al.: Characteristics of familial breast cancer in Sweden: Absence of relation to age and unilateral versus bilateral disease. Cancer, *48*:1688–1695, 1981.

Al-Jurf, A. S., Jochmisen, P. R., Urdaneta, L. F., et al.: Factors influencing survival in bilateral cancer. J. Surg. Oncol., *16*:343, 1981.

Amichetti, M., Perani, B., and Boi, S.: Metastases to the breast from extramammary malignancies. Oncology, *47*:257–260, 1990.

Andersen, J. A.: Lobular carcinoma in situ of the breast: An approach to rational treatment. Cancer, *39*:2597, 1977.

Anderson, D. E.: A high-risk group for breast cancer. Cancer Bull., *25*:23, 1973.

Andersson, M., Storm, H. H., and Mouridse, H. T.: Incidence of new primary cancers after adjuvant tamoxifen therapy and radiotherapy for early breast cancer. J. Natl. Cancer Inst., *83*:1013–1017, 1991.

Baker, R. R., and Kuhajda, F. P.: The clinical management of a normal contralateral breast in patients with lobular breast cancer. Trans. Am. Surg. Assoc., *107*:188–192, 1989.

Benfield, J. R., Jacobson, M., and Warner, N. E.: In situ lobular carcinoma of the breast. Arch. Surg., *91*:130, 1965.

Berg, J. W., Hutter, R. V. P., and Foote, F. W. Jr.: The unique association between salivary gland and breast cancer. J.A.M.A., *204*:771, 1968.

Berndt, V. H., Borrmann, C., and Klein, K.: Zweitkarzinom der Brustdruse. Arch. Geschwulstforsch., *36*:51, 1970.

Black, M. M.: Cell-mediated response in human mammary cancer. *In* Stoll, B. A. (Ed.): Host Defense in Breast Cancer. Chicago, Year Book Medical Publishers, 1975, p. 48.

Black, M. M., Cutter, S. J., and Barclay, T. H. C.: Post biopsy breast carcinoma: A natural experiment in cancer immunology. Cancer *29*:61, 1972.

Bloodgood, J. C.: The pathology of chronic cystic mastitis of the female breast. Arch. Surg., *3*:445, 1921.

Boice, J. D., Harvey, E. B., Blettner, M., et al.: Cancer in the contralateral breast after radiotherapy for breast cancer. N. Engl. J. Med., *326*:781–785, 1992.

Boivin, J. F.: Second cancers and other late side effects of cancer treatment: A review. Cancer, *66*:770–775, 1990.

Boring, C. C., Squires, T. S., and Tong, T.: Cancer Statistics—1993. C.A. Cancer J. Clin., *43*:7–41, 1993.

Cook, G. B.: A comparison of single and multiple primary cancers. Cancer, *19*:959, 1966.

Curtis, R. E., Hankey, B. F., Myers, M. H., et al.: Risk of leukemia associated with the first course of cancer treatment: An analysis of the surveillance, Epidemiology, and End Results Program experience. J. Natl. Cancer Inst., *72*:531, 1984.

Davis, N., and Baird, R. M.: Breast cancer in association with lobular carcinoma in situ: Clinicopathologic review and treatment recommendation. Am. J. Surg., *147*:641, 1984.

DiBonito, L., Luchi, M., Giaretti, L., et al.: Metastatic tumors to the female breast: An autopsy study of 12 cases. Pathol. Res. Pract., *187*:432–436, 1991.

Donegan, W. L.: Patterns and prognosis of advanced breast carcinoma. Mo. Med., *67*:853, 1970.

Donegan, W. L., and Perez-Mesa, C. M.: Lobular carcinoma: An indication for elective biopsy of the second breast. Ann. Surg., *176*:178, 1972.

Donnell, M. S., Meyer, G. A., and Donegan, W. L.: Estrogen-receptor protein in intracranial meningiomas. J. Neurosurg., *50*:499–502, 1979.

Dorr, F. A., and Coltman, C. A., Jr.: Second cancers following antineoplastic therapy. Curr. Probl. Cancer, *9*:1, 1985.

Drinkwater, N. R., and Klotz J. H.: Statistical methods for the analysis of tumor multiplicity data. Cancer Res., *41*:113, 1981.

Dunn, J. E. Jr., Bragg, K. U., Sautter, C., et al.: Breast cancer risk following a major salivary gland carcinoma. Cancer, *29*:1343, 1972.

Egan, R. L.: Bilateral breast carcinomas: Role of mammography. Cancer, *38*:931, 1976.

Einhorn, J., and Jakobsson, P.: Multiple primary malignant tumors. Cancer, *17*:1437, 1964.

Fenig, J., Arlen, M., Livingston, S. F., et al.: The potential for carcinoma existing synchronously on a microscopic level within the second breast. Surg. Gynecol. Obstet., *141*:394, 1975.

Fisher, B., Bauer, M., Margolese, R., et al.: Five-year results of a randomized clinical trial comparing total mastectomy and segmental mastectomy with or without radiation in the treatment of breast cancer. N. Engl. J. Med., *312*:665, 1985*b*.

Fisher, B., Redmond, C., Fisher, E. R., et al.: Ten-year results of a randomized clinical trial comparing radical mastectomy and total mastectomy with or without radiation. N. Engl. J. Med., *312*:674–681, 1985*c*.

Fisher, B., Rockette, H., Fisher, E. R., et al.: Leukemia in breast cancer patients following adjuvant chemotherapy or postoperative radiation: The NSABP experience. J. Clin. Oncol., *3*:1640, 1985*a*.

Fisher, B., Redmond, C., Poisson, R., et al.: Eight-year results of a randomized clinical trial comparing total mastectomy and lumpectomy with or without irradiation in the treatment of breast cancer. N. Engl. J. Med., *320*:822–828, 1989.

Fisher, E. R., and Fisher, B.: Lobular carcinoma of the breast: An overview. Ann. Surg., *185*:377, 1977.

Fisher, E. R., Gregorio, R. M., and Fisher, B.: The pathology of invasive breast cancer: A syllabus derived from findings of the NSABP (Protocol No. 4). Cancer, *36*:1, 1975*a*.

Fisher, E. R., Gregorio, R., Redmond, C., et al.: Pathological findings from the National Surgical Adjuvant Breast Project (Protocol No. 4): I. Observations concerning the multicentricity of mammary cancer. Cancer, *35*:247, 1975*b*.

Fitts, W. T. Jr., and Patterson, L. T.: Symposium on applied physiology in modern surgery: Spread of mammary cancer. Surg. Clin. North Am., *35*:1539, 1955.

Fraas B. A., Roberson, P. L., and Lichter, A. S.: Dose to the contralateral breast due to primary breast irradiation. Int. J. Radiat. Oncol. Biol. Phys., *11*:485–497, 1985.

Gallager, H. S., and Martin, J. E.: Early phases in the development of breast cancer. Cancer, *24*:1170, 1969.

Geller, R. B., Boone, L. B., Karp, J. E., et al.: Secondary acute myelocytic leukemia after adjuvant therapy for early stage breast carcinoma. Cancer, *64*:629–634, 1989.

Griswold, M. H., Wilder, C. S., Cutler, S. J., et al.: Cancer in Connecticut 1935–1951. Hartford, CT, Connecticut State Department of Health, 1955.

Haagensen, C. D.: Diseases of the Breast. Philadelphia, W. B. Saunders, 1971, p. 503.

Haagensen, C. D., Lane, N., and Bodian, C.: Coexisting lobular neoplasia and carcinoma of the breast. Cancer, *51*:1468, 1983.

Harrington, S. W.: Survival rates of radical mastectomy for unilateral and bilateral carcinoma of the breast. Surgery, *19*:154, 1946.

Harris, J. R., Botnick, L., Bloomer, W. D., et al.: Primary radiation therapy for early breast cancer: The experience at the joint center for radiation therapy. Int. J. Radiat. Oncol. Biol. Phys., *7*:1549, 1981.

Harrist, T. J., and Kalisher, L.: Breast metastasis: An unusual manifestation of a malignant carcinoid tumor. Cancer, *40*:3102, 1977.

Hébert, G., Quimet-Oliva, D., Paquin, F., et al.: Diffuse metastatic involvement of the breast. Can. Assoc. Radiol. J., *42*:353–356, 1991.

Hermann, R. E., Esselstyn, C. B., Jr., Cooperman, A. M., et al.: Partial mastectomy without radiation therapy. Surg. Clin. North Am., *64*:1103, 1984.

Hicken, N. F.: Mastectomy: Clinical pathological study demonstrating why most mastectomies result in incomplete removal of mammary gland. Arch. Surg., *40*:6, 1940.

Holdener, E. E., Osterwalder, J., Senn, H. J., et al.: Second malignancy after surgery for breast cancer: Comparison of retrospective and prospective experiences. Schweiz. Med. Wochenschr., *112*:1800, 1982.

Holland, R., Hendriks, J. H. C. L., Verbeek, A. L. M., et al.: Extent, distribution, and mammographic/histological correlations of breast ductal carcinoma in situ. Lancet, *335*:519–522, 1990.

Holleb, A. I., and Farrow, J. H.: St. Agatha and inadequate simple mastectomy. A.J.R. Am. J. Roentgenol., *99*:962, 1967.

Howarth, C. B., Caces, J. N., and Pratt, C. B.: Breast metastases in children with rhabdomyosarcoma. Cancer, *46*:2520, 1980.

Huff, L.: Bilateral carcinoma of the breast. Am. J. Surg., *118*:550, 1969.

Jackson, C. F., Palmquist, M., Swanson, J., et al.: The effectiveness of prophylactic subcutaneous mastectomy in Sprague-Dawley rats with 7,12-dimethylbenzanthracene. Plast. Reconstr. Surg., *73*:249–260, 1984.

Jouin, H., Baumann, R., Derlon, A., et al.: Is there an increased incidence of adenomatous polyps in breast cancer patients? Cancer, *63*:599–603, 1989.

Kapsinow, R.: Multiple primary cancer: A classification with report of cases. La. Med. Soc., *114*:194, 1962.

Kardinal, C. G., and Donegan, W. L.: Second cancers after prolonged adjuvant thiotepa for operable breast cancer. Cancer, *45*:2042, 1980.

Kesseler, H. J., Seidman, I., Grier, N., et al.: Bilateral primary breast cancer. J.A.M.A., *236*:278, 1976.

Khafagy, M. M., Schottenfeld, C., and Robbins, G. F.: Prognosis of the second breast cancer: The role of previous exposure to the first primary. Cancer, *35*:596, 1975.

Kilgore, A. R.: The incidence of cancer in the second breast. J.A.M.A., *77*:454, 1921.

Klamer, T. W., Donegan, W. L., and Max, M. H.: Breast tumor incidence in rats after partial mammary resection. Arch. Surg., *118*:933–935, 1983.

Kramer, W. M., and Rush, B. F.: Mammary duct proliferation in the elderly: A histopathologic study. Cancer, *31*:130, 1973.

Lanzafame, R. J., Kurchin, A., and Shermirani, M.: Metastatic melanoma presenting as a primary breast lesion. Contemp. Surg., *25*:47, 1984.

Lee, Y. M.: Additional malignant neoplasms in patients with breast carcinoma. J. Surg. Oncol., *31*:199–204, 1986.

Leis, H. P. Jr., Mersheimer, W. L., Black, M. M., et al.: The second breast. N. Y. State J. Med., *65*:2460–2468, 1965.

Leis, H. P. Jr.: Prophylactic removal of the second breast. Hosp. Med., *4*:45, 1968.

Leis, H. P. Jr.: Selective, elective, prophylactic contralateral mastectomy. Cancer, *28*:956, 1971.

Lesser, M. L., Rosen, P. P., and Kinne, D. W.: Multicentricity and bilaterality in invasive breast carcinoma. Surgery, *91*:234, 1982.

Lewis, T. R., Casey, J., Buerk, C. A., et al.: Incidence of lobular carcinoma in bilateral breast cancer. Am. J. Surg., *144*:635, 1982.

Lewison, E. F.: The management of the contralateral breast. Hosp. Pract., *5*:181, 1970.

Li, F. P., Corkery, J., Vawter, G., et al.: Breast carcinoma after cancer therapy in childhood. Cancer, *51*:521, 1983.

McDivitt, R. W., Hutter, R. V. P., Foote, F. W. Jr., et al.: In situ lobular carcinoma. J.A.M.A., *201*:96, 1967.

Martin, J. K. Jr., van Heerden, J. A., and Gaffey, T. A.: Synchronous and metachronous carcinoma of the breast. Surgery, *91*:12, 1982.

Masters, A.: Hypernephroma presenting as a lump in the breast. Aust. N. Z. J. Surg., *60*:305–306, 1990.

Michowitz, M., Noy, S., Lazebnik, N., et al.: Bilateral breast cancer. J. Surg. Oncol. *30*:109–112, 1985.

Miller, R. E.: Breast cancer and meningioma. J. Surg. Oncol., *31*:182–183, 1986.

Moertel, C. G., and Elvebeck, L. R.: The association between salivary gland cancer and breast cancer. J.A.M.A., *210*:306, 1969.

Moffat, F. L., Ketcham, A. S., Robinson, D. S., et al.: Breast cancer: Management of the opposite breast. Oncology 2:25–33, 1988.

Nance, F. C., MacVaugh, H., and Fitts, W. T. Jr.: Metastatic tumor to the breast simulating bilateral primary inflammatory carcinoma. Am. J. Surg., *112*:932–935, 1966.

Newman, W.: In situ lobular carcinoma of the breast: Report of 26 women with 32 cancers. Ann. Surg., *157*:591, 1963.

Nielsen, M., Andersen, J. A., Henriksen, F. W., et al.: Metastases to the breast from extramammary carcinomas. Acta Pathol. Microbiol. Scand. [A], *89*:251, 1981.

Nielsen, M., Christensen, L., and Andersen, J.: Contralateral cancerous breast lesions in women with clinical invasive breast carcinoma. Cancer, *57*:891–903, 1986.

Nunez, D. A., Sutherland, C. G., Sood, R. K.: Breast metastasis from a pharyngeal carcinoma. J. Laryngol. Otol., *103*:227–228, 1989.

Pack, G. T.: Argument for bilateral mastectomy. Surgery, *29*:929, 1951.

Parker, R. G., Frimm, P., and Enstrom, J. E.: Contralateral breast cancers following treatment for initial breast cancers in women. Am. J. Clin. Oncol., *12*:213–216, 1989.

Pennell, V.: Primary carcinoma multiplex: A series of 17 cases with review of the literature. Br. J. Surg., *46*:108, 1958.

Peters, T. G., Donegan, W. L., and Burg, E. A.: Minimal breast cancer: A clinical appraisal. Ann. Surg., *186*:704, 1977.

Pomerantz, R. A., Murad, T., and Hines, J. R.: Bilateral breast cancer. Am. J. Surg., *55*:441–444, 1988.

Pressman, P. I.: Selective biopsy of the opposite breast. Presented at the 38th Annual Cancer Symposium of the Society of Surgical Oncology. Houston, TX, May 1985.

Qualheim, R., and Gall, E.: Breast carcinoma with multiple sites of origin. Cancer, *10*:460, 1957.

Ratzer, E. R., Holleb, A. K., and Farrow, J. H.: The technique of bilateral simultaneous radical mastectomy. Surg. Gynecol. Obstet., *123*:601, 1966.

Robbins, G. F., and Berg, J. W.: Bilateral primary breast cancers. Cancer, *17*:1501, 1964.

Robinson, E., Rennert, G., Rennert, H. S., et al.: Survival of first and second primary breast cancer. Cancer, *71*:172–176, 1993.

Rosen, P. P., Groshen, S., Kinne, D. W., et al.: Contralateral breast carcinoma: An assessment of risk and prognosis in stage I (T1N0M0) and stage II (T1N1M0) patients with 20-year follow-up. Surgery, *106*:904–910, 1989b.

Rosen, P. P., Greshen, S., Kinne, D. W., et al.: Nonmammary malignant neoplasms in patients with stage I (T1N0M0) and stage II (T1N1M0) breast carcinoma. Am. J. Clin. Oncol., *12*:369–374, 1989a.

Rosen, P. P., Braun, D. W. Jr., Lyngholm, B., et al.: Lobular carcinoma in situ of the breast: Preliminary results of treatment by ipsilateral mastectomy and contralateral breast biopsy. Cancer, *47*:813, 1981.

Rosen, P. P., Fracchia, A. A., Urban, J. A., et al.: ''Residual'' mammary carcinoma following simulated partial mastectomy. Cancer, *35*:739, 1975.

Rubinstein, A. B., Schein, M., and Reichenthal, E.: The association of carcinoma of the breast with meningioma. Surg. Gynecol. Obstet., *169*:334–336, 1989.

Schenker, J. G., Levinsky, R., and Ohel, G.: Multiple primary malignant neoplasms in breast cancer patients in Israel. Cancer, *54*:145, 1984.

Schoenberg, B. S.: Multiple Primary Malignant Neoplasms. The Connecticut Experience. 1935–1964. Berlin, Springer-Verlag, 1977.

Schoenberg, B. S., Christine, R. W., and Whisnant, J. P.: Nervous system neoplasms and primary malignancies of other sites: The unique association between meningiomas and breast cancer. Neurology, *25*:705–712, 1975.

Schwartz, G. F., Patchefsky, A. S., Feig, S. A., et al.: Multicentricity of non-palpable breast cancer. Cancer, *45*:2913, 1980.

Shellito, J. G., and Bartlett, W. C.: Bilateral carcinoma of the breast. Arch. Surg., *94*:489, 1967.

Silverman, E. M., and Oberman, H. A.: Metastatic neoplasms in the breast. Surg. Gynecol. Obstet., *138*:26, 1974.

Slack, N. H., Nemoto, T., and Fisher, B.: Experiences with bilateral primary carcinoma of the breast. Surg. Gynecol. Obstet., *136*:433, 1973.

Spratt, J. S.: Multiple primary cancers: Review of clinical studies from two Missouri hospitals. Cancer, *40*:1806, 1977.

Spratt, J. S., and Hoag, M.: Incidence of multiple primary cancers per man-year of follow-up. Ann. Surg., *164*:775, 1966.

Spratt, J. S., and Spratt, T. L.: Correlation of the rates of growth of pulmonary metastases and host survival. Ann. Surg., *159*:161, 1964.

Sterns, E. E., and Fletcher, W. A.: Bilateral cancer of the breast: A review of clinical, histologic, and immunohistologic characteristics. Surgery, *110*:617–622, 1991.

Tagart, R. E. B.: Partial mastectomy for breast cancer. Br. Med. J., *2*:1268, 1978.

Tinnemans, J. G. M., Wobbes, T., van der Sluis, R. F.: Multicentricity in nonpalpable breast carcinoma and its implications for treatment. Am. Surg., *151*:334–338, 1986.

Trevor, W.: Bilateral breast cancer. N. Y. State J. Med., *54*:1937, 1954.

Urban, J. A.: Bilaterality of cancer of the breast: Biopsy of the opposite breast. Cancer, *29*:1867, 1967.

Urban, J. A.: Biopsy of the ''normal'' breast in treating breast cancer. Surg. Clin. North Am., *49*:291, 1969*a*.

Urban, J. A.: Bilateral breast cancer. Cancer, *24*:1310, 1969*b*.

Vergier, B., Trojani, M., de Mascarel, I., et al.: Metastases to the breast: Differential diagnosis from primary breast cancer. J. Surg., *104*:227–228, 1991.

Vitale, G. C., and Spratt, J. S.: The adenoma-carcinoma sequence: An update. Probl. Gen. Surg., *4*:24–38, 1987.

Wanebo, H. J., Senofsky, G. M., Fechner, R. E., et al.: Bilateral breast cancer: Risk reduction by contralateral biopsy. Ann. Surg., *201*:667, 1985.

Warren, S., and Gates, O.: Multiple primary malignant tumors: A survey of the literature and statistical study. Am. J. Cancer, *16*:1358, 1932.

Webber, B. L., Heise, H., Neifeld, J. P., et al.: Risk of subsequent contralateral breast carcinoma in a population of patients with in-situ breast carcinoma. Cancer, *47*:2928, 1983.

Wilson, N. D., and Alberty, R. E.: Bilateral carcinoma of the breast. Am. J. Surg., *126*:244, 1973.

28 Local and Regional Recurrence

William L. Donegan

Recurrence is reappearance of an original cancer in a patient after a period of clinical cure. The period between treatment and recurrence is known as the *disease-free interval* (DFI). This period is different from *persistence*, in which there is no DFI. Recurrence follows primary treatment for two reasons, either (1) because the cancer was occultly disseminated before treatment or (2) because it was incompletely eliminated from local and regional tissues. It was to prevent the latter that Halsted advocated radical mastectomy in 1894, and it cannot be doubted that recurrence of cancer on the chest wall was reduced by his operation (Table 28–1). Recurrence was further reduced by the introduction of postoperative irradiation to the chest wall and the regional lymph nodes. Nevertheless, local-regional recurrence continues to be a vexing problem and is frequently the earliest and most obvious sign of the failure of therapy.

DEFINITIONS

Local-regional recurrence is recurrence in the breast or anterior chest and in its regional lymph nodes. Recurrences elsewhere are considered "distant." It is important to distinguish between local and regional recurrence. This distinction is not always made in the literature and accounts for some inconsistencies in data regarding frequency of recurrence and treatment results. *Local recurrence* may be

defined as recurrence within the soft tissues of the ipsilateral anterior chest—that is, the skin, breast or residual breast tissue, subcutaneous tissue, or underlying muscles. This zone includes a region bounded by the sternum medially, the clavicle superiorly, the posterior axillary line laterally, and the costal margin inferiorly. *Regional recurrence* refers to recurrence in unremoved regional lymph nodes—that is, the axillary nodes, internal mammary nodes (IMNs), and supraclavicular nodes.

It may be difficult to distinguish local from regional recurrences. Fixed subcutaneous mounds of tumor that appear between rib spaces along the sternal border seem to be within the local area, but they often represent involved IMNs and are therefore regional recurrences (Fig. 28–1). The same is true for deep masses located just inferior to the medial end of the clavicle, which often signify involvement of the apical axillary, or "infraclavicular," nodes. Masses apparently within the pectoralis major muscle may be metastases in unremoved interpectoral (Rotter's) nodes rather than truly local recurrences (Fig. 28–2) (Chen, et al., 1985). Lymph nodes can be found within the breast, and breast tissue can overlap node-bearing regions, especially in the axilla. Often, the origin of recurrence from nodal or nonnodal tissues can only be surmised. Identifying specific sites of failure is important for improving future treatment, but it is not surprising that local and regional recurrences often are reported together because of these problems.

MECHANISMS

Some or all of the following factors probably account for local-regional recurrence:

1. Retrograde embolization through transected lymphatics.

2. Incomplete removal of the primary tumor or its local extensions (Fig. 28–3) (Peters et al., 1977).

3. Progression of metastases in regional nodes.

4. Transection of a tumor, with surgical implantation in the wound.

5. Implantation of circulating cells as a part of general dissemination (Dao and Nemoto, 1963).

6. Growth of cancer cells trapped in stagnant lymphatics after regional node dissection, that is, "in transit" metastases (Spratt et al., 1965).

The close association of local-regional recurrence and distant recurrence is well known and suggests common

Table 28–1. RESULTS OF OPERATIONS FOR THE CURE OF CANCER OF THE BREAST

Surgeon	Dates	No. of Cases	Local Recurrence (%)
Bergman	1882–87	114	51–60
Billroth	1867–76	170	82
Czerny	1877–86	102	62
Fischer	1871–78	147	75
Gussenbauer	1878–86	151	64
Konig	1875–85	152	58–62
Kuster	1871–85	228	59.6
Lucke	1881–90	110	66
Volkman	1874–78	131	60
Halsted	1889–94	50	6

(From Halsted, W. S.: The results of operations for the cure of cancer of the breast performed at the Johns Hopkins Hospital from June 1889 to January 1984. Medical Classics, 3:441, 1938.)

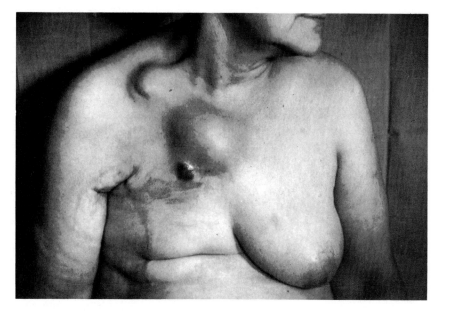

Figure 28-1. Recurrent mammary carcinoma after radical mastectomy. Disease is confined clinically to local and regional sites. The supraclavicular nodes are enlarged, and the large mass at the upper sternal border is characteristic of tumor growth in internal mammary lymph nodes. A dermal recurrence is present in the medial skin flap.

mechanisms (Fig. 28–4) (Spratt, 1967; and Bruce, 1970). Extensive local recurrence confined to a previously irradiated area of the chest often features erythema, skin thickening, and myriad small nodules that enlarge and coalesce. Diehl and coworkers (1984) postulated that in patients with such features, irradiation-induced vascular endothelial cell damage leads to the increased trapping, survival, and growth of tumor cells. Evidence for this is based on animal models in which preferential tumor cell trapping and persistence has been demonstrated in traumatized or irradiated tissues.

FREQUENCY AND DISTRIBUTION

Local Recurrence

Local recurrence may occur any time after initial treatment. Danckers and colleagues (1960) found in the literature 26 cases of local recurrence that appeared 15 years after mastectomy. Others have reported local recurrences after 25 years (Meltzer, 1990) and 30 years (McCormack, et al., 1989). Local recurrence is most likely within the first 2 years after treatment, with a peak incidence in the second

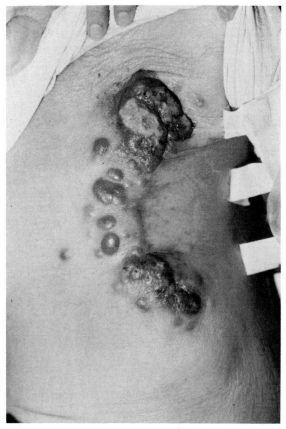

Figure 28-3. Recurrence concentrated around the scar of a limited mastectomy suggests incomplete removal of the primary cancer's local extensions.

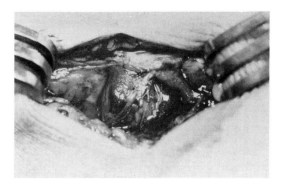

Figure 28-2. Recurrence in an interpectoral node (Rotter's node) masquerading as local recurrence. The mass was palpable on the anterior chest but was located deep to the pectoralis major muscle.

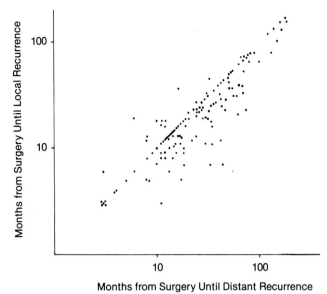

Figure 28–4. A logarithmic plot of time from mastectomy to local and distant recurrence for 139 patients with both events illustrates a good temporal correlation between the two. In 45% of cases, distant recurrence preceded local recurrence or was diagnosed simultaneously. (Ellis Fischel State Cancer Hospital cases reviewed by the author.)

year, after which the annual rate steadily declines (Fig. 28–5).

Slightly more than one-sixth of 704 patients (17.4%) treated at Ellis Fischel State Cancer Hospital (EFSCH) in Columbia, Missouri, with radical mastectomy and without adjuvant irradiation or systemic therapy developed local recurrence within 5 years. Eighty seven per cent of the local recurrences that occurred within 10 years had appeared before the fifth year. The problem is cumulative with time: 24.5% of 1296 women treated with radical mastectomy at EFSCH for unilateral carcinomas and observed for up to 24 years developed local recurrences (Donegan, 1972). Similarly, the rate of local failure in Halsted's original 50 patients rose from an initial 6% in 1894 to 32% when the

cases were reviewed in 1931 by Lewis and Rienhoff (1932). Thus, the interval of observation is an important variable in determining local treatment failure and must be uniform to permit valid comparisons of alternative treatments (see Fig. 28–5).

Despite various periods of observation, a more or less constant proportionality is maintained among local, regional, and distant recurrences (Table 28–2). Local recurrences do not predominate early and distant recurrences later. The cumulative rate of recurrence is approximately the same at all sites—that is, the same proportion of all recurrences that are to occur at local-regional or distant sites will have appeared after each interval of observation (Fig. 28–6). It is as if the risk of spread beyond the primary location varies, but not the pattern.

The frequency of local recurrence after mastectomy correlates with a number of clinical variables. Prominent among these are the number of axillary nodes that contain metastases at the time of treatment and the size of the primary tumor. Local recurrence within 5 years of radical mastectomy (without postoperative radiotherapy) is greater when axillary nodes are involved (26%) than when they are not (6.5%) (Donegan et al., 1966) and is directly related to the number of involved nodes (Table 28–3). It is also directly related to the size of the primary tumor, reaching 33% for tumors that are 8 cm in diameter or larger (Table 28–4). It is a function of tumor-node-metastasis (TNM) clinical stage at the time of mastectomy (Fig. 28–7), increases with signs of local and regional advancement, and is particularly likely after treatment of inflammatory breast cancer (Donegan and Padrta, 1990). All other factors being equal, the risk of local recurrence is not influenced by whether the mastectomy wound is closed primarily or with a skin graft (Fig. 28–8). The author has found that surgical skin margins that were too narrow increased the rate of local recurrence. Dao (1963) was unable to confirm this, but few margins were less than 3.0 cm, and follow-up periods were short. The proximity of a tumor to the retromammary fascia is not a strong determinant of local recurrence provided that the areolar plane between the breast and the underlying fascia is uninvolved (Ahlborn et al., 1988). Ewers and associates (1992) were unable to relate local

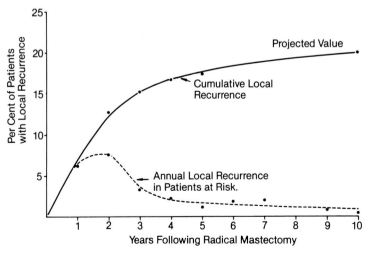

Figure 28–5. Local recurrences in 704 patients treated with radical mastectomy (no irradiation or systemic adjuvants) for unilateral breast carcinoma. The annual rate reaches a maximum the second year following mastectomy and diminishes thereafter. (Data from Donegan, W. L., Perez-Mesa, C. M., and Watson, F. R.: A biostatistical study of locally recurrent breast carcinoma. Surg. Gynecol. Obstet., *112*:529, 1966.)

Table 28–2. DISTRIBUTION OF LOCAL AND REGIONAL RECURRENCE AFTER VARIOUS MASTECTOMIES—MEDICAL COLLEGE OF WISCONSIN

Operation	Axillary Metastases	Local	Axilla	Supraclavicular
Auchincloss modified radical mastectomy (axillary Levels I and II)	All	10 (56%)	5 (28%)*	3 (17%)
	Ax 0	5 (56%)	3 (33%)	1 (11%)
	Ax +	5 (55%)	2 (22%)	2 (22%)
Patey modified radical mastectomy (axillary Levels I, II, III)	All	13 (68%)	1 (5%)*	5 (26%)
	Ax 0	6 (67%)	1 (11%)	2 (22%)
	Ax +	7 (70%)		3 (30%)
Halsted radical mastectomy (axillary Levels I, II, III)	All	36 (70%)	7 (13%)	9 (17%)
	Ax 0	11 (58%)	4 (21%)	4 (21%)
	Ax +	25 (76%)	3 (9%)	5 (15%)

*Difference is not significant; P = .08
Shown are not the absolute but the relative frequencies of recurrence. Local recurrence is more frequent than regional even when the axilla was pathologically involved. Axillary recurrence is less frequent than supraclavicular after a complete axillary dissection is performed.

recurrence to ploidy, S-phase fraction, or estrogen receptor content of the primary tumor independently of node status. Postoperative irradiation reduces future recurrence in treated areas (Fisher et al., 1985, 1989), but its effectiveness declines with increasing numbers of involved axillary nodes. After a median follow-up of almost 5 years, Ewers and associates (1992) found that local-regional control in 235 irradiated mastectomy cases versus 271 nonirradiated mastectomy cases was 100% versus 91% in node-negative cases, 94% versus 71% in cases with 3 positive nodes, 93% versus 65% in cases with 4 to 9 positive nodes, and an identical 67% in cases with 10 or more positive nodes.

Variations in primary treatment can change the pattern of local-regional recurrence. Recurrence after six different treatments are shown in Tables 28–5 and 28–6. Table 28–5, which compares radical mastectomy, total mastectomy, and total mastectomy combined with local and regional irradiation for clinical Stage I and Stage II breast cancers,

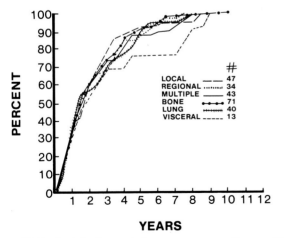

Figure 28–6. A plot of cumulative recurrence after modified mastectomy indicates that local or regional recurrence is not uniquely early or delayed compared with recurrence at other locations. (From Tomin, R., and Donegan, W. L.: Screening for recurrent breast cancer—Its effectiveness and prognostic value. J. Clin. Oncol., 5:62, 1987. Reprinted with permission.)

clearly shows a 75% reduction in local recurrence produced by postoperative irradiation in both Stage I and Stage II; however, this reduction was not accompanied by a corresponding reduction in distant dissemination. The table also shows a high frequency of recurrence (18%) in the axillary nodes if these nodes are not removed or radiated in patients with clinical Stage I cancers. Recurrence in axillary lymph nodes is largely prevented by complete dissection or irradiation of the nodes; in the presence of adenopathy (Stage II), this is perhaps more effectively achieved by dissection alone. Recurrence in supraclavicular nodes is infrequent but is reduced by prophylactic irradiation. IMN involvement is rarely recognized as a first sign of failure whether the nodes are treated or not. Table 28–6 presents a comparison of modified radical mastectomy, segmental mastectomy and axillary dissection in combination with breast irradiation, and segmental mastectomy and axillary dissection without breast irradiation. Irradiation reduced recurrences in the breast by 80% (from 40% to 8%). Recurrences in the axillae were equally low after axillary dissection in all three treatments, and IMN and supraclavicular node recurrences were a low risk despite no treatment to these nodes. Again, distant dissemination was not influenced by variations in local treatment.

Agreement is not uniform on the most frequent site of local recurrences. Demaree (1951) and Pawlias and co-workers (1958) reported a predominance medial to diagonal mastectomy scars. Haagensen (1971) found the greatest number to be located at the site of skin grafts, as did Danckers (1960). At EFSCH, 42% of 146 local recurrences were found in the scar or grafted area (Fig. 28–9). Twenty-two per cent occurred in the medial flap, and 15% within the lateral flap. The remainder occurred in various other locations.

Overall, the prognosis of patients with local recurrence after mastectomy is bleak; only 23% of 47 patients reviewed by Tomin and Donegan (1987) were alive 5 years later. However, this rate is somewhat more favorable than that of patients with recurrence in regional nodes or distant sites (Fig. 28–10). The prognosis is also more favorable when local recurrence is isolated rather than concurrent

Table 28–3. NUMBER OF INVOLVED AXILLARY LYMPH NODES AND LOCAL RECURRENCE WITHIN 5 YEARS*

No. of Involved Nodes	No. of Patients	No. of Patients with Local Recurrence	Per Cent with 5-Year Local Recurrence
0	308	20	6.5
1	93	9	10.3
2	56	7	12.3
3	34	6	17.6
4	30	8	26.7
5	26	9	34.6
6	18	6	33.3
7	13	5	38.5
8	16	9	56.3
9	15	7	46.7
10–12	30	9	30.0
13–19	36	16	44.4
20 or more	28	12	42.9
(Number of nodes not given in one patient—no recurrence)			

(From Donegan, W. L., Perez-Mesa, C. M., and Watson, F. R.: A biostatistical study of locally recurrent breast carcinoma. Surg. Gynecol. Obstet., *112*:529, 1966. Reprinted with permission.
*A chi-squared test indicates that values for local recurrences with increasing numbers of involved axillary lymph nodes are not the same at a level of significance of $P < .01$.

Table 28–4. PRIMARY TUMOR DIAMETER AND LOCAL RECURRENCE WITHIN 5 YEARS*

Tumor Diameter (cm)	No. of Patients	No. with Local Recurrence	Per Cent with Local Recurrence
0.0–0.9	7	0	0
1.0–1.9	66	5	7.6
2.0–2.9	120	15	12.5
3.0–3.9	159	25	15.8
4.0–4.9	119	26	21.8
5.0–5.9	51	14	27.4
6.0–6.9	36	11	30.6
7.0–7.9	24	8	33.3
8.0 and greater	24	8	33.3
Unmeasured	98	11	11.2

(From Donegan, W. L., Perez-Mesa, C. M., and Watson, F. R.: A biostatistical study of locally recurrent breast carcinoma. Surg. Gynecol. Obstet., *112*:529, 1966. Reprinted with permission.)
*A chi-squared test indicates that the incidences of local recurrence for the nine categories of size are not the same ($P < .01$).

Table 28–5. SITES OF INITIAL RECURRENCE AFTER DIFFERENT TREATMENT OF REGIONAL LYMPH NODES: NSABP PROTOCOL B-04 10-YEAR RESULTS

	Axilla Clinically Negative for Cancer			Axilla Clinically Positive for Cancer	
	RM	*TM + RT*	*TM*	*RM*	*TM + RT*
Total Cases	362	352	365	292	294
Sites of Recurrence					
Local	4.4%	1.1%	7.7%	7.2%	1.7%
Regional	2.5%	3.4%	4.1%	7.5%	11.9%
Axilla	1.4%	3.1%	17.8%*	1.0%	10.5%
Supraclavicular	1.1%	0.3%	2.7%	5.1%	0.0%
Parasternal	0.0%	0.0%	0.0%	0.0%	0.0%
Distant	27.1%	32.7%	30.1%	37.1%	40.8%
Combinations	3.3%	2.6%	3.4%	7.5%	5.7%

*This represents initial treatment failure in the axilla that were treatable with axillary dissection. Failures of treatment in the axilla that were either not treatable or after delayed therapeutic axillary dissection occurred in 1.1% of cases. All figures are per cent of the total number of patients.
Abbreviations: RM = radical mastectomy (axillary nodes removed); TM = total mastectomy (axillary nodes not treated); TMR + RT = total mastectomy combined with chest wall and regional irradiation (axillary nodes irradiated).

Cumulative Local-Regional Recurrence after Mastectomy with Level II vs Level III Axillary Dissection

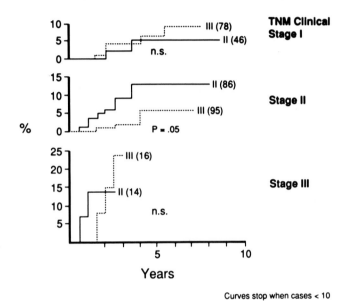

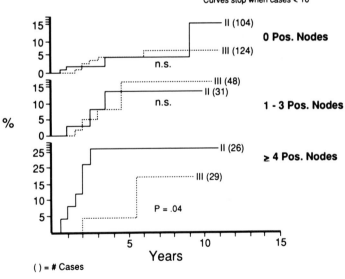

Figure 28–7. Local-regional recurrence is cumulative over time and increases directly with clinical stage and number of axillary metastases. In patients with clinically involved axillary lymph nodes and in those with four of more pathologically involved nodes, local-regional recurrence was increased when a more limited axillary dissection was performed (i.e., Level II rather than Level III), largely owing to an increase in axillary recurrences. A Level III dissection is more effective in these patients.

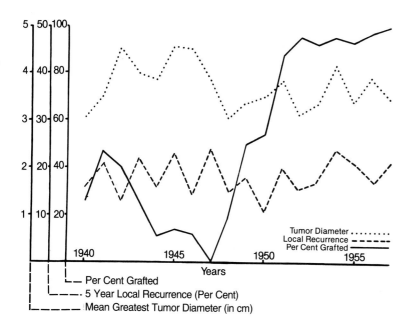

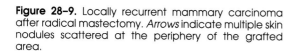

Per Cent Grafted

5 Year Local Recurrence (Per Cent)

Mean Greatest Tumor Diameter (in cm)

Figure 28–8. Relationship between skin grafting and local recurrence within 5 years after mastectomy. Skin grafting did not reduce the rate of local recurrence. (From Donegan, W. L., Perez-Mesa, C. M., and Watson, F. R.: A biostatistical study of locally recurrent breast carcinoma. Surg. Gynecol. Obstet., *112*:529, 1966. Reprinted with permission of Surgery, Gynecology, & Obstetrics.)

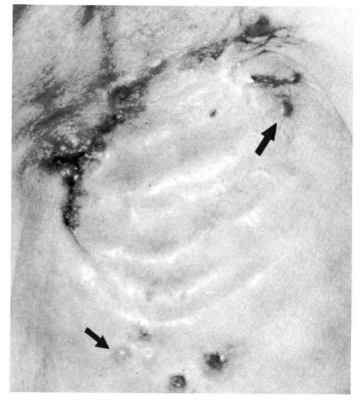

Figure 28–9. Locally recurrent mammary carcinoma after radical mastectomy. *Arrows* indicate multiple skin nodules scattered at the periphery of the grafted area.

Table 28–6. SITES OF INITAL RECURRENCE AFTER DIFFERENT TREATMENT OF THE BREAST: NSABP PROTOCOL B-06 8-YEAR RESULTS*

	TM	Seg M	Seg M + RT
Total No. of Patients	590	636	629
Sites of Recurrence			
Local or Breast	8.1%	39.0†	10.0%‡
Regional	3.9%	7.2%	4.5%
Distant§	18.8%	21.9%	22.7%
Combination/Unknown	0.8%	1.3%	1.0%

*All patients had axillary lymph node dissection, and patients with axillary metastases received adjuvant chemotherapy (Fisher et al., 1989).
†Unresectable or recurrent after salvage mastectomy = 7.2%.
‡Unresectable or recurrent after salvage mastectomy = 1.1%.
§Includes second primary tumors in the opposite breast.
Abbreviations: TM = total mastectomy; Seg M = segmental mastectomy (lumpectomy); Seg M + RT = segmental mastectomy (lumpectomy) combined with breast irradiation.

with distant metastases (Patanaphan et al., 1984) (Fig. 28–11).

A number of factors are predictors for dissemination and for survival after local-regional recurrence (Ames and Balch, 1990; and Kennedy and Abeloff, 1993). Local recurrence usually comprises about 60% of such cases, but prognosis is not always determined separately for local versus regional disease. Favorable indicators are a long DFI, single rather than multiple tumor nodules, a small rather than a large recurrent tumor, early stage, and negative axillary nodes at the time of original treatment (Janjan et al., 1986; and Crowe et al., 1991), the presence of tumor estrogen and progesterone receptors (Schwaibold et al., 1991), and local rather than regional recurrence.

Extent of the recurrence and the DFI are two particularly potent influences on prognosis (Bedwinek et al., 1981*b*; Chen et al., 1985; Probstfeld and O'Connell, 1989; Crowe et al., 1991; and Halverson et al., 1992*b*). Bedwinek and associates found the most favorable outlook to be associated with a single nodule, no nodule greater than 1.0 cm in size, and a DFI longer than 24 months. Five-year survival

exceeded 50% in the presence of any two of these factors. Reporting on 106 patients treated with irradiation at Kaiser Permanente Medical Center (Los Angeles, CA), Probstfeld and O'Connell found that after a median follow-up of 5.5 years 84% of patients whose DFI was 24 months or longer had distant metastases compared with only 38% of those whose DFI was shorter than 24 months. According to Halverson and colleagues (1992*b*), the 5-year survival associated with a DFI of longer than 24 months was 50% compared with a survival of 35% for a DFI shorter than 24 months. Survival reached 61% for patients who had a combination of a long DFI, excisional biopsy, and local disease control. Other associations with favorable prognosis include ability to control the chest wall disease (Janjan et al., 1986; Ames and Balch, 1990; and Schwaibold et al., 1991) and a solitary site of local or regional recurrence rather than both (Halverson et al., 1992*b*). Elevated levels of carcinoembryonic antigen or CA 15-3 suggest simultaneous distant recurrence and an unfavorable prognosis (O'Dwyer et al., 1990).

Recurrence in the Breast

The breast is a potential site of local treatment failure after primary treatment with breast conservation. Failure rates as high as 40% are reported in the absence of breast irradiation (Fisher et al., 1989). With breast irradiation, the failure rate is reduced, and with irradiation combined with chemotherapy, it possibly is reduced further (Fisher et al., 1989; and Haffty et al., 1991); however, recurrences can still be expected to occur at an average rate of 1% to 3% per year, and some appear more than 10 years after initial treatment. Young age, incomplete tumor resection, high nuclear tumor grade, the presence of multiple primary tumors, and tumors with an extensive intraductal component (EIC) place patients at a higher-than-average risk for this problem (Schnitt et al., 1984; Kurtz et al., 1990; and Vicini et al., 1992). The majority of breast recurrences appear in or adjacent to the site of the original primary tumor (Kurtz et al., 1989; Stotter

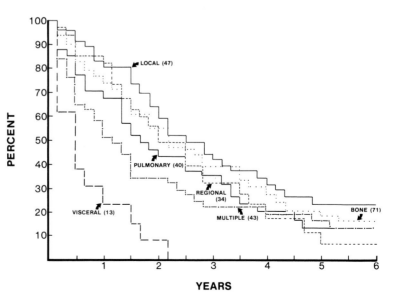

Figure 28–10. Survival following recurrence at various sites indicates the relatively favorable prognosis associated with isolated local recurrence. (From Tomin, R., and Donegan, W. L.: Screening for recurrent breast cancer—Its effectiveness and prognostic value. J. Clin. Oncol., 5:62, 1987. Reprinted with permission.)

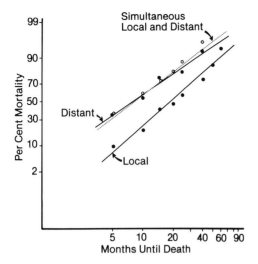

Figure 28–11. Logarithmic plots of mortality after recurrence are shown for EFSCH patients treated with radical mastectomy who had local recurrence alone, distant recurrence followed by local recurrence, and both types of recurrence simultaneously. The survival of patients whose first sign of recurrence was restricted to the surgical area was superior to that of others at all points. The prognosis of patients with local recurrence as the first sign of treatment failure, therefore, is more favorable than that of those who first exhibit dissemination.

et al., 1989; Osborne et al., 1992); in addition, most are detected as a palpable mass, and less often recurrent tumors are identified as a change on a mammogram (Solin et al., 1990; and Sardi et al., 1991). Mammographic signs of recurrence are most frequently a new or enlarging mass or the development of suspicious microcalcifications (Dershaw et al., 1990) (Fig. 28–12). Kurtz and coworkers (1989) reported detection with ultrasound and thermography.

The breast is the most frequent site of local-regional treatment failure after breast conservation but is often accompanied by recurrence in the dermis and regional lymph nodes and can be associated with inflammatory changes. Sixty-seven per cent of 49 cases reported by Stotter and colleagues (1990) were isolated to the breast, and 84% to the breast and axillary lymph nodes. Recurrence was isolated to the breast in 46% of cases reported by Clarke and coworkers (1985), and in 8% of cases it was associated with distant dissemination. Kurtz and associates (1991) reported that 13 of 70 (18.6%) local-regional recurrences were inoperable, sometimes because of supraclavicular node or IMN involvement but most often owing to extensive involvement of the breast and to inflammatory changes. Patients who had invasive cancers with poor prognostic features presented in this fashion, and despite chemohormonal therapy, only 22% of them lived 2.5 years. In eight series reviewed by Kurtz and associates (1991), from 84% to 94% of patients with local-regional recurrence were considered treatable with resection.

Regional Recurrence

Axillary Lymph Nodes

In the presence of an invasive tumor, axillary nodes that are clinically negative for cancer contain metastases in al-

most 40% of cases (Fisher et al., 1985). If these metastases are undisturbed, regional failure of treatment at this site after mastectomy can be expected as the first sign of recurrence in a substantial number of patients.

According to Fisher and coworkers (1985), 17.8% of 365 patients treated with simple mastectomy for invasive cancers and having axillary nodes that were clinically negative for cancer had initial treatment failure in ipsilateral axillary lymph nodes within 10 years. The majority of failures occurred in the first 2 years after mastectomy, but adenopathy continued to appear more than 9 years later. Development of axillary adenopathy had the same ominous implications as when it was present initially. Dissemination occurred in three-quarters of these patients following axillary dissection, but few of them had further recurrence in the axilla.

Elimination of tumor progression in the axillary nodes is an important objective even when it is for palliation. Brachial plexus involvement is a particularly morbid and disabling complication of uncontrolled metastasis in the axillary nodes. This complication developed in 4% of 74 cases of uncontrolled local-regional recurrence reported by Bedwinek and coworkers (1981*a*). Symptoms include unremitting pain in the arm and shoulder and progressive paralysis. Pain is not always present; sometimes, increasing loss of motor and sensory sensation in the arm and hand are the only signs. Metastases to the cervical spine and irradiation-related neuropathy can produce similar symptoms and should be considered in the differential diagnosis. Computed tomography or magnetic resonance imaging can be helpful for evaluating the axillary nodes; however, in the

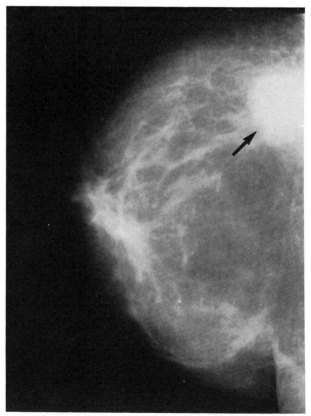

Figure 28–12. Recurrence in the breast after lumpectomy and breast irradiation is seen as a density in a mammogram.

absence of obvious recurrence, exploration of the brachial plexus may be necessary for diagnosis. This can be performed through the axilla, and if metastases are found, expeditious treatment is important to prevent further functional impairment of the arm. If it has not been previously used, irradiation provides effective palliation. Management includes pain control and physical therapy.

■ Case Report

A 63-year-old woman underwent modified radical mastectomy for an invasive carcinoma of the right breast with four nodal metastases. She received adjuvant chemotherapy postoperatively. After a DFI of 14 years, she developed multiple small asymptomatic pulmonary metastases. Treatment with tamoxifen produced a brief period of stability, following which her therapy was changed to treatment with megestrol acetate (Megace); this resulted in regression. After 1 year of hormonal therapy, and with the pulmonary metastases still in regression, she began to have progressive weakness of the entire right upper extremity associated with numbness in some fingers but not with pain. The result of her physical examination was otherwise normal as was a radiograph of her chest; however, electromyography showed nerve damage, and magnetic resonance imaging of the right axilla and neck suggested the presence of a mass involving the brachial plexus. Exploration of the right brachial plexus via the axilla found diffuse tumor involvement that was histologically confirmed. The patient received radiotherapy to the axilla and supraclavicular areas and underwent physical therapy for the arm, with some return of function but with persistent wrist drop and little motion of the fingers. She remained active with the aid of a wrist splint. Seventeen months after diagnosis of the axillary recurrence, and almost 18 years after her original diagnosis, she developed rapidly increasing levels of carcinoembryonic antigen and CA 15-3, progression of pulmonary metastases, and a left pleural effusion.

Supraclavicular Lymph Nodes

The supraclavicular dissections of Dahl-Iversen (1963) showed that 8% of patients with operable tumors already had metastases in this node group. Haagensen (1971) found that an almost identical proportion (8.7%) of 356 carefully selected surgical patients developed clinical evidence of supraclavicular metastases within the 5-year period after radical mastectomy.

Supraclavicular adenopathy is usually a sign of impending distant dissemination. Fentiman and associates (1986) reviewed 35 cases of isolated supraclavicular recurrences after radical mastectomy at Guy's Hospital in London, England. The patients had been diagnosed after a mean DFI of 37 months, which is greater than the 22-month mean of patients with isolated local recurrences. Axillary nodes had tested positive for carcinoma at the time of mastectomy in 74% of the patients.

Internal Mammary Lymph Nodes

Metastases in the IMNs become clinically apparent less frequently than do nodal treatment failures at other sites because of these nodes' location deep to the ribs. It can be estimated from the findings of surgeons who included IMN dissections with mastectomy that approximately one-third

of patients deemed suitable for mastectomy already have IMN metastases, the probability of which depends on the location and size of the primary tumor (Donegan, 1977). In patients with axillary nodes that are pathologically negative for cancer, the IMNs are involved in 9% of cases; this constitutes a sizable error when nodal staging is limited only to evaluation of the axilla (Veronesi et al., 1984). This error can reach 20% in patients with medial primary tumors (Morrow and Foster, 1981). IMN metastases, which are beyond the boundaries of modified or radical mastectomy, contribute to regional treatment failure. Ten per cent of patients with untreated IMN metastases can be expected to develop clinically detectable parasternal recurrences after 9 to 24 years of observation (Donegan, 1977). Veronesi and Valagussa (1981) reported parasternal recurrences in 3.7% of patients treated with radical mastectomy; this was reduced to 0.3% in patients whose treatment had included prophylactic resection of these nodes.

Recurrence in the IMNs after mastectomy is made obvious by the development of a deep, fixed mass in an intercostal space at the ipsilateral sternal border. Before a mass is appreciated, it is often heralded by persistent pain and tenderness at the site. The ominous nature of persistent parasternal pain was recognized as early as 1779 by Petrus Camper, who considered it a sure sign of incurable breast cancer (Camper, 1779). The author has seen several patients in whom parasternal recurrence was detected on computed tomography after several months of parasternal pain, usually in the second or third intercostal space (Fig. 28–13). The differential diagnosis includes Tietzie's syndrome (costochondritis), neuroma, and bone metastases, but this clinical symptom complex should raise the suspicion of parasternal recurrence and lead to the performance of appropriate imaging studies (e.g., bone scanning, magnetic resonance imaging, and computed tomography) and, for definitive diagnosis, even in the absence of physical signs, to surgical exploration of the interspace.

MANAGEMENT

Recurrence on the chest wall or in regional nodes is deserving of prompt diagnosis and vigorous treatment. Effective

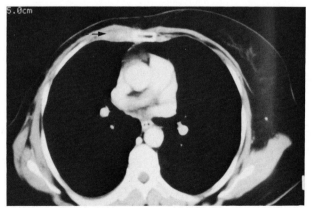

Figure 28–13. Computed tomography of the chest shows recurrence in the internal mammary lymph nodes on the side of a previous mastectomy *(arrow)*.

control not only spares the patient much discomfort and embarrassment from weeping, bleeding, and odoriferous ulceration but also may retard the development of dissemination (Donegan et al., 1966). In a few cases, treatment appears to be curative.

Histologic analysis is essential if misdiagnosis is to be avoided. Fat necrosis, cutaneous cysts, nodal hyperplasia, and other processes can mimic recurrence and precipitate unnecessary treatment. Suspicious nodules in the surgically treated area or enlarged regional nodes should be biopsied. Excisional biopsy is preferable when it is feasible. Analysis of estrogen receptors and progesterone receptors as well as tumor kinetic studies are performed on the tumor tissue. Previous irradiation can reduce the number of hormone receptors, so tumor tissue from regions beyond the irradiated areas is preferable if this is an option (Janssens et al., 1981). Confirmation of chest wall recurrence should be followed by restaging to detect distant dissemination. The latter has been found present in 17% to 32% of patients (Chu et al., 1984; and Crowe et al., 1991), indicating the need for systemic as well as local treatment.

Local Excision

After mastectomy, complete excision of a small, isolated nodule of local recurrence is occasionally sufficient for control. This is particularly useful when recurrence occurs in a previously irradiated site. Four of 15 patients (27%) who were so treated at EFSCH remained tumor-free with regard to the chest wall; however, metastases did progress elsewhere. Surgical excision was successful in controlling local disease in 6 of 11 such patients, according to Humphrey and coworkers (1990).

Salvage Mastectomy

In the absence of dissemination or inoperability, the current practice is to treat recurrences in the breast or in the breast and axilla after breast-conserving therapy with ''salvage mastectomy''—that is, with total mastectomy in combination with axillary dissection if nodes are palpable or if axillary dissection was not performed originally. Recurrences of in situ carcinoma are treated with total mastectomy alone. Wide local excision or partial mastectomy is used for selected cases of breast recurrence at some centers, but experience with this approach is still limited (Stotter et al., 1989; Veronesi et al., 1990; and Nemoto et al., 1991). Kurtz and coworkers (1988b) selected patients with small (<2 cm), mobile, indolent recurrences for partial mastectomy; of these, 20% to 30% developed further recurrence in the breast.

The prognosis of cases treated with salvage mastectomy is generally favorable: the 5-year survival rate ranges from 48% to 84%, and some clinicians report that 55% to 59% of patients remain disease-free at 5 years (Harris et al., 1984; Kurtz et al., 1988a; Stotter et al., 1989; Ames and Balch, 1990; Fowble et al., 1990; and Osborne, et al., 1992). Survival is directly related to the DFI and indirectly to the original clinical stage (Kurtz et al., 1988a; and Kurtz et al., 1989), but prognosis is also influenced by the pattern of recurrence. An isolated parenchymal recurrence has a more favorable prognosis than recurrence in the skin of the breast or recurrence in multiple sectors of the breast (Price et al., 1988).

Local-regional recurrence after breast conservation has a detrimental influence on prognosis. Estimates are that it reduces survival to the same extent as an asynchronous primary tumor of similar stage in the second breast (Stotter et al., 1990). Fisher and colleagues (1991) reported that breast recurrence was associated with an increased risk of dissemination, and Clark (1983) found that the prognosis of patients with recurrence only in the breast to be inferior to that of patients who remained recurrence-free. Others have found no difference (Clarke et al., 1985; and Stotter et al., 1989). Recurrence strictly limited to the breast does have a prognosis superior to that of recurrence in the axilla or in the axilla and breast, which in turn is less ominous than distant dissemination (Clark 1983; and Clarke et al., 1985). Recurrence in the retained breast has a more favorable prognosis than recurrence in the chest wall after mastectomy, which provides some reassurance about treatment with breast conservation. The two, however, are not comparable. The latter reflects extensive infiltration of the tissues of the chest wall or involvement of nodes rather than regrowth in the tumor bed. Although the same factors that influence local-regional failure may promote dissemination, the possibility cannot be discounted that the former provides a second opportunity for dissemination (Hayward and Caleffi, 1987). If it is not prevented, then early detection and vigorous treatment should be the objectives. Retreatment with irradiation is usually not an option in patients with recurrence in the conserved breast unless the recurrence is in an nonirradiated area. Surgical resection is employed when possible and usually is supplemented with systemic adjuvant therapy (Clarke et al., 1985; Kurtz et al., 1988a; and Stotter et al., 1990).

Data on the ultimate success of local-regional control in patients treated initially with breast conservation are few. More than 80% of patients treated with salvage mastectomy obtain long-lasting local control; in one report, survival was 88% at 5 years (Kurtz et al., 1989; and Clarke et al., 1985). Barr and coworkers (1989) reported that at 5 years uncontrolled local-regional disease was present in 2% of 356 patients with Stage I and II tumors treated with breast conservation and that it was present in 11% of those who died. The corresponding figures for patients initially treated for Stage III and IV cancers were 16% and 36%. It is speculated that the proportions of patients who ultimately die with persistent local-regional cancer are similar whether treatment is initiated with lumpectomy and irradiation or with mastectomy (Barr et al., 1989).

Irradiation

Irradiation is the therapy of choice for local and regional recurrence in previously nonirradiated sites. Successful and durable control of recurrences can be expected in a high proportion of cases, particularly if the recurrences are detected and treated while still minimal (Madoc-Jones et al., 1976), and it has a higher probability of success than chemotherapy alone (Janjan et al., 1986). Irradiation may also improve local-regional control in patients receiving systemic therapy for simultaneous distant metastases (Bedwinek et al., 1983). Overall, irradiation can be expected to produce at least temporary control of chest wall recurrence in 41% to 72% of cases, but the probability of attaining ultimate control with radiation therapy may be substantially less (Chu et al., 1976; Bedwinek et al., 1983; Patanaphan et al., 1984; and Chen et al., 1985).

The ability to control local disease is strongly related to the amount of tumor present and to the volume and dose of radiation given. Microscopic disease is more likely to be eradicated by irradiation than is gross disease. Hence, treatment is more often successful when gross recurrence is removed surgically prior to irradiation (Loprinzi et al., 1984; Probstfeld and O'Connell, 1989; and Halverson et al., 1992b). Although this may reflect bias in that less extensive disease can be removed surgically, it suggests that excisional biopsy rather than incisional biopsy for diagnosis of local recurrence when feasible may be advantageous. Comprehensive irradiation is also superior to "spot" irradiation. Ports limited to the gross disease can achieve remarkable results (Fig. 28–14), but progression to beyond the treated area becomes apparent in 27% to 46% of patients (Bedwinek et al., 1983; and Chen et al., 1985); this creates a problem with regard to the juxtaposition of ports and to the necessity for additional periods of treatment. The preferred approach is comprehensive treatment of the involved site and all adjacent uninvolved sites at risk for local-regional failure (Janjan et al., 1986; Bedwinek, 1990; and Halverson et al., 1990). This includes the chest wall as well as the supraclavicular and internal mammary areas. The uninvolved axilla is an exception, as it is rarely a site of treatment failure after complete dissection, and irradiation superimposed on dissection increases the risk of disabling lymphedema. Halverson and associates (1990) reported that "optimal" irradiation of 109 patients resulted in a 5-year local-regional control rate of 75% compared with a rate of only 44% in 116 patients without optimal treatment. "Optimal irradiation" was defined as the irradiation of large fields encompassing the entire region of recurrence and elective irradiation of the chest wall and supraclavicular areas. Radiation doses in excess of 4500 cGy are required for adequate treatment (Bedwinek et al., 1983). Administration of doses between 4500 and 5000 cGy is standard for patients with subclinical disease and are supplemented with electron boosts of 1000 to 1500 cGy to bulky tumors, if present (Janjan et al., 1986).

If breast reconstruction has preceded local recurrence, the presence of an implanted prosthesis does not compromise therapy, particularly if the recurrence has been excised. But if recurrence is extensive or deep to the prosthesis, the latter should be removed prior to the initiation of treatment (Shank, 1988).

Unresectable local-regional recurrences that persist after irradiation and systemic therapy represent a difficult problem. The threat of radionecrosis of the chest wall places a limit on the use of further irradiation (Zimmerman et al., 1966). The application of hyperthermia combined with low-dose irradiation (DuBois et al., 1990) as well as the use of photodynamic therapy employing light-activated hemato-

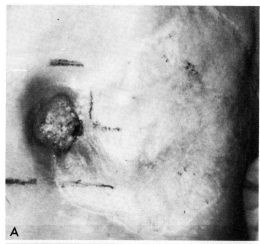

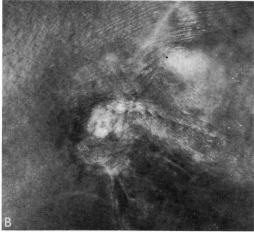

Figure 28-14. *A,* Cancer recurred on the medial chest wall 3 years after a radical mastectomy in a 51-year-old woman for an adenocarcinoma metastatic to 4 of 24 axillary lymph nodes. *B,* She underwent irradiation to a limited port (marked) encompassing the lesion and was well, with no further evidence of metastasis 55 months later. Irradiation controlled progressive growth of cancer in what was apparently an isolated internal mammary node.

porphyrin derivatives are being explored (Kennedy and Abeloff, 1993).

Axillary Node Dissection

Regional failure of treatment in the axilla in the absence of metastases elsewhere can be treated with axillary node dissection or with irradiation. Judging from the results of National Surgical Adjuvant Breast Project Protocol B-04 (see Table 28–5), a complete axillary dissection appears to provide more lasting local control of resectable clinical adenopathy. The frequency of axillary recurrence was 10-fold greater when clinically positive axillary metastases were treated with irradiation than when they were treated with dissection. Axillary dissection is also recommended for isolated axillary recurrence after breast conservation when no sign of breast tumor recurrence is present (Wilson, 1984; Kurtz et al., 1988a; Barr et al., 1989; and Ames and Balch,

1990). If nodes are fixed or if distant metastases are present, radiotherapy is preferable to dissection.

Axillary recurrence, however, signals a poor prognosis. At least 71% of patients who had axillary dissection for isolated failure at this site after total mastectomy in Protocol B-04 of the National Surgical Adjuvant Breast Project subsequently had further disease progression (Fisher et al., 1977). Thirty-eight per cent of 13 patients managed with dissection for axillary recurrence at EFSCH were alive 5 years after the original mastectomy.

Therapeutic dissection of the supraclavicular area for isolated recurrence at this site is unproductive. After biopsy confirmation, treatment generally consists of irradiation with or without systemic therapy. Fentiman and associates (1986) reported good control of supraclavicular metastases in patients after excision for diagnosis and treatment with irradiation; however, within 12 months, 50% of the patients had further signs of recurrence, and 80% had recurrence in 4 years. The 5-year survival rate after supraclavicular recurrence was 30%, and the 10-year survival rate was 20%.

Systemic Therapy

Since the presence of occult dissemination is highly likely in patients with clinically isolated local regional recurrence, the addition of systemic therapy as an adjuvant to local treatment has a logical basis. Nevertheless, no randomized trials are available to confirm its value, and after a review of retrospective studies, Ames and Abeloff (1993) concluded that benefits of such adjuvant therapy remain uncertain.

In a pilot study, Buzdar and coworkers (1979) used fluorouracil, doxorubicin, cyclophosphamide, and bacille Calmette-Guérin (BCG) to treat 68 patients who had been rendered disease-free by local treatment of isolated recurrences; this treatment prolonged the DFI of these patients in comparison with that of a historical control group. Thirty-nine patients with chest wall recurrences were included, and 66% of these remained disease-free up to 2 years; in contrast, only 25% of 38 historical controls survived 2 years free of disease. Survival of the two groups at 2 years, however, was not significantly different (91% and 84%, respectively). Beck and coworkers (1983) observed superior 5-year survival and disease-free survival rates in 42 patients who received systemic therapy for local-regional recurrence compared with 43 patients who received radiotherapy alone. They recommended systemic therapy for those with DFIs shorter than 24 months and with initially advanced stages of disease.

Other researchers had different findings. Janjan and associates (1986) reviewed 164 patients treated for local-regional recurrence at M.D. Anderson Cancer Center in Houston, Texas, and found no significant difference in survival or local control of patients who received chemotherapy in addition to radiotherapy compared with those who did not. They considered chemotherapy without radiotherapy to be inappropriate. In a retrospective study of 230 patients with local-regional recurrence, all of whom were treated with irradiation, Halverson and associates (1992a) found no survival benefits associated with adjuvant chemo-

therapy. Adjuvant hormonal therapy (tamoxifen or megestrol acetate administration, oophorectomy) did increase survival and deterred dissemination, but it did not improve local-regional control. The benefits of hormonal therapy were particularly prominent in postmenopausal patients. These authors favored the use of adjuvant hormonal therapy. Kurtz and colleagues (1989) found no survival benefit from chemohormonal therapy, but patients treated with hormonal therapy fared better than those treated with chemotherapy.

The uncontrolled influences on the results of retrospective studies leave the value of adjuvant systemic therapy in doubt, and until this issue is resolved definitively, many clinicians will favor adjuvant systemic therapy in patients with signs of poor prognosis (Bedwinek et al., 1981b; Janjan et al., 1986; Probstfeld and O'Connell, 1989; and Halverson et al., 1992a). Crowe and coworkers (1991) considered systemic therapy appropriate for patients with nodal recurrence, a short DFI, and axillary nodes previously positive for cancer. Ames and Abeloff (1993) recommended systemic therapy for those with extensive local relapse and a brief DFI. In prognostically favorable cases, deferring systemic therapy spares morbidity for a few patients who will never need it and conserves treatment until it is clearly appropriate.

Chest Wall Resection

In selected patients, radical resection is appropriate for the treatment of persistent local and parasternal recurrences. It may be the only recourse for those with isolated or symptomatic recurrences that have failed treatment with irradiation and systemic therapy. When performed by an experienced surgeon, chest wall resection can be achieved with low mortality; in addition, it can offer palliation for most patients as well as an opportunity for cure or long-term freedom from disease for a few. The best results are achieved when the recurrence is completely encompassable, preceded by a prolonged DFI, and unaccompanied by distant dissemination; however, the presence of these three factors are not necessarily contraindications.

Sauerbruch is credited as being the first to remove recurrent mammary carcinoma with chest wall resection in 1907; however, Schede preceded him in 1886 and, in turn, credited Kolaczek for using it even earlier for the removal of other tumors. Urban used this method for the treatment of parasternal recurrences beginning in 1951—a prelude to his development of the extended mastectomy.

Most reports of chest wall resection include few cases, but patients up to 73 years of age have undergone the procedure. Hospitalization durations average between 18 and 20 days, and mortality from the procedure is low or nonexistent. Resections involve the removal of partial or full thicknesses of the chest wall, with the latter including ribs (average of three); part or all of the sternum; and, sometimes, part or all of the clavicle or underlying lung. Large defects are stabilized with the placement of synthetic materials—most often Marlex or Prolene mesh that is sometimes combined with methyl methacrylate in a composite "sandwich"—to prevent paradoxical motion (Mc-

Cormack et al., 1989; and Nash et al., 1991). Bridging defects with rigid material has reduced or eliminated the need for prolonged postoperative ventilation. Small defects usually require no stabilization. Soft tissue coverage is accomplished with a variety of methods, the most popular being the placement of transverse rectus abdominis myocutaneous flaps (TRAM) or latissimus dorsi flaps or free flaps; or, when cosmetic considerations are not paramount, advancement of the contralateral breast (Fig. 28–15). When only deep tissues require resection, primary closure occasionally is possible.

Case selection undoubtedly accounts for variations in results. Snyder and associates (1969) reported 24 patients treated with chest wall resection, and of these, 17% were long-term survivors and free of disease. The results were particularly good when the DFI exceeded 48 months. Shah and Urban (1975) reported 52 cases performed between 1950 and 1972 at Memorial-Sloan Kettering Cancer Center in New York City, New York, primarily for the treatment of parasternal recurrences. The indications in most instances were failure to respond to irradiation, recurrence in irradiation ports, radionecrosis, and irradiation-induced cancers of the chest wall. The 5-year survival rate of patients treated for recurrence was higher when resection was the initial treatment (43%) than when the tumor had proved resistant to irradiation (16%). From the same institution, McCormack and coworkers (1989) reviewed the disease histories of 35 patients so treated specifically for recurrent breast cancer that was resistant to multimodality therapy and found that 20 of the 35 patients were living a median of 50 months later.

For recurrence or radionecrosis, McKenna and associates (1984) included as indications (1) local symptoms of pain, infection, and ulceration; (2) tumor recurrence despite radiotherapeutic intervention; and (3) the presence of infection that precluded chemotherapy. As contraindications, they identified tumor en cuirass, brain metastasis, bone marrow involvement, and the presence of bulky cancerous disease in two or more organs. They did not consider liver, lung, bone, or malignant pleural effusions to be absolute contraindications. The surgical mortality among their 43 cases was 5%. Tumors recurred on the chest in 12.5% of patients, but 72% of patients lived longer than 1 year, and three patients for longer than 40 months.

Twenty-seven extensive resections with no in-hosptial deaths were reported from M.D. Anderson Cancer Center (Ames and Balch, 1990). Eighteen of these included the removal of a full thickness of the chest wall. Complete tumor resection in nine of the patients resulted in an average survival of 46 months. The average survival was longer than 20 months in 18 patients with dissemination or in whom resection margins were not free of tumor; for those in the latter group, palliation was judged as being "fair to good." Twelve cases treated at Rush-Presbyterian–St. Lukes Medical Center in Chicago included no operative deaths (Kluiber et al., 1991), and in four cases, complications were limited to pneumonia or flap necrosis. Four of the patients were alive and free of disease from 3 to 71 months after the resection, but only one had survived at least 5 years. Five (38.5%) of 13 cases reported by Nash and associates (1991) survived for 5 years after chest wall resection, only 1 of whom was alive and tumor-free.

SUMMARY

Local-regional recurrence has many manifestations and a variable prognosis. In general, it is a harbinger of dissemination; however, this is not always the case, nor is dissemination always imminent. Control of this problem offers considerable benefit to patients, and for this reason, recurrence deserves vigorous treatment. The following guidelines are offered. In general, after mastectomy, the optimal treatment is local excision of the gross recurrence when feasible; this is followed by comprehensive irradiation to the chest wall and regional nodes. After breast conservation, when irradiation has already been used, a salvage mastectomy is the preferred treatment when disease is limited to the breast and axillary lymph nodes. Because the failure rate remains high after both of these measures are taken, systemic chemotherapy or hormonal therapy, or

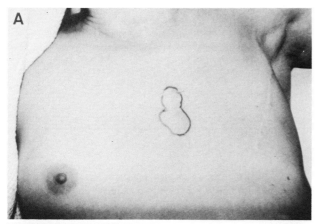

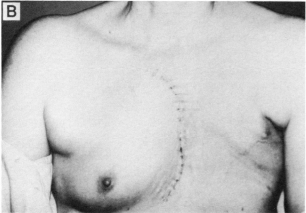

Figure 28–15. Chest wall resection for local recurrence. Fifteen years after mastectomy, cancer reappeared as a subcutaneous nodule superficial to the sternum. Local excision, irradiation, and tamoxifen therapy resulted in a disease-free period of 23 months, after which tumor recurred at the same site, involved the skin, and became fixed to the sternum *(A)*. The lesion was widely resected en bloc with the outer table of the sternum, and the defect was closed by advancing the medial portion of the right breast *(B)*. Twenty-four months later, the patient remained disease-free.

both, are often added, particularly for patients who are likely to have prompt relapse. However, justification of the value of the latter requires better documentation, and in favorable cases, systemic therapy might be held in reserve. Chest wall resection is appropriate for selected patients with persistent local-regional recurrence when other measures have failed.

References

Ahlborn, T. N., Gump, F. E., Bodian, C., et al.: Tumor to fascia margin as a factor in local recurrence after modified radical mastectomy. Surg. Gynecol. Obstet., *166*:523–526, 1988.

Ames, F. C., and Balch, C. M.: Management of local and regional recurrence after mastectomy or breast-conserving treatment. Surg. Clin. North Am., *70*:1115–1124, 1990.

Barr, L. C., Brunt, A. M., Goodman, A. G., et al.: Uncontrolled local recurrence after treatment of breast cancer with breast conservation. Cancer, *64*:1203–1207, 1989.

Beck, T. M., Hart, N. E., Woodard, D. A., et al.: Local or regionally recurrent carcinoma of the breast: Results of therapy in 121 patients. J. Clin. Oncol., *1*:400, 1983.

Bedwinek, J. M., Fineberg, B., Lee, J., and Ocwieza, M.: Analysis of failures following local treatment of isolated local-regional recurrence of breast cancer. Int. J. Radiat. Oncol. Biol. Phys., *7*:581–585, 1981*a*.

Bedwinek, J. M., Lee, J., Fineberg, B., et al.: Prognostic indicators in patients with isolated local-regional recurrence of breast cancer. Cancer, *47*:2232, 1981*b*.

Bedwinek, J.: Radiation therapy of isolated local regional recurrence of breast cancer: Decisions regarding dose, field size, and elective irradiation of uninvolved sites. Int. J. Radiat. Oncol. Biol. Phys., *19*:1093–1095, 1990.

Bedwinek, J. M., Munro, D., and Fineberg, B.: Local-regional treatment of patients with simultaneous local-regional recurrence and distant metastases following mastectomy. Am. J. Clin. Oncol., *6*:295–300, 1983.

Bruce, J., Carter, D. C., and Fraser, J.: Patterns of recurrent disease in breast cancer. Lancet, *i*:453, 1970.

Buzdar, A. U., Bluenschein, G. R., Smith, T. L., et al.: Adjuvant chemoimmunotherapy following regional therapy for isolated recurrences of breast cancer (Stage IV NED). J. Surg. Oncol., *12*:27, 1979.

Camper, P.: Over denwaren aart der kankervorming en over een zeer zakelijk en onfeilbaar teken van onherstelbaaren horstkanker. Genees, Nat Huishoudk Kabinet, *2*:193–208, 1779.

Chen, K. K. Y., Montague, E. D., and Oswald, M. J.: Results of irradiation in the treatment of locoregional breast cancer recurrence. Cancer, *56*:1269, 1985.

Chu, F. C. J., Lin, F. J., Kim, J. H., et al.: Locally recurrent carcinoma of the breast: Results of radiation therapy. Cancer, *37*:2677, 1976.

Chu, A. M., Cope, O., Russo, R., and Lew, R.: Patterns of local-regional recurrence and results in Stages I and II breast cancer treated by irradiation following limited surgery: An update. Am. J. Clin. Oncol., *7*:221–229, 1984.

Clark, R. M.: Alternatives to mastectomy: The Princess Margaret Hospital Experience. *In* Harris, J. R., Hellman, S., and Silen, W. (Eds.): Conservative Management of Breast Cancer. Philadelphia, J. B. Lippincott, 1983, pp. 35–46.

Clarke, D. H., Le, M. G., Sarrazin, D., et al.: Analysis of local-regional relapses in patients with early breast cancers treated by excision and radiotherapy: Experience of the Institut Gustave-Roussy. Int. J. Radiat. Oncol. Biol. Phys., *11*:137–145, 1985.

Crowe, J. P. Jr., Gordon, N. H., Antunez, A. R., et al.: Local-regional breast cancer recurrence following mastectomy. Arch. Surg., *126*:429–432, 1991.

Dahl-Iversen, E.: An extended radical operation for carcinoma of the breast. J. R. Coll. Surg. Edinb., *8*:81, 1963.

Danckers, V. F., Hamann, A., and Savage, J. L.: Postoperative recurrence of breast cancer after thirty-two years: A case report and review of the literature. Surgery, *47*:656, 1960.

Dao, T. L., and Nemoto, T.: The clinical significance of skin recurrence after radical mastectomy in women with cancer of the breast. Surg. Gynecol. Obstet., *117*:447, 1963.

Demaree, E. W.: Local recurrence following surgery for cancer of the breast. Ann. Surg., *134*:863, 1951.

Dershaw, D. D., McCormack, B., Cox, L., et al.: Differentiation of benign and malignant local tumor recurrence after lumpectomy. A. J. R. Am. J. Roentgenol., *155*:35–38, 1990.

Diehl, L. F., Jurwitz, M. A., Johnson, S. A., et al.: Skin metastases confined to a field of previous irradiation: Report of two cases and review of the literature. Cancer, *53*:1864, 1984.

Donegan, W. L.: Mastectomy in the primary management of invasive mammary carcinoma. Adv. Surg., *6*:1–101, 1972.

Donegan, W. L.: The influence of untreated internal mammary metastases upon the course of mammary cancer. Cancer, *39*:533, 1977.

Donegan, W. L., Perez-Mesa, C. M., and Watson, F. R.: A biostatistical study of locally recurrent breast carcinoma. Surg. Gynecol. Obstet., *112*:529, 1966.

Donegan, W. L., and Padrta, B.: Combined therapy for inflammatory breast cancer. Arch. Surg., *125*:578–582, 1990.

DuBois, J. B., Hay, M., and Bordure, G.: Superficial microwave-induced hyperthermia in the treatment of chest wall recurrences in breast cancer. Cancer, *66*:848–852, 1990.

Ewers, S. B., Attewell, R., Baldetorp, B., et al.: Flow cytometry, DNA analysis and prediction of loco-regional recurrence after mastectomy in breast cancer. Acta Oncol., *31*:733–740, 1992.

Fentiman, I. S., Lavelle, M. A., Caplan, D., et al.: The significance of supraclavicular fossa node recurrence after radical mastectomy. Cancer, *57*:908, 1986.

Fisher, B., Montague, E., Redmond, C., et al.: Comparison of radical mastectomy with alternative treatments for primary breast cancer: A first report of results from a prospective randomized clinical trial. Cancer, *39*:2827–2839, 1977.

Fisher, B., Redmond, C., Fisher, E. R., et al.: Ten year results of a randomized clinical trial comparing radical mastectomy and total mastectomy with or without radiation. N. Engl. J. Med., *312*:674–681, 1985.

Fisher, B., Anderson, S., Fisher, E. R., et al.: Significance of ipsilateral breast tumor recurrence after lumpectomy. Lancet, *338*:327–331, 1991.

Fisher, B., Redmond, C., Poisson, R., et al.: Eight-year results of a randomized clinical trial comparing total mastectomy and lumpectomy with or without irradiation in the treatment of breast cancer. N. Engl. J. Med., *320*:822–828, 1989.

Fowble, B., Solin, L. J., Schultz, K. J., et al.: Breast recurrence following conservative surgery and radiation: Patterns of failure, prognosis, and pathologic findings from mastectomy specimens with implications for treatment. Int. J. Radiat. Oncol. Biol. Phys., *19*:833–842, 1990.

Haagensen, C. D.: Diseases of the Breast. Philadelphia, W. B. Saunders, 1971, pp. 710.

Haffty, B. G., Fischer, D., Rose, M., et al.: Prognostic factors for local recurrence in the conservatively treated breast cancer patient: A cautious interpretation of the data. J. Clin. Oncol., *9*:997–1003, 1991.

Halsted, W. S.: The results of operations for the cure of cancer of the breast performed at the Johns Hopkins Hospital from June 1889 to January 1894. Johns Hopkins Hosp. Rep., *4*:297, 1894.

Halverson, K. J., Perez, C. A., Kuske, R. R., et al.: Locoregional recurrence of breast cancer: A retrospective comparison of irradiation alone versus irradiation and systemic therapy. Am. J. Clin. Oncol., *15*:93–101, 1992*a*.

Halverson, K. J., Perez, C. A., Kuske, R. R., et al.: Survival following locoregional recurrence of breast cancer: Univariate and multivariate analysis. Int. J. Radiat. Oncol. Biol. Phys., *23*:285–291, 1992*b*.

Halverson, K. J., Perez, C. A., Kucke, R. R., et al.: Isolated local-regional recurrence of breast cancer following mastectomy: Radiotherapeutic management. Int. J. Radiat. Oncol. Biol. Phys., *19*:851–858, 1990.

Harris, J. R., Recht, A., Amalric, R., et al.: Time course and prognosis of local recurrence following primary radiation therapy for early breast cancer. J. Clin. Oncol., *2*:37, 1984.

Hayward, J., and Caleffi, M.: The significance of local control in the primary treatment of breast cancer. Arch. Surg., *122*:1244–1247, 1987.

Humphrey, L. J., Moore, D. L., and Lytle, G. H.: Postmastectomy locally recurrent breast cancer. J. Surg. Oncol., *43*:88–91, 1990.

Janjan, N. A., McNeese, M. D., Buzdar, A. L. U., et al.: Management of locoregional recurrent breast cancer. Cancer, *58*:1552–1556, 1986.

Janssens, J. P., Teuwen, D., Bonte, J., et al.: Effect of radiotherapy on steroid receptors in breast cancer. Lancet, *ii*:1108, 1981.

Kennedy, M. J., and Abeloff, M. D.: Management of locally recurrent breast cancer. Cancer, *71*:2395–2409, 1993.

Kluiber, R., Bines, S., Bradley, C., et al.: Major chest wall resection for recurrent breast carcinoma. Am. Surg., *57*:523–530, 1991.

Kurtz, J. M., Jacquemier, J., Brandone, H., et al.: Inoperable recurrence after breast conserving surgical treatment and radiotherapy Int. J. Surg. Gynecol. Obstet., *172*:357–361, 1991.

Kurtz, J. M., Amalric, R., Brandone, H., et al.: Local recurrence after breast-conserving surgery and radiotherapy: Frequency, time course, and prognosis. Cancer, *63*:1912–1917, 1989.

Kurtz, J. M., Amalric, R., Brandone, H., et al.: Results of salvage surgery for mammary recurrence following breast-conserving therapy. Ann. Surg., *207*:347–351, 1988*a*.

Kurtz, J. M., Amalric, R., Brandone, H., et al.: Results of wide excision for mammary recurrence after breast-conserving therapy. Cancer, *61*:1969–1972, 1988*b*.

Kurtz, J. M., Jacquemier, J., Amalric, R., et al.: Risk factors for breast recurrence for premenopausal and postmenopausal patients with ductal cancers treated by conservation therapy. Cancer, *65*:1867–1878, 1990.

Lewis, D., and Rienhoff, W. F. Jr.: Study of results of operations for cure of breast cancer performed at Johns Hopkins Hospital from 1889–1931. Am. Surg., *95*:336, 1932.

Loprinzi, C. L., Carbone, P. P., Tormey, D. C., et al.: Aggressive combined modality therapy for advanced local-regional breast carcinoma. J. Clin. Oncol., *2*:157–163, 1984.

Madoc-Jones, H., Nelson, A. J. III, and Montague, E. D.: Evaluation of the effectiveness of radiotherapy in the management of early nodal recurrences from adenocarcinoma of breast. Breast, *2*:31, 1976.

McCormack, P. M., Bains, M. S., Burt, M. E., et al.: Local recurrent mammary carcinoma failing multimodality therapy. Arch. Surg., *124*:158–161, 1989.

McKenna, R. J. Jr., McMurtrey, M. J., Larson, D. L., et al.: A perspective on chest wall resection in patients with breast cancer. Ann. Thorac. Surg., *38*:482, 1984,

Meltzer, A.: Dormancy and breast cancer. J. Surg. Oncol., *43*:181–188, 1990.

Morrow, M., and Foster, R. S. Jr.: Staging of breast cancer. Arch. Surg., *116*:748, 1981.

Nash, A. G., Tuson, J. R. D., Andrews, S. M., et al.: Chest wall reconstruction after resection of recurrent breast tumours. Ann. R. Coll. Surg. Engl., *73*:105–110, 1991.

Nemoto, T., Patel, J. K., Rosner, D., et al.: Factors affecting recurrence in lumpectomy without irradiation for breast cancer. Cancer, *678*:2079–2082, 1991.

O'Dwyer, P. J., Duffy, M. J., O'Sullivan, F., et al.: CEA and CA 15-3 in primary and recurrent breast cancer. World J. Surg., *14*:562–566, 1990.

Osborne, M. P., Borgen, P. I., Wong, G. Y., et al.: Salvage mastectomy for local and regional recurrence after breast-conserving operation and radiation therapy. Surg. Gynecol. Obstet., *174*:189–194, 1992.

Patanaphan, V., Salazar, O. M., and Poussin-Rosillo, H.: Prognostications in recurrent breast cancer: A 15 year experience with irradiation. Cancer, *54*:228, 1984.

Pawlias, K. T., Dockerty, M. B., and Ellis, F. H. Jr.: Late local recurrent carcinoma of the breast. Ann. Surg., *148*:192, 1958.

Peters, T. F., Donegan, W. L., and Burg, E. A.: Minimal breast cancer: A clinical appraisal. Ann. Surg., *186*:704, 1977.

Price, P., Walsh, G., McKinna, A. J., et al.: Patterns of breast relapse after local excision +/- radiotherapy for early stage breast cancer. Radiother. Oncol., *13*:53–60, 1988.

Probstfeld, M. R., and O'Connell, T. X.: Treatment of locally recurrent breast carcinoma. Arch. Surg., *124*:1127–1130, 1989.

Sardi, A., Eckholdt, G., McKinnon, W. M., et al.: The significance of mammographic findings after breast-conserving therapy for carcinoma of the breast. Surg. Gynecol. Obstet., *173*:309–312, 1991.

Sauerbruch, F.: Beitrag zur Resektion der Brustwand mit Plastik auf die Freigelegte Lunge. Dtsch. Z. Chir., *86*:275, 1907.

Schede: Aerzlicher Verein zu Hamburg. Dtsch. Med. Wochenschr., *37*:646, 1886.

Schnitt, S. J., Connolly, J. L., Harris, J. R., et al.: Pathologic predictors of early local recurrence in stage I and II breast cancer treated by primary radiation therapy. Cancer, *53*:1049–1057, 1984.

Schwaibold, F., Fowble, B. L., Solin, L. J., et al.: The results of radiation therapy for isolated local regional recurrence after mastectomy. Int. J. Radiat. Oncol. Biol. Phys., *21*:299–310, 1991.

Shah, J. P., and Urban, J. A.: Full thickness chest wall resection for recurrent breast carcinoma involving the bony chest wall. Cancer, *35*:567, 1975.

Shank, B.: Breast irradiation for recurrence in a patient with a silicone implant. Oncology, *2*:58, 1988.

Snyder, A. F., Farrow, G. M., Masson, J. K., et al.: Chest wall resection for locally recurrent breast cancer. C. A. Cancer J. Clin., *19*:282, 1969.

Solin, L. J., Fowble, B. L., Schultz, D. J., et al.: The detection of local recurrence after definitive irradiation for early stage carcinoma of the breast. Cancer, *65*:2497–2502, 1990.

Spratt, J. S.: Locally recurrent cancer after radical mastectomy. Cancer, *20*:1051, 1967.

Spratt, J. S., Shieber, W., and Dillard, B. M.: Anatomy and Surgical Technique of Groin Dissection. St. Louis, C. V. Mosby, 1965, pp. 69.

Stotter, A., Atkinson, E. N., Fairston, B. A., et al.: Survival following locoregional recurrence after breast conservation therapy for cancer. Ann. Surg. *212*:166–172, 1990.

Stotter, A. T., McNeese, M. D., Ames, F. C., et al.: Predicting the rate and extent of locoregional failure after breast conservation therapy for early breast cancer. Cancer, *64*:2217–2225, 1989.

Tomin, R., and Donegan, W. L.: Screening for recurrent breast cancer: Its effectiveness and prognostic value. J. Clin. Oncol., *5*:62–67, 1987.

Urban, J. A.: Radical excision of chest wall for mammary cancer. Cancer, *4*:1263, 1951.

Veronesi, U., and Valagussa, P.: Inefficacy of internal mammary node dissection in breast cancer surgery. Cancer, *47*:170, 1981.

Veronesi, U., Cascinelli, N., Bufalino, R., et al.: Risk of internal mammary lymph node metastases and its relevance on prognosis of breast cancer patients. Ann. Surg., *198*:681, 1984.

Veronesi, U., Salvadori, B., Luini, A., et al.: Conservative treatment of early breast cancer: Long-term results of 1232 cases treated with quadrantectomy, axillary dissection and radiotherapy. Ann. Surg., *211*:250–259, 1990.

Vicini, F. A., Recht, A., Abner, A., et al.: Recurrence in the breast following conservative surgery and radiation therapy for early stage breast cancer. Monogr. Natl. Cancer Inst., *11*:33–39, 1992.

Wilson, R. E.: Surgical management of locally advanced and recurrent breast cancer. Cancer, *53*:752–757, 1984.

Zimmerman, K. W., Montague, E. D., and Fletcher, G. H.: Frequency, anatomical distribution and management of local recurrences after definitive therapy for breast cancer. Cancer, *19*:67, 1966.

29

Orthopedic Management of Skeletal Metastases

John Mahan
David Seligson

Let us now see what is the case as regards the bones in cancer of the breast.

SIR JAMES PAGET, 1889

Bone is the most common site of metastasis of breast cancer (Joo et al., 1979; Kamby et al., 1987) (Fig. 29–1). Skeletal metastases are detected in 2% of patients at the time of primary diagnosis, whereas one-third of patients with recurrent breast cancer have detectable osseous metastases. Approximately 70% of patients with breast cancer have skeletal metastases at autopsy (Abrams et al., 1950; Meissner and Warren, 1971; Galasko, 1972; Viadana et al., 1973; Bunting et al., 1976; Cifuentes and Pickren, 1979; Cho and Choi, 1980; Hagemeister et al., 1980; Nikkanen, 1981; Sears et al., 1982; Lee, 1984; and Kamby and Rasmussen, 1991).

Bone metastases can be the first evidence of metastatic disease in many patients with breast cancer. Indeed, a pathologic fracture due to a metastasis may be the first manifestation of the malignant disease and must be considered whenever a patient fractures a major bone such as the femur owing to a less traumatic insult than would normally be expected to produce a fracture (Koskinen and Nieminen, 1973; Gerber et al., 1977; and Heinz et al., 1989). Although pathologic fractures or bony metastases can occur with many cancers, breast cancer is the most common cause (Fig. 29–2).

Pathologic fractures occur in approximately 33% of patients with radiographic evidence of skeletal metastases (Bunting et al., 1976; Nikkanen, 1981; Sears et al., 1982; Lee, 1984; and Kamby et al., 1987). The morbidity associated with pathologic fracture includes not only the loss of function from the broken limb but also the trauma to surrounding tissues, the morbidity of fracture treatment, and loss of independence during convalescence and rehabilitation (Higinbotham and Marcove, 1965). Patients with metastatic breast cancer have diminished physiologic reserves. Treatment is associated with more complications and greater morbidity than the usual care of broken bones. Therefore the detection of skeletal metastases prior to pathologic fracture is worthwhile. The primary investigations for bone metastases in a patient with breast cancer are the skeletal x-ray survey and the technetium bone scan (Habermann and Lopez, 1989). Today, new methods are becoming available that seem promising (Kamby and Rasmussen, 1991).

The treatment of skeletal metastases of breast cancer depends on the particular patient, the specific bone affected, the location of the metastatic lesion, the degree of osseous destruction, and the likelihood of fracture (Klein et al., 1989). In this chapter, guidelines for preventive, nonoperative treatment and prophylactic fixation are outlined, as well as current methods for treating pathologic fractures.

HISTORY OF TREATMENT OF BREAST CANCER METASTATIC TO BONE

Surgeons once regarded pathologic fractures without hope. Reviewing the literature from 1886 through 1904, Grunert stated, ''We are justified in saying that in carcinomatous, that is to say, in true carcinomatous metastases, union of the fragments can never occur.'' Cotton stated, ''Fractures through carcinoma do not heal.'' Pancoast was more optimistic, citing a 40% rate of healing in his treatment of pathologic fractures (Eliason, 1933). Pancoast, however, was the exception. In general, a tone of pessimism permeated early accounts, which catalogued the extent of bone involvement in patients dying from breast cancer.

A systematic review of a larger series of pathologic fractures was conducted at the Massachusetts State Hospital for Cancer at Pondville (Welch, 1936). Of 637 patients with breast cancer, 151 (24%) had radiographic evidence of osseous metastasis, and 26 (17%) suffered pathologic fractures. Various methods were used to treat these pathologic fractures, including x-irradiation, skeletal fixation, and traction. Nine pathologic fractures were judged to have healed with firm union. Six of these had been treated with moderate doses of x-irradiation. Welch concluded that bone metastases could be treated with radiation therapy to achieve healing.

Bouchard at McGill reviewed 24 cases of breast cancer with skeletal metastases treated with radiation therapy. Repeat physical and radiologic examinations were often positive in patients with ''neuralgic'' or ''rheumatic'' complaints. Bouchard found that 66% of patients experienced subjective improvement while 26% had objective radiographic improvement following radiation therapy. According to Bouchard (1945), ''No case is so hopeless as to warrant discard without a trial of therapeutic irradiation.''

Thus, metastatic bone disease secondary to breast cancer was regarded with more optimism as larger series of cases were compared and systematically analyzed.

In 1945, the Küntscher method of intramedullary nailing was described for treatment of pathologic fractures (Küntscher, 1945). Böhler (1948) observed, "Spontaneous fractures after malignant bone tumors are very well suited for closed medullary nailing."

Küntscher's successors at the University of Kiel performed nailings not only for pathologic fractures but also for two cases of impending fracture of the femur. The nailings were followed by radiation therapy. They reported that the patients had no complaints and were able to walk again and the metastases were no longer observable on radiographs (Griessmann and Schüttemeyer, 1947). Intramedullary nailing gradually became an accepted mode of therapy for pathologic fractures, but it was not without its hazards (Ehrenhaft and Tidrick, 1949; Lehmann, 1951; and Altman, 1953). Fat embolism, shock, soft tissue injury, and mechanical failure of the intramedullary device were some of the problems described by Küntscher (1967) in using his method. Peltier (1951a) performed experiments to delineate the local and systemic effects of inserting a nail into the marrow cavity. Peltier's experimental conclusions were that tumor cells could be spread locally and to distant sites by the process of reaming and placing an intramedullary nail in animals, but this mode of dissemination of cancer cells in bone has not proved clinically significant. In the late 1970s, Zickel, Harrington, and Habermann established the open operative treatment of pathologic fractures with polymethylmethacrylate acrylic cement and metal constructs. Today, techniques of percutaneous fixation using flexible or interlocking nails and aggressive resection and reconstructive surgery are available to treat fractures as the lon-

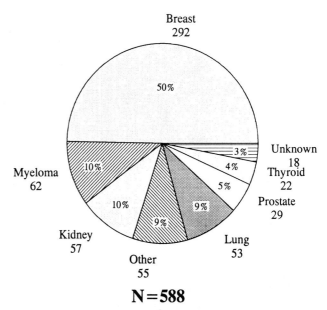

Figure 29–2. Distribution of metastatic cancer to bone. (From Habermann, E.T., and Lopez R.A.: Metastatic disease of bone and treatment of pathological fractures. Orthop. Clin. North Am., *20*:469–486, 1989.)

gevity of patients with breast cancer continues to increase (Fey, 1981).

BASIC PATHOPHYSIOLOGIC BEHAVIOR OF SKELETAL METASTASES

"The microenvironment of the bone marrow tissue, rather than the cortical bone, is the primary soil of metastatic disease in human breast cancer" (Kamby and Guldhammer, 1987). In breast cancer, hematogenous embolization appears to be more important than lymphatic spread in the production of distant metastases. The metastatic deposit that becomes established in the marrow cavity may be quite large before it is detected by conventional radiography. The appearance of x-ray changes in patients with metastatic breast carcinoma therefore indicates an advanced process affecting the radiodense lamellar bone of the cortex. The image reflects what the metastatic cancer has done to the bone and the bone's response to it (Enneking, 1982).

Skeletal metastases of breast cancer have a consistent distribution (Abrams and Spiro, 1950) (see Fig. 29–2). This distribution is independent of primary cell type. The three characteristic types of breast cancer metastasis are distinguished primarily by their respective radiographic appearances: lytic, blastic, or mixed lesions (Bouchard, 1945; Bachman and Sproul, 1955; and Mootoosamy et al., 1985). These categories reflect the ultimate outcome in the balance between osteoclast-mediated bone resorption and osteoblast-mediated bone formation. The mixed lesions represent to a large extent uncoupling of the normally integrated process of remodeling that occurs in living bone (Fig. 29–3). Bone is an exquisitely designed material. The layers of the cortex are arranged around interlocked cables of collagen strategically oriented to bear load. Depending on the interaction between the deposit and the bone there is more

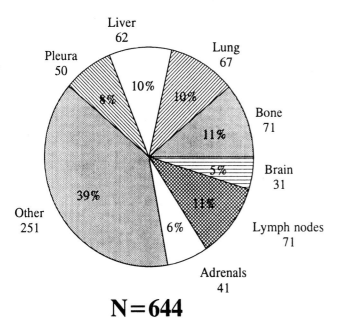

Figure 29–1. Distribution of metastatic breast cancer. (From Cifuentes, N., and Pickren, J.W.: Metastases from carcinoma of mammary gland: an autopsy study. J. Surg. Oncol., *11*:193–205, 1979. Copyright © 1979, John Wiley & Sons, Inc. Reprinted by permission of John Wiley & Sons, Inc.)

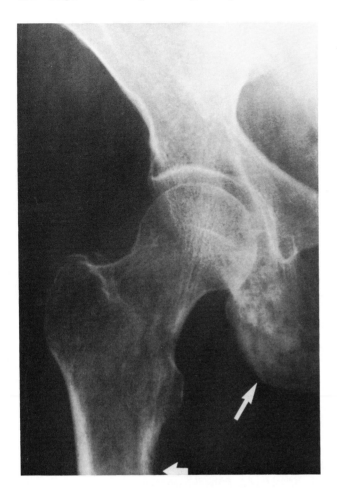

Figure 29–3. Right hip with metastatic cancer from the breast. Two patterns can be seen: the lesion in the ischium is 'mixed,' lytic, and blastic; and the lesion in the lesser trochanter is lytic.

or less loss of strength (Fig. 29–4). The presence of increased x-ray density, as in sclerotic lesions, is not necessarily equivalent to increased mechanical capacity: the arrangement is critical.

Cancer cells shed from the primary lesion and secondaries are found in the bloodstream of patients with breast cancer. The fate of these circulating tumor cells is determined by their ability to survive transport through the bloodstream, survive host defense mechanisms, and attach to the endothelium of distant vessels and then establish their

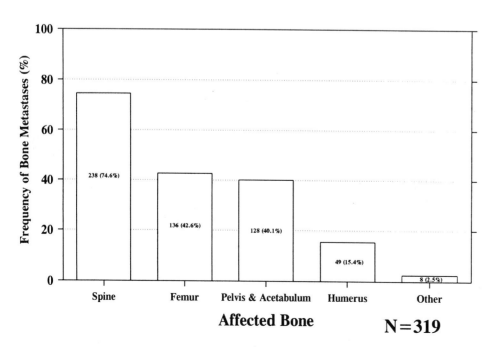

Figure 29–4. The frequency of bone metastases in patients with breast cancer. (From Miller, F., and Whitehill, R.: Carcinoma of the breast metastatic to the skeleton. Clin. Orthop., *184*:121–127, 1984.)

own blood supply (Hart, 1982; and Mansi et al., 1989). Circulating tumor cells, in and of themselves, do not ensure the occurrence of metastatic disease in bone, but small colonies of tumor cells can establish themselves in bone marrow (micrometastasis). Markers for these micrometastases have been detected by iliac crest biopsy in at least one-third of patients with Stage IV disease (Singletary et al., 1991). In patients without evidence of metastases, immunocytochemical techniques demonstrate a substantial number of cells with tumor markers. The presence of these cells correlates with tumor size and vascular invasion (Berger et al., 1988; and Taha et al., 1989). The presence of these micrometastases, however, does not necessarily mean that colonies will form that lead to structurally significant changes.

Chemotactic factors seem to have an important role in the establishment of osseous metastases. A certain factor may be released during the turnover of bone. Tumor emboli may be organ specific, and some homing mechanism may be based on specific cell organ receptors that allow tumors to establish their own pattern of metastases (Mansi et al., 1989). Clearly, humoral and enzymatic factors play a role in creating an environment suitable for metastases. New bone formation is seen in most skeletal metastases, but this is dependent on the formation of a suitable fibrous stroma. Breast cancer metastases tend to establish poor fibrous stroma, resulting in little new bone formation. Osteoinductive factors such as the bone morphogenetic protein isolated by Urist and colleagues, as well as humoral factors secreted by tumor cells, may regulate the formation and resorption of bone near an osseous metastasis (Fig. 29–5). Prostaglandin E_2 secreted by osteoblasts has been shown to stimulate bone formation and resorption, and it is thought to be a local regulator as well as a mechanism that couples resorption and formation (Habermann et al., 1989).

Galasko conducted experiments to delineate the pathophysiology of progressive bone destruction associated with metastatic disease from tumors. He believed two mechanisms in bone were responsible for destruction by skeletal metastases. Galasko based his opinions on autopsy studies of spines with metastatic deposits and on a series of exper-

iments in which tumor cells were injected into rabbits. In the first mechanism, tumors secrete a humoral factor that stimulates osteoclast production and local migration. This was demonstrated by injecting a tumor cell suspension into rabbit thigh muscle. The number of osteoclasts observed in femora at progressive intervals distal to the site of these injections decreased, indicating osteoclast migration. The corresponding contralateral bone exhibited none of these effects, suggesting that the humoral osteoclast activator does not act systemically. The second mechanism, which Galasko believed to be quantitatively less important, involves the removal of bone rendered ischemic, and eventually necrotic, by local overgrowth of cancer cells. This ''osteocyclic osteolysis'' was observed in a few rabbit tibial cortices after direct injection of the tumor suspension but was not seen in the human autopsy material (Galasko, 1976). There is also evidence in vitro that breast cancer cells resorb bone directly without the intervention of osteoclasts (Kulenkampff, 1986; and Elion and Mundy, 1978).

The effect of radiation therapy on the normal biology of fracture healing and the abnormal process of tumor growth provides a unique illustration of the pathophysiology of metastatic disease. Bonarigo and Rubin created an animal model for pathologic fracture in rats (Bonarigo and Rubin, 1967). The experimental design consisted of three groups. The first group was subjected to fracture of the tibia, which was then irradiated and followed for evidence of fracture healing. A second group underwent ulnar fracture. The corresponding intact radius served as a splint; tumor cells were implanted at the ulna fracture site, and subsequent tumor growth was observed. The third group underwent tibial fracture, tumor cell implantation, internal fixation, and radiation therapy. The experimental results demonstrate, first, that nonunion occurs if a fracture site is irradiated; second, that tumor growth inhibits fracture healing with subsequent nonunion; and finally, that fractures that contain tumor cells will heal if treated with secure internal fixation and radiation therapy. These results were explained by the authors, who first point out that metastatic tumor growth and radiation therapy cause pathologic fracture because they are deleterious to cartilage formation. Fracture healing by callus

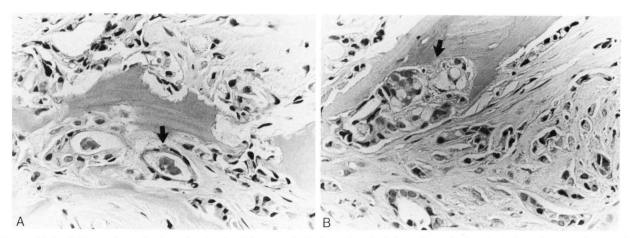

Figure 29–5. *A,* Resorption of a lamellar (mature) bone spicule by osteoclasts in a deposit of metastatic adenocarcinoma. *B,* New bone formation (osteoblasts) and absorption in metastatic breast cancer.

formation involves an intermediate phase of cartilage, which eventually ossifies and is remodeled into lamellar bone. A lytic metastasis without a fracture heals by direct osteogenesis, since chondrogenesis is radiosensitive but osteogenesis is not. Thus, lytic lesions respond to radiotherapy, whereas pathologic fractures, which heal by callus formation and a cartilaginous phase, do not. Pathologic fractures treated with secure internal fixation heal with radiation therapy because the callus structure that ordinarily is necessary to provide fracture site stability is replaced by the internal fixation device. This explains why radiation, a cause of nonunion (Bonfiglio, 1951), is effective in treating metastatic deposits, provided there is skeletal stability (Bonarigo and Rubin, 1967).

DIAGNOSTIC MODALITIES

Early detection of bone metastases is important in patients with breast cancer since the most common site of distant metastases is the skeleton (Gerber et al., 1977; and Joo et al., 1979). Since radical mastectomy is usually deferred in the presence of distant metastasis, an accurate diagnosis of metastatic disease is needed to plan treatment. The technetium bone scan is the most sensitive method of demonstrating occult osseous lesions (Galasko, 1969; Charkes et al., 1975; and Galasko, 1975). Bone metastases can be visualized by bone scan, on average, 4 months before they are evident on standard skeletal radiographs (Bachman and Sproul, 1955; Hoffman and Marty, 1972; Lentle et al., 1975; and Baker, 1977).

The technetium bone scan combined with ultrasonography of the liver is 95% sensitive in detecting metastatic disease at an early stage (Glynne-Jones et al., 1991), but it lacks specificity in eliminating other causes of increased radioisotopic uptake (Sklaroff and Sklaroff, 1976; and Perez, 1983). It is thus crucial to obtain a radiograph of the area that is "hot" on bone scan, to rule out other causes of this finding, such as a healing fracture, bone infection, or Paget's disease. The detection of metastases to bone by x-ray depends on the crystalline density of the affected bone. Serial bone and liver scans are useful in evaluating response to therapy (Citrin et al., 1975; Citrin et al., 1976; Bitran et al., 1980; Arnstein et al., 1984; Blomqvist et al., 1987; Coleman et al., 1990; and Glynne-Jones et al., 1991). The radiograph cannot distinguish a difference in bone density before a change in bone calcium content of at least 30% has occurred (Babaïantz, 1947). Bone scans reflect changes in metabolic activity from a variety of causes and thus reveal earlier disease (and smaller lesions) than radiographs do (Charkes et al., 1975).

Pain generally heralds the presence of osseous metastases and can precede x-ray changes by several weeks (Nussbaum et al., 1977; and Scher and Yagoda, 1987). A thorough history, physical examination, serum biochemical markers, technetium bone scan, x-ray evaluation, and surgical biopsy in selected instances are important means of evaluating suspicious osseous lesions in a patient with breast cancer (Joo et al., 1979).

Several investigators have proposed radiographic criteria for identifying metastatic lesions at risk of fracture (Fidler,

1973). In the opinion of some authors, these criteria have not consistently demonstrated the likelihood of fracture. This is because the distribution of stress in bone is not uniform. A small lesion in an area of high stress such as the subtrochanteric region of the femur is more likely to fracture than a similar-sized lesion in a low-stress area (Buturla et al., 1985; and Hipp et al., 1989). Keene and colleagues reported that 57% of metastatic lesions in their series could not be adequately measured on standard radiographs (Keene et al., 1986). Overall, however, measurable lesions showed a definite propensity toward fracture (81%) when the metastasis occupied more than two-thirds of the affected bone's diameter (Mirels, 1985).

Pain at the site of a metastatic lesion is also predictive of impending fracture. As an isolated symptom, however, pain is nonspecific, and not useful as a single predictor of pathologic fracture (Front et al., 1979; and Blomqvist et al., 1987). Combined methods that integrate the symptom of pain with radiographic criteria are superior for the assessment of lesions at risk for fracture.

Biochemical markers have a specific role in the screening and diagnosis of metastatic breast cancer, specifically osseous lesions (Hortobagyi et al., 1982; and Kamby et al., 1991). The serum level of carcinoembryonic antigen, and to a lesser degree of serum alkaline phosphatase, is helpful when used in combination with the clinical symptom of musculoskeletal pain and bone scan results to screen and follow osseous deposits (Perez, 1982; and Blomqvist et al., 1987). Isolated elevations in carcinoembryonic antigen or alkaline phosphatase level, without correlation with other diagnostic criteria, are of minimal help in diagnosing metastatic breast cancer. Hortobagyi and coworkers recommend baseline determinations of biochemical markers with repeat serum levels every 3 months to detect metastases and to assess response to treatment (Hortobagyi et al., 1982; and Coleman et al., 1988).

Estrogen receptor–bearing tumors have a predilection for osseous metastasis (Stewart et al., 1980; Campbell et al., 1981; Samaan et al., 1981; Budd, 1983; and Kamby and Rasmussen, 1991). It is of interest that patients with estrogen receptor–positive tumors also tend to have a more favorable prognosis and response to therapy than patients with a similar stage of estrogen receptor–negative disease. However, neither the estrogen receptor status of the primary tumor nor the receptor status of osseous metastases significantly alters the treatment plan of an orthopaedist confronted with an impending fracture or a pathologic fracture secondary to breast cancer. With current therapy, the orthopaedic problem is primarily mechanical, not biological. Skeletal failure demands an immediate mechanical treatment to restore quality of life. Biological methods retard tumor growth and prevent fracture in the longer run.

When the source of a skeletal lesion cannot be discerned with diagnostic imaging techniques, biopsy of the lesion becomes necessary (Fig. 29–6). Several techniques are described in the literature for acquiring a sample of an osseous lesion for histologic examination (Hebert et al., 1980; Frisch, 1984; and Smith et al., 1986).

An indirect method of biopsy is the sampling of bone marrow. Frisch and coworkers examined 504 patients with known or suspected metastatic breast cancer and performed

Known Breast Cancer

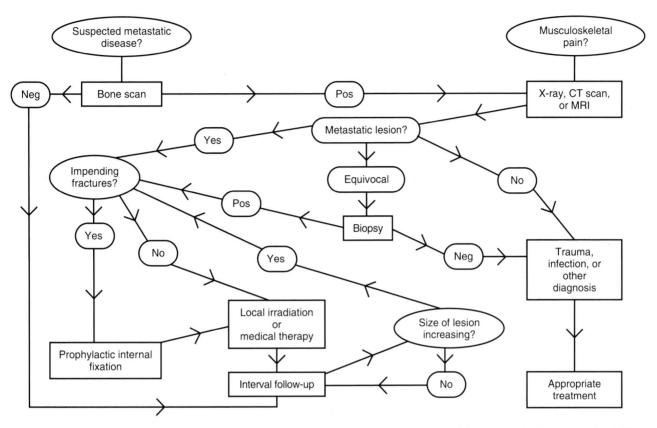

Figure 29–6. Flow diagram for work-up of bone metastasis in a breast cancer patient. CT = computed tomography; MRI = magnetic resonance imaging; Pos = positive; Neg = negative.

either anterior or posterior iliac crest biopsy to obtain samples of the marrow. Forty-two per cent of patients had metastatic breast cancer in the marrow of the ilium. The authors emphasized the likelihood of metastatic infiltration in the marrow of several bones in a given patient when the iliac crest is randomly sampled and micrometastases are present (Frisch et al., 1984). This particular method of biopsy would signal the need for further investigation for osseous metastases but would not be useful for identifying lesions at risk for pathologic fracture at specific locations.

Ridell and Landys (1979) examined 532 women with unilateral breast cancer and reported a lower rate (10%) of positive samples in patients with known breast cancer, employing a method of biopsy similar to that of Frisch's group. Since most patients (97%) in their series with positive biopsies did not have radiographically demonstrable lesions, iliac bone marrow biopsy is not recommended for routine investigation of metastatic breast cancer.

Ceci and colleagues (1988) performed bone marrow biopsy from the posterior iliac crest in 173 patients with breast cancer. In 99% of patients with negative bone scans and skeletal radiographs, the bone marrow biopsy specimen was also negative. The authors believe that this confirms that there is no correlation between metastatic involvement of bone and involvement of the bone marrow. They did not find this method of biopsy useful for discovering metastatic foci in breast cancer patients when findings of both technetium bone scan and radiography were negative.

Methods for biopsy of suspicious skeletal lesions are described in the literature. Hebert and coworkers (1982) report the diagnostic value of closed medullary biopsy. The 31 biopsies in their series were obtained by reaming of the medullary canal for nail placement. A long bronchial biopsy forceps was inserted to the site of the lesion under fluoroscopic guidance and a sample of the lesion was grasped and removed. This method produced adequate tissue specimens at a rate (70%) that was comparable to that of open bone biopsy (75%).

Smith and coworkers report a different method of closed intramedullary biopsy. A large-bore plastic catheter is advanced to the lesion in an unreamed intramedullary canal and biopsy material is suctioned out with a syringe. In their series of 27 biopsies, 92.5% were positive.

Biopsy specimens can also be taken by making a cortical window directly over a lesion. In high-stress areas such as the subtrochanteric region of the femur, direct biopsy has a substantial risk of causing a fracture, since increased local bone resorption is a preliminary step to repair of the defect. Once the diagnosis of osseous breast cancer metastasis is established and appropriate therapy is outlined, continuous follow-up is crucial (Fig. 29–6). Scanlon and colleagues (1980) recommended a physical examination with appropriate radiography of symptomatic areas every 3 months for the first 4 years after diagnosis.

The accurate diagnosis of a skeletal deposit in the axial or acral skeleton requires coordination between oncologist, radiologist, and surgeon. In this way, most testing can be done on an outpatient basis and procedures coordinated for short hospital stays.

CURRENT RECOMMENDATIONS FOR THERAPY

Although the diagnosis of metastatic breast cancer may provoke a dreadful reaction from patient and family, it carries a more favorable prognosis than other forms of disseminated malignancy (Habermann and Lopez, 1989). The longevity of patients who suffer from metastatic breast cancer continues to improve. It is, therefore, a challenge for physicians confronted with osseous metastases from breast cancer to preserve function and improve the woman's quality of life (Yazawa et al., 1990). It is also desirable, when possible, to diagnose impending fractures secondary to metastatic lesions and to spare patients the morbidity of pathologic fracture.

Orthopedic Care

The primary goal of orthopedic care is to restore musculoskeletal integrity and facilitate a patient's rehabilitation (Parrish and Murray, 1970; Lewallen et al., 1982; Ganz et al., 1984). The basic principles of restoring and preserving function, and thus enhancing a patient's quality of life, are specific to each skeletal location (Coran et al., 1968; Gilbert et al., 1977; and Friedl and Krebs, 1986).

Secure internal fixation is an effective method of stabilizing a bone at risk of fracture from a metastatic lesion, especially when nonoperative methods prove to have limited value (Higinbotham and Marcove, 1965; Parrish and Murray, 1970; Perez and Bradfield, 1972). Patients must be carefully selected on the basis of the particular lesion (Yablon, 1977). The severity of the underlying disease, the overall operative risk, and the rehabilitation potential are the other factors that are important in the selection of internal fixation as optimal therapy for individual patients. The importance of a strong coordinated team approach involving oncologists, orthopedic surgeons, radiotherapists, and physical and occupational therapists is emphasized in the literature (Habermann and Lopez, 1989).

There is a characteristic distribution of bone metastases from cancer of the breast (Bouchard, 1945; Abrams et al., 1950). The sites, in decreasing order of frequency, are spine, pelvis, femur, humerus, and the acral skeleton. This distribution reflects the distribution of the bone marrow in the skeleton (see Fig. 29–2).

The spine is the most common site of metastasis (Krishnamurthy et al., 1977). In the spine, the marrow-bearing vertebral body is the most frequent target and is affected in most cases (85%). Because the incidence of involvement at specific levels is proportional to the percentage a segment occupies in the vertebral column (Black, 1979), the thoracic spine is most frequently affected (Schaberg and Gainor, 1985). Spinal canal metastases may be divided into epidural, leptomeningeal, and intramedullary lesions. Extension of tumor locally in the spine from the vertebral body

to the spinal canal is thought to occur via the venous plexuses of Batson (Batson, 1940; Boland and Lane, 1982). When a metastasis affects the epidural regions, recognition and treatment are urgent to avoid cord compression and paraplegia (Nussbaum et al., 1977). The lesions that most commonly cause neurologic compromise are in the thoracic spine (70%) (Boland and Lane, 1982; Byrne, 1992). When radiation and chemotherapy do not halt the progression of neurologic symptoms, vertebral body resection and anterior cord decompression are advisable. Posterior laminectomy creates instability and is not, therefore, recommended for treating these lesions. The anterior approach to the vertebral body permits tumor resection and surgical exposure of the dural canal (Harrington, 1981, 1984, 1988). This is preferable, as decompressing the canal posteriorly leaves the metastatic lesion to grow anteriorly. Special diagnostic imaging techniques (computed tomography with or without myelography, magnetic resonance imaging) are undertaken to locate precisely the metastatic lesion before the operative procedure.

Harrington and coworkers described a classification scheme that is useful for identifying which lesions are most amenable to operative intervention (Harrington, 1986) (Table 29–1). Patients with Class IV or V lesions benefit most from early operative intervention. In most cases a procedure is planned to resect the tumor anteriorly with vertebral body resection, anterior decompression, and bone grafting or methylmethacrylate placement around spinal instrumentation (Fig. 29–7). Autologous bone grafting requires at least 3 to 6 months for osseous consolidation to occur. Radiation therapy cannot be used after an autologous bone graft since the graft will be resorbed. Metal instrumentation with polymethylmethacrylate reinforcement can provide immediate stability that facilitates recovery, ambulation, and subsequent radiation treatment (Harrington, 1981; and Sim et al., 1974). Radiation therapy with doses as large as 4000 rad does not affect the structural integrity of metal-acrylic composites.

Conservative treatment applied to lesions of the femur cannot be relied upon to produce satisfactory results on a consistent basis (Bremner and Jelliffe, 1958; and Snell and Beals, 1964). This statement expresses a long-held belief and has retained its validity for the current treatment of

Table 29–1. CLASSIFICATION AND TREATMENT SCHEME FOR SPINAL METASTASES

Class	Definition	Therapy
I	No symptoms	Radiotherapy
II	Stable vertebrae, minor neurologic symptoms	Radiotherapy
III	Stable vertebrae, major neurologic symptoms	Radiotherapy ± corticosteroids
IV	Unstable vertebrae, minor neurologic symptoms	Surgical intervention
V	Unstable vertebrae, major neurologic symptoms	Surgical intervention

(From Harrington, K. D.: Anterior decompression and stabilization of the spine as a treatment for vertebral collapse and spinal cord compression from metastatic malignancy. Clin. Orthop., *233*:177–197, 1988.)

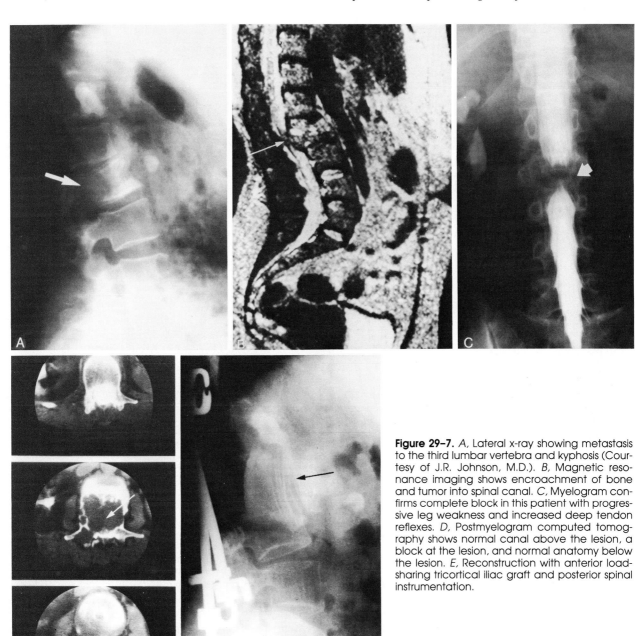

Figure 29–7. *A,* Lateral x-ray showing metastasis to the third lumbar vertebra and kyphosis (Courtesy of J.R. Johnson, M.D.). *B,* Magnetic resonance imaging shows encroachment of bone and tumor into spinal canal. *C,* Myelogram confirms complete block in this patient with progressive leg weakness and increased deep tendon reflexes. *D,* Postmyelogram computed tomography shows normal canal above the lesion, a block at the lesion, and normal anatomy below the lesion. *E,* Reconstruction with anterior load-sharing tricortical iliac graft and posterior spinal instrumentation.

femoral metastases (Coran and Banks, 1968; and Maatz et al., 1986).

The appropriate treatment for metastatic lesions of the femur varies according to what part of the bone is affected (Gristina et al., 1983). Pathologic fractures and impending fractures of the femoral head and neck are treated by resection and replacement with an endoprosthesis (Habermann and Lopez, 1989). Nail-plate devices can also be used for the treatment of the femoral head and neck, but this method requires a phase of fracture healing before rehabilitation and ambulation. The use of an endoprosthesis for complete replacement of the femoral head and neck may require a special or custom implant. This technique has grown in acceptance since it removes the metastatic lesion and stabi-

lizes the hip joint (Habermann et al., 1982). Prosthetic replacement facilitates immediate ambulation, nursing care, and rehabilitation for the patient. The surgeon who decides to employ an endoprosthesis in the proximal femur must carefully examine the entire femur radiographically to avoid locating the stem of an endoprosthesis at the site of another metastatic lesion. If a more distal femoral metastasis is associated with a femoral head or neck lesion, an endoprosthesis with a longer stem is required to bypass the distal metastasis (Nussbaum et al., 1977; and Habermann et al., 1982). It is important to assess the acetabular region for metastatic disease at the time of femoral head replacement, since the acetabulum often does not show metastatic disease on standard imaging techniques. It may nonetheless be

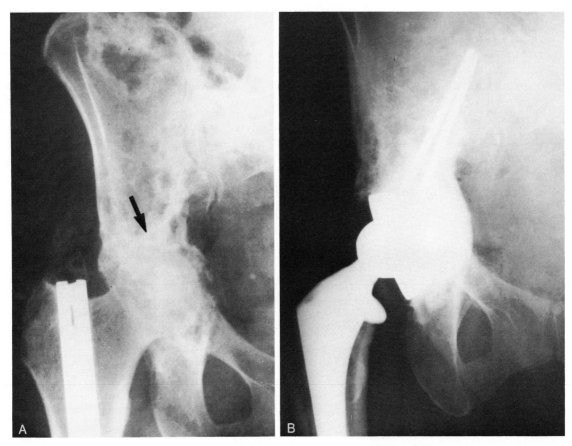

Figure 29–8. *A,* Exclusive acetabular destruction by metastasis in a patient with prior prophylactic nailing of the femur. *B,* Long stem total hip replacement. Methylmethacrylate and Steinmann pin reconstruction for deficient superior and medial acetabulum.

compromised by osseous metastases at the time the corresponding femoral head and neck are involved (Kramer et al., 1987). Biopsy examination of the acetabulum at the time of surgery for the femoral head has often yielded metastasis. With significant acetabular involvement, both sides of the joint should be replaced (Fig. 29–8) (Harrington, 1981). Habermann and coworkers (1989) recommend replacing both the acetabulum and the femoral head with an appropriate prosthetic device at the time of surgery, regardless of the radiologic appearance of the acetabulum.

Intertrochanteric lesions are also approached with devices designed to replace the affected portion of the femur. The intertrochanteric region of the femur, an area of high stress (Buturla et al., 1985; and Mirels, 1985), is particularly at risk for fracture when breast cancer deposits are present. The affected intertrochanteric region should be resected and replaced by an endoprosthesis when the metastatic disease affects a substantial percentage of the intertrochanteric region or proximal femur (Habermann and Lopez, 1989). Koskinen and Nieminen (1973) recommended the use of nail-plate fixation for stabilizing isolated intertrochanteric lesions. This method provides less stability than replacement procedures but can nonetheless be expected to maintain the structural integrity of the proximal femur when the metastatic deposit is small. Use of a fracture implant avoids loosening of the endoprosthesis.

The abductor mechanism must be addressed when the metastatic deposit replaces the greater trochanter. This can be accomplished by a trochanteric mesh that, when secured to the endoprosthesis, transmits the forces of the abductor group to the proximal femur (Habermann and Lopez, 1989).

Metastatic disease in the subtrochanteric region of the femur is treated with an intramedullary device. Historically, the Zickel device has been employed for this purpose with good results (Zickel and Mouradian, 1976; Nussbaum et al., 1977; and Habermann and Lopez, 1989). The device may be used with or without methylmethacrylate. Proper preparation is necessary to avoid malrotation. As with intertrochanteric lesions, surgical manipulation of the subtrochanteric femur requires attention to the abductor mechanism. Today, closed tubular interlocking nails that can be inserted over guidewires are available for the treatment of pathologic subtrochanteric fractures. These can be combined with other internal fixation devices and bone cement to provide stable load-bearing constructs (Burny et al., 1976; and Isler, 1990).

Fractures and impending fractures of the femoral shaft are treated optimally with an intramedullary device (Bennish and Hammond, 1955; Beals et al., 1971; and Habermann et al., 1989) (Fig. 29–9). A Küntscher nail or Enders nail is recommended for prophylactic internal fixation of

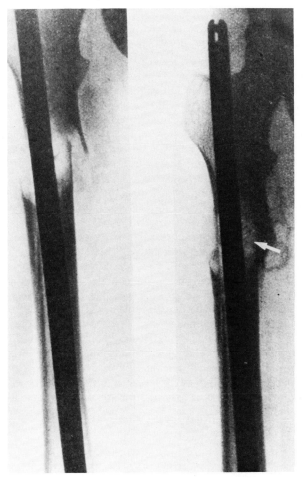

Figure 29–9. *Left,* Intramedullary nailing for pathologic fracture of the femur. *Right,* After subsequent radiation therapy with healing. (From Küntscher, G., and Matz, R.: Teknique der Marknagelung. Leipzig, Georg Thieme Verlag, 1945, p. 82.)

ton, 1976; and Flemming and Beals, 1986). In the case of impending fracture, however, a trial of radiotherapy is warranted, since the risk of pathologic fracture is less than with similar involvement at other sites (Cheung et al., 1980). Finally, when a metastatic deposit in the humerus fails to resolve, prosthetic replacement (Frassica, 1986), open reduction with internal fixation, or closed rodding is the optimal mode of therapy (Lewallen and Pritchard, 1980; and Flemming and Beals, 1986).

Specific radiographic and clinical indices have been described when internal fixation of a metastatic lesion at risk of fracture is considered: "(1) a painful lytic destructive lesion involving greater than 2.5 cm of the cortex; (2) a painful intramedullary lytic lesion greater than 50% of the cross-sectional diameter of the bone; and (3) a progressively painful lesion not relieved by radiotherapy" (Fidler, 1973). Once the decision has been made to operate, the method and device employed must be tailored to the specific bone and lesion (Beals et al., 1971; Allen and Watson, 1976).

Systemic Therapy

Hormone therapy has been the traditional mode of treating disseminated breast cancer (Bhardwaj and Holland, 1982; and Smith and Macaulay, 1985). A 30% response rate is expected in the treatment of bone metastases with hormone manipulations. These modalities include oophorectomy, estrogen, androgen, and tamoxifen pharmacotherapy (Legha et al., 1978). The status of estrogen receptors in breast cancer–related metastatic disease is a useful prognosticator of the response to hormonal manipulations (Asbury et al., 1981); estrogen receptor–bearing lesions respond in 45% to 60% of cases, whereas fewer than 10% of estrogen receptor–negative lesions improve with hormone therapy (McQuire et al., 1975). In lieu of estrogen receptor status, L-dopa has been used successfully to predict responsiveness to hormone therapy (Dickey and Minton, 1972; Minton, 1976; and Davies, 1979). L-Dopa inhibits pituitary production of prolactin, which alleviates symptomatic bone pain. Therapy has also been directed toward inhibiting adrenal function. Agents such as aminoglutethimide and megesterol

impending fractures. When extensive destruction of the femoral shaft is present, methylmethacrylate is useful to reinforce and maintain femoral length (Heppenstall, 1980; and Isler, 1990).

Metastatic lesions to the acetabulum from breast cancer can be divided into four classes based on location and patterns of structural deformation (Table 29–2). The acetabulum is often involved when the femoral head and neck have radiographic evidence of metastatic disease (Harrington, 1981; and Kramer et al., 1987). When the acetabulum is affected it is necessary to restore the structural integrity to the entire hip joint (Isler, 1990). Most authors currently recommend replacement of the hip joint with a prosthetic cup device that transmits the forces from the femur upward into the ilium. This device is also the optimal method of preventing and treating protrusion of the femoral head into the pelvic cavity for Class II lesions.

Metastatic breast disease may involve the humerus. These lesions result in pathologic fracture only 10% of the time. This is because, unlike the spine, pelvis, and femur, the upper extremities do not participate in weight bearing. When pathologic fracture occurs through the humerus, surgical methods are superior to nonoperative ones (Harring-

Table 29–2. CLASSIFICATION AND TREATMENT SCHEME FOR ACETABULAR METASTASES

Class	Definition	Surgical Method
I	Isolated defects	Total hip arthroplasty
II	Deficient medial cortex	Protrusio acetabuli ring
III	Deficient superior, medial, and lateral cortices	Steinmann pins (ilium), methylmethacrylate, protrusio acetabuli ring
IV	Diffuse structural defect	Resection en bloc, Steinmann pins (ilium), methylmethacrylate, protrusio acetabuli ring

(From Harrington, K. D.: The management of acetabular insufficiency secondary to metastatic malignant disease. J. Bone Joint Surg., 63A:653–664, 1981.)

acetate achieve a 20% response rate of osseous metastases (Asbury et al., 1981; and Lipton and Santen, 1974). The agent biphosphonate pamidronate, an inhibitor of osteoclast function, has shown promise in inhibiting osteolysis of bony metastases from breast cancer (Dodwell et al., 1990).

Dichloromethylene diphosphonate has been used successfully to decrease pain from breast cancer metastases in bone (Scher and Yagoda, 1987; and Martoni et al., 1991). Chemotherapy for the treatment of metastatses in bone includes 5-fluorouracil, which produces a modest response rate (Donaldson and Horsley, 1970).

Radiation Therapy

Radiation therapy is effective for long-term management of localized bony metastases (Allen and Watson, 1976; and Cheung and Driedger, 1980). In one study, moderate doses of radiotherapy—2000 to 2500 rad over a 2-week interval—produced symptomatic relief in 96% of cases and recalcification of osseous lesions in 78% (Gilbert et al., 1977). Patients in one study exhibited a rise in calcium-47 uptake lasting as long as 2 months and strontium-85 retention lasting a year. These changes in mineral uptake and retention are indicative of the recalcification process in a previously destructive metastatic lesion (Garmatis and Chu, 1978). Shorter courses of treatment have also been recommended (Jensen and Rosendahl, 1976). Regardless of the dosage regimen, a moderate dose consistently results in palliation of metastases (Penn, 1976). Irradiating the entire affected bone is important, since tumor cells are assumed to be present throughout a bone involved with metastases (Perez et al., 1972; and Salazar et al., 1986).

FUTURE DIRECTIONS

Historically, the treatment of skeletal metastases from breast cancer began with desperate cases. Patients with extensive metastases sustained spontaneous fractures and were hospitalized in the caring but fearful atmosphere of institutions for the terminally ill. There patients with incurable pain, seizures, large fungating masses, and amputated limbs and body parts were sheltered from public view, and death was the mode of discharge. In this setting, physicians came to realize that pathologic fractures could be treated with surgical stabilization or radiation therapy to improve quality of life and offer some chance of healing. The basic principles continue today. Bone destroyed by metastases is reinforced with constructs of metal and acrylic. The vitality of tumor cells is altered by radiation therapy. The concept is similar to that of reinforcing scaffolding applied to a collapsing building. Patients with metastatic carcinoma are close to the end of their lives. The objective of treatment is palliation; the approach is to temporize. With improved understanding of surgical physiology, extensive extirpation of tumor has been possible, and extensive reconstruction has been added to the therapeutic armamentarium for the treatment of symptomatic metastases. *Replacement* has been added to the strategy of *reinforcement* for significant tumor deposits. Oncologists have improved the prognosis

of patients with breast cancer (Fey, 1981). Breast cancer metastatic to bone is susceptible to chemotherapy. Responses confer increased activity, decreased pain, increased bone density, decreased size of lytic metastasis, and a restoration of more normal bony architecture (Gilbert et al., 1977; Friedl and Krebs, 1988; and Friedel et al., 1986). In the future investigators will develop a better understanding of which chemotherapy routines are most beneficial for patients with bony metastases. The physiology of cancer cells that grow vigorously in the skeletal system must be radically different from that of those that do not. The environment of calcified tissue is substantially different from that of liver, lung, brain, and other sites. Improved understanding of the biology of metastatic cells and of osteocytes will doubtless result in regimens that favorably alter the relationship between cancer cells and the skeletal system.

With the increased availability of new materials for repairing the skeleton (e.g., new metals, new plastics, and absorbable materials) there will doubtless arise markedly improved strategies for dealing with skeletal metastases in specific locations. The thrust of this therapy will shift from reinforcement to a strategy of *renovation* of bone infested with tumor deposits. One can conceive of bioactive implants that inhibit tumor growth and restore skeletal integrity. In recent years excision of cancerous deposits and replacement with plastics from which methotrexate leaches out can be seen as a first step toward implementation of this strategy. Newer metals will not only match the mechanical properties of bone but will be more refractory to infection because they combine materials with bioactive properties. Real advances will come with information about oncogenesis. Cancer cells metastatic to bone are cells with special tastes. The future of genetic engineering offers the possibility of inhibiting these cells with specific forms of nucleic acid that reprogram them for decline and death. Metastatic tumors with special affinities, such as cancer of the breast has for bone, may be ideal for testing new therapeutics.

References

Abrams, H. L., Spiro, R., and Goldstein, N.: Metastases in carcinoma: Analysis of 1000 autopsied cases. Cancer, *3*:74–85, 1950.

Allen, K. L., Watson, T. W., and Hibbs, G. C.: Effective bone palliation as related to various treatment regimens. Cancer, *37*:984–987, 1976.

Altman, H.: Metallic fixation for pathologic fracture and impending fracture of long bones. J. Int. Coll. Surg., *19*:612–617, 1953.

Arnstein, N. B., Harbert, J. C., and Byrne, P. J.: Efficacy of bone and liver scanning in breast cancer patients treated with adjuvant chemotherapy. Cancer, *54*:2243–2247, 1984.

Asbury, R. F., Bakemeier, R. F., Folisch, E., et al.: Treatment of metastatic breast cancer with aminoglutethimide. Cancer, *47*:1954–1958, 1981.

Babaiantz, P. L.: Les ostéoporoses. Radiologie Clinica, *16*:291–322, 1947.

Bachman, A. L., and Sproul, E. E.: Correlation of radiographic and autopsy findings in suspected metastases in the spine. Bull. NY Acad. Med., *31*:146–148, 1955.

Bagshaw, M. A.: Presumptive palliative irradiation in metastatic carcinoma of the breast. Cancer, *28*:1692–1694, 1971.

Baker, E. R.: The indications for bone scans in the preoperative assessment of patients with operable breast cancer. Breast, *3*:43–45, 1977.

Batson, O. V.: The function of the vertebral veins and their role in the spread of metastases. Ann. Surg., *112*:138–149, 1940.

Beals, R. K., Lawton, G. D., and Snell, W. E.: Prophylactic internal fixation of the femur in metastatic breast cancer. Cancer, *28*:1350–1354, 1971.

Bennish, E. L., and Hammond, G.: Treatment of actual and imminent pathological fractures of the femur by intramedullary nailing. Surg. Clin. North Am., *35*:865–872, 1955.

Berger, U., Bettelheim, R., Mansi, J. L., et al.: The relationship between micrometastases in the bone marrow. Histopathologic features of the primary tumor in breast cancer and prognosis. Am. J. Clin. Pathol., *90*:1–6, 1988.

Bhardwaj, S., and Holland, J. F.: Chemotherapy of metastatic cancer in bone. Clin. Orthop., *169*:28–37, 1982.

Bitran, J. D., Bekerman, C., and Desser, R. K.: The predictive value of serial bone scans in assessing response to chemotherapy in advanced breast cancer. Cancer, *45*:1562–1568, 1980.

Black, P.: Spinal metastasis: Current status and recommended guidelines for management. Neurosurgery, *5*:726–746, 1979.

Blomqvist, C., Elomma, I., Virkkunen, P., et al.: The response evaluation of bone metastases in mammary carcinoma: The value of radiology, scintigraphy, and biochemical markers of bone metabolism. Cancer, *60*:2907–2912, 1987.

Böhler, L.: Medullary Nailing of Küntscher. Baltimore, Williams & Wilkins, 1948.

Boland, P. J., Lane, J. M., and Sundaresan, N.: Metastatic disease of the spine. Clin. Orthop. *169*:95–102, 1982.

Bonarigo, B. C., and Rubin, P.: Nonunion of pathologic fracture after radiation therapy. Radiology, *88*:889–898, 1967.

Bonfiglio, M.: The pathology of fracture of the femoral neck following irradiation. Radiation, *70*:449–459, 1953.

Bouchard, J.: Skeletal metastases in cancer of the breast: Study of the character, incidence, and response to roentgen therapy. Am. J. Roentgenol., *54*:156–171, 1945.

Bremner, R. A., and Jelliffe, A. M.: The management of pathological fracture of the major long bones from metastatic cancer. Br. J. Bone Joint Surg., *40B*:652–659, 1958.

Brewin, T.: The cancer patient—too many scans and x-rays? Lancet, *2*:1098–1099, 1981.

Budd, G. T.: Estrogen receptor profile of patients with breast cancer metastatic to bone marrow. J. Surg. Oncol., *24*:167–169, 1983.

Bunting, J. S., Hemsted, E. H., and Kremer, J. K.: The pattern of spread and survival in 596 cases of breast cancer related to clinical staging and histological grade. Clin. Radiol., *27*:9–15, 1976.

Burny, F., Moulart, F., and Hinsenkamp, M.: Treatment of metastatic fractures in the subtrochanteric region. Acta Orthop. Belg., *42*:31–41, 1976.

Buturla, E., Hawkins, C., Seligson, D., et al.: The use of finite element modelling in the pathologic fracture in patients with metastatic cancer. Automedica, *6*:147–157, 1985.

Byrne, T. N.: Spinal cord compression from epidural metastasis. N. Engl. J. Med., *327*:614–619, 1992.

Campbell, F. C., Blamey, R. W., Elston, C. W., et al.: Oestrogen-receptor status and sites of metastasis in breast cancer. Br. J. Cancer, *44*:456–469, 1981.

Ceci, G., Granciosi, V., Nizzoli, R., et al.: The value of bone marrow biopsy in breast cancer at time of diagnosis. Cancer, *1*:96–98, 1988.

Charkes, N. D., Malmud, L. S., Caswell, T., et al.: Preoperative bone scans: Use in women with early breast cancer. J.A.M.A., *233*:516–518, 1975.

Cheung, A., and Driedger, A.: Evaluation of palliation of metastatic bone lesions from carcinoma of the breast and prostate. Radiology, *134*:209–212, 1980.

Cheung, D. S., Seitz, C. B., and Eyre, H. J.: Nonoperative management of femoral, humeral, and acetabular metastases in patients with breast cancer. Cancer, *45*:1533–1537, 1980.

Cho, S. Y., and Choi, H. Y.: Causes of death and metastatic patterns in patients with mammary cancer: Ten-year autopsy study. Am. J. Clin. Pathol., *73*:232–234, 1980.

Cifuentes, N., and Pickren, J. W.: Metastases form carcinoma of mammary gland: An autopsy study. J. Surg. Oncol., *11*:193–205, 1979.

Citrin, D. L., Bessent, R. G., Greig, W. R., et al.: The application of the $^{99}Tc^m$ phosphate bone scan to the study of breast cancer. Br. J. Surg., *62*:201–204, 1975.

Citrin, D. L., Furnival, C. M., Bessent, R. G., et al.: Radioactive technetium phosphate bone scanning in preoperative assessment and follow-up study of patients with primary cancer of the breast. Surg. Gynecol. Obstet., *143*:360–364, 1976.

Coates, G., Bowen, B. M., Nahmias, C., et al.: An analysis of factors which influence the local accumulation of bone seeking radiopharmaceuticals. J. Nucl. Med., *16*:520, 1975.

Coleman, R. E., Fogelman, I., and Rubens, R. D.: Hypercalcaemia and breast cancer—an increased humoral component in patients with liver metastases. Eur. J. Surg. Oncol., *14*:423–428, 1988.

Coleman, R. E., Fogelman, I., Habibollahi, F., et al.: Selection of patients with breast cancer for routine follow-up bone scans. Clin. Oncol., *2*:328–332, 1990.

Coleman, R. E., Mashiter, G., Fogelman, I., et al.: Osteocalcin: A potential marker of metastatic bone disease and response to treatment. Eur. J. Cancer Clin. Oncol., *24*:1211–1217, 1988.

Coombs, R., and Friedlaender, G.: Bone Tumour Management. Boston, Butterworths, 1987.

Coran, A. G., Banks, H. H., Aliapoulios, M. A., et al.: The management of pathological fractures in patients with metastatic carcinoma of the breast. Surg. Gynecol. Obstet., *127*:1225–1230, 1968.

Davies, J., Trask, C., and Souhami, R. L.: Effect of mithramycin on widespread painful bone metastases in cancer of the breast. Cancer Treat. Rep., *63*:1835–1838, 1979.

Dickey, R. P., and Minton, J. P.: Levodopa relief of bone pain from breast cancer. N. Engl. J. Med., *286*:843, 1972.

Dodwell, D. J., Howell, A., and Ford, J.: Reduction in calcium excretion in women with breast cancer and bone metastases using oral bisphosphonate pamidronate. Br. J. Cancer, *61*:123–125, 1990.

Donaldson, M. H., and Horsley, J. S. III: Nonhormonal chemotherapy of tumors metastatic to bone. Clin. Orthop., *73*:64–72, 1970.

Ehrenhaft, J. L., and Tidrick, R. T.: Intramedullary bone fixation in pathological fractures. Surg. Gynecol. Obstet., *88*:519–527, 1949.

Eliason, E. L.: Pathological fractures. Surg. Clin. North Am., *10*:1335, 1930.

Elion, G., and Mundy, G. R.: Direct resorption of bone by human breast cancer cell *in vitro*. Nature, *276*:726–728, 1978.

Enneking, W. F.: Metastatic carcinoma. *In* Enneking, W. F. (Ed.): Musculoskeletal Tumor Surgery. New York, Churchill Livingstone, 1982.

Fey, M. F., Brunner, K. W., and Sonntag, R. W.: Prognostic factors in metastatic breast cancer. Cancer Clin. Trials, *4*:237–247, 1981.

Fidler, M.: Prophylactic internal fixation of secondary neoplastic deposits in long bones. Br. Med. J., *1*:341–343, 1973.

Flemming, J. E., and Beals, R. K.: Pathologic fracture of the humerus. Clin. Orthop., *203*:258–260, 1986.

Francis, K. C., Higinbotham, N. L., Carroll, R. E., et al.: The treatment of pathological fractures of the femoral neck by resection. J. Trauma, *2*:465–473, 1962.

Frassica, F. J., Sim, F. H., and Chao, E. Y. S.: Primary malignant bone tumors of the shoulder girdle: Surgical technique of resection and reconstruction. Am. Surgeon, *53*:264–269, 1987.

Friedl, W., and Krebs, H.: Die operative Stabilisierung pathologischer Frakturen: Einfluß auf Überlebenszeit und Lebensqualität. Versicherungsmedizin, *4*:104–107, 1988.

Friedl, W., Ruf, W., and Krebs, H.: Funktionelle Ergebnisse nach konservativer und operativer Therapie pathologischer Frakturen bei malignen Erkrankungen. Langenbecks Arch. Chir., *368*:185–196, 1986.

Frisch, B., Bartl, R., Mahl, G., et al.: Scope and value of bone marrow biopsies in metastatic cancer. Invasion Metastases, *4*:12–30, 1984.

Front, D., Schneck, S. O., Frankel, A., et al.: Bone metastases and bone pain in breast cancer: Are they closely associated? J.A.M.A., *242*:1747–1748, 1979.

Galasko, C. S. B.: The detection of skeletal metastases from mammary cancer by gamma camera scintigraphy. Br. J. Surg., *56*:757–764, 1969.

Galasko, C. S. B.: Skeletal metastases and mammary cancer. Ann. R. Coll. Surg. Engl., *50*:3–28, 1972.

Galasko, C. S. B.: The significance of occult skeletal metastases, detected by skeletal scintigraphy, in patients with otherwise apparently 'early' mammary carcinoma. Br. J. Surg., *62*:694–696, 1975.

Galasko, C. S. B.: Mechanisms of bone destruction in the development of skeletal metastases. Nature, *263*:507–510, 1976.

Ganz, R., Isler, B., and Mast. J.: Internal fixation technique in pathological fractures of the extremities. Arch. Orthop. Trauma Surg., *103*:73–80, 1984.

Garcia-Morteo, D., Lema, B., Maldonnado-Cocco, J. A., et al.: Carcinomatous arthritis of the elbow caused by metastatic breast carcinoma. Clin. Rheumatol., *6*:273–275, 1987.

Garmatis, C. J., and Chu, F. C. H.: The effectiveness of radiation therapy in the treatment of bone metastases from breast cancer. Radiology, *126*:235–237, 1978.

Gerber, F. H., Goodreau, J. J., Kirchner, P. T., et al.: Efficacy of preoperative and postoperative bone scanning in the management of breast carcinoma. N. Engl. J. Med., *297*:300–302, 1977.

Gilbert, H. A., Kagan, A. R., Nussbaum, H., et al.: Evaluation of radiation therapy for bone metastases: Pain relief and quality of life. Am. J. Roentgenol., *129*:1095–1096, 1977.

Glynne-Jones, R., Young, T., Ahmed, A., et al.: How far investigations for occult metastases in breast cancer aid the clinician. Clin. Oncol., *3*:65–72, 1991.

Griessmann, H., and Schüttemeyer, W.: Weitere Erfahrungen mit der Marknagelung nach Küntscher an der Chirurgischen Universitätsklinik Kiel. Chirurg., *17–18*:316–333, 1947.

Gristina, A. G., Adair, D. M., and Spur, G. L.: Intraosseous metastatic breast cancer treatment with internal fixation and study of survival. Ann. Surg., *197*:128–134, 1983.

Habermann, E. T., and Lopez, R. A.: Metastatic disease of bone and treatment of pathological fractures. Orthop. Clin. North Am., *20*:469–486, 1989.

Habermann, E. T., Sachs, R., Stern, R., et al.: The pathology and treatment of metastatic disease of the femur. Clin. Orthop., *169*:70–82, 1982.

Hagemeister, F. B. Jr., Buzdar, A. U., Luna, M. A., et al.: Causes of death in breast cancer: A clinicopathologic study. Cancer, *46*:162–167, 1980.

Harrington, K. D.: The management of acetabular insufficiency secondary to metastatic malignant disease. J. Bone Joint Surg., *63A*:653–664, 1981.

Harrington, K. D.: The use of methylmethacrylate for vertebral-body replacement and anterior stabilization of pathological fracture-dislocations of the spine due to metastatic malignant disease. J. Bone Joint Surg., *63A*:36–46, 1981.

Harrington, K. D.: Anterior cord decompression and spinal stabilization for patients with metastatic lesions of the spine. J. Neurosurg., *61*:107–111, 1984.

Harrington, K. D.: Impending pathologic fractures from metastatic malignancy: Evaluation and management. *In* Anderson, L. D. (Ed.): AAOS Instructional Course Lectures. Vol. 35. St. Louis, C. V. Mosby, 1986, pp. 357–381.

Harrington, K. D.: Anterior decompression and stabilization of the spine as a treatment for vertebral collapse and spinal cord decompression from metastatic malignancy. Clin. Orthop., *223*:177–197, 1988.

Harrington, K. D., Sim, F. H., Enis, J. E., et al.: Methylmethacrylate as an adjunct in internal fixation of pathological fractures: Experience with three hundred and seventy-five cases. J. Bone Joint Surg., *58A*:1047–1055, 1976.

Hart, I. R.: 'Seed and soil' revisited: Mechanisms of site-specific metastasis. Cancer Metastasis Rev., *1*:5–16, 1982.

Hebert, J., Couser, J. A., and Seligson, D.: Closed medullary biopsy for disseminated malignancy. Clin. Orthop., *163*:214–217, 1982.

Heinz, T., Stoik, W., and Vecseei, V.: Behandlung und Ergebnisse von pathologischen Fraktuern: Sammelstudie aus den Jahren 1965 bis 1985 aus 16 osterreichischen Krankenhausen. Unfallchirurg., *92*:477–485, 1989.

Heppenstall, R. B.: Pathological fractures secondary to metastatic disease. *In* Fracture Treatment and Healing. Philadelphia, W.B. Saunders, 1980.

Higinbotham, N. L., and Marcove, R. C.: The management of pathological fractures. J. Trauma, *5*:792–798, 1965.

Hipp, J. A., McBroom, R. J., Cheal, E. J., et al.: Structural consequences of endosteal metastatic lesions in long bones. J. Orthop. Res., *7*:828–837, 1989.

Hoffman, H. C., and Marty, R.: Bone scanning: Its value in the preoperative evaluation of patients with suspicious breast masses. Am. J. Surg., *124*:194–199, 1972.

Hortobagyi, G. N., Libshitz, H. I., and Seafold, J. E.: Osseous metastases of breast cancer: Clinical, biochemical, radiographic, and scintigraphic evaluation of response to therapy. Cancer, *53*:577–582, 1984.

Isler, B.: Chirurgische Massnahmen bei metastatischen Läsionen des Extremitäten- und des Beckenskelettes. Unfallchirurg., *93*:449–456, 1990.

Jensen, N. H., and Rosendahl, K.: Single-dose irradiation of bone metastases. Acta Radiol. Ther. Phys. Biol., *15*:337–339, 1976.

Joo, K. G., Parthasarathy, K. L., Bakshi, S. P., et al.: Bone scintigrams: Their clinical usefulness in patients with breast carcinoma. Oncology, *36*:94–98, 1979.

Kamby, C., Guldhammer, B., Vejborg, I., et al.: The presence of tumor cells in bone marrow at the time of first recurrence of breast cancer. Cancer, *60*:1306–1312, 1987.

Kamby, C. Rasmussen, B. B., and Kristensen, B.: Prognostic indicators of metastatic bone disease in human breast cancer. Cancer, *68*:2045–2050, 1991.

Kamby, C., Vejborg, I., Daugaard, S., et al.: Clinical and radiologic characteristics of metastases in breast cancer. Cancer, *60*:2524–2531, 1987.

Keene, J. S., Sellinger, D. S., McBeath, A. A., et al.: Metastatic breast cancer in the femur: A search for the lesion at risk of fracture. Clin. Orthop., *203*:282–288, 1986.

Klein, J. P., Keiding, N., and Kamby, C.: Semiparametric Marshall-Olkin models applied to the occurrence of metastases at multiple sites after breast cancer. Biometrics, *45*:1073–1086, 1989.

Koskinen, E. V. S., and Nieminen, R. A.: Surgical treatment of metastatic pathological fracture of major long bones. Acta Orthop. Scand., *44*:539–549, 1973.

Kramer, W., Gaebel, G., Stuhldreyer, G., et al.: Ergebnisse der Behändlung pathologischer Frakturen langer Röhrenknochen. Unfallchirurgie, *13*:22–26, 1987.

Krishnamurthy, G. T., Tubis, M., Hiss, J., et al.: Distribution pattern of metastatic bone disease: A need for total body skeletal image. J.A.M.A., *237*:2504–2506, 1977.

Kulenkampff, H. A., Dreyer, T., Kersjes, W., et al.: Histomorphic analysis of osteoclastic bone resorption in metastatic bone disease from various primary malignomas. Virchows Arch. (Pathol. Anat.), *409*:817–828, 1986.

Küntscher, G.: Practice of Intramedullary Nailing. Springfield, IL, Charles C Thomas, 1967.

Lee, Y.-T.N. Breast carcinoma: Pattern of recurrence and metastasis after mastectomy. Am. J. Clin. Oncol. *7*:443–449, 1984.

Legha, S. S., Davis, H. L., and Muggia, F. M.: Hormonal therapy of breast cancer: New approaches and concepts. Ann. Intern. Med., *88*:69–77, 1978.

Lehmann, O.: Problems of pathological fractures. Bull. Hosp. Joint Dis., *12*:90–102, 1951.

Lentle, B. C., Burns, P. E., Dierich, H., et al.: Bone scintiscanning in the initial assessment of carcinoma of the breast. Surg. Gynecol. Obstet., *141*:43–47, 1975.

Lewallen, R. P., Pritchard, D. J., and Sim, F. H.: Treatment of pathological fractures or impending fractures of the humerus with Rush rods and methylmethacrylate. Clin. Orthop., *166*:193–198, 1982.

Lipton, A., and Santen, R. J.: Medical adrenalectomy using aminoglutethimide and dexamethasone in advanced breast cancer. Cancer, *33*:503–512, 1974.

Maatz, R., Lentz, W., Arens, W., et al.: Intramedullary Nailing and Other Intramedullary Osteosyntheses. Philadelphia, W.B. Saunders, 1986.

Mansi, J. L., Berger, U., McDonnell, T., et al.: The fate of bone marrow micrometastases in patients with primary breast cancer. J. Clin. Oncol., *7*:445–449, 1989.

Martoni, A., Guaraldi, M., Camera, P., et al.: Controlled clinical study of the use of dichloromethylene diphosphate in patients with breast carcinoma metastasizing to the skeleton. Oncology, *48*:91–101, 1991.

McQuire, W. L., Carbone, P. P., Sears, M. E., et al.: Estrogen receptors in human breast cancer: An overview. *In* McQuire, W. L., Carbone, P. P., and Vollmer, E. P. (Eds.): Estrogen Receptors in Human Breast Cancer. New York, Raven Press, 1975.

Meissner, W., and Warren, S.: Distribution of metastases in 4012 cancer patients. *In* Anderson, W. A. D. (Ed.): Pathology. 6th ed. Vol. 1. St. Louis, C. V. Mosby, 1971, p. 538.

Miller, F., and Whitehill, R.: Carcinoma of the breast metastatic to the skeleton. Clin. Orthop., *184*:121–127, 1984.

Minton, J. P.: Precise selection of breast cancer patients with bone metastasis for endocrine ablation. Surgery, *80*:513–517, 1976.

Mirels, H.: Metastatic disease in long bones: A proposed scoring system for diagnosing impending pathologic fractures. Clin. Orthop., *249*:256–264, 1989.

Mootoosamy, I. M., Anchor, S. C., and Dacie, J. E.: Expanding osteolytic bone metastases from carcinoma of the breast: An unusual appearance. Skeletal Radiol., *14*:188–190, 1985.

Nikkanen, T. A. V.: Recurrence of breast cancer: A retrospective study of 569 cases in clinical stages I–III. Acta Chir. Scand., *147*:239–245, 1981.

Nussbaum, H., Allen, B., Kagan, A. R., et al.: Management of bone metastasis—multidisciplinary approach. Semin. Oncol., *4*:93–97, 1977.

Parrish, F. F., and Murray, J. A.: Surgical treatment for secondary neoplastic fractures. J. Bone Joint Surg., *52*:665–686, 1970.

Patterson, A. H. G., Lees, A. W., Hanson, J., et al.: Impact of chemotherapy on survival in metastatic breast cancer. Lancet, *2*:312, 1980.

Peltier, L. F.: Theoretical hazards in the treatment of pathological fractures by the Küntscher intramedullary nail. Surgery, *29*:466–472, 1951*a*.

Peltier, L. F.: Further observations upon intramedullary pressures during the fixation of fractures by Küntscher's method. Surgery, *30*:964–966, 1951*b*.

Penn, C. R. H.: Single dose and fractionated palliative irradiation for osseous metastases. Clin. Radiol., *27*:405–408, 1976.

Perez, C. A., Bradfield, J. S., and Morgan, H. C.: Management of pathological fractures. Cancer, *29*:684–693, 1972.

Perez, D. J., Milan, J., Ford, H. T., et al.: Detection of breast carcinoma metastases in bone: Relative merits of x-rays and skeletal scintigraphy. Lancet, *10*:613–616, 1983.

Ridell, B., and Landys, K.: Incidence and histopathology of metastases of mammary carcinoma in biopsies from the posterior iliac crest. Cancer, *44*:1782–1788, 1979.

Salazar, O. M., Rubin, P., Hendrickson, F., et al.: Single-dose half-body irradiation for palliation of multiple bone metastases from solid tumors: Final Radiation Therapy Group report. Cancer, *58*:29–36, 1986.

Samaan, N. A., Buzdar, A. U., Aldinger, K. A., et al.: Estrogen receptor: A prognostic factor in breast cancer. Cancer, *47*:554–560, 1981.

Scanlon, E. F., Oviedo, M. A., Cunningham, M. P., et al.: Preoperative and follow-up procedures on patients with breast cancer. Cancer, *46*:977–979, 1980.

Schaberg, J., and Gainor, B. J.: A profile of metastatic carcinoma of the spine. Spine, *10*:19–20, 1985.

Scher, H. I., and Yagoda, A.: Bone metastases: Pathogenesis, treatment, and rationale for use of resorption inhibitors. Am. J. Med., *82*:6–28, 1987.

Schwarzenbach, O., Boos, N., and Aebi, M.: Metastasen und durch Metastasen bedingte pathologische Frakturen der Wirbelsäule. Unfallchirurgie, *93*:457–466, 1990.

Sears, H. F., Janus, C., Levy, W., et al.: Breast cancer without axillary metastases: Are there high-risk biologic subpopulations? Cancer, *50*:1820–1827, 1982.

Sim, F. H., Daugherty, T. W., and Ivins, J. C.: The adjunctive use of methylmethacrylate in fixation of pathological fractures. J. Bone Joint Surg., *56A*:40–48, 1974.

Singletary, S. E., Larry, L., Tucker, S. L., et al.: Detection of micrometastatic tumor cells in bone marrow of breast carcinoma patients. J. Surg. Oncol., *47*:32–36, 1991.

Sklaroff, R. B., and Sklaroff, D. M.: Bone metastases from breast cancer at the time of radical mastectomy as detected by bone scan: Eight-year follow-up. Cancer, *38*:107–111, 1976.

Smith, D. G., Behr, J. T., Hall, R. F., et al.: Closed flexible intramedullary biopsy of metastatic carcinoma. Clin. Orthop., *229*:162–164, 1988.

Smith, I. E., and Macaulay, V.: Comparison of different endocrine therapies in management of bone metastases from breast carcinoma. J. R. Soc. Med., *78*:15–17, 1985.

Snell, W., and Beals, R. K.: Femoral metastases and fractures from breast cancer. Surg. Gynecol. Obstet., *119*:22–24, 1964.

Stewart, J. F., King, R. J. B., Sexton, S., et al.: Oestrogen receptors, sites of metastatic disease and survival in recurrent breast cancer. Eur. J. Cancer, *17*:449–453, 1981.

Sundaresan, N., and Galicich, J. H.: Treatment of spinal metastases by vertebral body resection. Cancer Invest., *2*:383–397, 1984.

Suzuki, S., Nomizu, T., Nihei, M., et al.: Clinical evaluation of serum osteocalcin in patients with bone metastasis of breast cancer. J. Jpn. Soc. Cancer Ther., *24*:2386–2393, 1989.

Taha, M., Ordonez, N. G., Kulkarni, S., et al.: A monoclonal antibody cocktail for detection of micrometastatic tumor cells in the bone marrow of breast cancer patients. Bone Marrow Transplant., *4*:297–303, 1989.

Theriault, R. L.: Management of hypercalcemia in breast cancer. Oncology, *4*:43–46, 1990.

Tofe, A. J., Francis, M. D., and Harvey, W. J.: Correlation of neoplasms with incidence and localization of skeletal metastases: An analysis of 1355 diphosphonate bone scans. J. Nucl. Med., *16*:986–989, 1975.

Tong, D., Gillick, L., and Hendrickson, F. R.: The palliation of symptomatic osseous metastases: Final results of the study by the Radiation Therapy Oncology Group. Cancer, *50*:893–899, 1982.

Usui, M., Seiichi, I., Matsuyama, T., et al.: Orthopedic local treatment for metastatic bone tumor. Jpn. J. Cancer Chemother., *15*:1365–1369, 1988.

Vargha, Z. O., Glicksman, A. S., and Boland, J.: Single-dose radiation therapy in the palliation of metastatic disease. Radiology, *93*:1181–1184, 1969.

Viadana, E., Bross, I. D. J., and Pickren, J. W.: An autopsy study of some routes of dissemination of cancer of the breast. Br. J. Cancer, *27*:336–340, 1973.

Welch, C. E.: Pathological fractures due to malignant disease. Surg. Gynecol. Obstet., *62*:735–744, 1936.

White, von R. R., and Seligson, D.: Operative Stabilisierung pathologischer Frakturen. Beitr. Orthop. Traumatol., *30*:567–571, 1983.

Winchester, D. P., Sener, S. F., Khandekar, J. D., et al.: Symptomatology as an indicator of recurrent or metastatic breast cancer. Cancer, *43*:956–960, 1979.

Yablon, I. G.: Recent advances in the treatment of pathologic fractures. J. Fam. Pract., *4*:45–48, 1977.

Yamashita, K., Ueda, T., Komatsubara, Y., et al.: Breast cancer with bone only metastases: Visceral metastases-free rate in relation to anatomic distribution of bone metastases. Cancer, *68*:634–637, 1991.

Yazawa, Y., Frassica, F. J., Chao, E. Y. S., et al.: Metastatic bone disease: A study of the surgical treatment of 166 pathologic humeral and femoral fractures. Clin. Orthop., *251*:213–219, 1990.

Zickel, R. E., and Mouradian, W. H.: Intramedullary fixation of pathological fractures and lesions of the subtrochanteric region of the femur. J. Bone Joint Surg., *58*:1061–1066, 1976.

Thoracic Surgical Problems in Breast Cancer Therapy

George B. Haasler

Patients with a history of breast carcinoma may develop complex and sometimes devastating intrathoracic and chest wall problems. Although these problems are usually due to recurrent or metastatic carcinoma, skin ulceration and radionecrosis of ribs and soft tissue may also represent consequences of therapy. The management of these problems can be complex, requiring the combined expertise of radiologists, cardiologists, plastic surgeons, and cardiothoracic surgeons. The purpose of this chapter is to outline some of the more common thoracic surgical problems and their management. The improvement of imaging techniques and new technical developments, particularly in the field of video-assisted thoracic surgery, have significantly altered both the diagnostic approaches and management of pleural and pericardial diseases. Hormonal manipulation and advanced chemotherapeutic techniques impact significantly on the usual, rapidly fatal outcome of many of these conditions. Careful attention to the diagnosis and management of these problems is therefore paramount.

Thoracic pathology secondary to breast cancer occurs most commonly in the following four areas: (1) the pulmonary parenchyma, (2) the pleural cavity, (3) the pericardium, and (4) the chest wall.

PULMONARY METASTASES

Pulmonary nodules can be found either synchronously during the initial presentation of a breast cancer or at a later time. The analysis of these nodules should be guided by the same basic principles as that for nodules presenting in the absence of a breast cancer. The solitary pulmonary nodule appears less likely to represent a metastatic lesion than a new primary cancer or granuloma; however, in our experience, 56% of patients with new nodules and a history of breast cancer are found to have an adenocarcinoma. Pathologically, the presence of these lesions is usually interpreted as being ''consistent with'' metastasis from the breast, even though this cannot always be confirmed. Assays for determining whether estrogen receptors are present in these nodules are available. These assays can be performed even on fixed tissues at a time remote from that of the resection.

In the past 5 years in our institution, 11 patients with a history of breast carcinoma have undergone operations for the treatment of pulmonary nodules. Of these patients, nine were noted to have solitary nodules on radiography, and two were found to have multiple nodules. Seven of the 11

nodules proved to be carcinoma, although only 3 were found unequivocally to be metastatic breast carcinoma. Three of the other four patients had adenocarcinoma (two of these bronchoalveolar adenocarcinoma), and one had a squamous cell carcinoma (presenting within a radiation field of this nonsmoker 18 years after treatment of breast cancer). Of the patients with pulmonary nodules that were identified as solitary on preoperative radiographs, one had multiple breast cancer metastases at the time of surgery. Of the two patients with multiple nodules, one had multiple granulomas, and the other had multifocal bronchoalveolar carcinoma.

In Cahan and Castro's series of 72 patients with a solitary pulmonary nodule and a history of breast cancer (1973), 43 were found to have primary lung cancers, 23 had metastatic breast cancer, and 6 benign lung lesions. The metastatic lesions of nine patients were associated with lymphatic involvement in the lung, and radical operations (at least lobectomy) were considered the treatment of choice.

Diagnosis and Resection

The work-up of a patient with a solitary pulmonary nodule should include a carefully recorded history and physical examination to determine whether she has predisposing factors for lung carcinoma. Chief among these factors are smoking, advanced age, and the presence of respiratory symptoms such as cough and hemoptysis. The presence of fever, chills, or night sweats or a positive reaction to a tuberculin test are more suggestive of an infectious etiology such as tuberculosis or fungal disease. Patients who live in areas endemic for fungal disorders such as histoplasmosis (the Midwest) or coccidioidomycosis (the Southwest) should be suspected of having these disorders, but the diagnosis can be confirmed with certainty only on biopsy analysis. Dense calcification within lesions supports a diagnosis of benign disease.

Based on the data of Cahan and Castro's series and on this author's own experience, a solitary noncalcified nodule presenting within the lung of a patient with a history of breast cancer should always be viewed as a possible second primary malignancy or as a single metastasis. Generally, it is not possible to be certain that a lesion is infectious in nature or otherwise benign without removing it. The one exception to this might be the case of a patient whose reaction on a tuberculin skin test has changed from negative to positive simultaneously with the development of one or more nodular densities. For such a patient, a trial of therapy with antituberculosis drugs (to learn whether the nodules shrink in size) is reasonable.

The presence of metastatic disease is most likely when multiple pulmonary nodules are found in the absence of tuberculous or fungal exposure; however, a complete work-up for infectious disease should not be omitted in patients with such a finding. Open biopsy of at least two nodules is almost always required to establish a tissue diagnosis of metastatic disease. A long disease-free interval is not re-assuring; this author has found recurrent breast cancer in pleura as late as 25 years after management of an original tumor.

Work-up prior to a thoracotomy should include screening for metastatic breast cancer with a bone scan as well as screening of the liver, adrenal glands, and the entire thorax with computed tomography. Pulmonary function studies should also be performed as for patients who are to undergo any other lung operation. Because adenocarcinoma is the prevailing histology in patients with pulmonary nodules, preoperative magnetic resonance imaging or computed to-mography of the head is usually recommended to determine whether silent metastases are present.

The role of preoperative needle biopsy in patients with pulmonary nodules is controversial. Although needle bi-opsy makes it possible to ascertain whether malignancy is present, it may not be used to confirm the absence of malig-nancy. A finding of adenocarcinoma is not proof that a lesion is metastatic rather than primary. The physician must still decide whether the lesion should be treated as a pri-mary lung cancer or as a metastasis.

Excision of a pulmonary nodule needs to be carried out in the same manner in patients with and those without an antecedent history of breast cancer. Patients are prepared for a thoracotomy by blood cross-matching and obtaining routine laboratory tests, as with any major operation. Op-erations are performed with the patient in the lateral decu-bitus position and with intubation with a double-lumen tube. A limited thoracotomy (or thoracoscopy) is then car-ried out, and the nodule is removed by wedge resection, if possible. Specimens for frozen section as well as for estro-gen and progesterone receptor analysis are obtained. If the results of frozen section analysis demonstrate the presence of an adenocarcinoma or are believed to be highly consis-tent with the presence of metastatic breast cancer, the op-tions are (1) to terminate the operation if margins appear to be adequate, (2) to re-excise a somewhat wider margin of tissue in the hope that better local control will be achieved, or (3) to carry out a formal segmentectomy or lobectomy. Generally, with indications that a nodule is metastatic, the surgeon should be less inclined to carry out a lobectomy, which would be more appropriate for the treatment of a primary lung cancer. However, the series by Cahan and Castro (1973) suggests that lymphatic involvement is fre-quent with metastatic tumors; thus, a lobectomy may be appropriate even for the treatment of solitary metastases. Regional lymph nodes should be assessed carefully both to help determine the appropriate degree of resection and to stage a cancer after a lobectomy or segmentectomy has been carried out. Factors favoring a diagnosis of metastasis

over primary lung carcinoma include histologic evidence of adenocarcinoma, a short interval between recognition of the breast cancer and the detection of lung lesions (0–5 years), and positive determination of estrogen receptor markers. Sometimes, it may be technically impossible to excise a nodule without carrying out a lobectomy or even a pneu-monectomy. In this case, the surgeon must judge whether the location of the pulmonary lesion is the only apparent site of disease, whether it is part of a more complex picture, and whether a patient's pulmonary function and general medical condition are suitable for a larger resection.

Role of Video-Assisted Resection

Thoracoscopy with video-assisted resection is an alternative to performing a large incision for diagnostic purposes. With this technique, an entire nodule can be removed for patho-logic examination if necessary. When patients are subjected to a thoracotomy, a surgeon may be influenced by the magnitude of the incision to carry out a definitive resection (even if lobectomy is required) at the initial procedure with-out having all the pathologic data. In contrast, with thora-coscopic approaches, it is possible to remove nodules from many locations with a wedge resection (which involves making three small surgical ports) for pathologic study. If a lesion is found to represent a primary lung cancer, a decision can be made later as to whether a more extensive operation should be carried out. Also, if a nodule is found to be a granuloma, a large incision can be avoided. Signifi-cant advances in the development of video-assisted tech-niques and in the pathologic examination of specimens make this technique superior to other diagnostic methods whenever it is technically possible. Lung nodules that are near the edge of lobes are more accessible to biopsy by this technique than are those that are centrally located within lobes. Although the general consensus among thoracic sur-geons is that finding a cancer in a thoracoscopic wedge resection should prompt a thoracotomy for definitive man-agement, thoracotomy may not always be the wisest course of action, particularly if a patient has poor pulmonary func-tion or if metastatic disease is suspected. A third approach to resection of these nodules is with a small incision di-rectly over the nodules if their location can be identified on radiography and computed tomography. A small rib seg-ment is excised subperiosteally, and a small window is made into the chest. Excision using standard techniques is easy with this approach, and patients recover rapidly.

At the Medical College of Wisconsin, the approach to patients with solitary pulmonary nodules is to perform ini-tial laboratory screening to rule out metastatic disease. If the results of the laboratory studies are negative and the patient's pulmonary function is adequate, open or thoraco-scopic biopsy is carried out. At the time of biopsy, the remaining lung and the pleura are carefully examined for signs of metastases. The nodule is removed by wedge re-section, and frozen sections of it are prepared and exam-ined. Any abnormal lymph nodes found in the mediastinum or hilum are also biopsied. If the findings are more consis-tent with the presence of a primary lung carcinoma than with a metastatic lesion, a definitive resection can be performed at this time. If doubt exists, if the lesion clearly suggests breast carcinoma, if multiple lesions are found, or if the patient has severely limited pulmonary reserve, the wedge resection (by either open or video techniques) is considered definitive. After recovery, patients may be treated with chemotherapy or local radiation therapy to decrease local recurrence. Although local resection combined with radiation therapy represents an approach borrowed from the treatment of primary lung cancers (in which radiation therapy after wedge resection has been found to lower the local recurrence rate), the technique may also be applicable to the treatment of solitary metastases. In addition, this approach acknowledges the ability of metastases to metastasize further.

When multiple pulmonary lesions are present, it is wise to remove at least two for analysis so that the presence of metastatic disease can be convincingly established or disproved. At this time, the physician should clearly be cognizant of future therapeutic options. A patient who is not a candidate for further chemotherapy or radiation may require a more definitive resection at the outset. Randomized or integrated group protocols may mandate the sampling of mediastinal nodes or performing specific analyses of a specimen; and in the near future, it may be desirable to perform chemosensitivity assays. Although commercial assays to determine chemosensitivity have been available for several years, their usefulness is limited. Specimens usually require special processing and handling, and a physician should determine in advance whether these assays are available and would have a role in decision making.

Resection of Pulmonary Metastases

Whether resection of metastatic nodules of breast carcinoma improves survival is not completely answered by the current literature. Patients with breast cancer who have had pulmonary metastases removed surgically have 5-year survival rates of between 14% and 36% (Cahan and Castro, 1973; Benfield and Hammond, 1983; Mountain et al., 1984; and Staren et al., 1992). In Cahan and Castro's series (1973), 5 of the 23 patients (21%) who underwent removal of solitary pulmonary metastases (some with lymphatic involvement) survived 5 years or longer. In the series of Mountain and coworkers (1984) of 30 patients, the 5-year survival rate was 27.4%, and 50% of the patients survived 3 years or longer. Whether these rates are a function of the slow natural history of these cancers or a result of surgical debulking is not known.

One retrospective, matched-pair analysis carried out on medically (versus surgically) treated patients with pulmonary metastases from breast cancer attempted to answer this question. Staren and associates (1992) showed a 36% 5-year survival rate in 33 patients treated by resection of metastatic lesions compared with an 11% rate for a medically treated group of patients selected and matched for initial disease stage, age, and the distribution of metastases. The majority of the patients had solitary nodules, but 3 of 6 patients with multiple nodules also had prolonged survivals after resection (30–80 months). The major problems with this series are that it does not represent a prospective

randomized trial and that the selection criteria were not controlled. In addition, since many of the patients had solitary lesions, it is uncertain how many of the tumors were new primary Stage I lung cancers and not metastases. Nevertheless, the study's results suggest that resection of limited pulmonary metastases may improve survival.

If complete surgical removal of limited pulmonary metastases is contemplated, the basic requirements for removal should be satisfied: (1) the primary disease site should be controlled; (2) the patient should be able to tolerate the resection in terms of pulmonary function and general medical condition; (3) it should appear possible to remove all pulmonary metastases; and (4) no other distant metastases should remain. Patients should be carefully screened for this approach. Clearly, solitary nodules are amenable to resection with some optimism about the results. On the other hand, the existence of multiple nodules suggests the presence not only of extensive pulmonary involvement but also of other widespread disease.

PLEURAL METASTASES

The most common thoracic surgical problem in patients with breast cancer is the presence of malignant pleural effusions. A variety of pleural effusions that are the result of inflammatory causes or cardiac disorders can be seen in patients who have had breast carcinoma. Radiation therapy may lead to pleural and pericardial effusions. This author's belief is that all patients with a history of breast cancer who present with a new pleural effusion should be assessed for the presence of pleural metastases. Only in this way can one hope to minimize the debilitating problems that result from the neglect of malignant pleural effusions. These include dyspnea, malaise, a heavy feeling in the chest, pneumonia from compressive atelectasis, and, in the worst case, a lung trapped by a thick tumor peel that can never expand. In addition, the availability of new chemotherapeutic approaches such as bone marrow transplantation increases the importance of early diagnosis of recurrent malignancy.

Diagnosis

Diagnosis of an unresolved or recurring pleural effusion in patients with breast carcinoma is essential. When a pleural effusion is first seen, thoracocentesis should be performed to ascertain its nature. Malignant effusions are exudative and usually straw-colored; however, they may occasionally be bloody. Cytologic confirmation of malignancy must be unequivocal. If only suspicious or atypical cells are seen, additional study should be undertaken. In the presence of an exudative effusion but no signs of infection, metastases should be suspected until their absence is proven. Although blind, closed pleural biopsy may occasionally reveal carcinoma, false-negative results are obtained in as many as 30% of cases (Martin and Newhouse, 1986). Diagnostic pleuroscopy makes it possible to perform directed biopsy of abnormal areas and is recognized as the procedure of choice. Small, nodular implants may be present. Such implants can

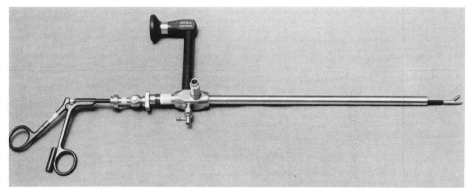

Figure 30–1. An operating thoracoscope of the type used for diagnostic pleuroscopy. The optical elements are positioned at an angle for easy viewing or for attachment of the thoracoscope to a camera. A biopsy forceps can be placed through the coaxial operating channel, allowing direct visualization of the area to be biopsied as well as sampling through the operating port with a single thoracostomy wound.

escape diagnosis with either fluid analysis or random closed pleural biopsy. Thoracoscopic techniques have evolved sufficiently that diagnoses can be made with limited trauma to the patient, a high degree of reliability, and, often, only local or regional anesthesia (Martin and Newhouse, 1986; and Thomas, 1986). In addition, thoracoscopy allows sclerosant agents such as talc to be instilled easily and uniformly (Weissberg, 1981; and Weissberg and Ben-Zeev, 1993).

Technique of Thoracoscopy

Thoracoscopy is usually performed with a patient under general anesthesia if the patient is able to tolerate it. A double-lumen endotracheal tube or a single-lumen endotracheal tube equipped with a bronchial blocker is utilized (Ginsberg, 1981; Inoue et al., 1982; Kamaya and Krishna, 1985). The patient is placed in a lateral decubitus position. After standard skin preparation and sterile draping, a small incision is made over the effusion (at the sixth or seventh interspace in the midaxillary line), and a thoracoscope in-

serted into the pleural cavity. Care must be taken to make the initial incision in an area where fluid can be aspirated with a needle; this ensures that the pleural cavity is not obliterated by tumor or adhesions in the area of incision. If the effusion moves freely on radiologic examination of the chest with the patient in different positions, this is not a problem. If the pleural fluid shows signs of being loculated (based on radiographic criteria), then the point of entry needs to be determined carefully on the basis of inspection of decubitus radiographs and, in some cases, computed tomography of the chest.

Several types of thoracoscopes (both rigid and flexible) are available for use. Older traditional tools such as mediastinoscopes (which provide a more limited field of view) may still prove adequate, especially for talc insufflation (Weissberg, 1981). The newer-generation thoracoscopes are coupled to a high-resolution video monitor via a color camera, and the rigid scopes offer far better resolution than do the flexible instruments. Thoracoscopes are available with or without a coaxial instrument channel (Figs. 30–1 and 30–2). Thoracoscopes without a coaxial biopsy channel offer the best visibility for a given diameter, but the "operat-

Figure 30–2. A thoracoscope and three trocars of different sizes that allow placement of instruments and scopes. In some patients, a trocar may not be necessary to maintain a wound opening and may in fact interfere with manipulation. However, in patients who are more muscular or are obese, the trocars become essential for maintaining wound channels through the chest wall.

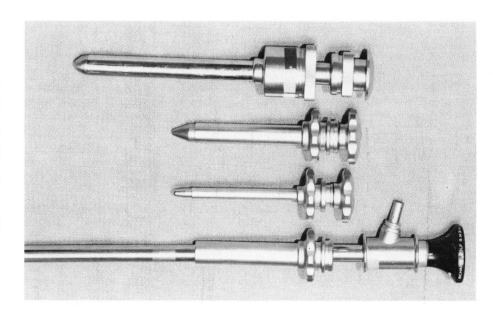

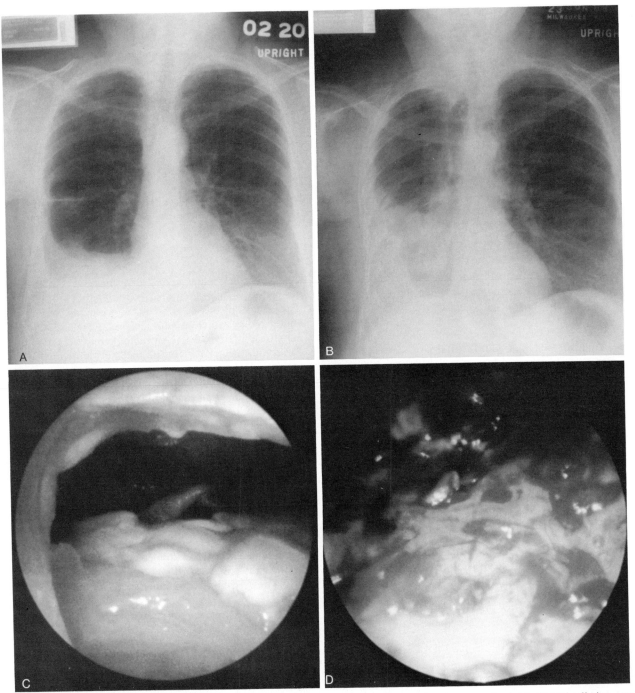

Figure 30-3. *A* and *B,* Radiographs of one patient taken 2 years apart. Progressive increase in right pleural effusion and compression of the lung with a thickened process that is both intrapleural tumor and fluid are demonstrated. *C,* A view through the thoracoscope into the pleural space. Sheets of tumor can be seen. *D,* Multiple biopsy sites where tissue has been taken for sampling. Tissue analysis demonstrated the presence of recurrent adenocarcinoma that was consistent with the patient's previous breast carcinoma.

ing thoracoscopes'' (see Fig. 30–2) (with a built-in channel) are the most useful for diagnostic pleural biopsy. Biopsy instruments are passed easily through the operating channel to sample those areas where lesions are visible (Fig. 30–3). The lung can also be biopsied through such a channel if necessary. If an operating thoracoscope is not used, then the single incision may be enlarged slightly to allow inser-

tion of a biopsy forceps adjacent to the thoracoscope. Alignment of these two tools can be difficult; however, with good light sources and the wide-angle dispersion of most of the thoracoscopic lenses available, biopsy can be readily accomplished.

Thoracoscopy offers a more panoramic view of the pleural space than is possible with conventional open incisions owing to the excellent lighting, magnification, and optical resolution made available with modern video technology. The magnification alone allows assessment of subtle pathologic changes that were not previously visualized with other techniques.

In over 100 thoracoscopic biopsy procedures carried out since 1985 for diagnosis of persistent pleural effusions, this author has been able to determine the presence or absence of malignancy with 98% accuracy. Only two patients with pleural effusions that were initially considered benign were subsequently diagnosed as having malignancy. One patient was shown to have adenocarcinoma of the lung 2 years after the original thoracoscopic procedure was performed, and the second patient developed pulmonary lymphoma 1 year after initial thoracoscopy was conducted. In all other cases, malignancy was reliably confirmed or excluded.

Chylothorax is an occasional finding in patients with a history of prior breast irradiation or other thoracic irradiation. Thoracoscopic biopsy can be useful to identify the source of lymphatic congestion or pleural tumor. In the single case of chylothorax after treatment for breast cancer in the author's review, no tumor was found.

After identifying malignant effusions, our approach has been to instill sterilized talc (USP) through a thoracoscopic port with the patient under general anesthesia if the lung is expandable. Other options are discussed in the section on sclerotherapy. A chest tube is inserted through the thoracoscopy incision, secured in place, and attached to a drainage device with an airtight seal. The lung is then re-expanded by the anesthesiologist.

Case History 1

A 49-year-old woman who had breast cancer 25 years earlier presented with slowly progressive shortness of breath and a persistent pleural effusion that had begun 4 years earlier (see Fig. 30–3). Several thoracocentesis procedures, including closed pleural biopsy, demonstrated the presence of exudate but no obvious malignancy. The pleural effusion was loculated, and the lung apparently fixed. The patient had been receiving supplemental estrogen therapy for postmenopausal symptoms for several years. Thoracoscopic examination revealed a thick pleural peel; a biopsy of this peel was clearly consistent with the presence of metastatic carcinoma of the breast. The thick peel and extensive tumor precluded re-expansion of the lung. The patient's estrogen therapy was stopped, and tamoxifen therapy was initiated. Her disease subsequently regressed. This case history emphasizes the problem that can result from inadequate study of a persistent pleural effusion. In this case, major therapeutic changes resulted from proper diagnosis.

Case History 2

A patient with a history of breast and ovarian carcinoma developed a right pleural effusion. Cytologic results demonstrated malignancy; however, whether the pleural effusion was secondary to metastatic ovarian carcinoma or breast carcinoma could not be clearly defined. Because different therapies would

be considered, thoracoscopic examination was undertaken so that larger tissue samples could be obtained. Samples were obtained from pleural nodules, and the patient was definitively diagnosed as having metastatic ovarian carcinoma. Chemotherapy was directed toward the treatment of ovarian carcinoma. This demonstrates the utility of thoracoscopy for identifying a specific malignancy.

Treatment of Pleural Effusions

When possible, effusions due to metastatic breast cancer should be treated aggressively. This involves re-expansion of the lung through pleural drainage (with the use of a needle or chest tube) followed by sclerotherapy. To reduce the likelihood of recurrence of symptomatic pleural effusions (Anderson et al., 1974), this author advocates definitive management at the time of diagnosis. The effect of leaving the lung unexpanded is entrapment of the lung. This process becomes more difficult to reverse the longer it is allowed to progress because the dense intrapleural tumor aggressively invades the visceral pleura and lung parenchyma. Patients with malignant pleural effusion frequently describe shortness of breath, malaise, poor exercise tolerance, and a feeling of heaviness in the chest (Ruckdeschel and Thurer, 1989). These symptoms contribute substantially toward an overall lack of well-being. Dyspnea is one of the most distressing of all terminal symptoms and whatever measures are necessary to relieve it should be taken (Cohen et al., 1992).

The options for controlling pleural effusions include chemical sclerotherapy, permanent mechanical drainage (placement of a pleuroperitoneal shunt or permanent chest tube), and pleural decortication and parietal pleurectomy. For many years, pleural drainage with a chest tube followed by the instillation of tetracycline was considered the standard therapy. Success rates ranged from 33% to 95% (Rubinson and Bolooki, 1972; Wallach, 1975; Bayly et al., 1978; Friedman and Slater, 1978; Narang et al., 1980; Opfell et al., 1980; Light, 1983; Zaloznik et al., 1983; and Ruckdeschel et al., 1990). A variety of other sclerosant agents have also been utilized; of these, the most important are bleomycin (Paladine et al., 1976; Friedman and Slater, 1978; Opfell et al., 1980; and Ostrowski, 1989), nitrogen mustard (Leininger et al., 1969; Friedman and Slater, 1978; and Fentiman et al., 1983), talc (Friedman and Slater, 1978; Harley, 1979; Weissberg, 1981; Fentiman et al., 1983; Weissberg, 1986; and Weissberg and Ben-Zeev, 1993), quinacrine (Borda and Krant, 1967; Kattwinkel et al., 1973; Bayly et al., 1978; and Friedman and Slater, 1978), and doxycycline (Mansson, 1988; and Vaughan et al., 1992). In the late 1980s and early 1990s, when tetracycline became unavailable owing to manufacturing problems, the use of bleomycin became popular because success rates were as high as 100% after a single intrapleural dose of the drug (Austin and Flye, 1979). A major advantage of using bleomycin was a relative lack of associated pain on intrapleural administration when compared with the use of tetracycline or its analogues. However, with increasing use of the drug, it became evident that the success rate for preventing recurrent effusions was only 67% (Ruckdeschel et al., 1990). The high cost of bleomycin also reduced the drug's popularity (a sclerosing dose can range in price from $800 to over $2000).

Although tetracycline is no longer available for sclerotherapy, its analogues doxycycline and minocycline have been used in its place (Mansson, 1988; and Vaughan et al., 1992). Doxycycline (500 mg) exhibits sclerosing effects similar to those produced by tetracycline but is not as effective as tetracycline after administration of a single dose. Multiple instillations are often required (Mansson, 1988; and Vaughan et al., 1992). It causes substantially more pain than other agents, including tetracycline. Minocycline is minimally painful when given intrapleurally with lidocaine, but its effectiveness for the treatment of malignant pleural effusions is not well documented (Vaughan et al., 1992). Quinacrine, which also must be administered for several doses (usually 3–4), is associated with markedly less pain than doxycycline.

Talc, instilled either as a spray powder or in a saline slurry, is emerging as the sclerosant of choice (Friedman and Slater, 1978; Harley, 1979; Weissberg, 1981; Fentiman et al., 1983; Weissberg, 1986; and Weissberg and Ben-Zeev, 1993). It has long been recognized as a highly effective sclerosant and was initially discarded only because its purity (particularly with respect to asbestos fibers) could not be ensured by manufacturers. Although this issue may be a minor concern to patients whose expected survival is short, it was an important issue for younger patients with benign conditions. Concern about pleural restriction due to overly vigorous pleural reaction also prevented the use of talc. The availability of purified talc led to renewed interest. Administration in a saline slurry is particularly convenient (Rusch, 1989). Preparations for a randomized trial to compare powder insufflation and saline slurry administration of talc are underway in multi-institutional cancer study groups.

The goals of treatment for patients with malignant pleural effusions are (1) to re-expand the lung, (2) to prevent re-accumulation of the effusion, and (3) to optimize lung function. No technique of treating malignant pleural effusions is cytoreductive, and thus treatment is palliative. Therefore, patient care must be carefully individualized to offer cost-effective, expeditious, and, if possible, single-step therapy.

Technique of Sclerosis with Doxycycline (or Other Chemical Agents)

A chest tube is inserted through a 1-cm incision at a lateral point from which pleural fluid can be aspirated and where dependent drainage is ensured. Prior to this, decubitus radiographs should have been obtained to ascertain whether the effusion layers out. After sterile skin preparation and draping, the shortest possible incision that provides a subcutaneous tunnel into the pleura is made. Because of the potential for disseminating tumor within the tube tract and within the chest wall, as little dissection as possible should be carried out in the muscular and subcutaneous planes. A Kelly clamp or one with a more pointed tip (e.g., a Crile hemostat) should be used to punch the initial hole into the pleura. The puncture wound should open sufficiently to allow digital palpation of the lung, diaphragm, and pleural space (with the fifth finger) to ensure that entry into the lung or under the diaphragm has not been made. A chest tube (size 28 to 32 French) is then directed into the pleural space posteriorly. This is secured in place with a 2–0 or 0 Dacron or silk suture.

Depending on how long a patient has had an effusion, 500 to 1000 mL may be drained initially; the tube is then clamped. The tube is clamped in order to avoid causing excessive symptoms related to pulmonary re-expansion (cough, pain, dyspnea) and re-expansion pulmonary edema with its resultant hypoxemia. Should a patient begin to cough intractably or complain of significant pain prior to removal of the initial 500 to 600 mL, the tube can be clamped earlier to allow the symptoms to dissipate. Although up to 2000 mL have been removed at one time without complications, removal of such amounts from long-standing effusions may cause pain to the patient. The tube can be unclamped every 1 to 2 hours, and 200 to 300 mL of fluid released at a time. This process is repeated until the drainage becomes minimal or until the chest is empty of fluid on radiography. The tube can then remain unclamped with a water seal or be connected to a source of low-level suction (-10 to -20 cm H_2O). If the chest tube has a water seal alone, chest radiography should be used to determine whether the lung is expanded. If the lung does not expand fully, gentle suction should be applied. Great care should be taken in chest tube placement and manipulation so that damage to the lung with leakage of air is avoided; an unexpanded lung in the presence of malignancy can be extremely troublesome.

When the chest tube drains less than 150 mL per 24 hours, the chest can be considered sufficiently empty to instill a sclerosant. Situations do occur in which an effusion continues to drain at rates higher than this despite radiographic evidence of an empty chest. Sclerosant agents can be safely and effectively instilled at this time so that pleural loculations and gradual plugging of the tube by proteinaceous debris do not develop. If doxycycline is to be used, the patient should be premedicated with 250 mg of intrapleurally administered lidocaine as a 0.5% or a 1% solution (25 or 50 mL), and the patient should be rotated with the chest tube clamped to ensure that the drug comes in contact with the entire pleura. Some practitioners prefer to instill the lidocaine at the same time as the doxycycline rather than sequentially. This probably does not decrease the effectiveness of the doxycycline, but simultaneous instillation does not offer the same analgesia as preparatory lidocaine administration. Supplementary systemic analgesia (with either intravenous morphine or meperidine hydrochloride [Demerol]) is usually helpful.

Doxycycline (500 mg) is then instilled into the chest tube, and the tube is clamped close to the chest wall. The patient is rotated into supine, prone, and right and left lateral decubitus positions while lying flat. Each position is maintained for 15 to 30 minutes to allow adequate distribution and contact of the drug with the pleural surface. The chest tube is left clamped for an additional 4 hours. The chest tube is then unclamped and coupled to a source of suction (-20 cm H_2O). Administration of the same dose of doxycycline is usually repeated on the 2nd and 3rd day of treatment. Drainage from the chest tube is closely monitored during the day following administration, and administration of the dose is repeated if the volume of drainage is greater than 50 mL per 8-hour period.

It is not at all uncommon for patients to have body temperatures as high as 102° F on the night after sclerotherapy. Such temperatures are undoubtedly due to the combination of pleuritis, splinting of the chest to relieve pain, and atelectasis. It is important to maintain systemic pain control, encourage the patient's respiratory efforts through the use of incentive spirometry, and use chest physiotherapy for as long as the chest tube is in place. After the chest tube is removed, the wound is covered with a sterile, occlusive pressure dressing for 24 hours. Chest radiographs are performed and assessed immediately after treatment and then monthly (or more frequently, as symptoms dictate).

Bleomycin in a single sclerosing dose of 60 mg is administered into the pleural space exactly as is doxycycline but without analgesia. Whether the patient is hypersensitive to bleomycin is first tested with administration of a subcutaneous intradermal skin dose of 1 mg. Significant fever or skin reaction indicates the need to use an alternate agent. Quinacrine (100–150 mg) may be used in the same manner as doxycycline but, as with bleomycin, its administration is relatively pain-free.

Controversy in the literature concerns the importance of rotating the patient after a sclerosant has been instilled. Nuclear medicine tracer studies (Lorch et al., 1988) demonstrate diffusion of the sclerosant throughout the pleural space, suggesting that there is no need to rotate the patient. However, computed tomography of the chest frequently demonstrates pleural effusions in a dependent location. This suggests that contact of the fluid with the pleura is not uniform if only a single position is maintained.

When it is to be instilled through a thoracoscope, 5 to 10 g of USP talc is sprayed into the pleural cavity with an insufflation device (Weissberg, 1981; Weissberg, 1986; and Haasler, 1994). The use of thoracoscopic insufflators is not absolutely essential. Insufflation with a bulb syringe through a mediastinoscope is advocated by Weissberg (Weissberg, 1981; Weissberg, 1986; and Weissberg and Ben-Zeev, 1993). A 16- or 18-French suction catheter attached to a bulb syringe filled with talc (Fig. 30–4) can be used with visual guidance. This system is inexpensive, and if the catheter should become plugged owing to humidity or contact with the moist pleural surface, it can simply be changed. With thoracoscopic guidance, the talc may be applied uniformly to the entire pleural surface.

A talc-containing slurry prepared using 250 and 500 mL of normal saline can be instilled into the chest tube using a standard Toomey or bulb syringe. The patient should be rotated into different positions following instillation, as previously described. A somewhat larger volume of solution provides a better distribution of talc throughout the pleural space.

Sterile preparation of the talc requires special arrangements with hospital pharmacies. This product is now available in the United States and is guaranteed to be asbestos-free.* Sterilization of talc can be carried out by heating and

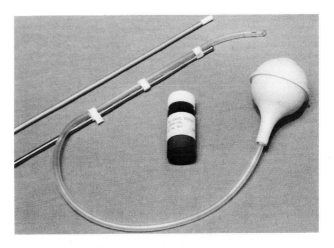

Figure 30–4. A bulb syringe that has been cut off and attached to a 16-French polyvinyl chloride suction catheter and made rigid by attachment to a probe. This system allows easy introduction of sterilized USP talc (shown bottled after heat drying). If the ports on the suction catheter become plugged, the suction catheter can be easily replaced. The use of the rigid probe allows even insufflation to all parts of the pleural space. Otherwise, uneven clumping of talc might occur.

drying in the hospital pharmacy (with subsequent packaging in 5-g bottles), or heat-sealed packets of talc can be prepared and sterilized with irradiation. Both processes are effective. It has been our practice to culture 1 or 2 bottles of talc out of each 10-bottle batch prepared by our pharmacy. In Europe, a sterile aerosolized talc preparation has been available that can be sprayed through a thoracoscope with a nozzle that is supplied.

Contraindications to Pleural Sclerotherapy

The most important contraindication to sclerotherapy is non-expansion of the lung. The parietal pleura and visceral pleura need to come together so that they can adhere. Occasionally, the lung largely re-expands, but a small residual space at the bottom or at the top of the chest remains. Clearly, significant improvement might be envisioned if the majority of the lung can be made to adhere to the chest wall. However, if the lung is trapped and a large residual space exists, instillation of a sclerosant agent is likely to be unsuccessful and could lead to space infection. In this situation, four options are available. The first is to remove the tube and palliate the patient with oxygen. Second, a pleural peritoneal shunt can be inserted. Third, an open procedure such as a pleural decortication or parietal pleurectomy can be considered (Martini et al., 1975). The fourth option is simply to leave the patient with a permanent chest tube connected to a sterile drainage bag that the patient can empty. Although this final option is not ideal, it may be reasonable if the patient's life expectancy is short.

A second relative contraindication to chemical sclerotherapy is an inability to document the malignant nature of a pleural effusion. A recurrent effusion, regardless of its

---

*Bryan Corporation, Woburn, MA.

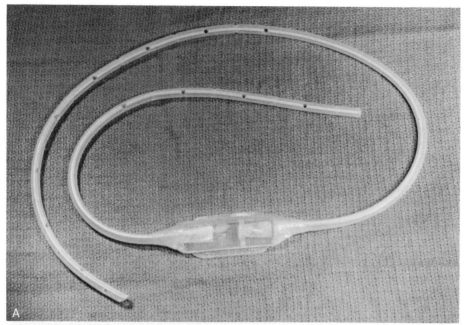

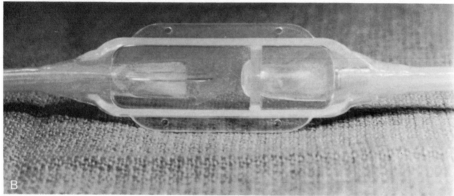

Figure 30–5. *A*, A Denver shunt (see acknowledgment). The unidirectional compressible valve and the shorter intrapleural arm with multiple side holes can be seen. The longer arm is for insertion into the peritoneum. The flat portion of the shunt is anchored external to a rib and in an anterior position to allow easy access by the patient for compression. *B*, A close-up view of the valve apparatus.

etiology, may eventually require sclerotherapy to alleviate a patient's symptoms; however, obliteration of the pleural space may impede future diagnostic efforts. With the multiple treatment options now available to patients with metastatic breast cancer, the need for a precise diagnosis must be weighed against a patient's need for relief of symptoms.

Pleurectomy and Decortication for Malignant Pleural Disease

Pleurectomy is only rarely of benefit in the management of malignant pleural effusions. Two notable exceptions are breast cancer and mesothelioma (Martini et al., 1975). In the study by Martini and coworkers (1975), 106 patients who underwent parietal pleurectomy between 1966 and 1973 were reviewed. Thirty-three had metastatic breast cancer to the pleura, and many had undergone several attempts to control the effusions by other means. Parietal pleurectomy, including decortication and a pericardial window, was carried out; this usually left some tumor along the diaphragmatic portion of the pleura. Blood loss ranged from minimal to 3500 mL. One hundred per cent control of

effusions was obtained in all patients. Thirty-day mortality was 3%. Of the surviving patients, nearly two-thirds were alive at 1 year, and one-third were alive at 2 years. Four patients survived longer than 3 years. Median survival for the entire group was 14 months.

Although the poor condition of patients with malignant effusions may preclude a major thoracotomy, the occasional patient who does not respond to other measures and has a good performance status may benefit from pleurectomy. Careful selection must be utilized.

Pleural Peritoneal Shunt

The pleural peritoneal shunt can be used for patients who have recurrent malignant pleural effusions despite previous sclerotherapy. Periodically, someone who has a residual space and only incomplete pulmonary expansion develops recurrent effusions under tension; such effusions cause discomfort and require drainage. The most popular shunt is a completely implantable silicone system (Fig. 30–5) with an intrapleural portion that contains multiple side holes and a pumping chamber placed external to a rib, and with an outflow portion (also a multiple-hole catheter) that is inserted into the peritoneum (Little et al., 1988; Tsang et al., 1990; and Ponn et al., 1991). A requirement for this system is that the patient be able to depress the pumping chamber (which has a one-way valve) several times each day to move fluid from the pleural space to the peritoneal cavity. The pressure gradient from the pleura to the abdomen is from negative to positive; thus, flow into the abdomen is not spontaneous. Approximately 1.5 mL of fluid is transported with each depression of the pumping chamber. Patients must be lucid and sufficiently reliable to manage the pump. The silicone pumping chamber must be implanted anteriorly and low enough on the chest (usually overlying the sixth or seventh rib in the midclavicular line, or in a somewhat more medial location) to be easily accessible for manipulation. The experience with this technique indicates that short-term success rates are high (Little et al., 1988; Tsang et al., 1990; and Ponn et al., 1991). One aspect of this technique that makes it undesirable to many patients is that cancer cells are transferred from the pleural space to the peritoneal space. Although the survival of patients with a malignant pleural effusion is usually short, the possibility of spreading cancer cells in this way is unappealing to them if they become aware of it. The same possibility of spreading cancer cells from one body cavity to another exists for patients who undergo pericardial-pleural window operations; however, these patients seem less concerned about the risk. Abdominal carcinomatosis caused by pleuroperitoneal shunts has yet to be recognized in published series.

Technique of Insertion

Before implanting a pleural-peritoneal shunt, the surgeon should carefully discuss the advantages and disadvantages of the device with the patient. Once it has been agreed that the procedure will be performed, a small incision is made anteriorly over an accessible rib and low in the chest while the patient is under local anesthesia. Access to the pleural space is secured with a Seldinger technique so that air bubbles are not introduced and fluid is maintained within the chest. The surgeon should try not to lose all the pleural fluid during insertion so that the shunt can be pumped early to maintain patency. The afferent arm of the catheter is placed into the pleural space with a tunnel of skin sufficient to maintain the pumping chamber in place over the rib. The pump is positioned slightly away from the incision to avoid causing the patient pain and disrupting the wound when the pump is pressed in the early postoperative period. The peritoneal surface is isolated through a separate small incision, and the distal end of the catheter placed into the peritoneal cavity. Fascial sutures are used to close the space around the catheter. Pumping is begun immediately to keep the system open. The chamber must be pumped frequently by the patient or by a family member in order to keep the drainage system working. For short-term control of pleural effusions, the success rate of the technique is in the range of 80%. Failure of the pumping system may occur secondary to progressive tumor growth, blood clotting, or fluid loculation.

An example of a patient with a difficult course in whom a pumping system was employed is described in the following case history.

Case History 3

A 37-year-old woman with a history of breast cancer was found to have a malignant effusion and metastases to the right sixth rib. Insertion of a chest tube resulted in an air leak and failure of the lung to expand. After an additional chest tube was placed, pleural drainage became purulent and the lung remained unexpanded. Bronchoscopy revealed extrinsic narrowing of the right upper lobe bronchus that contributed to the lung's continued collapse. The location of the chest tube was changed but without success, and it was believed that a more definitive procedure would be needed to control the empyema and persistent leakage of air, especially since chemotherapy and potential bone marrow transplantation were considered necessary for treatment. The patient underwent a partial decortication, with rotation of a flap consisting of the latissimus dorsi and serratus anterior muscles, as well as thoracoplasty of several lower ribs to close all spaces. The postoperative course was complicated by the need for additional chest tubes, multiple bronchoscopic procedures, and prolonged chest tube drainage over the next several weeks. The patient underwent multidrug chemotherapy and bone marrow transplantation 6 months later; however, the patient died as a result of metastatic disease 9 months afterwards.

PERICARDIAL METASTASES

The most common problem involving the pericardium in patients with breast cancer is the development of malignant pericardial effusions and cardiac tamponade. Multiple options (catheter drainage, thoracoscopic drainage, creating a subxyphoid window) are now available for treatment of this problem, and the physician must decide which option is best for each patient. As all of the options may produce similar results, the selection of one over the others depends on the expertise of individual physicians. Patients with malignant pericardial effusions have dyspnea, orthopnea, and peripheral edema and present signs of hemodynamic compromise. The characteristic signs of cardiac tamponade are narrowed pulse pressure, distention of the jugular veins, muffled heart tones, and a paradoxic pulse. A patient's chest radiograph is often suggestive of the problem, demonstrating an enlarged cardiac silhouette and the classic "water bottle" appearance (Fig. 30–6). An echocardiogram can demonstrate the amount of fluid present and can suggest the possibility of early tamponade by showing the presence of right ventricular outflow tract compression in diastole. If the presence of a significant pericardial effusion is confirmed, the effusion should be aspirated under ultrasound guidance using a subxyphoid approach or under fluoroscopic guidance in the cardiac catheterization laboratory. Collected samples are sent for cytology. Opinions differ on the advisability of leaving a catheter in the pericardial sac, but several soft catheters are available for short-term use.

Pericardial metastases generally indicate a grim prog-

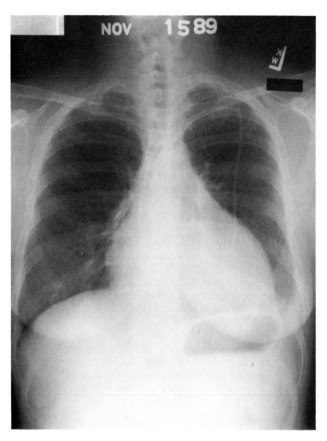

Figure 30–6. The typical appearance of a large pericardial effusion is shown. The heart has the appearance of a water bottle, with flattened side areas over the right atrium and left atrial portions and a large lower aspect along the diaphragm. This patient underwent an open pericardial window procedure.

nosis for a patient, with survivals ranging from several weeks to a few months. With this in mind, the practitioner should manage pericardial effusions quickly and effectively, leaving little chance for recurrence. Ideally, patients who have undergone treatment leave the hospital within a few days. A large pericardial window handles the acute problem of fluid accumulation and prevents recurrence very effectively. The window can be created by several surgical approaches: (1) partial pericardiectomy (Levin and Aaron, 1982) or pleuropericardial communication (Dabir and Warren, 1984) by an extrapleural subxyphoid approach; (2) thoracoscopically guided pericardial window creation (right or left); (3) limited anterior left thoracotomy (Gregory et al., 1985); and (4) the subcostal approach (Steiger et al., 1985). Although a median sternotomy can be considered, the less invasive approaches are preferable, especially since many patients have received irradiation and are cachectic, and the healing of a sternal wound might be impaired. Surgical approaches are highly successful.

Instillation of sclerosant agents into the pericardial sac through a catheter has been utilized by some authors with favorable results. Shepherd and associates utilized 500 to 1000 mg of tetracycline hydrochloride (after lidocaine) in 58 patients (Shepherd et al., 1987). Pain was described as

moderate to severe in nine patients (16%) and was worse after instillation of 1 g than after administration of 500 mg. A mean of 2.9 doses per patient was required. Catheters were left in place, and additional doses of tetracycline were used if the drainage volume exceeded 25 mL in 24 hours. In the series of Davis and coworkers (35 patients), catheters were in place for a mean of 8.8 days (Press and Livingston, 1987; and Davis et al., 1984). Control of pericardial effusions was reported in 91% of Davis and coworkers' patients and in 86% of Shepherd's patients. Criteria for success were a decrease in or the disappearance of the effusion for 30 days, absence of cardiac tamponade, and no requirement for repeat pericardiocentesis. In this author's experience, the instillation of tetracycline caused such great pain in patients (despite the systemic use of narcotics and the instillation of lidocaine) that we stopped utilizing it as a palliative measure.

Van der Gaast and associates (1989) utilized 20 to 30 mg of bleomycin dissolved in 30 mL normal saline as a single dose to treat five patients and waited until drainage decreased to less than 25 mL over 12 hours before removing the catheter. A repeat of the dose was required for only one patient. All five patients had resolution of their effusions and survived for 1 to 29 months. Cormican and Nyman (1990) described a single patient who survived 65 days without recurrence after receiving an intrapericardial dose of 5 mg diluted in 20 mL saline. The low cost of these small doses of bleomycin compared with that of those utilized in the treatment of malignant pleural effusions makes this a reasonable modality.

Recently, a technique involving percutaneous balloon catheter pericardiostomy under fluoroscopic guidance has been described and may be an option for certain patients (Ziskind et al., 1993).

Surgical Drainage of the Pericardial Sac

Before anesthesia is administered, the volume of fluid in the pericardium and whether tamponade is present must be ascertained. In the presence of tamponade, a patient's blood pressure may rapidly decrease when sedatives or general anesthesia is given. The patient's skin is prepared for incision prior to induction of anesthesia, and the surgeon must be prepared to operate quickly. Emergency subxyphoid needle pericardiocentesis may be required. A safer alternative involves needle or catheter drainage of the pericardial effusion using fluoroscopy or echocardiography prior to performing the surgical procedure.

A limited left anterior thoracotomy (Levin and Aaron, 1982; Gregory et al., 1985; and Press and Livingston, 1987) and the subxyphoid technique are standard approaches for pericardial access. An anterior left thoracotomy permits quick access into the chest and may be readily employed in an emergency. An incision in the fourth or fifth interspace gives good exposure of the pericardium anterior to the phrenic nerve. A portion of the pericardium (as large as feasible), including that part which extends to the right, can be easily excised. The left phrenic nerve should be visualized and protected. Frequently, considerable prepericardial fat is present on the left side, and bleeding from the vessels in this fat must be carefully controlled. Removal of a large piece of pericardium is best. Usually, as much anterior pericardium as possible is removed from between the phrenic nerves. Chest tubes are left in place, and the incision is closed in a standard manner. A separate pericardial drain is not necessary, but if one is desired, a soft Silastic or rubber drain represents the best option.

An equally popular approach that can be carried out using local anesthesia is creation of a subxyphoid window (Levin and Aaron, 1982; and Press and Livingston, 1987). For many practitioners, this technique is becoming the procedure of choice (Levin and Aaron, 1982; Press and Livingston, 1987; and Graeber et al., 1989). It is very useful for patients who have not had previous drainage (because of the possibility of loculations) and when it is desirable to avoid general anesthesia. The patient's chest is prepared and draped, and the patient is lightly sedated. A short upper midline abdominal incision is made overlying the xyphoid process and extending 2 to 3 inches below the xyphoid process (Fig. 30–7). The xyphoid process is removed, and the branches of the internal mammary artery on each side of the xyphoid process are cauterized. This allows access to the space just anterior to the diaphragm and cephalad to the peritoneum. The diaphragm is mobilized from the sides of the incision. Fat anterior to the pericardium can then be separated bluntly to allow exposure of the pericardial sac. The pericardium is grasped with a small clamp, and a small button of tissue excised to allow entry into the pericardial sac. The incision is then widened, and a section of pericar-

dium measuring several square centimeters can be removed. The pleura on either the right or the left side can be entered to allow pleural-pericardial communication; however, this is not essential for continued pericardial decompression. The diaphragmatic pericardium is explored posteriorly with suction to break up loculations. A soft rubber drain is placed through the defect in the pericardium and brought out through the lower portion of the abdominal incision or through a separate stab wound. Use of a soft rubber tube (size 28 to 32 French) or one of the many silicone mediastinal drains is preferred. The drain is left in place until drainage ceases; it is then removed.

Steiger and colleagues (1985) described a variation on both of these techniques in which a left subcostal approach via a small incision parallel to the left costal margin is used. This technique was as efficacious as other surgical approaches and was well tolerated by patients.

Video-assisted thoracoscopy can be used to form a pericardial window. The approach is easier from the right side owing to the posterior position of the phrenic nerve. The greater distance between chest wall and pericardium than on the left side allows easier visualization and manipulation of instruments (Caccavale, 1993). The patient is anesthetized as for diagnostic thoracoscopy with either a double-lumen endotracheal tube (to allow decompression of the right lung) or with a single-lumen tube and a bronchial blocker. The patient is placed in the left lateral decubitus position. Two or three thoracoscopic ports are made in a triangular fashion, the camera is inserted, the lung is collapsed, and the pericardium is visualized. The lung may

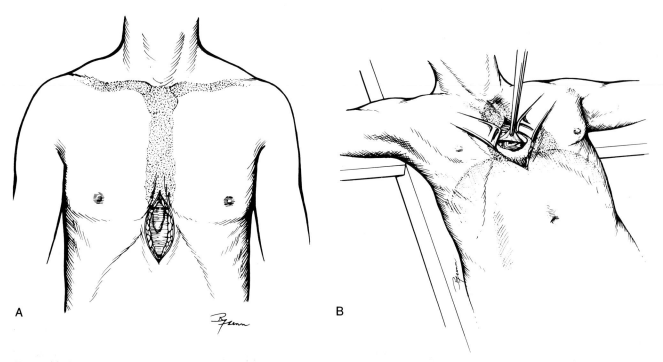

Figure 30–7. The subxyphoid approach to the pericardium. *A,* The xyphoid process has been excised and the small blood vessels on each side of it cauterized. The diaphragm has been reflected medially and away from the costal cartilages to allow exposure of the pericardium. *B,* A hole is made into the pericardium (this hole tends to enlarge after it has been made). The pleura may be entered (if easily accessible) to allow additional drainage. If the pleural space is entered, chest tubes are placed. A small rubber drain is brought out through a separate incision or at the bottom of the wound at the completion of the procedure.

need to be retracted posteriorly with an endoscopic retractor or by positioning the patient obliquely so that the lung falls backwards against the posterior chest wall. The pericardium is grasped, and an incision made into the pericardium, with care taken to avoid injuring the atrium beneath. Ideally, a portion of the pericardium is grasped with a ring forceps, and the portion within the clamp incised. After the pericardial fluid is drained, the opening is enlarged. Electrocautery is used for hemostasis, with care taken to avoid damaging the phrenic nerve.

A technique to manage excess pericardial fat has been described. After the initial incision is made in the pericardium, an endoscopic linear cutter (two to three staple lines with a blade between them) is used to enlarge the pericardial opening. This results in an opening with the fat on each side of the staple line securely controlled. This allows manipulation of blood vessels close to the phrenic nerve with less risk of injury to the nerve from the heat of the cautery. After a window has been made and the pericardial fluid has been drained, a chest tube is placed, and the incisions are closed. Recovery is rapid, and the patient is usually discharged within several days.

Pericardiectomy for Constrictive Pericarditis

Occasionally, patients who previously underwent radiation therapy present with pericardial fibrosis and constriction. The pericardium is thickened and often calcified, and signs of hemodynamic compromise are present. Although malignancy or radiation therapy can be responsible, one must remember other possible causes, most notably tuberculosis. The treatment of symptomatic pericardial constriction is excision of as much of the pericardium as possible, including that region posterior to the phrenic nerves. This is accomplished best through a bilateral anterior thoracotomy with the patient in the supine position; however, a sternotomy approach is also feasible (Graeber et al., 1987). The bilateral thoracotomy allows easier access to the left posterior pericardium, which must be freed if the operation is to be successful. The left atrium and ventricle should be released before the right ventricle and atrium to avoid flooding the lungs with blood before the increased flow can be accommodated by the left side of the heart. Constrictive pericarditis is more difficult to treat surgically than is pericardial tamponade because the pericardium is often adherent to the epicardium and must be carefully dissected away. In addition, fibrosis may require partial stripping or careful cross-hatching of the epicardium to release the inflammatory process. Cardiopulmonary bypass may need to be performed emergently in the event that the patient cannot tolerate elevation of the heart for dissection of the posterior pericardium.

Patients who have undergone pericardiectomy are often extremely ill postoperatively and exhibit a myocardial dysfunction that is still poorly understood. This dysfunction can be sufficiently severe to require hemodynamic support with pressor agents or an intra-aortic balloon pump. At present, no role for thoracoscopic approaches to constrictive pericarditis has been defined.

CARDIAC ARRHYTHMIAS

Patients with a history of irradiation for breast cancer can exhibit a variety of arrhythmias, including atrioventricular block (Janjan et al., 1989). These patients occasionally require ventricular pacemakers.

CHEST WALL PROBLEMS

Breast cancer can lead to several chest wall problems. Probably the best known is extensive lymphangitic spread throughout the skin in patients with advanced metastatic disease. Not much can be done for the patient when spread is truly extensive except for pain control, symptomatic treatment of open wounds, and, in some patients, additional chemotherapy. When a chest tube must be placed for drainage of pleural fluid, it is wise to place the tube in an unirradiated area and away from disease.

Local recurrence of cancer in mastectomy sites can lead to involvement of underlying ribs and intercostal muscles. Previous radiation therapy further complicates the problem (Larson and McMurtrey, 1987; and Larson, 1991). Recurrences in an irradiated field can result in nonhealing wounds or in necrosis of underlying ribs (Figs. 30–8 and 30–9). The areas ulcerate and become infected. The sternum may be involved in addition to ribs. It is not uncommon for the pleura and the lung to be involved. Such situations are often cosmetically and functionally devastating to patients.

The work of Larson and McMurtrey has addressed the problem of cancer recurrence in mastectomy sites (Larson and McMurtrey 1987; and Larson, 1991). The general approach involves radical débridement of the involved skin and underlying chest wall. Cultures are taken preoperatively to plan appropriate perioperative antibiotic coverage. For many reconstructions, a contralateral rectus muscle myocutaneous flap is utilized if the internal mammary arteries are intact. If the patient has not had cardiac surgery, thoracic surgery, or a mastectomy involving internal mammary dissection, the internal mammary artery is assumed to be intact. Since atherosclerosis of the internal mammary artery is rarely a concern, one need not study it angiographically.

After excision of the involved portion of chest wall and underlying rib cage, reconstruction is performed using a latissimus dorsi muscle myocutaneous flap or a contralateral rectus muscle myocutaneous rotation flap (see Fig. 30–9). The size of the defect must be anticipated so that the appropriate skin preparation and reconstruction can be planned. If the underlying lung has become attached to the parietal pleura where the chest wall is removed, the involved portion of lung can be stapled and removed en bloc with the specimen.

Postoperatively, a moderate degree of flail chest is tolerated. Sometimes, mechanical ventilation is required for several days until the chest wall stabilizes. Antibiotics are continued perioperatively, depending on the degree of bacterial contamination of the skin and the operative field. Radical operative débridement of chest wall and involved tissues followed by muscle flap reconstruction has improved the management of both selected chest wall recur-

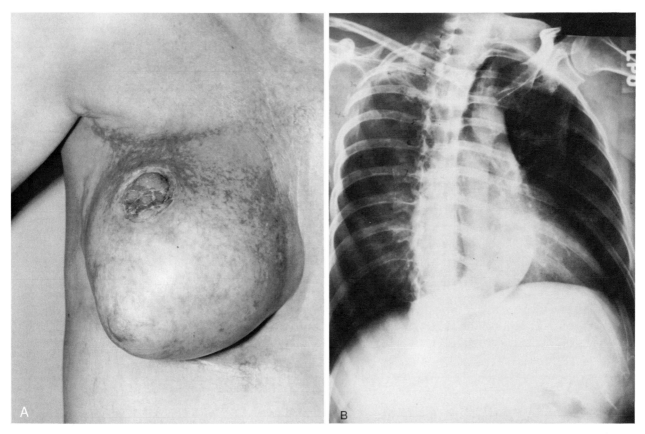

Figure 30–8. *A,* A locally recurrent breast tumor in a patient after lumpectomy and irradiation. *B,* A radiograph of the same patient shows necrosis of the underlying ribs. (Photographs courtesy of David Larson, M.D.)

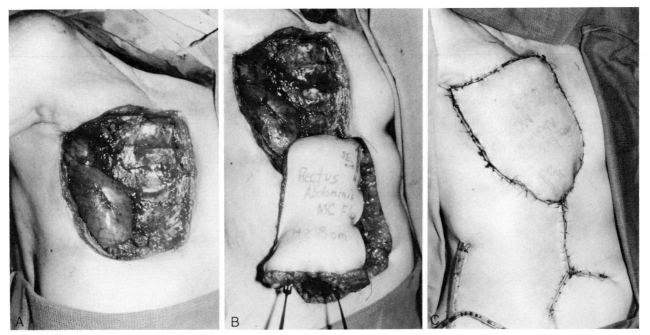

Figure 30–9. *A,* The remaining breast and underlying chest wall of the patient shown in Figure 30–8 have been removed to the point at which tissue was believed to be viable and not involved with either tumor or radiation necrosis. The chest wall was attached to the lung, and a stapled lung surface is seen. The pericardium can also be seen. *B,* The left rectus muscle myocutaneous flap is based on the left internal mammary artery and its perforating branches. This has been prepared as a rotation flap to cover the defect. *C,* The rotated rectus muscle flap and all wounds have been closed. No prosthetic material has been employed in the reconstruction. (Photographs courtesy of David Larson, M.D.)

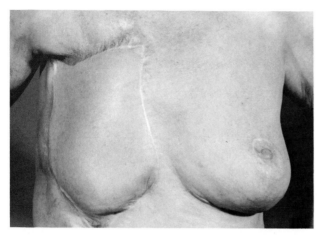

Figure 30-10. Reconstruction of the breast of the patient shown in Figure 30-9 is shown after 6 months of healing. The patient had excellent functional and cosmetic results. (Photograph courtesy of David Larson, M.D.)

rences and radionecrosis (Fig. 30-10; see also Figs. 30-8 and 30-9).

SUMMARY

Multiple thoracic complications can be seen in patients with a history of breast cancer. Lesions of the pulmonary parenchyma, when solitary, need to be managed with the same approach as for any solitary pulmonary nodule. In patients with multiple nodules, the likelihood of metastasis is great, and the usual role of the chest surgeon is to obtain biopsy specimens so that other treatments can be evaluated and employed. There may be benefit from removing multiple metastases in selected patients. The most common problems requiring thoracic surgical intervention are those that occur in the pleural and pericardial spaces. Several new options for treatment of pleural-pericardial disease exist, including video-assisted thoracic surgical techniques and trans-catheter sclerotherapy. For the treatment of disease involving the chest wall caused by either tumor recurrence or radiation therapy, wide surgical resection combined with muscle flap reconstruction benefits some patients. Although the objectives of wide surgical resection are largely palliative, patients are provided with improved comfort and, sometimes, prolonged survival.

Acknowledgments

Denver Pleuro-Peritoneal Shunts for pleural effusions are manufactured and sold by DENVER BIOMATERIALS, INC., 6851 Highway 73, Evergreen, CO 80439, tel.: (303) 674-5294.

The help of Mrs. Mary Lynne Koenig in typing the manuscript is gratefully acknowledged. Ms. Becky Varley and Mrs. Patricia Schopp also completed numerous errands vital to this chapter's completion. Finally, I offer my thanks to Dr. David Larson, Professor and Chairman of Plastic and Reconstructive Surgery at the Medical College of Wisconsin, who shared his time, expertise, and photographic collection with me so that I could prepare this chapter's section on chest wall problems and reconstruction.

References

Anderson, C. B., Philpott, G. W., and Ferguson, T. B.: Pretreatment of malignant pleural effusions. Cancer, *33:*916–922, 1974.

Austin, E. H., and Flye, M. W.: The treatment of recurrent malignant pleural effusion. Ann. Thorac. Surg., *28:*190–203, 1979.

Bayly, T. C., Kisner, D. L., Sybert, A., et al.: Tetracycline and quinacrine in the control of malignant pleural effusions. Cancer, *41:*1188–1192, 1978.

Benfield, J. R., and Hammond, W. G.: Surgery for lung metastasis. Contemp. Surg., *22:*31–36, 1983.

Borda, I., and Krant, M.: Convulsions following intrapleural administration of quinacrine hydrochloride. J.A.M.A., *201:*173–174, 1967.

Caccavale, R. J.: Video assisted thoracic surgery for pericardial disease. Chest Surg. Clin. North Am., 3:271–281, 1993.

Cahan, W. G., and Castro, E. B.: Significance of a solitary lung shadow in patients with breast cancer. Ann. Surg., *181:*137–143, 1973.

Cohen, M. H., Johnston-Anderson, A., Krasnow, S. H., et al.: Treatment of intractable dyspnea: Clinical and ethical issues. Cancer Invest., *10:*317–321, 1992.

Cormican, M. C., and Nyman, C. R.: Intrapericardial bleomycin for the management of cardiac tamponade secondary to malignant pericardial effusion. Br. Heart J., *63:*61–62, 1990.

Dabir, R., and Warren, S. E.: Drainage of pericardial effusions using the peritoneal and pericardial window technique. Surg. Gynecol. Obstet., *159:*485–486, 1984.

Davis, S., Rambotti, P., and Grignani, F.: Intrapericardial tetracycline sclerosis in the treatment of malignant pericardial effusion: An analysis of 33 cases. J. Clin. Oncol., *2:*631–636, 1984.

Fentiman, I. S., Rubens, R. D., and Hayward, J. L.: Control of pleural effusions in patients with breast cancer. Cancer, *52:*737–739, 1983.

Friedman, M. A., and Slater, E.: Malignant pleural effusions. Cancer Treat. Rev., *5:*49–66, 1978.

Ginsberg, R. J.: New technique for one lung anesthesia using an endobronchial blocker. J. Thorac. Cardiovasc. Surg., *82:*542–546, 1981.

Ginsberg, R. J.: Lung-sparing operations for cancer. *In* Roth, J. A., Cox, J. D., and Hong, W. K. (Eds.): Lung Cancer. Boston, Blackwell Scientific Publications, 1993, p. 138.

Graeber, G. M.: Complications of therapy of malignant tumors involving the pericardium. *In* Roth, J. A., Ruckdeschel, J. C., Weisenburger, T. H. (Eds.): Thoracic Oncology. Philadelphia, W. B. Saunders, 1989, pp. 504–512.

Graeber, G. M., Macon, M. G., Heric, B. R., et al.: Pericardiectomy through a median sternotomy. Surg. Rounds, November 1987, pp. 17–27.

Gregory, J. R., McMurtrey, M. J., and Mountain, C. F.: A surgical approach to the treatment of pericardial effusions in cancer patients. Am. J. Clin. Oncol., *8:*319–323, 1985.

Haasler, G. B.: Video-assisted thoracic surgery: Thoracoscopy revisited. St. Louis, Mosby-Yearbook (in press).

Harley, H. R. S.: Malignant pleural effusions and their treatment by intercostal talc pleurodesis. Br. J. Dis. Chest, *73:*173–177, 1979.

Inoue, H., Shohtsu, A., Ogawa, J., et al.: New device for one lung anesthesia: Endotracheal tube with moveable blocker. J. Thorac. Cardiovasc. Surg., 83:940–941, 1982.

Janjan, N. A., Gillin, M. T., Prows, J., et al.: Dose to the cardiac vascular and conduction systems in primary breast irradiation. Med. Dosim., *14:*81–87, 1989.

Kamaya, H., and Krishna, P. R.: New endotracheal tube (Univent tube) for selective blockade of one lung. Anesthesiology, *63:*342–343, 1985.

Kattwinkel, J., Taussig, L. M., McIntosh, C. L., et al.: Intrapleural instillation of quinacrine for recurrent pneumothorax. J.A.M.A., *226:*557–559, 1973.

Larson, D. L.: Surgical management of complications of cancer therapy. Adv. Plast. Reconstr. Surg., *7:*167–189, 1991.

Larson, D. L., and McMurtrey, M.: Chest wall reconstruction. Adv. Plast. Reconstr. Surg., *4:*217–244, 1987.

Leininger, B. J., Barker, W. L., and Langston, H. T.: A simplified method for management of malignant pleural effusions. J. Thorac. Cardiovasc. Surg., *58:*758–763, 1969.

Levin, B. H., and Aaron, B. L.: The subxyphoid pericardial window. Surg. Gynecol. Obstet., *155:*804–806, 1982.

Light, R. W.: Malignant pleural effusions. *In* Light, R. W. (Ed.): Pleural Diseases. Philadelphia, Lea & Febiger, 1983, pp. 77–88.

Little, A. G., Kadowaki, M. H., Ferguson, M. K., et al.: Pleuro-peritoneal shunting: Alternative therapy for pleural effusions. Ann. Surg., *208:*443–450, 1988.

Lorch, D. G., Gordon, L., Wooten, S., et al.: Effect of patient positioning on distribution of tetracycline in the pleural space during pleurodesis. Chest, *93:*527–529, 1988.

Mansson, T. Treatment of malignant pleural effusion with doxycycline. Scand. J. Infect. Dis. Suppl., *53:*29–34, 1988.

Martin, D. H., and Newhouse, M. T.: Thoracoscopy: A clinical perspective. *In* Kittle, C. F. (Ed.): Current Controversies in Thoracic Surgery. Philadelphia, W.B. Saunders, 1986, pp. 107–112.

Martini, N., Bains, M. S., and Beattie, E. J. Jr.: Indications for pleurectomy in malignant effusion. Cancer, *35:*734–738, 1975.

Mountain, C. F., McMurtrey, M. J., and Hermes, K. E.: Surgery for pulmonary metastasis: A 20-year experience. Ann. Thorac. Surg., *38:*323–330, 1984.

Narang, R. K., Mital, O. P., and Kumar, A.: Intrapleural tetracycline in management of malignant pleural effusions. Indian J. Chest. Dis. Allied Sci., *22:*166–168, 1980.

Opfell, R. W., Padova, J., Margileth, D., et al.: Intrapleural bleomycin vs. tetracycline for control of malignant pleural effusion: A randomized study. Proceedings of the American Association for Cancer Research, American Society of Clinical Oncology, 1980, p. 366.

Ostrowski, M. J.: Intracavitary therapy with bleomycin for the treatment of malignant pleural effusions. J. Surg. Oncol. Suppl., *1:*7–13, 1989.

Paladine, W., Cunningham, T. J., Sponzo, R., et al.: Intracavitary bleomycin in the management of malignant effusions. Cancer, *38:*1903–1908, 1976.

Ponn, R. B., Blancaflor, J., D'Agostino, R. S., et al.: Pleuroperitoneal shunting for intractable pleural effusions. Ann. Thorac. Surg., *51:*605–609, 1991.

Press, O. W., and Livingston, R.: Management of malignant pericardial effusion and tamponade. J.A.M.A., *257:*1088–1092, 1987.

Rubinson, R. M., and Bolooki, H.: Intrapleural tetracycline for control of malignant pleural effusion: A preliminary report. South. Med. J., *65:*847–849, 1972.

Ruckdeschel, J. C., Moores, D. W. O., Lee, J. Y., et al.: Management of malignant pleural effusions (MPE): A randomized comparison of tetracycline (TETRA) and bleomycin (BLEO) (Abstract). Proc. Am. Soc. Clin. Oncol., *9:*323, 1990.

Ruckdeschel, J. C., and Thurer, R.: Malignant pleural effusions. Contemp. Surg., *35:*79–104, 1989.

Rusch, V. W., and Haper, G. R.: Pleural effusions in patients with malignancy. *In* Roth, J. A., Ruckdeschel, J. C., and Weisenburger, T. H. (Eds.): Thoracic Oncology. Philadelphia, W.B. Saunders, 1989, pp. 594–608.

Shepherd, F. A., Morgan, C., Evans, W. K., et al.: Medical management of malignant pericardial effusion by tetracycline sclerosis. Am. J. Cardiol., *60:*1161–1166, 1987.

Staren, E. D., Salerno, C., Rongione, A., et al.: Pulmonary resection for metastatic breast cancer. Arch. Surg., *127:*1282–1284, 1992.

Steiger, Z., McAlpin, G., and Wilson, R. F.: Left subcostal approach to the pericardium. Surg. Gynecol. Obstet., *160:*414–416, 1985.

Thomas, P.: Thoracoscopy: An old procedure revisited. *In* Kittle, C. F. (Ed.): Current Controversies in Thoracic Surgery. Philadelphia, W.B. Saunders, 1986, pp. 101–116.

Tsang, V., Fernando, H. C., and Goldstraw, P.: Pleuroperitoneal shunt for recurrent malignant pleural effusions. Thorax, *45:*369–372, 1990.

van der Gaast, A., Kok, T. C., Hoogerbrugge van der Linden, N., et al.: Intrapericardial instillation of bleomycin in the management of malignant pericardial effusion. Eur. J. Cancer Clin. Oncol., *25:*1505–1506, 1989.

Vaughan, L. M., Walker, P. B., and Sahn, S. A.: Alternatives to tetracycline pleurodesis (Letter). Ann. Pharmacother., *26:*562–563, 1992.

Wallach, H. W.: Intrapleural tetracycline for malignant pleural effusions. Chest, *68:*510–512, 1975.

Weissberg, D.: Talc pleurodesis: A controversial issue. Poumon-Coeur, *37:*291–294, 1981.

Weissberg, D.: The surgical management of recurrent or persistent pneumothorax: Pleuroscopy and talc poudrage. *In* Kittle, C. F. (Ed.): Current Controversies in Thoracic Surgery. Philadelphia, W.B. Saunders, 1986, pp. 46–50.

Weissberg, D., and Ben-Zeev, I.: Talc pleurodesis: Experience with 360 patients. J. Thorac. Cardiovasc. Surg., *106:*689–695, 1993.

Zaloznik, A. J., Oswald, S. G., and Langin, M.: Intrapleural tetracycline in malignant pleural effusions. Cancer, *51:*752–755, 1983.

Ziskind, A. A., Pearce, A. C., Lemmon, C. C., et al.: Percutaneous balloon pericardiotomy for the treatment of cardiac tamponade and large pericardial effusions: Description of technique and report of the first 50 cases. J. Am. Coll. Cardiol., *21:*1–5, 1993.

31

Metastasis to the Eye and Ocular Adnexa

John W. Gamel
Arthur H. Keeney

Many malignancies metastasize to ocular structures. Among women, most of these lesions originate in the breast. Although ocular involvement usually follows other clinical manifestations of disseminated disease, occasionally it may provide the first clinical evidence of dissemination. For a small fraction of patients, this evidence precedes diagnosis of the primary tumor, and thus breast carcinoma must be included in the differential diagnosis of a mass lesion discovered in the eye or orbit of a woman. Life expectancy is limited for most patients with metastatic disease, but ophthalmic lesions usually respond well to palliative therapy, especially when detected early.

INCIDENCE OF OPHTHALMIC METASTASIS

The incidence of ocular metastasis varies from approximately 10% to 40% among patients with breast cancer (Table 31–1). The breast predominates as the primary site among women, and the breast rivals the lung as the primary site among unselected patients (Bloch and Gartner, 1971; and Hutchinson and Smith, 1979). Weiss (1993) examined published data on several primary carcinomas and concluded that, allowing for the relative blood flow to various metastatic sites, the uveal tract is the most highly favored target organ. Ophthalmic metastasis occurs most commonly in the fifth, sixth, and seventh decades of life, paralleling the incidence of primary breast carcinoma (Usher, 1923; Hart, 1962; Jaeger et al., 1971; Henderson, 1973; Thatcher and Thomas, 1975; Hutchinson and Smith, 1979; Bullock and Yanes, 1980; and Mewis and Young, 1982).

Occasionally, metastatic ocular disease appears first in a patient with clinically undetected breast carcinoma or in a patient with known primary disease but no other evidence of dissemination. The incidence of such occurrences is difficult to ascertain, as findings are greatly influenced by methods of patient selection and evaluation. Nevertheless, various studies suggest that of all patients with breast malignancy metastatic to various ocular sites, from 3% to 9% have previously undiagnosed primary disease (Ferry and Font, 1974; Stephens and Shields, 1979; and Bullock and Yanes, 1980). Arnold and associates (1985) found a much higher incidence of occult primary cancers (30%) among patients with tumors that involve the eyelid, suggesting that the eyelid may be an especially likely site for metastasis

from occult breast carcinoma. For approximately one-fourth of all patients with primary breast malignancy, ocular structures are the first clinically detected site of metastasis (Hart, 1962; Henderson, 1973; Thatcher and Thomas, 1975; and Maor et al., 1977), although some authors have derived a much lower (Mewis and Young, 1982) or much higher estimate (Stephens and Shields, 1979).

More often, ocular involvement affects patients with known metastases. Of particular interest is the observation of Mewis and Young (1982) that, among patients suffering from Grade IV metastatic breast carcinoma, those with ocular complaints had an incidence of intraocular metastasis that was fourfold greater than that of patients with no visual symptoms (see Table 31–1). Combining these results with those of Albert and associates (1977), one can expect to find ocular involvement in roughly 10% of all patients with metastatic breast malignancy and in a much higher percentage of patients within this group that report eye-related symptoms.

LOCATION, SIGNS, AND SYMPTOMS OF OPHTHALMIC METASTASIS

Breast carcinoma disseminates to the eye more often than to the eyelids or orbit, and within the globe the posterior uvea (choroid) is more commonly involved than the ciliary body or iris (Ferry and Font, 1974). The data of Hutchinson and Smith (1979) suggest that approximately two-thirds of ophthalmic metastasis from breast cancer involves the globe and that approximately 90% of all intraocular lesions involve the choroid. Similar findings were reported by Ratanatharathorn and colleagues (1991). In addition, individual reports can be found of breast cancer metastatic to the optic nerve, meninges, vitreous, sclera, and retina (Leys et al., 1990).

A substantial fraction of ophthalmic patients have bilateral metastases; among patients with unilateral disease, some investigators report that the left eye is involved more often than the right (Table 31–2). These findings suggest that structural differences in vasculature between the left and right cranial circulation may affect the ocular dissemination of malignancy. A substantial fraction of patients with choroidal metastasis have more than one tumor in the same eye (Stephens and Shields, 1979; and Mewis and Young, 1982).

Table 31-1. INCIDENCE OF OPHTHALMIC METASTASIS IN PATIENTS WITH BREAST CARCINOMA

Author	Number of Patients with Breast Carcinoma	Patients with Ophthalmic Metastasis	Incidence of Ophthalmic Disease (%)
Albert et al. (1977)	52	7	13
Bloch and Gartner (1971)	52	19	37
Nelson et al. (1983)	31	3	10
Mewis and Young (1982)	250	67	27
Ophthalmic Symptoms:			
No	98	9	9
Yes	152	58	38

The signs and symptoms of ophthalmic metastasis are determined primarily by the structures involved. Patients with choroidal metastasis most commonly experience decreased or distorted vision, diplopia, or blind spots as manifestations of tumor-related retinal detachment (Fig. 31–1) (Mewis and Young, 1982). Such detachment may reflect direct tumor involvement, subretinal hemorrhage, or subretinal serous transudation from leaky tumor vessels.

Orbital lesions from breast carcinoma most often are manifested by proptosis, periorbital swelling, or a palpable mass (Fig. 31–2). Also noted in some patients are pain from nerve invasion, decreased acuity from distortion of the globe, and diplopia from infiltration of the extraocular muscles or their nerve supply (Henderson, 1973; and Font and Ferry, 1976). Of particular interest is enophthalmos, an uncommon sign that has been reported only with scirrhous carcinoma of the breast that is metastatic to the orbit. Retraction of the globe and eyelids is the result of scirrhous infiltration of orbital tissues, which also causes progressive ophthalmoplegia (Henderson, 1973).

Additional uncommon manifestations of metastatic ocular disease include iritis and glaucoma from invasion of the iris and ciliary body (Ferry and Font, 1975) and nodules or diffuse infiltration from involvement of the eyelids (Arnold et al., 1985).

LOCATION AND HISTOLOGY OF THE PRIMARY TUMOR

Most authors have found an equal likelihood of ophthalmic metastasis from the right and the left breasts (Usher, 1923; and Thatcher and Thomas, 1975), although one study has reported a predominance of primary tumors in the right

breast (Jaeger et al., 1971). The majority of breast tumors that metastasize to ocular structures are classified histologically as adenocarcinoma. The authors are aware of no study that establishes a correlation between histologic type of breast cancer and site or incidence of ophthalmic metastasis.

DIAGNOSIS

Any patient with ocular complaints who is at risk for metastatic cancer should first undergo a complete eye examination, including evaluation of visual acuity, ocular motility, and pupillary response as well as inspection of the lids and slit-lamp examination of the anterior segment. For orbital lesions, exophthalmometry provides an objective measure of the extent of protrusion of each eye. Measurement of the width of the lid fissures and position of each lid with respect to the cornea also provides useful information. Given the propensity of metastatic disease for the posterior choroid, examination of the fundus is indispensable. Serous retinal detachment from a metastasis in the peripheral choroid can cause visual symptoms in an eye, but examination by direct ophthalmoscopy discloses no abnormality. Thus, a widely dilated pupil and an indirect ophthalmoscope are essential for adequate visualization of the entire choroid. All fundus lesions should be drawn in the medical record.

For medical and legal documentation, appropriate photographs may be taken using a macrolens for the lids and orbit, a specially adapted slit-lamp camera for the anterior segment, and a fundus camera for posterior lesions. Additional diagnostic procedures include the following:

1. *Transillumination*, which may in some instances al-

Table 31-2. LATERALITY OF OPHTHALMIC METASTASIS FROM BREAST CARCINOMA

Author	Bilateral Number (%)	Right Eye Only	Left Eye Only	Overall Ratio Left/Right
Usher (1923)	26 (48)	12	16	1.33
Hutchinson and Smith (1979)	4 (13)	10	16	1.60
Mewis and Young (1982)	27 (40)	18	22	1.22
Thatcher and Thomas (1975)	17 (40)	12	13	1.08
Maor et al. (1977)	15 (36)	10	17	1.70
Henderson (1973)	1 (5)	7	11	1.57
Total	80 (33)	69	95	1.38

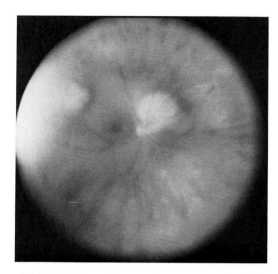

Figure 31–1. Breast carcinoma with multiple choroidal metastases (wide angle photograph). A large lesion can be seen invading the disc with a second lesion temporal to the macula.

low the examiner to distinguish pigmented from nonpigmented lesions of the uvea.

2. *Fluorescein angiography*, which can be used to assess the vascular status of a mass involving the posterior choroid or iris. In particular, this test may distinguish vascular from avascular lesions and may determine the extent of plasma leakage from vascular spaces within a tumor. These findings are of little value, however, in distinguishing primary malignancies from metastatic ones (Davis and Robertson, 1973).

3. *Ultrasonography*, which provides an acoustic profile of intraocular and retrobulbar lesions. Two-dimensional ultrasonography is especially useful for evaluating tumors contained in eyes with opaque media that preclude ophthalmoscopic examination. One-dimensional ultrasonography can also provide a measure of "acoustic texture," which in some instances allows metastatic lesions with adenomatous structures or mucinous spaces to be distinguished from primary melanomas, which are histologically homogeneous (Coleman et al., 1974).

4. *Radiography, computed tomography, and magnetic resonance imaging*, which can provide essential informa-

tion on the size, shape, location, and infiltrative characteristics of orbital lesions (Fig. 31–3). Because of the high density of vital and delicate structures within the orbit, it is important to localize a lesion as precisely as possible before attempting diagnostic or therapeutic surgical intervention. High resolution computed tomographic scanning has also been used to characterize intraocular lesions (Jacobs et al., 1980). Unfortunately, in most instances these techniques do not allow metastases of the eye or orbit to be distinguished from primary malignancy. Some authors suggest that magnetic resonance imaging can be used to distinguish choroidal melanomas from metastatic lesions (Chambers et al., 1987). In at least one instance, however, a lesion with classic magnetic resonance imaging features of a melanoma proved to be metastatic breast cancer (Davidorf et al., 1992).

5. *Radioactive phosphorus uptake*, which provides a differential measure of the metabolic activity of an intraocular lesion compared with that of an uninvolved choroid. Thus, a hematoma or cyst can generally be detected because of minimal phosphorus uptake. On the other hand, metastatic and primary malignancies share a similar level of metabolic activity and thus cannot be distinguished with this method (Shields, 1978).

6. *Needle biopsy*, which can be performed on intraocular and orbital lesions. Although this procedure offers the opportunity for histologic diagnosis, occasionally the resulting diagnosis has been proved incorrect by subsequent surgical biopsy (Krohel et al., 1985). Furthermore, the potential exists for injury to ocular structures or for local dissemination of tumor cells. Needle biopsy should be reserved for those patients whose diagnosis cannot be determined with less invasive procedures (Shields, 1983; Karcioglu et al., 1985; and Liu, 1985).

7. *Aspiration of fluid* from the anterior chamber, vitreous, or subretinal space, which also offers the opportunity for histologic diagnosis of malignant cells (Piro et al., 1982; Scholz et al., 1983; and Sternberg et al., 1984). Although this procedure is potentially less dangerous than direct needle biopsy of a tumor, opportunity for serious complications still exists, and the material obtained is sometimes insufficient for cytologic analysis. This technique should also be reserved for selected cases.

A special diagnostic dilemma is presented by patients

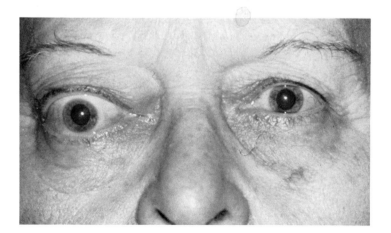

Figure 31–2. Breast carcinoma metastatic to the orbit, displacing the right eye forward, downward, and temporally.

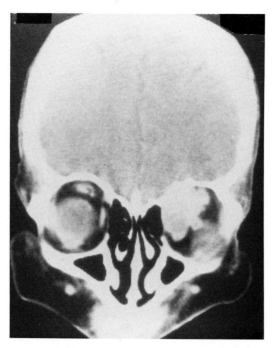

Figure 31–3. Computed tomographic scan of patient in Figure 31–2, showing large metastatic lesion in the superonasal portion of the orbit.

with a mass in the orbit or choroid who have no known primary tumor. Pigmented choroidal malignancies almost always represent either metastatic melanoma or primary intraocular disease, but a nonpigmented tumor may represent primary amelanotic melanoma, metastatic carcinoma, or one of a number of uncommon lesions (e.g., choroidal hemangioma, sarcoid granuloma). Patients with a known primary tumor but with no extraocular metastasis also present a dilemma, as the ocular lesions might represent an independent process. When confronted with such dilemmas, it is often best for one to perform a systemic evaluation in search of an occult primary cancer or other metastases before resorting to invasive procedures on the eye or orbit.

Important insight is provided by Doig and associates (1992), who examined 21 breast cancer patients with symptoms of visual loss from choroidal metastasis. Of these, seven had no known extraocular metastasis at the time. Upon systemic evaluation, however, all but one of the seven had metastatic extraocular lesions not previously diagnosed. This suggests that a thorough evaluation discloses the systemic nature of their disease for most patients with visual loss as the first symptom of metastases. Thus, for a patient with visual loss from a choroidal lesion of uncertain origin, a negative result on breast examination combined with negative results on systemic work-up provides substantial evidence excluding metastatic breast cancer as the etiology.

Given the prevalence of breast carcinoma and its propensity for ocular metastasis, all women with an unexplained orbital or intraocular nonpigmented lesion should be examined for occult breast cancer.

TREATMENT

Irradiation is well established as the most effective treatment for a variety of ophthalmic malignancies, including metastatic adenocarcinoma of the breast. Several workers report improvement or stabilization in a majority of eyes with intraocular metastasis (Wilmer, 1934; Jaeger et al., 1971; Thatcher and Thomas, 1975; Maor et al., 1977; Mewis and Young 1982; Panizzoni et al., 1990; Ratanatharathorn et al., 1991; and Doig et al., 1992). It should be noted that some therapists recommend prophylactic treatment to fellow eyes that do not demonstrate clinically detectable lesions (Panizzoni et al., 1990). Radiation therapy also benefits patients with orbital metastasis (Henderson, 1973; and Huh et al., 1974). The standard regimen includes 2500 to 3000 cGy delivered in 10 sessions over 2 to 3 weeks from a lateral port that spares the cornea and the lens. Serious complications are relatively uncommon, in part because of the limited life expectancy of these patients.

Chemotherapy, although less consistently effective than radiation for ophthalmic metastasis, may stabilize some lesions (Mewis and Young, 1982). Logani and colleagues (1992) suggest that high titers of estrogen receptors may indicate high susceptibility to chemotherapy. As patients with metastatic ocular disease often have extraocular dissemination, systemic therapy may be indicated, even though dissemination is not clinically apparent.

Palliative surgery should be limited to patients with blind or nearly blind eyes that are painful and unresponsive to radiation therapy, in whom enucleation can lead to prompt relief of pain. Surgery with curative intent can be justified in two clinical settings, provided that no evidence of extraocular disease is present: (1) partial iridectomy when the lesion involves only the iris; and (2) enucleation when the lesion involves only the ciliary body or choroid. Such intervention, however, rarely is justified in clinical practice.

SURVIVAL

On the average, patients survive approximately 1 year beyond the diagnosis of metastatic cancer to the eye or ocular adnexa (Hart, 1962; Jaeger et al., 1971; Thatcher and Thomas, 1975; Maor et al., 1977; Stephens and Shields, 1979; and Mewis and Young, 1982). Some encouraging information is provided by Bullock and Yanes (1980), who found that a patient with occult breast carcinoma survived a diagnosis of ocular metastasis for 36 months. Seven patients with known breast cancer survived the diagnosis of a first metastasis to the eye for an average of 27 months. Six of the seven patients were still living at the time of publication. In contrast, 22 patients who developed ocular metastases subsequent to the discovery of extraocular metastases survived for an average of only 3 months. These findings suggest that metastases confined to ophthalmic structures carry a substantially better prognosis than cancer disseminated to multiple sites.

The work of Ratanatharathorn and associates (1991) offers a more pessimistic picture. For 18 patients with choroidal metastasis, median survival was only 6 months from the time of diagnosis of ocular metastasis, whereas for 11 patients with orbital metastasis median survival was only 2 months. Furthermore, for those seven patients with ophthalmic metastasis as the first sign of dissemination, survival was no better than for the remaining patients.

SUMMARY

Among women, the breast is the predominant source of metastasis to the eye and ocular adnexa. Ophthalmic metastasis may represent the first clinical manifestation of breast carcinoma, and this malignancy should be included in the differential diagnosis of all women who have an infiltrative lid lesion, a mass lesion of the orbit, or a nonpigmented lesion of the choroid. Women with breast cancer who develop ocular signs or symptoms should be referred promptly to an ophthalmologist. Although survival is limited following the development of ophthalmic metastases, timely diagnosis and treatment can greatly enhance the quality of life for these patients.

References

Albert, D. M., Rubenstein, R. A., and Scheie, H. G.: Metastases to the eye: Part I. Incidence in 213 adult patients with generalized malignancy. Am. J. Ophthalmol., 63:723, 1977.

Arnold A. C., Bullock, J. D., and Foos, R. Y.: Metastatic eyelid carcinoma. Ophthalmology, 92:114, 1985.

Bloch, M. S., and Gartner, S.: Incidence of ocular metastatic carcinoma. Arch. Ophthalmol., 85:673, 1971.

Bullock, J. D., and Yanes, B.: Ophthalmic manifestations of metastatic breast carcinoma. Ophthalmology, 87:961, 1980.

Chambers, R. B., Davidorf, F. H., McAdoo, J. F., et al.: Magnetic resonance imaging of uveal melanomas. Arch. Ophthalmol., 105:917, 1987.

Coleman, D. J., Abramson, D. H., Jack, R. L., et al.: Ultrasonic diagnosis of the choroid. Arch. Ophthalmol., 91:344, 1974.

Davidorf, F. H., Chambers, R. B., and Gresak, P.: False-positive magnetic resonance imaging of a metastatic carcinoma simulating a malignant melanoma. Ann. Ophthalmol., 24:391, 1992.

Davis, D. L., and Robertson, D. M.: Fluorescein angiography of metastatic choroidal tumors. Arch. Ophthalmol., 89:97, 1973.

Doig, R. G., Jeal, P. N., Oliver, I. N., et al.: Symptomatic choroidal metastases in breast cancer. Aust. N. Z. J. Med., 22:349, 1992.

Ferry, A. P., and Font, R. L.: Carcinoma metastatic to the eye and orbit: I. A clinicopathological study of 227 cases. Arch. Ophthalmol., 92:276, 1974.

Ferry, A. P., and Font, R. L.: Carcinoma metastatic to the eye and orbit: II. A clinicopathological study of 26 patients with carcinoma metastatic to the anterior segment of the eye. Arch. Ophthalmol., 93:472, 1975.

Font, R. L., and Ferry, A. P.: Carcinoma metastatic to the eye and orbit: III. A clinicopathologic study of 28 cases metastatic to the orbit. Cancer, 38:1326, 1976.

Hart, W. M.: Metastatic carcinoma of the eye and orbit. Int. Ophthalmol. Clin., 2:465, 1962.

Henderson, J. W.: Orbital Tumors. Philadelphia, W. B. Saunders, 1973.

Huh, S. H., Nisce, L. Z., Simpson, L. D., et al.: Value of radiation therapy in the treatment of orbital metastasis. A. J. R. Am. J. Roentgenol., 120:589, 1974.

Hutchinson, D. S., and Smith, T. R.: Ocular and orbital metastatic carcinoma. Ann. Ophthalmol., 11:869, 1979.

Jacobs, L., Weisberg, L. A., and Kinkel, W. R.: Computerized Tomography of the Orbit and Sella Turcica. New York, Raven Press, 1980.

Jaeger, E. A., Frayer, W. C., Southard, M. E., et al.: Effects of radiation therapy on metastatic choroidal tumors. Trans. Am. Acad. Ophthalmol. Otol., 75:94, 1971.

Karcioglu, A. A., Gordon, R. A., and Karcioglu, G. L.: Tumor seeding in ocular fine needle aspiration biopsy. Ophthalmology, 92:1763, 1985.

Krohel, G. B., Tobin, D. R., and Chavis, R. M.: Inaccuracy of fine needle aspiration biopsy. Ophthalmology, 92:666, 1985.

Leys, A. M., Van Eyck, L. M., Nuttin, B. J., et al.: Metastatic carcinoma to the retina: Clinicopathologic findings in two cases. Arch. Ophthalmol., 108:1448, 1990.

Liu, D.: Complications of fine needle aspiration biopsy of the orbit. Ophthalmology, 92:1768, 1985.

Logani, S., Gomez, H., and Jampol, L. M.: Resolution of choroidal metastasis in breast cancer with high estrogen receptors. Arch. Ophthalmol., 110:451, 1992.

Maor, M., Chan, R. C., and Young, S. E.: Radiotherapy of choroidal metastases: Breast cancer as primary site. Cancer, 40:2081, 1977.

Mewis, L., and Young, S. E.: Breast carcinoma metastatic to the choroid: Analysis of 67 patients. Ophthalmology, 89:147, 1982.

Nelson, C. C., Hertzberg, B. S., and Klintworth, G. K.: A histopathologic study of 716 unselected eyes in patients with cancer at the time of death. Am. J. Ophthalmol., 95:788, 1983.

Panizzoni, G. A., Gasparini, G., Fior, S. D., et al.: Radiotherapeutic treatment for breast cancer choroidal metastases. Tumori, 76:563, 1990.

Piro, P., Pappas, H. R., Erozan, Y. S., et al.: Diagnostic vitrectomy in metastatic breast carcinoma in the vitreous. Retina, 2:182, 1982.

Ratanatharathorn, V., Powers, W. E., Grimm, J., et al.: Eye metastasis from carcinoma of the breast: Diagnosis, radiation treatment and results. Cancer Treat. Rev., 18:261, 1991.

Scholz, R., Green, R., Baranao, E. C., et al.: Metastatic carcinoma to the iris: Diagnosis by aqueous paracentesis and response to irradiation and chemotherapy. Ophthalmology, 90:1524, 1983.

Shields, J. A.: Accuracy and limitations of the ^{32}P test in the diagnosis of ocular tumors: An analysis of 500 cases. Ophthalmology, 85:950, 1978.

Shields, J. A.: Diagnosis and Management of Intraocular Tumors. St. Louis, C. V. Mosby, 1983.

Stephens, R. F., and Shields, J. A.: Diagnosis and management of cancer metastatic to the uvea: A study of 70 cases. Ophthalmology, 86:1336, 1979.

Sternberg, P., Tiedman, J., Hickingbotham, D., et al.: Controlled aspiration of subretinal fluid in the diagnosis of carcinoma metastatic to the choroid. Arch. Ophthalmol., 102:1622, 1984.

Thatcher, N., and Thomas, P. R. M.: Choroidal metastases from breast carcinoma: A survey of 42 patients and the use of radiation therapy. Clin. Radiol., 26:549, 1975.

Usher, C. H.: Cases of metastatic carcinoma of the choroid and iris. Br. J. Ophthalmol., 7:10, 1923.

Weiss, L.: Analysis of the incidence of intraocular metastasis. Br. J. Ophthalmol., 77:149, 1993.

Wilmer, W. H.: Atlas Fundus Oculi. New York, Macmillan, 1934.

32

Neurologic Aspects of Breast Cancers

Christopher B. Shields
George H. Raque
Paul K. Gardner

The central nervous system (CNS) is a frequent site of spread of metastatic breast cancer. This may be due either to direct involvement of neural tissue, as in the case of cerebral metastasis, or to compression of neural structures from metastasis to surrounding tissues, as in the case of spinal cord compression from vertebral or epidural tumor. The most frequent sites of CNS metastases are the cerebrum (58%), leptomeninges (21%), cerebellum (16%), brain stem (3%), optic nerve (3%), and spinal cord (2%) (Kiricuta et al., 1992). As the treatment of systemic disease has improved, central nervous system metastases have increased in frequency, owing to the prolonged exposure of the brain, spinal cord, and vertebral axis to viable circulating tumor cells.

Because of the blood-brain barrier, once a metastasis has seeded the CNS it is relatively secluded, which diminishes the effects of systemically administered chemotherapeutic agents. The presence of CNS metastases affects prognosis in a negative fashion, and requires aggressive, often multimodal therapy, especially in cases where systemic disease is well controlled. The therapeutic challenges may include (1) surgical and nonsurgical treatment of cerebral and spinal metastasis, (2) relief of intractable pain, and (3) differentiation of the effects of complications of therapy from those of recurrent CNS metastases. In this chapter we address areas of neurologic involvement in breast cancer (i.e., intracranial and spinal metastasis, leptomeningeal carcinomatosis, neurologic complications of therapy, and pain control).

INTRACRANIAL METASTASIS

The CNS is the first site of metastatic involvement in 61% of patients with breast cancer (Kiricuta et al., 1992). Cerebral metastases are recognized clinically in some 5% to 16% of all victims of breast cancer (Gamache et al., 1982; and Patanaphan et al., 1988) and in 10% to 34% of autopsy series (Yap et al., 1978; DiStefano et al., 1979). Metastasis to the brain may be hematogenous, though direct compression of neural tissue from cranial metastasis may occur. Only rarely, however, does tumor invade cerebral tissue through intact dura. Cerebellar metastasis occasionally arises through Batson's venous plexus, located in the spinal epidural space, which serves as a direct line of communi-

cation from the spine to the intracranial contents (Boogerd et al., 1991). The frontal lobes of the cerebrum are the most frequent site of metastatic deposits; the prevalence is proportional to the greater cerebral blood flow to that area. The hallmark of cerebral metastases is their multiplicity, but single lesions do occur. Metastatic deposits tend to be well demarcated from adjacent brain tissue, both grossly and microscopically, though there is often considerable surrounding edema, which can magnify the neurologic deficit. An estimated 50% of presumed single lesions have unrecognized multiple cerebral metastases (Gamache et al., 1982). The advent of gadolinium-enhanced magnetic resonance imaging (MRI) has greatly facilitated the detection of multiple metastatic deposits and currently is the examination of choice for evaluation of metastatic disease. Metastases to the brain are more likely to occur in association with Stage IV breast tumors, especially when axillary lymph nodes are involved, and less frequently with Stage I disease (Korzeniowski et al., 1987).

Symptoms of cerebral metastases are related to their location and growth rate. The interval from diagnosis of the primary lesion to cerebral involvement ranges from 3 to 192 months (median = 37 months) (Gamache et al., 1982). Headaches, confusion, disorientation, focal or generalized seizures, hemiparesis, and visual field defects constitute the commonly recognized symptoms that suggest cerebral metastasis in patients with breast cancer. Posterior fossa deposits may cause limb or gait ataxia and signs of increased intracranial pressure from obstruction of the fourth ventricle or aqueduct of Sylvius. The median survival time from the first symptom of cerebral metastasis is 4 to 6 months (DiStefano et al., 1979; Kiricuta et al., 1992), although long-term survival (more than 18 months) does occur (DiStefano et al., 1979). Longer survival is noted when the interval between the onset of primary tumor and the first cerebral signs is greater (Kamby et al., 1988). Survival is greater in patients with "negative" axillary lymph nodes (12 months) than in those with involved lymph nodes (3 months) (Patanaphan et al., 1988). No patient in Kiricuta's series survived more than 10 years with CNS metastases (Kiricuta et al., 1992).

Plain radiographs of the skull may reveal an osteolytic or osteoblastic deposit lodged in the diploic space. Unenhanced computed tomography (CT) may show a decreased attenuation coefficient, with a shift of the midline structures away from the side of the tumor. Both tumor mass and cerebral edema around the tumor cause the mass effect. Contrast enhancement with a nonionic agent usually results in tumor enhancement in the form of a solid, homogeneous mass (Fig. 32–1*A*) or a ring-enhancing lesion (Fig. 32–1*B*). Multiple enhancing deposits tend to confirm the diagnosis of metastatic tumor.

Unenhanced MRI (T1-weighted) of metastatic breast tumors reveals an area of low intensity to isointensity of the lesion relative to the normal brain. Much of the low intensity on this scan may be due to surrounding cerebral edema; however, the tumor nodule may be slightly more intense than the edema. Unenhanced T2-weighted MR images show marked hyperintensity, which represents vasogenic edema surrounding a nodule of tumor. On T1-weighted MRI there may be a line isointense with gray matter that separates the hyperintense nodule from the hyperintense edema (Latchaw et al., 1991). Contrast-enhanced T1-weighted MRI demonstrates a hyperintense enhancing nodule (see Fig. 32–1*A*) surrounded by low-intensity or isointense edema. There is little difference in the demonstration of intracranial metastases comparing enhanced and unenhanced CT and plain MRI (Taphoorn et al., 1989), though gadolinium-enhanced MRI has significantly increased the detection of small metastatic deposits as compared to CT

(Healy et al., 1987). Plain radiographs of the skull may reveal an osteolytic or osteoblastic deposit.

A diagnostic challenge may occasionally arise if a solitary mass lesion is detected. Primary brain tumors, meningiomas, brain abscesses, or resolving strokes can all present in a clinically identical fashion and may be differentiated from a solitary metastasis by interval CT and MRI (T1 and T2). If doubt persists, stereotactic biopsy of the lesion may be necessary to confirm the diagnosis.

Before treatment is instituted, the extent of systemic involvement must be assessed with a chest radiograph, bone scan, and a liver-spleen scan to provide information on prognosis. Intensive treatment may be justified for patients whose Karnofsky score (a measure of neurologic function) is 60 or better.

Treatment

Treatment of cerebral metastases may include surgery, radiotherapy, chemotherapy, or a combination of several modalities. Therapy must be individualized, but decisions are based on the presence of a single—versus multiple—intracranial tumor or of widespread systemic metastases, neuro-

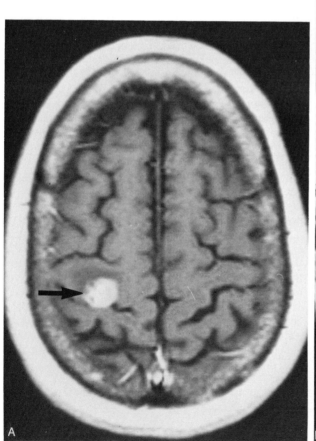
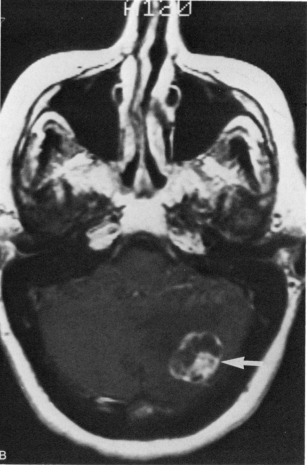

Figure 32–1. MRI scan that demonstrates multiple metastases of breast cancer (*arrows*) affecting the right parietal lobe (*A*) and the left cerebellar hemisphere (*B*).

logic status, age of the patient, and whether prior therapy was administered (Black, 1979*a*).

Patients who harbor a single cerebral metastasis may be treated by craniotomy and surgical removal. Surgery is indicated when the nature of the intracranial mass is in doubt and the tumor is larger than 3 cm in diameter and located in an accessible site. Posterior fossa metastatic tumors can cause rapid deterioration and death from hydrocephalus and cerebral herniation or direct pressure on the brain stem, and should be treated aggressively, usually with combined surgical resection and radiotherapy. In general, surgical therapy is recommended only if there is minimal evidence of systemic disease and the prognosis for survival is greater than 1 year. Whole brain radiotherapy lengthens mean survival by 3 to 6 months (Salvati et al., 1992). A high correlation between carcinoma of the breast and cerebral meningiomas has been documented, which further increases the risk of misdiagnosis of a single intracranial lesion (Mehta et al., 1983). The mortality rate following removal of a solitary metastasis is approximately 10% to 15% (Black, 1979*a*); however, the cause of death in 84% of patients was related to progression of the systemic disease and not directly to the surgical procedure (Salvati et al., 1992).

If the patient is comatose owing to increased intracranial pressure from one or more intracranial deposits, intravenous administration of dexamethasone, 10 mg initial dose followed by 6 mg every 6 hours, may significantly reduce peritumoral edema and result in marked neurologic improvement. The favorable response to the first dose of dexamethasone can be dramatic; the patient's condition may change from comatose to alert and conversant. Megadose steroids (dexamethasone up to 100 mg per day) may be administered for multiple cerebral metastases near the end of a terminal course. If the patient exhibits focal neurologic deficits (such as hemiparesis, hemianopia, aphasia) but is awake and alert, has multiple intracranial deposits, or has widespread systemic metastases, management is nonsurgical. Corticosteroid therapy may produce dramatic alleviation of symptoms in 70% to 75% of patients. The mechanism of action of steroids is ill understood, but the degree of cerebral edema does appear to be diminished on sequential CT or MRI scans. Often, the symptoms resolve within hours of initiating steroid therapy. If used in combination with radiotherapy, corticosteroid therapy is maintained for 1 week following completion of radiotherapy and then the dose is gradually tapered. Antacids (aluminum hydroxide [Amphojel] or histamine H2 antagonists [Cimetidine]) are administered with steroids to diminish the risk of gastrointestinal ulceration and subsequent hemorrhage. Anticonvulsant medications (phenytoin, 300 mg at bedtime) decrease the risk of seizures; however, both steroid withdrawal and hepatic metastases may induce phenytoin toxicity, so close monitoring of plasma levels is required for several months.

Cerebral metastases from breast cancers are moderately radiosensitive, so if multiple intracranial deposits exist and the patient's general condition is stable, radiotherapy is the treatment of choice. Several radiotherapeutic regimens exist. Gamache and associates (1982) recommend 5 Gy on days 1 to 3, no radiation on days 4 to 7, 3 Gy on days 8 to 12, no radiation on days 13 and 14, and 3 Gy on days 15 to 17. This provides a total dose of 39 Gy in 17 days. Total head radiotherapy (3900 rad in 17 days) is widely practiced following removal of a single mass or for multiple metastases. Even following craniotomy for mass removal, the likelihood of total removal of microscopic deposits from the tumor bed is remote, and the likelihood that multiple microscopic deposits remain is 15% to 50% (Gamache et al., 1982). The roles of surgery and radiotherapy are complementary, and provide an optimal chance for prolonged survival.

New hope has been provided within the past 5 years to patients with deep-seated gray matter or brain stem metastases that are not amenable to direct surgical removal. Focused beam irradiation (radiosurgery) has been utilized with great success to treat these metastatic tumors. This treatment consists of administration of multiple beams of highly focused radiation to intracranial deposits. Common delivery systems include the LINAC scalpel (x-ray), γ-knife (gamma rays), and heavy-particle units (helium or proton beam). Rather than depending on the differential radiosensitivity of normal brain tissue and tumor to create a therapeutic effect, radiosurgery creates an area of tissue destruction where the multiple noncoplanar radiation sources intersect.

This technique is performed on an outpatient basis. A stereotactic head ring is applied, followed by enhanced CT (or MRI) to allow precise localization of the intracranial metastasis. Following a treatment-planning session in which the optimal dose plan is developed, the patient undergoes a single treatment of focused irradiation, using a precisely focused collimator aimed at the metastatic deposit. Up to 0.2 mm precision is available with some radiosurgery units. Up to three intracranial deposits can be treated at a single session, each lesion receiving as much as 1500 cGy to the 80% isodose curve.

Early results following radiosurgery are favorable. In a series of 33 patients with a variety of intracranial metastases, 50% of the deposits were significantly reduced in size, 12% had stabilized in size, and 29% had disappeared (Adler et al., 1992). If the patient has had prior whole brain radiotherapy, radiosurgery may pose a problem owing to the possibility of radionecrosis of normal brain adjacent to the metastatic tumor.

Chemotherapy may also play a part in the treatment of cerebral metastases. Standard doses of cyclophosphamide, methotrexate, and 5-fluorouracil (CMF), or cyclophosphamide, doxorubicin, and 5-fluorouracil (CAF), combined with corticosteroids initially produced clinical improvement in 75% of patients with breast cancer with cerebral metastases; however, this response is not associated with improved survival because most patients die from progressive systemic disease (Boogerd et al., 1991).

Rosner and colleagues (1986), used several combinations of chemotherapeutic agents, and noted that 40% of the patients had a partial neurologic response and 10% had complete resolution (median duration, 7 months and more than 10 months, respectively). There was also a favorable response of systemic disease using this regimen. In addition, competitive endocrine therapy using tamoxifen may provide long-term remission of metastases in the brain (Pors et al., 1991).

SPINAL METASTASIS

Some 37% to 53% of all breast cancers metastasize to the spinal column, particularly to the thoracic spine (Black, 1979b), and less often to the lumbar or the cervical spine. Metastatic deposits usually involve either the vertebral body or the epidural space (Livingston and Perrin, 1978). Spread along the spinal axis is facilitated by Batson's plexus, a valveless network of veins in the epidural space of the spinal canal. Direct extension to the thoracic spine may also occur from a posterior mediastinal metastasis through the intervertebral foramina. Breast tumors rarely metastasize to the spinal cord (intramedullary) (Fig. 32–2). It is also unusual for metastatic cancer to traverse the dura, as it usually serves as an effective barrier to tumor cells (Black, 1979b).

Symptoms of spinal metastases depend on both the level of spinal involvement and the rate of expansion of the metastatic deposit. Back pain that is more severe at night is the hallmark of spinal metastasis. Metastatic disease to the spine is noted in 38% of patients known to have cancer who complain of back pain alone (Maranzano et al., 1992). Numbness and weakness of the arms and legs may occur with cervical metastases, and similar symptoms in the legs may be associated with thoracic or lumbar metastases. Objective evidence of a neurologic deficit is present in 50% to 70% of patients at the time an epidural metastasis is diagnosed. Bladder and bowel dysfunction are present in half the patients at the time of diagnosis (Gilbert et al., 1978). The sensory level is a more reliable indicator of the segmental level of metastasis than is loss of motor function. Symptoms frequently "evolve" over the course of several

weeks, during which time recognition of the symptoms affords the alert diagnostician an opportunity to prevent a downhill course from weakness to quadriplegia in the case of cervical cord compression, or paraplegia with thoracic and lumbar lesions. The earlier the spinal metastasis is recognized, the sooner treatment can be instituted, resulting in a better prognosis. Neurologic deficits resulting from spinal cord compression should be treated emergently, as even long-standing symptoms can progress rapidly. Acute progression of paraplegia in less than 24 hours carries an extremely poor prognosis, as spinal cord infarction has likely occurred and there is no hope of neurologic recovery.

Radiologic confirmation is sought once the diagnosis is suspected. As 17% of patients have multiple spinal lesions, the entire spine requires evaluation (Gilbert et al., 1978). Plain radiographs of the spine may reveal pathologic compression fractures, osteoblastic infiltration, subluxation, kyphosis, or paravertebral soft tissue swelling at the site of the metastasis. Involvement of bone does not invariably signify the presence of an epidural deposit, nor are epidural deposits invariably associated with adjacent bony metastases. CT is ideal for identifying bony abnormalities and can define osteoblastic lesions in the vertebral body and neural arch more clearly than plain radiographs. Furthermore, enhanced CT often demonstrates the relative contribution of bone or epidural tumor at a site of narrowing of the spinal canal.

MRI can also be used to evaluate spinal metastasis, and it has major diagnostic advantages over both myelography and CT by visualizing both bony elements and neural structures. Spinal puncture, with its inherent discomfort and risk of infection or sudden neurologic deterioration, is also avoided. If the needle is placed below a complete or nearly complete spinal block, myelography may convert an incomplete neurologic defect to a complete and permanent one. MRI of the spine may demonstrate collapse of the vertebral body, tumor involvement of the vertebra, epidural metastasis (with or without spinal cord compression), leptomeningeal seeding, or intramedullary metastasis. In many cases, MRI has replaced myelography as the procedure of choice for evaluating metastatic disease of the spine.

Treatment

Once spinal metastasis has occurred, total cure is unlikely and the treatment is mainly palliative. Decompressive laminectomy used to be the standard therapy for epidural deposits, but Posner and coworkers asserted that radiotherapy was superior to surgery (Gilbert et al., 1978; and Slatkin and Posner, 1983).

Metastatic tumors from the breast are moderately radiosensitive, so most spinal deposits are treated with a course of local tumor radiotherapy. If the lesion remains entirely intraosseous (without expansion of the periosteum), pain is unlikely; however, once the pain-sensitive periosteum is stretched, back pain becomes a major symptom. Conventional radiotherapy of the metastatic tumor is the treatment of choice for such lesions. Ten days of divided doses for a total of 3000 cGy is provided to relieve the pain and achieve radiographic resolution of the lesion.

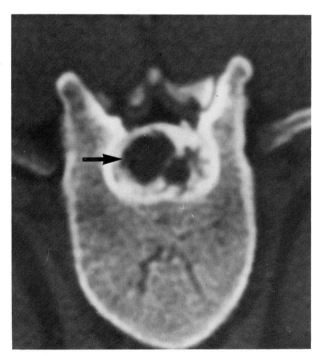

Figure 32–2. Intradural metastases of breast tumors involving the conus medullaris (*arrow*) at the level of the L-1 vertebral body.

For metastatic deposits in the epidural space (with or without vertebral involvement), radiotherapy to the spine is usually recommended. If the decision is made to treat an intraspinal metastasis by radiotherapy, close monitoring of neurologic status is mandatory. Should the patient's neurologic condition deteriorate, emergency laminectomy may be necessary. Clinical results of radiotherapy alone versus surgery plus radiotherapy for metastasis to the spine are difficult to assess. Black (1979*b*) reviewed the results for metastatic tumors from various primary sites and noted that the rate of improvement following surgery alone was 30%, following radiotherapy alone 46%, and following a combination of surgery and radiotherapy 51%. The only prospective randomized study performed to date showed no significant difference between the effectiveness of radiotherapy alone and that of surgery plus radiotherapy, with respect to pain relief, improved ambulation, or improved sphincter function. As expected, patients with a complete myelographic block (Tomita et al., 1983) fared less well than those with an incomplete block.

Maranzano and colleagues (1992) studied the effect of radiotherapy alone on 56 patients with metastatic disease and spinal cord compression, with or without a neurologic deficit. Their regimen consisted of a split-course program: 5 Gy to the affected area of spine each day, then a break for 4 days. Patients who showed some response to initial treatment received an additional 5-day course of radiation. The target volume covered two vertebrae above and two vertebrae below the site of neural compression, and laterally included the entire mass as demonstrated by MRI. Eighty-nine percent of patients with back pain showed improvement or elimination of their symptoms, and four of six patients with urinary dysfunction responded to treatment. Of 35 patients with motor dysfunction at the onset of treatment, 60% regained the ability to walk and the condition of 14% who were able to walk with support did not deteriorate. All 21 patients without motor deficits before treatment maintained normal strength after treatment (Maranzano et al., 1992).

Surgical intervention is indicated for patients who present with rapidly progressive motor weakness, when there is doubt about the etiology of the tumor, or when spinal cord compression is caused by bone fragments from a pathologic fracture. Surgical decompression is performed on an emergent basis, as the chance of recovery of function in the face of a complete neurologic lesion is small. Surgical intervention may also be beneficial for selected patients who have previously received maximal radiotherapy to the spine. In any of these situations, wide decompressive laminectomy providing access to the dural tube is required. This approach allows exposure for multiple-level, bilateral nerve root decompression and for intradural exploration if it is needed. If the spine is unstable, either owing to tumor invasion or secondary to surgical decompression, instrumented fusion is performed with either autogenous or banked bone graft. If extensive destruction of the bony spine exists and the life expectancy is very limited, a posterior spinal approach with the application of Luque rectangles encased in methylmethacrylate often provides adequate spinal stability (Fig. 32–3); however, if a pathologic compression fracture of a vertebral body or an anteriorly situated tumor causes anterior spinal cord compression, an anterior approach is the procedure of choice, particularly if the patient is in good medical condition and disease is limited to one or two segments. The involved vertebral bodies are removed, and the tumor is debulked, if feasible. Once decompression of the neural elements is achieved, stability of the spine is restored by insertion of autogenous iliac crest graft, banked fibular bone strut, or methylmethacrylate reinforced with Steinmann pins. Owing to the difficulty of spinal reconstruction, anterior techniques are limited to no more than three segmental levels. More extensive disease is best treated through a posterior approach. Occasionally, a combined (anterior and posterior) procedure may be indicated, either in a single operation or separated by several days (Fig. 32–4).

A corticosteroid (usually dexamethasone) is used as adjuvant therapy, but the role of this class of drugs is less well established than it is for cerebral metastasis. The standard dosage of dexamethasone is 16 to 24 mg per day, though megadoses of methylprednisolone (1 g/day) occasionally are required to achieve the desired results (Slatkin and Posner, 1983).

Hormonal therapy has been used effectively to treat painful spinal metastases from breast tumors, but its role in relieving neurologic dysfunction is not established (Slatkin and Posner, 1983). Boogerd and colleagues (1988) showed that chemotherapy and/or hormonal therapy can occasionally be of value for treatment of spinal epidural metastases. Chemotherapy has consisted of tamoxifen, aminoglutethimidine, cyclophosphamide (CTX), methotrexate, and 5-fluorouracil.

LEPTOMENINGEAL CARCINOMATOSIS

The incidence of leptomeningeal carcinomatosis has increased as a result of prolonged survival of patients with systemic cancer, increased awareness of this condition, and the recognition that most chemotherapeutic drugs fail to cross the blood-brain barrier. This allows the subarachnoid space to serve as a sanctuary where tumor cells escape the cytotoxic effects of chemotherapeutic agents. Breast cancer is the most frequent cause of leptomeningeal seeding of tumor cells (Sondak et al., 1981; and Horton, 1984). Leptomeningeal carcinomatosis is rarely the presenting symptom of breast cancer; however, the cerebrospinal fluid pathway was the site of recurrent disease following remission in 11 of 25 patients in one series (Yap et al., 1978; and Harris et al., 1984). As many as 5% of patients with breast cancers developed clinical evidence of leptomeningeal carcinomatosis (Yap et al., 1978), and as many as 75% in autopsy series were found to have it (Lesse and Netsky, 1954). The interval from identification of the first evidence of metastatic disease to the diagnosis of leptomeningeal carcinomatosis averaged 15 months (range = 1 to 37 months) (Yap et al., 1978; and Sondak et al., 1981).

Leptomeningeal carcinoma should be suspected when a patient with a history of breast cancer develops symptoms of cerebral, cranial nerve, spinal root, or meningeal involvement. Headache, confusion, dementia, seizures, visual and auditory symptoms, and cranial nerve abnormalities (Black,

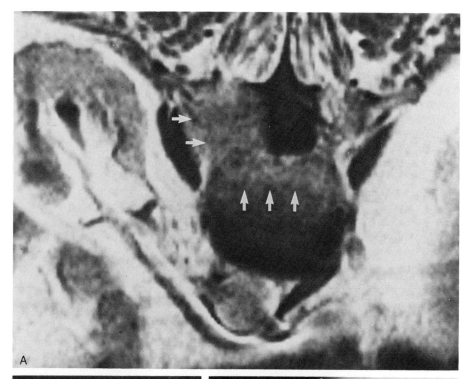

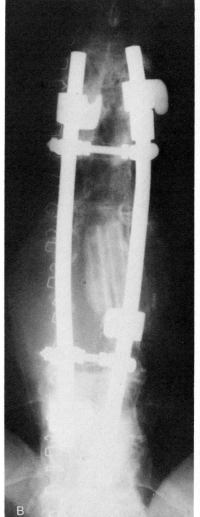

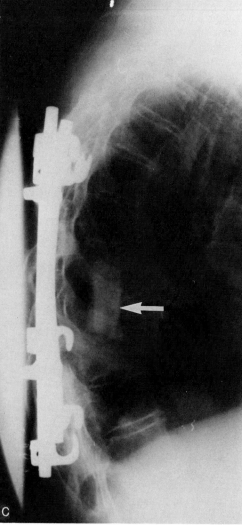

Figure 32–3. *A,* Preoperative MRI scan that demonstrates a metastasis from a breast cancer affecting the T-8 vertebral body and right pedicle *(arrows)*. Postoperative anteroposterior *(B)* and lateral *(C)* thoracic radiographs of the spine following vertebrectomy of the T-8 vertebral body, pediculotomy, autogenous strut graft placement *(arrow)*, and posterior spinal fusion with instrumentation.

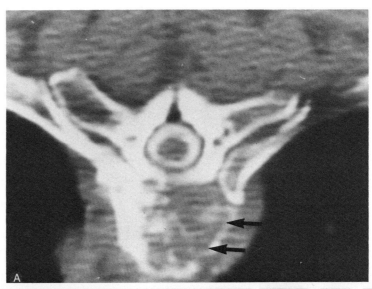

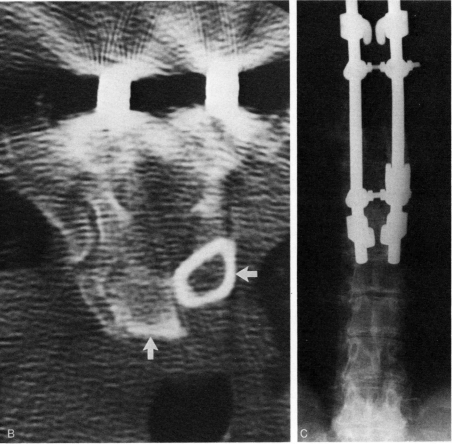

Figure 32–4. *A,* This preoperative postmyelographic CT scan shows a metastasis from breast cancer infiltrating the T-4 vertebral body *(arrows).* A postoperative CT scan *(B)* and an anteroposterior radiograph of the spine *(C)* following partial vertebrectomy, placement of two autogenous strut grafts between T-3 and T-5 *(arrows),* and posterior spinal stabilization with bone and instrumentation.

1979*a*; and Cantillo et al., 1979) characterize this disorder. Sudden onset of blindness (Cantillo et al., 1979) and acute bilateral hearing loss (Houck et al., 1992) are rare presentations of leptomeningeal carcinomatosis. Meningeal symptoms, such as neck pain and stiffness, and photophobia are common. Patients are usually afebrile, in contrast to those with infectious meningitis. Cerebral and spinal metastases must be excluded by gadolinium-enhanced MRI. The diagnosis of leptomeningeal carcinomatosis is confirmed by examination of cerebrospinal fluid (CSF), which is characterized by a decreased glucose level (less than 40 mg/dl), increased protein concentration (greater than 100 mg/dl), positive cytologic test for malignant cells (Yap et al., 1978), and negative cultures for bacteria and fungi. Levels of the biomarkers creatine kinase (CK) and its BB isoenzyme (CK-BB) in the CSF are frequently elevated above 0.2 U/L. This level was significantly higher in patients with leptomeningeal carcinomatosis than in patients with either

CNS metastases or parenchymal brain metastases only (Bach et al., 1990). Elevated CSF myelin basic protein was used as an indicator of disease activity in leptomeningeal carcinomatosis (Siegal et al., 1987). Cerebrospinal fluid also shows elevation of β-glucuronidase (above 27 mU/L) and of lactate dehydrogenase in leptomeningeal carcinomatosis (Twijnstra et al., 1987). Tissue polypeptide antigen elevation in CSF is a reliable marker of CNS metastasis of breast cancer. For CSF values of tissue polypeptide antigen above 95 U/L the sensitivity was 74% for breast cancer with CNS metastases and the specificity 100% (Bach et al., 1991). Tissue polypeptide antigen and BB isoenzyme may be elevated in leptomeningeal carcinomatosis, even if the cell count in CSF is normal (Bach et al., 1989, 1991).

Therapy of leptomeningeal carcinomatosis consists of combination radiotherapy, intrathecal chemotherapy (methotrexate, thiotepa, or cytosine arabinoside), and large doses of corticosteroids. Radiotherapy to the head (3900 rad over 2 weeks) has provided long-term improvement in many instances; however, the most widely accepted therapy is intrathecal methotrexate (25 mg twice per week). This is administered via an intraventricular cannula in the anterior horn of the right lateral ventricle or a lumbar subarachnoid cannula connected to an Ommaya reservoir placed subcutaneously. Rarely, this has been complicated by blindness and coma (Boogerd et al., 1989). Untreated, leptomeningeal carcinomatosis results in death in approximately 6 to 8 weeks (Sondak et al., 1981). Aggressive therapy consisting of combined radiotherapy and intrathecal methotrexate improves the median survival time to approximately 22 weeks (Sondak et al., 1981). Boogerd pointed out that the median survival time for chemotherapy responders is 5 months, versus 1 month for nonresponders (Boogerd et al., 1991). The longest reported survival was more than 3 years after the diagnosis of leptomeningeal carcinomatosis was made (Boogerd et al., 1991). Late neurotoxicity following aggressive treatment leads to impairment of the quality of life in more than 50% of long-term survivors (Boogerd et al., 1991).

NEUROLOGIC COMPLICATIONS OF CHEMOTHERAPY

Metastatic breast carcinoma is sensitive to chemotherapy. Various chemotherapeutic agents, including methotrexate and cyclophosphamide (Cytoxan), chlorambucil (Leukeran), thiotepa, and hormone therapy, have been used.

Chemotherapeutic agents (such as vincristine, cyclophosphamide, methotrexate, 5-fluorouracil, and prednisone), administered singly or in combination, may cause neurotoxicity in 65% of patients (McCarthy et al., 1992). Symptoms of neurotoxicity (particularly with vincristine) include pain, numbness, paresthesia, and involuntary movements. Voice changes occur with involvement of the trigeminal and glossopharyngeal nerves. Such changes were most frequent in patients younger than 50 years. Tamoxifen retinopathy has been reported as a rare occurrence of the administration of this drug, in either large or normal-sized doses (Bentley et al., 1992).

Methotrexate, an antimetabolite, interferes with purine metabolism by binding the enzyme dihydrofolate reductase, resulting in inhibition of the synthesis of purine and thymidylic acid. Standard doses of methotrexate given intravenously are frequently toxic to bone marrow, the gastrointestinal tract, and the liver, but they are not considered neurotoxic. Methotrexate is poorly transported across the blood-brain barrier, so its CSF concentration is less than 10% of that in plasma following conventional administration. Administration of methotrexate in innovative ways has been advocated—for example, intravenous administration of extremely large doses of methotrexate, direct instillation of methotrexate into the cerebral ventricles or lumbar subarachnoid space via an Ommaya reservoir; direct bolus administration into the internal carotid artery; and intratumor infusion. When these routes of administration are used neurotoxicity may be immediate or delayed. Manifestations of CNS toxicity from methotrexate are the following (Young, 1982):

Acute transient side effects of intrathecal injection of methotrexate may develop shortly following injection, reach maximum intensity at 6 to 12 hours, and last 2 to 3 days. The clinical picture mimics that of aseptic meningitis, manifested by meningismus, headaches, photophobia, nausea, vomiting, dizziness, and fever, along with a modest granulocytic pleocytosis on CSF examination. CSF cultures are all negative. It is not known whether this reaction is caused by the drug itself or by preservatives and impurities in the preparation. The disease is self-limited and resolves in 1 to 2 weeks, regardless of whether intraventricular methotrexate is continued.

Transient radiculopathy, which follows inadvertent injection into the lumbar epidural or subdural space, is of minor consequence and resolves spontaneously.

Acute transverse myelopathy, with transient or permanent paraplegia, is a rare complication of intrathecal methotrexate administration and presumably represents an idiosyncratic reaction to the drug (Gagliano et al., 1976).

Intrathecal methotrexate may also cause a *delayed methotrexate encephalopathy (disseminated necrotizing leukoencephalopathy)* manifested by a progressive personality change, apathy, confusion, lethargy, blindness, dementia, motor abnormalities (tremor, ataxia, hemiparesis), and seizures. The course may progress rapidly to a permanent vegetative state or death, though the majority of patients experience partial or complete recovery when the drug is withdrawn. Predisposing factors include multiple injections of methotrexate intrathecally or systemically, previous whole-brain radiotherapy, hydrocephalus, and concomitant use of vincristine and cytosine arabinoside (Boogerd et al., 1990). Variability exists in the clinical presentation, CT appearance, and histopathologic picture. The incidence of methotrexate leukoencephalopathy after intrathecal methotrexate therapy is 2%. CT may disclose multiple areas of lucency involving the white matter, periventricular enhancement with contrast administration, and ventriculomegaly, though some patients' CT scan is normal. Histologic examination of white matter reveals gliosis, spongiform changes, extensive demyelination with axonal swelling, and focal calcification. Treatment consists of discontinuing methotrexate and administering arabinoside-C and citrovorum factor. The median survival time of patients with leukoencephalopathy is 9 months (range = 6 to 41 months) (Boogerd et al., 1991).

Intraventricular administration of γ-interferon for the treatment of leptomeningeal carcinomatosis causes progressive neurologic deterioration that culminates in a vegetative state. Patients become unresponsive to verbal commands but open their eyes to auditory or tactile stimulation. They gradually return to their baseline level within 3 weeks following discontinuation of therapy (Meyers et al., 1991).

Tamoxifen (an antiestrogen compound) is effective in treating breast cancers that have estrogen receptors. Its neurologic complications are indirect and are caused by the development of hypercalcemia.

COMPLICATIONS OF RADIOTHERAPY FOR BREAST CANCER

Neurologic complications may follow radiotherapy of the primary lesion or metastases. Total head irradiation may be complicated by early or delayed reactions. *Early reactions* arise 3 to 10 weeks after completion of radiotherapy and are characterized by nausea, vomiting, ataxia, dysarthria, or cerebellar signs. This syndrome resolves spontaneously and completely over the course of several weeks. If the patient dies from unrelated causes, postmortem examination reveals changes consistent with disseminated demyelination and vasculitis in the radiation field (Rider, 1963).

Delayed cerebral radiation necrosis usually occurs 1 to 3 years after completion of radiotherapy but can appear as early as 3 months or as late as 12 years afterward. The clinical syndrome consists of headaches, seizures, personality changes, focal motor weakness, papilledema, dysphagia, and unconsciousness. The total radiation dose is usually between 5000 and 6000 rad. Sheline (1980) reported that 45 of 83 patients with radionecrosis received more than 7000 rad, and only 22 received less than 4500 rad. Total head irradiation of 5000 rad in 5 weeks is a relatively safe dose; however, higher doses may be justified for tumor control. Recurrent tumor and cerebral radionecrosis may be indistinguishable on clinical and radiographic grounds. Intracranial pressure may be elevated in both. The appearance of radionecrosis on enhanced CT is a hypodense mass lesion with peripheral enhancement. Such changes in the field of radiotherapy support the diagnosis of radionecrosis, but biopsy is often required to rule out residual or recurrent tumor.

The mechanism of radiation damage is controversial. Neural or vascular elements may be damaged primarily by radiation, or secondarily by the patient's immune system. Delayed radiation damage is a function of the total dose, individual fraction size, overall duration of treatment, volume of tissue irradiated, and modifying factors, such as oxygen supply, status of the vascularity, and type of radiation used (Berger, 1982). The role of prophylactic steroids during and following radiotherapy is unknown, but once radionecrosis develops, large doses of steroids (dexamethasone, 24 mg/day in divided doses) seem to be of value. If this is ineffective in reversing clinical deterioration, surgical extirpation of the focus of radionecrosis may be justified.

Following radiosurgery, there is a low incidence of radiation necrosis surrounding the area of treatment. Smaller-diameter lesions can be treated with a larger dose of radiation, but smaller doses are administered to large-diameter lesions. Should radiation necrosis develop, prolonged treatment with dexamethasone must be instituted.

Radiation myelitis may result from radiotherapy of the primary breast lesion or of spinal metastasis if the radiation portals include the spinal cord. *Acute transverse myelopathy* may be manifested several weeks after completion of radiotherapy as numbness and paresthesia of the arms or legs (or both) and a shocklike sensation in the trunk and extremities following neck flexion (Lhermitte's sign). Although Lhermitte's sign is a benign entity without associated objective signs, if it is present the patient must be monitored carefully for evidence of delayed *chronic progressive myelopathy,* the most frequent and devastating complication of spinal cord irradiation. Though it is most common within 1 year after radiotherapy, it may appear as long as 10 to 12 years after treatment. Initially, sensory symptoms predominate (paresthesia, hypesthesia, numbness), followed by spastic paraparesis or quadriparesis and sphincter disturbance. The clinical defects gradually progress over several months, followed by stabilization of the neurologic signs. Once they develop, these signs rarely regress. If the damaged cord was in the radiation field and MRI reveals an atrophic cord shadow, without evidence of spinal metastasis, radiation myelopathy is likely the diagnosis. Radiation myelopathy has no effective therapy; however, administration of large doses of steroids may alleviate progressive neurologic symptoms and signs. On histologic examination, necrosis of white matter exceeds that of gray matter. Vascular changes include hyalinization and fibrinoid degeneration of the arterial walls (Berger, 1982). The thoracic spinal cord is more susceptible to radiation myelopathy, as it contains a ''watershed area'' (T4–T6), which lies between the abundant blood supply of the upper thoracic segments and the thoracolumbar ones.

Vocal cord paralysis due to recurrent laryngeal nerve damage has been reported following radiation for breast cancer. Of 37 patients with vocal cord paralysis reported by Westbrook and coworkers (1974), radiation fibrosis was responsible in 2 patients, metastasis in 32, and miscellaneous causes in 3 others.

Radiotherapy of breast cancer may cause a *radiation-induced brachial plexus injury* (Killer and Hess, 1990). The incidence of plexopathy is dose related: 73% are associated with doses greater than 55 Gy and 15% with doses of 5100 Gy (Stoll and Andrews, 1966). The onset of symptoms varies from 5 months to 18 years (average, 4.2 years) following completion of radiotherapy (Killer and Hess, 1990). Symptoms consist of numbness, paresthesia, pain, and muscle weakness, all of which may level off in severity or progress until the arm is totally paralyzed and anesthetic. In some patients, pain becomes the major complaint late in the course of the disease. Once symptoms are fully developed, resolution does not occur. Radiation plexopathy is not painful, whereas malignant tumor infiltration causes severe pain soon after invasion of the brachial plexus (Kori et al., 1981). Such a distinction is critical because effective therapy for plexus infiltration includes total radiotherapy. Surgical treatment for radiation-induced brachial plexus injury in 8 of 12 patients in Killer's series (Killer and Hess, 1990) consisted of neurolysis plus omental grafting to obviate progression of the symptoms. None of the patients in this series experienced improvement in muscle strength, whether they were operated on or not. In fact, 8 of 12 patients were left with severe or total paresis of the arm. The investigators suggested that surgery might have a beneficial effect only for pain relief.

PAIN MANAGEMENT

Breast cancer may cause pain as a result of (1) bony metastasis, (2) compression or infiltration of the peripheral nerves, brachial plexus, or nerve roots, (3) swelling within a structure invested by fascia or periosteum, (4) necrosis, infection, inflammation, and ulceration of pain-sensitive structures, or (5) the effects of treatment (surgery, radiation) (Onofrio, 1983). Radiation, surgery, or chemotherapy may relieve pain by decreasing tumor size; however, adjuvant analgesic therapy is usually required. By adjusting the dose, the analgesic therapy most effective for pain relief is found. Recent advances in neuropharmacology and neurophysiology have revolutionized pain management.

Simple, peripherally acting, nonsteroidal anti-inflammatory drugs usually are not effective in treating cancer pain. They act peripherally to irreversibly block the action of cyclo-oxygenase on the arachidonic acid metabolic cycle, which diminishes prostaglandin synthesis. Prostaglandins serve as sensitizers of pain receptors to the effects of histamine and bradykinin. Nonsteroidal anti-inflammatory drugs may be effective for mild pain, but severe pain requires narcotics.

Three classes of opioid receptors have been identified (alpha, mu, and kappa), for which morphine and enkephalin are antagonists (Slatkin and Posner, 1983). Morphine and other narcotic analgesics produce their analgesic effect by central uptake by opioid receptors. Parenteral doses of morphine required to relieve pain may be 300 to 400 mg per day, which causes somnolence, nausea, vomiting, constipation, and respiratory depression. Neurosurgical ablative procedures, such as dorsal horn rhizotomy or cordotomy, avoid these undesirable side effects (Onofrio, 1983); however, dorsal horn rhizotomy requires a major neurosurgical procedure and may leave an extremity useless from lack of position sense while effective analgesia lasts less than 6 months. High thoracic or cervical percutaneous cordotomy is effective in relieving unilateral pain, although dysesthesia develops some months later and limits its long-term value. Bilateral percutaneous cordotomy fails to relieve midline deep pain and bilateral lower extremity pain and frequently is associated with postoperative bladder disturbances and motor weakness. Nearly 50% of all patients with breast carcinoma eventually develop bony metastases. There has been interest in the use of strontium-89 for treatment of bone pain after conventional treatment modalities have failed. The overall response rate, in terms of decreased pain or improved quality of life, was 80% (Robinson et al., 1987).

Frequently, thoracic pain is a major disabling symptom that does not respond to customary methods. Initial treatment may consist of intercostal blocks or epidural anesthesia. Alternatively, intermittent intrapleural injection of bupivacaine and methylprednisolone for relief of thoracic pain can be highly effective (Klein and Klein, 1991). This technique is performed by injecting 20 mL of 0.5% bupivacaine and 40 mg methylprednisolone into the involved pleural space through a catheter placed at the third or fourth anterior intercostal space. Klein has reported successful relief of pain for as long as 6 months following a single injection.

On the other hand, intermittent administration of intrathecal or intraventricular morphine was used successfully in the management of intractable cancer pain (Onofrio, 1983). Intraspinal administration of preservative-free morphine (Duromorph) relieves lower extremity, pelvic, and trunk pain, whereas head, neck, and upper extremity pain is best treated by intraventricular injection of Duromorph via an Ommaya reservoir. A trial of intrathecal Duromorph is given percutaneously to assess the candidate for implantation of an Ommaya reservoir. Patients who survive less than 1 year have the best results. Long-term administration has not yet been assessed. Injection into the reservoir is carried out by a nurse, the patient, or a family member. One milligram of Duromorph is usually effective for 12 to 24 hours, but the dosage may be increased to 3 mg every 12 hours, as needed. These intrathecal doses provide an analgesic effect superior to that of 100 to 200 mg of intravenous morphine per day, but tolerance can develop to morphine or other analgesics that have a similar chemical structure. Temporarily decreasing or discontinuing them can reverse tolerance and allow reinstitution of the drug in smaller doses.

Side effects of intrathecal Duromorph are pruritus, sedation, nausea, and respiratory depression, which may necessitate decreasing the morphine dose. Acute respiratory depression can be reversed by naloxone, by competitively inhibiting the effects of morphine. Malignant disease may progress, so any significant increase in analgesic requirements should prompt a careful reassessment of tumor size. Optimal treatment for cancer pain is removal of the tumor that is compressing pain-sensitive structures. Metastases from breast cancer are moderately radiosensitive, so that focal radiation therapy to the tumor or to painful osteolytic lesions may be very effective for pain relief. Furthermore, hormone therapy may be effective in relieving pain, particularly if the tumor is estrogen receptor positive. No hard and fast rules can be set for pain relief, and what turns out to be the most effective therapy varies in individual cases.

References

Adler, J. R., Cox, R. S., Kaplan, I., et al.: Stereotactic radiosurgical treatment of brain metastasis. J. Neurosurg., 76:444–449, 1992.

Bach, F., Soletormos, G., and Dombernowsky, P.: Tissue polypeptide antigen activity in cerebrospinal fluid: A marker of central nervous system metastases of breast cancer. J. Natl. Cancer Inst., 83:779–784, 1991.

Bentley, C. R., Davies, G., and Aclimandos, W.A.: Tamoxifen retinopathy: A rare but serious complication. Br. Med. J., 304:495–496, 1992.

Berger, P. S.: Neurological complications of radiotherapy. In Silverstein, A. (Ed.): Neurological Complications of Therapy: Selected Topics. Mount Kisco, NY, Futura, 1982, p. 137.

Black, P.: Brain metastasis: Current status and recommended guidelines for management. Neurosurgery, *5*:617, 1979*a*.

Black, P.: Spinal metastasis: Current status and recommended guidelines for management. Neurosurgery, *5*:726, 1979*b*.

Boogerd, W., Hart, A. A. M., van der Sande, J. J., et al.: Meningeal carcinomatosis in breast cancer. Cancer, *67*:1685–1695, 1991.

Boogerd, W., Moffie, D., and Smets, L. A.: Early blindness and coma during intrathecal chemotherapy for meningeal carcinomatosis. Cancer, *65*:452–457, 1990.

Boogerd, W., van der Sande, J. J., and Moffie, D.: Acute fever and delayed leukoencephalopathy following low dose intraventricular methotrexate. J. Neurol. Neurosurg. Psychiatry, *51*:1277–1283, 1988.

Boogerd, W., van der Sande, J. J., Kroger, R., et al.: Effective systemic therapy for spinal epidural metastases from breast carcinoma. Eur. J. Cancer Clin. Oncol., *25*:149–153, 1989.

Cantillo, R., Fain, I., Singhakowinta, A., et al.: Blindness as initial manifestations of meningeal carcinomatosis in breast cancer. Cancer, *44*:755, 1979.

DiStefano, A., Yap, H. Y., Hortobagyi, G. N., et al.: The natural history of breast cancer patients with brain metastases. Cancer, *44*:1913, 1979.

Gagliano, R. G., and Costanzi, J. J.: Paraplegia following intrathecal methotrexate. Cancer, *37*:1663–1668, 1976.

Gamache, F. W. Jr., Posner, J. B., and Patterson, R. H. Jr.: Metastatic brain tumors. *In* Youmans, I. R. (Ed.): Neurological Surgery. Vol. 5. Philadelphia, W.B. Saunders, 1982, p. 2872.

Gilbert, R. W., Kim, I. H., and Posner, I. B.: Epidural spinal cord compression from metastatic tumor: Diagnosis and treatment. Ann. Neurol., *3*:40, 1978.

Harris, M., Howell, A., Chrissohou, M., et al.: A comparison of the metastatic pattern of infiltrating lobular carcinoma and infiltrating duct carcinoma of the breast. Br. J. Cancer, *50*:23–30, 1984.

Healy, M. E., Hesselink, J. R., Press, G. A., et al.: Increased detection of intracranial metastases with intravenous gd-DTPA. Radiology, *165*:619–624, 1987.

Horton, J.: Diagnosis and treatment of meningeal carcinomatosis. Curr. Concepts Oncol., *6*:10, 1984.

Houck, J. R., and Murphy, K.: Sudden bilateral profound hearing loss resulting from meningeal carcinomatosis. Otolaryngol. Head Neck Surg., *106*:92–97, 1992.

Kamby, C., and Sorensen, P. S.: Characteristic of patients with short and long survivals after detection of intracranial metastasis from breast cancer. J. Neurooncol., *6*:37–45, 1988.

Killer, H. E., and Hess, K.: Natural history of radiation-induced brachial plexopathy compared with surgically treated patients. J. Neurol., *237*:247–250, 1990.

Kiricuta, I. C., Kolbl, O., Willner, J., et al.: Central nervous system metastases in breast cancer. J. Cancer Res. Clin. Oncol., *118*:542–546, 1992.

Klein, D. S., and Klein, P. W.: Intermittent interpleural injection of bupivicaine and methylprednisolone for analgesia in metastatic thoracic neoplasm. Clin. J. Pain, *7*:232–236, 1991.

Kori, S. H., Foley, K. M., and Posner, I. B.: Brachial plexus lesions in patients with cancer: 100 cases. Neurology, *31*:45, 1981.

Korzeniowski, S., and Szpytma, T.: Survival of breast cancer patients with brain metastasis treated by irradiation. J. Eur. Radiother., *8*:25–30, 1987.

Latchaw, R. E., Johnson, D. W., and Kanal, E.: Metastasis. *In* Latchaw, R. E. (Ed.): MR and CT imaging of the head, neck, and spine. St. Louis: Mosby–Year Book, 1991, pp. 597–626.

Lesse, S., and Netsky, M. G.: Metastasis of neoplasms to central nervous system and meninges. Arch. Neurol. Psychiatry, *72*:133, 1954.

Livingston, K. E., and Perrin, R. G.: The neurosurgical management of spinal metastasis causing cord and cauda equina compression. J. Neurosurg., *49*:839, 1978.

Maranzano, E., Latini, P., Checcaglini, F., et al.: Radiation therapy of spinal cord compression caused by breast cancer: Report of a prospective trial. Int. J. Radiation Oncol. Biol. Phys., *24*:301–306, 1992.

McCarthy, G. M., and Skillings, J. R.: Orofacial complications of chemotherapy for breast cancer. Oral Surg. Oral Med. Oral Pathol., *74*:172–178, 1992.

Mehta, D., Khatib, R., and Patel, S.: Carcinoma of the breast and meningioma: Association and management. Cancer, *51*:1937, 1983.

Meyers, C. A., Obbens, E. A. M. T., Scheibel, R. S., et al.: Neurotoxicity of intraventricularly administered alpha-interferon for leptomeningeal disease. Cancer, *68*:88–92, 1991.

Onofrio, B. M.: Treatment of chronic pain of malignant origin with intrathecal opiates. Clin. Neurosurg., *31*:304, 1983.

Patanaphan, V., Salazar, O. M., and Risco, R.: Breast cancer: Metastatic patterns and their prognosis. South. Med. J., *81*:1109–1112, 1988.

Pors, H., von Eyben, F. E., Sorensen, O. S., et al.: Long-term remission of multiple brain metastases with tamoxifen. J. Neuro-Oncol., *10*:173–177, 1991.

Rider, W. D.: Radiation damage to the brain: A new syndrome. J. Can. Assoc. Radiol., *14*:67, 1963.

Robinson, R. G., Spicer, J. A., Preston, D. F., et al.: Treatment of metastatic bone pain with strontium-89. Nucl. Med. Biol., 14:219–222, 1987.

Rosner, D., Nemeto, T., and Lane, W.: Chemotherapy induces regression of brain metastasis in breast carcinoma. Cancer, *58*:832–839, 1986.

Salvati, M., Capoccia, G., Orlando, E. R., et al.: Single brain metastasis from breast cancer: Remarks on clinical patterns and treatment. Tumori, *78*:115–117, 1992.

Sheline, G. E.: Irradiation injury of the human brain: A review of clinical experience. *In* Gilbert, H. A., and Kagan, A. R. (Eds.): Radiation Damage to the Nervous System. New York, Raven, 1980, p. 39.

Siegal, T., Ovadia, H., Yatsiv, I., et al.: CSF myelin basic protein levels in leptomeningeal metastasis: Relationship to disease activity. J. Neurol. Sci., *78*:165–173, 1987.

Slatkin, N. E., and Posner. J. B.: Management of spinal epidural metastases. Clin. Neurosurg., *30*:698, 1983.

Sondak, V., Deckers, P. J., Feller, J. H., et al.: Leptomeningeal spread of breast cancer: Report of case and review of the literature. Cancer: *48*:395, 1981.

Stoll, B. A., and Andrews, J. T.: Radiation-induced peripheral neuropathy. Br. Med. J., *1*:834, 1966.

Taphoorn, M. J. B., Heimans, J. J., Kaiser, M. C. R. L. E., et al.: Imaging of brain metastases: Comparison of computerized tomography (CT) and magnetic resonance imaging (MRI). Neuroradiology, *31*:391–395, 1989.

Tomita, T., Galicich, J. H., and Sundaresan, N.: Radiation therapy for epidural metastasis with complete block. Acta Radiol. Oncol., *22*:135–143, 1983.

Twijnstra, A., Ongerboer de Visser, B. W., and van Zanten, A. P.: Diagnosis of leptomeningeal metastasis. Clin. Neurol. Neurosurg., *89*:79–85, 1987.

Westbrook, K. C., Ballantyne, A. J., Eckles, N. E., et al.: Breast cancer and vocal cord paralysis. South. Med. J., *67*:805–807, 1974.

Westling, P., Svensson, H., and Hele, P.: Cervical plexus lesions following post-operative radiation therapy of mammary carcinoma. Acta Radiol. [Ther.], *11*:209, 1972.

Yap, H. Y., Yap, B. S., Tashima, C. K., et al.: Meningeal carcinomatosis in breast cancer. Cancer, *42*:283, 1978.

Young, D. F.: Neurological complications of cancer chemotherapy. *In* Silverstein, A. (Ed.): Neurological Complications of Therapy: Selected Topics. Mount Kisco, NY, Futura, 1982, p. 57.

33

Management of Pain

David E. Weissman

Principles of modern pain management include performance of a thorough and well-documented pain assessment and frequent reassessments, timely use of antineoplastic therapy and liberal use of multiple classes of analgesics with a reliance on oral medications (Agency for Health Care Policy and Research, 1994). Analgesic drug therapy, combined with antineoplastic therapy and other noninvasive treatments such as behavioral treatments, heat, cold and massage, can effectively control more than 90% of breast cancer–related pain (Agency for Health Care Policy and Research, 1994). For the remaining patients, more invasive treatments such as spinal opioid infusions, neurolytic blocks, and other neurodestructive procedures may be indicated and can control most of the remaining pain.

PAIN ETIOLOGY AND ASSESSMENT

Establishing a cause for pain is critical, so that diagnosis-specific treatment can be instituted, though failure to establish a cause should not necessarily limit analgesic therapy. Furthermore, there is usually no reason to withhold analgesics during the pain evaluation period. Common causes of breast cancer–related pain are listed in Table 33–1. Bony metastases and their complications (hypercalcemia, fracture, spinal cord compression) represent the most common cause of pain for breast cancer patients.

A thorough pain assessment includes the basic pain history (i.e., location, duration, quality, intensity, response to treatments), an understanding of the impact of pain on a patient's activities of daily living, and, for certain patients, the personal meaning of pain. Two particularly important aspects of the pain history are pain intensity and quality. Patients should be asked to rate their pain using one of a variety of verbal or written pain scales (e.g., zero to 10 verbal scale). This value can be charted and used as a future indicator of pain relief. Obtaining the patient's report of pain quality can help establish a diagnosis and determine treatment. Characteristics of the three common types of pain are listed in Table 33–2. Important questions that help determine the impact of pain on activities of daily living include effects on sleep, movement, eating, and mood. Patients who are reluctant to discuss their pain or to accept pain treatment should be questioned about their belief system concerning pain and pain treatment, as it is common for patients to view pain from cancer as a punishment from which they do not deserve relief or as inevitable and untreatable. For others, fear of pain therapy, especially opioids, inhibits acceptance of treatment.

PAIN THERAPY

Options for pain therapy include antineoplastic treatment, drug therapy, behavioral treatments, anesthetics, and, rarely, neurosurgery. Drug therapy is the mainstay of treatment, and is used most effectively when integrated with a comprehensive plan that includes other pain treatment modalities. The following sections focus on drugs and other noninvasive treatments; antineoplastic and invasive pain treatments are covered elsewhere in this book.

Drug Therapy

General principles of pharmacologic therapy of breast cancer pain include (1) using oral preparations whenever possible, (2) basing the initial choice of analgesic on the patient's report of pain, (3) administering drugs around the clock rather than p.r.n. for continuous pain, (4) anticipating and aggressively treating side effects, (5) re-evaluating the patient's report of pain frequently, and (6) ensuring a continuous supply of analgesics.

Nonopioid Analgesics

Mild pain initially is treated with a nonopioid such as aspirin, acetaminophen, or a nonsteroidal anti-inflammatory drug (NSAID). NSAIDs may be preferable to acetaminophen for bony metastases, whereas acetaminophen is used when there is thrombocytopenia or another bleeding risk. All NSAIDs have analgesic activity, and a specific preparation should be chosen on issues of cost and ease of administration. The nonopioids all have an analgesic ceiling; thus, above a certain dose, no further analgesic activity is to be expected.

Opioid Analgesics

Opioids are indicated when pain is not adequately controlled by nonopioids alone. Obtaining a careful pain history is important before using opioids, since neuropathic pain may not be opioid responsive. Other concerns before starting opioids include assessment of respiratory, renal, and hepatic function.

Opioids of the morphine agonist type (morphine, oxycodone, hydromorphone, fentanyl, meperidine, methadone, levorphanol, hydrocodone, propoxyphene) all share certain

Table 33-1. COMMON CAUSES OF PAIN IN BREAST CANCER

Pain due to direct tumor involvement
 Bone metastases
 Neural metastases
  Brachial plexopathy
  Spinal cord compression
  Meningeal carcinomatosis
 Visceral metastases
  Pleura
  Liver
  Bowel
  Peritoneum
Pain due to anti-neoplastic treatment
 Procedure-related pain
 Postmastectomy pain
 Peripheral neuropathy
 Mucositis
 Osteoporosis or aseptic necrosis
 Dermatomal herpes zoster
Pre-existing conditions

pharmacologic features: (1) There is no standard dose. (2) Equianalgesic doses of different morphine-like agonists produce equipotent analgesia. (3) There is no ceiling analgesic effect and no ceiling dose. Mild to moderate pain can be treated with codeine, hydrocodone, or oxycodone, as single agents or, more commonly, as fixed-dose products combined with aspirin or acetaminophen. These drugs have analgesic activity for 3 to 4 hours. The dose of combination products can be escalated until side effects from the non-narcotic substances (e.g., tinnitus, gastrointestinal pain, hepatic toxicity) appear. If pain still is not well controlled, a more potent opioid is indicated (Weissman et al., 1994).

Morphine is the opioid of choice for severe pain. It is available in numerous formulations including tablet and liquid short-acting preparations (active 3 to 4 hours), long-acting preparations (active 8 to 12 hours), rectal suppositories, and parenteral dosing formulations for intravenous, subcutaneous, intramuscular, spinal, or ventricular administration. Before starting oral morphine, a dose equal in analgesia to opioids already being used should be calculated to avoid serious overdosing or underdosing. Oral morphine can be started by using either a short-acting preparation given every 3 to 4 hours or a long-acting preparation administered every 8 or 12 hours. The dose of short-acting preparations can be escalated 25% to 50% every 8 to 12 hours. The dose of long-acting preparations can be escalated every 24 hours or the dosing interval can be reduced, the limit being no more frequently than every 8 hours. Patients receiving a long-acting preparation need to be supplied with a short-acting opioid, such as immediate-release morphine, that can be taken every 2 to 4 hours for breakthrough pain. Oxycodone and hydromorphone are both excellent alternatives to morphine. Hydromorphone has a similar duration of analgesia, 3 to 4 hours, as morphine but is four to six times more potent, milligram for milligram, and may be tolerated better in the presence of renal failure, since morphine has an active metabolite that accumulates in patients with renal failure (Portenoy et al., 1991). Levorphanol and methadone are also reasonable alternatives to morphine, having a more variable duration of analgesia, 4

to 6 hours, or even 8 to 12 hours in some patients. The major disadvantage of these drugs is their long elimination half-life, up to 36 hours for methadone. This feature makes rapid dose adjustments impractical and potentially dangerous owing to drug accumulation and central nervous system toxicity. Methadone is a very inexpensive analgesic and a good choice for patients with normal renal function for whom an established dose of opioid has been determined.

One of the morphine-like drugs not indicated for chronic pain is meperidine. Meperidine has both a toxic metabolite and a very short-lived activity (2 to 3 hours), so it is inappropriate for long-term use (Inturrisi et al., 1986). Opioids with mixed agonist-antagonist properties such as pentazocine, nalbuphine, or butorphanol are not indicated for chronic pain as they can cause psychotomimetic effects with long-term administration and may induce opioid withdrawal if given to a patient already receiving opioids (Weissman et al., 1994).

The oral route is preferred for administration of opioids (Agency for Health Care Policy and Research, 1994; and Weissman et al., 1994). Liquid preparations of several opioids are available for patients who are unable to swallow pills or who have a feeding tube. Rectal opioids are equianalgesic to oral preparations and are a good alternative for patients who are unable to swallow (Weissman et al., 1994). Yet another option is the transdermal fentanyl patch. This product is best used for patients with an established opioid requirement (not for acute crisis management) who cannot take oral medications. After patch placement (on nonirradiated, hairless skin) it takes 24 hours for the patch to reach full effectiveness, after which analgesic activity lasts for 48 to 72 hours. Active drug remains in the subcutaneous tissue and circulation as long as 24 hours after removal of the patch (Payne, 1992).

Patients with severe pain or those for whom the oral, rectal, or transdermal route is not appropriate may benefit from a parenteral infusion, either intravenous or subcutaneous (Portenoy, 1986). To avoid the complications of a chronic indwelling venous catheter, a chronic subcutaneous infusion is a well-tolerated method of drug delivery (Braera et al., 1988). The dose in subcutaneous infusions is the same as in intravenous infusions and is administered through a 25- or 27-gauge butterfly needle. The concentration is set so that the infusion rate is less than 2.0 mL per hour using short-acting opioids such as morphine or hydromorphone. Spinal (epidural or intrathecal) opioid administration is useful for carefully selected patients with severe trunk or lower body pain (Coombs, 1988). Spinal opioids can be administered as repeated bolus injections or as a continuous infusion.

Opioid Toxicity

The most common side effects from opioids are dry mouth, constipation, nausea, and sedation. Sedation and nausea are usually short-term problems that resolve with long-term administration. Patients frequently report nausea following opioid use, described as an ''allergy.'' Nausea is not an allergic manifestation of opioids and is not to be considered a contraindication to future use of opioids. True opioid

Table 33–2. TYPES OF CANCER PAIN

	Somatic	Visceral	Neuropathic
Quality	Dull, aching	Dull, aching, throbbing	Sharp, lancinating, burning
Location	Focal	Focal, or diffuse or referred	Radicular
Example	Bone metastases	Intestinal obstruction	Brachial plexopathy
Drug treatment	NSAIDs, opioids	Acetaminophen, opioids	NSAIDs, opioids, adjuvants

allergy, manifested as an anaphylactoid reaction, is uncommon. Sedation can usually be controlled by careful dose adjustment, or, in more refractory cases, small doses of stimulants can be used (Bruera et al., 1989). Constipation is a problem that does not improve over time, so all patients receiving opioids need measures to ensure regular bowel movements. A common approach is to use stool softeners daily and intermittent laxatives such as senna or milk of magnesia. Respiratory depression is very uncommon in patients who routinely take oral opioids since tolerance to the respiratory depressant effects of opioids develops rapidly. Risk factors for respiratory depression include rapid intravenous administration, rapid dose escalation of levorphanol or methadone, and new hepatic or renal dysfunction (Weissman et al., 1994).

Tolerance and Physical and Psychologic Dependence

Tolerance to opioids is defined as the need to increase the amount of drug to produce the same pharmacologic effect. Tolerance is heralded by a decrease in the duration of effect and is managed by increasing the dose. Since there is no ceiling dose for most opioids, the development of tolerance rarely limits opioid therapy. It should be noted that many patients remain on stable doses of opioids for weeks to months with no evidence of tolerance (Foley, 1989). Physical dependence is a condition in which withdrawal symptoms develop if opioids are discontinued or an opioid antagonist is administered. Like tolerance, it is a pharmacologic property of opioids and it occurs in all patients who routinely take these drugs. Withdrawal can be avoided by ensuring a continuous supply of analgesics. If patients no longer need opioids because the cancer has been reduced by antineoplastic treatment or because other analgesic therapies have been effective, opioids can be gradually tapered off over several days to avoid acute withdrawal symptoms.

Psychologic dependence (addiction) is a behavioral condition characterized by overwhelming involvement with the acquisition and use of opioids for nonmedical purposes. The fear of iatrogenic addiction is a major barrier to appropriate prescribing and dispensing of opioids by health professionals and a significant limiting factor in patients' acceptance of opioids. Although both health professionals and the public are afraid that patients will become addicted to opioids, studies indicate that iatrogenic addiction is rare when opioids are used for legitimate medical reasons (Porter et al., 1980; Taub, 1982).

Adjuvant Analgesics

Antidepressants, anticonvulsants, and systemic local anesthetics are used to treat neuropathic pain that is unresponsive to nonopioids or opioids. Amitriptyline, the most extensively studied antidepressant for neuropathic pain (Spiegel et al., 1983; and Max et al., 1987), has analgesic activity separate from antidepressant activity in doses of 25 to 150 mg per day. Other tricyclic antidepressants, with side effects different from amitriptyline's, can also be used. The newer antidepressants that act by inhibiting release of serotonin do not seem to have analgesic effects. Carbamazepine and phenytoin are anticonvulsants used for neuropathic pain, in standard anticonvulsant doses. Blood levels are monitored to avoid toxicity (Weinberger et al., 1976; and Swerdlow, 1984). Carbamazepine is particularly useful for patients experiencing shooting or lancinating, rather than burning, pain. Glucocorticoids have analgesic effects in cases of nerve compression or bony metastases; however, they have a myriad of side effects that limit their long-term usefulness (Weissman et al., 1987). Finally, hydroxyzine can be administered with opioids to provide sedative and antiemetic activity, but they probably have little intrinsic analgesic activity (Runmore et al., 1986). Muscle relaxants, benzodiazepines, and other sedative-hypnotics should be avoided in patients with poorly controlled pain, as they generally provide sedation without analgesia (Weissman et al., 1994).

Behavioral Treatments

Behavioral treatments can be used at any phase of pain management. They should be considered as additive rather than alternative treatments to drugs, antineoplastic therapy, or more invasive treatments (Agency for Health Care Policy and Research, 1994). Simple procedures such as progressive muscle relaxation or imagery are easily taught to motivated patients and can result in an increased sense of self-control. Hypnosis, biofeedback, music therapy, and individual or group psychotherapy may be helpful for carefully selected patients. All behavioral treatments work best initially in cases with mild to moderate pain, but they can be of value in cases of severe pain if they are already integrated into a patient's coping system.

OTHER TREATMENTS

Simple physical modalities, such as applications of heat or cold and massage, are routinely used by patients, often with excellent results. Transcutaneous electric nerve stimulation (TENS) is a noninvasive, relatively inexpensive treatment that may benefit 25% or more of cancer patients with focal pain (Agency for Health Care Policy and Research, 1994). Acupuncture has been of benefit to selected patients, but, like TENS, it has been the focus of little systematic research to define which patients and what types of pain respond best (Patel et al., 1989).

For the minority (fewer than 20%) of patients with pain that responds poorly to antineoplastic, drug, behavioral, and physical treatments, invasive pain treatments may be indicated (Patt, 1993). These include procedures of low to moderate cost and low morbidity (peripheral or autonomic nerve block, non-neurolytic block, spinal opioid infusions) and high-cost and high-morbidity procedures (cordotomy, central neuraxis block, implantable spinal infusion pump, implantable spinal stimulators). Decisions about the specific indications for a particular procedure should be made in consultation with specialists in pain management.

References

Agency for Health Care Policy and Research: Management of Cancer Pain, Clinical Practice Guideline. Washington, D.C., U.S. Department of Health and Human Services, Public Health Service, 1994, pp. 1–245.

Bruera, E., Brenneis, C., Michaud, M., et al.: Use of subcutaneous route for the administration of narcotics in patients with cancer pain. Cancer, 62:407–411, 1988.

Bruera, E., Brenneis, C., Paterson, A. H., et al.: Use of methylphenidate as an adjuvant to narcotic analgesics in patients with advanced cancer. J. Pain Symptom Management, 4:3–6, 1989.

Coombs, D. W.: Intraspinal narcotics for intractable cancer pain. In Abram, S. E. (Ed.): Cancer Pain. Boston, Kluwer Academic Publishers, 1988, pp. 77–96.

Foley, K. M.: Controversies in cancer pain: Medical perspectives. Cancer, 63:2257–2265, 1989.

Inturrisi, C. E., and Umans, J. G.: Meperideine biotransformation and central nervous system toxicity in animals and humans. In Foley, K. M., and Inturrisi, D. E. (Eds.): Advances in Pain Research and Therapy: Opioid Analgesics in the Management of Clinical Pain. New York, Raven Press, 1986, pp. 143–153.

Max, M. B., Culname, M., Schafer, S. C., et al.: Amitriptyline relieves diabetic neuropathy pain in patients with normal or depressed mood. Neurology, 37:589–594, 1987.

Patel, M., Gutzwiller, F., Paccaud, F., et al.: A meta-analysis of acupuncture for chronic pain. Int. J. Epidemiol., 18:900–906, 1989.

Patt, R. B.: Cancer Pain. Philadelphia, J. B. Lippincott, 1993, pp. 275–460.

Payne, R.: Transdermal fentanyl: Suggested recommendations for clinical use. J. Pain Symptom Management, 7:S40–S43, 1992.

Portenoy, R. K.: Continuous infusion of opioid drugs in the treatment of cancer pain: Guidelines for use. J. Pain Symptom Management, 1:223–228, 1986.

Portenoy, R. K., Foley, K. M., Stulman, J., et al.: Plasma morphine and morphine-6-glucuronide during chronic morphine therapy for cancer pain: Plasma profiles, steady-state concentrations and the consequences of renal failure. Pain, 47:13–19, 1991.

Porter, J., and Jick, H.: Addiction rate in patients treated with narcotics (Letter). N. Engl. J. Med., 302:123, 1980.

Runmore, M. M., and Schlichting, D. A.: Clinical efficacy of antihistamines as analgesics. Pain, 25:7–22, 1986.

Spiegel, K., Kalb, R., and Paternak, G. W.: Analgesic activity of tricyclic antidepressants. Ann. Neurol., 13:462–465, 1983.

Swerdlow, M.: Anticonvulsant drugs and chronic pain. Clin. Neuropharmacol., 7:51–82, 1984.

Taub, A.: Opioid analgesics in the treatment of chronic intractable pain of non-neoplastic origin. In Kitahata, L. M., and Collins, D. (Eds.): Narcotic Analgesics in Anesthesiology. Baltimore, Williams & Wilkins, 1982, pp. 199–208.

Weinberger, J., Nicklas, W. J., and Beri, S.: Mechanism of action of anticonvulsants. Neurology, 26:162–173, 1976.

Weissman, D., Duffer, D., Vogel, V., et al.: Corticosteroid toxicity in neurooncology patients. J. Neurooncol., 5:125–128, 1987.

Weissman, D., Buchman, S., Dinndorf, P., et al.: Handbook of Cancer Pain Management. Madison, WI, Wisconsin Cancer Pain Initiative, 1994, pp. 1–35.

34 Breast Carcinoma and Pregnancy

William L. Donegan

The association of pregnancy with breast cancer raises special issues. The curability of this disease when it coincides with pregnancy, the proper therapy, and the risks of future pregnancies have long been subjects of debate. Because the problem is infrequent, the experience of individuals or even institutions is generally limited, and conclusions are often based on assumptions and small numbers of cases. A few large series have been reported. (Westberg, 1946; Holleb and Farrow, 1964; Clark and Reid, 1978; Deemarsky and Neishtadt, 1981). The subject has been reviewed by others (Wallack et al., 1983; Theriault and Hortobagyi, 1989; Jones, 1992; Shapiro and Mayer, 1992).

From the biologic standpoint, concern about the effect of pregnancy on malignancy of the breast appears justified. Many of the systemic changes that favor fetal development appear equally to favor the promotion of tumor growth (Fig. 34–1). During both pregnancy and lactation the breasts are under intense hormonal stimulation. To varying degrees, breast cancers retain the hormonal dependence of their parent tissue, remaining potentially responsive to the same physiologic changes that stimulate the mammary parenchyma. Laboratory and clinical evidence indicates that estrogens and prolactin, both of which increase in amount dramatically during pregnancy, can enhance the growth of mammary carcinoma. So might the increased levels of growth hormone or of corticosteroids, which impair cell-mediated immunity and favor the implantation and spread of tumors in animal models. In view of the important role attributed to cell-mediated immunity in maintaining resistance to cancer, the evidence for depression of T lymphocytes in early pregnancy (Strelkauskas et al., 1975), the impaired mitogen response of lymphocytes (Purtilo et al., 1972; Nelson et al., 1973), depressed natural killer cell activity (Koshi et al., 1989), and the depletion of germinal centers in pelvic lymph nodes would seem to represent disadvantages for the gravid host. Add to this the rich blood supply and enhanced lymphatic drainage of the breast during pregnancy, and it would seem that ideal circumstances for the growth and spread of cancer are present. Past experience has, in fact, generally confirmed a poor outlook for the pregnant patient. The opinions expressed by 35 authorities in this field, compiled by Cheek in 1953, reflected pessimism and a lack of unanimity regarding management.

Notwithstanding the aforementioned biologic considerations, and in contrast to the pessimism of early publications on this subject, the trend in recent years has been toward an attitude of optimism, a change based largely on the awareness that poor results may have been due in no small measure to delay in diagnosis and procrastination or compromise in treatment. Overall, there is a growing tendency to minimize the significance of the pregnancy and to aggressively diagnose and treat patients much as nonpregnant women are treated. Byrd and colleagues (1962) summed up this attitude after a review of material at Vanderbilt University: "In the face of general enthusiasm for terminating the pregnancy, we believe the evidence is that the cancer should be terminated."

FREQUENCY

The problem under consideration is infrequent because breast cancer favors an older population, women past the childbearing years, and there is no reason to believe that a woman is especially susceptible to breast cancer during pregnancy. The coincidence exists only because the age-specific incidence of breast cancer begins to rise early (i.e., at age 25 years), and by age 35 years it has become the most frequent cancer of women (Donegan, 1983). As fertility declines in the fourth decade of life, women who are affected with breast cancer when pregnant are youthful, with ages ranging from 21 to 44 years, averaging 32 to 35 years in recent series (Table 34–1).

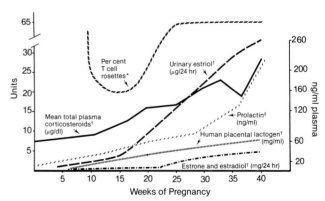

*Strelkauskas et al., 1975
†Hytten and Leitch, 1971
‡Vorrgerr, 1974

Figure 34–1. Hormonal and immunologic changes of pregnancy that are potentially important with respect to the growth of mammary carcinoma. (Adapted from Donegan, W. L.: Pregnancy and breast cancer. Obstet. Gynecol., *50*:244, 1977. Reprinted with permission.)

Table 34–1. ESTIMATED AGE-SPECIFIC FREQUENCY OF BREAST CANCER CONCURRENT WITH PREGNANCY PER 100,000 WOMEN IN THE UNITED STATES FOR 1970*

Age Category (y)	Incidence of Breast Cancer	Incidence of Live Births and/or Abortions	Estimated Coincidence of Breast Cancer and Pregnancy
15–19	0.1	8080	0.008
20–24	1.2	19870	0.248
25–29	8.8	17180	1.512
30–34	23.0	8680	1.996
35–39	53.3	3750	1.999
40–44	102.8	960	0.986

*Derived from the Third National Cancer Survey and Statistical Abstracts of the United States. Both are necessary to calculate the total incidence of pregnancies.

Examination of the breasts is a routine of obstetric care, but practicing obstetricians can expect to discover relatively few cases of breast cancer. Finn (1952) reported 46 breast cancers among 62,561 patients observed during pregnancy at the New York Lying-In Hospital between 1932 and 1951, approximately 1 case per 1360 patients. White (1955) found only 74 in a collected series of 238,299 pregnancies, or 1 per 3200 pregnancies. More recently Parente and co-workers (1988) found 8 cases among 12,500 pregnancies, or 1 per 1563 pregnancies.

Although breast cancer is relatively uncommon among the youthful, pregnancy is sufficiently frequent in this population that it is not unusual for the few young women who develop this cancer to be pregnant at the time. Among 45,881 cases of breast cancer, White found 1296 with a coincident or recent pregnancy, a prevalence of 2.8%. More recent reports have since set this figure between 0.75% and 3.1% (Rosemond, 1964; Peters, 1968; Applewhite et al., 1973; Sahni et al., 1981). Considering only women of childbearing age, the frequency of coincidence is considerable. Applewhite found that 7.3% of 655 women with breast cancer who were younger than 45 years of age were pregnant or lactating. Among 549 women younger than 35 years of age, Treves and Holleb (1958) reported a remarkable 14%. Horsley and associates (1969) also confirmed the high coincidence among young women, reporting that 10% of 67 patients less than 35 years of age were pregnant at the time of diagnosis, and an additional 15% had been pregnant within the previous year. Nugent and O'Connell (1985) pointed out that the 11% pregnancy rate found in their patients 25 to 40 years old was almost identical to the 10% expected in a similar age group without breast cancer based on an average of two pregnancies. This infers a coincidental rather than a causal relationship.

DIAGNOSIS

Pregnancy makes diagnosis of breast cancer more difficult. The enlargement of the breasts during pregnancy and lactation tends to obscure parenchymal masses. When masses are appreciated, they are often erroneously attributed to normal hypertrophy of the gland or they are lost in surrounding tissues as pregnancy progresses, creating the illusion that they have resolved. The effectiveness of mammography is also compromised by the full development and function of mammary parenchyma. These changes, with the accompanying hyperemia and increased water content of the breasts, contribute to a generalized radiographic density with loss of the contrasting fatty tissue that usually helps to define tumor masses (Hoeffken and Lanyi, 1977) (Fig. 34–2). For this reason, and because of potential exposure of the fetus to irradiation, mammography ordinarily is not used during pregnancy (Canter et al., 1983). The obscuring physical changes of pregnancy may also cause breast cancers to be clinically understaged and as a consequence to appear unusually aggressive in behavior.

The literature confirms that the clinical course of gravid women with mammary carcinoma is marked by unusual delays. Applewhite (1973), reporting on women seen at Louisiana State University between 1948 and 1967, documented an average duration of symptoms of 11 months, versus 4 months for nonpregnant women. Diagnosis was delayed an additional month after the first visit to a physician, and the delay from diagnosis to treatment averaged 8 days, versus 3 days for the nonpregnant woman. Westberg (1946) found the mean delay between discovery of a lump and treatment to be 2 months longer for pregnant women than for others, and this finding was confirmed by Bunker and Peters (1963). Byrd and coworkers (1962) attributed three-fourths of the delay in treatment directly to physician procrastination. Contributory factors have included failure to examine the breasts regularly at prenatal clinics (Montgomery, 1961), reluctance to obtain tissue for a histologic diagnosis, and failure to treat known carcinomas promptly.

The practice of "watching" a lump in the breast during pregnancy is unjustified. Indications for biopsy of breast lesions are the same as those for nonpregnant women. Aspiration of masses with a fine needle serves to differentiate cysts or galactoceles from solid tumors quickly and innocuously. Biopsy of solid tumor masses with incision or needle under local anesthesia on an outpatient basis is expeditious and involves minimal risk (Saltzstein et al., 1974). Byrd and colleagues (1962) point out that if general anesthesia is necessary for biopsy or mastectomy, it entails minimal risk to the fetus. Of 134 cases so managed, including 29 with malignant disease, only one resulted in fetal death (0.75%). This menopausal woman aborted spontaneously 3 weeks after removal of a benign cyst. Although the risk of fetal loss is small, well below the 5% reported by Westberg before 1946, it is important that the patient be

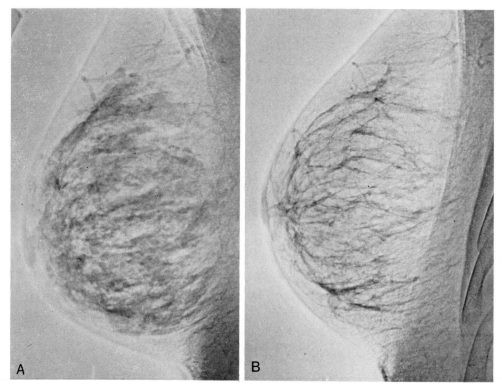

Figure 34–2. The increase in parenchymal density of the breast of a 36-year-old woman during lactation *(A)* is shown in these mammograms. This change tends to obscure carcinomas. *B*, Same breast without pregnancy or lactation.

advised of it before the physician proceeds with surgery under either general or local anesthesia.

No spontaneous abortions have followed 13 breast biopsies performed by the author during pregnancy. Two were done with general anesthesia and the remainder with local anesthesia. Diazepam (Valium), which is often used for sedation during local anesthesia, is avoided during pregnancy. This and other minor tranquilizers (e.g.. meprobamate, chlordiazepoxide) have been associated with increased risk of congenital malformations when used during the first trimester.

The indication for biopsy during pregnancy or lactation is almost always a palpable mass. In a series of 247 consecutive breast biopsies in women younger than 40 years performed by the author, 6.9% of the women were gravid or lactating at the time. Ninety-three percent of this group had palpable masses. Other indications are not frequent. Bloody nipple discharge during pregnancy is usually due to ductal epithelial hyperplasia (Lefreniere, 1990) Typically this involves multiple ducts and disappears after delivery. Suspicious mammographic signs are an infrequent indication for biopsy, as screening is not routine in this young population.

Lactation need not be interrupted to perform a biopsy of the breast of a nursing mother, but postoperative galactoceles and milk fistulas are potential complications. The former respond to aspiration; fistulas eventually close with local care. Closure can be hastened by discontinuing nursing or by suppressing lactation. The risk of postoperative galactocele or milk fistula probably is reduced by meticulously closing transected ducts with fine absorbable suture during biopsy.

PATHOLOGIC FINDINGS

Biopsies reveal cancer no less often in pregnant women than in nonpregnant women of similar age (Byrd et al., 1962) In the author's series of breast biopsies involving nonpregnant patients younger than 40 years cancers were found in 11.7% of cases. Among 29 biopsies during pregnancy or lactation cancer was found in 17.2%. The most frequent benign mass is lactating adenoma, and this is true during pregnancy or lactation. If lactating adenoma is excluded, the spectrum of benign lesions is similar to that found in nonpregnant women of comparable age, fibroadenomas and fibrocystic changes being the most frequent (Table 34–2).

The cancers that are found are not notably different in

Table 34–2. FINDINGS IN BIOPSY SPECIMENS DURING PREGNANCY OR LACTATION—AUTHOR'S SERIES OF 29 CASES

Diagnosis	No.	%
Lactating adenoma	11	37.9
Fibroadenoma	6	20.7
Carcinoma*	5	17.2
Fibrocystic changes	3	10.3
Duct papilloma	1	3.4
Infarction	1	3.4
Fat necrosis	1	3.4
Duct ectasia	1	3.4
Total	29	(100%)

*Ductal carcinoma in situ = 20%; invasive carcinoma = 80%.

character or distribution from those in nonpregnant women, nor is inflammatory carcinoma a more frequent occurrence. Rosemond (1964) reported one inflammatory carcinoma among 56 cases (1.8%), Montgomery (1961) found three among 70 cases (4.3%), and Clark and Reid (1978) discovered five among 201 (2.5%) cases of breast cancer during pregnancy or lactation. Save for the unusually high figure of 13% found at the Mayo Clinic by King and associates (1985), this is comparable to the 1.5% to 4% reported among nonpregnant women. Inflammatory cancer has the same poor prognosis during pregnancy as at other times (Zeigerman et al., 1968). As might be expected in young women, 71% of the tumors lack estrogen receptors (Nugent and O'Connell, 1985), a factor that would seem to negate any influence of pregnancy on prognosis. Receptor negativity may be less frequent during lactation, but confirmation of this is needed (Holdaway et al., 1984). Breast cancers in pregnant or lactating Nigerian women were found by Chiedozi and coworkers (1988) to be of higher histologic grades than those of other young women, suggesting that they may be inherently more aggressive.

STAGING DURING PREGNANCY

Staging during pregnancy is modified to avoid exposing the fetus to ionizing irradiation. (Theriault and Hortobagyi, 1989; Shapiro and Mayer, 1992). With appropriate shielding a radiograph of the chest can be obtained with negligible exposure (i.e., 0.008 cGy). Serologic tests of liver function are appropriate, and if they are abnormal the liver can be examined for metastases with ultrasonography. Magnetic resonance imaging is an effective alternative to computed tomography of the head or liver. Isotope scans and CT are avoided as much as possible, but it is important to confirm distant metastases if symptoms suggest them. Risk to the fetus can be minimized and is tempered by the fact that effective palliation will likely necessitate a therapeutic abortion unless the fetus has reached viability (Baker et al., 1987). The fetal dose from a bone scan is estimated to be 0.194 cGy, and that from radiography of the pelvis 0.04 cGy. The fetal irradiation associated with most nuclear scans is less than 5 cGy, a dose unlikely to result in abnormalities.

TREATMENT AND PROGNOSIS

Early reports on the association of breast cancer with pregnancy emphasized rapid spread of the tumor and early demise of the patient. Delayed discovery of cancers because of increased breast size, early dissemination due to increased vascularity of the breast, and unfavorable hormonal factors operative during pregnancy have been blamed for the poor prognosis (Costarides and Theofanides, 1963). After review of the discouraging experience at the Presbyterian Hospital from 1915 to 1935, Haagensen and Stout (1943) considered the pregnant patient categorically incurable and not a candidate for surgery. In the face of mounting evidence to the contrary, this opinion was revised in 1949 (Haagensen, 1956). Harrington (1937) is given credit

for reviving optimism about treatment. He reported on 92 patients operated on at the Mayo Clinic whose 5-year survival rate was 61.5% for women without axillary metastases. This report emphasized the favorable results achievable when the disease was detected and treated when still confined to the breast. Unfortunately, spread beyond the confines of the breast is frequent, and many carcinomas arising during pregnancy have been in advanced stages when treated (Table 34–3). Three-fourths (74%) of Montgomery's 70 patients had metastases, and in 20% the metastases were systemic. Seventy-two per cent of Holleb and Farrow's (1964) and 75% of Applewhite and colleagues' (1973) operable groups had axillary metastases. This high incidence of metastatic disease has marked each trimester of pregnancy as well as the postpartum period.

There is reason to believe, however, that the prognosis of pregnant patients is equal to that of others of comparable age and with tumors at the same stage if they are managed as expeditiously. Rissanen (1968) found early cancers not appreciably less curable in pregnant women than in other women of similar age. Peters (1968) found that 187 pregnant patients survived equally well as a control group matched for age and stage of disease. No more than a 10% to 15% deficit in 5-year survival could be discerned in any clinical stage, and women 36 to 40 years of age fared altogether as well as their nonpregnant counterparts. During a 10-year period of follow-up, the difference in actuarial survival of the two groups was unimpressive. In a small series, Nugent and O'Connell (1985) found the 5-year survival rate of women under 40 years of age comparable by stage, whether or not they were pregnant at diagnosis.

Treatment during pregnancy has the objectives of providing uncompromised care for the patient and delivering an undamaged infant. Treatment should be initiated without unnecessary delay and should conform as closely as possible to that appropriate for the patient were she not pregnant. The patient's obstetrician should be involved with the plan at the outset. For early stages of invasive cancer optimal therapy ordinarily involves local treatment with either modified radical mastectomy or lumpectomy and axillary dissection followed by irradiation to the breast, and for most patients systemic adjuvant chemotherapy, with or without tamoxifen, is also indicated. For patients with noninvasive cancers or small (<1.0 cm) invasive cancers with uninvolved axillary lymph nodes systemic therapy is not routine. Breast irradiation and systemic therapy are customarily initiated within 5 weeks after an operation.

Risk for the fetus varies with the trimester of the pregnancy and the form of treatment. In all trimesters an operation can produce spontaneous abortion, but it does not increase the risk of birth defects. Several surveys of fetal outcome after general anesthesia during pregnancy have failed to identify any anesthetic as a teratogen, but information is scant (Shnider and Levinson, 1985). The risk of spontaneous abortion is probably less than 1%; the patient should be advised of this.

In all trimesters ionizing irradiation is potentially damaging to the pregnancy (Wallack et al., 1983, p. 28). Before implantation (at 2 weeks), it may prove fatal to the conceptus, but it infrequently results in malformations. Irradiation is most damaging during the period of organogenesis (2 to

Table 34–3. RESULTS OF TREATMENT—BREAST CANCER WITH PREGNANCY OR LACTATION

Period Reviewed	Number of Cases	5-Year Survival (%)	Resected for Cure (%)	Axillary Metastases (%)	5-Year Survival of Operable Cases			Reference
					All (%)	Ax+ (%)	Ax− (%)	
1910–1933	92		92	85	15	6	62	Harrington (1937)
1915–1959	48	(33)*	65	55	(45)	(24)	(71)	Haagensen (1971)
1920–1953	133	31	90	72	30	17	65	Holleb and Farrow (1964)
Pre-1956	37		37	68	22	8	50	White and White (1956)
1921–1962	17		71	67	100	100	100	Horsley et al. (1969)†
1925–1960	29	55	72	—	71	33	100	Byrd et al. (1962)
1926–1972	100	48	91	67	54	43	73	Deemarsky and Neishtadt (1981)
1930–1964	46	39	83	50		28	68	Earley et al. (1969)
1931–1975								
Pregnancy	121	31		83		(22)	(35)	Clark and Reid (1978)
Lactation	80	26		80		(18)	(69)	
1931–1964	14	36	79	64	45	29	75	Peete et al. (1966)
1932–1946	6	17	33	100	50	50	—	Brooks and Proffitt (1949)
1938–1961	187	33						Peters (1968)
1940–1965	50	34	48	71	48	31	86	Donegan (1979)
1940–1961	33	42	90	75	47			Rissanen (1969)
1941–1983	121	37		72			79	Ribeiro et al. (1986)
1948–1967	48	25	69	50	36	18	56	Applewhite et al. (1973)
Pre-1953	20	40	90	75	50	42	75	Hochman and Schreiber (1953)
1950–1980	63	53	100	62	53	36	82	King et al. (1985)
1954–1961	35	13	17‡	—	100			Heiman and Bennett (1963)
1960–1973	33		88	75		27	33	Cheek (1973)
1960–1980	56	61	100	61	61	47	82	Petrek et al. (1991)
1970–1980	19	57	95	78	61	50	100	Nugent and O'Connell (1985)

A chronologic summary is shown of selected reports on the results of treating breast cancer during pregnancy or lactation. No trend is evident. Patients without metastases in axillary lymph nodes have a relatively favorable prognosis.
*Parentheses indicate 10-year survival.
†Only patients 35 years of age or younger.
‡Clinical Stages I and II.

8 weeks; Fig. 34–3). Malformations are produced as well as retardation of growth and mental development. Microcephaly, hydrocephaly, microphthalmia, and spina bifida are the most frequent abnormalities, but Down's syndrome and malformed extremities and genitals are seen. Exposure later during fetal development can result in central nervous system defects, but these are unlikely after 30 weeks of gestation. The risk of childhood malignancies may be increased, particularly leukemia.. It is not possible to completely shield the fetus during therapeutic irradiation to the breast because of scatter within the patient's body and leakage from the source of irradiation. The fetal dose increases as the pregnancy progresses, bringing the fetus closer to the field of irradiation (Wallack et al., 1983, p. 26). With fetal exposure of 10 cGy malformations become detectable, and they are dependable at 100 or more cGy.

DEATHS AND ABNORMALITIES AT TERM AFTER RADIATION EXPOSURE*

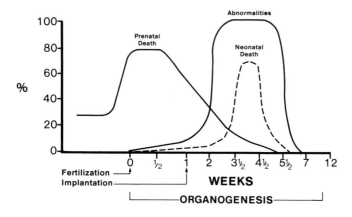

Figure 34–3. Animal experiments demonstrate that irradiation in the first trimester of pregnancy during the period of organogenesis can be expected to result in a high frequency of fetal deaths and abnormalities. This risk is not expressed later in pregnancy, but as the uterus enlarges it becomes more difficult to shield the fetus, and long-term effects become a matter of concern. (Redrawn from Brill, A. B., and Forgotson, E. H.: Radiation and congenital malformations. Am. J. Obstet. Gynecol., *90*:1149, 1964.)

*Estimated for humans based on animal data.

Tamoxifen given during pregnancy may cause fetal harm. Most information is from animal studies; there are no adequate or well-controlled studies of pregnant women. In rats tamoxifen produces nonteratogenic skeletal changes. In rabbits, reduced implantation, fetal death, and retarded growth in utero are documented. There are reports of fetal deaths, birth defects, spontaneous abortions, and vaginal bleeding in pregnant women.

Cytotoxic chemotherapy is mutagenic and can produce developmental defects in the fetus. This is clearly a risk in the first trimester, during organogenesis. Experience to date suggests little or no risk during the late second and the third trimester (Nicholson, 1968; Raich and Curet, 1975).

Early Clinical Stages

A strategy of treatment for early stages (I, II, IIIA) of invasive breast carcinoma during pregnancy may be summarized as follows:

First Trimester (1 to 13 Weeks)

Local Treatment. Modified radical mastectomy may be used without disturbing the pregnancy. If breast conservation is desired, therapeutic abortion is necessary to avoid fetal irradiation.

Systemic Treatment. If it is necessary to initiate chemotherapy during the first trimester, therapeutic abortion is advisable.

Second Trimester (14 to 26 Weeks)

Local Treatment. Modified radical mastectomy is appropriate. If breast conservation is desired, therapeutic abortion is necessary to avoid fetal irradiation.

Systemic Treatment. Adjuvant chemotherapy may be given if indicated.

Third Trimester (27 to 39 Weeks)

Local Treatment. Modified radical mastectomy is appropriate. If breast conservation is desired and the patient is near term, lumpectomy and axillary dissection can be performed and irradiation begun after delivery.

Systemic Treatment. Adjuvant chemotherapy can be given if indicated. If adjuvant chemotherapy is instituted during pregnancy, the last dose should be given 4 weeks before delivery to avoid neutropenia in the infant. Tamoxifen, if indicated, should begin after delivery.

Post Partum and During Lactation

Local Treatment. Modified radical mastectomy or breast conservation should be considered. Breast feeding should be discontinued, and operations are facilitated by suppressing lactation to reduce vascularity.

Systemic Treatment. Systemic treatment can be given as indicated. Breast feeding should not be practiced during adjuvant chemotherapy, since most agents are secreted in breast milk and can cause cytopenia in the infant. It is not known whether tamoxifen is excreted in human milk, but because of the potential for serious reactions in the nursing infant breast feeding is not advised.

As shown in Table 34–3, the results of treatment generally are poor when metastases are present in lymph nodes, whereas when disease is confined to the breast the survival rate is gratifying, frequently comparable to that expected in nonpregnant patients. Five-year survival rates are 75% (Peete et al., 1966), 100% (Byrd et al., 1962), 82% (King et al., 1985), and 75% for patients without axillary metastases (Hochman and Schreiber, 1953). Petrek and coworkers (1991) compared 56 cases of operable breast cancer treated during or within a year of pregnancy with 166 cases in other young patients. A logistic regression analysis indicated that nodal status was a highly significant predictor of survival whereas pregnancy was not. The trimester in which cancer is diagnosed and treated is not a significant determinant of prognosis (Ribeiro et al., 1986; Zemlickis et al., 1992). The fact that stage of the cancer is the major determinant of survival provides reason to believe that prompt diagnosis and treatment during pregnancy improve overall chances for survival.

Postoperative radiotherapy has not had a demonstrable effect on survival. The arguments for and against its use to prevent local recurrence in high-risk cases can be found in Chapter 19. The hazard to the fetus posed by ionizing irradiation would discourage its use during pregnancy as either primary or adjuvant therapy (see Fig. 34–3) (Dekaban, 1968; Covington and Baker, 1969).

The use of cytotoxic agents as adjuvant chemotherapy is hazardous to normal fetal development in the first trimester of pregnancy (Nicholson, 1968; Raich and Curet, 1975). Both antimetabolites and alkylating agents are associated with developmental anomalies. Methotrexate and aminopterin pose a special risk, shared to a lesser degree by chlorambucil, cyclophosphamide, and busulfan. Murray and coworkers (1984) reviewed collected results from 164 patients treated during the first trimester and found an 11.6% rate of fetal malformations (e.g., cleft palate, hydrocephalus). This is approximately a fivefold increase over the expected prevalence (Schapira and Chudley, 1984). When patients treated with aminopterin were omitted, the rate fell to 8%. Several of the patients received irradiation as well, and this combination is considered particularly teratogenic. No malformed fetuses followed treatment of 76 women during the second or third trimester. Although exposure of the fetus during the second or third trimester of pregnancy is not likely to interfere with normal organ development, long-term effects are unknown. In a more recent experience Zemlickis and coworkers (1992) at the Princess Margaret Hospital in Toronto confirmed the hazard of first trimester chemotherapy. Five of thirteen women treated during the first trimester went to term, and two of the five infants had major malformations. One stillbirth resulted among four women treated during the second trimester, but no malformations were observed. Four women treated during the third trimester delivered normal infants. If it is considered desirable to undertake this form of treatment in the first trimester, serious consideration should be given to terminating the pregnancy.

Despite the theoretical advantages of reversing the hormonal changes of pregnancy, therapeutic abortion in operable cases has not improved the results of treatment. In 1953, Adair published the results with a small group of patients who appeared to survive longer when termination of pregnancy was as part of therapy. More than two-thirds (69.5%) of a group of 23 patients whose pregnancies were simultaneous with or subsequent to initial therapy and who underwent therapeutic abortion lived 5 years. Only 44% of 25 patients who had not had abortions survived as long. A difference was also present when the patients were considered on the basis of axillary lymph node involvement. The differences, however, were not statistically significant, and subsequent reports by others have been similarly inconclusive. Holleb and Farrow (1962) reported on 24 patients treated with radical mastectomy, half of whom underwent abortions and half of whom did not. The 5-year clinical cure rate for the patients whose pregnancies were terminated in this instance was inferior (17%) to that of those who were allowed to deliver normally (33%), but, again, the difference was not significant. At the Princess Margaret Hospital, Toronto, the results were similar (Clark and Reid, 1978). Ninety-three women allowed to deliver spontaneously had 5-year and 10-year survival rates of 29% and 23%, respectively, superior to those with therapeutic abortion (15% and 8%, respectively) (Table 34–4). Selection obviously was involved in a decision for or against abortion, and the cases are not staged, but the figures suggest no benefit, and authorities now agree that abortion does not improve prognosis (Hubay et al., 1978). Many authorities agree, however, that other indications for termination of pregnancy may exist and that a decision can be individualized, taking into consideration factors of risk, prognosis, religious beliefs, size of family, or personal desires of the patient.

The chance of metastatic spread of cancer to the concep-

tus during continued pregnancy is small. No instance of transplacental metastasis of breast cancer to a fetus has been documented, although six cases are known in which cancer of the breast has metastasized to the placenta (Donegan, 1983). Following delivery, the child remained healthy in each case.

Advanced and Disseminated Cancer

The outlook for patients with advanced cancers (TNM Stage IIIB [locally advanced] or IV [disseminated]) generally is bleak. For 73 inoperable patients, Holleb and Farrow (1964) found a median survival time from admission to death of only 7 months (range 1 month to 3 years). Seventy-three per cent of patients died within 1 year, and 93% within 2 years from the date of admission. None of Haagensen's nine patients with Columbia clinical Stage D lesions treated with radical mastectomy survived 10 years, and only one of eight with Stage C lesions did so (Haagensen, 1971). In the series of Zemlickis and coworkers (1992) 20% of TNM Stage III and 12% of Stage IV patients survived 5 years (though none of the latter 10 years).

Effective palliation for patients with disseminated cancer is usually an urgent need; prognosis is poor. Elimination of estrogens from endocrine sources is a primary consideration in premenopausal women. In the absence of estrogen receptors in tumor tissue, however, oophorectomy and therapeutic abortion have little therapeutic value. Whether a decision is for endocrine ablation or cytotoxic chemotherapy, continuation of the pregnancy is undesirable. In the first trimester, dilation and suction curettage of the uterus is sufficient for termination of pregnancy; later, therapeutic abortion can be accomplished by the instillation of prostaglandin $F_{2\alpha}$ or 20% hypertonic saline into the amniotic fluid, or alternatively, by surgical evacuation of the uterus or hysterectomy. Whether a pregnancy near term is interrupted depends much on the urgency of initiating palliative measures and on the patient's wishes. A brief delay in the interest of delivering a viable fetus may not be accompanied by significant deterioration of the patient's condition. Chemotherapy late in pregnancy entails little risk to normal fetal development.

The results of endocrine therapy in patients younger than 35 years are poor. Despite castration and termination of pregnancy, Holleb and Farrow's seven patients died within 2 years. None of 32 patients reported by Bunker and Peters (1963) who were castrated for palliation demonstrated measurable improvement, and only two benefited subjectively. King and associates (1985) treated 8 of 12 pregnant patients with advanced local or disseminated disease with therapeutic abortion, and only one lived 5 years.

SUBSEQUENT PREGNANCIES

Pregnancies are not unusual among women treated for mammary carcinoma who remain fertile. In Treves and Holleb's series (1958), 5.5% of women 35 years of age or younger had subsequent pregnancies. Ten per cent of Pe-

Table 34–4. RESULTS OF THERAPEUTIC ABORTION IN CONJUNCTION WITH MASTECTOMY FOR EARLY STAGES OF BREAST CANCER*

5-Year Survival		
Abortion	No Abortion	Reference
4/6	4/10	Hochman and Schreiber (1953)
2/12	4/12	Holleb and Farrow (1962)†
4/7	3/3	Helman and Bennett (1963)
2/7	3/6	Peete et al (1966)
3/4	8/10	Rissanen (1968)
15.4%/13	28.9%/93	Clark and Reid (1978)
6/14	7/8	Deemarsky and Neishtadt (1981)
9/21	22/37	King et al. (1985)

*Listed are reports in which therapeutic abortion was used in conjunction with mastectomy (usually radical) in selected cases of clinically early breast cancer. Cases in each are few; no advantage in 5-year survival is apparent overall in conjunction with the procedure.

†Figures available for first trimester only.

ters' 221 patients (1968) and 15% of Rissanen's 27 patients (1968) who were treated initially during pregnancy or lactation and who retained their ovaries became pregnant again. Seventy per cent of these conceptions occurred within the first 5 years of treatment.

With increasing numbers of women receiving adjuvant chemotherapy as a component of initial treatment, the effect of cytotoxic drugs on the fertility of patients and on their offspring is a matter of interest. Ovarian failure after chemotherapy is age dependent. After age 30 years permanent amenorrhea is frequent, whereas before age 25 the majority of women continue to menstruate normally. To date, no increase in congenital anomalies or abnormal pregnancies has been noted in women who received chemotherapy for a variety of malignancies (Averette et al., 1990). In a review of 227 consecutive patients with breast cancer 35 years of age or younger treated with adjuvant chemotherapy containing doxorubicin, Sutton and coworkers (1990) noted that 11% later became pregnant after a median interval of 12 months. Twenty-eight per cent of those who became pregnant developed recurrence. Ten of the pregnancies were terminated, two ended in spontaneous abortion, and nineteen resulted in the birth of normal infants. Survival and disease-free survival did not appear to be adversely affected by pregnancy. Jochimsen and colleagues (1981) reported two patients who became pregnant while receiving adjuvant chemotherapy and recommended that contraception be practiced during such treatment.

Of importance is whether the pregnancies influence the patient's prognosis and whether they should be prevented or terminated. The fact is that patients with pregnancies fare very well. On review they prove to have a low incidence of axillary node involvement at the time of their original mastectomy, and their survival does not appear to be curtailed (Holleb and Farrow, 1962). Survival is often remarkably long; for example, 5-year and 10-year survival rates amounting to 67% and 57%, respectively, were reported by White and White (1956), and 77.4% (5-year) and 69.5% (10-year) by Rissanen (1969). Selection undoubtedly is involved, as women with aggressive tumors tend to have recurrence early and die, allowing those with a more favorable prognosis to survive and become pregnant. Reports that control for this bias, however, lend support to the thesis that pregnancy is not deleterious. Peters (1968) matched the age and clinical stage of 96 such patients with an equal number of patients who had no further conceptions. Those who became pregnant not only lived longer but also had longer recurrence-free survival times (Peters, 1968). Even when pregnancy occurred during a high-risk period—that is, within 6 months of mastectomy—54% lived 5 years. A case-matching study by Cooper and Butterfield (1970) with 40 pairs of patients matched for age, stage of tumor, status of axillary nodes, and equivalent survival at least to the time of conception, found superior survival in the group with subsequent pregnancies. At Memorial Sloan-Kettering Cancer Center, New York City, Harvey and colleagues (1981) reviewed 41 patients with subsequent pregnancies and found no detrimental effect, overall or selectively, for their patients with positive nodes or with early pregnancies. Abortion also had no beneficial effect.

In a survey by the Société Française de Gynécologie,

Mignot and coworkers (1986) collected 68 cases of pregnancy following mastectomy: 41 of these women had at least one uninterrupted pregnancy. The 10-year survival rate for these patients was not significantly different from that of 136 matched patients who did not become pregnant when compared overall, by node status, or by interval to pregnancy. Therapeutic abortion in 27 cases did not influence survival. These authors concluded that there were no therapeutic grounds for recommending avoidance or termination of pregnancy in patients who were free of recurrence.

Thus, a pregnancy after treatment does not provoke recurrence or jeopardize continued well-being of the patient (Helman and Bennett, 1963; Holleb and Farrow, 1964; Cheek, 1973; Ariel, 1989). It should be appreciated, however, that one or more successful pregnancies without difficulty provide no assurance against a subsequent recurrence.

In an era of planned parenthood, pregnancies are becoming a matter of choice rather than accident. Patients treated for breast cancer who desire to become pregnant must make this decision with a full appreciation of the circumstances of their case. Figure 34–4 shows annual risk of recurrence for young women in Milwaukee after mastectomy over a period of 10 years. It is evident that the interval after treatment and the presence or absence of metastases to axillary lymph nodes are important determinants of risk. The highest morbidity is within the first 2 years; pregnancies during this time are most likely to coincide with recurrence. Treat-

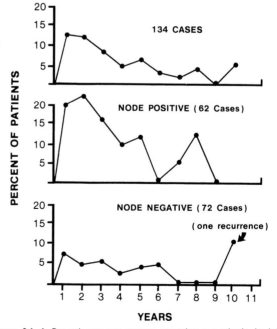

Figure 34–4. Breast cancer recurs over long periods, but the highest risk is in the first 2 years after treatment and is of considerably greater magnitude in patients with axillary nodal metastases.

ment failures occurred in 13% of the total number of patients at risk in the first year. The annual morbidity declined progressively thereafter, until at 10 years the figure approximated 5% or less.

The failures each year were considerably higher for those who had metastases in axillary lymph nodes. On the other hand, the figure never exceeded 7% for patients without nodal metastases even in early years, and after 8 years it had fallen to negligible levels. As cumulative recurrence rises progressively to claim an increasing number of previously healthy women, it might be concluded in these circumstances that the best chance of having a child and enjoying motherhood for as long as possible would be provided by a pregnancy as soon after mastectomy as possible. Conversely, maximum assurance of an uncomplicated pregnancy and of continued health lies in lengthening the period between treatment and conception. Most authorities discourage conception for 2 years to several years to pass the period of highest risk and to improve the chances of a woman's remaining healthy to care for her child. Decisions are best made on an individual basis with concern for the patient's wishes, circumstances, prognosis, and other prevailing factors.

The complexities created by legal issues relating to the therapy of pregnant women have been discussed by Theriault and colleagues (1992). The current climate of opinion has served to erode the pregnant pateint's autonomy and, potentially, to polarize divergent interests of mother and fetus. Intervention by the state on behalf of fetal welfare is evident in instances of court-ordered cesarean section and detention of women for unhealthy prenatal conduct. The ability of children to bring suit against parents for prenatal injury and for wrongful life adds to the hazards of decision making and childbearing. Knowedge of laws pertaining to the pregnant patient and a complete explanation of the potential consequences of treatment alternatives are essential to serving the interests of all.

SUMMARY

Among premenopausal women, approximately 10% of newly diagnosed breast cancers are associated with pregnancy, most patients being in the fourth decade of life. The prognosis for these patients, and for those whose cancers are diagnosed soon after pregnancy, generally is less favorable than that for nonpregnant females, but if age and stage of disease are comparable, pregnancy per se has little influence on prognosis. Mastectomy is as effective for pregnant patients as for other women, and the chance of spontaneous abortion is small. Therapeutic abortion does not improve the chances for cure of patients with clinically localized cancer. Effective endocrine therapy or chemotherapy for advanced or disseminated breast cancer does require therapeutic abortion, and an early pregnancy is best terminated. For pregnancies near term, the decision depends greatly on the desire of the patient. Unless therapeutic needs are urgent, intervention can sometimes be delayed without significant deterioration of the patient's condition.

Pregnancies subsequent to a mastectomy have little bearing on continued well-being, and as long as the patient is clinically free of cancer, no therapeutic benefit can be expected from interrupting them. A decision for future pregnancies should be individualized, with due regard for the risk of recurrence and the desirability of the patient's completing her family while still reasonably young.

Progress with the treatment of breast cancer depends in part on the appreciation that cancers do occur during pregnancy and lactation, that they are best diagnosed early, and that they are curable. Pregnancy should neither deter a prompt diagnosis nor delay definitive treatment.

References

Adair, F. E.: Cancer of the breast. Surg. Clin. North Am., *33:*313, 1953.

Applewhite, R. R., Smith, L. R., and DiVincenti, F.: Carcinoma of the breast associated with pregnancy and lactation. Am. Surg., *39:*101, 1973.

Ariel, I. M., and Kempner, R.: The prognosis of patients who become pregnant after mastectomy for breast cancer. Int. Surg., *74:*185–187, 1989.

Averette, H. E., Boike, G. M., Jarrell, M. A.: Effects of cancer chemotherapy on gonadal function and reproductive capacity. CA Cancer J. Clin., *40:*199–209, 1990.

Baker, J., Ali, A., Groch, M. W., et al.: Bone scanning in pregnant patients with breast carcinoma. Clin. Nucl. Med., *12:*519–524, 1987.

Brill, A. B., and Forgotson, E. H.: Radiation and congenital malformations. Am. J. Obstet. Gynecol., *90:*1149, 1964.

Brooks, B., and Proffitt, J. N.: The influence of pregnancy on cancers of the breast. Surgery, *25:*1, 1949.

Bunker, M. L., and Peters, M. V.: Breast cancer associated with pregnancy or lactation. Am. J. Obstet. Gynecol., *85:*312, 1963.

Byrd, B. F. Jr., Bayer, D. S., Robertson, J. C., et al.: Treatment of breast tumors associated with pregnancy and lactation. Ann. Surg., *155:*940, 1962.

Canter, J. W., Oliver, G. C., and Zaloudek, C. J.: Surgical diseases of the breast during pregnancy. Clin. Obstet. Gynecol., *26:*853, 1983.

Cheek, J. H.: Survey of current opinions concerning carcinoma of the breast occurring during pregnancy. Arch. Surg., *66:*664, 1953.

Cheek, J. H.: Cancer of the breast in pregnancy and lactation. Am. J. Surg., *126:*729, 1973.

Chiedozi, L. C., Iweze, F. I., Aboh, I. F., et al.: Breast cancer in pregnancy and lactation. Trop. Geogr. Med., *40:*26–30, 1988.

Clark, R. M., and Reid, J.: Carcinoma of the breast in pregnancy and lactation. Int. J. Radiation Oncol. Biol. Phys., *4:*693, 1978.

Cooper, D. R., and Butterfield, J.: Pregnancy subsequent to mastectomy for cancer of the breast. Ann. Surg., *171:*429, 1970.

Costarides, J., and Theofanides, C.: Carcinoma of the breast during pregnancy or lactation. J. Int. Coll. Surg., *40:*146, 1963.

Covington, E. E., and Baker, A. S.: Dosimetry of scattered radiation to the fetus. J.A.M.A., *209:*414, 1969.

Deemarsky, L. J., and Neishtadt, E. L.: Breast cancer and pregnancy. Breast, *7:*17, 1981.

Dekaban, A. S.: Abnormalities in children exposed to x-radiation during various stages of gestation: Tentative timetable of radiation injury to the human fetus, part I. J. Nucl. Med., *9:*471, 1968.

Donegan, W. L.: Pregnancy and breast cancer. Obstet. Gynecol., *50:*244, 1977.

Donegan, W. L.: Mammary carcinoma and pregnancy. In Donegan, W. L., and Spratt, J. S. (Eds.): Cancer of the Breast. 2nd ed. Philadelphia, W. B. Saunders, 1979, p. 448.

Donegan, W. L.: Cancer and pregnancy. CA Cancer J. Clin., *33:*5, 1983.

Earley, T. K., Gallagher, J. Q., and Chapman, K. E.: Carcinoma of the breast in women under thirty years of age. Am. J. Surg., *118:*832, 1969.

Finn, W. F.: Pregnancy complicated by cancer. Bull. Margaret Hague Maternity Hosp., *5:*2, 1952.

Haagensen, C. D.: Diseases of the Breast. 1st ed. Philadelphia, W. B. Saunders, 1956, p. 538.

Haagensen, C. D.: Diseases of the Breast. 2nd ed. Philadelphia, W. B. Saunders, 1971, p. 662.

Haagensen, C. D., and Stout, A. P.: Carcinoma of the breast. II. Criteria for operability. Ann. Surg., *118:*859, 1943.

Harrington, S. W.: Carcinoma of the breast: Results of surgical treatment when the carcinoma occurred in course of pregnancy or lactation and when pregnancy occurred subsequent to operation, 1910–1933. Ann. Surg., *106:*690, 1937.

Harvey, J. C., Rosen, P. P., Ashikari, R., et al.: The effect of pregnancy on the prognosis of carcinoma of the breast following radical mastectomy. Surg. Gynecol. Obstet., *153:*723, 1981.

Helman, P., and Bennett, M. B.: Breast cancer and pregnancy. S. Afr. Med. J., *37:*1236, 1963.

Hochman, A., and Schreiber, H.: Pregnancy and cancer of the breast. Obstet. Gynecol., *2:*268, 1953.

Hoeffken, W., and Lanyi, M.: Mammography. Philadelphia, W. B. Saunders, 1977, p. 76.

Holdaway, I. M., Mason, B. H., and Kay, R. G.: Steroid hormone receptors in breast tumors presenting during pregnancy or lactation. J. Surg. Oncol., *25:*38, 1984.

Holleb, A. I., and Farrow, J. H.: The relation of carcinoma of the breast and pregnancy in 283 patients. Surg. Gynecol. Obstet., *115:*65, 1962.

Holleb, A. I., and Farrow, J. H.: Breast cancer and pregnancy. Acta Un. Int. Cancr., *20:*1480, 1964.

Horsley, J. S., III, Alrich, E. M., and Wright, C. B.: Carcinoma of the breast in women 35 years of age or younger. Ann. Surg., *196:*839, 1969.

Hytten, F. E., and Leitch, I.: The Physiology of Human Pregnancy. 2nd ed. Oxford, Blackwell, 1971.

Hubay, C. A., Barry, F. M., and Marr, C. C.: Pregnancy and breast cancer. Surg. Clin. North Am., *58:*819, 1978.

Jochimsen, P. R., Spaight, M. E., and Urdaneta, L. F.: Pregnancy during adjuvant chemotherapy for breast cancer. J.A.M.A., *245:*1660, 1981.

Jones, S. E.: Management of breast cancer in the pregnant patient. Contemp. Oncol. 216:19–24, 1992.

King, R. M., Welch, J. S., Martin, J. K. Jr., et al.: Carcinoma of the breast associated with pregnancy. Surg. Gynecol. Obstet., *160:*228, 1985.

Koshi, S., Egami, T., Isogai, M., et al.: Breast cancer associated with pregnancy. Nippon Geka Gakkai Zasshi, *90:*127–129, 1989.

Lefreniere, R.: Bloody nipple discharge during pregnancy: Rationale for conservative treatment. J. Surg. Oncol., *43:*228–230, 1990.

Mignot, L., Morvan, F., Berdah, J., et al.: Pregnancy after treated breast cancer. Results of a case-control study. Presse Med., *15:*1961–1964, 1986.

Montgomery, T. L.: Detection and disposal of breast cancer in pregnancy. Am. J. Obstet. Gynecol., *81:*926, 1961.

Murray, C. L., Reichert, J. A., Anderson, J., et al.: Multimodal cancer therapy for breast cancer in the first trimester of pregnancy. A case report. J.A.M.A., *252:*2607, 1984.

Nelson, J. H., Lu, T., Hall, J. E., et al.: The effect of trophoblast on immune state of women. Am. J. Obstet. Gynecol., *117:*689, 1973.

Nicholson, O. P.: Cytotoxic drugs in pregnancy. J. Obstet. Gynecol. Br. Commonw., *75:*307, 1968.

Nugent, P., and O'Connell, T. X.: Breast cancer and pregnancy. Arch. Surg., *120:*1221, 1985.

Parente, J. T., Amsel, K. M., Lerner, R., et al.: Breast cancer associated with pregnancy. Obstet. Gynecol., *71(1):*861–864, 1988.

Peete, C. H. Jr., Huneycutt, H. C. Jr., and Cherny, W. B.: Cancer of the breast in pregnancy. N. C. Med. J., *27:*514, 1966.

Peters, M. V.: The effect of pregnancy in breast cancer. *In* Forrest, A. P. M., and Kunkler, P. B. (Eds.): Prognostic Factors in Breast Cancer. Baltimore, Williams & Wilkins, 1968, p. 65.

Petrek, J. A., Dukoff, R., and Rogatko, A.: Prognosis of pregnancy-associated breast cancer. Cancer, *67:*869–872, 1991.

Purtilo, R. T., Hallgren, H. M., and Yunis, E. S.: Depressed maternal lymphocyte response to PHA in human pregnancy. Lancet, *1:*769, 1972.

Raich, P. C., and Curet, L. B.: Treatment of acute leukemia during pregnancy. Cancer, *36:*861, 1975.

Ribeiro, G., Jones, D. A., and Jones, M.: Carcinoma of the breast associated with pregnancy. Br. J. Surg., *73:*507–509, 1986.

Rissanen, P. M.: Carcinoma of the breast during pregnancy and lactation. Br. J. Cancer, *22:*663, 1968.

Rissanen, P. M.: Pregnancy following treatment of mammary cancer. Acta Radiol., *8:*415, 1969.

Rosemond, G. P.: Management of patients with carcinoma of the breast in pregnancy. Ann. NY Acad. Sci., *114:*851, 1964.

Sahni, K., Sanyal, B., Agrawal, M. S., et al.: Carcinoma of breast associated with pregnancy and lactation. J. Surg. Oncol., *16:*167, 1981.

Saltztein, E. C., Mann, R. W., Chua, T. Y., et al.: Outpatient breast biopsy. Arch. Surg., *109:*287, 1974.

Schapira, D. V., and Chudley, A. E.: Successful pregnancy following continuous treatment with combination chemotherapy before conception and throughout pregnancy. Cancer, *54:*800, 1984.

Shapiro, C. L., and Mayer, R. J.: Breast cancer during pregnancy. Adv. Oncol., *8:*25–29, 1992.

Shnider, S. M., and Levinson, G.: Obstetric anesthesia. *In* Miller, R. D. (Ed.): Anesthesia. 2nd ed. New York, Churchill Livingston, 1986, p. 1719.

Strelkauskas, A. J., Wilson, B. S., Dray, D., et al.: Inversion of levels of human T & B cells in early pregnancy. Nature, *258:*331, 1975.

Sutton, R., Buzdar, A. U., and Hortobagyi, G. N.: Pregnancy and offspring after adjuvant chemotherapy in breast cancer patients. Cancer, *65:*847–850, 1990.

Theriault, R. I., and Hortobagyi, G. N.: When breast cancer complicates pregnancy: What options are available? Prim. Care Cancer, *9:*27–32, 1989.

Theriault, R. L., Stallings, C. B., and Buzdar, A. U.: Pregnancy and breast cancer: Clinical and legal issues. Am. J. Clin. Oncol., *15:*535–539, 1992.

Third National Cancer Survey: Incidence Data. National Cancer Institute Monograph No. 41, March 1975. DHEW Publ. No. (NIH) 75-787. N, Bethesda, MD, U.S. Public Health Service, 1975.

Treves, N., and Holleb, A. I.: A report of 549 cases of breast cancer in women 35 years of age or younger. Surg. Gynecol. Obstet., *107:*271, 1958.

U.S. Bureau of the Census. Statistical Abstract of the United States 1990. 110th ed. Washington, DC, U.S. Government Printing Office, 1990.

Wallack, M. K., Wolf, J. A., Bedwinek, J., et al.: Gestational carcinoma of the female breast. Curr. Probl. Cancer, *7:*26, 1983.

Westberg, S. V.: Prognosis of breast cancer for pregnant and nursing women. Acta Obstet. Gynecol. Scand., *25*(Suppl. 4):179, 1946.

White, T. T.: Prognosis of breast cancer for pregnant and nursing women: Analysis of 1413 cases. Surg. Gynecol. Obstet., *100:*661, 1955.

White, T. T., and White, W. C.: Breast cancer and pregnancy, report of 49 cases followed five years. Ann. Surg., *144:*384, 1956.

Zeigerman, J. H., Honigman, F. H., and Crawford, R. W.: Inflammatory mammary cancer during pregnancy and lactation. Obstet. Gynecol., *32:*373, 1968.

Zemlickis, D., et al.: Cancer during pregnancy—maternal and fetal outcomes. Am. J. Obstet. Gynecol., *166:*781–787, 1992.

35

Sarcomas of the Breast

William L. Donegan

Nonepithelial cancers account for approximately 1% of all breast cancers. They represented 0.7% of all cases of breast cancer referred to the Ellis Fischel State Cancer Hospital (EFSCH) during a 25-year period. At Sinai Samaritan Medical Center (SSMC) in Milwaukee, they constituted 1.3% of 751 consecutive cases of breast cancer. They are disproportionately few in number compared with the large component of the breast devoted to mesenchymal supporting tissues, re-emphasizing the fact that cancer of the breast is predominantly a disease of epithelium. Phyllodes tumors (PTs) are the most frequent sarcomas of the breast, followed by lymphomas and a variety of pure soft tissue sarcomas. Classification of the latter is based on the cell of probable origin as determined by histologic examination, ultrastructural study, and immunocytochemical tests.

These tumors typically present as discrete masses, often large but only infrequently attached to the skin or deep tissues. Nipple discharge, peau d'orange changes, and skin invasion or retraction, seen with carcinomas, do occur but are infrequent. Palpable axillary lymph nodes are rarely a feature, and clinical adenopathy is more often due to hyperplasia than to tumor (Pollard et al., 1990). The predominantly hematogenous metastases are to the lungs, bones, and liver.

The mammographic features of sarcomas are deceptively similar to those of benign lesions such as cysts or fibroadenomas. They appear dense and well marginated, with little evidence of invasiveness. The radiographic dimensions correspond closely with the clinical and pathologic measurements (Berger and Gershon-Cohen, 1962; Elson et al., 1992).

Sarcomas of the breast tend to behave like sarcomas in other sites. No separate staging system exists for them in the breast. They are staged and treated as sarcomas, not as carcinomas. Prognosis is related to tumor grade, size, and anatomic extent.

The disposition of sarcomas toward extensive local infiltration, often well beyond what appear grossly to be well-encapsulated margins, and their inclination to metastasize through blood vessels rather than lymphatics support treatment with wide surgical removal without routine regional lymph node dissection, though local recurrence and distant dissemination continue to frustrate many attempts at cure.

PHYLLODES TUMORS (CYSTOSARCOMA PHYLLODES)

PTs, also known as cystosarcoma phyllodes, not only are unique to the breast but also are unique among sarcomas in containing a benign epithelial component. They probably develop from the benign and more familiar fibroadenoma and differ from it only in having a more cellular, often clearly malignant, stroma. PTs account for 55% of nonepithelial breast cancers at SSMC. They constitute 2.5% of fibroepithelial tumors of the breast (Lester and Stout, 1954). Treves (1964) reported 93 among 3200 fibroadenomas. At EFSCH 9 were diagnosed among 4001 women referred for breast disease between 1940 and 1965, a prevalence of 0.2%. Ariel (1961) derived from many reports that PTs represent 0.3% of all mammary neoplasms in patients admitted to general hospitals.

PT is known by many names and, as witnessed by the voluminous literature on the subject, has posed problems of definition, clinicopathologic correlation, and management. In a historical review of the subject, Fiks (1981) was able to collect 62 names from the literature. Cystosarcoma phyllodes (literally cystic, fleshy, leafy tumor), the name coined in 1838 by Muller on the basis of the large specimens familiar to him, is a misnomer propagated by popular use. The tumor is not regularly cystic or leafy in appearance and only occasionally expresses its deadly potential. Histologic features of the stroma vary from benign to malignant, and these tumors are so classified. Faced with the paradox of a ''benign sarcoma,'' the World Health Organization solved this dilemma by recommending that the term ''phyllodes tumor'' be used as a more appropriate designation, one that can be qualified as *benign, malignant,* or *borderline malignant* (WHO, 1981).

The present understanding of PTs has evolved through a long period of controversy. Probably the first description was that of Chelius in 1828, who described a large ''cystic hydatid'' of the breast and considered it a benign condition. Muller described the tumor 10 years later, and again emphasized its benign nature as well as the tendency to have large dimensions.

Lee and Pack (1931), who summarized 105 cases from the literature and reported six of their own, likened the histologic features to those of an intracanalicular fibroadenoma but considered metaplasia of the stroma into myxomatous tissue with cellular pseudosarcomatous regions as its distinguishing feature. They suggested the name ''giant intracanalicular fibroadenomyxoma.'' Among other features were large size, protracted symptoms, lobulation and mobility, slow growth initially followed by rapid acceleration, and probable development from a fibroadenoma. The tumor was also considered benign, although 6 of 91 patients had recurrence after the lesion was removed. Owens and Adams (1941) attributed the myxomatous changes simply to edema and recommended the name ''giant intracanalicular fibroadenoma." Accumulating reports of local recurrence and occasional distant metastases made it increasingly clear that a malignant variant existed. White (1940) documented dissemination to the lungs and mediastinum. Cooper and Ackerman (1943) were first to describe metastases to axillary lymph nodes. In 1950 McDonald and Harrington estimated that a sarcomatous stroma occurred in 10% of cases and considered this variant fibrosarcoma. Their report on 13 cases of cystosarcoma phyllodes was confined to benign cases, and large size was essential: the tumors had to involve at least four-fifths of the breast. Foote and Stewart (1946) disagreed. They pointed out that typical proliferative changes could be found in small tumors, which they dubbed miniature cystosarcoma phyllodes. Treves and Sunderland's review of 77 cases at Memorial Hospital, New York, in 1951 served to emphasize the tumor's malignant potential and to eliminate size as a criterion for diagnosis. These authors identified stromal overgrowth as the essential characteristic for differentiating cystosarcoma from fibroadenoma and included tumors as small as 1.0 cm in their report. Tumors were also divided into benign, malignant, and borderline malignant categories, depending on the character of the stroma. Fifty per cent of 18 malignant lesions metastasized to viscera and one to an axillary lymph node. Although four borderline tumors recurred locally, none disseminated. Wide local excision or simple mastectomy was recommended for benign cases, and radical mastectomy for those with a malignant stroma. Applying these criteria, however, has been a persistent problem. Lester and Stout (1954) found only a disappointing correlation between histologic findings and clinical outcome in their material at Presbyterian Hospital in New York. Not all of the tumors that metastasized appeared to be histologically malignant, and one tumor judged to be benign metastasized. They attributed the difficulty to pleomorphism of the stroma, and they warned against sampling error. Others identified the same problem. Oberman (1965*a*) was able to achieve reasonable clinicopathologic correlation in 18 cases at the University of Michigan, but at the Mayo Clinic 2 of 23 tumors judged benign eventually metastasized (West et al., 1971). Blichert-Toft and associates (1975) also found a disappointing correlation between tumor grade and clinical course and noted that with recurrences the character of tumors could become progressively more malignant. Four of twelve initially benign tumors recurred with a malignant stroma, and three of these patients died of disseminated disease. The problem of clinicopathologic correlation has persisted to the present day. In reality, the patient's clinical course serves to determine the true malignancy of a PT. The incidence of malignancy is uncertain. Most large series are reported from referral centers, where difficult cases tend to be concentrated. In addition to sampling problems, subtle biases may create differences in histologic classification. Table 35–1 shows the histologic classification of PTs in five sizable series.

Clinical Features

PTs appear later in life than fibroadenomas and earlier than carcinomas. Ages of affected women range from 9 to 88 years, but mean ages are narrowly distributed between 44 and 50, and 83% of patients are between 31 and 60 years of age (Palmer et al., 1990; Cohn-Cedermark et al., 1991; Cosmacini et al., 1992; Hawkins et al., 1992; Keelan et al., 1992). Asian women are younger; Chua and coworkers (1989) reported a mean age of only 30 years for 106 women in Singapore, 86% being between 15 and 44 years old, and Kario's group (1990) reported a mean age of 36 years for 34 Japanese women. It is exceptionally rare in men. Lee and Pack reported in 1931 that 3% of their patients were men, and Keelan and associates (1992) found 1 man among 60 cases at the Mayo Clinic. Ansah-Boateng and Tavassoli (1992) were able to find only five cases in men in the files of the Armed Forces Institute of Pathology and attributed this to the dearth in the male breast of lobules, the structure from which fibroepithelial tumors are believed to originate. As many as 12.5% of patients with PTs have a history of fibroadenomas, and as many as 20% have concurrent fibroadenomas (Zurrida et al., 1992; Rowell et al., 1993). The evidence that PTs originate in fibroadenomas has led some to suggest that removal of fibroadenomas may help to prevent PTs (Treves, 1964; Amerson, 1970).

A palpable, well-circumscribed, often lobulated mass with a rubbery consistency is the most frequent presenting sign of PT; a few are painful. These features, and the youth of patients, account for a preoperative diagnosis of fibroadenoma in most cases. Histories vary much, from 1 week to 20 years. Recent rapid growth is noted by many patients, and the tumor can reach great size: average diameters of 5.0 to 9.0 cm are reported (Palmer et al., 1990; Hawkins et al., 1992). Nine cases at EFSCH averaged 18 cm in diameter (Donegan, 1988) (Fig. 35–1). Some massive tumors are obviously cystic in places (Fig. 35–2). The overlying skin becomes attenuated, shiny, and erythematous and eventually ulcerates. Nipple discharge is unusual, as is adenopa-

Table 35–1. HISTOLOGIC CLASSIFICATION OF PHYLLODES TUMORS IN FIVE STUDIES

Investigation	Age (y)	Lesions (no.)	Classification		
			Benign	Borderline	Malignant
Rowell et al., 1993	9–68	18	11	4	3
Grimes, 1992	13–76	187	95	42	50
Zurrida et al., 1992	9–?	216	140	46	30
Chua et al., 1989	—	106	97	6	3
Cohn-Cedermark, 1991	18–85	77			35
Total		604			121 (20%)

*Consultation cases omitted.

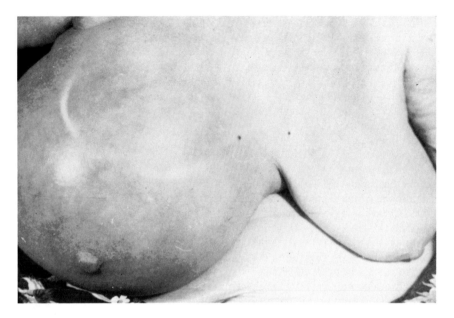

Figure 35-1. This phyllodes tumor developed in the breast of an 82-year-old woman over an 8-month period. Notable are the shininess and mild erythema of the tense overlying skin and absence of ulceration despite massive proportions of the tumor. No axillary lymph nodes were palpable.

thy. The latter deserves attention when it is found because nodal metastasis does occur, though the frequency may be no higher than 3% (Donegan, 1988; Palmer et al., 1990). These rare tumors occur with equal frequency in the right and left breasts. They are bilateral in 3% of cases, and rarely are multiple (Grimes, 1992; Hawkins et al., 1992). PTs have been reported in ectopic axillary breast tissue (Saleh and Klein, 1990).

Mammography may fail to visualize this tumor in a dense breast and cannot distinguish it from fibroadenoma or even a cyst, though large size suggests it (Fig. 35–3). The circumscribed density, often with a clear surrounding halo, is consistent with a benign tumor (Buchberger et al., 1991). Microcalcifications may be seen (Cosmacini et al., 1992). Characteristic sonographic features are a discrete structure with cystic spaces (Fig. 35–4). Fine-needle aspiration (FNA) cytologic examination is unreliable. Mixed stromal and epithelial elements suggest the lesion, but FNA examination is plagued by false positive and false negative diagnoses and misidentification as carcinoma (Buchberger et al., 1991; Rao and Jaganathan, 1992; Rowell et al., 1993). Core needle biopsy provided a correct diagnosis in only 50% of cases in one series (Chua et al., 1989). Excision is the usual means for accurate diagnosis and evaluation of the tumor.

Pathology

On gross examination PTs appear encapsulated. The surface is smooth and separates easily from surrounding tissues. The cut surface is gray-white and glistening and bulges outward. Many slitlike spaces are seen, and often cavities containing grapelike or leafy formations (Fig. 35–5). Larger

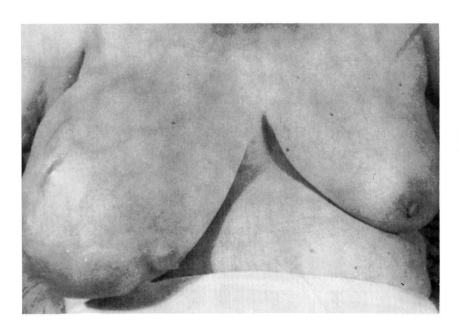

Figure 35-2. This phyllodes tumor in the right breast of a 66-year-old woman demonstrates the lobulation and cystic prominences that are frequently evident on clinical examination. The lesion was thought to be of borderline malignancy histologically. It recurred locally years after simple mastectomy.

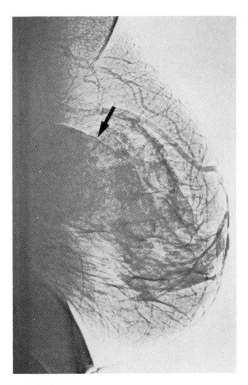

Figure 35–3. Mammogram showing a large phyllodes tumor deep within the breast as a well-marginated mass.

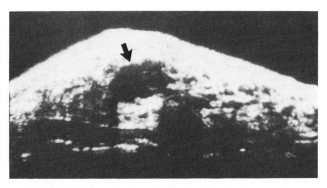

Figure 35–4. Sonogram of this phyllodes tumor *(arrow)* suggests a cystic structure with irregular walls and few internal echoes.

tumors are prone to hemorrhage and necrosis. Histologically they are composed predominantly of a stroma that is more densely cellular than that of a fibroadenoma and spaces lined by benign ductal epithelium (Fig. 35–6). The stroma varies histologically from benign to obviously malignant (Fig. 35–7). The probability of finding a malignant stroma increases with the size of the tumor and the age of the patient (Zurrida et al., 1992). Approximately 20% of PTs are histologically malignant (see Table 35–1). Malig-

nant stroma is anaplastic and shows much mitotic activity. It often has the appearance of fibrosarcoma or myxoliposarcoma, but less often osteosarcoma, chondrosarcoma, or even rhabdomyosarcoma is found. An infiltrating, rather than pushing, border indicates biologic aggressiveness (Bot and Donner, 1981). Stromal overgrowth (i.e., disappearance of benign epithelium from large areas of the tumor [at least one low-power field]) is also a strong indicator of malignancy (Hart et al., 1978; Ward and Evans, 1986). El-Naggar and colleagues (1990a) found ploidy to be a significant predictor of clinical outcome, but most investigators have found neither ploidy nor S-phase fraction to be a reliable prognostic marker (Layfield et al., 1989; Grimes, 1992; Keelan et al., 1992; Rowell et al., 1993). Most agree that stromal overgrowth, anaplasia, high mitotic rate, and an infiltrating border are the best predictors of metastasis. Cohn-Cedermark and associates found the presence of necrosis and stromal elements other than fibromyxoid tissue to be independent predictors of metastasis or death. Immunocytochemically PTs stain for vimentin and Type I and Type III collagen but not for cytokeratin or epithelial membrane antigen (Lewko et al., 1990). Both PTs and fibroadenomas regularly contain significant amounts of progeste-

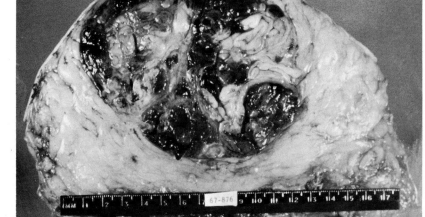

Figure 35–5. Cut section of a phyllodes tumor demonstrates pseudoencapsulation.

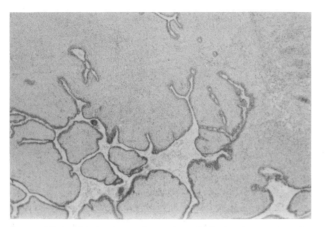

Figure 35–6. Histologic section of a phyllodes tumor showing dense cellular stroma and spaces lined with benign epithelium.

rone receptor protein but infrequently contain estrogen receptors (Rao et al., 1981). Brentani and colleagues (1982) studied seven cases and found 40% of five low-grade PTs to contain estrogen receptors and 60% glucocorticoid receptors.

Coincident adenocarcinoma of the breast, which is occasionally reported, affects the patient's prognosis independently. The incidence of one tumor does not influence that of the other (Richards and Way, 1963; Grimes, 1992).

Treatment

The only therapy for PTs that offers a chance of cure is wide surgical removal with tumor-free tissue margins. Enucleation is not adequate. In general, the choice of operation is guided by the size and histologic classification of the tumor. Vascular metastases are probably little affected by the extent of operation. The frequency of dissemination is more closely related to the degree of malignancy of the stroma than to the magnitude of resection. This is not the case for local recurrence. For tumors of comparable size and histologic appearance the probability of local recur-

rence appears to be inversely correlated with the magnitude of operation (Donegan, 1988; Palmer et al., 1990; Cohn-Cedermark et al., 1991). In the past, mastectomy, frequently radical mastectomy, was the operation chosen for treatment of PTs. Currently the operation most often recommended is wide local resection. Mastectomy is reserved for large tumors, malignant or borderline tumors, and those that are recurrent (Chua et al., 1989; Salvadori et al., 1989; Bartoli et al., 1990; Palmer et al., 1990; Grimes, 1992; Keelan et al., 1992; Zurrida et al., 1992). Axillary lymph node removal is not recommended in the absence of adenopathy. The trend to wide local excision rather than mastectomy is motivated by cosmetic concerns, an important consideration for young women, and that local recurrences usually can be controlled with further resection, particularly those of histologically benign tumors. This is largely true, but not routinely so. The behavior of this tumor remains unpredictable; benign tumors can be stubbornly persistent locally, and rarely can metastasize. In adolescents PTs have a reputation for not being aggressive, but Turalba and colleagues (1986) reported the third case of local recurrence, metastasis, and death of an adolescent girl.

Recurrences appear locally or at distant sites. Most are seen within the first 2 years of treatment, but they can appear many years later. Local recurrences are the most frequent form of treatment failure (Figs. 35–8 through 35–11). They are more likely after treatment of malignant than

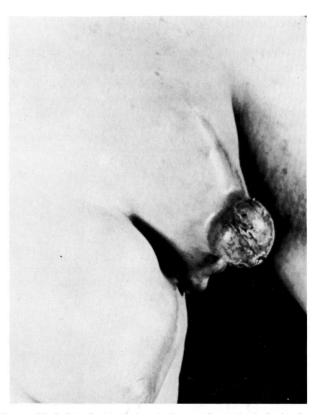

Figure 35–8. This Grade 2, borderline malignant phyllodes tumor recurred in the surgical scar 4 months after local excision. It persisted despite a subsequent simple mastectomy and several further attempts to treat it with local excision and radiotherapy.

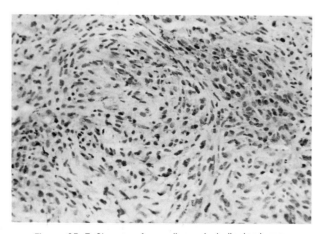

Figure 35–7. Stroma of a malignant phyllodes tumor.

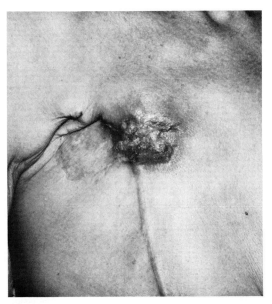

Figure 35–9. Recurrent phyllodes tumor at the medial edge of a skin graft after radical mastectomy.

of benign tumors (Table 35–2) and after limited operations (Table 35–3). Increased histologic malignancy is often apparent in recurrences (Chua et al., 1989; Grimes, 1992). Local recurrences are best treated by mastectomy or radical surgical excision when this is possible, even if it requires repeated attempts. Some can be controlled (Palmer et al., 1990).

Distant metastases are preceded by local recurrence in the majority of cases. Borderline malignant tumors and malignant ones pose far greater threats than benign tumors (see Table 35–2). When distant metastases appear, the survival time thereafter is usually less than 2 years. The lungs and mediastinum are favored sites for deposits, but metastases also seek the heart, bones, brain, and intra-abdominal organs (McCullough and Lynch, 1960; West et al., 1971).

Ariel (1961) found osseous involvement in 33% of a collected group with metastatic disease. Intractable heart failure may be the only sign of spread to the heart.

PTs are weakly radioresponsive. Adjuvant irradiation is not evaluable (Cohn-Cedermark et al., 1991), but radiation can produce local palliation (Burton et al., 1989).

Hormone therapy and chemotherapy have little effect. Cyclophosphamide has produced regression (Hoover et al., 1975). Allen and coworkers (1985) reported complete remission of pulmonary metastases in response to six cycles of doxorubicin and cisplatin, although the patient died of progression in the brain. Burton and colleagues (1989) reported two partial responses to cisplatin and etoposide and none to hormone therapy. Of interest are the in vitro studies of Lewko and associates (1990), in which PT cells were inhibited by theophylline, vitamin C, and tumor-infiltrating lymphocytes.

Case Reports

Two benign PTs treated by the author occurred in young white women. One, 44 years old, presented with a 3.5-cm mass in the upper midline of the left breast. Fibroadenoma was diagnosed on frozen section, but this was later revised to PT. Treatment was with wide re-excision, and the patient was free of recurrence 14 months later. The second patient was 49 years old and had required repeated attention for multiple, bilateral gross cysts. The PT presented as a 3.0-cm solid mass in the upper inner quadrant of the right breast. After removal for diagnosis it was widely re-excised, and the patient was without recurrence 12 months later.

Two malignant PTs occurred in older women, both of whom had previously had fibroadenomas. The first was a 54-year-old white woman who had had a fibroadenoma removed from the same breast 12 years earlier. The PT presented as a 2.0-cm discrete mass in the lower inner quadrant of the right breast and was suspected on the basis of aspiration cytology. A mammogram was normal. After excision of the tumor for diagnosis the patient was treated with total mastectomy and has been well for 17 months. One lymph node seen in the specimen was

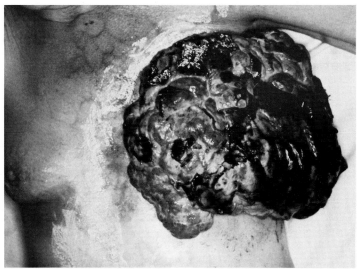

Figure 35–10. Exophytic growth of recurrent phyllodes tumor. (Courtesy of Harvey Lerner, M.D.)

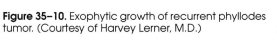

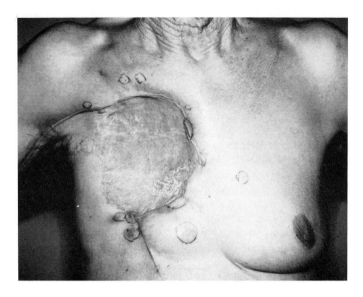

Figure 35-11. Multiple subcutaneous and dermal recurrences of phyllodes tumor around the site of chest wall resection performed in an effort to control local persistence. The patient later developed pulmonary metastases and died.

Table 35-2. LOCAL RECURRENCE AND DISSEMINATION OF PHYLLODES TUMORS BY HISTOLOGIC TYPE*

| Investigation | Follow-up (mo) | Histologic Classification | | | | Deaths |
		Total	Benign	Borderline	Malignant	
Local Recurrence						
Rowell, 1993	26 median	3/18	2/11	0/4	1/3	
Cohn-Cedermark, 1991	96 median	15/77				
Palmer, 1990	5–108	6/31				
Keelan, 1992	186 mean	4/58				
Layfield, 1989	46.5 median	7/10	3/4		4/6	
Grimes, 1992	79–152 mean	28/100	14/51	7/22	7/27	
Chua, 1989	41.5 mean	20/106	12/98	2/6	1/3	
Zurrida, 1992	118 mean	27/216	11/140	9/46	7/30	
Total no.		110/610	42/304	18/74	20/69	
Total (%)		(18.0%)	(13.8%)	(24.3%)	(29.0%)	
Dissemination						
Rowell, 1993	26 median	1/18				1/18
Cohn-Cedermark, 1991	96 median	16/77				
Palmer, 1990	5–108	4/31				4/31
Keelan, 1992	186 mean	2/58				2/58
Layfield, 1989	46.5 median	3/10			3/6	
Grimes, 1992	79–152 mean	8/100	0/51	2/22	6/27	5/100
Chua, 1989	41.5 mean	1/106	0/98	0/6	1/3	1/3
Total no.		35/370	0/149	2/28	10/36	13/201
Total (%)		(9.4%)	(0%)	(7.1%)	(27.8%)	(6.4%)

*Both local recurrence and dissemination of phyllodes tumors after surgical removal increase with increasing histologic malignancy of the stroma. Fractions refer to cases of local recurrence or dissemination over total cases in the category. In the series shown, 9.4% of cases had dissemination and 6.4% died of the tumors.

Table 35-3. RELATION OF LOCAL RECURRENCE TO TUMOR SIZE, HISTOLOGIC APPEARANCE, AND TYPE OF RESECTION

| Tumor Size (cm) | Histologic Type | | | | | | Total Cases (Two Series)* | |
| | Benign | | Borderline | | Malignant | | | |
	Ex	Mast	Ex	Mast	Ex	Mast	Ex	Mast
1–5	1/4	0/3	0/1		3/9	0/2	8/29	0/8
>5	0/6	1/8	1/1	1/6	4/6	1/5	6/17	4/28
Total no.	1/10	1/11	1/2	1/6	7/15	1/7	14/46	4/36
Local recurrence (%)	(10%)	(9%)	(50%)	(17%)	(47%)	(14%)	(30%)	(11%)

*Data from Donegan, W. L., Sarcomas of the breast. *In* Donegan, W. L., and Spratt, J. S. (Eds.): Cancer of the Breast. 3rd ed. Philadelphia, W. B. Saunders, 1988; and from Palmer, M.L., DeRisi, D. C., Pelikan, A., et al.: Treatment option and recurrence potential for cystosarcoma phyllodes. Surg. Gynecol. Obstet., *170:*193–196, 1990. Only cases from the first source could be categorized by histologic type. Length of follow-up varied.
Ex = wide local excision; Mast = mastectomy of various types.

hyperplastic. The second patient was a 70-year-old Black woman who had had fibroadenomas removed from both breasts when she was 18 years old. She had noted a gradually enlarging mass in the upper outer quadrant of the left breast for years. The tumor was firm and mobile and measured 6.0 cm in diameter. Her mammogram showed a second 1.8-cm mass in the lower inner quadrant of the same breast, which proved to be a fibroadenoma. With a biopsy diagnosis of malignant PT, she was treated with total mastectomy; two lymph nodes found in the specimen were normal. Two years later she required treatment for a carcinoma of the endometrium but was still recurrence-free 7 years after mastectomy.

LYMPHOMA

Lymphomas are considered primary in the breast only in the absence of widespread disease or of antecedent extra-mammary lymphoma. Lymphoma represents 0.1% of breast malignancies (DeLeon et al., 1961; Lamovec and Jancar, 1987; Giardini et al., 1992). It constitutes 10% of breast sarcomas and 2.2% of all extranodal non-Hodgkin's lymphomas (Misra et al., 1991). One man is affected for every 32 women, and the age frequency is similar to that of carcinoma (DeCosse et al., 1963; Sonnenblick and Abraham, 1976; Schouten et al., 1981). Lymphoma resembles carcinoma in presenting as a mass and in having the ability to produce skin retraction, erythema, or peau d'orange, but its growth is generally more rapid (Figs. 35–12 through 35–14). It may present as multiple masses. Axillary nodes are involved in 30% to 40% of cases, but adenopathy is softer than that associated with carcinoma. About 13% of patients have bilateral disease; almost as many eventually develop it. Night sweats, fever, and weight loss are associated in 6% to 20% of cases (El-Ghazawy and Singletary, 1992;

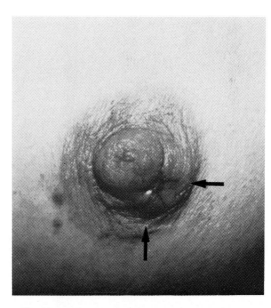

Figure 35–13. Histiocytic lymphoma appearing as a small subareolar mass with involvement of the nipple in a 67-year-old woman. She had been treated for an identical tumor of the opposite breast 3 years earlier.

Giardini et al., 1992). The disease is often more extensive than it first appears to be.

Histologically, lymphoma can be mistaken for medullary carcinoma of the breast or undifferentiated carcinoma, but epithelial markers are absent (Amadori et al., 1987). Monoclonal markers and electron microscopy can be helpful in differentiating it from pseudolymphoma and plasmacytoma (Lin et al., 1980). Primary mammary lymphomas have been characterized as having two divergent clinical patterns (Hugh et al., 1990). The first, a Burkitt's type lymphoma, affects both breasts of pregnant or lactating women and has a rapidly fatal course. The second arises unilaterally in most cases, affects women of a broad age spectrum, and has a variable course. Most of the latter cases are diffuse large cell lymphomas of B-cell origin and are of the immunoglobulin M heavy chain type (Cohen and Brooks, 1991) (Table 35–4). These are considered to be mucosa-associated lymphoid tissues and may have a tendency to spread to other mucosal sites (e.g., respiratory or gastrointestinal tract), with or without nodal dissemination. Diffuse histiocytic lymphoma has a less favorable prognosis than nodular forms. Estrogen receptors are sometimes expressed. Hodgkin's disease is occasionally reported (Schouten et al., 1981). One of thirteen cases of primary mammary lymphoma reported by Dao and coworkers (1992) was classified as nodular sclerosing Hodgkin's disease. Lymphomas that arise in the breast are classified as extranodal lymphoma, the prognosis of which is influenced by both histologic type and stage (Table 35–5).

Treatment

Lymphomas of the breast are managed like extranodal lymphomas at other sites. After a biopsy and histologic diag-

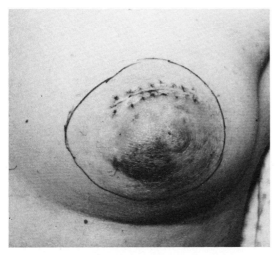

Figure 35–12. Diffuse histiocytic lymphoma of the left breast in a 50-year-old woman appearing as a large, isolated central mass of 3 months' duration associated with axillary adenopathy. Mammography showed a poorly defined, lobulated mass that was hypoechoic on ultrasonography. A CT scan revealed retroperitoneal involvement. Treatment consisted of breast irradiation and systemic combination chemotherapy. The size of the tumor is indicated by the circle drawn on the skin.

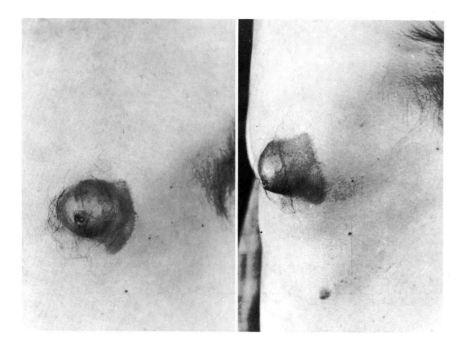

Figure 35–14. Lymphoma of the breast in a 66-year-old man. This lesion gradually enlarged over the course of 1 year. No axillary metastases were found, and the patient died without recurrence 7 years after radical mastectomy.

nosis, careful staging is performed to determine the full extent of disease. Radiographs of the chest, bone marrow biopsy, and computed tomography scans of the abdomen and chest are appropriate. Lymphangiography and a gallium scan may be useful (Armitage, 1993).

In the past, radical mastectomy with postoperative irradiation to the chest and regional nodes was widely used (DeCosse et al., 1962; Melander and Pack, 1963). Because these tumors respond readily to radiation and to chemotherapy, radical operations are no longer considered necessary. Local excision plus irradiation was recommended by Hof-

man and Goodman (1968). Ten of fourteen cases reported by Mambo and coworkers (1977) were managed with biopsy or local excision followed by radiation or chemotherapy, usually both. As a general therapeutic strategy Misra and colleagues (1991) recommended diagnostic surgery followed by adjunctive radiotherapy and combination chemotherapy. Mastectomy with node dissection was reserved for local failures. By analogy with treatment of other extranodal lymphomas a CHOP regimen (cyclophosphamide, doxorubicin, vincristine, and prednisone) of at least three cycles was preferred for systemic therapy. Others have added bleomycin to CHOP and continued every 3 weeks for 6 to 24 cycles (El-Ghazawy and Singletary, 1992).

It is said that the prognosis of mammary lymphoma is better than that of carcinoma or of other extranodal lymphomas, but this is not always evident. Small numbers and the vicissitudes of staging probably contribute to diverse outcomes. Forty-nine per cent of patients reported by Mambo and associates survived 5 years. Six of thirteen patients (46%) seen at the University of Wisconsin were free of disease from 11 to 48 months after treatment (Schouten et

Table 35–4. HISTOPATHOLOGIC TYPES OF LYMPHOMA

Hodgkin's disease
  Nodular sclerosis
  Lymphocyte predominance
  Mixed cellularity
  Lymphocyte depletion
  Unclassified
Non-Hodgkin's lymphoma
  Low-grade malignant lymphoma
    Small lymphocytic
    Follicular, predominantly small, cleaved cell
    Follicular, mixed, small and large cell
  Intermediate-grade malignant lymphoma
    Follicular, predominantly large cell
    Diffuse small, cleaved cell
    Diffuse mixed, small and large cell
    Diffuse large cell, cleaved/noncleaved
  High-grade malignant lymphoma
    Diffuse, large cell, immunoblastic
    Small noncleaved cell (Burkitt's/non-Burkitt's)
    Lymphoblastic (convoluted/nonconvoluted)
Miscellaneous
  Composite
  Mycosis fungoides
  Other

(Adapted from American Joint Committee on Cancer: Manual for Staging of Cancer. 4th ed. Philadelphia, J. B. Lippincott, 1992, pp. 255, 259.)

Table 35–5. STAGING FOR LYMPHOMAS OF THE BREAST

Stage	Findings
IE	Involvement of breast alone
IIE	Involvement of breast and one or more nodal sites above diaphragm
IIIE	Involvement of breast and nodal sites above and below diaphragm or of spleen
IVE	Involvement of breast and liver or of bone marrow, or extensive involvement of another extralymphatic organ

(Adapted from American Joint Committee on Cancer: Manual for Staging of Cancer. 4th ed. Philadelphia, J. B. Lippincott, 1992, pp. 255, 258.)
Qualifiers: A = No fever, night sweats or weight loss ≧ 10%; B = presence of fever, night sweats, or weight loss ≧ 10%; E = extranodal.

Table 35–6. SURVIVAL(S) AND DISEASE FREE SURVIVAL (DFS) OF PATIENTS WITH PRIMARY LYMPHOMA OF THE BREAST

Investigation	Total Cases	Overall S	Overall DFS	Stage I S	Stage I DFS	Stage II S	Stage II DFS
Giardinia, 1992	35	43	—	61	50	27	26
El-Ghazawy, 1992	10	60	—	75	—	0	—
Hugh, 1990	20	35	24	50	—	33	—
Lamovec, 1987	8	60	40	—	—	—	—

*Based on patients dead or followed at least 5 years.

al., 1981). In other small series 5-year survival rates of 72% and 85% are reported (Dixon et al., 1987; Dao et al., 1992). Table 35–6 shows 5-year survival data from four series.

The rare Burkitt's-like lymphoblastic lymphoma of the breast is important to recognize because of its strong tendency to disseminate, particularly to the ovaries, and to progress to lymphoblastic leukemia. Acute tumor lysis with renal failure is a particular hazard (Amadori et al., 1987). Aggressive chemotherapy is necessary (Carbone et al., 1982). Two cases of lymphoma of the breast seen at Sinai Samaritan Medical Center follow.

Case 1

A 66-year-old white woman had been treated for a Stage 1B histiocytic lymphoma of the right breast 4 years earlier with combination chemotherapy (C-MOPP) and irradiation to the breast and regional lymph nodes. One of her sisters had been treated for carcinoma of the breast. She presented with a 2.5-cm rubbery mass deep to the left nipple associated with enlarged ipsilateral axillary nodes. A mammogram demonstrated only thickening of the nipple. Biopsy of the mass again showed histiocytic lymphoma, and without evidence of disease elsewhere she was treated with irradiation of the breast and nodes. Two years later she developed fever, night sweats, and splenomegaly, and an exploratory laparotomy revealed extensive involvement of the stomach and other abdominal viscera. Combination chemotherapy with cyclophosphamide, doxorubicin, VP-16, and prednisone was used, but she died of progressive pulmonary involvement 3 months later. This patient developed lymphoma in both breasts but lived 6 years after the original diagnosis.

Case 2

A 50-year-old white woman presented with a 6.0-cm circumscribed mass deep to the left nipple associated with a 2.0-cm mobile node in the left axilla. Biopsy of the mass showed large cell lymphoma. No estrogen or progesterone receptors were present. The lesion was staged as IIEA and treated with a combination of bleomycin, doxorubicin, cyclophosphamide, vincristine, and dexamethasone with apparent success, but the tumor recurred in the same breast 15 months later. She was then treated with irradiation to the breast and regional lymph nodes and was well after 6 months, when last seen.

STROMAL SARCOMA

Stromal sarcomas differ from malignant PTs only in lacking a benign epithelial component. They were described by Berg and colleagues in 1962. The basic cell is a spindle cell resembling a poorly differentiated fibroblast but differing from the cells of a fibrosarcoma in having greater variation in cellular morphology, fewer reticular fibers, and more mitotic figures. Ultrastructural studies by Tang and associates (1979) suggest predominantly an undifferentiated mesenchymal cell. These authors believed that pure stromal sarcoma and malignant PTs represented neoplastic growth of the periductal mammary stromal cells. The incidence of this tumor is about 0.5% of primary breast cancers, and the ratio of stromal sarcomas to PTs is about 1:3.

The ages of patients range widely; women as young as 15 years and as old as 74 years are reported (El-Naggar et al., 1990b). Stromal sarcomas are well circumscribed, encapsulated, rubbery, and firm. Ulceration may be seen when they reach large size (Fig. 35–15). A bulging, pink to tan, somewhat trabecular pattern is typical on the cut surface. Like PTs, these sarcomas metastasize hematogenously to the lungs and only rarely to the lymph nodes. The propensity to metastasize is directly related to the number of mitotic figures in the tumor. Deoxyribonucleic acid analysis of seven cases seen at the M.D. Anderson Cancer Center between 1960 and 1982 found all to be aggressive aneuploid tumors with deoxyribonucleic acid indices between 1.2 and 2.0 (El-Nagger et al., 1990b). Three patients lived longer than 5 years, but only one was free of recurrence. Median survival time was 24 months.

Treatment of 105 cases collected from the English literature varied from local excision to radical mastectomy (Tang et al., 1979). Fifty-nine per cent of the patients survived a minimum of 5 years. Berg and associates (1962) reported a 60% five-year survival rate for 10 patients with

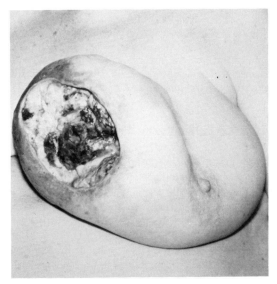

Figure 35–15. Stromal sarcoma. This 71-year-old white woman came to medical attention with a 20 × 16-cm centrally ulcerated tumor confined to the left breast. The patient had been aware of it for 5 months. The tumor was not fixed to the chest wall and was removed with a total mastectomy.

stromal sarcomas and no instance of local recurrence when treatment was either simple or radical mastectomy. By contrast, 9 of 15 patients had local recurrence when limited excision was performed. Recurrence generally occurs during the first 2 years after treatment. Local recurrences should be widely removed surgically when possible. Two cases at SSMC illustrate the varied course of patients with stromal sarcoma.

Case 3

A 71-year-old white woman was aware of a mass in the left breast for 5 months before she sought consultation. The tumor had enlarged rapidly and finally ulcerated, discharging foul material. It measured 20.0 cm in diameter, featured a deep necrotic crater, and was attached to the pectoralis major muscle. No regional or distant metastases were evident. Microscopically, the tumor consisted of pleomorphic malignant spindle cells with frequent mitoses (four or five per 10 high-power fields). Some areas looked like fibroadenoma, suggesting that it might have evolved from a PT, but there was no admixture of epithelial elements. Estrogen and progesterone receptors were absent. The tumor was removed with a total mastectomy including the pectoralis major muscle en bloc. Lymph nodes in the specimen were free of tumor. Within 5 months pulmonary metastases appeared that soon caused painful rib erosion. The patient developed spinal cord compression from metastases to the vertebrae, requiring laminectomy and irradiation, and she died 18 months after diagnosis.

Case 4

A 30-year-old white woman developed a 1.0-cm painless nodule in the upper outer quadrant of the left breast. Mammography showed an oval density at the site. The tumor was removed for diagnosis and showed spindle-shaped cells with abundant mitoses. Immunoperoxidase stains for cytokeratin were negative. With a diagnosis of stromal sarcoma, wide excision was performed. No residual sarcoma was found, but a small focus of ductal carcinoma in situ, cribriform type, was seen incidentally in the tissues. The patient received no further treatment, subsequently had a normal pregnancy, and has remained free of recurrence for 13 years.

FIBROSARCOMA

Fibrosarcomas originate from fibrocytes, and low-grade varieties must be differentiated from infiltrating fibromatosis, an indolent, less cellular lesion that lacks nuclear atypia and does not metastasize (Page et al., 1987). Fibrosarcomas, termed ''dermatofibrosarcoma protuberans,'' arise from the integument of the anterior chest, and it is often difficult to determine if advanced lesions originated in skin or mammary parenchyma. Fibrosarcomas are not always differentiated from malignant fibrous histiocytomas, but they may have a better prognosis than the latter (Jones et al., 1992). Histologically, they are said to have a herringbone pattern and can form metaplastic elements that include muscle,

cartilage, and bone. Some fibrosarcomas may originate in PTs.

Elson and coworkers (1992) reported five cases of fibrosarcoma of the breast in women aged 48 to 79 years. The tumors measured 1.5 to 7.0 cm in diameter, and three were thought to have arisen from PTs. All showed dense masses with indistinct margins on mammography, but the signs were nonspecific. Aspiration cytologic findings were suggestive of sarcoma in only two cases. Three of the four patients with follow-up were alive 4, 8, and 12 years later. These authors recommended simple mastectomy with removal of the deep pectoral fascia.

Four women seen at EFSCH were aged 37, 71, 75, and 79 years, respectively, and the right breast was involved in three instances. Two had noted a stationary mass for years with recent rapid growth of 2 and 5 months' duration. The other two patients reported a gradually enlarging mass, for 7 months and 18 months, respectively. All lesions had reached large size, and physical findings were emblematic of locally advanced sarcomas. The skin was stretched until it assumed a glazed appearance (Fig. 35–16). One tumor occupied half the breast, and the overlying skin was shiny and purple. Two measured 15 cm in diameter. One of these was associated with large overlying veins (Fig. 35–17). The second was fixed to the skin and chest wall and was associated with cutaneous erythema as well as a palpably enlarged axillary lymph node.

One of the patients was treated with a simple mastectomy and lived for 18 years without recurrence; the other three died from their tumors. Two of the latter had been referred for local recurrences after local excision and after multiple local resections including mastectomy, respectively. Both were treated with irradiation with little effect and died, one 2 months later and the other 3 years and 5 months after diagnosis. The remaining patient had pulmonary and bony metastases on presentation. A palliative simple mastectomy was followed by local recurrence 3 years later, and she died 2 months thereafter.

One patient with a dermatofibrosarcoma on the breast was 48 years old and claimed to have had the lesion for 14 years. It was treated with wide local excision and recurred locally on two occasions, 9 and 15 years later. The patient was living a year after the last removal.

MALIGNANT FIBROUS HISTIOCYTOMA

Malignant fibrous histiocytoma (MFH) may be the most frequent pure soft tissue sarcoma of the breast. It accounted for 44% of cases in one report (Pollard et al., 1990). Approximately 4% of MFHs occur in the female breast (O'Brien and Stout, 1964). These tumors may arise as a stromal component of PTs, in previously irradiated tissues, or in the skin. A few arise in mammary tissue without skin involvement.

Its histologic features, which are a mixture of fibroblasts, bizarre histiocytes, giant cells, and foam cells, suggest that it arises from a tissue histiocyte capable of acting as a facultative fibroblast, or from a primitive precursor of both. A storiform pattern is characteristic of MFH, and mitoses are frequent. By contrast, fibrosarcomas appear to arise

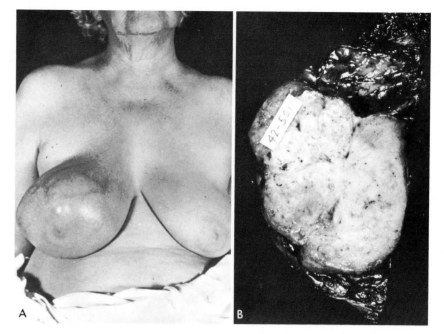

Figure 35-16. *A,* Fibrosarcoma of the right breast. Characteristic of large fibrosarcomas is the tense and mildly erythematous overlying skin. This case demonstrates the presence of prominent superficial veins, which often accompany these neoplasms. *B,* The resected tumor is grossly well marginated and presents a typical appearance.

from a mature fibroblast and generally have a herringbone pattern. With immunoperoxidase technique the cells stain positive for vimentin and negative for cytokeratin, confirming their mesenchymal origin. Some also stain positive for desmin and S-100 protein (Rossen et al., 1991). Ultrastructurally, the presence of both perinuclear filaments and fat in the same cell favors the diagnosis of MFH.

The tumor can reach large size and occasionally metastasizes to regional lymph nodes (vanNiekerk et al., 1987). None of 10 cases of mammary MFH reported by Pitts and coworkers (1991) metastasized to regional lymph nodes; though 1 of 11 did so in the series of Pollard and associates (1990) and 1 of 32 reviewed by Rossen's group (1991). In other locations MFH produces nodal metastases in 12% to 32% of cases. The prognosis for MFH in the breast is comparable to that of MFH in superficial tissues elsewhere. The degree of cellular atypia and number of mitoses are important prognostically. Jones and colleagues (1992) found that high-grade tumors were more likely than low-grade ones to disseminate and cause death.

Limited excision invites local recurrence, even of low-grade lesions (Rossen et al., 1991). Wide excision may be adequate for small superficial lesions, and quadrantectomy with axillary lymph node dissection has been employed (Tellin et al., 1990), but mastectomy is probably the best treatment for MFH arising in the substance of the breast. In

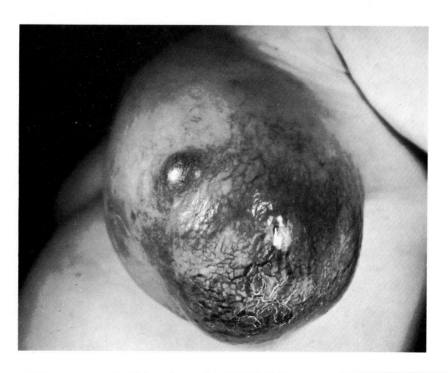

Figure 35-17. A massive fibrosarcoma of the breast near ulceration, with tortuous dilated overlying veins.

the absence of adenopathy, simple mastectomy is most often recommended as adequate therapy. The utility of axillary node dissection is unclear, but some consider it prudent considering the occasional discovery of nodal metastasis (vanNiekerk et al., 1987). Forty-one per cent of the 17 MFH cases reviewed by Jones and colleagues (1992) recurred after various operations within a mean follow-up of 5.5 years. Twenty-two per cent of patients had dissemination or died of their tumor in Rossen and associates' literature review. Langham and coworkers (1984) reported four cases that arose within mammary parenchyma. Local recurrence followed a simple mastectomy in one case, but not radical mastectomy in two others. The fourth patient, treated with excisional biopsy, had local recurrence 14 months later but was well 11 months after a modified radical mastectomy. In a fifth case (Liebert and Edwards, 1982) the tumor recurred locally 1 year after excisional biopsy, and the patient was treated with segmental mastectomy but developed pulmonary metastases. The lesion of a sixth patient (vanNiekerk et al., 1987) exhibited inflammatory changes and progressed rapidly; the patient died from dissemination to lungs and soft tissues a few weeks after irradiation and radical mastectomy. Irradiation can produce some regression of MFH, but its role and that of chemotherapy as adjuvants remain to be defined.

CARCINOSARCOMAS

True carcinosarcomas, "collision tumors," are mixtures of both malignant epithelial and malignant mesenchymal tissues. They are to be distinguished from carcinomas with spindle cell or "pseudosarcomatous" metaplasia. It is uncertain whether the sarcomatous element of carcinosarcomas arises as a change from epithelial to mesenchymal differentiation, independently by induction of tumor stroma, or from metaplasia of myoepithelial cells. Some may arise from malignant change in the epithelial component of PTs (Azzopardi, 1979). The carcinomatous element may be small in these tumors and can be missed if sampling is inadequate. It can consist of adenocarcinoma, undifferentiated carcinoma, or sometimes squamous carcinoma and can be invasive or in situ. Osteosarcoma is often a component of the sarcomatous element, but other histologic types have been reported, including rhabdomyosarcoma (Carstens and Cooke, 1990). They have the capacity to metastasize via both lymphatics and the bloodstream, and either or both elements may do so. The presence of carcinoma places the regional lymph nodes at higher than usual risk, but carcinoma and sarcoma can remain associated in nodal metastases (Curran and Dodge, 1962).

Carcinosarcomas in the breast present as large masses, not uncommonly as painful ones (Robb and MacFarlane, 1958; Williams and Diamonon, 1964; Wargotz and Norris, 1989). Clinical history ranges from 1 month to 20 years. Harris and Persaud (1974) contributed two cases and summarized fourteen from the literature. Ages ranged from 10 to 91 years (average = 58 years). In seven cases the tumors were believed to have arisen from pre-existing fibroadenomas or PTs. Only three of the sixteen patients lived 5 years after treatment, though others were alive for shorter periods. In five cases (31.3%) metastases were documented in axillary lymph nodes; other sites of spread included bone and lung. Two cases treated at SSMC are reported below.

▪ Case 5

An 85-year-old nursing home patient was found to have a 4.0-cm lobulated mass in the lower outer quadrant of the right breast on routine physical examination. It was partially cystic and yielded bloody fluid on aspiration, which cytologically suggested ductal carcinoma. The frozen section diagnosis was PT, but this was revised to carcinosarcoma on the basis of permanent section examination. The tumor was weakly estrogen-receptor positive (13 fmol/mg protein) and progesterone-receptor negative and was aneuploid with a high S-phase fraction. Treatment was with a modified radical mastectomy. All nodes were normal. She has remained recurrence free after short follow-up.

▪ Case 6

A 73-year-old white woman presented with an enlarging 10.0-cm mass in the central right breast of 8 months' duration. The tumor was firm, bosselated, and attached to the pectoral fascia, and a previous biopsy incision was unhealed (Fig. 35–18). The axilla contained a 1-cm soft node. Extensive bone formation within the tumor was demonstrated in a mammogram (Fig. 35–19). Initially the biopsy suggested stromal sarcoma, but carcinosarcoma was evident when the entire tumor was examined (Fig. 35–20). She was treated with mastectomy, including the underlying pectoralis major muscle and axillary nodes. All nodes were normal, and the tumor was estrogen-receptor and progesterone-receptor negative. Postoperatively she received chest wall irradiation and tamoxifen, 10 mg twice daily, but developed multiple pulmonary metastases after 7 months. Biopsy of the latter showed sarcoma. The metastases partially regressed on treatment with doxorubicin and dacarbazine, and the patient was alive 28 months after her original diagnosis.

Simple mastectomy would not seem appropriate treatment for these tumors. Their capacity to infiltrate the underlying pectoral muscles and to produce axillary metastases

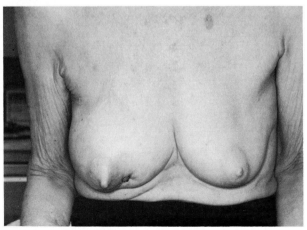

Figure 35–18. Large carcinosarcoma of the right breast. Ulceration is due to a previous biopsy.

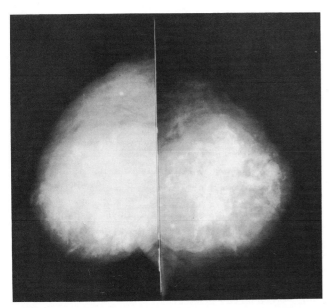

Figure 35-19. Mammogram of a carcinosarcoma shows extensive bone formation in the tumor.

argues for total mastectomy and axillary lymph node dissection, including the pectoral muscles if the tumor is large or if involvement seems likely. Systemic adjuvant therapy should also be considered. Cyclophosphamide, doxorubicin, and fluorouracil was suggested by Baker (1990) as a combination that promises to be active against both malignancies. The addition of tamoxifen seems logical if estrogen receptors are present. Large tumor size and predominance of the sarcomatous component imply a poor prognosis.

It must be noted that the rare squamous cell carcinoma of the breast is not confined to carcinosarcomas (Bogomoletz, 1982). Eggers and McChesney reviewed this subject in 1984 and found most cases to be associated with pure epithelial cancers. Cornog and associates (1971) found one well-differentiated pure squamous cell carcinoma in asso-

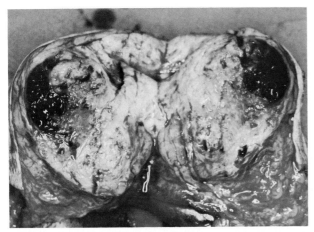

Figure 35-20. Cut surface of a bisected carcinosarcoma. The tumor is fleshy in appearance, is pseudoencapsulated, and shows internal hemorrhage.

ciation with a PT, and a few were thought to be of epidermal origin. Squamous cell carcinoma has the same prognosis as invasive adenocarcinoma of the breast at a similar stage.

GRANULOCYTIC SARCOMA (CHLOROMA)

Granulocytic sarcomas sometimes appear as primary tumors of the breast. These extramedullary tumors composed of myeloid or monocytoid precursor cells are regularly associated with acute myelocytic leukemia. The mass ordinarily develops adjacent to bone but less frequently occurs in the ovaries, breast, lymph nodes, and dura. If it precedes the diagnosis of acute leukemia, which happens occasionally by a month to more than a year, it can be mistaken for an eosinophilic granuloma. A characteristic green color accounts for the original designation chloroma, but this hue is not regularly present. Both the green color and red fluorescence in ultraviolet light are attributed to the enzyme myeloperoxidase. Several granulocytic sarcomas in the breast have been described (Wiernik and Serpick, 1970). Although the tumors respond to localized external radiation, and sometimes to chemotherapy, the course of acute myelocytic leukemia is one of uniformly short survival. Wiernik and Serpick described a 40-year-old woman with a 1-cm-by–0.5-cm gray-green, firm tumor in her right breast that proved to be a granulocytic sarcoma. Acute myelocytic leukemia was diagnosed during the same admission, and, despite therapy with hydroxyurea and daunomycin, the patient died within 1 month.

ANGIOSARCOMA

While angiosarcoma of the breast was reported in 1887 by Schmidt, the first well-documented case was that reported by Borrmann in 1907 as metastasizing hemangioma. Subsequently, such tumors have been reported as hemangiosarcoma (Shore, 1957), angiosarcoma (Scheid et al., 1964), hemangioendothelioblastoma (Edwards and Strouth, 1956), and hemangioblastoma (Patrick et al., 1957–1958). Angiosarcomas are highly lethal and, fortunately, are rare even among sarcomas. Only one can be expected among every 2000 carcinomas; two were reported from the Mayo Clinic among 36 cases of mammary sarcomas in more than 53 years (Barber et al., 1960; Lissoos et al., 1969). Chen and colleagues (1980) collected 87 cases. Twenty-nine cases were seen at Memorial Sloan-Kettering Cancer Center in the 25 years prior to 1992 (Liberman et al., 1992).

Clinical Features

Angiosarcomas of the breast are concentrated in young women (average age = 35 years) although the tumor has been reported in men. Clinically it is first manifested as a rapidly enlarging mass of relatively short duration that is occasionally tender or painful. As the patients are often young, they are sometimes pregnant (Rosen et al., 1988;

Kumar et al., 1990). The mass is generally poorly defined and deeply located, but when it is superficial a characteristic blue or purple discoloration of the skin is present that suggests an inflammatory condition or recent trauma. Skin fixation is unusual, and enlarged axillary lymph nodes are seldom a clinical feature. Nodal enlargement ordinarily proves to be due to hyperplasia. Ecchymosis may indicate hemorrhage within the tumor and may account for associated local discomfort. No predilection is evident for either breast. Bilateral breast involvement ultimately occurs in about 21% of cases, though only 3% are bilateral initially (Donnell et al., 1981). Metastasis to the opposite breast is frequent. Previous irradiation appears to be causal in some cases.

The mammographic appearance is most often a solitary mass, sometimes with calcification or skin thickening and occasionally multiple masses. Mammograms show no abnormalities in one-third of cases (Liberman et al., 1992). Ultrasonography usually demonstrates a solid mass.

Pathology

The tumor is spongy, soft, and unencapsulated (Fig. 35–21). Microscopically it may appear deceptively benign. Dilated vascular spaces combine with interstitial hemorrhage, and occasionally focal necrosis is present. The important features are irregularly intercommunicating vascular channels lined by atypical endothelial cells that pile up with foci of papillary intraluminal proliferation. Much variation in cellularity in different parts of the tumor is also seen. Infiltration of neoplastic elements tends to extend far beyond the gross limits of the tumor and to foster incomplete removal. Experience with cytologic diagnosis is scant (Gupta et al., 1991). Antman and coworkers (1982) found no estrogen receptors in one tumor. The degree of mitotic activity, the histologic differentiation of the tumor, and possibly its

size, are related to prognosis (Donnell et al., 1981; Merino et al., 1983). Rosen and associates (1988) found that prognosis was related to histologic differentiation (type) but not to tumor size. Type I tumors were well differentiated and had few mitotic figures and no papillary formations. Type II lesions showed sites of solid proliferation and papillary formations, and Type III ones were overtly sarcomatous with many mitoses, focal necrosis, and hemorrhage. Estimated 5-year disease-free survival rates were 76%, 70%, and 15%, respectively.

Because of histologic variability, vascular tumors of the breast should be removed totally for diagnosis. Although almost all are malignant, the occasional benign cavernous hemangioma or vascular anomaly must be distinguished from angiosarcoma. Banergee and coworkers (1992) described seven cases of carcinoma that had a pseudoangiosarcomatous pattern due to complex anastomosing channels and spaces, and emphasized the importance of not mistaking these for angiosarcoma. They yielded negative results with endothelial cell markers.

Therapy

Total mastectomy is generally recommended, and pectoral muscles are removed if necessary for margin (Hunter et al., 1985; Rainwater et al., 1986; Rosen et al., 1988). Axillary dissection is not routine, though it is indicated if nodes are enlarged, as nodal metastases are reported (Chen et al., 1980). Of 87 cases collected by Chen's group in 1980 only five patients (6%) were alive and free of recurrence at 5 years. More favorably, 33% of 40 patients reported by Donnell's group (1981) were disease free after 5 years, and in the Mayo Clinic series of 20 patients 30% were alive at 5 years and 5% at 10 years (Rainwater et al., 1986).

The place of systemic adjuvant therapy is uncertain because experience is anecdotal, but indications are that it

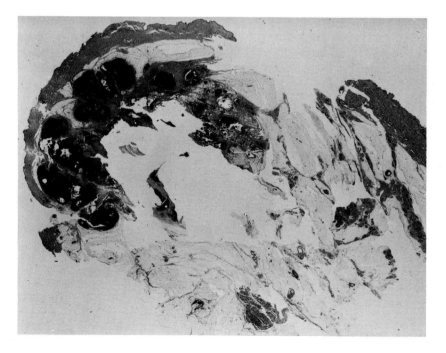

Figure 35–21. This whole organ histologic section of an angiosarcoma of the breast demonstrates the hemorrhagic and unencapsulated character of the tumor. This 43-year-old woman reported a mass of 1 year's duration. She was treated with radical mastectomy, and 12 axillary nodes were found to be free of metastases. She died 6 months later of metastases, principally in the lungs.

may be worthwhile. Antman and colleagues (1982) treated five cases with a combination of resection, chemotherapy (cyclophosphamide, doxorubicin hydrochloride, and dacarbazine), and irradiation without improving the median survival time, although two were disease free at 20 and 38 months, respectively. Five of eight patients who received actinomycin D in the report of Donnell and coworkers (1981) survived without recurrence for 5 to 15 years. A complete response of angiosarcoma to intralesional vinblastine was noted by Rosner (1988), who then used it, 4 mg intravenously per week for 24 to 33 courses, as a surgical adjuvant in two cases. Both patients were long-term survivors.

For the majority survival after diagnosis is brief (median 2.2 years). Most recurrences appear within 3 years. Local recurrence is frequent, and widespread hematogenous dissemination in lungs, skin, bones, brain, and abdominal viscera is the usual course. Hemoptysis signals the presence of pulmonary involvement; bone pain accompanies osseous metastases; and coma or hemiparesis is often a sequela of intracranial spread. Anemia supervenes from hemorrhage and bone marrow replacement. Thrombocytopenia is sometimes seen. Death frequently is the result of massive hemorrhage from an involved intra-abdominal organ, particularly the liver.

Chest wall recurrences or isolated recurrences elsewhere should be excised when possible. Occasionally long-term survival follows a salvage mastectomy (Donnell et al., 1981). Radiotherapy has little to offer in management, either as primary or as adjuvant therapy, but information is scant, and some palliation of advanced disease occasionally is claimed. Chemotherapy for recurrences is disappointing. The only patients cured of this tumor are those with small primary lesions; thus, the desirability of early detection.

■

Case 7

At 40 years of age a white woman was seen at the Milwaukee County Medical Complex for nodular sclerosing Hodgkin's disease in the left side of the neck and mediastinum. She was treated with irradiation in an upper mantle pattern, receiving 3500 cGy to the anterior mediastinum. Ten years later she presented with fullness in the left axilla. The left breast was enlarged and edematous and displayed erythematous angioma-like lesions on the medial aspect within the radiation port. A biopsy specimen demonstrated angiosarcoma, and simple mastectomy was performed. Within 8 months the tumor re-established itself on the left chest, and a fungating red tumor measuring 8 cm by 6 cm replaced the nipple of the right breast. The patient received multiple-drug chemotherapy, but it was soon apparent that the tumor was not controlled. The patient then received irradiation to the right breast (6000 cGy) and to the left chest (4500 cGy) that achieved partial regression. The patient survived an additional 13 months and died of her tumor 2 years after its onset.

CHONDROSARCOMA

Chondrosarcomas are among the rarest of pure sarcomas of the breast. Ladefoged and Nielsen reported only the fourth

case in 1984. This occurred in an 84-year-old woman as a 5-cm, slow-growing tumor in the upper midline of the right breast. The overlying skin was normal, and no nodes could be felt in the axilla. The tumor was excised widely, and the patient was free of recurrence 2 years later. In establishing this diagnosis, it is necessary to exclude metaplastic changes in PTs or in osteosarcomas with multiple sections of the tumor and to consider metastatic osteosarcomas from other sites. The lower extremities are the most frequent site of extraosseous chondrosarcomas. Furthermore, staining for S-100 protein is a useful marker for cells of chondrocytic origin and serves to rule out the possibility of metastatic carcinoma. Like other pure sarcomas of the breast, chondrosarcomas have the potential for hematogenous spread to the lungs and bones. One case may have produced hepatic metastases. Electron microscopic studies are useful (Ladefoged and Nielsen, 1984).

OSTEOGENIC SARCOMA

This unusual bone-forming sarcoma is thought to arise from the stroma of long-standing fibroadenoma, or possibly from mastopathy as progression of osseous metaplasia (France et al., 1970; Cole-Beuglet et al., 1976). The first report of a malignant mammary neoplasm composed of bone and cartilage is that of Bonet in 1700. From that time to 1963, 115 cases were reported (Jernstrom et al., 1963). Not unusual in the breast as a component of carcinosarcomas, osteogenic sarcomas also occasionally occur in a pure form. Jernstrom and coworkers observed one osteosarcoma among 3309 cases of mammary cancer during a period of 18 years. Middle-aged and older women are most susceptible, though it has been reported in the third decade of life. The tumor is composed of pleomorphic osteoblastic tissue with bone and cartilage as well as giant cells of the osteoclastic type. It produces a mass that is smooth, mobile, and understandably firm, but it may be cystic, fixed and occasionally ulcerated. Radiographs demonstrate bone formation in the breast (Teich and Brecher, 1985). The axilla is rarely involved. Hematogenous spread, usually to the lungs, is the rule. Treatment of potentially curable cases most often has been with radical mastectomy, which may be necessary to ensure wide margins of resection. The infrequency with which lymphatic spread is encountered would appear to justify a less extensive procedure in the absence of adenopathy. For advanced disease, cyclophosphamide and cortisone have proved useful for the temporary control of pulmonary metastases (Kolarsick, 1972).

A case reported by Aubrey and Andrews (1971) illustrates the features of this sarcoma.

■

Case 8

A 52-year-old woman presented with a mass in the lower outer quadrant of the left breast of 3 weeks' duration. A cyst had previously been removed from the same breast. The mass was 2.5 cm in diameter, hard, irregular, and not associated with adenopathy. Carcinoma was suspected, and she was treated with a left radical mastectomy. The diagnosis was low-grade malignant osteogenic sarcoma. The patient was well for 8 years but then developed weakness, weight loss, and a chronic cough. A radiograph of the chest showed multiple metastases in both lungs, and subsequently metastases appeared in the subcutaneous tissues of the buttocks, in a finger, and within the abdomen. Thiotepa, testosterone, and prednisolone produced no response, and the patient died 9 years and 2 months after the mastectomy. An autopsy revealed firm, gritty masses of tumor with areas of cystic necrosis; metastases were found invading the chest wall, the bodies of the thoracic vertebrae, the left adrenal gland, the brain, the peritoneum, and the myocardium.

LEIOMYOSARCOMA

Experience with leiomyosarcoma is scant. The first report is attributed to Crocker and Murad in 1968. Other reports include those of Hill and Stout (1942), Haagensen (1971), Pardo-Midan and coworkers (1974) and Chen's group (1981). Five cases have arisen in nipples, one of which was ectopic (Neuman and Fletcher, 1991; Alessi and Sala, 1992). The fact that two cases were found among 265 male breast cancers by Visfeldt and Sheike (1973) suggests that it is more frequent among men than among women.

Eleven cases of leiomyosarcoma of the breast were collected by Waterworth and colleagues (1992), and Parham and coworkers (1992) added a twelfth. The average age was 53 years (range = 24 to 59 years), and 82% of the patients were women. The tumors reached 9.0 cm in diameter.

Clinical features suggest a benign lesion but are typical of sarcoma; the tumor is soft to firm, lobulated, and circumscribed. Histologically it is easily recognizable. The neoplasm is highly cellular, composed of elongate cells with blunt ends, caricaturing smooth muscle cells. Mitoses are frequent, and multinucleate giant cells occasionally are present. The tumors usually stain positive for muscle-specific antigen (Arista-Nasr et al., 1989; Parham et al., 1992). The case described by Pardo-Midan and colleagues is representative.

■ ▨▨▨▨▨▨▨▨▨▨▨▨▨▨▨▨▨▨▨▨▨▨▨▨

Case 9

A 49-year-old woman had a 7.5-cm firm, mobile, smooth nodule that appeared clinically benign in the inferior lateral region of the left breast, near the nipple. The axilla was free of adenopathy. On biopsy the tissues were firm and white, with irregular, reddish areas. Microscopically, it was considered a Grade IV leiomyosarcoma, according to the Silverberg classification of uterine leiomyosarcomas. Small areas of necrosis were present, and the tumor had invaded vascular walls. A simple mastectomy was performed, and the patient was living without recurrence 6 months later.

Haagensen described a similar case in a 77-year-old woman who had been aware of the tumor for only 2 weeks although it measured 8.0 cm in diameter and occupied most of the upper portion of the breast. Treatment was with complete mastectomy (probably radical mastectomy), and the patient was surviving without recurrence 14 years later.

Leiomyosarcomas are thought to be less aggressive biologically than other sarcomas of the breast, but this is difficult to verify. Almost all cases reported to date have been treated with simple or radical mastectomy. In Waterworth's group's (1992) 11 collected cases, survival for longer than 5 years was documented in four cases, but two of these women had not been cured. All but two were treated with mastectomy. One of the two treated with local excision had a local recurrence. Cellular atypia appeared to have some prognostic value, more so than tumor size or mitotic activity.

LIPOSARCOMA

Liposarcomas constitute 0.3% of all sarcomas of the breast; only 20 cases were found in the files of the Armed Forces Institute of Pathology in 1986 (Austin and Dupree, 1986). Neuman made the earliest report in 1862, and Hummer and Burkart were able to collect 28 cases in 1967. The tumors may arise as pure liposarcomas or as a component of malignant PTs.

The majority of patients are women; a small fraction are men, and ages range from young adult to advanced (mean = 47 years). The tumor presents as an enlarging lobulated mass that is sometimes painful. The overlying skin may be erythematous and display dilated veins when the tumor reaches large size. Bilaterality has been reported.

Grossly the tumor is well circumscribed, though some are lobulated, irregular, or infiltrative. The color is yellow or tan, and the myxoid variety, which accounted for three of the six cases seen by Pollard's group (1990), has a gelatinous appearance. A diagnosis of liposarcoma requires the demonstration of characteristic lipoblasts, which must not be confused with vacuolated cells found in other lesions such as fat necrosis or granulomatous inflammations. The tumor is classified histologically into one of four categories: well-differentiated, myxoid, round cell, and pleomorphic, the last being the most aggressive. Margins of the tumor can appear pushing or infiltrative; axillary nodes are seldom, if ever, involved.

■ ▨▨▨▨▨▨▨▨▨▨▨▨▨▨▨▨▨▨▨▨▨▨▨▨

Case 10

A 60-year-old white woman presented at EFSCH with a tender right breast mass she had first noticed 7 weeks earlier. The tumor measured 12 cm in diameter, filling both upper quadrants. Overlying skin was discolored by topical ointments. No fixation to skin or deep tissues was noted, and no axillary nodes were palpable. At the time of biopsy the hard, nodular tumor was found to lie between the pectoralis major and pectoralis minor muscles. It involved the deep fascia but not obviously the mammary parenchyma. On cut section the tumor was light tan and was composed predominantly of solid fibrous tissue with many tiny cysts, and it contained a large amount of mucinous material. Histologically, the tissues were myxomatous and contained elongated, spidery cells and vacuolated cells resembling adult lipocytes, which were moderately well differentiated. In some areas the cells had bizarre nuclei, and scattered mitoses were evident. The patient was treated with radical mastectomy, but within the specimen tumor was noted close to the deep margin. Five years and three months later a recurrence was noted fixed to the chest wall in the vicinity of the scar. This was widely excised in continuity with a full thickness of the chest wall, using a pedicle flap to cover the defect. No reappearance of the tumor was noted 15 months after this resection.

Surgery and irradiation, alone and in combination, have been advised for treatment of liposarcomas of the breast (Geschickter, 1943; Stout and Bernanke, 1946; Homes and Leis, 1962; Hare and Cerny, 1963; Menon and van Velthoven, 1974). Wide surgical removal takes the form of local excision, total mastectomy, or radical mastectomy, depending on the size of the tumor and its local extent. A wide margin of normal tissue is the best assurance against local recurrence. While many liposarcomas are radiosensitive, radiotherapy alone is not reliable treatment, though irradiation may be of value as an adjuvant. Wide resection, if possible, is also the treatment of choice for recurrences, but radiation can be palliative when resection is not possible. Local recurrence is a continuing threat, and dissemination to lungs, heart, bones, and abdominal viscera is the usual course of uncontrolled liposarcoma.

Two of the 20 patients with liposarcomas reviewed by Austin and Dupree (1986) had local recurrences, and three had developed blood-borne dissemination after short-term follow-up. Thirteen (65%) were alive and well 3 months after resection and two others were well after shorter periods.

RHABDOMYOSARCOMA

Rhabdomyosarcomas are not unusual among nonepithelial cancers of the breast. Oberman (1965*b*) observed 3 among 13 mammary sarcomas and Botham 4 among 23. Sugar and Sapi (1988) reported one in a 14-year-old girl and Altomare's group (1990) another concurrent with pregnancy in a 15-year-old. Rapid growth, indefinite borders, and large size characterized these aggressive neoplasms. Cure was infrequent.

Histologically these tumors feature cells with sarcoplasmic cross-striations. Multinucleate neoplastic giant cells, racquet cells, and strap cells are characteristic. Immunohistochemical study is useful. Skeletal muscle actin is a reliable marker for identifying rhabdomyosarcomas and can be complemented with desmin, myosins, and myoglobin (Bussolati et al., 1987). As the mammary parenchyma lacks striated muscles, from which tissues rhabdomyosarcomas arise is not known. The case for origin from pectoral muscles is frustrated by lack of regularly demonstrable continuity (Hill and Stout, 1942). Oberman noted that three rhabdomyosarcomas infiltrated skeletal muscle, but the tumors were centered in the mammary gland.

Hematogenous dissemination is the most frequent mode of spread of rhabdomyosarcomas, but metastasis to regional nodes is relatively frequent, especially from the alveolar type. Horn (1963) reported nodal metastasis in 19% of rhabdomyosarcomas.

■

Case 11

A poorly differentiated rhabdomyosarcoma was treated at EFSCH. The same case was reported by Haagensen (1971), along with another seen in consultation by Stout. The 75-year-old white woman related that a large cystic mass had been present in her left breast for 1½ years and had burst 2 weeks earlier, draining blood and pus. A large, fungating mass with a deep central sinus was present in the outer portion of the breast (Fig. 35–22). A few small nodes were palpable in the axilla. A simple mastectomy was initially performed to remove the mass, and when the wound was healed a radical mastectomy followed. The tumor measured 9 cm by 10 cm by 7 cm. On section it was soft and light gray and featured small zones of necrosis. Microscopically, undifferentiated tumor cells with faintly acidophilic cytoplasm were found, displaying a large number of abnormal mitotic figures. Many large tumor giant cells, frequently with vacuolated cytoplasm, populated the tumor. Metastases were seen in 4 of 17 axillary lymph nodes. On consultation, Dr. A. P. Stout said, "The large elongated syncytial masses with many nuclei strongly resemble the way rhabdomyoblasts grow in vitro." Sixteen months after the radical operation a radiograph showed a metastatic nodule in the left lung. The tumor followed a surprisingly indolent course, and the patient died at home 3 years and 4 months after the pulmonary metastases were discovered.

Mastectomy is the treatment of choice for these aggressive tumors, including the pectoral muscles if necessary to

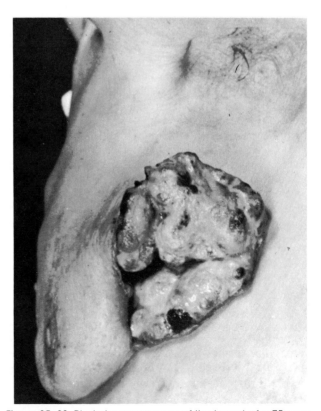

Figure 35–22. Rhabdomyosarcoma of the breast of a 75-year-old woman. This advanced tumor appeared as a fungating mass associated with a sinus tract. Metastases were present in 4 of 17 axillary lymph nodes.

provide a safe margin around larger tumors. Because metastasis to regional nodes is more frequent than with most sarcomas, removal of axillary nodes is included. Radiotherapy, and radiotherapy combined with chemotherapy, produce temporary regression (del Regato, 1963). Response of rhabdomyosarcomas to chemotherapy is becoming more frequent with drug combinations (Morton, 1974; Delaney et al., 1976).

MELANOMA

Melanoma may arise in the skin of the breast or the nipple. It may also metastasize to the breast. Primary melanoma of the glandular tissue of the breast is so rare that involvement of the subcutaneous tissues or the parenchyma should suggest metastasis from another primary site (Gatch, 1956; Stephenson and Byrd, 1959). It has been suggested that clear cell sarcoma of the breast is a soft tissue form of malignant melanoma since melanosomes have been seen on electron microscopic examination (Pollard et al., 1990). When the nipple is involved the differential diagnosis includes Paget's disease of the nipple and Bowen's disease, as they can be histologically similar but their treatment is considerably different. Use of immunocytochemical studies to detect the S-100 protein indicative of melanoma and cytokeratin characteristic of epithelial cancer can be helpful (Reed et al., 1990). High–molecular weight melanoma-associated antigen can also identify melanoma of the nipple (D'Aluto et al., 1991). Pigmented invasive carcinoma of the nipple, in which an abundance of benign melanocytes produces a dark color, can mimic melanoma (Sau et al., 1989).

Melanoma of the skin of the breast or nipple accounts for 1.8% to 6.4% of cutaneous melanomas (Lee et al., 1977; Roses et al., 1979; Papachristou et al., 1979). Patients are predominantly male, perhaps because the male breast is more often exposed to sunlight, and ages range from 16 to 72 years, the median age being late in the fourth or early in the fifth decade of life. Since only in advanced cases do the tumors reach the mammary parenchyma, they behave like cutaneous malanomas elsewhere. In the absence of distant dissemination or regional adenopathy, the probability of lymphatic metastasis and prognosis depend on the depth of invasion into the skin as measured by Clark's levels or the Breslow depth in millimeters. Lymph nodes at risk are primarily the axillary ones, which Papachristou and colleagues (1979) found involved in 60% of 103 cases. They were more often involved by lateral than by medial primaries. These investigators also found supraclavicular nodes involved in some cases when primaries were located within 3 cm of the clavicle. Internal mammary lymph nodes contain metastases less often than might be expected. None of 19 internal mammary dissections reported by Papachristou's group showed metastases, despite the fact that involvement was found in 38% of autopsies after death from disseminated melanoma. Although the breast is an organ of the skin, it is possible that cutaneous lymphatics, unlike those within the breast, do not drain into these nodes. In a large series of 115 cases at Memorial Sloan-Kettering Cancer Center the disease-free survival rates at 5 years, by Clark's level, were as follows: I, 90%; II, 80%; III, 60%; IV, 30%; and V, 22% (Papachristou et al., 1979). In the presence of node involvement the figure was 23%; in its absence more than 71% of patients were alive and well. Two of twenty-one patients treated at New York University Medical Center had histologically involved axillary nodes. Nine patients followed more than 5 years remained disease free (Roses et al., 1979).

Surgical resection is the preferred treatment for melanoma involving the nipple or skin of the breast (D'Aluto 1991). Formerly, mastectomy was believed necessary, but retrospective studies indicate that local excision and axillary node dissection produces comparable 5-year disease-free survival (Papachristou et al., 1979). Melanoma of the breast is treated like cutaneous melanoma elsewhere on the trunk. The primary lesion is encompassed with a margin of normal tissue appropriate for the depth of invasion. For in situ melanomas 1.0 cm is adequate; for invasive lesions 1.0 mm or less in thickness 1.0 to 2.0 cm is considered adequate. For invasive melanomas 1 to 4 mm thick a minimum margin of 3.0 cm is acceptable (Urist et al., 1985). Primary closure is preferred to skin grafting, and mastectomy is not necessary unless it is required to adequately encompass a large lesion. Regional lymph node dissection is performed in the presence of adenopathy. The role of prophylactic lymph node dissection is controversial (Urist et al., 1985). Sentinel node biopsy as described by Morton and coworkers (1992) may prove useful.

LYMPHANGIOSARCOMA OF THE EDEMATOUS ARM

Lymphangiosarcoma is a calamitous complication of chronic arm edema following axillary lymph node dissection. A significant association between carcinoma of the breast and soft tissue sarcomas reported by Schoenberg (1975) was largely attributable to this tumor. When radical mastectomy and postoperative irradiation was routine therapy for mammary carcinoma, lymphedema was a common sequel. Lymphangiosarcoma of the arm was originally described by Stewart and Treves in 1948 and subsequently became known as the Stewart-Treves syndrome. The prevalence was estimated at between 0.45% and 0.07% of patients treated for early carcinoma of the breast (Fitzpatrick, 1969).

Typically, the patient gives a history of persistent arm edema following a mastectomy. After an average interval of 10 years (1 to 24) small, pigmented nodules (often mistaken for insect bites) appear on the arm. The onset was vividly described by Stewart and Treves (1948):

After an interval of years, a purplish red, subdermal, slightly raised, macular or polypoid lesion appears. The primary site is in the skin of the arm or antecubital area. The lesion occurs as a solitary tumor followed by similar satellite areas that sometimes become confluent to form a larger lesion, or remain as distinct and later partially bullous areas. The larger lesions appear almost as papillomatous growths colored by shiny, tense, atrophied epithelium. It has a tendency to ulcerate and discharge a serous or serosanguinous fluid. They heal spontaneously only to break down again and discharge. As new lesions appear, all stages of imminent ulceration, discharge, and healing can be seen. Once the process is initiated, the discrete nodules continue to grow, and new ones appear on the forearm, dorsum of the hand, and finally the skin of the adjacent thorax.

Local infection becomes a problem and eventually the lesion disseminates, most reliably to the lungs but also to bones, brain, lymph nodes, and skin. The characteristic purple-red color and distribution of the lesions suggest the diagnosis (Fig. 35–23). The lesions do not resemble the cutaneous nodules of recurrent mammary carcinoma and do not have their origin in the surgical or irradiated areas, though they may extend to them. Histologically, the lesions can easily be mistaken for Kaposi's sarcoma or for highly anaplastic recurrent carcinoma, but the features usually permit a definitive diagnosis.

The prognosis of the patient is poor (median survival = 1.3 years); in most cases the tumor is unresponsive to all forms of treatment. Radiotherapy to the involved arm may produce some regression, but only three cases of long-term survival are recorded (Tong and Winter, 1974). Both local excision of isolated nodules and amputation of the arm have been used, with occasional success (Barnett et al., 1969; Fitzpatrick, 1969; Haagensen, 1971). Two of eight patients treated at M.D. Anderson Cancer Center with forequarter amputation lived 5 years without recurrence (Yap et al., 1981). At the time of Herrmann and Ariel's report in 1967, 83 cases were in the literature. Only 5 of the 75 patients had survived longer than 5 years free of recurrence after an attempted cure. One had been treated with external irradiation, one by wide excision, and three by amputation. The additional 5-year survivor was treated with external irradiation followed by intra-arterial yttrium microspheres. Herrmann and Ariel suggested initial treatment with irradiation followed by radical amputation of the extremity if irradiation was unsuccessful. For disseminated disease, most forms of chemotherapy are ineffective or produce only brief benefit. In one report systemic chemotherapy with fluorouracil, methotrexate, or various combinations produced complete or partial responses in 42% of cases (median duration = 6 months) (Yap et al., 1981). Temporary remission has attended regional perfusion with nitrogen mustard (Tragus and Wagner, 1969) and melphalan and methotrexate (Yap et al., 1981), and Tong and Winter (1974) reported dramatic, though temporary, response in two patients to cyclophosphamide. Prompt progression occurred when the drug was discontinued because of leukopenia.

The fact that this tumor rarely affects extremities rendered lymphedematous by other causes raises speculation that it is uniquely associated with a constitutional disposition to cancer of the breast or with a common carcinogen. Some speculate, further, that an immunocompromised extremity is favored. Whatever the inciting factor, its dismal prognosis is an additional incentive for preventing lymphedema of the arm and for taking action to treat it effectively when it occurs. Mastectomy wound complications and irradiation of the axilla after axillary dissection both promote fibrotic obstruction of lymphatics and edema, so avoiding these presumably could help prevent this neoplasm.

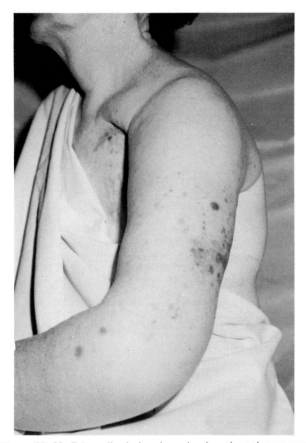

Figure 35–23. This patient developed a lymphangiosarcoma on the upper extremity 5 years after a left radical mastectomy. The arm had been chronically lymphedematous from the time of her original surgery. The characteristic purple lesions can be seen on the arm and the adjacent chest wall, and osteolytic lesions were present in vertebrae. The neoplasm progressed rapidly, and she died several months later with widespread dissemination.

RADIATION-INDUCED SOFT TISSUE SARCOMAS IN BREAST CANCER PATIENTS

Some soft tissue sarcomas are a consequence of irradiation to treat breast cancer (Ferguson et al., 1985; Kuten et al., 1985; Wiklund et al., 1991). These tumors appear in irradiation ports after a latent period of 4 to 26 years in about 1% to 1.5% of patients, and they are highly lethal. Wiklund and coworkers (1991) reported seven cases of postirradiation sarcoma in breast cancer patients from the Finnish Cancer Registry. These lesions appeared from 3.4 to 15.8 years after treatment. Most (three) were osteosarcomas or malignant fibrous histiocytomas (two), but a fibrosarcoma and a malignant schwannoma were also observed. Osteosarcomas involved the sternum, scapula, or humerus. A review at the Institut Gustave Roussy revealed nine sarcomas in irradiated areas of breast cancer patients (Taghian et al., 1991). Most lesions in this series were malignant fibrous histiocytomas or fibrosarcomas. The mean latent period was 9.5 years. The risk of sarcoma following irradiation was clearly elevated: cumulative incidence was 0.2% at 10 years and the observed-expected incidence ratio was 1.81:1. Thirty-eight cases of angiosarcoma in irradiation ports are documented in the literature, 13 of which followed treatment of breast cancer (Edeiken et al., 1992). Seven that followed breast conservation developed after a latent period of 4 to 12½ (average = 8½) years. Four of these appeared in the skin of the breast, but two developed in the parenchyma, and one in the underlying lung.

Wide resection of postirradiation sarcomas is the preferred therapy when this is possible, though successes are few. Further irradiation is rarely feasible. Chemotherapy provides a few partial responses. Kuten and associates (1985) reported two partial responses among seven patients treated with the four-drug combination cyclophosphamide, vincristine, doxorubicin, and dacarbazine. Two of the seven patients reported by Wiklund's group (28.6%) survived longer than 5 years. All but two of Taghian and associates' (1991) cases died of their sarcomas. Median survival time was 2.4 years.

In the past, chest wall irradiation was frequently used after mastectomy when the risk for treatment failure was great. This served to reduce local recurrences, but since it did little to improve survival, the long-range morbidity of irradiation frequently was not appreciated. Though the use of irradiation after mastectomy has declined, breast irradiation is currently widely employed as a more "cosmetic" alternative to mastectomy for early breast cancer. Patients so treated are likely to be cured and have good prospects for becoming long-term survivors. Consequently, the absolute number of radiation-induced sarcomas can be expected to increase (Badwe et al., 1991). Prolonged follow-up with early recognition and treatment of these tumors is the most promising means of management.

References

Alessi, E., and Sala, F.: Leiomyosarcoma in ectopic areola. Am. J. Dermatopathol., *14*:165–169, 1992.

Allen, R., Nixon, D., York, M., et al.: Successful chemotherapy for cystosarcoma phyllodes in a young woman. Arch. Intern. Med., *145*:1127, 1985.

Altomare, D. F., Sbisa, G., DePalo, R., et al.: Fatal breast rhabdomyosarcoma in a 15 year old primigravida. Eur. J. Gynaecol. Oncol., *11*:149–151, 1990.

Amadori, G., Brigato, G., Cordiano, V., et al.: Pelvic and mammary Burkitt-like lymphoma with simultaneous development of leukemia. Gynecol. Oncol., 26:246–250, 1987.

American Joint Committee on Cancer: Manual for Staging of Cancer. 4th ed. Philadelphia, J.B. Lippincott, 1992, pp. 255–263.

Amerson, J. R.: Cystosarcoma phyllodes in adolescent females: A report of seven patients. Ann. Surg., *171*:849, 1970.

Ansah-Boateng, Y., and Tavassoli, F. A.: Fibroadenoma and cystosarcoma phyllodes of the male breast. Mod. Pathol., *5*:114–116, 1992.

Antman, K. H., Corso, J., Greenberger, J., et al.: Multimodality therapy in the management of angiosarcoma of the breast. Cancer, *50*:2000, 1982.

Ariel, L.: Skeletal metastases in cystosarcoma phyllodes. A case report and review. Arch. Surg., *82*:275, 1961.

Arista-Nasr, J., Gonzalez-Gomez, I., Angeles-Angeles, A., et al.: Primary recurrent leiomyosarcoma of the breast: Case report with ultrastructural and immunohistochemical study and review of the literature. Am. J. Clin. Pathol., *92*:500–505, 1989.

Armitage, J. O.: Treatment of non-Hodgkin's lymphoma. N. Engl. J. Med., *328*:1023–1030, 1993.

Aubrey, D. A., and Andrews, G. S.: Mammary osteogenic sarcoma. Br. J. Surg., *58*:472, 1971.

Austin, R. M., and Dupree, W. B.: Liposarcoma of the breast: A clinicopathologic study of 20 cases. Hum. Pathol., *17*:906–913, 1986.

Azzopardi, J. G.: Problems in Breast Pathology. Philadelphia, W.B. Saunders, 1979, pp. 373–376.

Badwe, R. A., Hanby, A. M., Fentiman, I. S., et al.: Angiosarcoma of the skin overlying an irradiated breast. Breast Cancer Res. Treat., *19*:169–172, 1991.

Baker, R. R.: Unusual lesions and their management. Surg. Clin. North Am., *70*:963–975, 1990.

Banergee, S. S., Eyden, B. P., Wells, S., et al.: Pseudoangiosarcomatous carcinoma: A clinicopathological study of seven cases. Histopathology, *21*:13–23, 1992.

Barber, K. W. Jr., Harrison, E. G., Clagett, O. T., et al.: Angiosarcoma of the breast. Surgery, *48*:869, 1960.

Barnett, W. O., Hardy, J. D., and Hendrix, J. H.: Lymphangiosarcoma following post-mastectomy lymphedema. Ann. Surg., *169*:960, 1969.

Bartoli, C., Zurrida, S., Veronesi, P., et al.: Small sized phyllodes tumor of the breast. Eur. J. Surg. Oncol., *16*:215–219, 1990.

Berg, J. W., DeCosse, J. J., Fracchia, A. A., et al.: Stromal sarcomas of the breast. A unified approach to connective tissue sarcomas other than cystosarcoma phyllodes. Cancer, *15*:418, 1962.

Berger, S. M., and Gershon-Cohen, J.: Mammography of breast sarcoma. AJR, *87*:76, 1962.

Blichert-Toft, M., Hansen, J. P. H., Hansen, O. H., et al.: Clinical course of cystosarcoma phyllodes related to histologic appearance. Surg. Gynecol. Obstet., *149*:929, 1975.

Bogomoletz, W. V.: Pure squamous cell carcinoma of the breast. Arch. Pathol. Lab. Med., *106*:57, 1982.

Borrmann, R.: Metastasenbildung bei histologisch gutartigen Geschulsten (Fall von metastasierendem Angiom). Beitr. Pathol. Anat., *40*:372, 1907.

Bot, F. J., and Donner, R.: Metastatic cystosarcoma phyllodes. Report of a case with a ten-year interval. Neth. J. Surg., *33*:34, 1981.

Botham, R. J., McDonald, J. R., and Clagett, O. T.: Sarcoma of the mammary gland. Surg. Gynecol. Obstet., *107*:55, 1958.

Brentani, M. M., Nagai, M. A., Oshima, C. T. F., et al.: Steroid receptors in cystosarcoma phyllodes. Cancer Detect. Prevent., *5*:211, 1982.

Buchberger, W., Strasser, K., Heim, K., et al.: Phyllodes tumor: Findings on mammography, sonography, and aspiration cytology in 10 cases. AJR, *157*:715–719, 1991.

Burton, G. V., Hart, L. L., Leight, G. S. Jr., et al.: Cystosarcoma phyllodes. Effective therapy with cisplatin and etoposide chemotherapy. Cancer, *63*:2088–2092, 1989.

Bussolati, G., Papotti, K. M., Foschini, M. P., et al.: The interest of actin immunocytochemistry in diagnostic histopathology. Basic Appl. Histochem., *31*:165–176, 1987.

Carbone, A., Volpe, R., Tirelli, U., et al.: Primary lymphoblastic lymphoma of the breast. Clin. Oncol., *8*:367, 1982.

Carstens, H. B., and Cooke, J. L.: Mammary carcinosarcoma presenting as rhabdomyosarcoma: An ultrastructural and immunocytochemical study. Ultrastruct. Pathol., *14*:537–544, 1990.

Chelius, M. J.: Teleangiektasie. Heidelberg. Klin. Ann., *4*:499, 517, 1828.

Chen, K. T. K., Kirkegaard, D. D., and Bocian, J. J.: Angiosarcoma of the breast. Cancer, *46*:368, 1980.

Chen, K. T. K., Kuo, T. T., and Hoffmann, K. D.: Leiomyosarcoma of the breast. A case of long survival and late hepatic metastasis. Cancer, *47*:1883, 1981.

Chua, C. L., Thomas, A., Ng, B. K.: Cystosarcoma phyllodes: A review of surgical options. Surgery, *105*:141–147, 1989.

Cohen, P. L., and Brooks, J. J.: Lymphomas of the breast. A clinicopathologic and immunohistochemical study of primary and secondary cases. Cancer, *67*:1359–1369, 1991.

Cohn-Cedermark, G., Rutqvlist, L. E., Rosendahl, I., et al.: Prognostic factors in cystosarcoma phyllodes. Cancer, *68*:2017–2022, 1991.

Cole-Beuglet, C., Kirk, M. E., Selouan, R., et al.: Bone within the breast. Radiology, *119*:643, 1976.

Cooper, W. G. Jr., and Ackerman, L. V.: Cystosarcoma phyllodes: With a consideration of its more malignant variant. Surg. Gynecol. Obstet., *77*:279, 1943.

Cornog, J. L., Mobini, J., Steiger, E., et al.: Squamous carcinoma of the breast. Am. J. Clin. Pathol., *55*:410, 1971.

Cosmacini, P., Surrida, S., Veronesi, P., et al.: Phyllode tumor of the breast: Mammographic experience in 99 cases. Eur. J. Radiol., *15*:11–14, 1992.

Crocker, D. J., and Murad, T. M.: Ultrastructure of fibrosarcoma in a male breast. Cancer, *23*:891–899, 1969.

Curran, R. C., and Dodge, O. G.: Sarcoma of breast, with particular reference to its origin from fibroadenoma. J. Clin. Pathol., *15*:1, 1962.

D'Aluto, G., Del Vecchio, S., Mansi, L., et al.: Malignant melanoma of the nipple: A case studied with radiolabeled monoclonal antibody. Tumori, *77*:449–451, 1991.

Dao, A. H., Adkins, R. B. Jr., Glick, A. D.: Malignant lymphoma of the breast: A review of 13 cases. Am. Sur., *58*:792–796, 1992.

DeCosse, J. J., Berg, J. W., Fracchia, A. A., et al.: Primary lymphosarcoma of the breast. Cancer, *15*:1264, 1962.

Delaney, W. E., Orossi, C., and Nealon, T. F. Jr.: The soft tissues. *In* Nealon, T. F. Jr. (Ed.): Management of the Patient with Cancer. 2nd ed. Philadelphia, W.B. Saunders, 1976, p. 851.

DeLeon, D. M., Viallafria, L., and Crisostomo, C.: Nonsystemic reticulum cell sarcoma of the breast: A case report. Philip. J. Surg., *16*:149, 1961.

del Regato, J. A.: Radiotherapy of soft-tissue sarcomas. J.A.M.A. *185*:216, 1963.

Dixon, J. M., Lumsden, A. B., Krajewski, A., et al.: Primary lymphoma of the breast. Br. J. Surg., *74*:214–217, 1987.

Donegan, W. L.: Sarcomas of the breast. *In* Donegan, W. L., and Spratt, J. S. (Eds.): Cancer of the Breast. 3rd ed. Philadelphia, W.B. Saunders, 1988, pp. 692.

Donnell, R. M., Rosen, P. P., Lieberman, P. H., et al.: Angiosarcoma and other vascular tumors of the breast. Pathologic analysis as a guide to prognosis. Am. J. Surg. Pathol., *5*:629, 1981.

Edeiken, S., Russo, D. P., Knecht, J., et al.: Angiosarcoma after tylectomy and radiation therapy for carcinoma of the breast. Cancer, *70*:644–647, 1992.

Edwards, J. A., and Strouth, B. P.: Hemangioendothelioblastoma of the breast. Northwest. Med., *55*:788, 1956.

Eggers, J. W., and Chesney, T. M.: Squamous cell carcinoma of the breast: A clinicopathologic analysis of eight cases and review of the literature. Hum. Pathol., *15*:526, 1984.

El-Ghazawy, I. M. H., and Singletary, S. E.: Surgical management of primary lymphoma of the breast. Ann. Surg., *214*:724–724, 1992.

El-Naggar, A. K., Ro, J. Y., Mclemore, D., et al.: DNA content and proliferative activity of cystosarcoma phyllodes of the breast. Potential prognostic significance. Am. J. Clin. Pathol., *93*:480–485, 1990*a*.

El-Naggar, A. K., Mackay, B., Sneige, N., et al.: Stromal neoplasms of the breast: A comparative flow cytometric study. J. Surg. Oncol., *44*:151–156, 1990*b*.

Elson, B. C., Ikeda, D. M., Andersson, I., et al.: Fibrosarcoma of the breast: Mammographic findings in five cases. AJR, *158*:993–995, 1992.

Ferguson, D. F., Sullon, H. G., and Dawson, P. J.: Long effects of adjuvant radiotherapy for breast cancer. Cancer, *54*:2319, 1985.

Fiks, A.: Cystosarcoma phyllodes of the mammary gland—Muller's tumor. Virchows Arch. (Pathol. Anat.), *392*:1, 1981.

Fitzpatrick, P. J.: Lymphangiosarcoma in breast cancer. Am. J. Surg., *12*:172, 1969.

Foote, F. W., and Stewart, F. W.: A histologic classification of carcinoma of the breast. Surgery, *19*:74, 1946.

France, C. J., and O'Connell, J. P.: Osseous metaplasia in the human mammary gland. Arch. Surg., *100*:238–239, 1970.

Gatch, W. K.: A melanoma, apparently primary, in a breast. Arch. Surg., *73*:266, 1956.

Geschickter, C. F.: Diseases of the Breast. Philadelphia, J. B. Lippincott, 1943, p. 386.

Giardini, R., Piccolo, C., and Rilke, F.: Primary non-Hodgkin's lymphomas of the female breast. Cancer, *69*:725–735, 1992.

Grimes, M. M.: Cystosarcoma phyllodes of the breast: Histologic features, flow cytometric analysis, and clinical correlations. Mod. Pathol., *5*:232–239, 1992.

Gupta, R. K., Naran, S., Dowle, C.: Needle aspiration cytology and immunocytochemical study in a case of angiosarcoma of the breast. Diagn. Cytopathol., *7*:363–365, 1991.

Haagensen, C. D.: Diseases of the Breast. Philadelphia, W.B. Saunders, 1971, p. 300.

Hare, H. F., and Cerny, J. J., Jr.: Soft tissue sarcoma. Review of 200 cases. Cancer, *16*:1332, 1963.

Harris, M., and Persaud, V.: Carcinoma of the breast. J. Pathol., *112*:99, 1974.

Hart, W. R., Bauer, R. C., and Oberman, H. A.: Cystosarcoma phyllodes. A clinicopathologic study of twenty-six hypercellular periductal stromal tumours of the breast. Am. J. Clin. Pathol., *70*:211–216, 1978.

Hawkins, R. E., Schofield, J. B., Fisher, C., et al.: The clinical and histologic criteria that predict metastases from cystosarcoma phyllodes. Cancer, *69*:141–147, 1992.

Herrmann, J. B., and Ariel, I. M.: Therapy of lymphangiosarcoma of the chronically edematous limb. Five year cure of a patient treated by intraarterial radioactive yttrium. AJR, *99*:393, 1967.

Hill, F. P., and Stout, A. P.: Sarcoma of the breast. Arch. Surg., *44*:723, 1942.

Hofman, W. I., and Goodman, M. L.: Primary lymphosarcoma of the breast. Arch. Surg., *96*:410, 1968.

Homes, R. S., and Leis, H. P. Jr.: Liposarcoma of the female breast. Review of the literature and report of a case. Ann. Geriatr. Soc. J., *10*:355, 1962.

Hoover, H. C., Trestioreanu, A., and Ketcham, A. S.: Metastatic cystosarcoma phyllodes in an adolescent girl: An unusually malignant tumor. Ann. Surg., *181*:279, 1975.

Horn, R. C. Jr.: Sarcomas of soft tissue. J.A.M.A., *1283*:511, 1963.

Hugh, J. C., Jackson, F. I., Hanson, J., et al.: Primary breast lymphoma. An immunohistologic study of 20 new cases. Cancer, *66*:2602–2611, 1990.

Hummer, C. D. Jr. and Burkart, T. J.: Liposarcoma of the breast. A case of bilateral involvement. Am. J. Surg., *113*:558, 1967.

Hunter, T. B., Martin, P. C., Dietzen, C. D., et al.: Angiosarcoma of the breast. Two case reports and a review of the literature. Cancer, *56*:2099–2106, 1985.

Jernstrom, P., Lindberg, A. L., and Meland, O. N.: Osteogenic sarcoma of the mammary gland. Am. J. Clin. Pathol., *40*:521, 1963.

Jones, M. W., Norris, H. J., Wargotz, E. S., et al.: Fibrosarcoma—malignant fibrous histiocytoma of the breast—a clinicopathological study of 32 cases. Am. J. Surg. Pathol., *16*:667–674, 1992.

Kario, K., Maeda, S., Mizuno, Y., et al.: Phyllodes tumor of the breast: A clinicopathologic study of 34 cases. J. Surg. Oncol., *45*:46–51, 1990.

Keelan, P. A., Myers, J. L., Wold, L. E., et al.: Phyllodes tumor: A clinicopathologic review of 60 patients and flow cytometric analysis in 30 patients. Hum. Pathol., *23*:1048–1054, 1992.

Kolarsick, A. J.: Primary sarcoma of the breast. J. Med. Soc. N. J., *69*:243, 1972.

Kumar, A., Gupta, S., Chopra, P., et al.: Bilateral angiosarcoma of the breast: An overview. Aust. N. Z. J. Surg., *60*:341–345, 1990.

Kuten, A., Sapir, D., Cohen, Y., et al.: Postirradiation soft tissue sarcoma occurring in breast cancer patients: Report of seven cases and results of combination chemotherapy. J. Surg. Oncol., *28*:168, 1985.

Ladefoged, C., and Nielsen, B. B.: Primary chondrosarcoma of the breast: A case report and review of the literature. Breast, *16*:26, 1984.

Lamovec, J., and Jancar, J.: Primary malignant lymphoma of the breast. Lymphoma of the mucosa-associated lymphoid tissue. Cancer, *60*:3033–3041, 1987.

Langham, M. R., Mills, A. S., DeMay, R. M., et al.: Malignant fibrous histiocytoma of the breast. A case report and review of the literature. Cancer, *54*:558, 1984.

Layfield, L. J., Hart, J., Neuwirth, H., et al.: Relation between DNA ploidy and the clinical behavior of phyllodes tumors. Cancer, *64*:1486–1489, 1989.

Lee, B. J., and Pack, G. T.: Giant intracanalicular fibroadenomyxoma of the breast—the so-called cystosarcoma phyllodes of Johannes Mueller. Am. J. Cancer, *15*:2583, 1931.

Lee, Y-T. N., Sparks, F. C., and Morton, D. L.: Primary melanoma of skin of the breast region. Ann. Surg., *185*:17–22, 1977.

Lester, J., and Stout, A. P.: Cystosarcoma phyllodes. Cancer, *7*:335, 1954.

Lewko, W. M., Vaghmar, R., Maleckar, J. R., et al.: Cultured breast cystosarcoma phylloides cells and applications to patient therapy. Breast Cancer Res. Treat., *17*:131–138, 1990.

Liberman, L., Dershaw, D. D., Kaufman, R. J., et al.: Angiosarcoma of the breast. Radiology, *183*:649–654, 1992.

Liebert, C. W. Jr., and Edwards, D. K.: Malignant fibrous histiocytoma of the breast. South. Med. J., *75*:1281, 1982.

Lin, J. J., Farha, G. J., and Taylor, R. J.: Pseudolymphoma of the breast. I. In a study of 8,654 consecutive tylectomies and mastectomies. Cancer, *45*:973–978, 1980.

Lissoos, I., Schmann, A., Path., M. C., et al.: Haemangiosarcoma of the breast. S. Afr. Med. J., *43*:1229, 1969.

Mambo, N. C., Burke, J. S., and Butler, J. J.: Primary malignant lymphomas of the breast. Cancer, *39*:2003, 1977.

McCullough, K., and Lynch, J. M.: Metastatic sarcoma of heart from cystosarcoma phyllodes of the breast. Md. State Med. J., *9*:66, 1960.

McDonald, J. R., and Harrington, S. W.: Giant fibroadenoma of the breast—cystosarcoma phyllodes. Ann. Surg., *133*:243, 1950.

Melander, D. W., and Pack, G. T.: Lymphosarcoma—choice of treatment and end results in 567 patients. Role of surgical treatment for cure and palliation. Rev. Surg., *20*:3, 1963.

Menon, M., and van Velthoven, P. C. M.: Liposarcoma of the breast. Arch. Pathol., *98*:370, 1974.

Merino, M. J., Berman, M., and Carter, D.: Angiosarcoma of the breast. Am. J. Surg. Pathol., *7*:53, 1983.

Misra, A., Kapur, B. M. L., Rath, G. K.: Primary breast lymphoma. J. Surg. Oncol., *47*:265–270, 1991.

Morton, D. L.: Soft tissue sarcomas. *In* Holland, J. F., and Frei, E. (Eds.): Cancer Medicine. Philadelphia, Lea & Febiger, 1974, p. 1845.

Morton, D., Wen, D., and Cochran, A.: Management of early-stage melanoma by intraoperative lymphatic mapping and selective lymphadenectomy: An alternative to routine elective lymphadenectomy or "watch and wait." Surg. Oncol. Clin. North Am., *1*:247–259, 1992.

Neumann, E.: Beitrage zur Casuistik der Brustdrusengeschwulste. Virchows Arch. (Pathol Anat.), *24*:316, 1862.

Newman, P. L., and Fletcher, C. D.: Smooth muscle tumours of the external genitalia: Clinicopathological analysis of series. Histopathology, *18*:523–529, 1991.

van Niekerk, J. L. M., Wobbes, T., Holland, R., et al.: Malignant fibrous histiocytoma of the breast with axillary lymph node involvement. J. Surg. Oncol., *34*:32, 1987.

O'Brien, J. E., and Stout, A. P.: Malignant fibrous xanthomas. Cancer, *17*:1445, 1964.

Oberman, H. A.: Cystosarcoma phyllodes, a clinicopathologic study of hypercellular periductal stromal neoplasm of breast. Cancer, *18*:697, 1965a.

Oberman, H. A.: Sarcomas of the breast. Cancer, *18*:1233, 1965b.

Owens, F. M. Jr., and Adams, W. E.: Giant intracanalicular fibroadenoma of the breast. Arch. Surg., *43*:588, 1941.

Page, D. L., Anderson, T. J., Johnson, R. L.: Sarcomas of the breast. *In* Page, D. L., and Anderson, T. J. (Eds.): Diagnostic Histopathology of the Breast. New York, Churchill Livingstone, 1987, p. 350.

Palmer, M. L., DeRisi, D. C., Pelikan, A., et al.: Treatment options and recurrence potential for cystosarcoma phyllodes. Surg. Gynecol. Obstet., *170*:193–196, 1990.

Papachristou, K. N., Kinne, D. W., Rosen, P. P., et al.: Cutaneous melanoma of the breast. Surgery, *85*:322–328, 1979.

Pardo-Midan, J., Garcia-Julian, G., and Altuna, M. A.: Leiomyosarcoma of the breast. Am. J. Clin. Pathol., *72*:477, 1974.

Parham, D. M., Robertson, A. J., Hussein, K. A., et al.: Leiomyosarcoma of the breast: Cytological and histological features, with a review of the literature. Cytopathology, *3*:245–252, 1992.

Patrick, R. S., Jarvis, J., and Miln, D. C.: Hemangioblastoma of one breast—a report of three cases. Br. J. Surg., *45*:188, 1957–58.

Pitts, W. C., Rojas, V. A., Gaffey, M. J., et al.: Carcinomas with metaplasia and sarcomas of the breast. Am. J. Clin. Pathol., *95*:623–632, 1991.

Pollard, S. G., Marks, P. V., Temple, L. M., et al.: Breast sarcoma. A clinicopathologic review of 25 cases. Cancer, *66*:941–944, 1990.

Rainwater, L. M., Martin, J. K. Jr., Gaffrey, T. A., et al.: Angiosarcoma of the breast. Arch. Surg., *121*:669–676, 1986.

Rao, B. R., Meyer, J. S., and Fry, C. G.: Most cystosarcoma phyllodes and fibroadenomas have progesterone receptor but lack estrogen receptor: Stromal localization of progesterone receptor. Cancer, *47*:2016, 1981.

Rao, C. R., and Jaganathan, K.: Cystosarcoma phyllodes. Diagnosis by fine needle aspiration cytology. Acta Cytol., *36*:203–207, 1992.

Reed, W., Oppedal, B. R., Eeg-Larsen, T.: Immunohistology is valuable in distinguishing between Paget's disease, Bowen's disease and superficial spreading malignant melanoma. Histopathology, *16*:583–588, 1990.

Richards, W. G., and Way, R. W.: Co-existent cystosarcoma phyllodes and scirrhous adenocarcinoma of one breast. Wis. Med. J., *62*:425, 1963.

Robb, P. M., and MacFarlane, A.: Two rare breast tumors. J. Pathol., *75*:293, 1958.

Rosen, P. P., Dimmel, M., and Ernsberger, D.: Mammary angiosarcoma. The prognostic significance of tumor differentiation. Cancer, *62*:2145–2151, 1988.

Roses, D. F., Harris, M. N., Stern, J. S., et al.: Cutaneous melanoma of the breast. Ann. Surg., *189*:112–115, 1979.

Rosner, D.: Angiosarcoma of the breast: Long-term survival following adjuvant chemotherapy. J. Surg. Oncol., *39*:90–95, 1988.

Rossen, K., Stamp, I., and Sorensen, I. M.: Primary malignant fibrous histiocytoma of the breast. A report of four cases and review of the literature. Acta Pathol. Microbiol. Immunol. Scand., *99*:696–702, 1991.

Rowell, M. D., Perry, R. R., Hsiu, J-G., et al.: Phyllodes tumors. Am. J. Surg., *163*:376–379, 1993.

Saleh, H. A., and Klein, L. H.: Cystosarcoma phyllodes arising synchronously in right breast and bilateral axillary ectopic breast tissue. Arch. Pathol. Lab. Med., *114*:624–626, 1990.

Salvadori, B., Cusumano, F., DelBo, R., et al.: Surgical treatment of phyllodes tumors of the breast. Cancer, *63*:2532–2536, 1989.

Sau, P., Solis, J., Lupton, G. P., et al.: Pigmented breast carcinoma. A clinical and histopathologic simulator of malignant melanoma. Arch. Dermatol., *125*:536–539, 1989.

Scheid, M. F., Cogan, J. E., and Waldron, G. W.: Angiosarcoma of the breast. Texas J. Med., *60*:488, 1964.

Schoenberg, B. S.: Multiple primary neoplasms. *In* Fraumeni, J. F. (Ed.): Persons at High Risk of Cancer. New York, Academic Press, 1975, p. 103.

Schouten, J. T., Weese, J. L., and Carbone, P. P.: Lymphoma of the breast. Ann. Surg., *194*:749, 1981.

Shore, J. H.: Hemangiosarcoma of the breast. J. Pathol. Bacteriol., *74*:289, 1957.

Sonnenblick, M., and Abraham, A. S.: Primary lymphosarcoma of the breast: Review of the literature on occurrence in elderly patients. J. Am. Geriatr. Soc., *24*:225, 1976.

Stephenson, S. E., and Byrd, B. F.: Malignant melanoma of the breast. Am. J. Surg., *97*:232, 1959.

Stewart, F. W., and Treves, N.: Lymphangiosarcoma in postmastectomy lymphedema. A report of six cases in elephantiasis chirurgica. Cancer, *1*:64, 1948.

Stout, A. P., and Bernanke, M.: Liposarcoma of the female mammary gland. Surg. Gynecol. Obstet., *83*:216, 1946.

Sugar, J., and Sapi, Z.: Alveolar rhabdomyosarcoma—a case report. Arch. Geschwulstforschung., *58*:445–448, 1988.

Taghian, A., de Vathaire, F., Terrier, P., et al.: Long-term risk of sarcoma following radiation treatment for breast cancer. Int. J. Radiat. Oncol. Biol. Physics., *21*:361–367, 1991.

Tang, P. H., Petrelli, M., and Robechek, P. J.: Stromal sarcoma of breast. A light and electron microscopic study. Cancer, *43*:209, 1979.

Teich, S., and Brecher, I. N.: Osteogenic sarcoma of the breast. A case report. Breast, *11*:11, 1985.

Tellin, A., Walzbard, E., Levine, T., et al.: Malignant fibrous histiocytoma of the breast. Int. Surg., *75*:63–66, 1990.

Tong, D., and Winter, J.: Postmastectomy lymphangiosarcoma—temporary response to cyclophosphamide chemotherapy in two cases. Br. J. Surg., *61*:76, 1974.

Tragus, E. T., and Wagner, D. E.: Current therapy for postmastectomy lymphangiosarcoma. Arch. Surg., *97*:839, 1969.

Treves, N.: A study of cystosarcoma phyllodes. Ann. N. Y. Acad. Sci., *114*:922, 1964.

Treves, N., and Sunderland, D. A.: Cystosarcoma phyllodes of the breast. Cancer, *4*:1286, 1951.

Turalba, C. I. C., El-Mahdi, A. M., and Ladaga, L.: Fatal metastatic cystosarcoma phyllodes in an adolescent female: Case report and review of treatment approaches. J. Surg. Oncol., *33*:176, 1986.

Urist, M. M., Balch, C. M., Milton, G. W.: Surgical management of the primary melanoma. *In* Balch, C. M., and Milton, G. W. (Eds.): Cutaneous Melanoma. Philadelphia, J. B. Lippincott, 1985, pp. 75, 85.

Urist, M. M., Balch, C. M., Maddox, W. A., et al.: Management of regional metastatic melanoma. *In* Balch, C. M., and Milton, G. W. (Eds.): Cutaneous Melanoma. Philadelphia, J. B. Lippincott, 1985, p. 155.

Visfeldt, J., and Sheike, O.: Male breast cancer. Cancer, *32*:985, 1973.

Ward, R., and Evans, H.: Cystosarcoma phyllodes. A clinicopathologic study of 26 cases. Cancer, *58*:2282–2289, 1986.

Wargotz, E., and Norris, H. Metaplastic carcinomas of the breast. Cancer, *64*:1490–1499, 1989.

Waterworth, P. D., Gompertz, R. H. K., Hennessy, M. C., et al.: Primary leiomyosarcoma of the breast. Br. J. Surg., *79*:169–170, 1992.

West, T. L., Weiland, L. H., and Clagett, O. T.: Cytosarcoma phyllodes. Ann. Surg., *173*:520, 1971.

White, J. W.: Malignant variant of cystosarcoma phyllodes. Am. J. Cancer, *40*:458, 1940.

WHO 1981 International Histological Classification of Tumors. Histologic Typing of Breast Tumours. 2nd ed. Geneva, World Health Organization, 1981.

Wiernik, P. H., and Serpick, A. A.: Granulocytic sarcoma (chloroma). Blood, *35*:361, 1970.

Wiklund, T. A., Blomqvist, C. P., Raty, J., et al.: Postirradiation sarcoma. Cancer, *58*:524–531, 1991.

Williams, B. V., and Diamonon, J.: Carcinosarcoma of the breast. South. Med. J., *57*:462, 1964.

Yap, B. S., Yap, H. Y., McBride, C. M., et al.: Chemotherapy for postmastectomy lymphangiosarcoma. Cancer, *47*:853, 1981.

Zurrida, S., Bartoli, C., Galimberti, V., et al.: Which therapy for unexpected phyllodes tumour of the breast? Eur. J. Cancer, *28*:654–657, 1992.

36

Cancer of the Male Breast

William L. Donegan

In men the breast is a vestigial organ, and the development of cancer in it is unusual. Only 1% of all breast cancers develop in men, and it accounts for no more than 0.17% of cancers in the male population (Cancer Facts and Figures, 1994). An estimated 1000 new cases and 300 deaths occur each year in the United States, which represent 0.5% and 0.7% of morbidity and mortality from breast cancer, respectively. Because of this low frequency the experience of individual physicians with male breast cancer is limited, and principally in referral centers does experience with more than a few cases accumulate. Furthermore, screening and clinical trials, now so much a part of management of female breast cancer, are nonexistent for men. Nevertheless, the widespread educational and scientific efforts to control the disease in women has also benefited male victims. Breast cancer in men is fundamentally identical to breast cancer in women except for being less frequent, occurring at an older age, arising more regularly beneath the nipple, and being more hormonally sensitive.

The Edwin Smith surgical papyrus, which dates from 3000 B.C., records the case of a man with a bulging tumor in his breast (Breasted, 1930). The writer indicated, ''There is no treatment.'' This is the earliest reference to what may have been breast cancer. The first clinical description of breast cancer in a male is attributed to John of Arderne, who practiced in England in the 14th century (Holleb et al., 1968). The Spanish surgeon Francisco Arceo (1493–1571) noted that breast cancer was less frequent in men than in women, and Fabricius Hildanus (1537–1619) also mentioned the problem. Until the 19th century this curiosity was addressed principally in isolated reports. In 1886, Schuchart was able to collect 406 cases, and in 1927, Wainwright reported on 418 collected cases. Wainwright observed that men were affected at an older age than women and were not as often cured (Wainwright, 1927). Sizeable series are now available from numerous sources (Holleb et al., 1968; Crichlow, 1972; Meyskens et al., 1976; Gupta, 1981; Adami, 1989; and Borgen et al., 1992).

EPIDEMIOLOGY

The incidence of breast cancer in males varies in synchrony with that of females throughout the world, suggesting a common cause. The incidence is low in Japan and high in the United States and Great Britain (Waterhouse et al., 1982). Close correspondence was noted in different Scandinavian countries by Ewertz and colleagues (1989). The incidence is not rising appreciably, perhaps because males

do not participate in screening programs and the tumor is underreported. Risk for the disease is strongly age related. Although it has been reported in a 5-year-old boy (Crichlow, 1972), in 1989 Fodor could find only three cases in males younger than 21 years. It is sufficiently rare in the young that no average annual age-specific incidence for persons under 30 years old was provided by the Third National Cancer Survey in the United States. Beginning at age 30 the incidence rises steadily throughout life, from 0.1 per 100,000 population at ages 30–34 to 6.5 at age 85 and thereafter. The decreased rise seen in women after menopause is not seen in men (Ewertz et al., 1989). In the United States the difference in incidence between males and females decreases as the population ages. As illustrated in Figure 36–1, at ages 35 to 39, breast cancer is 572 times more frequent in females than in males; by age 85 it is only 34 times more frequent (Donegan, 1991).

Risk factors other than age are less well established than in females, but they suggest similar influences. A high prevalence has been noted in Jewish males (Lin and Kessler, 1980; and Mabuchi et al., 1985). A familial tendency is also evident. Affected males often report a male or female family member with breast cancer (Bagley, 1987). Breast cancer in related males has been appreciated since 1889 (Williams, 1889). Kozak and coworkers (1986) summarized 13 reports. Six of these involved brothers, and four a father and son. Three others involved a father, son, and the father's brother. In two additional cases a generation was skipped. Demeter and colleagues (1990) reported an instance in which a man's sister and both maternal grandparents also had the disease. Because of scant information the risk for relatives of men with breast cancer has not been accurately determined; however, transmission through the male line can be demonstrated in rodents. It has been suggested that the breasts of other members of a patient's family should be examined (Siddiqui et al., 1988).

The possibility of a viral cause has not been excluded. Using antisera to the mouse mammary tumor virus and to the gp52 glycoprotein of its envelope, Lloyd and colleagues (1983) identified related antigen in cancer tissue sections of 88% of 34 males with breast cancers. The same antigen has been found in human milk and in the serum of women with breast cancer.

Ionizing radiation is a well-known breast carcinogen, and Eldar and colleagues (1989) reviewed 10 cases of men who developed breast cancer following radiation to the chest. Virtually all were exposed early in life, five before age 20 years, variously for thymic enlargement, lymphoma, prepubertal gynecomastia, eczema, and osteogenic sarcoma

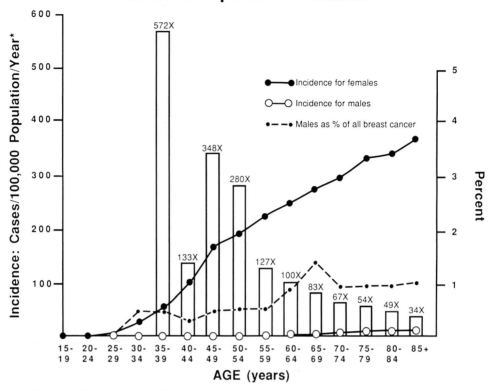

Figure 36–1. The incidence of breast cancer in both sexes increases with age, but the difference in incidence decreases. Men represent 1% of all new cases of breast cancer after age 60 years. (Compiled from Surveillance, Epidemiology and End Results (SEER) data collected from 1973 to 1977 and published in 1981, and from the Third National Cancer Survey of the U.S. *Vertical bars* represent the incidence of breast cancer in females as multiples of the incidence in males at each age. (Reprinted with permission from Donegan, W.L.: Cancer of the breast in men. CA Cancer J. Clin., 41:339–354, 1991.)

(Thompson et al., 1979). Tumors appeared as early as 12 years after exposure; the median latency period was 30 years.

Feminization appears to increase risk, whether it is brought about genetically, by hormone administration, or by hypogonadism. Men with Klinefelter's syndrome (i.e., gynecomastia, small testes, aspermatogenesis, hypoleydigism, increased follicle-stimulating hormone, and an XXY sex chromosome genotype) are suspected of having an increased risk of breast cancer (Klinefelter et al., 1942). Dodge and associates (1969) found this syndrome in three of 21 cases of male breast cancer and estimated the associated risk of breast cancer to be 66.5 times the usual risk for men. This is probably exaggerated, as no case of Klinefelter's syndrome was mentioned in five other reports since 1978 totaling 357 cases (Heller et al., 1978; Yap et al., 1979; Axelsson and Andersson, 1983; Erlichman et al., 1984; and Vercoutere and O'Connell, 1984). Evans and Crichlow (1987) estimated that about 3% of males with Klinefelter's syndrome develop breast cancer. Three cases of breast cancer have been reported in transsexual males after prolonged treatment with estrogens (Pritchard et al., 1988). The mother of one had died of metastatic breast cancer. Primary carcinomas occasionally develop in the breasts of men treated with estrogens for cancer of the

prostate (Crichlow, 1972; and Wilson and Hutchinson, 1976). In this circumstance metastases to the breast from the prostate also occur, but they can be distinguished with stains for prostate-specific antigen. Olsson and colleagues (1984) observed breast cancer in a male with an hypophyseal prolactinoma and estrogen excess. Case-control studies associating male breast cancer with orchitis, inguinal herniorrhaphy, gonadal injury, undescended testes, late marriage with no children, and with occupations involving exposure to high temperatures, all raise the possibility of testicular damage (Lin and Kessler, 1980; Mabuchi et al., 1985; McLaughlin et al., 1988; and Olsson and Ranstam, 1988). Casagrande and colleagues (1988) found obesity at a young age more frequent among men with breast cancer than among controls and suggested that excess bio-available estrogens were influential. The increased proportion of breast cancers found in males in Egypt and Zambia (15% of cases) is attributed to hyperestrogenism caused by bilharziasis and malnutrition (Fodor, 1989).

Feminization of the male breast (gynecomastia) might be expected to carry a risk for breast cancer comparable to that of women, but proof remains elusive. The increased frequency associated with Klinefelter's syndrome is the most compelling evidence for an association between gynecomastia and breast cancer. Gynecomastia is common among males, and the age-specific frequency rises during life coincidentally with that of breast cancer, but they are not always associated clinically (Sirtori and Veronesi, 1957). Gynecomastia is found histologically in 1% to 40% of males with breast cancer (Scheike and Visfeldt, 1973; and Heller et al., 1978). This may be no higher than expected, since gynecomastia is clinically detectable in 57% of the general male population older than 44 years (Nuttal, 1979). Cole and Quizelbash (1979) investigated 233 cases of gynecomastia and found no cases of malignant change; however, the same might be true for an equal number of females chosen at random. Epithelial proliferation and atypia can be found with gynecomastia; nevertheless, it has been difficult to demonstrate direct histologic transition to invasive cancer (Scheike and Visfeldt, 1973). This may be limited to a single report (Lyall, 1947).

Elevated endogenous estrogen production is not regularly found in men with breast cancer, nor is it clear that estrogens are metabolized differently. Dao (1973) found higher than expected urinary estrogen levels in seven male patients, but Calabresi and coworkers (1976) found no consistent elevation of plasma estrogens. Studies of estradiol metabolism have given inconsistent results (Zumoff, 1966; and Sheike et al., 1973).

CLINICAL PRESENTATION

Historically men with breast cancer have averaged 5 to 10 years older than women with breast cancer. The average age in 1888 cases reported prior to 1972 was 59.6 years (Crichlow, 1972). Ages vary with the population served. In a medically indigent population the author found the average age of 27 male patients to be 71.2 years (10.6 years older than that of 2370 women with the disease) (Donegan and Perez-Mesa, 1973). Among 48 military personnel the average was only 49 years (Panettiere, 1974). Whether the age at diagnosis is declining is uncertain. Between 1945 and 1975 the median age of 87 patients seen at Memorial Hospital in New York was 61 years (Yap et al., 1979); for 104 cases seen between 1975 and 1990 it was only 58 years (Borgen et al., 1992). The long-range trend, however, may reflect an aging population; a relatively youthful 54.2 years was the average age of 401 cases collected by Wainwright in 1927.

In men breast cancers are rarely found when they are asymptomatic or in the absence of physical signs. Men are not screened for breast cancer and are said to be slow to seek medical consultation. The duration of symptoms in various reports on males varies widely, with median values from 3 to 18 months (Panettiere, 1974). A firm lump in the breast is the presentation in almost all cases, and signs of local advancement are often present (Table 36–1). Consistent with the limited distribution of breast tissue in men, the lump is closely associated with the nipple. In 90% of the cases reported by Hodson and colleagues (1985) it was beneath or within 1 cm of the areola. Eccentric tumors favor the upper outer quadrant; in one report the tumor was beneath the areola in 76% of cases, in the upper outer quadrant in 6%, in the upper inner quadrant in 4%, and in the lower inner quadrant in 2% (Ouriel et al., 1984). The

Table 36-1. PRESENTING SIGNS AND SYMPTOMS OF MALE BREAST CANCER

Sign or Symptom	Prevalence (%)
Mass	43–92
Painful mass	2
Nipple involvement	38–39
Nipple retraction	8–31
Nipple discharge	3.7–9
Bloody nipple discharge without a mass	2
Bloody nipple discharge	8–15
Itching of the nipple	2
Nipple ulceration	7.9–31.6
Ulceration of the breast	9–10
Breast swelling	4
Edema of the breast	5.3
Erythema, inflammatory changes	7.9–10.5
Skin retraction	16
Skin nodules	3.4
Local pain	5.1–16
Fixed or ulcerated axillary nodes	16
Enlarged axillary nodes	5.1–22
Axillary mass only	2
Supraclavicular metastases	7.7
Bone pain	2.2

(Data from Vercoutere and O'Connell, 1984; Donegan and Perez-Mesa, 1973; Axelsson and Andersson, 1983; Yap et al., 1979; Borgen et al., 1992; Erlichman et al., 1984; and Hodson et al., 1985.)

tumor may be associated with nipple retraction. Less frequent presentations are bloody nipple discharge, generalized swelling of the breast, itching of the nipple, and axillary mass (Vercoutere et al., 1984). Paget's disease of the nipple (Fig. 36–2) has been reported in at least 28 cases (Serour et al., 1988). In locally advanced cases, skin or nipple ulceration, satellite nodules, and inflammatory signs are seen (Figs. 36–3 and 36–4). The left breast is affected minimally more often than the right one; Crichlow (1972) found a ratio of 1.07 favoring the left breast. Simultaneous involvement of both breasts was present in two of 104 cases (1.9%) reported by Borgen's group (1992), and, ultimately,

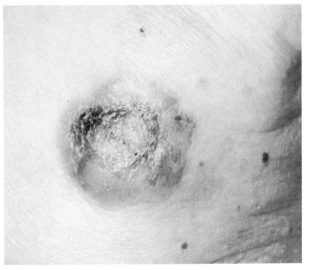

Figure 36-2. Paget's disease of the male breast. (Courtesy of Carlos M. Perez-Mesa, M.D.)

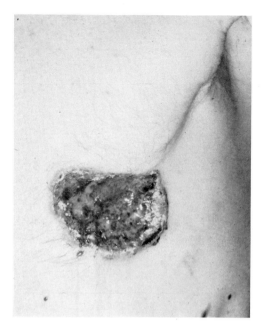

Figure 36–3. Locally advanced breast cancer in a 59-year-old man that has destroyed the nipple and become attached to the pectoral fascia. Local advancement is a frequent finding in men.

As most of the benign mass-producing lesions of the female breast are rare in men, the differential diagnosis of a breast mass in males is generally limited to unilateral gynecomastia, carcinoma (primary or metastatic), and a few other lesions such as adenoma of the nipple (Richards et al., 1973) and rare sarcomas. Mammography has limited diagnostic utility. Mammograms may demonstrate a spiculated mass at the site of a cancer (Fig. 36–5), but this can be obscured in the presence of dense gynecomastia. In 50 cases Borgen's group (1992) found that mammograms demonstrated a mass in 58%, microcalcifications alone in 8%, an architectural deformity in 28%, and no abnormality in 8%. Occasionally, mammograms reveal an unsuspected cancer in the opposite breast, and can serve for early diagnosis in this respect, both on initial evaluation and during follow-up (Dershaw, 1986).

Definitive diagnosis is accomplished with biopsy and histologic examination; core needle biopsy of large masses and excisional biopsy of small ones are standard methods of diagnosis (Fig. 36–6). Experience with fine-needle aspiration and cytologic examination of the male breast is still limited, and its reliability is uncertain (Gupta et al., 1988; and Bhagat & Kline, 1990). Cancerous tissues are routinely assayed for estrogen receptor (ER) and progesterone receptor (PR) proteins. ERs and PRs are present more often than in women: prevalence was 83% to 89% and 76% to 86%,

as many as 5% of patients develop bilateral involvement (Heller et al., 1978). In most reports primary tumors average 4 to 5 cm in diameter, and approximately 50% of surgically treated cases have axillary metastases. Physical examination of the axilla for metastases is no more accurate in men than in women. Some 18% to 38% of clinically "negative" axillae contain metastases; the nodes in clinically positive cases are tumor free in 8% to 21% (Heller et al., 1978; and Ouriel, 1984). Supraclavicular adenopathy may be evident in advanced cases. No information is available on the frequency of internal mammary metastases. As in females, distant metastases most often seek bones, lungs, pleura, and liver. Bone pain, cough, or chest pain suggests metastases.

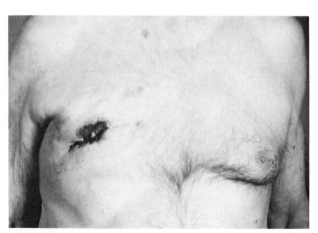

Figure 36–4. Contraction of the skin and nipple of an 81-year-old male with a locally advanced carcinoma of the right breast. (Courtesy of Stuart Wilson, M.D.)

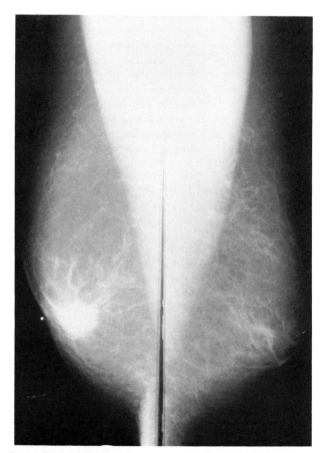

Figure 36–5. Mammogram (right and left oblique views) showing a dense 1.5-cm spiculated invasive carcinoma in the right breast of a 63-year-old man.

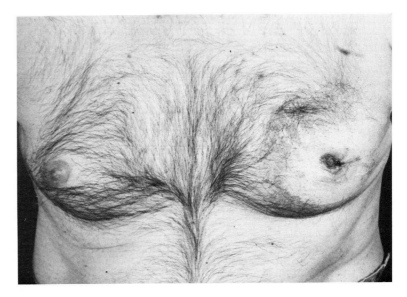

Figure 36–6. Cancer of the left breast associated with bilateral gynecomastia. The firm tumor is in a typical location beneath the nipple, which it has invaded and retracted. A suture marks the site of biopsy. Gynecomastia is often associated with breast cancer in men and is usually bilateral (see Yap et al., 1979).

respectively, in two recent series (Morimoto et al., 1990; and Borgen et al., 1992). Experience with flow cytometry in men is still limited.

It should be kept in mind that some 0.5% to 2% of cancers in the male breast are metastatic rather than primary. The most frequent sources of these metastases are melanoma, lymphoma, and lung cancer (Sneige et al., 1989). An unusual histologic picture should prompt further evaluation with electron microscopy and appropriate tumor markers. Concurrent second extramammary primaries are not unusual in this elderly population. In a collected series of 328 male breast cancers Panettiere (1974) found that 7.9% had at least one additional noncutaneous primary cancer, most often in the large bowel or prostate. Almost 20% of Scheike's 26 patients (1973) with a second cancer had cancer of the stomach, an unusually high frequency. Only 6% of one series in the United States had stomach cancer (Vanderbilt and Warren, 1971). Men with multiple primaries tend to be older and to have family members with cancer (Yap et al., 1979).

HISTOLOGIC APPEARANCE

Carcinomas account for 96% of male breast cancers; the remainder are sarcomas. The majority of carcinomas are invasive ductal carcinomas, but all histologic types are reported. In four reports totaling 357 cases, 89% were invasive ductal carcinomas, 5% were ductal carcinoma in situ, and the remainder were special histologic types (Visfeldt and Scheike, 1973; Gupta et al., 1981; Vercoutere and O'Connell, 1984; and Borgen et al., 1992): Paget's disease (1%) and mucinous (1.4%), medullary (1.4%), papillary (2%), and tubular carcinomas (0.3%). Secretory carcinoma has been observed, as has an oncocytic carcinoma (Roth et al., 1988; and Costa and Silverberg, 1989). Nine cases of intracystic papillary carcinoma have been reported, a histologic variety associated with favorable prognosis (Chinn et al., 1989). Although lobules are rare in the male breast, they can be found (Fig. 36–7), and it is therefore not sur-

prising that invasive lobular carcinoma and lobular carcinoma in situ have been reported (Sanchez et al., 1986; and Nance and Reddick, 1989).

Among sarcomas are phyllodes tumors (Reingold and Ascher, 1970; and Pantoja et al., 1976) and a variety of others, most often fibrosarcoma or leiomyosarcoma (Visfeldt and Scheike, 1973). Neurogenic sarcomas and lymphosarcomas also occur. Panettiere (1974) reported a liposarcoma, and Yadaw and colleagues (1976) reported an angiosarcoma. These tumors spread hematogenously and infrequently involve axillary nodes.

STAGING

Staging (i.e., establishing the extent of disease) serves to identify cases that are potentially curable and to estimate prognosis. Staging is similar for men and women and is determined by physical examination and appropriate supplementary examinations. These include a mammogram of

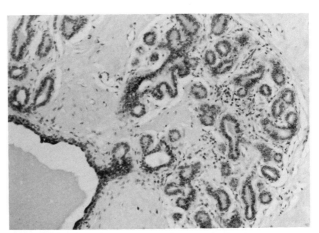

Figure 36–7. Lobule formation around a central duct in a male breast. Lobules are rare in men, and lobular carcinoma is far less frequent in men than in women.

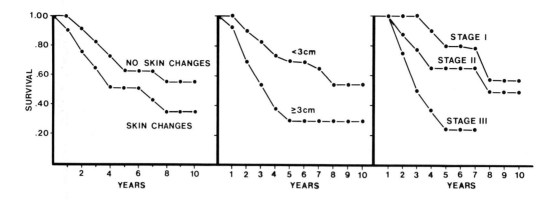

From Ouriel et al 1984

Figure 36-8. Survival of men with breast cancer. (From Ouriel, K., Lotze, M.T., and Hinshaw, J.R.: Prognostic factors of carcinoma of the male breast. Surg. Gynecol. Obstet., *159*:373, 1984. Reprinted with permission of SURGERY, GYNECOLOGY, and OBSTET-RICS.)

both breasts, a radiograph of the chest, and a hemogram. Experience with women indicates that bone scans often do not detect metastases in the absence of bone pain, but they may serve as a baseline against which to evaluate future symptoms. Abnormalities may require computed tomography of the chest or abdomen for further evaluation. In men measures are taken to detect excess estrogen production. If Klinefelter's syndrome is suspected, karyotyping is performed.

The most important parameters of stage are defined by the international TNM system, which is increasingly used for reporting results of treatment. Distant dissemination (M1) is synonymous with incurability and for this reason should be documented histologically. In cases without dissemination the histologic status of the axillary lymph nodes and the extent of their involvement are the most important determinants of prognosis. The size of the primary lesion also has prognostic value (Fig. 36-8).

MASTECTOMY

For surgical treatment of Stage I, II, and sometimes III lesions, radical mastectomy has largely been replaced by modified radical mastectomy. Earlier diagnosis and clinical trials in women showing comparable results with the two operations have influenced this change to the more aesthetically acceptable modified radical mastectomy (Fig. 36-9). This trend is clearly evident in recent reports. At various institutions modified radical mastectomy was used for 9% of cases treated between 1949 and 1976 (Erlichman et al., 1984), for 40% between 1961 and 1981 (Ouriel et al., 1984), for 54% between 1967 and 1981 (Heller et al., 1978), and for 67% between 1975 and 1990. Lefor and Numann (1988) found no significant difference in the 8-year actuarial survival of nine potentially curable patients treated with modified radical mastectomy and 16 treated with the radical procedure.

In a retrospective study, Ouriel and coworkers (1984) found no significant difference in 5-year survival between 19 men with Stage I and Stage II cancer treated with radical

mastectomy (76%) and 18 men treated with modified mastectomy (80%). The same was found by Hodson and colleagues (1985) among potentially curable cases, although 5-year survival rates were lower (44% and 43%, respectively). Patients deemed unable to tolerate major surgery, or those with locally advanced tumor, usually are managed with simple mastectomy or local excision combined with postoperative irradiation to the chest wall and regional nodes (Robison and Montague, 1982).

A frequent observation is that men fare worse than women overall, particularly in the presence of metastases in axillary lymph nodes, but evidence is growing that cancer of the male breast is as curable, at any given stage, as that in women (Lefor and Numann, 1988; Morimoto et al., 1990; and Borgen et al., 1992). The poor record of the past is likely attributable to the typically advanced age and stage associated with most cases, and probably the greater extent of axillary involvement in operable cases though this is difficult to document. Scheike (1973) documented that

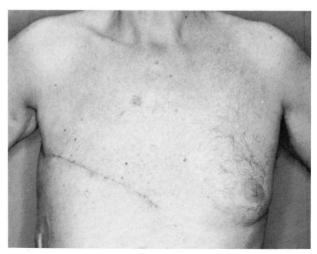

Figure 36-9. Postoperative appearance of a man treated with modified radical mastectomy for carcinoma of the right breast. Except for absence of the nipple, the operation results in little change of the anterior chest.

cases had become clinically more favorable in Denmark when those seen during 1943 to 1957 were compared with those seen between 1958 and 1972. TNM Stage I or II cases among 253 patients had increased from 39% to 53%, and Stage IV cases had decreased from 18% to 5%.

Factors that have an important influence on prognosis are histologic features of the tumor, the presence of axillary metastases, the size of the tumor, and the stage (see Fig. 36–8). Duration of symptoms was found to be important by Borgen and coworkers (1992), but any influence of gynecomastia or of hormone receptors has not been demonstrated. In a large series reported by Spence and coworkers (1985) none of four variables—the location of the tumor, postoperative hormone therapy, postoperative irradiation, or type of local operation—influenced prognoses. Gattuso and colleagues (1992) found that 78.1% of 32 men had aneuploid tumors, but ploidy was not correlated with mean survival time after mastectomy. Noteworthy is the great diversity in survival despite comparable stage and axillary node status, an indication of the complex interplay of other influences within these categories.

Men with noninvasive ductal cancers and intracystic papillary carcinomas have excellent prospects for cure; recurrence is unusual (Heller et al., 1978; and Axelsson and Andersson, 1983). The special histologic types, such as medullary, colloid, and papillary carcinomas, have a prognosis more favorable than that of the ductal type. Yap and coworkers (1979) found median survivals closely correlated with the size of invasive ductal carcinomas—that is, 59.8 months for 2 cm or less, 50.8 months for 2 to 5 cm, and 15 months for greater than 5 cm. Corresponding 5-year survival rates were 53%, 44%, and 25%.

It can be demonstrated that clinical stage (TNM) correlates well with prognosis. Among 214 cases collected by Crichlow (1976), 5-year and 10-year survival rates, respectively, after all treatments were as follows: Stage I, 58% and 38%; Stage II, 38% and 10%; Stage III, 29% and 9%; and Stage IV, 4% and 0%.

The most important prognosticator among surgically treated patients is the presence of axillary metastases. The 5-year and 10-year survival rates for 143 patients collected by Crichlow (1976) were 79% and 62% for those without axillary metastases, as opposed to a much reduced 28% and 4.3% for those with metastases. More recent reports cited in Table 36–2 provide survival ranges based on stage and axillary nodal status. The extent of axillary involvement in node-positive cases affects prognosis and contributes to the variable results in small series. Prognoses based on quantitations of nodal involvement are now available (Guinee et al., 1993).

In three series, including the author's, 31 (57%) of 54 men treated specifically with radical mastectomy (Cortese and Cornell, 1970; Crichlow et al., 1972; and Donegan and Perez-Mesa, 1973), all of whom had been at risk for at least 5 years, survived the period; 42% of 24 patients with axillary metastases survived 5 years, as did 84% of 25 patients without such metastases.

In the surgical management of men with breast cancer, it is fair to say that modified radical mastectomy is now the surgical procedure most appropriate for those with relatively small tumors that spare the pectoralis major muscle

Table 36–2. SURVIVAL OF MEN WITH BREAST CANCER

TNM Stage	Survival	
	5 Yr (%)	10 Yr (%)
0 (TIS)	88–100	
I	75–100	57–89
II	63–83	12
III	25–70	
IV	0	
Axillary metastases		
Absent	77–100	79–80
Present	38–60	11–36
Overall	42–85	2–60

(Data from Heller et al., 1978; Robison & Montague, 1982; Axelsson & Andersson, 1983; Ouriel et al., 1984; Patel et al., 1984; and Borgen et al., 1992.)

and that are associated with limited axillary involvement. The improved appearance over radical mastectomy is welcome, and the stronger arm it leaves is an advantage for the working man. Segmental resection combined with axillary dissection and high-dose irradiation of the breast has provided survival equal to that afforded by modified radical mastectomy for women in selected cases, and while the same might be true for men, the central location of tumors in men, which ordinarily requires nipple removal for complete excision, greatly reduces its cosmetic advantages.

ADJUVANT THERAPY

Postoperative irradiation to the chest wall and remaining regional lymph nodes has often been used to supplement mastectomy in the treatment of men, particularly in cases in which there are signs of local advancement or with proven axillary metastases, for which prognosis is poor. By analogy with females the result is probably a decreased chance of recurrence in the fields of treatment but no improvement in survival. Irradiation would seem most appropriate for those at high risk specifically for local recurrence, or perhaps preoperatively to improve operability in locally advanced cases.

The success of adjuvant chemotherapy in women translates to men with some uncertainty. It is reasonable to consider adjuvant chemotherapy for men with metastases in axillary lymph nodes, but the fund of available information is fragmentary and inconclusive (Ouriel et al., 1984; and Vercoutere and O'Connell, 1984). Nevertheless, because the majority of recurrences in men are at distant sites (79% according to Yap and colleagues [1979]) and because prospective studies in males are unlikely, clinicians generally support the use of adjuvant chemotherapy or hormone therapy (or both) with the same indications as in women (Yap et al., 1979; Erlichman et al., 1984; and Vercoutere and O'Connell, 1984).

Kinne (1991) recommended systemic adjuvant therapy for all males with axillary node involvement and for selected patients without it who were judged to be at high risk for recurrence. Combination chemotherapy is preferred, and at Memorial Sloan-Kettering Cancer Center in New York, tamoxifen was added to the chemotherapy when ERs were present. Whether the combination of tamoxifen with chemotherapy is superior to tamoxifen alone (or to chemotherapy alone) for men with ER-positive tumors is uncertain. Experience with systemic adjuvant therapy in men is still limited, and its success can only be inferred by comparison with historical controls.

Bagley and colleagues (1987) treated 24 males with axillary metastases with 12 cycles of adjuvant cyclophosphamide, methotrexate, and 5-fluorouracil (CMF). None received postoperative irradiation. Four patients had disease recurrence, and the 5-year actuarial survival was projected to be 90%, much higher than is ordinarily expected. Adjuvant tamoxifen was used to treat 23 men with pathologic Stage II and Stage III breast cancers after surgery and irradiation at the Christie Hospital and Holt Radium Institute in Manchester, U.K. (Ribeiro, 1985). The 5-year survival rate of 55% was improved over the historical 28%.

Patel and associates (1989) treated 11 men with TNM Stage II or III cancer, all with axillary metastases, using principally the combination of 5-fluorouracil, doxorubicin, and cyclophosphamide (FAC). After a median follow-up of 52 months the projected 5-year survival rate was 85%.

RECURRENCE AND DISSEMINATION

The initial sites of distant metastases are similar to those in women: bone, lungs, and lymph nodes are the principal sites (Erlichman et al., 1984). Seventy-one cases reported by Huggins and Taylor (1955) were distributed as follows: bone, 23; lungs and pleura, 16; supraclavicular lymph nodes, 12; liver, 7; brain, 3; and other, 10. Fifty-five per cent of the cases reported by Treves (1959) had initial metastasis to bones, followed in order by lymph nodes in 21.4%, lungs in 19%, skin in 14%, and soft tissues in 5%. Bone metastases are most often lytic but may also be blastic. Scilletta and coworkers (1989) reported a case with bilateral ocular metastases.

Median survival time after recurrence is approximately 22 months (Heller et al., 1978). One (12.5%) of eight patients with Stage IV cancer reported by Siddiqui and colleagues (1988) was known to be alive after a mean follow-up of 64.6 months. Twenty per cent of Erlichman and associates' patients (1984) lived 5 years. Local-regional recurrence usually indicates incurability, but with further treatment, ordinarily irradiation, survival times can range from 4 to 92 months (Robison and Montague, 1982) (Fig. 36–10).

ENDOCRINE ABLATIONS

The endocrine responsiveness of male breast cancer has been known since 1942, when Farrow and Adair demonstrated reduction in size of an advanced primary cancer and recalcification of osteolytic metastases after castration of a 72-year-old man. Subsequently, bilateral adrenalectomy (Huggins and Bergenstal, 1952) and hypophysectomy (Luft et al., 1956) proved effective in temporarily reversing the

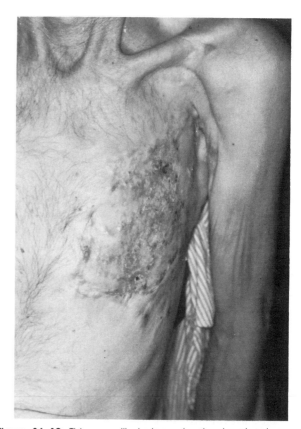

Figure 36–10. This case illustrates extensive local cutaneous recurrence of carcinoma following treatment with radical mastectomy. Although mastectomy is the treatment of choice for potentially localized carcinoma of the male breast, the relatively advanced status of most tumors contributes to a high failure rate after surgical treatment. Adjuvant irradiation in selected cases can help to reduce this problem. Local failures can also be treated by irradiation with good effect.

progress of this cancer. Bilateral orchiectomy, bilateral adrenalectomy, and hypophysectomy have produced regression of metastases in bone, lungs, skin, and lymph nodes as well as reduction of osseous pain.

In general, endocrine ablations have proved more effective in men than in women, but the critical hormonal changes involved remain uncertain. Endocrine ablation is the primary method of management for disseminated carcinoma of the male breast; orchiectomy has been considered the appropriate initial procedure although recently tamoxifen has had increasing use as an alternative. Erlichman and coworkers (1984) found no correlation between disease-free interval and the likeliness of benefit from castration, but this was not the experience of Kraybill and associates (1981), who observed increased success after 12 months. In contrast to the case in women, the success of castration in men is not age related. Metastases are seldom found in testes, in contrast with the approximately 25% occurrence in the ovaries of women.

Orchiectomy produces tumor regressions in 45% to 88% of cases, with durations averaging 16 to 29 months (Fig. 36–11) (Neifield et al., 1976). In four reports since 1981 totaling 62 orchiectomies, the overall response rate was 45% (Kraybill et al., 1981; Erlichman et al., 1984; Ouriel

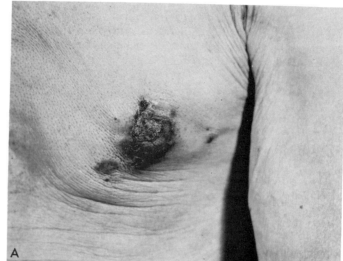

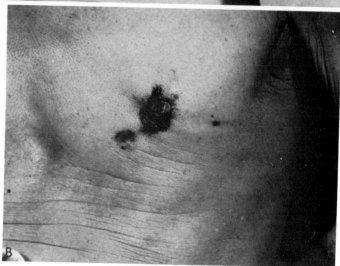

Figure 36–11. This advanced cancer of the breast *(A)* had destroyed the areola and produced cutaneous satellite nodules. It responded to orchiectomy with partial regression *(B)* 3 months later. Bilateral orchiectomy frequently provides successful palliation, more often than does oophorectomy for women, and its success is not age dependent, as is oophorectomy in women.

et al., 1984; and Patel et al., 1984). Meyskens and associates (1976) reviewed the endocrine treatment of male breast cancer and defined a response as disappearance of all lesions lasting 3 months or longer. Using this criterion 67% of 70 collected evaluable patients responded to orchiectomy, with a median response duration of 22 months. Median survival of responders and nonresponders from the time of primary diagnosis was 56 months versus 38 months. Nineteen of 25 patients treated with adrenalectomy responded to the procedure, four of whom had not benefited from a previous castration. The response to adrenalectomy had a mean duration of 32 months if an earlier castration had been helpful; if not, the duration was shorter. Thus, a total of 76% of individuals treated with adrenalectomy had complete responses of 3 months' duration or longer. Men can respond to adrenalectomy despite a failure of orchiectomy (Li et al., 1970), but an earlier response to castration enhances the probability of success. Among 17 evaluable patients collected from the literature who had had hypophysectomies, 10 responders (60%) were found, and the median duration of response was 20 months. A short disease-free interval, that is, less than 24 months, does not preclude

a good response (Izuo et al., 1972; and Stephens and Muggia, 1974).

Although the experience with ERs in men is far less extensive than that with women, positive levels of ER serve as a guide for hormone and endocrine therapy. The tumors of men frequently contain ERs. In some reports, 80% or more had ER-bearing tumors (Gupta et al., 1980; and Friedman et al., 1981). This is in contrast with approximately 60% prevalence in women measured similarly. It has been suggested that men's lower estrogen environment leaves receptor sites more often available for binding. The quantitative levels of ER, however, are not notably higher. The fact that so few men are ER negative diminishes but does not negate the value of this test; the limited information available indicates that high rates of response follow endocrine therapy in ER-positive patients. In two reports, two of three and four of five men with disseminated ER-positive tumors responded to orchiectomy (Gupta et al., 1980; and Patel et al., 1984). In another, two of four patients with ER-positive tumors responded to endocrine manipulations (Ouriel et al., 1984). Two ER-positive patients both responded to adrenalectomy, according to Patel and coworkers (1984). Information is almost nonexistent on the response rates of men with ER-negative cancers, and although cytoplasmic PRs are often present (in six of nine patients in one report), their influence on tumor responsiveness or on prognosis remains to be determined (Pegoraro et al., 1982).

HORMONE THERAPY

Hormone therapy has assumed increasing importance in the palliative treatment of male breast cancer since the introduction of the antiestrogen agent tamoxifen. This agent has proved highly successful in producing tumor regression, and this fact, combined with the reluctance of men to accept orchiectomy, has prompted some authors to advocate tamoxifen as the most appropriate initial endocrine manipulation, replacing orchiectomy (Becher et al., 1981; Pegoraro et al., 1982). Patterson and associates (1980) reported an objective response rate of 48% to treatment with tamoxifen in 31 patients; an additional five patients exhibited stabilization. In 33 additional cases summarized from four reports, tamoxifen produced tumor regressions in 51% of patients, with durations of 5 to 60 months (median 21 months) (Becher et al., 1981; Ribeiro, 1983; Hilliard et al., 1984; and Patel et al., 1984). Metastases in soft tissues, bones, liver, and lungs have shown regression. Tamoxifen has been effective in patients without orchiectomy, after orchiectomy failure or progression, and after adrenalectomy. Complete and partial responses are approximately equally distributed (Ribeiro, 1983). Hilliard and associates (1984) reported an objective response to tamoxifen of 17 months' duration of a patient with an ER-positive tumor that had been unaffected by orchiectomy. As in women, it appears that ER-positive tumors may respond to secondary endocrine manipulation when the initial one proves ineffective. Orchiectomy can still prove effective after a period of benefit from tamoxifen followed by relapse (Aisner et al., 1979).

Two of 14 patients treated with estrogens by Treves (1959) responded for 2 and for 7 months, respectively. Regressions were limited to metastases in soft tissues and lung. The author's experience is somewhat better; osseous and soft tissue metastases regressed for 16 to 25 months in two of five cases treated with estrogens (Donegan and Perez-Mesa, 1973).

The luteinizing hormone–releasing hormone (LHRH) agonist buserelin (6-D-ser-(BU1)-LHRH-(1-9)-ethylamide) represents another means of reducing testicular function. This drug stimulates a surge of follicle-stimulating hormone and luteinizing hormone from the pituitary during the first week of therapy, followed by a rapid and sustained reduction. The interruption of gonadotropic stimulation to the testes results in a drop in the testosterone level comparable to that subsequent to castration. The estradiol levels also decline, presumably from reduced peripheral aromatization of testosterone. Buserelin is conveniently given by nasal spray, and the effects are reversible. Side effects include hot flashes, weight gain, decreased libido, and impotence. The androgen blocker flutamide is used in conjunction with

buserelin to prevent disease flare from the initial surge of androgens. Complete regression of a 60-year-old man's pulmonary metastases for 44 weeks produced by buserelin was reported by Vorobiof and Falkson (1987). Using 1.2 mg of buserelin daily for induction and 0.4 mg daily for maintenance, Doberauer and coworkers (1988) reported partial responses in 33% of 15 patients. One of 10 treated with buserelin alone had regression for 12 months, and four of five treated with the combination of buserelin and flutamide had partial responses lasting a median of 15 months.

Experience has also been gained with antiandrogens, which block androgen receptors in target tissues. Two that have proved useful are cyproterone acetate and flutamide. Cyproterone acetate has a steroidal structure and, in addition to blocking androgen receptors, has progestational and glucocorticoid actions, so it also produces pituitary inhibition. Flutamide is a pure androgen receptor blocker and is nonsteroidal (Namer, 1988). If flutamide is used alone, the compensatory increase in gonadal testosterone under pituitary stimulation eventually overcomes the block; therefore, the testes must be removed or defunctionalized (e.g., as with buserelin). Potential side effects of flutamide include diarrhea, gynecomastia, and occasionally chemical hepatitis. A further disadvantage is its short half-life and the need for frequent administration. Cyproterone acetate does not share these limitations and was used by Lopez (1985) to treat 10 male patients with advanced breast cancers. On a dose of 100 mg orally twice daily, seven had objective remissions lasting 3 to 52 months. Two remissions were complete. Remissions were independent of age, duration of free interval, and site of metastasis. One responder had suffered a relapse after earlier exhibiting a response to castration; another had not responded to medroxyprogesterone. The patients experienced fatigue, gynecomastia, and weight gain as side effects.

Progesterones were identified as potentially useful for men with breast cancer by Geller and colleagues (1961), who reported a response in one case to 17α-hydroxyprogesterone caproate (Delalutin). Subsequently, Kennedy and Kiang (1972) used estrogen combined with progesterone in one case with good effect and suggested that this combination be used in advance of chemotherapy. Subsequently, a number of progesterone preparations have shown activity against male breast cancer. These have included cyproterone acetate, medroxyprogesterone acetate (Provera), megestrol acetate, and combinations of Provera and stilbestrol as well as combinations of Provera and prednisolone. Eight of 12 patients in recent reports responded positively to these agents (Kraybill et al., 1981; Lopez and Barduagni, 1982; and Patel et al., 1984). Mitsuyasu and colleagues (1981) observed regression of a pulmonary metastasis in a patient receiving megestrol (40 mg orally four times daily) after relapse of an ER-positive tumor treated with orchiectomy. In women, megestrol is often effective for tamoxifen relapses (Ross et al., 1982).

In the past, androgens were considered contraindicated for carcinoma of the male breast, largely because of a few early experiences in which they appeared to aggravate the disease. Farrow and Adair (1942) observed such an event in one case, as did Huggins and Taylor (1955) in two cases.

A response to androgens was reported by Donegan and Perez-Mesa (1973) when cutaneous metastases at a mastectomy site in a 72-year-old man regressed on treatment with fluoxymesterone (Halotestin), 10 mg orally three times daily. The benefit lasted 16 months. Subsequently, Horn and Roof (1976) observed responses in two cases to the androgen calusterone. Responses to androgen therapy were also observed in a review of experience with metastatic male breast cancer at the M.D. Anderson Hospital and Tumor Institute, in Houston (Kantarjian et al., 1983).

Adrenal suppression with aminoglutethimide was used successfully in one case by Patel and coworkers (1984) following orchiectomy failure. After progression of the disease the patient also responded to adrenalectomy.

Adrenocorticosteroids (prednisone, cortisone) often produce a sense of well-being and are indicated specifically for the management of symptomatic intracranial metastases and hypercalcemia. Remission of osseous and pulmonary metastases for brief periods was observed in three of five cases by Treves and Holleb (1955) during treatment with corticosteroids.

A summary of responses to endocrine ablative and hormone therapy is shown in Table 36–3. It should be noted that rebound regressions that sometimes follow sudden withdrawal of hormone therapy in women have also been noted in men (Kennedy and Kiang, 1972; Mitsuyasu et al., 1981; and Harris et al., 1986) If the course of disease is slow, it may be worthwhile to delay initiating alternative therapy until it can be determined if the patient will have a rebound regression.

CHEMOTHERAPY

In view of the frequent and substantial benefit men obtain from endocrine therapy, chemotherapy has a secondary role in palliation. With more information on ERs, however, it may become apparent that patients lacking tumor ERs are best treated initially with chemotherapy. Cancer of the male breast yields to agents known to be useful for mammary carcinoma of women. Drug combinations are probably more often effective than single agents; soft tissue, lung, and bone metastases are most responsive to treatment. Meyskens and associates (1976) reviewed four cases in which chemotherapy proved of value in three patients. A patient with painful osseous metastases initially responded subjectively to a course of fluorouracil for 18 months. Recurrent pain was then palliated for an additional 5 months with courses of methotrexate and thiotepa repeated every 6 to 8 weeks. A second patient with osseous metastases failed to benefit from the same course of methotrexate and thiotepa. Objective regression of pulmonary lesions, lymph nodes, and skin nodules for a period of 14 months was observed in a third patient treated with cyclophosphamide (Cytoxan). The final patient responded with reduction of cutaneous, nodal, and bony metastases for 12 months to combination chemotherapy with Cytoxan, doxorubicin hydrochloride (Adriamycin), and fluorouracil (CAF). Chlorambucil has also been of value (Holleb et al., 1968). Cyclophosphamide alone produces a response rate of 50% (Griffith and Muggia, 1989).

Vercoutere and O'Connell (1984) reported "good" responses to combination chemotherapy in five of eight cases (63%); cyclophosphamide, methotrexate, and fluorouracil (CMF) was used in four cases and cyclophenylamide, vincristine (Oncovin), methotrexate, and prednisone in another. Fifty per cent of eight cases reported by Ouriel and coworkers (1984) responded to CMF or CAF. Kraybill and associates reported that four cases in 11 treated with various agents responded with complete regressions (25%) or partial regression (75%) for 7 to 32 months. The successful agents were Cytoxan plus prednisone; Cytoxan, fluorouracil, and prednisone (CFP); and leukeran.

SUMMARY

Cancer of the male breast is infrequent but not rare. In contrast to women with breast cancer, men with breast cancer are older and have more advanced disease. The disease is biologically similar, however, and in comparable circumstances men are equally curable. Mastectomy is the mainstay of treatment. The tumor is sensitive to radiation and often responds to endocrine and hormone therapy, making the latter exceptionally useful for palliation of systemic metastases. Chemotherapy can also be beneficial.

Table 36–3. RESPONSE OF MALES TO ENDOCRINE ABLATION AND HORMONE THERAPY

Therapy	Cases (No.)	Responses Prevalence (%)	Median Duration (mo.) (%)
Oophorectomy	92	44	17.5
Adrenalectomy	18	78	15
Hypophysectomy	11	64	13
Estrogens	84	32	6
Androgens	5	60	7
Progestins	13	31	7
Tamoxifen	77	45	21
Cyproterone acetate	10	70	8
Buserelin/±flutamide	11	55	15
Corticosteroids	19	37	11
Aminoglutethimide	1	100	

(Data from Ouriel et al., 1984; Kantarjian et al., 1983; Kraybill et al., 1981; Bezwoda et al., 1987; Patel et al., 1984; Ribeiro, 1983; Houttuin et al., 1967; Kennedy and Kiang, 1972; Horn and Roof, 1976; Patterson et al., 1980; Becher et al., 1981; Lopez, 1985; Vorobiof and Falkson, 1987; and Doberauer et al., 1988.)

References

Adami, H. O., Hakulinen, T., Ewertz, M., et al.: The survival pattern in male breast cancer: An analysis of 1429 patients from the Nordic countries. Cancer, 64:1177–1182, 1989.

Aisner, J., Ross, D. D., and Wiernik, P. H.: Tamoxifen in advanced male breast cancer. Arch. Intern. Med., 139:480, 1979.

American Joint Committee on Cancer. Manual for Staging of Cancer. 3rd Ed. Philadelphia, J.B. Lippincott, 1988, pp. 145–150.

Axelsson, J., and Andersson, A.: Cancer of the male breast. World J. Surg., 7:281, 1983.

Bagley, C. S., Wesley, M. N., Young, R. C., et al.: Adjuvant chemotherapy in males with cancer of the breast. Am. J. Clin. Oncol., *10*:55, 1987.

Becher, R., Hoffken, K.., Page, H., et al.: Tamoxifen treatment before orchiectomy in advanced breast cancer in men. N. Engl. J. Med., *305*:169, 1981.

Bezwoda, W. R., Hesdorffer, C., Dansey, R., et al.: Breast cancer in men. Clinical features, hormone receptor status, and response to therapy. Cancer, *60*:1337–1340, 1987.

Bhaget, P., and Kline, T. S.: The male breast and malignant neoplasms. Diagnosis by aspiration biopsy cytology. Cancer, *65*:2338–2341, 1990.

Borgen, P. I., Wong, G. Y., Vlamis, V., et al.: Current management of male breast cancer. A review of 104 cases. Ann. Surg., *215*:451–459, 1992.

Breasted, J. H.: The Edwin Smith Surgical Papyrus. Chicago, The University of Chicago Press, 1930, pp. 403–406.

Calabresi, E., DeGiuli, G., Becciolini, A., et al.: Plasma estrogens and androgens in male breast cancer. J. Steroid Biochem., 7:605–609, 1976.

Cancer Facts and Figures—1994. Atlanta, American Cancer Society, 1994.

Casagrande, J. T., Hanisch, R., Pike, M. C., et al.: A case-control study of male breast cancer. Cancer Res., *48*:1326–1330, 1988.

Chinn, K., Kalisher, L., and Rickert, R. R.: Intracystic papillary breast carcinoma in a 55-year-old man: Radiologic and pathologic correlation. Can. Assoc. Radiol. J., *40*:40–42, 1989.

Cole, F. M., and Quizelbash, A. J.: Carcinoma in situ of the male breast. J. Clin. Pathol., *32*:1128, 1979.

Cortese, A. F., and Cornell, G. N.: Carcinoma of the male breast. Ann. Surg., *173*:275, 1971.

Costa, M. J., and Silverberg, S. G.: Oncocytic carcinoma of the male breast. Arch. Pathol. Lab. Med., *113*:1396–1399, 1989.

Crichlow, R. W.: Carcinoma of the male breast. Surg. Gynecol. Obstet., *134*:1011, 1972.

Crichlow, R. W.: Breast cancer in males. Breast, 2:12, 1976.

Crichlow, R. W., Kaplan, E. L., and Kearney, W. H.: Male mammary cancer: An analysis of 32 cases. Ann. Surg., *175*:489, 1972.

Dao, T. L., Morreal, C., and Nemoto, T.: Urinary estrogen excretion in men with breast cancer. N. Engl. J. Med., *289*:138, 1973.

Demeter, J. G., Waterman, N. G., and Verdi, G. D.: Familial male breast carcinoma. Cancer, *65*:2342–2343, 1990.

Dershaw, D. D.: Male mammography. Am. J. Roentgenol., *146*:127–131, 1986.

Doberauer, C., Niederle, N., and Schmidt, C. G.: Advanced male breast cancer treatment with the LH-RH analogue buserelin alone or in combination with the antiandrogen flutamide. Cancer, *62*:474–478, 1988.

Dodge, O. G., Jackson, A. W., and Muldal, S.: Breast cancer and interstitial cell tumor in a patient with Klinefelter's syndrome. Cancer, *24*:1027, 1969.

Donegan, W. L.: Cancer of the breast in men. CA Cancer J. Clin., *41*:339–354, 1991.

Donegan, W. L., and Perez-Mesa, C. M.: Carcinoma of the male breast. A 30-year review of 28 cases. Arch. Surg., *106*:273, 1973.

Eldar, S., Nash, E., and Abrahamson, J.: Radiation carcinogenesis in the male breast. Eur. J. Surg. Oncol., *15*:274–278, 1989.

Erlichman, C., Murphy, K. C., and Elhakim, T.: Male breast cancer: A 13-year review of 89 patients. J. Clin. Oncol., 2:903, 1984.

Evans, D. B., and Crichlow, R. W.: Carcinoma of the male breast and Klinefelter's syndrome: Is there an association? CA Cancer J. Clin., *37*:246–251, 1987.

Ewertz, M., Homnberg, L., Kajjalainen, S., et al.: Incidence of male breast cancer in Scandinavia 1943–1982. Int. J. Cancer, *43*:27–31, 1989.

Farrow, J. H., and Adair, F. E.: Effect of orchidectomy on skeletal metastases from cancer of the male breast. Science, *95*:654, 1942.

Fodor, P. B.: Breast cancer in a patient with gynecomastia. Plast. Reconstr. Surg., *84*:976–979, 1989.

Friedman, M. A., Hoffman, P. G., Jr., Dandolos, E. M., et al.: Estrogen receptors in male breast cancer: Clinical and pathologic correlations. Cancer, *47*:134, 1981.

Gattuso, P., Reddy, V. B., Green, L., et al.: Prognostic significance of DNA ploidy in male breast carcinoma. Cancer, *70*:777–780, 1992.

Geller, J., Volk, H., and Lewin, M.: Objective remission of metastatic breast carcinoma in a male who received 17-alpha hydroxy progesterone caproate (Delalutin). Cancer Chemother. Rep., *14*:77, 1961.

Griffith, H., and Muggia, F. M.: Male breast cancer: Update on systemic therapy. Rev. Endocrine Related Cancer, *31*:5–11, 1989.

Guinee, V. P., Olsson H., Mollert, T., et al.: The prognosis of breast cancer in males. Cancer, *71*:154–161, 1993.

Gupta, N., Cohen, J. L., Rosenbaum, C., et al.: Estrogen receptors in male breast cancer. Cancer, *46*:1781, 1980.

Gupta, R. K., Naran, S., and Simpson, J. The role of fine needle aspiration cytology (FNAC) in the diagnosis of breast masses in males. Eur. J. Surg. Oncol., *13*:317–320, 1988.

Gupta, S., Pant, G. C., and Gupta, S.: Male breast cancer. J. Surg. Oncol., *16*:149, 1981.

Harris, A. L., Dowsett, M., Stuart-Harris, R., et al.: Role of aminoglutethimide in male breast cancer. Br. J. Cancer, *54*:637–660, 1986.

Heller, K. S., Rosen, P. P., Schottenfeld, D., et al.: Male breast cancer: A clinicopathologic study of 97 cases. Ann. Surg., *188*:60, 1978.

Hilliard, D. A., Wilbur, D. W., and Camacho, E. S.: Tamoxifen response following no response to orchiectomy in metastatic male breast cancer: A case report. J. Surg. Oncol., *25*:42, 1984.

Hodson, G. R., Urdaneta, L. F., Al-Jurf, A. S., et al.: Male breast carcinoma. Am. Surg. *51*:47, 1985.

Holleb, A. I., Freeman, H. P., and Farrow, J. H.: Cancer of male breast. I and II. N.Y. State J. Med., *68*:544, 656, 1968.

Horn, Y., and Roof, B.: Male breast cancer: Two cases with objective regressions from calusterone (7α,17β-dimethyltestosterone) after failure of orchiectomy. Oncology, *33*:188, 1976.

Houttuin, E., VanProhaska, J., and Taxman, P.: Response of male mammary carcinoma metastases to bilateral adrenalectomy. Surg. Gynecol. Obstet., *125*:279–283, 1967.

Huggins, C., Jr., and Bergenstal, D. M.: Inhibition of human mammary and prostatic cancer by adrenalectomy. Cancer Res., *12*:134, 1952.

Huggins, C., Jr., and Taylor, G. W.: Carcinoma of the male breast. Arch. Surg., *70*:303, 1955.

Izuo, M., Ishida, T., and Fujimori, M.: Carcinoma of the male breast with metastases treated by adrenalectomy: A case report and review of the literature. J. Clin. Oncol. (Jpn.), 6:77, 1972.

Kantarjian, H., Yap, H. Y., Hortobagyi, G., et al.: Hormonal therapy for metastatic male breast cancer. Arch. Intern. Med., *143*:237, 1983.

Kennedy, B. J., and Kiang, D. T.: Hypophysectomy in the treatment of advanced cancer of the male breast. Cancer, *29*:1606, 1972.

Kinne, D. W.: Management of male breast cancer. Oncology, 5:45–48, 1991.

Klinefelter, H. F., Jr., Reifenstein, E.C., Jr., and Albright, F.: Syndrome characterized by gynecomastia, aspermatogenesis without A-Leydigism, and increased excretion of follicle stimulating hormone. J. Clin. Endocrinol., 2:615–627, 1942.

Kozak, F. K., Hall, J. G., and Baird, P. A.: Familial breast cancer in males: A case report and review of the literature. Cancer, *58*:2736–2739, 1986.

Kraybill, W. G., Kaufman, R., and Kinne, D.: Treatment of advanced male breast cancer. Cancer, *47*:2185, 1981.

Lefor, A. T., and Numann, P. J.: Carcinoma of the breast in men. N. Y. State J. Med., *88*:293–296, 1988.

Li, M. C., Janelli, D. E., Kelly, E. J., et al.: Metastatic carcinoma of the male breast treated with bilateral adrenalectomy and chemotherapy. Cancer, *25*:678, 1970.

Lin, R. S., and Kessler, I. I.: Epidemiologic findings in male breast cancer. Proc. Am. Assoc. Cancer Res., *21*:72, 1980.

Lloyd, R. V., Rosen, P. P., Sarkar, N. H., et al.: Murine mammary tumor virus related antigen in human male mammary carcinoma. Cancer, *51*:654, 1983.

Lopez, M.: Cyproterone acetate in the treatment of metastatic cancer of the male breast. Cancer, *55*:2334–2336, 1985.

Luft, R., Olivecrona, H., Ikkos, D., et al.: Hypophysectomy in the treatment of malignant tumors. Ann. J. Med., *21*:728, 1956.

Lyall, A.: Choriocarcinoma of the testis with gynecomastia. Report of a case with early breast cancer. Br. J. Surg., *34*:278–280, 1947.

Mabuchi, K., Bross, D. S., and Kessler, I. I.: Risk factors for male breast cancer. J. N. C. I., J. Natl. Cancer Inst., *74*:371, 1985.

McLaughlin, J. K., Malker, H. S. R., Blot, W., Jr., et al.: Occupational risks for male breast cancer in Sweden. Br. J. Indust. Med., *45*:275–276, 1988.

Meyskens, F. L., Jr., Tormey, D. C., and Neifield, J. P.: Male breast cancer: A review. Cancer Treat. Rev., 3:83, 1976.

Mitsuyasu, R., Bonomi, P., Anderson, K., et al.: Response to megestrol in male breast carcinoma. Arch. Intern. Med., *141*:809, 1981.

Morimoto, T., Komaki, K., Yamakawa, T., et al.: Cancer of the male breast. J. Surg. Oncol., *44*:180–184, 1990.

Namer, M.: Clinical applications of antiandrogens. J. Steroid Biochem., *31*:719–729, 1988.

Nance, K. V., and Reddick, R. L.: In situ and infiltrating lobular carcinoma of the male breast. Hum. Pathol., *20*:1220–1222, 1989.

Neifield, J. P., Meyskens, F., Tormey, D. C., et al.: The role of orchiectomy in the management of advanced male breast cancer. Cancer, *37*:992, 1976.

Nuttall, F. Q.: Gynecomastia as a physical finding in normal man. J. Clin. Endocrinol. Metab., *48*:338, 1979.

Olsson, H., and Ranstam, J.: Head trauma and exposure to prolactin-elevating drugs as risk factors for male breast cancer. J. Natl. Cancer Inst., *80*:679–683, 1988.

Olsson, H., Alm, P., Kristoffersson, U., et al.: Hypophyseal tumor and gynecomastia preceding bilateral breast cancer development in a man. Cancer, *53*:1974, 1984.

Ouriel, K., Lotze, M. T., and Hinshaw, J. R.: Prognostic factors of carcinoma of the male breast. Surg. Gynecol. Obstet., *159*:373, 1984.

Panettiere, F. J.: Cancer in the male breast. Cancer, *34*:1324, 1974.

Pantoja, E., Lobet, R. E., and Lopez, E.: Gigantic cystosarcoma phyllodes in a man with gynecomastia. Arch. Surg., *111*:611, 1976.

Patel, H. Z., Buzdar, A. U., and Hortobagyi, G. N.: Role of adjuvant chemotherapy in male breast cancer. Cancer, *64*:1583–1585, 1989.

Patel, J. K., Nemoto, T., and Dao, T. L.: Metastatic breast cancer in males. Assessment of endocrine therapy. Cancer, *53*:1344, 1984.

Patterson, J. S., Battersby, L. A., and Balch, B. K.: Use of tamoxifen in advanced male breast cancer. Cancer Treat. Rep., *64*:801, 1980.

Pegoraro, R. J., Nirmul, D., and Joubert, S. M.: Cytoplasmic and nuclear estrogen and progesterone receptors in male breast cancer. Cancer Res., *42*:4812, 1982.

Pritchard, T. J., Pankowesky, D. A., Crowe, J. P., et al.: Breast cancer in a male-to-female transsexual. J.A.M.A., *259*:2278–2280, 1988.

Reingold, I. M., and Ascher, G. S.: Cystosarcoma phyllodes in a man with gynecomastia. Am. J. Clin. Pathol., *53*:852, 1970.

Ribeiro, G. G.: Male breast carcinoma—a review of 301 cases from the Christie Hospital and Holt Radium Institute, Manchester. Br. J. Cancer, *51*:115, 1985.

Ribeiro, G. G.: Tamoxifen in the treatment of male breast carcinoma. Clin. Radiol., *34*:625, 1983.

Richards, A. T., Jaffe, A., and Hunt, J. A.: Adenoma of the nipple in a male. S. Afr. Med. J., *47*:575, 1973.

Robison, R., and Montague, E. D.: Treatment results in males with breast cancer. Cancer, *49*:403, 1982.

Ross, M. B., Buzdar, A. U., and Blumenschein, G. R.: Treatment of advanced breast cancer with megestrol acetate after treatment with tamoxifen. Cancer, *49*:413, 1982.

Roth, J. A., Discafani, C., and O'Malley, M.: Secretory breast carcinoma in a man. Am. J. Surg. Pathol., *12*:150–154, 1988.

Sanchez, A. G., Villanueva, A. G., and Redondo, C.: Lobular carcinoma of the breast in a patient with Klinefelter's syndrome. Cancer, *57*:1181, 1986.

Scheike, O.: Male breast cancer. Clinical manifestations in 257 cases in Denmark. Br. J. Cancer, *28*:552, 1973.

Scheike, O., and Visfeldt, J.: Male breast cancer. Acta Pathol. Microbiol. Scand., *81*:359–365, 1973.

Scheike, O., Svenstrup, B., and Fraudsen, V. A.: Male breast cancer: 2. Metabolism of oestradiol-17β in men with breast cancer. J. Steroid Biochem., *4*:489, 1973.

Scilletta, B., Racalbuto, A., Russello, D., et al.: Carcinoma of the male breast and ocular metastases. Ital. J. Surg. Sci., *19*:93–96, 1989.

Serour, F., Birkenfeld, S., Amsterdam, E., et al.: Paget's disease of the male breast. Cancer, *62*:601–605, 1988.

Siddiqui, T., Weiner, R., Moreb, J., et al.: Cancer of the male breast with prolonged survival. Cancer, *62*:1632–1636, 1988.

Sirtori, C., and Veronesi, U.: Gynecomastia. A review of 218 cases. Cancer, *10*:645–854, 1957.

Sneige, N., Zachariah, S., Fanning, T.V., et al.: Fine-needle aspiration cytology of metastatic neoplasms in the breast. Am. J. Clin. Pathol., *92*:27–35, 1989.

Spence, R. A. J., Mackenzie, G., Anderson, J. R., et al.: Long-term survival following cancer of the male breast in northern Ireland. A report of 81 cases. Cancer, *55*:648, 1985.

Stephens, R. L., and Muggia, F. M.: Breast cancer in men. Report illustrating the value of endocrine ablation. Am. J. Med., *57*:679, 1974.

Thompson, D. K., Li, F. P., and Cassady, J. R.: Breast cancer in a man 30 years after radiation for metastatic osteogenic sarcoma. Cancer, *44*:2362, 1979.

Treves, N.: The treatment of cancer, especially inoperable cancer, of the male breast by ablative surgery (orchiectomy, adrenalectomy, and hypophysectomy) and hormone therapy (estrogens and corticosteroids). An analysis of 43 patients. Cancer, *12*:820, 1959.

Treves, N., and Holleb, A. I.: Cancer of the male breast; report of 146 cases. Cancer, *8*:1239, 1955.

Vanderbilt, P. C., and Warren, S. E.: Forty year experience with carcinoma of the male breast. Surg. Gynecol. Obstet., *133*:629, 1971.

Vercoutere, A. L., and O'Connell, T. X.: Carcinoma of the male breast. An update. Arch. Surg., *119*:1301, 1984.

Visfeldt, J., and Scheike, O.: Male breast cancer: I. Histologic typing and grading of 187 Danish cases. Cancer, *32*:985–990, 1973.

Vorobiof, D. A., and Falkson, G.: Nasally administered buserelin inducing complete remission of lung metastases in male breast cancer. Cancer, *59*:688–689, 1987.

Wainwright, J. M.: Carcinoma of the male breast. Arch. Surg., *14*:836, 1927.

Waterhouse, J., Muir, C., Shanmugaratnam, K., et al.: Cancer Incidence in Five Continents. Vol. IV. IARC, Lyon, 1982.

Williams, W. R.: Cancer of the male breast. Lancet 2:261, 1889.

Wilson, S. E., and Hutchinson, W. B.: Breast masses in males with carcinoma of prostate. J. Surg. Oncol., *8*:105–112, 1976.

Yadaw, R. V. S., Sahariah, S., Mittal, V. K., et al.: Angiosarcoma of the male breast. Int. Surg., *61*:463, 1976.

Yap, H. Y., Tashima, C. K., Blumenschein, G. R., et al.: Male breast cancer. A natural history study. Cancer, *44*:748, 1979.

Zumoff, B., Fishman, J., Cassouto, J., et al.: Estradiol transformation in men with breast cancer. J. Clin. Endocrinol. Metab., *26*:960–966, 1966.

37

Psychosocial Factors

Danielle M. Turns

Cancer is one of the major health problems facing today's industrialized society. Breast cancer is now the second leading cause of cancer-related death in women, and the age-adjusted breast cancer rate is about the same today as it was 60 years ago. It is estimated that in 1994, 182,000 women were diagnosed with breast cancer and that 46,000 died of the disease (*Cancer Facts and Figures*, 1994). The 5-year relative survival rate now stands at 76%, but for many the surviving years are marred by varying degrees of distress or disability. Many vivid media accounts of women's encounters with breast cancer have raised public awareness of how trying such an experience can be. Such a concern is reflected in the abundant and growing literature on breast cancer and psychosocial factors. Psychosocial factors not only relate to treatment, rehabilitation, and terminal care; they also operate in earlier stages of the disease, before it is detected, and at the time of detection.

PSYCHOSOCIAL FACTORS PRIOR TO THE DIAGNOSIS OF BREAST CANCER

Psychosocial Factors and Pathogenesis

Personality characteristics, depression, and stressors such as life events have been implicated in the pathogenesis of breast cancer. Since Galen's observation that "melancholic" women were more prone to cancer than those identified as "sanguine," the search for a "cancer personality" has proven elusive. Despite contradictory findings generated by studies from 1950 to 1980, the working hypothesis was that the inability to express emotions and to have meaningful relationships with others was the hallmark of the cancer-prone personality (Type C).

Persky and coworkers (1987) used the Minnesota Multiphasic Personality Inventory and the Cattel Personality Factor Inventory in a cohort of 2018 middle-aged men, and found no association between personality characteristics, among them psychologic repression, and incidence or mortality from cancer. Jasmin and coworkers (1990), however, gave open-ended interviews to a group of 77 women who presented for a breast lump biopsy and found that the best predictor of cancer was a "poorly organized neurotic structure." Other factors such as "excessive self-esteem," "hysterical disposition," and "unresolved recent grief" were also associated with breast cancer, but depression was not. Of note is a recent report by Faragher and Cooper (1990), who reported the unexpected finding that, even though women with breast cancer exhibited Type B personality characteristics, Type A traits were also present. As to

depression, Shekelle and colleagues (1981) found evidence of an association with cancer in their epidemiologic study of Western Electric male workers, and Persky and coworkers (1987), using the same population at a 20-year follow-up, confirmed this finding but showed a declining relationship over time. Helsing and associates (1981) showed that bereavement in men was associated with increased morbidity and mortality from a variety of diseases, but not specifically from cancer. Whereas Linkins and Comstock (1988) found a relationship between depression and cancer in smokers, Kaplan and Reynolds (1988) found none in their cohort, nor did Hahn and Petitti (1987) for breast cancer, or Zonderman and colleagues (1989) in a nationally representative sample.

Hurny (1990) was intrigued by the fact that small sample studies using open-ended interviews found positive correlations between cancer and personality traits or depression, whereas large-scale studies using standardized instruments did not. He hypothesized that reliance on a linear "cause-effect model" may be an inappropriate method of investigation because it does not take into consideration the complexity and circularity of mind-body-environment interactions. Neither the open-ended psychologic investigation nor the traditional epidemiologic method is adequate in this respect, and he advocated a system theory approach. Fox (1989) reviewed the literature specific to depression and risk of cancer and concluded from the combined evidence that the correlation is, at best, weak and certainly not consistent with a strong relationship between depression and cancer.

The investigation of stressful life events has been similarly frustrating. While Cooper and colleagues (1989) found that death of a husband or death of a close friend was associated with breast disease incidence and severity in a series of 1596 women attending a breast screening clinic and of 567 control subjects, Edwards and coworkers (1990), studying 1052 women with and without breast cancer, found no significant relationship. The findings of Sherg and Blohmke (1988) of a positive but weak relationship with historical life events such as death of a mother in childhood, loss of a spouse, or traumatic World War II experiences were undermined by the retrospective nature of the study.

At this point there is no definite body of research that formally establishes a cause-and-effect relationship between personality characteristics, depression or stress-inducing life events, and cancer risk. Though psychoimmunologic studies have found evidence that stressors may increase susceptibility to disease by altering the immune response, there is no definitive evidence of a clearly identified mechanism for cancer in general or breast cancer in particular.

It is clear that, though the popular belief that stress, certain personality traits, and depression are causally linked to cancer is well-entrenched, there is little scientific evidence to support it. Future research in this domain would have to combine a complex array of large sample, prospective design, validated psychologic scales as well as exhaustive clinical evaluations and immunologic markers to put the matter to rest.

Psychosocial Factors and Detection

Though there is evidence of racial and cultural factors that predispose to breast cancer, for example, diet, exposure to carcinogens, early menarche, number of pregnancies, and marital status, these are not relevant to psychiatry. More germane are the factors that mediate secondary prevention, that is, early detection and treatment.

Because breast self-examination (BSE), yearly physician breast examination, and mammography are known to be effective methods of detection, it is somewhat disheartening to note that even physicians who recommend BSE do not always give adequate training to their patients, an approach shown by Dorsay and associates (1988) and Olson and Mitchell (1989) to increase competence and compliance. Fox and coworkers (1988) found that fewer than a fifth of women over age 50 years were referred for screening mammography by their physicians. Even more dramatic, the cancer control objectives for the year 2000 include: ''Increase percentage of women aged 50 to 70 years who have an annual physical examination coupled with mammography to 80%, from 45% for physical examination alone and 15% for mammography'' (Greenwald and Sondik, 1986). This means that, in spite of intensive public and medical education efforts, the number of women receiving adequate screening still represents a minority of those who are candidates. What are the obstacles to more systematic adherence to principles of early detection?

Some women, particularly older ones, are often reluctant to avail themselves of the screening technology. Women of higher socioeconomic status and higher educational level are more likely to practice BSE, undergo yearly physical and mammographic examinations, stop smoking, or adopt a reasonable diet. They also may be more attuned to a rational health belief model and less captive to the overvaluation of the breast as a symbol of femininity.

The much publicized accounts of celebrity bouts with cancer do not appear to change attitudes about breast cancer prevention in most of the population, nor for very long. Lane and associates (1989) conducted a community-based mail survey of women over 50 just before and in the wake of Nancy Reagan's experience. Knowledge about lifetime risk of cancer increased, but perception of personal risk did not. Only a minority of respondents reported consulting a health professional or having a mammogram as a result of the publicity. The authors concluded that publicized events may trigger preventive action but that only community-based intervention specifically aimed at maintaining knowledge, promoting long-term behavior changes, and removing barriers to care can have a lasting effect.

In her study of rural women, Gray (1990) confirmed the association between health belief model factors and compliance with BSE reported by others: Perceived personal susceptibility, perceived seriousness of the illness, perceived benefits of early detection, and few perceived barriers to screening correlate with compliance, but these factors account for only 26% of the variance, a finding also reported by Champion (1988) and Burack and Liang (1989) in a study of black women. While a relationship between sociodemographic variables, personal experience of breast disease, and BSE practice was not observed in those two studies, others have reported decreasing frequency of BSE with increasing age and better compliance in more educated and married women (Hugueley and Brown, 1981). Redeker (1989), however, was able to explain 47% of the variance by combining health beliefs, internal health locus of control, occupation, and religion, and to predict accurately BSE nonpractice and high practice. In their 1986 study, Walker and colleagues showed that a woman's recent experience in the health care system was a stronger predictor of BSE practice than were health beliefs.

Women likely to undergo regular mammography are more knowledgeable about the disease, have a pattern of compliance with other preventive measures, are younger, of higher socioeconomic and educational status, and are more likely to live in urban areas and to be of the Jewish faith. Rimer and colleagues (1989) conducted telephone interviews with 600 randomly selected women, offering free mammography. Of the 484 nonsymptomatic women, 328 (68%) accepted the offer and 156 (32%) did not. No statistical difference between compliers and noncompliers was identified in the sociodemographic variables. Among health behaviors, perception of lifetime risk and BSE practice did not distinguish between the two groups, but compliant women were statistically more likely than noncompliers to remember receiving a pre–telephone call pamphlet (95% vs. 87%), more likely previously to have had a mammogram (100% vs. 26%), and less likely to be smokers (22% vs. 32%). In terms of perceived barriers to the procedure, noncompliant women reported more inconvenience, lack of time, being nonsymptomatic (and therefore not *needing* mammography), a physician's having recommended against it, and fear of radiation.

Some women who have symptoms delay seeking care. In their 1978 study, Todd and Magarey postulated that certain types of ego defenses can facilitate or hinder compliance. They interviewed 90 women with breast symptoms and determined the length of the delay between the appearance of symptoms and the seeking of treatment. The delayers displayed more anxiety and depression and used denial and suppression as coping mechanisms, while the nondelayers used intellectualization-isolation. They concluded that public health education programs relying on cognitive messages were effective with the intellectualization-isolation–oriented women but probably were not reaching women who use denial and suppression. Perhaps the more effective health educators would be primary care physicians, though we know that not all discharge that responsibility. The role of the physician as educator should be emphasized in medical school.

PSYCHOSOCIAL FACTORS AT THE TIME OF DIAGNOSIS

Few diagnoses generate as much turmoil as breast cancer. The emotions generated by the word "cancer"—and the prospect of mutilating surgery—potentiate each other, and this effect is even more pronounced when the woman has been asymptomatic and is not psychologically prepared to cope with a life-threatening condition. It is also a time when hard-nosed decision making is required within a relatively short period of time. Since the early 1970s it has become clear that mastectomy is not the only treatment for breast cancer and that, for small lesions, less mutilating procedures, such as lumpectomy with radiotherapy, are as effective as radical mastectomy. Though some women prefer to "leave it up to the physician," many others welcome the opportunity to participate in their care, in spite of the psychologic burden of sorting through the options. Whether or not reconstructive surgery would be appropriate, and whether it should be done at the time of surgery or later, must be considered. The array of information that must be integrated is overwhelming for some, and support systems are summoned to action. Family members are the first line of defense, but often they are also engaged in psychologic turmoil: concern, fear, anger, role shifts in the familial nexus, the impact on any healthy family and even more so on a dysfunctional one. The physician is the person who is expected to restore balance and perspective, but the patient's expectations are not free of ambivalence, as the physician is both potential savior and mutilator. In discussing the treatment choices, the patient and family may hear different recommendations from physicians of different specialties, which increases their confusion. Perhaps more unsettling is the fact that no one can give a full assurance of survival or cure. Are such factors measurably reflected in symptoms? Hughson and coworkers (1988) compared 91 patients awaiting breast biopsy and 30 awaiting cholecystectomy. They found that women subsequently found to have breast cancer were, as a group, no more anxious or depressed than the cholecystectomy patients or those with benign breast disease. (The latter group had the highest distress score.) Markedly more anxious *were* the women with cancer who were younger than 45 years. The results of this study were congruent with those of other studies conducted in the United Kingdom though not with those of older studies in the United States. Whether cultural factors, different sample selection, and control groups are responsible for the differences is open to question.

Coping styles have been related to psychopathology at the time of diagnosis by Burgess and colleagues (1988): A positive and confronting stance and a strong internal locus of control were associated with a lower rate of psychiatric morbidity than a hopeless and helpless response and a weak internal locus of control.

Tulman and Fawcett (1990) have proposed a more comprehensive assessment of women diagnosed with breast cancer. Based on Roy's Adaptation Model (1984), the elements of the patient's functional status include the level of performance in the woman's multiple roles as wife, parent, homemaker, community member, and worker. In future research this approach may provide a more substantive and systematic method of evaluation than psychologic measures of adaptation alone.

The diagnosis of breast cancer carries distress for both the patient and her family. Whether it also precipitates measurable psychopathologic responses depends on a variety of factors, such as age, pre-existing psychologic makeup and coping style, and familial support. Physicians must be prepared to provide advice and support.

PSYCHOSOCIAL ISSUES AND TREATMENT

Surgical Treatment

The impact of mastectomy has been studied extensively. Studies of the early 1950s described long-lasting and severe distress related to the mutilating surgery. Later studies gave a better picture of the depth, prevalence, and duration of the postmastectomy depressive syndrome. Miller (1980) reviewed the literature and concluded that depressed mood and sexual dysfunction affect as many as 25% of mastectomy patients during the first year after surgery. Gottschalk and Hoigaard-Martin (1986) showed significantly more psychopathology after mastectomy than after cholecystectomy or benign breast disease, or than in healthy women. Anxiety, death- and mutilation anxiety, ambivalence, hostility, depression, and general well-being were the most differentiating variables. Dean (1987) reported that after mastectomy about 8% of patients experience depression or an anxiety state that is severe enough to warrant treatment and 17% have a moderate depression or anxiety reaction. A study by the Breast Cancer Study Group (1987) compared women who had modified radical mastectomy for Stage I and II breast cancer with those who had cholecystectomy or benign breast disease and with healthy women. None of the women selected had a pre-existing psychiatric disorder. Three months after surgery, the mastectomy group reported greater psychologic distress related to social and interpersonal relationships, and women with Stage II cancer more distress than those with Stage I disease. At 1 year there was no difference in psychiatric morbidity or need for psychiatric intervention. The investigators concluded that mastectomy did not induce severe or long-lasting psychopathology in previously psychologically healthy women. Jones and Reznikoff (1989) highlighted the particular susceptibility of unmarried women to poor body image and self-image, sexual dysfunction, and negative affect; divorced women were most at risk. They emphasized the importance of support during postoperative adjustment.

Maguire (1990) listed the most common psychiatric disorders: depression, anxiety, body image problems (leading in some cases to social phobia or agoraphobia), and sexual problems. He felt that there is inadequate recognition of the need for psychologic help for women with breast cancer. He attributed some of this lack of recognition to the patients' acceptance of their psychiatric reactions as "par for the course"; one result was that they failed to report their distress to caregivers. He also contended that physicians and nurses have learned to avoid uncomfortable subjects, particularly psychologic ones, and that some use distancing techniques to that end. The actual extent and severity of psychopathology induced by mastectomy remains ill-defined. A consistent finding, however, is that women with a previous psychiatric history are at high risk for severe distress when confronted with breast cancer.

Assessing which personality characteristics are associated with postmastectomy psychopathology, Grassi and Molinari (1988) reported that women who did not express their anger or depression reported less anxiety at the time of the biopsy but were more likely to express depression, irritability, and hostility immediately after mastectomy and 6 months later. They thought that such personality characteristics should be included in the presurgery assessment as risk factors for psychoreactive problems.

Feather and Wainstock (1989), in their survey of 933 women after mastectomy, made the point that adjustment to mastectomy is more than just a psychologic issue. They took into account the interaction between social support, providers of such supports, adjustment, and sociodemographic variables. They concluded that women's attitudes toward mastectomy related less to social support than to self-esteem. Zenmore and Shepel (1989) found that emotional support from significant others correlated with better adjustment.

As to the type of support and its source, Neuling and Winefield (1988) concluded that both empathic and informational support were needed for 3 months postoperatively and that surgeons were often found wanting in empathy. Family members were relied upon for solace, but their support tended to wane over time. If social support was associated with better adjustment, the author cautioned that one cannot infer causality, because better-adjusted people elicit adequate support more easily.

Mastectomy is no longer the only surgical treatment for breast cancer; breast preservation, as well as breast reconstruction, are prevalent. Three questions arise: First, What are the elements of choice? Second, Are women who were given a choice faring better than those who were not? Third, Is the type of surgery related to different psychologic outcome and sexual adaptation?

To afford choice of treatment, access to factual information is paramount, but integration of the knowledge is influenced by a variety of factors: anxiety level, quality of the doctor-patient relationship, capacity for critical thinking, and decision-making style (Scott, 1983). It is clear that informed consent forms (Penman et al., 1984) and legislative fiats such as two-stage biopsy procedure mandate (Fischer, 1985) do little to inform decisions. Overall, only a minority of women have inordinate difficulty making a decision, and the majority accept their physician's recommendation.

Levy (1989) addressed the second issue. He found that, contrary to expectations, women who participated in decisions about treatment fared no better than those who did not. Fallowfield and colleagues (1990) conducted a prospective study of 269 women under the age of 75 years whose diagnosis was Stage I or II breast cancer and followed them for 1 year. On admission patients were given a self-assessment questionnaire and a semistructured psychiatric interview. They were also asked whether they felt they had been offered a choice of treatment and sufficient information to make a choice. The 22 surgeons in charge of the cases indicated whether the treatment was based on the patient's preference, the surgeon's preference, or technical reasons. Three surgeons whose policy was to offer treatment choice whenever that was technically appropriate provided their consultation tapes for review, so that agreement between them and their patients' perception could be evaluated. Two weeks postoperatively 42% of mastectomy patients and 37% of lumpectomy patients reported anxiety. This was still true 3 months later, the percentages being, respectively, 32% and 31%; at 1-year follow-up the percentages had declined to 28% and 27%. Some 15% to 29% of the entire group were found to be depressed at some point during the year, regardless of the treatment modality. The patients of surgeons who favored choice, overall, had less psychiatric morbidity than those of mastectomy-oriented or lumpectomy-oriented surgeons. The women were then classified in one–real choice group and no–real choice. There were no significant differences in anxiety and depression at 3-month follow-up. Women who had been given a choice and who opted for mastectomy were less frequently anxious or depressed at 12 months' follow-up, but the difference was not significant. It should be noted that before surgery most women had identified fear of cancer as their main concern and only 12% listed fear of losing a breast as worse than having cancer. Deadman and coworkers (1989) found that after mastectomy women were more likely to be depressed at their 12-month follow-up while after breast conservation patients were more anxious. They discuss the role of mediating factors such as control of treatment, feelings of competence to make a decision, concern for appearance, and adjuvant chemotherapy. There is, therefore, little compelling evidence that patients who were given a choice fared psychologically better than those who were not. There was, likewise, no evidence that they fared worse.

As to the third issue—that is, whether lumpectomy is associated with less psychopathology than mastectomy—again, we find conflicting conclusions. According to Sachs' (1983) and Margolis' (1983) groups, breast-preserving procedures induce less psychologic hardship. Other investigators found conservative techniques less psychologically burdensome than mastectomy (Sanger and Resnikoff, 1981; Schain et al., 1984; Ashcroft et al., 1985; Bartelink et al., 1985; Steinberg et al., 1985; deHaes et al., 1986; Lasry et al., 1987; and Kemeny et al., 1988). Margolis and colleagues (1990) reported that half of the mastectomy patients expressed regret about not having chosen the breast-conserving alternative, but others (Olschewski et al., 1988; Meyer and Aspegren, 1989; Kiebert et al., 1991; and Wolberg et al., 1989, 1990) found no distinct psychologic advantage to breast conservation. Even in those studies, however, a common finding is that women who receive conservative surgery have a better self-image (Meyer and Aspegren, 1989; and Wellisch et al., 1989) and better sexual adjustment (Kemeny et al., 1988; and Kiebert et al., 1991). Baider and colleagues (1986) examined couples' adjustment to lumpectomy versus mastectomy and found little difference in family relations, in either wives or husbands.

It is obvious from these observations that no treatment

method is free of psychologic distress or is clearly superior. The reason for such rather discouraging findings may be that no effort is being made to identify study groups at high or low risk for psychiatric difficulties. Younger women, unmarried women, women who wish to procreate, and women who have pre-existing psychiatric problems, marital maladjustment, or sexual difficulties bring to their ordeal a different set of issues than other women. It would be irrational to expect clear-cut responses from the heterogeneous populations described in the studies.

Breast reconstruction is viewed by Luce and Romm (1986) as a procedure that enhances self-esteem, restores body image, and instils a sense of hope and purpose. Schain and colleagues (1985) hold that immediate or ''early'' reconstruction (within 1 year) significantly reduces the recall of postmastectomy distress when compared with ''delayed'' reconstruction (after 1 year). They also found the early reconstruction group to be more symptomatic on depression, anxiety, psychoticism, and interpersonal sensitivity scales of the Brief Symptom Inventory and speculate that the early- and delayed reconstruction groups are psychologically different in their ability to tolerate the delay before reconstruction. They state further that for certain subjects the recommendation for reconstruction may be carried out ''the sooner the better,'' to minimize the emotional morbidity associated with mastectomy. It seems that some women adjust poorly to wearing a prosthesis, and wanting to get rid of it is the reason most frequently recorded for reconstruction. It should be noted, however, that all women are not candidates for breast reconstruction, nor are all interested in the procedure. Only about 10% of patients request breast reconstruction. Pasqualin and coworkers (1988) explored the reasons for refusal. The two principal causes were traumatization from the initial treatment and little understanding of the reconstruction procedure. All refusers reported high anxiety levels, lack of psychologic support during the early treatment phase, and being shocked by the mutilation of mastectomy and discouraged by the side effects of adjuvant therapy. The hospital had become an object of fear and loathing, and they did not wish to be re-exposed to it for what they regarded as an optional procedure. They also felt that surgeons gave scant information about the procedure, its length, or its cost. Some had more personal reasons: guilt feelings through the amputation, fear of recurrence if the scar was disturbed by further surgery, or feeling that they were ''too old'' for the procedure. The authors felt that detailed information and individualized emotional support at the time of mastectomy would help patients make more rational decisions about reconstruction.

Frischenschlager and colleagues (1990) failed to verify the assumption that reconstructive surgery of the breast has a supportive function, and Goin and Goin (1988) made the point that reconstruction itself can be psychologically traumatic, requiring emotional support before and after the procedure.

In earlier studies, women who chose reconstruction were described, as a group, as psychologically well adjusted, well informed, and realistic in their expectations. The most frequent reasons for reconstruction were to ''get rid of the prosthesis,'' to be ''whole again,'' and ''appearance'' (Jacobs et al., 1983; Schain et al., 1984). Eighty percent of the women were satisfied with the result of the surgery and their level of psychologic, sexual, and social function.

Adjuvant and Systemic Therapy

Chemotherapy, radiotherapy (Meyerowitz et al., 1983; Nerenz, 1986; Love et al., 1989), antiestrogen treatment, and oophorectomy induce side effects that tax the patients' adaptive resources. Anemia, bleeding, anorexia, nausea and vomiting, dysphagia, constipation, diarrhea, xerostomia, stomatitis and taste alteration, alopecia, rashes and other skin reactions, pruritus, and asthenia are the hallmarks of the first two; sexual and reproductive problems reflect the premature menopause induced by systemic therapy (Schover, 1991).

Some patients develop intense anxiety in anticipation of chemotherapy infusions or other procedures, including anticipatory nausea and vomiting and insomnia. Anticipatory reactions may become so pervasive that they occur in response to environmental clues that are only remotely connected with the treatment but are so intense as to end the treatment protocol prematurely (Redd et al., 1989).

Yasko and Green (1987) and Glasgow and colleagues (1987) adressed the sexual issues that may confront the patient. Unless the patient is asked specifically about sexual history, changes in sexual desire, obstacles to sexual intercourse, she and her partner may be deprived of appropriate counseling. Then, loss of intimacy, shame, and feelings of abandonment add their burden to an already trying experience. Hurny (1989) reviewed the psychosocial aspects of adjuvant therapy and their impact on patients' quality of life. He suggested that a patient's subjective experience be considered part of the treatment evaluation.

Recurrences and Terminal Phase

A recurrence of cancer precipitates a great deal of anxiety for the patient and her family: lack of control over life events or symptoms, loss of function, family role alterations, pain, side effects of treatment, and the prospect of death. This is the time for a tailored home care program that addresses the medical, financial, and emotional needs of the patient and her family. Grief reactions are common, and often intense and prolonged. Spiritual needs require attention. Referral to social agencies and hospice care is often needed. Pain management is of the utmost importance, narcotic analgesics being the drugs of choice. Group therapy and hypnosis have been found by Spiegel and Bloom (1983) to reduce the pain induced by metastatic breast cancer.

Factors Associated with Survival

Whether environmental stress adversely affects the course of breast cancer is as controversial as its role in the pathogenesis of the disease. Ramirez and colleagues (1989) suggest an association between profoundly affecting life events and recurrence, but methodologic issues such as small sample size and retrospective design weaken the validity of the findings. There is also little evidence that a positive attitude or a determination to "beat the disease" increases chances of survival, though these may promote compliance with treatment and improve the quality of life. They may also prompt a search for treatment methods outside the purview of conventional medicine (Cassileth, 1988, 1989). Hurny and Bernhard (1989) reviewed the literature on coping styles and survival and found no conclusive evidence of a positive correlation. The report by Spiegel and coworkers (1989) that group therapy could increase the survival of women with metastatic cancer has generated a great deal of interest. The sample included 86 women aged 49 to 54 years whose diagnosis was metastatic breast cancer and who were aware of the terminal nature of their condition. They were randomly assigned to a "How to Die" therapy group or no group. The group participants survived an average of 18 months longer than the controls (about 36 months) and three survived 10 years or longer. A more recent cohort study found no evidence for a clear association between psychologic intervention and survival (Gellert et al., 1993).

PSYCHOSOCIAL INTERVENTIONS

Routine Management

A variety of psychosocial interventions are available to today's practitioners. The most important are the establishment of a therapeutic alliance between primary physician and patient and an experienced and resourceful treatment team. Appraisal of the patient's support system and interventions aimed at preserving its integrity during the course of the illness should also be considered. Patient education about the disease and available treatment methods should begin early and in a supportive, nonthreatening atmosphere. An effort should be made to elicit a patient's idiosyncratic concerns. Patterns of coping with past stresses, psychiatric disorders, familial situation, presence of stress in the environment, and sexual functioning need to be ascertained to get a better appreciation for the patient's present and potential difficulties. This detailed anamnesis enhances communication and facilitates the patient's participation in treatment. Whenever possible, family members and significant others should be encouraged to participate in the process, and the mate's concerns should be addressed also. This type of interaction is most often initiated at the stage of diagnosis and is nurtured throughout the immediate postoperative period. To accomplish this long, hard task, reliance on trusted team members is usual. Nursing personnel and social workers participate in patient and family education, providing emotional support and referrals to social agencies to ensure help with finances, arranging for the assistance of a homemaker when needed, or helping to meet other needs. Physical therapists teach exercises designed to prevent limitation of motion and postmastectomy edema (Gaskin et al., 1989). An organization frequently called upon to help is Reach to Recovery, a self-help group composed of women who have been treated for breast cancer. These volunteers act as role models and give practical advice on acquiring and wearing a prosthesis (Rogers et al., 1985).

In recent years, group therapy has been used as a treatment method, not only for postmastectomy patients but also for patients at other stages of the disease. A study by Spiegel and colleagues (1981) provides objective evidence that group intervention for these patients is effective in reducing tension, depression, fatigue, and phobias.

To summarize, it is clear that a variety of interventions are at the disposal of the patient's primary physician to lessen the psychosocial consequences of the disease and its treatment. They rely not only on the patient herself but on trained health professionals who help meet emotional, social, familial, and psychiatric needs. The true impact of these interventions on the patient's quality of life is hard to objectify. The major hurdles in such research were the focus of the 1983 American Cancer Society workshop conference on methodology in behavioral and psychosocial cancer research (American Cancer Society, 1986). More recently, a special issue of Oncology (Tchekmedyian & Cella, 1990) was devoted to quality-of-life evaluation in clinical practice and research. That such concerns are now in the mainstream of cancer research is a welcome development.

Such concerns may seem esoteric to patients who are suffering, struggling with unwelcome aspects of treatment, and facing their own mortality. For them, alternative medicine may be powerfully attractive. Cassileth and Brown (1988) described such patients and offered useful suggestions to clinicians involved in their care.

Psychiatric Conditions

A certain degree of emotional distress is to be expected in any woman with breast cancer. An experienced surgeon and treatment team quickly recognize when this distress is so severe or prolonged that specialized intervention is necessary. Requesting a psychiatric consultation is then appropriate. Severe anxiety, depression, delirium, excessive somatic complaints, and lack of response to pain management are the most frequent indications.

A psychiatric evaluation should include, at least, a thorough history, including prior treatments for psychiatric and addictive disorders, response to medication, sexual adjustment, present social situation, and familial network and mental status.

Generalized anxiety disorders and panic attacks may require the prescription of anxiolytics; benzodiazepines are safe and effective, alone or in combination with antidepressants. Caution must be exercised lest tolerance and dependency develop, a concern particularly valid in patients with a history of alcoholism or drug abuse. Buspirone may be more appropriate for these patients. Psychotherapy should be instituted, and the psychiatrist may make recommendations to the treatment team.

Anticipatory anxiety, on the other hand, should be conceptualized as a respondent conditioning response. Behavioral techniques such as relaxation training and systematic desensitization are effective, and probably preferable to medication or traditional psychotherapy.

Depression, with its symptom constellation of sadness, pessimisim, helplessness, hopelessness, crying spells, insomnia, and anorexia, is easily diagnosable in the early phases of treatment. This condition is eminently treatable and responds well to the combination of psychotherapy and antidepressants such as tricyclics or fluoxetine. The diagnosis of depression may be more difficult in later stages of the disease, when physical debilitation or treatment side effects are expected. Gentle questioning, however, elicits the psychic component of depression, and treatment achieves appreciable improvement in the patient's emotional and physical symptoms. Chronic illness is bound to increase the risk of suicide, and missing a diagnosis of depression may have tragic results at this stage.

Multiple somatic complaints and poor response to appropriate pain management may or may not be the consequence of masked depression. In either case, antidepressants, and tricyclics in particular, may be valuable adjuncts to treatment. The prescription of amitriptyline for chronic pain may allow smaller doses of narcotics.

The causes of delirium may be multifactorial: electrolyte imbalance, medications, neurotoxicity, fever, metabolic disorders, excessive amounts of narcotics, anxiolytics, or hypnotics (alone or in combination), and brain metastasis result in disorientation, memory deficit, hallucinations, sleep disruption, agitation, and sometimes violent behavior. Physicians should be able to diagnose delirium in its early stages by routinely performing a mini–mental status examination. Too often, however, early signs are missed, and the patient may hurt herself or others as symptoms go unchecked. Specific treatment should be aimed at remedying the cause of the condition, and psychoactive drugs such as haloperidol or lorazepam in small doses are effective in reducing agitation. Restraints may have to be used to prevent the patient from harming herself until the symptoms resolve.

CONCLUSION

The systematic study of psychosocial factors in breast cancer patients is a relatively new field of scientific inquiry. Many answers still elude us, among them, the role of psychosocial factors in cancer pathogenesis, the obstacles to effective secondary prevention (early detection and treatment), and the complex interaction of quality of life and psychosocial therapeutic interventions. While the doctor-patient relationship remains the cornerstone of the therapeutic outcome, a multidisciplinary treatment team's involvement is important in managing the patient's psychosocial needs.

References

American Cancer Society: Cancer Facts and Figures—1994. Atlanta, American Cancer Society, 1994, p. 6.

Ashcroft, J. J., Leinster, S. J., and Slade, P. D.: Breast cancer—patient choice of treatment. Preliminary communication. J.R. Soc. Med., 78:43–46, 1985.

Baider, L., Rizel, S., and Kaplan De-Nour, A.: Comparisons of couples' adjustment to lumpectomy and mastectomy. Gen. Hosp. Psychiatry, 8:251–257, 1986.

Bartelink, H., van Dam, F., and van Donegen, J.: Psychological effects of breast conserving therapy in comparison with radical mastectomy. Int. J. Radiation Oncol. Biol. Phys., 11:381–387, 1985.

Breast Cancer Study Group: Psychological responses to mastectomy. A prospective comparison study. Psychological aspects of Breast Cancer Study Group. Cancer, 59:189–196, 1987.

Burack, R. C., and Liang, J.: The acceptance of mammography by older black women. Am. J. Public Health, 79:721–726, 1989.

Burgess, C., Morris, T., and Pettingale, K. W.: Psychological response to cancer diagnosis II. Evidence for coping styles (coping styles and cancer diagnosis). J. Psychosomat. Res., 32:263–272, 1988.

Cassileth, B.: The social implications of mind-body cancer research. Cancer Invest, 7:361–364, 1989.

Cassileth, B., and Brown, H.: Unorthodox cancer medicine. Cancer, 38:176–186, 1988.

Cassileth, B., Walsh, W. P., and Lusk, E. J.: Psychosocial correlates of cancer survival. J. Clin. Oncol., 6:1753–1759, 1988.

Champion, V. L.: Attitudinal variables related to intention, frequency and proficiency of breast self-examination in women 35 and over. Res. Nurs. Health, 11:283–291, 1988.

Cooper, C. L., Cooper, R., and Faragher, E. B.: Incidence and perceptions of psychological stress: The relationship with breast cancer. Psychol. Med., 19:415–422, 1989.

Deadman, J. M., Dewey, M. S., Owens, R. G., et al.: Threat and loss in breast cancer. Psychol. Med., 19:677–681, 1989.

Dean, C.: Psychiatric morbidity following mastectomy. J. Psychosomat. Res., 31:385–389, 1987.

de Haes, J. C. J. M., Van Oostsom, M. A., and Welvaart, K.: The effect of radical and conserving surgery on the quality of life of early breast cancer patients. Eur. J. Surg. Oncol., 12:337–342, 1986.

Dorsay, R. H., Cunco, W. D., Somkin, C. P., et al.: Breast self-examination: Improving competence and frequency in a classroom setting. Am. J. Public Health, 78:520–522, 1988.

Edwards, J. R., Cooper, C. L., Pearl, S. G., et al.: The relationship between psychosocial factors and breast cancer: Some unexpected results. Behav. Med., 16:5–14, 1990.

Fallowfield, L. J., Hall, A., Maguire, G. P., et al.: Psychological outcomes of different treatment policies in women with early breast cancer outside a clinical trial. Br. Med. J., 301:575–580, 1990.

Faragher, E. B., and Cooper, C. L.: Type A prone behavior and breast cancer. Psychol. Med., 20:663–670, 1990.

Feather, B. L., and Wainstock, J. M.: Perceptions of postmastectomy patients. Cancer Nurs., 12:293–300; 301–309, 1989.

Fischer, B.: Choice of surgery in early breast cancer. Presented at the Conference on Early Breast Cancer. The psychological perspective. Long Island Jewish Medical Center and Memorial Hospital Sloan Kettering Cancer Center, New York, October 11, 1985.

Fox, B. H.: Depressive symptoms and cancer (1989). J.A.M.A., 262:1231, 1989.

Fox, S. A., Klos, D. S., and Tsou, C. V.: Underuse of screening mammography by family physicians. Radiology, 166:431–433, 1988.

Frischenschlager, O., Balogh, B., and Predovic, M.: Psychosocial benefits of breast reconstruction after mastectomy in patients with benign or malignant tumors. Psychother. Psychosomat. Med. Psychol., 40:441–447, 1990.

Gaskin, T. A., LoBuglio, A., Kelly, P., et al.: STRETCH: A rehabilitative program for patients with breast cancer. South. Med. J., 82:467–469, 1989.

Gellert, G. A., Maxwell, R. M., and Siegel, B.: Survival of breast cancer patients receiving adjunctive psychosocial support therapy: A 10-year follow-up study. J. Clin. Oncol., 11:66–69, 1993.

Glasgow, M., Halfin, V., and Althausen, A. F.: Sexual response and cancer. Cancer, 37:322–333, 1989.

Goin, K. M., and Goin, J. M.: Growing pains: The psychological experience of breast reconstruction with tissue expansion. Ann. Plast. Surg., 21:217–222, 1988.

Gottschalk, L. A., and Hoigaard-Martin, J.: The emotional impact of mastectomy. Psychiatry Res., 17:153–167, 1986.

Grassi, L., and Molinari, S.: Pattern of emotional control and psychological reactions to breast cancer: A preliminary report. Psychol Rep., 62:727–732, 1988.

Gray, M. E.: Factors related to practice of breast self-examination in rural women. Cancer Nursing, 13:100–107, 1990.

Greenwald, P., and Sondik, E. (Eds.): Cancer Control Objectives for the

Nation: 1985–2000. Bethesda, MD, National Cancer Institute, 1986, pp. 586–2880.

Hahn, R. C., and Petitti, D. B.: Minnesota Multiphasic Personality Inventory–rated depression and the incidence of breast cancer. Cancer, *61:*845–848, 1988.

Helsing, K. J., and Szklo, M.: Mortality after bereavement. Am. J. Epidemiol., *114:*41–52, 1981.

Helsing, K. J., Comstock, G. W., and Szklo, M.: Causes of death in a widowed population. Am. J. Epidemiol., *116:*524–532, 1981.

Hughson, A. V. M., Cooper, A. F., McArdle, C. S., et al.: Psychosocial morbidity in patients awaiting breast biopsy. J. Psychosomat. Res., *32:*173–180, 1988.

Hugueley, C. M., and Brown, R. L.: The value of breast self-examination. Cancer, *47:*989–995, 1981.

Hurny, C.: Critical review of quality of life. Psychosocial aspects of adjuvant therapy in breast cancer. Recent Results Cancer Res., *115:*279–282, 1989.

Hurny, C.: Psyche and cancer. Ann. Oncol., *1:*6–8, 1990.

Hurny, C., and Bernhard, J.: Coping and survival with primary breast cancer. A critical analysis of current research strategies and proposal of a new approach integrating biomedical, psychological and social variables. Rec. Res. Ca. Res., *115:*255–271, 1989.

Jacobs, E., et al.: Who seeks breast reconstruction? A controlled psychological comparison (Abstract). Psychosomat. Med., *45:*80, 1983.

Jasmin, C., Le, M. G., Marty, P., et al.: Evidence for a link between certain psychological factors and the risk of breast cancer in a case-control study. Ann. Oncol., *1:*22–29, 1990.

Jones, D. N., and Reznikoff, M.: Psychosocial adjustment to mastectomy. J. Nerv. Ment. Dis., *177:*624–630, 1989.

Kaplan, G. A., and Reynolds, P.: Depression and cancer mortality and morbidity: Prospective evidence from the Alameda County Study. J. Behav. Med., *111:*1–12, 1988.

Kemeny, M. M., Wellish, D. K., and Schain, W. S.: Psychosocial outcome in a randomized surgical trial for treatment of primary breast cancer. Cancer, *62:*1231–1237, 1988.

Kiebert, G. M., de Haes, J. C. J. M., and van de Velde, C. H. J.: The impact of breast conserving treatment and mastectomy on the quality of life of early-stage breast cancer patients: A review. J. Clin. Oncol., *9:*1059–1070, 1991.

Lane, D. S., Polednak, A. P., and Burg, M. A.: The impact of media coverage of Nancy Reagan's experience on breast cancer screening. Am. J. Public Health, *79:*1551–1552, 1989.

Lasry, J. C.-M, Margolese, R. G., Poisson, E., et al.: Depression and body image following mastectomy and lumpectomy. J. Chronic Dis., *40:*529–534, 1987.

Levy, S. M., Herberman, R. B., Lee, J. K., et al.: Breast conservation versus mastectomy: Distress sequelae as a function of choice. J. Clin. Oncol., *7:*367–375, 1989.

Linkins, R. W., and Comstock, G. W.: Depressed mood and development of cancer (Abstract). Am. J. Epidemiol., *128:*894, 1988.

Love, R. R., Leventhal, H., Easterling, D. V., et al.: Side effects and emotional distress during cancer chemotherapy. Cancer, *63:*604–612, 1989.

Luce, E. A., and Romm, S.: Breast reconstruction after mastectomy. J. Kentucky Med. Assoc., *82:*183, 1984.

Maguire, P.: Psychologic consequences of the surgical treatment of cancer of the breast. Surg. Annu., *22:*77–91, 1990.

Margolis, G. J., Carabell, S. C., and Goodman, R. L.: Psychological aspects of primary radiation therapy for breast carcinoma. Am. J. Clin. Oncol., *6:*533–538, 1983.

Margolis, G., Goodman, R. L., and Rubin, A.: Psychological effects of breast-conserving cancer treatment and mastectomy. Psychosomatics, *31:*33–39, 1990.

Meyer, L., and Aspegren, K.: Long term psychological sequelae of mastectomy and breast conserving treatment for breast cancer. Acta Oncol., *28:*13–18, 1989.

Meyerowitz, B. E., Watkins, I. K., and Sparks, F. C.: Psychosocial implications of adjuvant chemotherapy. Cancer, *52:*1541–1545, 1983.

Miller, P. J.: Mastectomy: A review of psychosocial research. Health Social Work, *4:*60–65, 1980.

Nerenz, D. R., Love, R. R., Leventhal, H., et al.: Psychosocial consequences of cancer chemotherapy for elderly patients. Health Serv. Res., *20:*961–976, 1986.

Neuling, S. J., and Winefield, H. R.: Social support and recovery after surgery for breast cancer frequency and correlates of supportive behaviors by family, friends and surgeon. Soc. Sci. Med., *27:*385–392, 1988.

Olschewski, M., Verres, R., Scheurlen, H., et al.: Evaluation of psychosocial aspects in a breast preservation trial. Rec. Res. Ca. Res., *111:*258–269, 1988.

Olson, R. L., and Mitchell, E. S.: Self-confidence as a critical factor in breast self-examination. J. Obstet. Gynecol. Neonatal Nurs., *18:*476–481, 1989.

Pasqualin, F., Wilk, A., Gros, D., et al.: Refusal of reconstruction after mastectomy for breast cancer. Ann. Chir. Plast. Esth., *33:*127–129, 1988.

Penman, D. T., Holland, J. C., Bahna, G. F., et al.: Informed consent for investigational chemotherapy. Patients' and physicians' perception. J. Clin. Oncol., *2:*849–852, 1984.

Persky, V. W., Kempthorne-Rawson, T., and Shekelle, R. B.: Personality and risk of cancer: 20 years follow up of the Western Electric Study. Psychosomat. Med., *49:*435–499, 1987.

Ramirez, A. J., Craig, T. K. J., Watson, J. P., et al.: Stress and relapse of breast cancer. Br. Med. J., *298:*291–293, 1989.

Redd, W. H.: Behavioral approaches to treatment-related distress. Cancer, *38:*138–145, 1988.

Redd, W. H., Jacobsen, P. B., and Andrybowski, M. A.: Behavioral side effects of adjuvant chemotherapy. Rec. Res. Ca. Res., *115:*272–278, 1989.

Redeker, N. S.: Health belief, health locus of control, and the frequency of breast self-examination in women. J. Obstet. Gynecol. Neonatal Nursing, *18:*45–51, 1988.

Rimer, B. K., Keintz, M. K., Kessler, H. B., et al.: Why women resist screening mammography: Patient-related barriers. Radiology, *172:*243–246, 1989.

Rogers, T. F., Bauman, L. J., and Metzger, L.: An assessment of the Reach to Recovery program. Cancer, 25:116–124, 1985.

Roy, C.: Introduction to Nursing. An Adaptation Model. 2nd ed. Englewood Cliffs, NJ, Prentice Hall, 1984.

Sachs, E. L., Gerstein, D. G., and Mann, S. G.: Conservative surgery and radiation therapy for breast cancer. Front. Radiation. Ther. Oncol., *17:*23–32, 1983.

Sanger, C. K., and Resnikoff, M.: A comparison of the psychological effects of breast saving procedures with the modified radical mastectomy. Cancer, *48:*2341–2346, 1981.

Schain, W. S., Jacobs, E., Wellish, D. K.: Psychosocial issues in breast reconstruction: Intrapsychic, interpersonal and practical concerns. Clin. Plast. Surg., *11:*237–244, 1984.

Schain, W., Wellisch, D. K., Pasnau, R. O., et al.: The sooner the better: A study of psychological factors in women undergoing immediate versus delayed breast reconstruction. Am. J. Psychiatry, *142:*40, 1985.

Schover, L. R.: The impact of breast cancer on sexuality, body image and intimate relationships. Cancer, *41:*112–120, 1991.

Scott, D. W.: Anxiety, critical thinking and information processing during and after breast biopsy. Nurs. Res., *32:*24–26, 1983.

Semson, D. H., and Elinson, J.: Cancer screening and prevention: Knowledge, attitudes and practices of New York City physicians. N.Y. State J. Med., *87:*643–645, 1987.

Shekelle, R. B., Raynor, W. J., Ostfeld, A. M., et al.: Psychological depression and the 17-year risk of death from cancer. Psychosomat. Med., *43:*117–125, 1981.

Sherg, H., and Blohmke, M.: Associations between selected life events and cancer. Behav. Med., *14:*119–124, 1988.

Sinsheimer, L. M., and Holland, J. C.: Psychological issues in breast cancer. Semin. Oncol., *14:*75–82, 1987.

Spiegel, D., and Bloom, J. R.: Group therapy and hypnosis reduce metastatic breast carcinoma pain. Psychosomat. Med., *45:*333, 1983.

Spiegel, D., Bloom, J. R., and Yalom, I.: Group support for patients with metastatic cancer. Arch. Gen. Psychiatr., *38:*527, 1981.

Spiegel, D., Gotheil, C. E., Kraemer, H. C., et al.: Effect of psychosocial treatment on survival of patients with metastatic breast cancer. Lancet, *ii:*888–891, 1989.

Stein, M., Schleifer, S. J., and Kellen, S. E.: Psychoimmunology in clinical psychiatry. *In* Hales, R. E., and Frances, A. J. (Eds.): Annual Review of Psychiatry: Neurosciences Techniques in Clinical Psychiatry. Washington, D. C., American Psychiatric Press, 1987, pp. 210–234.

Steinberg, M. D., Juliana, M. A., and Wise, L.: Psychological outcome of lumpectomy versus mastectomy in the treatment of breast cancer. Am. J. Psychiatry, *142:*32–39, 1985.

Tchekmedyian, N. S., and Cella, D. F. (Eds.): Quality of life in current oncology practice and research. Oncology, 4(Special issue):21–208, 1990.

Todd, P., and Magarey, C.: Ego defences and affects in women with breast symptoms: A preliminary measurement paradigm. Br. J. Med. Psychol., *51:*177–180, 1978.

Tulman, L., and Fawcett, J.: A framework for studying functional status after diagnosis of breast cancer. Cancer Nursing, *13:*95–99, 1990.

Walker, L. R., and Glaz, K.: Psychosocial determinants of breast self evaluation. Am. J. Prevent. Med., *2:*169–178, 1986.

Wellisch, D. K., DiMatteo, R., Silverstein, M., et al.: Psychosocial outcome of breast cancer therapies: Lumpectomy versus mastectomy. Psychosomatics, *30:*365–373, 1989.

Wolberg, W. H., Romsaas, E. P., Tanner, M. A., et al.: Psychosexual adaptation to breast cancer surgery. Cancer, *63:*1645–1655, 1989.

Yasko, J. M., and Greene, P.: Coping with problems related to cancer and cancer treatment. Cancer, *37:*106–125, 1987.

Zenmore, R., and Shepel, L. F.: Effect of breast cancer and mastectomy on emotional support and adjustment. Soc. Sci. Med., *28:*19–27, 1989.

Zonderman, A. B., Costa, P. T., and McCrae, R. R.: Depression as a risk for cancer morbidity and mortality in a nationally representative sample. J.A.M.A., *262:*1191–1195, 1989.

38

Community Resources for the Breast Cancer Patient

Becky J. Hollingsworth

Receiving a diagnosis of breast cancer is a life-changing event, not only for the woman with the diagnosis but also for her entire social support network. "Serious illness not only takes over the patient's life, it greedily expands to consume the energy and resources of the patient's family. Far from being tightly confined inside the individual's skin, serious illness invades the entire network of connections around the sick person" (McDaniel et al., 1993). This "network of connections" around the breast cancer patient immediately expands to include interaction with a specialized segment of the health care services (oncologists, hospitals, home health agencies, and specialized oncology treatment centers); for most patients, it also leads to connection with other community services. The patient's physician is often called upon to function as a "guide" or "gatekeeper" for the patient as she passes through this maze of services. Because the treatment of cancer requires a patient to move through a complex series of changes, the types of assistance needed at any given point in treatment are unique to each patient. Also unique are each community's resources, which differ in structure and in accessibility from those of other localities. The sections of this chapter (1) address the broad range of services that are often required by a woman with breast cancer and her family, (2) relate these services to the critical periods during which the resources are most likely to be needed, and (3) suggest preliminary steps for the physician to take in accessing these resources.

TYPES OF RESOURCES TYPICALLY NEEDED BY THE BREAST CANCER PATIENT

From the moment when a woman suspects that she has breast cancer, the acquisition of *information* and *education* about cancer becomes a primary need. It is critical that a woman's knowledge about cancer be sufficient to identify symptoms if early diagnosis of the disease is to be made and effective treatment initiated. Education for this purpose generally precedes a patient's contact with the oncologist; however, most physicians have seen many women who delayed in seeking treatment owing to their failure to recognize the changes that signal the possible presence of cancer. Education and access to informational resources continue to be needs throughout the patient's treatment course, and these needs vary with the stages of treatment. *Financial resources and assistance* are needed by every

woman with breast cancer. Those patients with adequate healthcare insurance and adequate income are the most fortunate, but this segment of the patient population is shrinking. Even those with adequate financial resources often request assistance to deal with the bewildering maze of insurance and disability claim forms that they must prepare and to understand how insurance coverage affects their treatment options. For a growing number of Americans, healthcare insurance is available from employers; however, sizable deductibles, limitations on amount of available coverage, loss of income during the period of treatment, and increased out-of-pocket expenses for uncovered items may substantially alter a breast cancer patient's and her family's financial stability. Finally, an increasing number of women have no healthcare insurance at all and must depend on public resources to support their treatment.

Americans are engaged in a lively social and political debate on healthcare financing. Information about an individual's treatment options and their timing (once the exclusive purview of the physician and patient) and about the cost of care have to be assessed before a treatment plan is implemented. In today's economic climate, these considerations are heavily influenced by the decisions of people who are outside of the physician-patient dyad. Managed care programs, whether implemented under the auspices of a private sector insurer or mandated in the regulations governing public funding for healthcare, are now prevalent. Patients and family members must integrate complex financial information with the information they receive about treatment options. Physicians must likewise integrate information about financial resources and limitations when devising a treatment plan for each woman. Undoubtedly, the national debate over healthcare policy will continue to bring rapid change in patterns of treatment for breast cancer patients.

The development of specialized regional cancer centers has increased the need for *housing* and *transportation* to serve women and their families. In the author's practice at one such center, it is not uncommon to encounter patients referred for treatment from hundreds of miles away who require lodging for periods of up to 6 weeks. Patients who reside in the local community may become dependent on community resources to provide transportation when side effects of treatment interfere with their ability to drive. A limited social support network means that no one is available to assist patients in getting to and from the treatment facility. Specialized transportation (via wheelchair-accessible vehicle or ambulance) may be required as patients' physical disabilities increase. Expenses for transportation and lodging are seldom "covered" items in most healthcare insurance plans and thus must be borne almost exclusively by the patients, adding to the financial burden of treatment.

Women frequently seek assistance from community resources for a wide variety of *practical assistance*. Needs range from the need to obtain tangible items, such as breast prostheses, hospital beds, and shower rails, to the need for engaging in-home services, such as those that provide housekeeping, home repair services, or companions.

Home healthcare and *hospice care* are other community resources frequently needed by breast cancer patients. These services are typically provided by licensed agencies. Availability of these services, particularly in rural areas, is often limited; however, when they are available, home healthcare services can frequently be utilized as an alternative to office visits for patients whose limited social support network or transportation difficulties make keeping appointments difficult. Nurses and healthcare aides form the core of most home healthcare agencies. However, agencies licensed to receive reimbursement through Medicare or state medical assistance programs must also provide a range of adjunctive services such as medical social work, physical therapy, speech therapy, and occupational therapy. Hospice care is a specialized home healthcare program that focuses on the terminal phase of life and emphasizes palliative rather than curative treatment. Hospice care is typically provided by an interdisciplinary team that includes nurses, social workers, and chaplains and is under the direction of the physician. Some hospice programs also provide inpatient facilities for the short-term management of patients with acute symptoms or for those patients who have no caregiver in the home.

Finally, a wide variety of community agencies provide *psychologic, emotional, and spiritual counseling* to patients and their families. As Hermann (1992) explained,

> People with cancer represent the full range of human personality and needs. Cancer by itself does not result in poor coping. It can, however, present problems that the individual and family have never encountered before, and the family systems that are otherwise intact can appear threatened, with sufficient stress. Counseling for cancer related problem solving does not require 'personality change,' but does require a willingness to experiment with different ways of solving problems or dealing with stress.

A wide range of interventions may be employed in providing psychologic, emotional, and spiritual support to a woman with breast cancer and her social support network. In general, these interventions can focus on the individual patient, her family, or a group of breast cancer patients. With reasonable emotional support from their physicians, most women mobilize sufficient psychologic and spiritual resources within themselves and their existing social support networks to cope with the challenges presented by their disease. Zabora and Smith (1991) observed that accurate assessment of the entire family system is a significant task of the physician in oncology care:

> Accurate assessment that differentiates between dysfunctional family systems and adaptively impaired family systems must be

followed by effective intervention geared to the needs of either problem.

Support groups that emphasize emotional and social support are most useful for enhancing patients' coping skills and for providing emotional support to patients and family members. These groups vary widely in content and format—for example, some utilize a time-limited, psychoeducational approach in which different, specific topics are addressed at each meeting; others may have an "open-ended" format and focus each session on the particular concerns brought by the participants. Leadership of these groups likewise varies, although social workers and nurses are most frequently called upon to provide supervision. Individual counseling or family counseling is most often the intervention of choice when a patient experiences prolonged or acute emotional distress or exhibits behavior that indicates maladaptive coping patterns (e.g., alcohol or other substance abuse), family dysfunction, or mental illness.

The range of resources that may be required is large. The availability of particular services varies from community to community. In addition, each community's service providers have their own eligibility requirements and application procedures. Maintaining current information about these resources is a responsibility of the physician and other members of a patient's treatment team.

Key Stress Periods and Commonly Needed Resources

Period of Diagnosis

The diagnostic period begins at the time a woman first notices symptoms that require medical intervention, and it continues through the formulation of an initial treatment plan. Christ (1993) described this period, noting that

> For all patients, the diagnostic process initiates a confrontation with the reality of one's mortality, even if the biopsy or test results prove to be negative. When a cancer is diagnosed, patients describe feeling shocked, stunned and emotionally overwhelmed.

During this stage, *information* and *emotional support* are the primary needs. Patients need to assimilate a large amount of information so that they are able to make decisions about treatment options and must do so in a heightened state of psychologic arousal. Physicians must provide clinical information but can do so most effectively by recognizing that patients will inevitably experience difficulty in processing information that is given verbally and may have no skill in independently locating information about cancer and their treatment options. Thus, making available information in a variety of formats (written, audiovisual, oral) assists patients in assimilating sufficient information to arrive at an informed decision regarding treatment options. The information should not be limited to the clinical aspects of breast cancer but should include details about where diagnostic tests are performed, when test results can be expected, how patients obtain results, and the choices of settings in which treatment is rendered.

Emotional and psychologic support during this period is

usually provided by several members of the oncology treatment team. Social workers or nurses are often in a better position than physicians to devote the amount of time needed by each patient and her family members to express their feelings and to think through the information that they have been given. Patients who have successfully completed treatment may also serve as resources at this time, and programs that assign a trained volunteer to a newly diagnosed patient do exist. Spouses and family members of a patient also need emotional and psychologic support, although their coping tasks are different from those of the patient. Resources that extend this support to a patient's significant others enhance the patient's ability to move through the diagnostic stage in a timely manner and lessen the demand on the physician and his or her office staff to repeat the same information to several family members.

Treatment Period

Community resources are most intensively used during a patient's treatment period. During this period, the patient may require assistance in any or all of the areas outlined in the first section of this chapter. The patient experiences the physiologic effects of treatment, and, in many cases, the side effects significantly compromise the patient's quality of life and sense of personal control. The patient and her partner must adjust to alterations in the patient's body image as a result of surgery or of the side effects of chemotherapy. Numerous studies have found that women who have had mastectomies commonly report feelings of decreased attractiveness as a sexual partner and of a loss of femininity as well as a sense that they have been mutilated. Additionally, the partner of the woman may experience alterations in sexual image. These changes in perception may significantly alter the frequency and quality of sexual activity and thus can result in interpersonal distress (Cohen and Cordoba, 1983).

Practical matters such as getting to and from a treatment facility, reorganizing tasks of daily living, and coping with a reduction in personal or family income contribute to a patient's sense of being "out of control." Coping with treatment and its side effects are unknown territory for the patient, and she and her family frequently underestimate the magnitude of the change from a "normal routine" out of a desire to "normalize" the experience as much as possible. Changes that can be predicted by healthcare professionals (and about which they may have attempted to inform the patient) frequently are experienced as "surprises" by the patient (Cassileth et al., 1985). Community resources, on the other hand, are seldom organized to respond to "surprises" and may instead require lengthy periods for application and determination of eligibility for services. For example, in the community in which this author practices, several services that provide transportation for elderly and disabled persons are available. Each provider, however, requires that a patient complete an application process that includes written certification of disability by a physician and that typically lasts 3 to 4 weeks. Once the process has been completed, each provider requires at least 1 week's

advance notice to schedule the necessary transportation. Thus, this is a resource for which a breast cancer patient undergoing daily radiation therapy may technically be eligible, but one that cannot be accessed in a convenient manner.

A patient who is experiencing vocational or financial problems during treatment often does not initiate discussion of these issues with her physician. Patients may be perceived by healthcare professionals as "noncompliant," when in fact financial barriers prevent their full participation in treatment regimens. Physicians can be helpful in uncovering these problems by simply inquiring about other sources of stress in the patient's life (Hermann, 1992). Specific questions such as, Do you think you will have any problems keeping your appointments? often reveal additional areas in which assistance from community resources may be required.

Termination of Treatment

As the number of cancer survivors increases, healthcare professionals have recognized that termination of treatment represents a key stress period for the cancer patient. Whereas the needs of the patient during treatment are frequently for practical types of assistance and for managing acute emotional distress, the challenges of this period involve adaptation to cancer as a chronic illness. Although active disease is not present, the patient must integrate a ongoing follow-up with healthcare professionals with resumption of social, vocational, and recreational activities, all of which have been changed by her experience. Needs for transportation, lodging, and home healthcare normally diminish as the woman recovers from treatment. Emotional, psychologic, and spiritual needs gain prominence as the patient addresses the task of rehabilitation. These tasks, as described by Christ (1993), include (1) grieving losses; (2) coping with fears of recurrence; (3) coping with the stigma of cancer; (4) building a positive self-image with a new sense of self; (5) developing a sense of competence, mastery, and control; (6) continuing satisfying relationships; (7) regaining a sense of normalcy; and (8) integrating changes in values, goals, and priorities.

The information needed for a successful transition from breast cancer "patient" to breast cancer "survivor" changes with the termination of treatment. Questions about physiologic aspects of the disease and its treatment normally give way to questions about the experiences of other survivors. Support groups and periodic counseling are often the most useful means of meeting both the informational and emotional needs of patients during this period.

Recurrence and Advanced Disease

Women who experience a recurrence of breast cancer face the challenge of (1) obtaining and understanding complex information about their prognoses, (2) assessing the relative costs and benefits of treatment options, (3) mobilizing psychic and personal resources to support them through the resumption of treatment, and (4) organizing daily activities. Community resources accessed during the initial treatment period are likely to be called upon to resume services during the period of recurrence. Needs unique to this stage are usually additional referrals. What is most likely to be different at this stage is that patients must deal with feelings of guilt, failure, or hopelessness that may have been less intense or largely absent during the initial treatment period. Short-term individual or family counseling often helps patients to cope. Having faced the fact that standard treatments were not effective in eradicating cancer, the patients, their families, and their physicians are all challenged to maintain a hopeful attitude. Other spiritual needs, such as life review, the need for reconciliation with loved ones, and examination of one's (or a loved one's) life, gain prominence during this period.

Terminal Illness

The woman with advanced breast cancer enters the terminal phase when she refuses further treatment or when treatment begins to focus only on management of symptoms. During this period, the pattern and frequency of interpersonal contact between the patient and her physician changes. The patient frequently requires more intensive medication and psychosocial support, and the location of care shifts from the ambulatory setting to the patient's home. Specialized hospice programs employ an interdisciplinary team of professionals to meet the physical care needs of the patient and to prepare for her approaching death. The physician continues to be an important source of emotional support and information, but the frequency of direct, face-to-face communications about treatment between physician and patient decreases. Instead, the physician communicates primarily with family members and with hospice or home healthcare professionals.

Bereavement

At the time of the patient's death, the tasks facing her survivors are (1) accepting the reality of the loss, (2) experiencing the pain of grief, (3) adjusting to an environment that does not include the deceased, and (4) redirecting and reinvesting emotional energy in other relationships (Christ, 1993). The needs of the patient's survivors are most often addressed by counseling and social service agencies that are outside the healthcare system, although an increasing number of comprehensive cancer care centers have begun to offer time-limited services through systematic bereavement programs. Survivors who have received services through hospice programs or who have participated in support groups often continue their linkage with these community resources for a period of up to 1 year following the death of the patient.

CONSTRUCTING A "RESOURCE MAP" FOR SERVICES IN THE COMMUNITY

Physicians who practice in urban areas or in regional cancer treatment centers most often have access to the services of a social worker or nurse who specializes in oncology. These members of the healthcare team generally assume the responsibility for psychosocial assessment and treatment planning. Physicians who lack access to these professionals must locate other resources to meet the needs of the patient and her family. National organizations such as the American Cancer Society* and the Cancer Information Service† of the National Cancer Institute provide an entry point by identifying the local contacts for patient assistance programs available in a particular physician's area. A number of national organizations that provide services tailored to the needs and concerns of women with breast cancer have become active in recent years. The American Cancer Society or Cancer Information Service can also provide information about these organizations (see Appendix to this chapter).

Information about resources for assistance with financial concerns can be obtained from the Social Security Administration (listed under "U.S. Government" in the telephone book) or from county or state offices that administer a state's medical assistance benefits. Agencies that provide transportation, lodging, or services designed to obviate hospitalization of a person with chronic illness can often be located by contacting agencies that provide services to the elderly and disabled. In sparsely populated areas, the number of community resources may be limited. In these areas, the physician must obtain information about resources to which patients may be referred.

In large urban areas, the number of independent agencies that focus specifically on providing emotional and psychologic support to the cancer patient is growing. Many of these agencies offer support groups and a blend of individual, group, and family counseling services. They operate outside the traditional healthcare system, following the model of counseling or social service agencies. Practitioners in rural areas find fewer counseling resources devoted specifically to the oncology patient than do practitioners in urban areas; however, they may have access to other mental healthcare agencies.

The provision of spiritual care is often seen as the purview of the patient's particular faith community, but clergy are often not knowledgeable about cancer. Hospital chaplains may be more able to assist the patient and her family by virtue of their familiarity with issues related to life-threatening illnesses. In rural areas, churches often provide the practical assistance that is provided by community agencies in large urban areas. Spiritual leaders in rural areas can often provide rural physicians with information on the help that is available in the community.

---

* American Cancer Society, National Office, 1599 Clifton Road NE, Atlanta, GA 30329-4251.

† Cancer Information Service may be reached at 1-800-4-CANCER.

References

Cassileth, B., Lusk, E., Bodenheimer, B., et al.: Chemotherapeutic toxicity: The relationship between patients' pretreatment expectations and post-treatment results. Am. J. Clin. Oncol., 8:419–425, 1985.

Christ, G.: Psychosocial tasks throughout the cancer experience. *In* Stearns, N. M., Lauria, M. M., Hermann, J. F., et al. (Eds.): Oncology Social Work. Atlanta, GA, American Cancer Society, 1993, pp. 79–99.

Cohen, J., and Cordoba, C.: Psychologic, social and economic aspects of cancer. *In* Nyhuys, L. (Ed.): Surgery Annual, 15. Norwalk, CT, Appleton-Century-Crofts, 1983, pp. 99–112.

Hermann, J.: The prevention of psychosocial distress: The physician's opportunity. Curr. Probl. Cancer, 16:379–391, 1992.

McDaniel, M. A., Hepworth, J., and Doherty, W. J.: The new prescription for family health care. Family Therapy Network, 17:19–25, 1993.

Zabora, J. R., and Smith, E. D.: Family dysfunction and the cancer patient: Early recognition and intervention. Oncology, 12:31–38, 1991.

National and Community Resources for Patients with Breast Cancer

American Cancer Society, Inc.
1599 Clifton Road NE
Atlanta, GA 30329-4251
tel.: 1-800-ACS-2345

Established in 1913, this large volunteer organization offers programs of service, education, and research. It has 57 state-level divisions (see Appendix II). In many areas, programs lend equipment and provide transportation services for patients. Among the programs are the following:

Cancer Response System (1-800-ACS-2345): An information resource for individuals diagnosed with or concerned about cancer.

Reach to Recovery: A volunteer visitation program for patients newly treated for breast cancer. Breast cancer survivors supply helpful information on a face-to-face basis.

Reach to Recovery II: A volunteer visitation program for women with recurrent breast cancer.

Look Good...Feel Better: A cosmetology program for women undergoing cancer treatment, in particular chemotherapy, to improve their appearance and sense of well-being.

I Can Cope: Group sessions to share information on cancer with patients and their families.

Road to Recovery: Volunteers provide transportation for patients having treatment at local hospitals and clinics.

The National Cancer Institute
Bethesda, MD
Cancer Information Service
Phone: 1-301-496-5223

This national government center provides on request a wide variety of informational materials about the diagnosis and treatment of breast cancer. Other services that it offers include the following:

PDQ: A computer access program that makes available a list of physicians who are specialists in oncology and of hospitals with cancer programs in each locality.

Combined Health Information Database (CHID): A computer access program that provides information to cancer patients on resources and contact persons at cancer centers.

A Clinical Center: Individuals with cancer-related problems on which research is being conducted may be eligible for treatment at this center.

Breast Cancer Advisory Center
P. O. Box 224
Kensington, MD 20895

Founded in 1975 as a service group for women with breast cancer, this agency makes referrals, provides information, and supports a library on breast cancer–related issues.

National Alliance of Breast Cancer Organizations (NABCO)
2nd Floor
1180 Avenue of the Americas
New York, NY 10036
tel.: 1-212-719-0154

This organization was established as a resource for persons concerned about breast cancer. It is a public advocate for breast cancer patients in matters concerning insurance coverage and healthcare legislation.

Susan G. Komen Breast Cancer Foundation
5005 LBJ, Suite 730
Dallas, TX 75244
tel.: 1-800 IM AWARE

Founded in 1982 as a breast cancer patient advocacy organization. Activities include providing the public with information on breast cancer, campaigning for legislative reform in the area of patient rights, and supporting breast cancer research.

Y-ME National Organization for Breast Cancer Information and Support
212 W. Van Buren St.
4th Floor
Chicago, IL 60607-3908
tel.: 1-312-986-8338 or 1-800-221-2141

Founded in 1978, this organization offers peer support and information to women with breast cancer or who think that they might have breast cancer. It offers counseling and referral service and maintains a library on breast cancer–related issues.

Medicare
Medicare pays for a screening mammogram at 2-year intervals for women 65 years of age or older.

Chartered Divisions of the American Cancer Society, Inc.

Alabama Division, Inc.
504 Brookwood Boulevard
Homewood, AL 35209
1-(205)-879-2242

Alaska Division, Inc.
406 West Fireweed Lane
Anchorage, AK 99503
1-(907)-277-8696

Arizona Division, Inc.
2929 East Thomas Road
Phoenix, AZ 85016
1-(602)-224-0524

Arkansas Division, Inc.
901 North University
Little Rock, AR 72207
1-(501)-664-3480

California Division, Inc.
1710 Webster Street
Oakland, CA 94612
1-(510)-893-7900

Colorado Division, Inc.
2255 South Oneida
Denver, CO 80224
1-(303)-758-2030

Connecticut Division, Inc.
Barnes Park South
14 Village Lane
Wallingford, CT 06492
1-(203)-265-7161

Delaware Division, Inc.
92 Read's Way
New Castle, DE 19720
1-(302)-324-4227

District of Columbia Division, Inc.
1875 Connecticut Avenue, N.W.
Washington, DC 20009
1-(202)-483-2600

Florida Division, Inc.
3709 West Jetton Avenue
Tampa, FL 33629-5146
1-(813)-253-0541

Georgia Division, Inc.
46 Fifth Street, NE
Atlanta, GA 30308
1-(404)-892-0026

Hawaii Pacific Division, Inc.
Community Services Center Bldg.
200 North Vineyard Boulevard
Honolulu, HI 96817
1-(808)-531-1662

Idaho Division, Inc.
2676 Vista Avenue
Boise, ID 83705
1-(208)-343-4609

Illinois Division, Inc.
77 East Monroe
Chicago, IL 60603
1-(312)-641-6150

Indiana Division, Inc.
8730 Commerce Park Place
Indianapolis, IN 46268
1-(317)-872-4432

Iowa Division, Inc.
8364 Hickman Road
Des Moines, IA 50325
1-(515)-253-0147

Kansas Division, Inc.
1315 SW Arrowhead Road
Topeka, KS 66604
1-(913)-273-4114

Kentucky Division, Inc.
701 West Muhammad Ali Blvd.
Louisville, KY 40201-1807
1-(502)-584-6782

Louisiana Division, Inc.
Fidelity Homestead Bldg.
837 Gravier Street
New Orleans, LA 70112-1509
1-(504)-523-2029

Maine Division, Inc.
52 Federal Street
Brunswick, ME 04011
1-(207)-729-3339

Maryland Division, Inc.
8219 Town Center Drive
Baltimore, MD 21236-0026
1-(410)-931-6868

Massachusetts Division, Inc.
247 Commonwealth Avenue
Boston, MA 02116
1-(617)-267-2650

Michigan Division, Inc.
1205 East Saginaw Street
Lansing, MI 48906
1-(517)-371-2920

Minnesota Division, Inc.
3316 West 66th Street
Minneapolis, MN 55435
1-(612)-925-2772

Mississippi Division, Inc.
1380 Livingston Lane
Lakeover Office Park
Jackson, MS 39213
1-(601)-362-8874

Missouri Division, Inc.
3322 American Avenue
Jefferson City, MO 65102
1-(314)-893-4800

Montana Division, Inc.
17 North 26th
Billings, MT 59101
1-(406)-252-7111

Nebraska Division, Inc.
8502 West Center Road
Omaha, NE 68124-5255
1-(402)-393-5800

Nevada Division, Inc.
1325 East Harmon
Las Vegas, NV 89119
1-(702)-798-6857

New Hampshire Division, Inc.
360 Route 101, Unit 501
Bedford, NH 03110-5032
1-(613)-472-8899

New Jersey Division, Inc.
2600 US Highway 1
North Brunswick, NJ 08902
1-(908)-297-8000

New Mexico Division, Inc.
5800 Lomas Blvd., NE
Albuquerque, NM 87110
1-(505)-260-2105

New York State Division, Inc.
6725 Lyons Street
East Syracuse, NY 13057
1-(315)-437-7025

□ **Long Island Division, Inc.**
75 Davids Drive
Hauppauge, NY 11788
1-(516)-436-7070

□ **New York City Division, Inc.**
19 West 56th Street
New York, NY 10019
1-(212)-586-8700

□ **Queens Division, Inc.**
112-25 Queens Boulevard
Forest Hills, NY 11375
1-(718)-263-2224

□ **Westchester Division, Inc.**
30 Glenn Street
White Plains, NY 10603
1-(914)-949-4800

North Carolina Division, Inc.
11 South Boylan Avenue
Raleigh, NC 27603
1-(919)-834-8463

North Dakota Division, Inc.
123 Roberts Street
Fargo, ND 58102
1-(701)-232-1385

Ohio Division, Inc.
5555 Frantz Road
Dublin, OH 43017
1-(614)-889-9565

Oklahoma Division, Inc.
3000 United Founders Blvd.
Oklahoma City, OK 73112
1-(405)-843-9888

Oregon Division, Inc.
0330 SW Curry
Portland, OR 97201
1-(503)-295-6422

Pennsylvania Division, Inc.
Route 422 & Sipe Avenue
Hershey, PA 17033-0897
1-(717)-533-6144

□ **Philadelphia Division, Inc.**
1422 Chestnut Street
Philadelphia, PA 19102
1-(215)-665-2900

Puerto Rico Division, Inc.
Calle Alverio #577,
Esquina Sargento Medina,
Hato Rey, PR 00918
1-(809)-764-2295

Rhode Island Division, Inc.
400 Main Street
Pawtucket, RI 02860
1-(401)-722-8480

South Carolina Division, Inc.
128 Stonemark Lane
Columbia, SC 29210
1-(803)-750-1693

South Dakota Division, Inc.
4101 Carnegie Place
Sioux Falls, SD 57106-2322
1-(605)-361-8277

Tennessee Division, Inc.
1315 Eighth Avenue, South
Nashville, TN 37203
1-(615)-255-1227

Texas Division, Inc.
2433 Ridgepoint Drive
Austin, TX 78754
1-(512)-928-2262

Utah Division, Inc.
941 East 3300 S.
Salt Lake City, UT 84106
1-(801)-322-0431

Vermont Division, Inc.
13 Loomis Street
Montpelier, VT 05602
1-(802)-233-2348

Virginia Division, Inc.
4240 Park Place Court
Glen Allen, VA 23060
1-(804)-527-3700

Washington Division, Inc.
2120 First Avenue North
Seattle, WA 98109-1140
1-(206)-283-1152

West Virginia Division, Inc.
2428 Kanawha Boulevard East
Charleston, WV 25311
1-(304)-344-3611

Wisconsin Division, Inc.
N19 W24350 Riverwood Drive
Pewaukee, WI 53072-0902
1-(608)-249-0487

Wyoming Division, Inc.
2222 House Avenue
Cheyenne, WY 82001
1-(307)-638-3331

Medical Malpractice Liability for Errors in Breast Cancer Diagnosis and Treatment

Randal N. Arnold
Russell A. Klingaman

Allegations of failure to properly diagnose and treat breast cancer comprise a significant proportion of all medical malpractice claims. Familiarity with the types of malpractice cases that have resulted in settlements and damage awards for the plaintiff can alert the clinician to diagnostic pitfalls and contribute to improvement in the quality of patient care. It can also serve to illustrate the unrealistic expectations of the public that mammography screening and appropriate early intervention can prevent all deaths from breast cancer. This chapter analyzes the available data on jury verdicts and settlements in malpractice cases arising from breast cancer diagnosis and treatment, provides an overview of the theories of legal liability that may be applied in such cases, and offers recommendations to physicians for minimizing malpractice liability exposure.

Medical malpractice is a civil tort arising from the breach of a duty owed by a physician to a patient. Depending on the circumstances, such claims may be governed by federal or state law, or by a combination of both. There is wide variation among the states on such crucial issues as statutes of limitation, presuit mediation procedures, limitation of damage awards, availability of punitive damages, and insurance coverage, to name only a few. A comprehensive review of these issues on a state-by-state basis is beyond the scope of this chapter. Specific questions should be referred to competent counsel in the appropriate jurisdiction.

SETTLEMENTS AND VERDICTS

Medical Malpractice Claims in General

There is no comprehensive database that tracks medical malpractice claims in the United States. Caution must therefore be used in evaluating various reports on the frequency and severity of such claims, because different sources use different assumptions, numerical bases, and definitions. Despite these limitations, it can generally be said that, from the 1970s until the mid-1980s, claim frequency and award severity increased sharply and continuously. One study indicates that between 1975 and 1985 malpractice claims more than doubled (Jacobson, 1989). The average verdict in medical malpractice cases has likewise drastically in-

creased (Nye et al., 1988). Malpractice verdicts increased at nearly twice the rate of the consumer price index between 1975 and 1984 (Danzon, 1985). The steady increase in claims moderated in the late 1980s and early 1990s. Insurance industry sources report a recent rise in claim frequency, which is largely attributable to a rise in claims alleging failure to diagnose, especially against primary care physicians (Snyder, 1994).

A study by one large medical malpractice insurance carrier of its overall claims experience in 1989 and 1990 indicated that diagnostic issues accounted for the highest percentage (27.4%) of medical liability costs and for the largest number of claims reported. Failure to diagnose cancer was the most frequent diagnostic failure alleged, and accounted for 31% of the cost of these claims. Failure to diagnose cancer was second among all categories of claims; only surgical and postoperative complications ranked higher (St. Paul Fire and Marine, 1991). A similar review of medical malpractice claims paid on behalf of primary care physicians in Florida in 1987 listed failure to diagnose cancer as the single most common category of claim, and failure to diagnose breast cancer was reported most often (Dewar et al., 1992).

It is important to keep in mind that data on "average" medical malpractice awards reflect a skewed distribution, for while multimillion dollar verdicts make up only a small fraction of total awards, they have a large impact on the average award (Peterson, 1987). Many malpractice claims are settled with no payment or modest payments, and defendants win a majority of the litigated cases (Jacobson, 1989). One survey indicates that the defendant prevailed in 81% of the litigated cases (Hatch, 1989). Other studies report similar findings (Jacobson, 1989). In urban areas, plaintiffs win a higher percentage of medical malpractice verdicts. One report by the Rand Corporation showed that plaintiffs in San Francisco and Cook County, Illinois (Chicago) prevailed at a rate of approximately 50% (Peterson, 1987).

No overview of medical malpractice liability compensation would be complete without noting reports that suggest that only a small proportion of the potentially compensable incidents of medical negligence result in malpractice claims. One widely cited study indicates that only one in 10 legitimate malpractice cases reaches the tort system

(Mills, 1977). The Harvard Medical Practice Study, commissioned by the New York State Department of Health and based on a review of over 31,000 hospital records, reached similar conclusions. The study found that only 1.5% of patients identified as having suffered an adverse event due to medical negligence filed a malpractice claim. The study's authors concluded that medical malpractice litigation infrequently compensates patients injured by medical negligence, and rarely identifies providers and holds them accountable for substandard care (Localio et al., 1991).

Breast Cancer Claims

The largest single study of breast cancer malpractice claims was performed by the Physician Insurers Association of America (PIAA, 1990). Data was compiled regarding malpractice claims reported to 21 PIAA member companies insuring nearly 96,000 physicians. The study identified and analyzed 273 paid claims involving an alleged delay in the diagnosis of breast cancer. These claims accounted for a total indemnity payment of $60.5 million, averaging $221,524 per claim (range $1000 to $2 million).

Women younger than 50 years represented 69% of claimants and 84% of indemnity dollars paid. Women under 40 comprised 40% of claimants and 58% of paid indemnity. These findings may seem surprising in view of the fact that breast cancer is far more common in older patients. The predominance of younger women among malpractice plaintiffs reflects the difficulty of diagnosing breast cancer in younger women, who have denser breast tissue and whose physicians are less likely to suspect the disease. It may also reflect the fact that damage awards are generally higher for younger women, making the claims of younger women more economically appealing to plaintiffs' attorneys. Younger claimants generally receive larger awards because they have been deprived of a larger portion of their average life expectancy (and therefore of their expected income) and also because younger women are more likely to be survived by minor children.

In the PIAA study 69% of the cases involved a lesion that was first found by the patient. Physicians were surveyed for their evaluation of the reason for delay in diagnosis. The physician's failure to be impressed by the physical findings at examination was the most commonly reported explanation for delay, suggesting that greater attention may need to be paid when the patient insists that a physical abnormality is present that cannot be palpated by the physician. Patients had negative or equivocal mammograms in 49% of the PIAA claims. The study authors pointed out that false negative or equivocal mammograms occur more frequently in patients under 40, and suggest that a biopsy should follow any suspicious findings.

The PIAA study found no correlation between length of delay and average payment value. A delay in diagnosis of less than 6 months was alleged in 25% of the paid claims, and of less than a year in 56% of claims. These data suggest the difficulty of defending breast cancer claims with scientific evidence that the delay made no significant difference in the patient's prognosis.

Many of the observations of the PIAA study have been borne out by other examinations of claim and lawsuit data. Kern (1992) studied 45 breast cancer malpractice cases tried to verdict in 20 states between 1971 and 1990. Of the 21 claimants whose age could be identified, 76% were younger than 50 years and 58% younger than 40. As in the PIAA study, most patients found the lesion first, the most common presenting complaint to the physician being a painless mass. The diagnostic workup in 51% of the cases was limited to visual observation and physical examination (i.e., no mammogram). Only 44% of patients had mammograms. Of the mammograms that were performed, 80% were read as normal.

The mean delay in diagnosis in Kern's cases was 15 months, and 67% of patients had a definitive diagnosis made within 1 year of their initial presentation. Kern found no statistically significant correlation between the length of delay in diagnosis and advancing tumor-node-metastasis (TNM) stage or tumor size at final diagnosis.

Average payment per case in the Kern group was $675,532 (range of $150,000 to $3,080,000). Kern found that the largest payments were made to the youngest patients, pregnant patients, patients who experienced the longest delay in diagnosis, and patients from the northeastern United States. Kern's average jury verdict ($675,532) is substantially higher than the average claim payment reported in the PIAA study ($221,524). This reflects the fact that Kern studied only cases that went to trial, whereas the PIAA study focused on insurers' claim files, many of which were presumably settled prior to trial.

A series of 34 cases selected from the *New York Jury Verdict Reporter* between 1985 and 1991 was studied by Mitnick and coworkers (1993). Their findings were strikingly similar to those reported by Kern. Patient age was less than 50 in 76% of cases. Palpable masses were present in 94% of cases, and 50% had a diagnostic work-up that did not include a mammogram. Thirty-eight per cent of cases included a mammogram which was read as normal or as fibrocystic changes.

A survey of breast cancer cases recorded in the Lexis Legal Database (Lexis-Nexis, Mead Data Central, Dayton, OH) suggests that average payments continue to rise. From this database 158 breast cancer malpractice cases were identified from 1987 to 1993, consisting of 119 jury verdicts and 39 settlements. Verdicts for the defendant were recorded in 56.3% (67 of 119) of cases. Verdict awards for the plaintiff averaged $889,000. Payments to plaintiffs in settlements averaged $595,000. The verdict and settlement studies indicate that gynecologists are the most frequent targets of breast cancer malpractice claims, followed by family practice physicians/internists and surgeons.

THE ELEMENTS OF A MEDICAL MALPRACTICE CLAIM

The plaintiff in a medical malpractice action has the burden of proving four basic elements: (1) that the physician owed a duty to the patient arising out of a physician-patient relationship, (2) that the physician breached the duty, (3) that the breach in duty was the proximate cause of injury to the patient, and (4) that ascertainable damages resulted. Though a physician's duty to a patient is characterized differently in different jurisdictions, the following formulation is typical: The physician has a duty to "exercise that degree of care, knowledge, and skill ordinarily possessed and exercised by the average member of the profession practicing in that physician's field under the same or similar circumstances" (*Borgren v. United States,* 716 F. Supp. 1378, 1381 [D. Kan. 1989]). If the defendant physician is a specialist in a particular medical field, he or she is generally held to the higher standard of a specialist rather than that of a general practitioner (*Morrison v. Stallworth,* 326 S.E.2d 387, 391 [N.C. 1985]). For example, a radiation oncologist would be held to the standard of care of the "average" radiation oncologist, rather than that of the average radiologist or the average physician.

Each of the elements of a malpractice claim must be proved "to a reasonable certainty by the greater weight of the credible evidence." This is sometimes referred to as the preponderance of the evidence standard and is the lowest burden of proof imposed upon litigants. By contrast, criminal cases must be proved beyond a reasonable doubt. Civil cases involving penal aspects or criminal type behavior such as fraud, must be proved by "clear and convincing" evidence, sometimes called the *middle burden of proof.* The burden of proof in a medical malpractice case is sometimes referred to as a *more likely than not* standard, meaning that the plaintiff need only establish a greater than 50% probability that a given claim is true (Wis. J.I. Civil 200, 1991).

Duty or Standard of Care: Some Appellate and Trial Court Decisions

Knowing that one has a general legal duty to exercise the degree of care, knowledge, and skill of the average physician is of little practical value to the clinician in determining how to render appropriate patient care. The specific duties that constitute average care are established on a case-by-case basis through the testimony of expert witnesses, and in some instances through texts and learned treatises. It is the job of the finder of fact in each case, usually the jury, to determine what the standard of care is and whether it was met by the defendant. Since trial court decisions have no binding precedential effect, it is difficult to draw conclusions from them about the specific duties of a physician. Appellate court decisions, which have binding precedential effect within the court's geographic jurisdiction, sometimes contain statements regarding a physician's duty in particular circumstances, though these statements tend to be broad and general, affording scant guidance in real-life situations. It is nevertheless highly instructive to review trial and appellate court decisions to understand the range of conduct that is alleged to constitute malpractice and to see how the facts of specific cases are translated into generic statements of duty. This section contains a discussion of general duties that have been identified in appellate breast cancer malpractice cases, supplemented by case histories taken from verdict and settlement reports.

Allegations of diagnostic errors resulting in delayed treatment constitute the most frequent basis for breast can-

cer malpractice claims. It has generally been said that a physician has a duty to avail himself or herself of all available scientific means and facilities to aid in the diagnosis of cancer (*Wilkinson v. Vesey,* 295 A.2d 676, 683 [R.I. 1972]). Encompassed within the duty of proper diagnosis is the duty to take a complete history from the patient (*Beckom v. United States,* 584 F. Supp. 1471, 1478 [N.D.N.Y. 1984]). Physicians also have a duty to properly perform visual examination and palpation of breasts (*Livengood v. Kerr,* 391 S.E.2d 371, 375 [W.V.a. 1990]; *Beckom,* 584 F. Supp. at 1478). There is also a duty to direct the patient to return for follow-up examination within an appropriate period (*Beckom,* 584 F. Supp. at 1478, *Livengood,* 391 S.E.2d at 375).

The examination must be geared to the specific complaint of the patient (*Hernandez v. United States,* 636 F.2d 704, 707–08 [D.C. Cir. 1980]). Physicians have a duty to make an effort to determine the cause of any changes in a breast noticed by the patient (*Truan v. Smith,* 578 S.W.2d 73, 76 [Tenn. 1979]). A physician who discovers a persistent lump should not allow it to continue undiagnosed without a biopsy, even in the face of a negative mammogram (*DeBurkarte v. Louvar,* 393 N.W.2d 131, 133 [Iowa 1986]).

Diagnostic errors can be alleged at virtually any stage in the valuative process, as the following case histories show.

■

Case History 1

The plaintiff underwent routine breast cancer screening. The defendant radiologist read the mammogram as negative. Twenty-three months after the earlier screening, the plaintiff was sent a reminder notice for another routine mammogram. Thereafter, plaintiff scheduled an appointment with a different radiologist in her area. The second mammogram revealed a 1.5-cm malignant mass. Plaintiff alleged that the defendant radiologist failed to diagnose breast cancer at the initial screening. The defendant denied any negligence and contended that he read the mammogram to the best of his judgment. The jury found for the plaintiff and awarded $275,000 in damages (*Gracias-Frias v. McKnight, M.D.,* Case No. 920551 [Cir. Ct. VA, July, 1993] [LRP Pub. No. 117418]).

■

Case History 2

The patient-plaintiff claimed that mammograms were performed for several years without noticing changes indicating the need for a biopsy. The plaintiff alleged that, had a biopsy been performed earlier, her chances for disease-free survival would have been better. The jury found for the plaintiff and awarded $900,000 in damages (*Borgren v. United States,* Case No. 87-2191-S [D.C. Kansas, June, 1989] [LRP Pub. No. 48589]).

■

Case History 3

The plaintiff, a 49-year-old woman, sought treatment for a lump in her breast. She alleged that the defendant negligently failed to perform a mammogram. The defendant contended that the breast showed no signs of abnormalities and that no bump was palpable. The jury found for the plaintiff and awarded $1 million in damages (*Doe v. Roe*, Case No. L-016902-85 [Super. Ct. N.J., April, 1987] [LRP Pub. No. 0013158]).

Case History 4

Plaintiff, a 29-year-old woman, presented to the defendant physician complaining of a lump in her breast. A mammogram with two views was taken but was found to be inconclusive owing to the density of the breast tissue. When the patient returned eight months later for her next visit, breast cancer was diagnosed which had metastasized to her brain. The plaintiff alleged that ultrasonography should have been performed because the mammogram was inconclusive and because the patient had a family history of breast cancer. Plaintiff also alleged that the defendant was negligent for assuring the patient that the lump was normal. The jury found for the plaintiff and awarded $263,531 in damages (*McDonald v. Garfield, M.D.*, Case No. 749 [Cir. Ct. PA, April, 1991] [LRP Pub. No. 73651]).

Case History 5

The plaintiff, a 35-year-old woman, presented to her gynecologist with a small lump in her right breast in January 1990. A mammogram was performed immediately and was read as negative. Several months later, plaintiff's gynecologist referred her to a general surgeon. The surgeon saw the plaintiff in May 1990 and attempted to aspirate the cyst. He did not obtain any fluid and asked the plaintiff to return in July 1990. He examined the lump again in July and instructed the plaintiff to return in October. Plaintiff did not return for the October visit. Thereafter, in March 1991, she noticed a lump underneath her right arm. She was referred to a breast surgeon, who immediately performed needle aspiration. A pathologist reviewed the results and determined that the plaintiff had Stage II metastatic breast cancer. The plaintiff alleged that the defendant surgeon should have considered a core needle or incisional biopsy in May 1990 when he encountered a hard, painful lump. Plaintiff also alleged that the defendant should have considered the fact that she had a family history of breast cancer. Defendant contended that the plaintiff was at fault for not returning for the October 1990 appointment. The jury found for the plaintiff and awarded damages of $300,000. Because the plaintiff was found to be 35% at fault, the award was reduced to $195,000 (*Warren v. Briggs*, No. 92-72-31 [Cir. Ct. Miss. 1993]).

In addition to the duties associated with diagnosis, a physician has the duty to advise the breast cancer patient to consult with a specialist or with a physician qualified in a method of treatment that the physician is not competent to give, if the patient might enjoy better results by such a referral (*Harris v. Gallaher*, 375 A.2d 456 [Del. 1977]). A gynecologist has been held to have a duty to refer a patient with a complaint of breast soreness to a surgeon or to a radiologist for mammography (*Grippe v. Momtazee*, 705 S.W.2d 551, 553 [Mo. App. 1986]). A physician who does no more than advise a patient to consult a specialist normally is not liable for any negligence by the recommended

physician absent a showing of a partnership or employment relationship between the physicians. After a referral to a surgeon, the operating physician, not the referring physician, has the obligation to provide non-negligent care and to explain the risks of treatment to the patient.

When the physician has a duty to refer, the referral must be done as quickly and efficiently as the circumstances may require (*Harris v. Gallaher*, 375 A.2d 456 [Del. 1977]). The physician may be liable for referring the patient to another physician who the original physician knows or should have known cannot provide the particular type of care needed. The original or referring physician may also have a continuing duty to supervise the care of the patient, especially if the referral is for a limited purpose (*Harris v. Gallaher*, 375 A.2d 456 [Del. 1977]).

A physician who prescribes or administers drugs to a breast cancer patient is required to use reasonable skill and care for the safety and well-being of the patient. Printed literature from the manufacturer of the drug regarding its proper use, limitations, and possible ill effects may be considered as objective evidence as to the applicable standard of care for the treating physician (*Mulder v. Parke, Davis & Co.*, 181 N.W.2d 882 [Minn. 1970]). A showing of departure from the warnings or recommendations of the manufacturer is evidence of the physician's negligence. To avoid liability, the physician must be able to justify such a departure (*DaRoca v. St. Bernard General Hosp.*, 347 So. 2d 933 [La. App. 1977]).

Physicians have a duty to use radiation therapy properly in the treatment of breast cancer. This includes the duty to avoid exposing a patient to an excessive dose of radiation or otherwise causing harm (e.g., from overlap of a dual-beam radiation field) (*Davis v. Moran*, 735 P.2d 1014, 1016 [Idaho 1987]).

Associated with the duty of proper treatment is the duty to continue attention to the breast cancer patient for so long as the patient requires it (*Glicklich v. Spievack*, 452 N.E.2d 287, 290 n.1 [Mass. App. 1983]). A physician's responsibility to a regular patient who continues under the physician's care for a particular ailment is not limited to the periods when the patient is in the physician's presence (*Ferrell v. Geigler*, 505 N.E.2d 137, 140 [Ind. App. 1987]). Breach of this duty constitutes abandonment. Abandonment is based on the severance of the professional relationship without notice, when some medical attention still is needed. There is no abandonment if a substitute physician is provided or if the patient is referred to another physician or a medical facility. Furthermore, there is no abandonment if the physician-patient relationship is terminated by mutual consent.

Although many breast cancer malpractice actions involve allegations that surgery was performed negligently, claims have also been made that no surgery should have been performed at all (i.e., that the physician was negligent for performing unnecessary surgery). A claim that surgery was unnecessary may be based upon evidence that surgery was contraindicated and not in accord with accepted medical practice in light of the nature of the patient's symptoms, or evidence that surgery should not have been performed without sufficient prior nonsurgical tests (*Davis v. Caldwell*, 429 N.E.2d 741 [N.Y. 1981]). Similarly, an unnecessary surgery claim may be based on the physician's incorrect diagnosis of a condition that subjected the patient to surgery that was later discovered to be unnecessary. Unnecessary surgery claims have also been based on allegations that the physician failed to properly inform the patient of the risks of the surgical procedure and the alternative nonsurgical procedures available (*Goodard v. Hickman*, 685 P.2d 530 [Utah 1984]). Finally, the claim may be that the surgery performed was too radical.

Case History 6

The defendant surgeon removed the breast of a 58-year-old woman. The plaintiff alleged that the surgery was unnecessary because the pathology reports of a needle biopsy were negative for breast cancer. The defendant presented evidence that the plaintiff refused to have an open biopsy, thus prohibiting him from making the correct diagnosis. The jury found for the plaintiff and awarded $250,000 in damages (*Berndt v. Tauber, M.D.*, Case No. 11888 [Cir. Ct. VA, June, 1988] [LRP Pub. No. 43896]).

Case History 7

The defendant physician performed a bilateral subcutaneous mastectomy on the plaintiff, a 35-year-old woman. The plaintiff maintained that the surgery was not necessary because she was not at high risk for breast cancer. The plaintiff also alleged that the defendant had failed to obtain her informed consent. The defendant contended that he performed the surgery to prevent breast cancer. The jury found for the plaintiff and awarded $150,000 in damages (*Aprile v. Ellenby, M.D., et al.*, Case No. 83-6348-CA-10 [Cir. Ct. FL, December, 1987] [LRP Pub. No. 24246]).

Case History 8

The plaintiff, a 42-year-old woman, noticed a lump on the lateral side of her left breast. A general surgeon recommended a mammogram and a biopsy. The general surgeon recommended that the plaintiff see a plastic surgeon for the biopsy because she desired a good cosmetic result. Instead of performing a biopsy, the plastic surgeon performed a bilateral subcutaneous mastectomy with submuscular implants. Plaintiff brought a medical malpractice action against the plastic surgeon, alleging that the surgery was unnecessary and of poor quality. Plaintiff also alleged that there was no informed consent. Defendants contended that the surgery was required because plaintiff was cancerphobic and at high risk for cancer. Defendant also contended the surgery was a prophylactic measure to prevent the development of breast cancer. The jury found for the plaintiff and awarded $213,000 in damages. (*Foley v. Plastic Surgery Associates Medical Group, Inc.*, Case No. NWC-06153 [Super. Ct. Cal. June 7, 1989]).

Establishing the Standard of Care: General Requirement of Expert Testimony

Expert testimony is generally required to establish the standard of care and the physician's departure from that standard (*Francisco v. Parchment Medical Clinic*, 285 N.W.2d 39, 40 [Mich. 1979]; *Henning v. Parsons*, 623 P.2d 574 [N.M. App. 1981]). This is because the standard of care against which the conduct of physicians is measured is a matter peculiarly within the knowledge of experts and beyond the scope of lay persons. In most cases this testimony comes from expert witnesses not connected with the plaintiff's care who are hired by the parties to review the case and render opinions about the appropriateness of the defendant's care (*Dettmann v. Flanary*, 273 N.W.2d 348, 354 [Wis. 1979]). Expert testimony may also come from the defendant or other treating doctors and experts. A malpractice action is usually dismissed if the patient cannot present expert testimony that a violation of the applicable standard of care occurred (*Caputo v. Taylor*, 403 So.2d 551 [Fla. App. 1981]).

The expert witness must establish familiarity with the methods of customary and proper medical diagnosis and treatment in that or a similar community. So long as the witness is a doctor of medicine, most jurisdictions hold that the expert need not be a specialist in the same field as the defendant (*Morrison v. Stallworth*, 326 S.E.2d 387, 391 [N.C. App. 1985]). In other words, a specialist may testify to the standard of care of a general practitioner or a different specialist as long as the witness is knowledgeable about the standard of care (*Ives v. Redford*, 252 S.E.2d 315 [Va. 1979]). Expert testimony is not necessarily limited to expert physicians. Qualified nonphysician experts may also be permitted to testify in certain circumstances. The question of whether a witness qualifies as an expert is a discretionary matter for the trial judge.

Evidence of the applicable standard of care may often be provided by the testimony of the defendant physician (*Beckom v. United States*, 584 F. Supp. 1471, 1478 n.6 [N.D.N.Y. 1984]). It is generally accepted that the testimony of the defendant may serve to prove the standard of care by which the defendant's treatment is to be judged (*Wilkinson v. Vesey*, 295 A.2d 676, 682 [R.I. 1972]). In a few jurisdictions, evidence as to the applicable standard of care may be provided through the introduction of medical treatises. It has been said that the medical profession may not set its own standards of care or conduct, which is a matter for the courts or the legislature (*Helling v. Carey*, 83 Wash. 2d 514, 519 P.2d 981 [1974]).

Although the general rule is that expert testimony is necessary to establish the standard of care, the courts have held that, where the negligence is sufficiently obvious as to lie within the common knowledge of a lay person, expert testimony is not required (*Wilkinson v. Vesey*, 295 A.2d 676, 682 [R.I. 1972]). The so-called common knowledge exception applies where the evidence suggests to people of ordinary intelligence the proper standard of care. A typical situation is where a foreign object such as a sponge or needle is left within the body of a patient. Another well-established application of the common knowledge exception is where the physician has disregarded the directions of the manufacturer in administering or prescribing a drug. An exception has also been applied to establish that a doctor's delay in taking tests, or in submitting them to a laboratory for analysis, constituted negligence (*O'Brien v. Stover*, 443 F.2d 1013 [8th Cir. 1971]; *Jeanes v. Millner*, 428 F.2d 598 [8th Cir. 1970]). Expert testimony may also be held unnecessary when the physician willfully abandons the patient.

The Locality Rule

Early in the development of medical malpractice law, the Supreme Judicial Court of Massachusetts held that a medical practitioner "was bound to possess that skill only which physicians and surgeons of ordinary ability and skill, practicing in similar localities, with opportunities for no larger experience, ordinarily possess; and he was not bound to possess that high degree of art and skill possessed by eminent surgeons practicing in large cities" (*Small v. Howard*, 128 Mass. 131 [1880]). For a long time, the locality rule was generally accepted throughout the country; however, in 1968, the same court that first announced the locality rule repudiated it (*Brune v. Belinkoff*, 354 Mass. 102, 235 N.E.2d 793 [1968]). Under the *Brune* rule, the medical resources available to the physician are to be but one circumstance in determining the skill and care required and some allowance is made for the type of community in which the physician carries on his or her practice (*Wentling v. Jenny*, 293 N.W.2d 76, 79 [Neb. 1980]). A number of jurisdictions have formally abandoned the locality rule, usually holding that the locality is but one of the elements of the standard of care to be considered. The general trend has been to relax the locality rule rather than to abandon it outright (*Ives v. Redford*, 252 S.E.2d 315, 318 [Va. 1979]). This result has been accomplished primarily by an expansion of the "similar locality" concept (*Wentling v. Jenny*, 293 N.W.2d 76, 78 [Neb. 1980]).

CAUSATION

Liability in tort is predicated on a causal connection between the alleged negligence and the claimed injury. To recover damages in a malpractice action, the patient must prove that the alleged injuries were proximately caused by the physician's negligence. Causation is contested in most malpractice cases. Many malpractice plaintiffs lose their cases because they fail to prove causation, even though they successfully establish that the defendant violated the applicable standard of care. To establish causation, the patient need not prove the physician's negligence was the only cause of the injury suffered. In most jurisdictions, the patient must merely prove that physician's conduct was "a cause" or "a substantial factor" resulting in the harm suffered (*Jones v. Montefiore Hospital*, 431 A.2d 920, 923 [Pa. 1981]; *Swartzlander v. Hunt Laboratory, Inc.*, 552 So.2d 1339, 1342 [La. App. 1989]). Causation is a special problem in malpractice cases because physicians treat people who already have illnesses or injuries. In each case, therefore, there is a question whether the negative result complained of was the normal and expected result from the disease or whether the patient's condition was made worse by the physician's negligence. In most failure to diagnose cases, there is a substantial possibility that the patient's condition, rather than the physician's negligence, was the cause of the alleged injury (*Ladner v. Campbell*, 515 So.2d 882, 888 [Miss. 1987]). Courts have struggled especially with the standard that should be applied proving causation in cases where the patient's medical condition by itself dictated a less than 50% chance of a favorable outcome. This struggle has given rise to the loss of chance doctrine and various hybrids derived from it.

Causation: Traditional Tort Standard

The traditional tort standard, still followed by a majority of jurisdictions, requires proof of causation in medical malpractice cases to a reasonable degree of medical probability. Courts have used various linguistic formulations to express this standard (e.g., "preponderance of the evidence," "substantial factor," "reasonable medical certainty"), but the essence of the standard is that the plaintiff must prove that it is more probable than not (i.e., a greater than 50% likelihood) that the physician's negligence was a cause of the harm complained of by the patient. Evidence demonstrating only a "possibility" that the physician's negligence was a cause of harm is considered to be "speculation." If evidence of "possibilities" is the only evidence introduced on the issue of causation, dismissal of the plaintiff's case will result.

Put another way, in a jurisdiction that follows the traditional approach, a patient is not entitled to compensation when she probably would have suffered the same harm even if the physician made a timely diagnosis or used proper treatment (*Cooper v. Sisters*, 272 N.E.2d 97 [Ohio, 1971]; *Kilpatrick v. Bryant*, 868 S.W.2d 594 [Tenn. 1993]). An example of a case following the traditional standard is *Fennell v. Southern Maryland Hosp. Center, Inc.*, 320 Md. 776, 550 A.2d 206 (1990). In *Fennell*, a claim was brought by the family of a woman who died of bacterial meningitis. The plaintiffs claimed that treatment should have been commenced to reduce the plaintiff's cerebral edema immediately after it was observed on a computed tomography (CT) scan. The plaintiff introduced evidence that if treatment had begun immediately the patient would have had a 40% chance of surviving the disease. The court upheld a dismissal of the plaintiff's claim, on the grounds that a 40% chance of survival represented a "mere possibility" that the physician's negligence was the cause of the patient's death.

Causation: Loss of Chance

Plaintiff's attorneys have argued that the traditional tort standard unfairly denies recovery to patients who have had their prospects for a successful recovery significantly diminished by a physician's negligence, simply because those prospects were poor to begin with. To a patient with a 40% chance of recovery, they argue, a decrease to a 10% chance of recovery is a significant injury, for which the law should provide a remedy.

This argument found support in the following language from *Hicks v. United States*, 368 F.2d 626, 632 (4th Cir. 1966):

> *When a defendant's negligent action or inaction has effectively terminated a person's chance of survival, it does not lie in the defendant's mouth to raise conjectures as to the measure of the chances that he has put beyond the possibility of realization. If there was any substantial possibility of survival and the defendant has destroyed it, he is answerable.*

Though *Hicks* did not actually involve a patient with a less than 50% chance of recovery, it is often cited for the creation of the lost chance doctrine. This doctrine expands traditional tort principles of causation to permit recovery to a patient who would probably have had the same outcome regardless of medical intervention.

The lost chance doctrine was adopted by the Supreme Court of Washington in *Herskovitz v. Group Health Cooperative*, 99 Wash. 2d 609, 664 P.2d 474 (1983), a wrongful death case involving delayed diagnosis of lung cancer. Expert witnesses for the plaintiff testified that with timely diagnosis the patient had a 39% chance of 5-year survival, which was reduced by the delay in diagnosis to a 25% chance. The court held that this evidence was sufficient to allow the jury to consider the possibility that the delayed diagnosis was a cause of the patient's death. To hold otherwise, the court stated, would provide a "blanket release from liability for doctors and hospitals any time there was less than a 50% chance of survival, regardless of how flagrant the negligence."

Though there is considerable confusion in the reasoning expressed by courts that have adopted the lost chance rationale, two basic conceptual approaches have emerged. The first approach has been to relax the reasonable medical *probability* standard for proving causation and to permit recovery upon proof that the physician's negligence deprived the patient of a *possibility* of a better result.

This relaxed standard has been labeled the "substantial possibility" standard. Under this standard, proximate cause may be established by proof that the physician's negligence effectively precluded the patient from a substantial possibility of a better result. If the patient shows that the physician's conduct increased the risk of harm suffered by the patient, such evidence provides a basis upon which a jury may find that the physician's conduct was a substantial factor or proximate cause in bringing about the harm—even if the patient would probably have suffered the same harm with ideal treatment (*Clayton v. Saber*, 594 A.2d 365, 366 [Pa. Super. 1991]; *Ebers v. Dollinger*, 471 A.2d 405, 415 [N.J. 1984]). Expert testimony need show only that the defendant's conduct increased the risk of the harm actually sustained, and not necessarily that it directly caused the harm complained of (*Jones v. Montefiore Hospital*, 431 A.2d 920, 924 [Pa. 1981]).

The second conceptual approach to the "lost chance" situation preserves the traditional "reasonable medical probability" standard of proving causation but expands liability by recognizing the loss of a less-than-even chance to survive as a distinct compensable injury (*DeBurkaste v. Louvar*, 393 N.W.2d 131 [Iowa 1986]). In other words, plaintiff must prove to a reasonable degree of medical probability that the defendant's conduct diminished the patient's chances of a successful recovery. It does not matter if those chances were less than 50% at the time the negligence occurred. This approach was followed by the Nevada Supreme Court in *Perez v. Las Vegas Medical Center*, 805 P.2d 589 (Nev. 1991). In that case, the patient informed physicians at the defendant hospital that he was experiencing persistent headaches. The examining physicians made no attempt to diagnose the cause of the headaches. A few days later, a nurse discovered the patient having seizures. The patient received no examination or treatment other than the administration of valium and phenobarbital. A few hours later the patient died of a massive brain hemorrhage due to an aneurysm or a congenital defect in an artery. The trial court entered summary judgment in favor of the defendants and the Supreme Court of Nevada reversed. The court adopted the theory of loss of chance and defined the actionable injury as the "loss of chance of survival."

The distinction between the two conceptual approaches to the loss of chance doctrine, while subtle, is more than academic. It can have a profound effect on the calculation of damages. In general, courts that follow the "substantial possibility" approach allow the plaintiff to recover the *full value* of the injuries (*see Kallenberg v. Beth Israel Hosp.*, 357 N.Y.S.2d 508 [Ct. App. 1974]; *Thompson v. Sun City Community Hosp.*, 688 P.2d 605 [Ariz 1984]; *Mays v. United States*, 608 F. Supp. 1476, 1482 [D. Colo. 1985]). When this approach is applied, a patient may recover all damages resulting from an injury for which the physician may be only partly responsible. By contrast, in jurisdictions that recognize loss of chance as a separate compensable injury, recovery is generally limited to the value of the diminished chance of survival, usually calculated as a percentage of the total damages. The reduction may be based either on the percentage chance of survival that the patient had at the time of the alleged negligent act, or on the degree to which the patient's chances of survival were reduced by the alleged negligence.

To appreciate the widely different results that can be produced by the various standards of proof or causation, consider the following example. A patient whose physician negligently failed to diagnose her condition had a 40% chance of survival at the time of misdiagnosis. When the diagnosis was actually made, her chances of survival had diminished to 30%. A jury determined that the total damages resulting from her wrongful death are $1 million. In a state that follows the traditional causation rule, the plaintiff recovers nothing, since the patient's outcome would probably have been the same regardless of the misdiagnosis. In a state that follows the substantial possibility version of the lost chance doctrine, the plaintiff recovers the full value of the injury, or $1 million. In a state that recognizes a lost chance as a separate compensable injury, the plaintiff's recovery will either be $400,000 (if damages are reduced by 40%, the patient's chances of survival at the time of misdiagnosis) or $100,000 (if the patient's damages are reduced by 10%, the degree to which her chances of recovery were diminished by the misdiagnosis).

INFORMED CONSENT

In the 20th century, the legal doctrine of informed consent emerged from lawsuits based on claims by patients that a physician failed to sufficiently inform them of the risks and alternatives prior to treatment (*Canterbury v. Spence*, 464 F.2d 772 [D.C. Cir. 1972], *cert den'd*, 409 U.S. 1064 [1972]; *Cobbs v. Grant*, 502 P.2d 1 [Cal. 1972]; *Natanson v. Kline*, 350 P.2d 1093 [Kan. 1960]; *Truman v. Thomas*, 611 P.2d 902 [Cal. 1980], (Appelbaum et al., 1987; and Shugrue et al., 1991). For a thorough discussion of informed consent and its exceptions see, Appelbaum et al. (1987).

A physician must obtain the patient's consent before the physician is legally entitled to begin diagnosis or treatment. The patient's consent is a prerequisite to the rendering of medical care as long as the patient is mentally and physically able to discuss her condition. From the physician's viewpoint, informed consent requires disclosure of material information to the patient. The patient in turn makes an informed choice and communicates this choice back to the physician. The physician should document that a discussion took place and indicate the patient's choice of treatment.

A physician has a duty to give the patient all information material to the decision to undergo the proposed diagnosis or treatment. To be effective, the patient's consent must stem from an understanding based on accurate information about the professional services proposed, available alternatives, benefits and risks, including known side effects (*Canterbury*, 464 F.2d at 72; *Cobbs*, 502 P.2d at 10; [Appelbaum, et al., 1987]).

Two physicians, one of whom is also a lawyer, have written:

> *Adequately informing women with breast cancer of therapeutic options and potential complications is critical, and the failure to do so may result in physician liability. This includes discussing the relative benefits and risks of extensive surgery, conservative surgery, radiation therapy, and adjuvant chemotherapy.*
>
> (DEWAR ET AL., 1992)

This communication process can be complex, owing in part to the existence of legal standards that define whether a patient has been "adequately informed" (Goldman, 1988). There are two legal standards that are the measures by which informed consent claims are proven at trial, the professional standard and the reasonable patient standard.

Under the professional standard, the duty of the physician to disclose "is limited to those disclosures which a reasonable medical practitioner would make under the same or similar circumstances" (*Natanson*, 350 P.2d at 1106). Because the physician's duty to disclose is defined by the medical community, expert testimony is required on what

the standard is and whether the doctor deviated from it (*Natanson*, 350 P.2d at 673; *Davis v. Caldwell*, 429 N.E.2d 741, 744 [N.Y. 1981]); (Shugrue et al., 1991).

The professional standard came under criticism in the 1970s. *Canterbury v. Spence* was the first case to establish a "patient-oriented standard of disclosure" (464 F.2d 772 [D.C. Cir. 1972]). The *Canterbury* court rejected the professional standard, holding that physicians were not free to impose their own standard, but that their duty should be defined by law, regardless of their own particular customs or standards (*Canterbury*, 464 F.2d at 785-87; *Henning v. Parsons*, 623 P.2d 574, 480 [N.M. App. 1980]).

The reasonable patient standard, enunciated in *Canterbury*, requires the physician to disclose all facts, risks, and alternatives that a reasonable person in the patient's situation would consider material in making the decision whether or not to undergo the recommended treatment (*Canterbury*, 464 F.2d at 787; *Wilkinson v. Vesey*, 295 A.2d 676, 689 [R.I. 1972]). Generally, the materiality or significance of the information about a potential complication is a function of both the severity of the complication and the likelihood that it will occur. For example, one court identified the material risks associated with a subcutaneous mastectomy to include hematoma, infection, capsule contracture, and skin necrosis. These risks must be disclosed to the patient (*Goddard v. Hickman*, 685 P.2d 530, 533 [Utah, 1984]).

State laws that specifically address informed consent for treatment of breast cancer generally require that physicians provide their patients with standardized written summaries of medically viable or efficacious alternative methods of treatment, along with the relative advantages, disadvantages, and risks of such treatments. These statutes were developed to provide women who have a suspected or confirmed diagnosis of breast cancer with informed alternatives to a mastectomy (McKenna et al., 1987). The statutes range from making compliance optional in Georgia to harsh penalties for noncompliance in Kansas (Table 39–1). Some of the laws are discussed below; however, this discussion is not meant to be an exhaustive analysis of each statute. Physicians should know the particular requirements of their state, but an overview of some of the statutory requirements nationwide is instructive.

For example, the Georgia law requires the Board of Medical Examiners to develop an informational booklet regarding prevailing methods of treatment for breast cancer. The Georgia legislation represents one of the most lenient breast cancer informed consent statutes because it imposes no mandatory duty on physicians, has no enforcement procedure, and contains no penalties for noncompliance.

Hawaii also has mandated that its Board of Medical Examiners establish standards for health care providers to follow in providing information to patients to ensure informed consent for mastectomy. This statute is similar to the Georgia statute in that no provisions exist for mandating physician compliance with the standards. The Hawaii statute is unique, however, in providing that the standards are admissible as evidence of the standard of care required of health care providers.

Table 39-1. STATE LAWS THAT ADDRESS INFORMED CONSENT FOR TREATMENT OF BREAST CANCER

California	Cal. Health & Safety Code §§ 1704.5; 1704.55 (West, 1993) Cal. Bus. & Prof. Code §§ 2234; 2257 (West, 1993)
Florida	Fla. Stat. Ann. §§ 240.5121(4)(m); 458.324; 459.0125 (West, 1993)
Georgia	Ga. Code Ann. § 43-34-21 (Michie, 1993)
Hawaii	Haw. Rev. Stat. § 671-3 (1993)
Illinois	20 ILCS 2310/55.49 (1993)
Kansas	Kan. Stat. Ann. § 65-2836 (1992)
Kentucky	Ky. Rev. Stat. Ann. § 311.935 (Michie, 1993)
Maine*	Me. Rev. Stat. Ann. tit. 24, § 2905-A (1990)
Maryland	Md. Health-Gen. Code Ann. § 20-113; Md. Health Occ. Code Ann. § 14-404(a)(26) (West, 1993)
Massachusetts	Mass. Gen. Laws Ann. ch. 111 § 70E (West, 1993)
Michigan	Mich. Comp. Laws Ann. § 333.17013 (West, 1993)
Minnesota	Minn. Stat. Ann. § 144.651(9) (West, 1993)
New Jersey	N.J. Stat. Ann. § 45:9-22.2 (West, 1993)
New York	N.Y. Pub. Health Law § 2404 (McKinney, 1993)
Pennsylvania	Pa. Stat. Ann. tit 35, § 5641 (1992)
Texas	Tx. Health & Safety Code § 86.001 et. seq. (West, 1992)
Virginia	Va. Code Ann. § 54.1-2971 (Michie, 1993)

*'''Screening mammography'' is one of the ''practice guidelines'' in the Maine Medical Liability Demonstration Project, which expires in 1997. Under this legislation, if it is undisputed that a physician adhered to the practice guidelines, a suit brought against the physician can be dismissed before trial.

Type of Information Required To Be Disclosed to Breast Cancer Patients

As part of the informed consent process, physicians in some states, including California, Florida, Kentucky, Maine, Maryland, and Michigan, are required to inform breast cancer patients of the advantages, disadvantages, and risks of alternative methods of treatment.

Some states, including California, Florida, Kentucky, Massachusetts, and New York, require physicians to inform patients by means of a standardized written summary, in laymen's language, of ''alternative efficacious methods of treatment that may be medically viable'' including surgical, radiological, and chemotherapeutic treatments or combinations thereof. New York includes hormonal treatments among the medically viable alternative methods of treatment that must be disclosed.

Several states do not use the term *medically viable*. Maine requires that standardized written information be provided about ''alternative efficacious methods of treatment of breast cancer.'' Maryland requires the physician to educate the patient about alternative methods of treatment that may be ''medically practicable'' though this expression is not defined.

In California, each person or entity who owns or operates a health facility or clinic or who is licensed as a physician and surgeon and rents or owns the premises where his or her practice is located, must post the following notice where a physician and surgeon performs breast cancer screening

or biopsy as an outpatient service. If the notice is posted at the patient registration area it is in compliance with the statute. The sign or notice must state in English, Spanish, and Chinese:

BE INFORMED

If you are a patient being treated for any form of breast cancer, or prior to performance of a biopsy for breast cancer, your physician and surgeon is required to provide you a written summary of alternative efficacious methods of treatment, pursuant to Section 1704.5 of the California Health and Safety Code.

The information about methods of treatment was developed by the State Department of Health Services to inform patients of the advantages, disadvantages, risks, and descriptions of procedures.

Many of the statutes are silent on ''when and if'' the written summaries are required to be updated, thus calling into question one primary benefit of a written summary. The Florida statute requires that the written summary be updated ''periodically.'' The Kentucky legislation allows updating to be optional. Maryland requires that the summary be updated on an annual basis, whereas Texas requires annual updating only if necessary. Illinois requires that its written summary be updated every 2 years. Kansas, Maine, Michigan, New York, Minnesota, and Massachusetts do not have an updating provision. California's written summary is undergoing a major revision at this time. This revision is expected from the California Department of Health Services in the fall of 1994.

Michigan and Maine require that patients be informed *both* verbally by the physician and by the written standardized summary of alternative methods of treatment. Florida gives a physician the option of informing a patient of treatment alternatives verbally, in writing, or by a combination of both. In Massachusetts and Minnesota the legislation requiring disclosure of alternative methods of treatment is encompassed within a patient bill of rights statute.

Types of Patients Who Receive Breast Cancer Treatment Summaries

States including California, Kentucky, Maine, Maryland, Minnesota, and New York require that the standardized information on breast cancer treatment be provided only to those patients undergoing treatment for a diagnosis of breast cancer. The Maine and Michigan statutes impose the duty to disclose standardized information only on physicians who are providing the primary treatment for breast cancer (i.e., the initial treatment following the breast cancer diagnosis).

Several states have broader categories of persons to whom physicians are required to disclose breast cancer treatment information. Florida requires that patients who are at ''high risk'' of being diagnosed as having breast cancer must receive the standardized summary. Kansas requires that the standardized information be given to patients suffering from any form of abnormality of breast tissue for which surgery is a recommended form of treatment.

The Illinois and Texas legislation places no limitation on the types of patients that must receive such information. Under the Illinois statute, the Department of Public Health distributes the standardized written summary to hospitals, public health centers and physicians who are likely to perform or order diagnostic tests for breast cancer or treat breast cancer by surgical or other medical methods. The statute simply states, ''Those hospitals, public health centers and physicians shall make the summaries available to the public.'' The Texas law allows physicians to distribute the summary to ''a patient'' when the physician determines in his/her professional judgment that it is in the best interests of the patient; however, the statute implies that it relates only to breast cancer patients.

Methods of Ensuring Compliance with Breast Cancer Legislation

Time Requirements

Several states specify a particular time frame in which the standardized information must be provided to the patient to ensure compliance with the statute. California requires that the standardized information be given before a biopsy and that this must be noted on the patient's chart. Kansas requires that the information be provided ''as soon as practicable and medically indicated following diagnosis.'' Maryland requires that the patient must receive the summary within 5 days of the start of treatment for breast cancer but allows for exceptions in the case of emergency treatment or where treatment occurred within 5 days of diagnosis. New York requires disclosure of information upon diagnosis or as soon thereafter as practicable. Texas requires disclosure when a physician determines in his or her professional judgment that it is in the best interest of the patient to receive the summary. Minnesota requires that a patient must be informed ''prior to or at the time of admission and during the hospital stay.'' Illinois, Florida, Kentucky, Maine, and Massachusetts do not specify any time for disclosure of the information.

Documentation

Compliance with the breast cancer treatment statute is required to be documented in the patient's medical record in California, Florida, Maine, and Michigan. In Maryland, patients who receive the standardized breast cancer information must sign a form acknowledging receipt of that information. Maine and Michigan also require that patients sign a form acknowledging receipt of the required information; however, these states are unique in that signing the form effectively bars the patient from bringing any civil action regarding failure to provide informed consent.

Illinois, Kentucky, New York, Minnesota, and Massachusetts do not have specific provisions on documenting compliance with the breast cancer treatment statutes. Nota-

bly, Texas does not require compliance with its breast cancer treatment statute. At the present time, providing patients with the standardized summary is optional for physicians in Texas.

Penalties for Noncompliance with Legislation

Most states with specific breast cancer treatment legislation have no penalty provision for violation of the statute; however, California provides that failure by a physician to give the required standardized written summary to the patient constitutes unprofessional conduct. The Massachusetts statute specifically allows a medical malpractice cause of action should a physician not comply with disclosure of treatment information. Failure of a physician in Kansas to inform patients with breast cancer of treatment options may result in revocation, suspension or limitation of that physician's license, or the licensee may be publicly or privately censured. Maryland has a similar provision in its statute.

To recover based on a claim for negligent nondisclosure a breast cancer patient must prove that a causal connection exists between the physician's failure to inform the patient and the injury the patient claims to have suffered. The causal connection exists ''when, but only when, disclosure of significant risks incidental to the treatment would have resulted in a decision against it'' (*Canterbury v. Spence*, 464 F.2d 772, 790 [D.C. Cir. 1972]). The issue is not what this particular patient would have chosen if there had been significant disclosure, but objectively, what a reasonably prudent person in the patient's position would have done if sufficiently informed (*Canterbury*, 464 F.2d at 791). The patient's testimony is relevant, but it is not the determining factor.

RECOMMENDATIONS FOR AVOIDING MALPRACTICE LIABILITY

The following recommendations are designed to help clinicians avoid or minimize their malpractice liability exposure for errors in breast cancer diagnosis and treatment. They are risk management recommendations, delivered from a medicolegal perspective, and are not intended to reflect or create standards of care, even though in some instances they may be consistent with existing standards of care. While optimal care that meets the highest standards of clinical practice may well be the best method of avoiding malpractice lawsuits, it is not the legal standard of care. Nor will optimal care eliminate the risk of malpractice liability. Breast cancer diagnostic methods are imperfect, and, even with optimal care, cancers which in retrospect are felt to have been detectable will be missed. The majority of breast cancer malpractice cases arise from a diagnostic dilemma that cannot be resolved by risk management guidelines. Biopsy is the only means of making a definitive diagnosis of breast cancer, but it is a disfiguring and costly procedure that cannot reasonably be performed for every breast abnormality. Clinicians must therefore balance the risk of harm to patients from false positive results and overuse of biopsy, with the risk of false negative results and missed diagnosis. Balancing these risks calls for the exercise of clinical judgment, which will always be subject to scrutiny from the vantage point of hindsight.

Medical Record Keeping

Good medical records are often the cornerstone of the successful defense of a malpractice claim. Records that document the physician's decision-making process or advice to a patient can be invaluable when disputes arise between patient and physician about what actually happened. In general, juries will be more inclined to believe a physician's account of events if it is supported by a written record made contemporaneously with the events. In the minds of many jurors, inadequate record keeping is often equated with substandard patient care, even though such a conclusion may not be justified.

Patient History

Plaintiffs often allege that a physician "ignored" a patient's increased risk of breast cancer associated with family history. All patients who present with a breast complaint or who will be routinely followed for their breast care should have a thorough family health history and personal breast history documented in their record. When documenting the evaluation of possible diagnostic steps for a breast complaint, physicians should note their awareness and consideration of any family history of breast cancer or other risk factors.

Findings on Examination

A patient's symptoms and physical findings on examination should be carefully documented. Physical appearance of the breasts should be described, as should the absence of such findings as asymmetry, skin changes, nipple discharge, dominant masses, and axillary adenopathy (Dewar et al., 1992). Preprinted breast diagrams should be used to accurately record the location of physical findings. A careful record of the location of a suspected mass can be extremely valuable in determining whether a cancer found at a later date represents progression of the first mass or a new lesion.

Decision Making

The reasoning behind diagnostic decisions should be clearly documented. The reasoning should also be discussed with the patient, and the fact of the discussion noted in the chart.

Follow-up Visits

All directions to the patient regarding follow-up care should be recorded. The timing of follow-up visits should be clearly established, and whenever possible a follow-up ap-

pointment should be established while the patient is still in the office. The appointment should then be recorded in the chart, along with the fact that the patient has been given instructions to return sooner if any change in her condition develops. Consideration should also be given to the use of a reminder or callback system to follow up on missed appointments.

Informed Consent

Careful attention should be paid to documenting all informed consent discussions with patients regarding breast cancer treatment options. The physician must be sure to comply with state regulations governing informed consent for breast cancer treatment, especially any requirements for written disclosures. Even if written disclosures are not required in a state, consideration should be given to the use of printed materials describing treatment options.

Consultants

All telephone or other oral communications with consulting or referring physicians should be noted in the chart.

Patient Phone Calls

All phone contacts or other oral communications with patients between office visits should be recorded. Such a policy serves a dual purpose. It ensures an accurate record of all calls, and the absence of a chart entry can be used as evidence that a claimed call did not occur.

Noncompliance

Any patient noncompliance with diagnostic or treatment records should be documented in the chart along with a note that the implications of noncompliance were discussed with the patient.

Screening Mammography

Primary care physicians should select a recognized protocol for the frequency and timing of screening mammograms and should refer their patients for mammograms in accordance with the protocol. Imaging facilities engaged in screening mammography should clearly define their role, to avoid confusion on the part of patients and referring physicians. Particular care should be taken in performing screening mammography on self-referred patients. More complete risk management recommendations for imaging centers engaged in screening mammography can be found in Brenner (1989).

Diagnostic Evaluation of Breast Complaints

Virtually every patient complaint involving a suspected breast lesion should be evaluated by mammography, even when the physical findings are unimpressive. Kern's study of malpractice verdicts found that fewer than half of plaintiffs who presented with a painless mass discovered by self-examination received a mammogram (Kern, 1992). The most common reason reported by physicians in the PIAA study for delay in diagnosis was that physical findings failed to impress.

By the same token, physicians must not rely on negative mammograms to rule out cancer. The PIAA study's second most frequently reported reason for delay in diagnosis was a negative mammogram. In one study, 22% per cent of women with a palpable cancer had normal mammograms (Eideken, 1988).

In equivocal cases, consideration should be given to supplemental mammography examinations, such as spot magnification or special views. Comparison with prior mammograms, if available, should be obtained. In appropriate cases, a second opinion regarding the interpretation of mammograms may be sought. Where the patient reports a mass that can be neither palpated by the physician nor detected by mammography, repeat follow-up examination and mammography should be scheduled and the patient should be instructed to return sooner if any change is noted. In such cases, consideration may be given to the use of ultrasound, or in cases where the suspicious area can be sufficiently localized, to fine-needle aspiration. If such additional investigative techniques are considered and rejected, this fact and the reasons for doing so should be noted in the chart. When a physician has been able to palpate a suspected lesion reported by the patient but has concluded that it is presumptively benign, follow-up examination should be scheduled after the next menstrual cycle, and in postmenopausal women within 2 to 3 months (Dewar et al., 1992).

Particular attention needs to be paid to distinguishing between regional nodularity or symmetric thickening and a dominant mass. There is universal agreement that a dominant mass not shown to be a simple cyst by fine-needle aspiration requires definitive diagnosis by biopsy (Dewar et al., 1992).

Patient Expectations

Most patients have unrealistic expectations about the effectiveness of screening and early detection in eliminating their risk of dying of breast cancer. Limitations of diagnostic methods, and the fact that some cancers metastasize before they are detectable, should be discussed frankly with patients. Patients should not be unreasonably reassured that findings are benign and should be encouraged to report promptly any changes or new findings in their breasts.

References and Related Readings

Abel, R. L.: The crisis is injuries not liability. *In* Olson, W. (Ed.): New Directions in Liability Law. New York, Academy of Political Science, 1988, p. 31.

Abraham, K. S.: Medical liability reform: A conceptual framework. J.A.M.A., *260*:68, 1988.

Annas, J. G.: Why the British courts rejected the American doctrine of informed consent. Am. J. Public Health, *74*:1286, 1984.

Appelbaum, P. S., Lidz, C. W., and Meisel, A.: Informed Consent: Legal Theory and Clinical Practice. New York, Oxford Univ. Press, 1987.

Ashton, D. P.: Comment: Decreasing the risks inherent in claims for increased risk of future disease. Univ. Miami Law Rev., *43*:1081, 1989.

Berlin, L.: Malpractice in radiologists, Update 1986: An 11.5-year perspective. A.J.R., *147*:1291, 1986.

Boisaubin, E. V.: Practice standards: Implications for the internist. Am. J. Med. Sci., *300*:173, 1990.

Bovbjerg, R. R.: Medical malpractice on trial: Quality of care is the important standard. Law Contemp. Probl., *49*:321, 1986.

Brennan, T. A., Leape, L. L., Laird, N. M., et al.: Incidents of adverse events and negligence in hospitalized patients: Results of the Harvard medical practice study I. N. Engl. J. Med., *324*:370, 1991.

Brenner, R. J.: Screening mammography, medical-legal considerations. Cancer, *105*:187, 1990.

Brenner, R. J., Medicolegal aspects of screening mammography. A.J.R., *153*:53–49, 1989.

Brenner, R. J.: Medicolegal aspects of breast imaging: Variable standards of care relating to different types of practice. A.J.R., *156*:719, 1991.

Brenner, R. J.: Medicolegal aspects of screening mammography. A.J.R., *153*:53, 1989.

Campenella, P. J.: Breast cancer: Staging, treatment, and the duty to inform. Med. Trial Tech. Q., *35*:17, 1988.

Cheney, F. W., Posner, K., Caplan, R. A., et al.: Standard of care and anesthesia liability. J.A.M.A., *261*:1599, 1989.

Cohn, C. D.: Delay in diagnosis of breast cancer: A professional liability risk. J. Nurse Midwifery, *36*:74, 1991.

Solin, O. H. (Ed.): Current Award Trends, Jury Verdict Research, 1991.

Daniels, S.: Verdicts in medical malpractice cases. Trial, *25*:23, 1989.

Danzon, P. M.: Medical malpractice: Theory, evidence, and public policy. Cambridge, Mass., Harvard University Press, 1985.

Darios, R. J.: Biopsy of occult breast lesions and professional liability (Letter). J.A.M.A., *264*:1948, 1990.

Derrick, J. H.: Annotation: Medical malpractice: Liability for failure of physician to inform patient of alternative modes of diagnosis or treatment. Am. Law Rep. 4th, 38:900, 1985.

Dewar, M. A., and Love, N.: Legal issues in managing breast disease. Postgrad. Med., *92*:137, 1992.

Director, J. J.: Annotation: Malpractice: Physician's failure to advise patient to consult specialist or one qualified in a method of treatment which physician is not qualified to give. Am. Law Rev. 3d, *35*:349, 1971.

Dobson, T.: Medical malpractice in the birth place: Resolving the physician-patient conflict through informed consent, standard of care, and assumption of risk. Nebraska Law Rev., *65*:655, 1986.

Eideken, S.: Mammography and palpable cancer of the breast. Cancer, *61*:263–265, 1988.

Ellis, L. R.: Notes: Loss of chance as technique, toeing the line at fifty percent. Texas Law Rev., *72*:369, 1993.

Feld, D. E.: Annotation: Necessity and sufficiency of expert evidence to establish existence and extent of physician's duty to inform patient of risks of proposed treatment. Am. Rev. 3d, *52*:1084, 1973.

Feldman, H. R.: Comment: Chances as protected interests: Recovery for the loss of chance and increased risk. U. Balt. Law Rev., *17*:139, 1987.

Frantz, L. B.: Annotation: Modern status of views as to general measure of physician's duty to inform patient of risks of proposed treatment. Am. Law Rev. 3d, *88*:1008, 1978.

Gebhard, P. J., and Feingold, S. G.: Legal aspects of mammography screening. Cancer, *60*:1692, 1987.

Gerughty, R. P., and Wilkinson, A. P.: Negligence in the diagnosis of cancer. Trial, p. 69, Feb. 1984.

Goldman, E. B.: Legal requirements of informed consent for treatment of breast cancer: Telling it all. *In* Harnes, J. K., Oberman, H. A., et al. (Eds.): Breast Cancer: Collaborative Management. Chelsea, Mich., Lewis Publishers, 1988.

Hamer, M. M., Morlock, F., Foley, H. T., et al.: Medical malpractice in diagnostic radiology: Claims, compensation and patient injury. Radiology, *164*:263, 1987.

Harvard Medical Practice Study: Patients, doctors and lawyers: Medical injury, malpractice litigation and patient compensation in New York: The report of the Harvard medical practice study to the State of New

York. Cambridge, Mass., President and Fellows of Harvard College, 1990.

Hatch, M. A.: Medical Malpractice Claim Study: 1982–1987. St. Paul, Minnesota Department of Commerce, 1989.

Henderson, I. C., and Danner, D.: Legal pitfalls in the diagnosis and management of breast cancer. Hematol. Oncol. Clin. North Am., *3*:823, 1989.

Hirshfeld, E. B.: Should practice parameters be the standard of care in malpractice litigation? J.A.M.A., *266*:2886, 1991.

Hirshfeld, E. B.: Practice parameters and the malpractice liability of physicians. J.A.M.A., *263*:1556, 1990.

Hodson, J. D.: Annotation: Medical malpractice: "Loss of chance" causality. Am. Law Rep. 4th, *54*:10, 1987.

Jacobson, P. D.: Medical malpractice in the tort system. J.A.M.A., *262*:3320–3327, 1989.

Jones, C. J.: Autonomy and informed consent in medical decision making: Toward a new self-fulfilling prophecy. Wash. & Lee Law Rev., *47*:379, 1990.

Jury Verdict Research. LRP Publications, (various issues) 1986–93.

Keeton, W., Dobbs, D., Keeton, R., et al.: Prosser & Keeton on the Law of Torts. 5th ed. St. Paul, West Pub., 1984.

Kern, K. A.: Causes of breast cancer malpractice litigation: A 20-year civil court review. Arch. Surg., *127*:542, 1992.

Ketcham, A. S., and Moffat, F. L.: Vexed surgeons, perplexed patients and breast cancers which may not be cancer. Cancer, *65*:387, 1990.

King, J.: Causation, valuation, and chance in personal injury torts involving preexisting conditions and future consequences. Yale Law J., *90*:1353, 1981.

Kraft, R. B.: The breast cancer controversy and its implications for the informed consent doctrine. J. Legal Med., *2*:47, 1980.

Kusserow, R. P., Handley, E. A., and Yessian, M. R.: An overview of state medical discipline. J.A.M.A., *256*:820, 1987.

Laska, L.: Medical Malpractice Verdicts, Settlements & Experts. Nashville, (various issues) 1994.

Localio, A. R., Lawthers, A. G., Brennan, T. A., et al.: Relation between malpractice claims and adverse events due to negligence: Results of the Harvard medical practice study III. N. Engl. J. Med., *325*:245, 1991.

Louisell, D. W., and Williams, H.: Medical Malpractice. New York, Matthew Bender and Co., 1988.

McKenna, R. J., and Toghia, N. J.: The law of informed consent and mastectomy. *In* Ariel I. M., and Cleary, J. B. (Eds.): Breast Cancer Diagnosis and Treatment. New York, McGraw-Hill, 1987.

McMahon, M. J.: Annotation: Medical malpractice: Measure and elements of damages in actions based on loss of chance. Am. Law Rep. 4th, *81*:485, 1990.

Meyers, A. R.: "Lumping it": The hidden denominator of the medical malpractice crisis. Am. J. Public Health, *77*:1544, 1987.

Miller, F. H.: Medical malpractice litigation: Do the British have a better remedy? Am. J. Law Med., *11*:433, 1986.

Mills, D. H., Boyden, J. S., Jr., and Rubsamen, D. S.: Report on the Medical Insurance Feasibility Study. San Francisco, Sutter, 1977.

Mitnick, J. S., Vazquez, M. F., Plesser, K. P., et al.: Breast cancer malpractice litigation in New York State. Radiology, *189*:673, 1993.

Neupauer, R.: 1990 California Medical Malpractice Large Loss Trend Study. Oakland, Medical Underwriters of California, 1990.

Neupauer, R.: 1991 California Medical Malpractice Large Loss Trend Study. Oakland, Medical Underwriters of California, 1991.

Neupauer, R.: 1992 California Medical Malpractice Large Loss Trend Study. Oakland, Medical Underwriters of California, 1992.

Note: The loss of chance theory in medical malpractice cases: An overview. Am. J. Trial Advoc., *13*:1163, 1990.

Nye, D. J., Gifford, D. G., Webb, D. L., et al.: The causes of the medical malpractice crisis: An analysis of claims data and insurance company finances. Georgetown Law J., *764*:1495, 1988.

Olcott, D. J.: Note: Torts: Medical malpractice: Informed consent as measured by an objective prudent patient's standard: *Largey v. Rothman*, 110 N.J. 204, 540 A.2d 504, 1988. Seton Hall Law Rev., 20:303, 1989.

Orloff, N., and Stedinger, J.: A framework for evaluating the preponderance-of-the-evidence standard. Univ. Penn. Law Rev., *131*:1159, 1983.

Parver, C. P.: Defense of delayed diagnosis in the treatment of breast cancer. Med. Trial Tech. Q., *30*:34, 1983.

Peterson, M. A.: Civil juries in the 1980's: Trends in jury trials and verdicts in California and Cook County, IL. Santa Monica, Calif., The Rand Corp., 1987.

Physicians Insurers Association of America: Breast Cancer Study. Lawrenceville, N. J., Physicians Insurers Association of America, 1990.

Plotkin, D., and Blankenberg, F.: Breast cancer: Biology and malpractice. J. Clin. Oncol., *14*:254, 1991.

Potchen, E. J., Bisesi, M. A., Sierra, A. E., et al.: Mammography and malpractice. A.J.R., *156*:475, 1991.

President's Commission for the Study of Ethical Problems in Medicine and Biomedical and Behavioral Research: Making Health Care Decisions: The Ethical and Legal Implications of Informed Consent in the Patient-Practitioner Relationship. Washington, D.C., U.S. Govt. Printing Office, 1982.

Prillaman, H. L.: A physician's duty to inform of newly developed therapy. J. Contemp. H. Law Policy, *6*:43, 1990.

Prosser, W. L.: Handbook of the Law of Torts. 4th ed. St. Paul, West Publishing Co., 1971.

Reisig, R. A.: The loss of chance theory in medical malpractice cases: An overview. Am. J. Trial Advocacy, *13*:1183, 1990.

Restatement (Second) of Torts, § 323(a), 1965.

Reynolds, R. A., Risso, J. A., and Gonzales, M. L.: The cost of medical malpractice liability. J.A.M.A., *257*:2776, 1987.

Rigelhaupt, J. L.: Annotation: What constitutes physician-patient relationship for malpractice purposes. Am. Law Rev. 4th, *17*:132, 1982.

Robertson, G.: Informed consent to medical treatment. Law Q. Rev., *97*:102, 1981.

Rossati, J.: Note: Causation in medical malpractice: A modified valuation approach. Ohio St. Law J., *50*:469, 1989.

Rozovski, F. A.: Consent to Treatment: A Practical Guide. Boston, Little, Brown, 1984.

Schultz, M. M.: From Informed Consent to Patient Choice, A New Protected Interest. Yale Law J., *95*:219, 1985.

Seidelson, D. E.: Medical malpractice actions based on lack of informed consent "full-disclosure" jurisdictions: The enigmatic affirmative defense. Duquesne Law. Rev., *29*:39, 1990.

Seltzer, M. H.: Breast cancer malpractice: Understanding diagnosis and treatment. Trial Lawyer Q., *20*:12, 1989.

Shoenberger, A. E.: Medical malpractice injury: Causation and valuation of the loss of chance to survive. J. Legal Med., *6*:51, 1985.

Shugrue, R. E., and Linstromberg, K.: The practitioner's guide to informed consent. Creighton Law Rev., *24*:881, 1991.

Sloane, F. A., Mergenhagen, P. M., Burfield, W. B., et al.: Medical malpractice experience of physicians: Predictable or haphazard? J.A.M.A., *262*:3291, 1989.

Smith, D. H.: Increased risk of harm: A new standard for sufficiency of evidence and causation in medical malpractice cases. Boston Univ. Law Rev., *65*:275, 1985.

Snider, H. D.: Jury of My Peers: A Surgeon's Encounter with the Malpractice Crisis. Greenwood, Fla., Penkevill Pub., 1989.

Snyder, J. H.: The industry catches its breath after unprecedented catastrophe-related losses in 1992. Best's Rev.: Property-Casualty Insur. Ed., *94*:28, 1994.

Spratt, J. S., and Spratt, S. W.: Legal perspectives on mammography and self-referral. Cancer, *69*:599, 1992.

Spratt, J. S., and Spratt, S. W.: Medical and legal implications of screening and follow-up procedures for breast cancer. Cancer, *66*:1351, 1990.

St. Paul Fire & Marine Insurance Company: Physicians & Surgeons Update, 1988. St. Paul, Minn., St. Paul Fire and Marine Insurance Co., 1988.

St. Paul Fire & Marine Insurance Company: Physicians & Surgeons Update, 1989. St. Paul, Minn., St. Paul Fire & Marine Insurance Co., 1989.

St. Paul Fire & Marine Insurance Company: Physicians & Surgeons Update, 1990. St. Paul, Minn., St. Paul Fire & Marine Insurance Co., 1990.

St. Paul Fire & Marine Insurance Company: Physicians & Surgeons Update, 1991. St. Paul, Minn., St. Paul Fire & Marine Insurance Co., 1991.

St. Paul Fire & Marine Insurance Company: Physicians & Surgeons Update, 1992. St. Paul, Minn., St. Paul Fire & Marine Insurance Co., 1992.

Taub, S.: Legal problems in medical practice: Cancer and the law of informed consent. Law Med. Health Care, *10*:61, 1982.

Taylor, K. M., Shapiro, M., Soskolne, C. L., et al.: Physician response to informed consent regulations for randomized clinical trials. Cancer, *60*:1415, 1987.

Taylor, K. M., and Kelner, M.: Informed consent: The physicians' perspective. Soc. Sci. Med., *24*:135, 1987.

Tranum, B. L., and Westbrook, K.: Informed consent and treatment of primary breast cancer. J. Arkansas Med. Soc., *81*:324, 1984.

United States, Department of Health and Human Services, Task Force of Medical Liability and Malpractice: Report of the Task Force on Medical Liability and Malpractice. Washington, D.C., Department of Health and Human Services, 1987.

Verdicts, Settlements & Tactics (various issues). Colorado Springs, CO, Shepards-McGraw-Hill, 1986–93.

Watts, C. F.: Malpractice defense: Breast cancer. Oradell, NJ, Medical Economics Books, 1990.

Willard, R. K.: Wheel of fortune: Stopping outrageous and arbitrary liability verdicts. Policy Rev., *36*:40, 1986.

Willging, K. J.: Case note: *Falcon v. Memorial Hospital*: A rational approach to loss-of-chance tort actions. J. Contemp. H. Law & Policy, *9*:545, 1993.

Williams, A. P.: Malpractice, Outcomes, and Appropriateness of Care. Sanata Monica, Calif., The Rand Corporation, 1988.

Wolfstone, L., and Wolfstone, T.: Recovery of damages for the loss of a chance. Med. Trial Tech. Q., *28*:121, 1982.

Wright, R.: Causation in tort law. Calif. Law Rev., *73*:1735, 1985.

Zitter, J. M.: Annotation: Standard of care owed to patient by medical specialist as determined by local, ''like community'' state, national, or other standards. Am. Law Rev. 4th, *18*:603, 1982.

Zuckerman, S.: Medical malpractice: Claims, legal costs, and the practice of defense of medicine. Health Aff., *3*:128, 1984.

Zupanec, D. M.: Annotation: Malpractice in connection with diagnosis of cancer. Am. Law Rev. 3d, *79*:915, 1977.

40

The Role of Exercise and Weight Control in Cancer Prevention and Rehabilitation

James W. Yates

As a rehabilitative and a preventive technique for cancer patients, exercise is a relatively new idea. Fifty years ago, people were amazed at the idea of cardiac patients exercising, but today rehabilitation programs are common and provide great benefit in prevention of and recovery from heart attacks. A wealth of information on the impact of exercise in reducing the incidence of cancer has been published in the past 10 years. The concept of exercise as a restorative technique has also begun to flourish in recent years and is gaining momentum.

One purpose of this chapter is to discuss the role of exercise in reducing the incidence of cancer. A second goal is to review information concerning the effects of exercise on control of the problems associated with cancer therapy and on recovery of the cancer patient's functional capacity. Finally, the proper way safely to begin an exercise program is outlined. The goal is to provide the physician who is unfamiliar with exercise the information needed to prescribe exercise, both as a preventive and a restorative technique in the fight against cancer. Emphasis is placed on improving overall fitness and on weight reduction. By following the program, patients can improve their fitness level without undue risk of injury.

It is not fitness that provides the health benefits but rather the impact that the exercise program has on risk factors associated with health problems. Most persons who begin an exercise program develop better eating habits, lose weight, and, if they smoke, reduce the number of cigarettes or stop altogether. Each of these factors has a beneficial effect on overall health.

THE ROLE OF PHYSICAL ACTIVITY IN REDUCING THE INCIDENCE OF CANCER

While the focus of this book is on breast cancer, physical activity has had an impact on a number of different cancers. Evidence has been collected from epidemiologic studies and from studies on animal models and humans. Perhaps the strongest link is between physical activity and colon cancer, but a number of studies have reported positive effects for exercise in the prevention of breast cancer. Not all study findings agree, and some observers suggest that the

data are preliminary and controversial (Eichner, 1987). In this chapter I focus on research dealing with exercise and breast cancer. For more complete information, a number of excellent review papers that deal with the overall impact of physical activity on cancer may be consulted (Gauthier, 1986; Eichner, 1987; Vena et al., 1987; Kohl et al., 1988; Albanes et al., 1989; Blair et al., 1989; Willett, 1989; and Shephard, 1990).

By far the greatest volume of data linking cancer to exercise in humans comes from epidemiologic research. These studies use estimates of physical activity based on the individual subject's occupation, classify subjects according to athletic participation in college, use self-reported exercise habits, and in one case measured fitness using a maximal treadmill test. Thus, most of the data are inferential; cause and effect have not been established. Nonetheless, the data offer a starting point for examining this important relationship.

Epidemiologic Studies

Frisch and her colleagues (1985, 1987, 1989) published a series of papers dealing with the incidence of breast cancer and cancers of the reproductive system among former college athletes. The subjects were 5398 living alumni from eight colleges and two universities who responded to a detailed questionnaire. The subjects were classified as athletes or nonathletes based on participation on a varsity team, house team, or intramural team for at least one year. Team training had to be regular—at least two practice sessions a week. Other subjects were classified as athletes if they trained regularly, such as running 2 miles per day 5 days a week. The concept of an athlete used for this study varies considerably from today's standards.

The prevalence rate for breast cancer was consistently lower for the athletes than for the nonathletes. The relative risk for nonathletes was 1.86 compared with that for athletes. Other significant risk factors for breast cancer included age, history of cancer in the family, and age at menarche. These data also showed athletes to have lower rates of reproductive system cancers than nonathletes. The relative risk of cancer of the uterus, ovary, cervix, and vagina was 2.53 for nonathletes, as compared with athletes. Frisch and her colleagues concluded that long-term athletic training established a lifestyle that somehow lowers the risk of breast cancer and cancers of the reproductive system (1985, 1987, 1989). Lifestyle changes may include consumption of less dietary fat and a smaller percentage of body fat. The authors suggested that intensive exercise may stimulate natural immunity via increased activation of natural killer cells (Frisch et al., 1989).

Investigators conducting epidemiologic studies are forced to classify individuals on certain characteristics based on self-reported data. This poses difficult problems when dealing with exercise or physical activity. Epidemiologists have classified individuals by the physical demands of their work as well as their participation in sports; however, these classifications could lead to false conclusions. Often, the studies ignore recreational activity, owing to inability to handle the information. The assumptions are that physical activity leads to some characteristic change, which then results in a reduced risk of cancer. A better method of classification may be to measure the cardiovascular fitness of the subjects.

Blair and his colleagues (1989) published data collected on 13,344 subjects who received a preventive medical examination at the Cooper Clinic in Dallas, Texas between 1970 and 1981. Subjects that did not achieve 85% of age-predicted heart rate during a maximal treadmill exercise test were excluded from the study. Time to exercise exhaustion was the variable used in the analysis. This variable is highly correlated with measured maximal oxygen uptake in men (r = .92) and women (r = .94) (Pollock et al., 1984). Patients were assigned to physical fitness categories based on their age, sex, and maximal time on the treadmill.

The results showed that the least fit persons had a higher risk of death than the more fit ones. More importantly, death rates for cardiovascular disease and cancer showed a strong gradient across fitness groups in both men and women, whereas none was seen for other causes of death. These relationships held after adjustments were made for age, serum cholesterol, smoking habit, blood pressure, fasting glucose level, and length of follow-up.

The study by Blair's group is particularly significant since they actually measured physical fitness. Other epidemiologic studies only infer fitness levels from job or leisure activities. It is reasonable to assume that as time spent exercising increases, so does fitness. A person can be very fit owing to genetic factors alone, so measuring fitness does not answer all of the questions. Nonetheless, measuring fitness provides a stronger link between exercise and cancer than do estimates of physical activity from questionnaires. Unfortunately, the data from Blair's group (1989) do not include information about specific types of cancer.

The relative risk of colon cancer increases with resting heart rate (Severson et al., 1989). The assumption is that as the fitness level increases, the resting heart rate decreases. Thus, a higher level of fitness affords some protection from colon cancer. These data were collected from men, so no information was available on the association with breast cancer.

Two studies reported the risk of cancer using data from the National Health and Nutrition Examination Survey (NHANES I) (Swanson et al., 1988; and Albanes et al., 1989) investigated the relationship between anthropometry

and cancer on 7149 women between age 25 and 74 years. They reported that body size, as defined by weight, relative weight, and skinfold thickness (subscapular and triceps), was not associated with increased risk of breast cancer, though they did find that risk increased for larger women as measured by stature and elbow width. The authors suggested that early nutrition may play a role in the development of stature and of cancer. Other data from the NHANES I suggested that very active persons had a lower risk for cancer than inactive ones (Swanson et al., 1988). Active men had a lower risk of colorectal and lung cancers, whereas active women were less likely to experience cancers of the breast and cervix. The impact of recreational activity on the prevention of cancer was not as strong as the impact of occupational activity.

A number of studies investigated the impact of occupational exercise on the risk of cancer. Vena and coworkers (1985) examined the lifetime occupational histories of patients admitted to a hospital with cancer of the colon or rectum. They found that as the number of work years, proportion of work years, or proportion of life in jobs with sedentary or light work increased so did the risk of colon cancer. No associations were found between job activity variables and risk of cancer of the rectum. Similar results for colon cancer were found in a study on occupation and cause of death on 430,000 Washington State males and 25,000 females (Vena et al., 1987). This second study suggested that the risk of breast cancer is slightly elevated for women who have sedentary jobs. These two studies used different means to collect the data yet yielded similar results.

Paffenbarger and colleagues (1987) reported the results of four studies involving energy expenditure and cancer. Two involved longshoremen. Jobs were rated as demanding high energy expenditure. (5.2 to 7.5 kcal per minute), moderate (2.4 to 5.0 kcal per minute), or low (1.5 to 2.0 kcal per minute). The risk of death increased with decreasing energy expenditure; however, the cancer risk was not related to energy expenditure. The second study on longshoremen showed a trend toward decreased risk of colorectal cancer and higher risk for lung or prostate cancer. Paffenbarger and coworkers (1987) also studied the records of male students from Harvard and female students from the University of Pennsylvania. Physical activity was assessed based on participation in sports as a college student. The more active students (at least 5 hours per week of college sports) were less likely to develop rectal cancer and more likely to develop prostate cancer. The risk of breast cancer was not associated with sports participation.

Finally, this group examined the medical records of Harvard alumni with special emphasis on postcollege physical activity. The risk of all-cause mortality became progressively lower as physical activity energy expenditure increased from less than 500 to about 3500 kcal per week. However, the risk of death from cancer decreased as exercise expenditure increased over 500 kcal per week, but the risk remained steady at higher levels of exercise. Data from the American Cancer Society's Cancer Prevention Study II also suggest that exercise generally reduces the risk of death from cancer (Garfinkel et al., 1988). However, subjects who were classified as heavy exercisers showed an increased risk of cancer. These data were the results from only the first 2 years of the study and should be viewed with caution.

Data from the Framingham study (Ballard-Barbash et al., 1990*a*) reported an increased risk of large bowel cancer among inactive men, but not among inactive women. The authors suggested that the narrow range of physical activity reported by women may have limited their ability to detect an association between cancer and physical activity.

Association Between Body Fat, Exercise, and Neoplasms

It has been known for almost 80 years that underfeeding animals inhibits the growth of transplanted and spontaneous sarcomas (Moreschi, 1909; and Rous, 1914, 1915). Later work suggested that the incidence of skin tumors and spontaneous mammary tumors was augmented in mice fed a high-fat diet (Tannenbaum et al., 1953; Hopkins et al., 1979; and Pariza, 1987) and has led many to believe that dietary fat has important implications for breast cancer in humans. Subsequent research has shown that mammary tumor development does not depend on the amount of fat consumed but instead depends on total energy intake and energy retention in the body (Boissonneault et al., 1986; Kritchevsky et al., 1987; and Simopoulos, 1987). Garfinkel (1985) reviewed data on excess weight and cancer in men and women and concluded that the association between obesity and cancer risk, as shown by a number of studies, implies that high calorie intake may be a risk factor for a number of cancer sites. A high calorie intake over an extended period leads to obesity and its resulting complications.

The increased risk of cancers of the reproductive tissues (including the breast) and obesity seems to be related to the higher estrogen level associated with obesity (Siiteri, 1987; and Simopoulos, 1987). Although the question of estrogen's direct carcinogenicity is not settled, much evidence suggests that it can act as a cocarcinogen or promoter. Adrenal and gonadal androgens are converted to estrogens in peripheral tissues, and this process is enhanced in obese persons (Siiteri, 1987). The percentage conversion of androstenedione to estrone rises from 1% or 2% in normal subjects to 12% to 15% in women who weigh 300 to 400 pounds (Siiteri, 1987). In fact, adipose tissue functions as the major source of estrogen in postmenopausal women (Simopoulos, 1987). Thus, obesity raises the level of estrogen and its neoplasm-promoting characteristics.

Epidemiologists have often used the body mass index (BMI = weight (kg)/height^2 (m^2) as a measure of obesity. This indicates obesity but tells nothing of the distribution of the fat. The waist-hip ratio (WHR) may be a better predictor of the development of cancer than the BMI (Bjorntorp, 1988). In a study of 41,837 Iowa women between age 55 and 69 years, it was found that WHR was highly correlated with mortality while BMI showed little association (Folsom et al., 1993). Women with an upper body fat distribution pattern (android obesity) have a higher risk of breast and endometrial cancer than women with lower body fat distribution (Ballard-Barbash et al., 1990*b*; Elliott et al., 1990; and Schapira et al., 1990, 1991), though

there is some disagreement in this area (Tonkelaar et al., 1992). Bjorntorp (1987) suggested that abdominal obesity leads to an increase in plasma free fatty acids (FFA). This in turn leads to peripheral hyperinsulinemia, hypertriglyceridemia, and insulin insensitivity in muscle. The link between these endocrine aberrations and cancer has not been established (Klurfeld et al., 1989).

An aggressive exercise program will result in a greater loss of abdominal fat than midthigh adipose tissue (Despres et al., 1991). Thirteen obese, premenopausal women participated in a 14-month aerobic exercise program. Their body mass index ranged from 27 to 42 kg/m^2. Body density was measured from a CT scan. Training included 90 minutes of walking, cycling, aerobic dance, or swimming, four or five times per week. Heart rate was monitored to ensure that exercise intensity was approximately 55% of maximum oxygen uptake. A significant volume of fat was lost from the abdomen as well as the thighs, but the abdominal loss was greater. In addition, subjects showed a significant reduction in the insulinogenic index (ratio of insulin area to glucose area) after training. These data suggest that exercise can play a significant role in reducing the upper body fat pattern and may influence cancer risk.

Mice and rats have been used to investigate the influence of dietary fat, calorie restriction, and exercise on tumor promotion. Extrapolation to humans has been questioned (Shephard, 1990), but several animal studies do suggest that exercise reduces the incidence and growth of cancer. Cohen and coworkers (1988) found that female rats that were fed a high-fat diet and exercised voluntarily had a lower tumor appearance rate than animals on a low-fat diet. Exercise also delays protein loss that usually accompanies tumor growth (Deuster et al., 1985). Thompson and colleagues (1988) reported that treadmill exercise increased the incidence and number of 7,12-dimethylbenz[*a*]anthracene–induced tumors in rats as compared with those of their sedentary counterparts, though the level of exercise used in this study was extremely low.

Exercise During Cancer Treatment and Rehabilitation

Progressive loss of function is commonly reported in cancer patients. This deterioration is probably due to the cancer itself, the treatment of the cancer, and the dehabilitating effects of inactivity. Even short periods of bed rest result in dramatic losses in strength and endurance (Taylor et al., 1949; and Convertino et al., 1982). Understanding this relationship led cardiac rehabilitation specialists to the practice of mobilizing patients within 1 or 2 days after coronary artery bypass. Continued bed rest made the rehabilitation process longer and more difficult (Pollock et al., 1984). Evidence is appearing that suggests that these same practices can be beneficial for cancer patients.

One of the first reports on the effects of exercise on cancer patients was given by Buettner and Gavron in 1981. They showed that an 8-week aerobic training program resulted in an improvement in estimated maximum oxygen uptake, resting heart rate, and skinfold thickness in men and women with a history of cancer; however, only two subjects were undergoing treatment at the time of the study.

Winningham and MacVicar (1988) reported on the effects of a 10-week cycle ergometer program on patients with Stage II breast cancer undergoing chemotherapy. Patients were randomly assigned to exercise or nonexercise groups. A third group of healthy, exercising, age-matched women was used for comparison. The exercising group showed a marked improvement in fitness levels on a graded exercise test when compared with the nonexercising cancer group. In addition, the exercising cancer patients showed improvement in fitness comparable to that of the healthy women. A survey also showed that exercise resulted in a significant reduction of tension in the cancer patients. The same authors reported the results of aerobic training programs. In each of these studies, the patients were undergoing chemotherapy for breast cancer. In one study, exercise resulted in a significant decrease in nausea caused by chemotherapy (Winningham et al., 1988). Aerobic exercise also attenuates the gain in body weight associated with chemotherapy (Winningham et al., 1988). More importantly, the subjects who performed aerobic exercises regularly for 10 weeks showed a decrease in body fat, whereas the control group increased their body fat by 2.2%. Thus, the weight gain of the exercise group was lean body weight. These data demonstrate that patients undergoing chemotherapy respond to aerobic training in the same way as healthy persons. A third study reported by this group (MacVicar et al., 1989) investigated the effects of aerobic training on functional capacity as measured by maximum oxygen uptake (VO$_2$max). A 10-week training program at 60% to 85% of VO$_2$max resulted in a 40% improvement in VO$_2$max as well as maximum workload and test time. These data, taken together, show that patients with Stage II breast cancer not only are able to tolerate aerobic training but respond in a manner similar to that of healthy adults. In addition, the aerobic exercise was helpful in attenuating the nausea often associated with chemotherapy.

Mastectomy can lead to loss in shoulder range of motion (Gaskin et al., 1989). A structured stretching program improves flexibility, self-esteem, attitude, and coping strategies. A rehabilitation program that involved aerobic conditioning, keeping a journal, and a 6-day wilderness experience also helped women cope with many of the fears associated with having cancer (Johnson and Wilde-Kelly, 1990).

Guidelines and Precautions

Winningham and coworkers (1986) suggest that exercise prescriptions should address the needs of two types of cancer patients: those accustomed to exercise and those who have been sedentary. Patients who have exercised regularly before being diagnosed often want to continue exercising during and after treatment to maintain their lifestyle and feeling of well-being. These patients need counseling about the effects of the disease as well as the side effects of treatment that may make exercise hazardous. In some cases, exercise may be contraindicated for a time, depending on the type of cancer and the effects of treatment. In contrast, sedentary patients may interpret fatigue as evidence of the

need to rest. Fatigue is an inevitable consequence of the illness and treatment; though the patient may use these feelings to reduce activity further, which results in even greater loss in functional capacity (Pfalzer, 1988). Such patients need encouragement to stay active and may profit from motivational programs. Both kinds of patients can benefit from supervised exercise programs to ensure that they receive optimal benefits.

In designing an exercise program one must realize that cancer patients may suffer anorexia, weight loss, and fatigue. Side effects of treatment such as nausea, vomiting, diarrhea, and decreased appetite may impair the patients' ability to maintain an exercise program. It is also important to understand that cancer patients undergoing chemotherapy or irradiation may not respond to exercise in the same way as healthy persons. Many of the drugs inhibit protein anabolism and could block the processes expected to produce results from training (Pfalzer et al., 1986). Chemotherapeutic agents are also associated with both cardiac and pulmonary toxicity (Watchie, 1992). The most common manifestations of acute toxicity, arrhythmias and conduction disturbances, in rare cases can lead to left ventricular dysfunction and congestive heart failure. Exercise might however be beneficial in preserving muscle mass that is typically catabolized during cancer treatment.

Patients' responses to treatment differ, so it is necessary to closely monitor and reevaluate the exercise program of patients undergoing treatment. Those who develop an irregular pulse, joint pain, shortness of breath or excessive fatigue should be referred to a physician immediately (Winningham et al., 1986). It may be necessary during certain phases of treatment to reduce or even eliminate exercise programs. Contraindications to exercise are listed in Table 40–1. During periods of reduced activity, range of motion activities and mild resistance exercises can help slow the loss of functional capacity.

Owing to the many complications associated with cancer treatment, and given the fact that few persons are trained in both principles of exercise prescription and clinical oncology, a team approach is recommended to establish safe, individualized exercise guidelines. Such a team could con-

Table 40–1. CONTRAINDICATIONS TO EXERCISE FOR CANCER PATIENTS

Unusual fatigability
Unusual muscular weakness
Development of irregular pulse
Leg pain or cramps
Chest pain
Acute onset of nausea during exercise
Vomiting within previous 24–36 hours
Severe diarrhea within previous 24–36 hours
Disorientation, confusion
Dizziness, blurred vision, faintness
Pallor, cyanosis
Sudden-onset dyspnea
Decreased heart rate and/or blood pressure with increased workload
IV chemotherapy within previous 24 hours

(From Winningham, M. L., MacVicar, M. G., and Burke, C. A.: Exercise for cancer patients: Guidelines and precautions. Phys. Sports Med., *14*:125–134, 1986. Reproduced with permission of McGraw-Hill, Inc.)

sist of an exercise physiologist, a clinical nurse specialist in oncology, a physical therapist, and a dietitian (Winningham et al., 1986). This team should work closely with physicians.

Exercise Screening

Screening should always precede an exercise test or an exercise program (Watchie, 1992). In the case of the cancer patient, one cannot ignore the possibility of pre-existing cardiovascular problems. In addition, chemotherapy and radiation therapy may affect the cardiopulmonary system and complicate exercise therapy (Pfalzer, 1988; and Watchie, 1992). Patients should be screened for orthopedic problems that could prevent them from participating in aerobic activities (Winningham et al., 1986). Compromised skeletal integrity may preclude weight bearing. Non–weight-bearing activities such as cycling, swimming, and rowing can still provide cardiovascular benefits.

The patient's fitness level is best assessed by a symptom-limited, graded exercise test on a treadmill or a cycle ergometer. In most cases, the subject will be unable to attain a true maximum heart rate owing to fatigue or some other problem (Winningham et al., 1986); however, the results of the symptom-limited test are sufficient to develop an exercise prescription. Using a rating of perceived exertion (RPE) scale is often helpful during the endurance evaluation as well as in the exercise prescription. A rating of 13 or ''somewhat hard'' on a 6- to 20-point scale is a desirable goal for cancer patients (Watchie, 1992). The patient's primary care physician should approve the exercise prescription. Clearance should also be obtained from a cardiologist familiar with the screening results.

EXERCISE GUIDELINES FOR HEALTHY PERSONS

A patient undergoing cancer therapy needs to be cautious when beginning or continuing an exercise program. A healthy person may lower the risk of cancer by engaging in a regular endurance or aerobic exercise program. The word *exercise* has many different meanings, and without the proper supervision or some guidelines, most persons will not be successful in establishing a long-term exercise habit. The purpose of the following information is to provide guidelines for beginning an exercise program safely. It discusses the concept of ''fitness'' and the parameters involved with improving fitness.

What Is Physical Fitness?

Physical fitness is best viewed as an ability to exercise vigorously without undue fatigue. Fit persons have *endurance* and are able to work harder with less effort than those who are not physically fit. The term *fitness* can be used to describe a variety of abilities. Fitness can be described as the ability to lift a heavy weight, sprint short distances, or flex to extreme ranges of motion. By far the most important component of fitness is the capacity to sustain continuous exercise such as walking, jogging, cycling, or swimming with only moderate stress and to recover quickly when the exercise is finished. While the lay person uses the terms *stamina* and *endurance*, the physician and exercise physiologist use the terms *cardiovascular* or *aerobic fitness*. These labels are more descriptive because they point out the important role of the heart and circulation of the blood in the delivery of oxygen to the muscles, which is used to produce energy. One can generate some energy without oxygen, but the amount is limited. The way to increase the capacity to sustain exercise is to increase aerobic fitness.

Aerobic exercise is the most effective way to exercise when trying to lose weight. Activities such as weight lifting and calisthenics can improve overall physical fitness, but they do not use up a significant number of calories. Therefore, in addition to improving aerobic fitness, aerobic exercise is a useful means of weight control.

The primary role of exercise for the cancer patient is to help prevent the loss of functional capacity. In addition, exercise may play a role in diminishing the side effects associated with treatment, including psychological burdens. Finally, much evidence now exists to suggest that exercise may prevent cancer. This is true not only for breast cancer but other types of cancer as well. The information that follows provides a basis for safely beginning an exercise program.

The Exercise Program

Four factors must be considered when beginning an exercise program: intensity, frequency, duration, and mode (i.e., type of exercise).

Intensity of Exercise: The Target Zone. A certain level of exercise must be reached and sustained in order to train the cardiovascular system effectively and improve aerobic fitness. This so-called target zone is between 70% and 85% of the maximum exercise heart rate. Below 70% of capacity, little fitness benefit is achieved. Above 85% of maximum there is little added benefit. The added intensity also increases the chance for injury. As long as training takes place in the target zone, fitness will improve. However, many cancer patients can benefit from less intense exercise (20% to 60% of maximum heart rate) that may not be as threatening or fatiguing (Winningham et al., 1986). The fact that many cancer patients are often deconditioned accounts for the training response to lower intensities.

The target zone is based on an age-predicted maximum heart rate. Maximum heart rate can be determined by 3 or 4 minutes of all-out exercise, but this may be inadvisable because intense exercise is difficult, requires strong motivation, and could be dangerous to persons predisposed to heart disease. Maximum heart rate can be estimated by subtracting the person's age from 220 (e.g., a 40-year-old man would have an age-predicted maximum heart rate of 180 beats per minute). With increasing age, maximum heart rate decreases and the target zone becomes lower. Figure 40–1 shows the relationship between heart rate, age, and target zone.

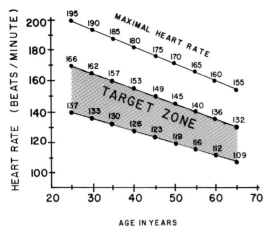

Figure 40–1. Relationship between maximum heart rate, target zone, and age.

For accuracy, it is important to count the pulse immediately upon stopping exercise because the rate changes very quickly when exercise is stopped or slowed down. The count for 10 seconds is multiplied by six to obtain the count for a full minute. Counting for a full minute, or even for 15 seconds, produces a false value because the heart rate drops off too fast.

By trial and error, the person develops an exercise pattern that seems easy for 5 to 10 minutes and then counts the pulse. It should be less than 50% of the age-predicted maximum heart rate. Then, the intensity of exercise is increased to achieve the *target zone.* After 3 to 5 minutes at the higher intensity the exerciser stops to check the heart rate again and adjusts the intensity if the rate is too high or too low. The high intensity workout is followed by one of lower intensity as a cool-down period. The exercise period should be increased progressively to 30 minutes; the length of the warm-up and cool-down basically stays the same. A typical exercise period should consist of (1) 10 to 15 minutes' warm-up, (2) 20 to 30 minutes' exercise with the heart rate in the target zone, and (3) 10 to 15 minutes of cool-down.

The intensity of the workout can easily be manipulated by changing the speed of walking or jogging. Some may find it difficult to achieve the target zone only by walking and will find it necessary to alternate walking with jogging. However, each individual must be cautioned about trying to do too much exercise in the initial stages of the program. They must *start slowly* and build up to the desired intensity. It is necessary to give the body time to adapt to the new demands placed on it by the exercise program. An early setback due to an injury may be the excuse someone needs to give up on exercise. In addition, persons undergoing cancer therapy may have to adjust the intensity level depending on the stage of treatment.

Frequency of Exercise. To make aerobic gains, exercise must be performed at least three times a week. It is true that persons who have been bedridden for some time can benefit from exercising twice a week, but their gains will be modest. It is best to space the intervals over a week's time rather than exercising on three consecutive days. Exercise on consecutive days tends to cause more injuries and may be counterproductive.

Duration of Exercise. It is a mistake to do too much too soon. Exercisers should start with 15 minutes, and gradually increase the duration of exercise to 30 minutes over a period of 5 to 6 weeks. The ankles, knees, and hips need time to adjust to the added workload.

Modes of Exercise. Not all types of exercise promote fitness equally. Exercises that result in cardiovascular fitness must (1) increase the heart rate to target zone and keep it there for at least 20 minutes, (2) involve large muscle masses, and be (3) rhythmic and (4) continuous.

Weight lifting and games such as tennis and racquetball are stop-and-go activities that generally cause peaks and valleys in the heart rate. Activities such as walking, jogging, swimming, cycling, rowing, cross-country skiing, and aerobic dancing are all highly aerobic and allow for continued improvement. Overall fitness is improved if the activities are varied. Rowing and jumping rope are examples of exercises that are aerobically demanding for both the arms and legs and therefore benefit both.

Getting Started

Guidelines to follow in beginning an aerobic exercise program are based on research and common sense.

Start slowly. Proceed carefully and do not hurry. For most people it is best to begin by walking. The intensity of the exercise can be varied by the speed of walking or by combining walking with short periods of jogging.

Dress sensibly. Do not begin an exercise program without proper footwear. No one shoe is right for everyone. Stores that deal exclusively in running apparel or athletic equipment are best when shopping for shoes. Wear loose-fitting clothing. The objective is to avoid excessive perspiration rather than encouraging it. Excessive sweating can lead to dehydration. Any weight that is lost by perspiration is quickly regained when the individual rehydrates with water or some other beverage.

Include a warm-up period. It is important to warm up for several minutes. This is perhaps the best time to include stretching exercises, which allow muscles and the circulatory system to adjust gradually.

Allow a cool-down period. Exercises should slow down gradually for at least 5 minutes before stopping. This allows the circulation and metabolism to return slowly to normal levels. During cool-down one must continue to walk slowly or stretch. A lukewarm shower, rather than a hot or a cold one, is in order.

After 2 to 3 weeks of regular exercise fitness begins to improve. The same workout feels easier. It is not uncommon, after 6 to 8 weeks of aerobic exercises, to observe a drop in heart rate of 20 to 30 beats per minute for the same running speed.

As fitness continues to improve the workload is increased if the heart rate is not in the target zone. Once a satisfactory fitness level is achieved, it is maintained by regular workouts. The amount of effort required to *maintain* fitness is considerably less than that required to *achieve* fitness.

FITNESS APPRAISAL

A fitness appraisal is used to test the effectiveness of the training program and to help set and achieve personal goals.

Fitness appraisal places rigorous demands on the body. Attempting to perform these tests after years of inactivity can result in more harm to the body than benefit. Therefore the cardiorespiratory endurance assessment is not recommended without clearance by a physician and until after a period of 4 to 6 weeks of regular exercise.

Cardiorespiratory Assessment

The ability of the body to utilize oxygen depends on the efficiency of the heart, lungs, blood, and muscles. The job of the heart, lungs, and blood is to deliver the oxygen to the muscles and to remove carbon dioxide. During vigorous activity, the muscles require increased amounts of oxygen and produce more carbon dioxide. Tests of cardiorespiratory endurance measure the ability of the system to deliver and utilize oxygen. The test estimates cardiorespiratory endurance and permits a comparison of the individual's fitness with recommended levels.

Step Test. The step test is suited for older adults or for those just beginning an exercise program. The test should be taken after 4 to 6 weeks of progressive conditioning. The following items are needed:

1. Box, step, or bench (15 3/4 inches high for men; 13 inches for women).

2. Clock or watch with a sweep second hand.

3. Metronome or other device programmed for 90 beats per minute.

4. A quiet room with a moderate temperature (65° to 75°F).

A pace of 90 beats per minute results in 22.5 steps per minute. With each signal from the pacing device, one step is taken, stepping up first with the left foot and then with the right and then down with the left foot and then with the right. The subject keeps pace with the tempo and straightens both legs when stepping up on the bench. The lead leg may be changed during the test if desired. If the subject is unable to keep pace with the timer, the test stops and another try is made after several weeks.

After 5 minutes of exercise the subject sits down, and the pulse is taken for a 15-second period starting exactly at 15 seconds after stopping the exercise and ending exactly at 30 seconds. Weight is measured in the outfit worn during the test.

The test is scored as follows:

1. Using Figure 40–2 for women, locate body weight.
2. Locate the postexercise pulse count in the extreme left column.

WOMEN　　　　　　　　　　　　　　　　　　　　　　　　　Fitness score ③

Post-exercise pulse count ②	80	90	100	110	120	130	140	150	160	170	180	190
45										29	29	29
44								30	30	30	30	30
43							31	31	31	31	31	31
42			32	32	32	32	32	32	32	32	32	32
41			33	33	33	33	33	33	33	33	33	33
40			34	34	34	34	34	34	34	34	34	34
39			35	35	35	35	35	35	35	35	35	35
38			36	36	36	36	36	36	36	36	36	36
37			37	37	37	37	37	37	37	37	37	37
36		37	38	38	38	38	38	38	38	38	38	38
35	38	38	39	39	39	39	39	39	39	39	39	39
34	39	39	40	40	40	40	40	40	40	40	40	40
33	40	40	41	41	41	41	41	41	41	41	41	41
32	41	41	42	42	42	42	42	42	42	42	42	42
31	42	42	43	43	43	43	43	43	43	43	43	43
30	43	43	44	44	44	44	44	44	44	44	44	44
29	44	44	45	45	45	45	45	45	45	45	45	45
28	45	45	46	46	46	47	47	47	47	47		
27	46	46	47	48	48	49	49	49	49			
26	47	48	49	50	50	51	51	51				
25	49	50	51	52	52	53	53					
24	51	52	53	54	54	55						
23	53	54	55	56	56	57						

① Body weight

Figure 40–2. Predicted fitness score for women based on weight and postexercise pulse count. (From Sharkey, B. J.: Physiology of Fitness. 2nd ed. Champaign, IL, Human Kinetics Publishers, 1984, p. 259. Copyright 1984 by Brian J. Sharkey. Reprinted by permission.)

3. Read across the pulse count row until it intersects with the column for body weight. Record the fitness score.

4. Using Figure 40–3, find the age-adjusted score opposite the nearest age.

5. With the adjusted fitness score find the physical fitness rating as compared with that of other persons of similar age in Figure 40–4. Properly administered, the test provides a reasonable estimate of aerobic fitness.

Body Composition Assessment

Although many people use the terms *overweight* and *obese* interchangeably, they have different meanings. Persons are *overweight* whose body weight is greater than that of the average person of their height. *Obesity* is defined as having an excess amount of body fat. It is possible to be obese and not overweight. The distinction between overweight and

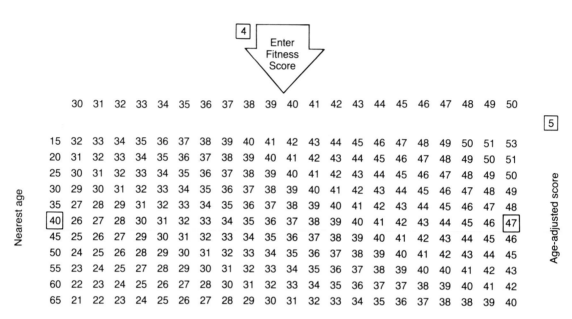

Example: If your age is 40 years and you score 50 on the step test, your age-adjusted score is 47.

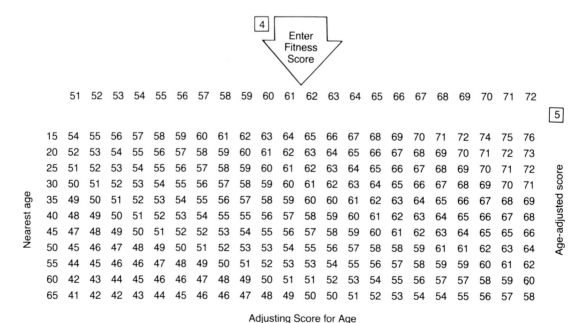

Example: If your age is 40 years and you score 50 on the step test, your age-adjusted score is 47.

Figure 40–3. Fitness score adjustment based on age. (From Sharkey, B. J.: Physiology of Fitness. 2nd ed. Champaign, IL, Human Kinetics Publishers, 1984, pp. 260–261. Copyright 1984 by Brian J. Sharkey. Reprinted by permission.)

PHYSICAL FITNESS RATING - WOMEN

(Use Age-Adjusted Score)   6   7

Nearest age	Superior	Excellent	Very good	Good	Fair	Poor	Very poor
15	54 +	53-49	48-44	43-39	38-34	33-29	28 –
20	53 +	52-48	47-43	42-38	37-33	32-28	27 –
25	52 +	51-47	46-42	41-37	36-32	31-27	26 –
30	51 +	50-46	45-41	40-36	35-31	30-26	25 –
35	50 +	49-45	44-40	39-35	34-30	29-25	24 –
40	49 +	48-44	43-39	38-34	33-29	28-24	23 –
45	48 +	47-43	42-38	37-33	32-28	27-23	22 –
50	47 +	46-42	41-37	36-32	31-27	26-22	21 –
55	46 +	45-41	40-36	35-31	30-26	25-21	20 –
60	45 +	44-40	39-35	34-30	29-25	24-20	19 –
65	44 +	43-39	38-34	33-29	28-24	23-20	19 –

Figure 40–4. Physical fitness rating for women. (From Sharkey, B. J.: Physiology of Fitness. 2nd ed. Champaign, IL, Human Kinetics Publishers, 1984, p. 262. Copyright 1984 by Brian J. Sharkey. Reprinted by permission.)

obese is an important one. When a large percentage of body weight is fat, it has a negative impact on health.

A variety of methods are used to assess body composition (Nieman, 1990). Height-weight tables have been used for well over 100 years, yet they do not distinguish between overweight and obesity. The BMI is used as a measure of body composition by a number of epidemiologists, but it still lacks the information needed to distinguish between fat and lean body weight. The WHR is a good predictor of cancer risk (Folsom et al., 1993). This simple measurement reveals the importance of abdominal fat for metabolic functions that may play a role in cancer risk. Guidelines suggest that for women WHR should not exceed 0.8 and for men it should be less than 0.9 (Howely et al., 1992).

Estimations of body composition by underwater weight or skinfold thickness are two of the better methods for estimating body composition. Another method that is almost as good requires only measurement of the circumference of various parts of the body. Each measurement should be performed twice, to the nearest 1/8 inch without indenting the skin, and then averaged. A woman's percentage of fat is estimated by taking these measurements:

1. Neck circumference just below the larynx
2. The circumference of the abdomen at the navel.
3. The largest circumference of the upper arm with the arm fully extended and parallel to the floor, palm facing up.
4. The largest circumference of the forearm with the arm fully extended and parallel to the floor, palm facing up.
5. The circumference of the thigh when the feet are approximately shoulder width apart, placing the tape just below the left buttock, parallel to the floor.

All measurements are converted to fat percentage points using Table 40–2. The points obtained from each of the five measurement sites are added and a correction factor of 54.598 is subtracted from the total. The difference is the percentage of fat.

What the percentage of body fat should be is sometimes difficult to answer. Goals of 24% for women and 18% for men will reduce risk for a variety of diseases and are reasonable expectations, in terms of weight control.

ENERGY BALANCE AND WEIGHT CONTROL

The most lasting form of weight reduction is achieved with a balance of diet and exercise. The energy balance relationship states that, in order to lose weight the number of calories expended must exceed the number of calories consumed. There are three ways to achieve a calorie deficit:

1. Eat less (i.e., reduce calorie intake below daily energy requirements).
2. Exercise more (i.e., increase calorie expenditure above daily intake).
3. Use a combination of items 1 and 2. (This is the best method.)

When weight is lost by dieting alone, much of the loss is muscle mass instead of fat. On the other hand, exercise alone is only slightly useful in short-term weight reduction. For example, it takes 26 minutes of walking at the rate of 3 miles per hour to burn off the calories in one doughnut or 11 minutes of jogging to spend the calories in 12 ounces of beer. An even more discouraging example is that only 1 pound of fat is used to run an entire marathon (26 miles). These examples point out the need to regard weight reduction as a long-term process.

Since most weight gains occur slowly as a result of a small positive calorie balance, exercise can help offset weight gain. Walking a mile a day (100 calories per mile) utilizes approximately 700 calories per week. Over a 1-year period this amounts to 36,400 calories, which is equivalent to 10.5 pounds of fat. This can add up over several years.

Reducing calorie consumption by 500 calories per day and increasing energy expenditure by 500 calories per day produces weight loss of 2 pounds per week. Over a period

Table 40–2. PREDICTING PERCENTAGE OF BODY FAT IN WOMEN

Neck*	PTS	Neck	PTS	Neck	PTS	Neck	PTS	Neck	PTS
15 5/8	0.1	13 7/8	4.1	12 1/8	8.0	10 3/8	11.9	8 5/8	15.4
15 4/8	0.4	13 6/8	4.3	12 0/8	8.2	10 2/8	12.1	8 4/8	16.1
15 3/8	0.7	13 5/8	4.6	11 7/8	8.5	10 1/8	12.4	8 3/8	16.3
15 2/8	1.0	13 4/8	4.9	11 6/8	8.8	10 0/8	12.7	8 2/8	16.7
15 1/8	1.3	13 3/8	5.2	11 5/8	9.1	9 7/8	13.0	8 1/8	16.9
15 0/8	1.5	13 2/8	5.4	11 4/8	9.4	9 6/8	13.3	8 0/8	17.2
14 7/8	1.8	13 1/8	5.7	11 3/8	9.6	9 5/8	13.5	7 7/8	17.4
14 6/8	2.1	13 0/8	6.0	11 2/8	9.9	9 4/8	13.8	7 6/8	17.7
14 5/8	2.4	12 7/8	6.3	11 1/8	10.2	9 3/8	14.1	7 5/8	18.0
14 4/8	2.7	12 6/8	6.6	11 0/8	10.6	9 2/8	14.4	7 4/8	18.3
14 3/8	2.9	12 5/8	6.8	10 7/8	10.8	9 1/8	14.7	7 3/8	18.6
14 2/8	3.2	12 4/8	7.1	10 6/8	11.0	9 0/8	14.9		
14 1/8	3.5	12 3/8	7.4	10 5/8	11.3	8 7/8	15.2		
14 0/8	3.8	12 2/8	7.7	10 4/8	11.6	8 6/8	15.5		

Biceps	PTS	Biceps	PTS	Biceps	PTS	Biceps	PTS	Biceps	PTS
5 7/8	0.1	7 5/8	4.8	9 3/8	9.4	11 1/8	14.1	12 7/8	18.8
6 0/8	0.4	7 6/8	5.1	9 4/8	9.8	11 2/8	14.5	13 0/8	19.1
6 1/8	0.8	7 7/8	5.4	9 5/8	10.1	11 3/8	14.8	13 1/8	19.5
6 2/8	1.1	8 0/8	5.8	9 6/8	10.4	11 4/8	15.1	13 2/8	19.8
6 3/8	1.4	8 1/8	6.1	9 7/8	10.8	11 5/8	15.5	13 3/8	20.1
6 4/8	1.8	8 2/8	6.4	10 0/8	11.1	11 6/8	15.8	13 4/8	20.5
6 5/8	2.1	8 3/8	6.8	10 1/8	11.4	11 7/8	16.1	13 5/8	20.8
6 6/8	2.4	8 4/8	7.1	10 2/8	11.8	12 0/8	16.5	13 6/8	21.1
6 7/8	2.8	8 5/8	7.4	10 3/8	12.1	12 1/8	16.8		
7 0/8	3.1	8 6/8	7.8	10 4/8	12.4	12 2/8	17.1		
7 1/8	3.4	8 7/8	8.1	10 5/8	12.8	12 3/8	17.5		
7 2/8	3.8	9 0/8	8.4	10 6/8	13.1	12 4/8	17.8		
7 3/8	4.1	9 1/8	8.8	10 7/8	13.5	12 5/8	18.1		
7 4/8	4.4	9 2/8	9.1	11 0/8	13.8	12 6/8	18.5		

Forearm	PTS	Forearm	PTS	Forearm	PTS	Forearm	PTS	Forearm	PTS
17 5/8	0.2	15 2/8	9.3	12 7/8	18.5	10 4/8	27.7	8 1/8	36.8
17 4/8	0.6	15 1/8	9.8	12 6/8	19.0	10 3/8	28.1	8 0/8	37.3
17 3/8	1.1	15 0/8	10.3	12 5/8	19.5	10 2/8	28.5	7 7/8	37.8
17 2/8	1.6	14 7/8	10.8	12 4/8	19.9	10 1/8	29.1	7 6/8	38.3
17 1/8	2.1	14 6/8	11.2	12 3/8	20.4	10 0/8	29.6	7 5/8	38.8
17 0/8	2.5	14 5/8	11.7	12 2/8	20.9	9 7/8	30.1	7 4/8	39.3
16 7/8	3.0	14 4/8	12.2	12 1/8	21.4	9 6/8	30.6	7 3/8	39.7
16 6/8	3.5	14 3/8	12.7	12 0/8	21.9	9 5/8	31.0	7 2/8	40.2
16 5/8	4.0	14 2/8	13.2	11 7/8	22.3	9 4/8	31.5	7 1/8	40.7
16 4/8	4.5	14 1/8	13.7	11 6/8	22.8	9 3/8	32.0	7 0/8	41.2
16 3/8	5.0	14 0/8	14.1	11 5/8	23.3	9 2/8	32.5	6 7/8	41.7
16 2/8	5.4	13 7/8	14.6	11 4/8	23.8	9 1/8	33.0	6 6/8	42.2
16 1/8	5.9	13 6/8	15.1	11 3/8	24.3	9 0/8	33.5	6 5/8	42.5
16 0/8	6.4	13 5/8	15.6	11 2/8	24.9	8 7/8	33.9	0 0/8	0.0
15 7/8	6.9	13 4/8	16.1	11 1/8	25.2	8 6/8	34.4		
15 6/8	7.4	13 3/8	16.6	11 0/8	25.7	8 5/8	34.9		
15 5/8	7.9	13 2/8	17.0	10 7/8	26.2	8 4/8	35.4		
15 4/8	8.3	13 1/8	17.5	10 6/8	26.7	8 3/8	36.0		
15 3/8	8.8	13 0/8	18.0	10 5/8	27.2	8 2/8	36.4		

Abdomen	PTS	Abdomen	PTS	Abdomen	PTS	Abdomen	PTS	Abdomen	PTS	Abdomen	PTS
17 5/8	0.0	23 0/8	4.4	28 3/8	8.9	33 6/8	13.3	39 1/8	17.8	44 4/8	22.3
17 6/8	0.1	23 1/8	4.5	28 4/8	9.0	33 7/8	13.4	39 2/8	17.9	44 5/8	22.3
17 7/8	0.2	23 2/8	4.6	28 5/8	9.1	34 0/8	13.5	39 3/8	18.0	44 6/8	22.4
18 0/8	0.3	23 3/8	4.7	28 6/8	9.2	34 1/8	13.6	39 4/8	18.1	44 7/8	22.5
18 1/8	0.4	23 4/8	4.8	28 7/8	9.3	34 2/8	13.7	39 5/8	18.2	45 0/8	22.6
18 2/8	0.5	23 5/8	4.9	29 0/8	9.4	34 3/8	13.8	39 6/8	18.3	45 1/8	22.7
18 3/8	0.6	23 6/8	5.0	29 1/8	9.5	34 4/8	14.0	39 7/8	18.4	45 2/8	22.8
18 4/8	0.7	23 7/8	5.2	29 2/8	9.6	34 5/8	14.1	40 0/8	18.5	45 3/8	22.9
18 5/8	0.8	24 0/8	5.3	29 3/8	9.7	34 6/8	14.2	40 1/8	18.6	45 4/8	23.1
18 6/8	0.9	24 1/8	5.4	29 4/8	9.8	34 7/8	14.3	40 2/8	18.7	45 5/8	23.2
18 7/8	1.0	24 2/8	5.5	29 5/8	9.9	35 0/8	14.4	40 3/8	18.8	45 6/8	23.3
19 0/8	1.1	24 3/8	5.6	29 6/8	10.0	35 1/8	14.5	40 4/8	18.9	45 7/8	23.4
19 1/8	1.2	24 4/8	5.7	29 7/8	10.1	35 2/8	14.6	0 5/8	19.0	46 0/8	23.5
19 2/8	1.3	24 5/8	5.8	30 0/8	10.2	35 3/8	14.7	40 6/8	19.1	46 1/8	23.6
19 3/8	1.4	24 6/8	5.9	30 1/8	10.3	35 4/8	14.8	40 7/8	19.2	46 2/8	23.7

Table 40–2. PREDICTING PERCENTAGE OF BODY FAT IN WOMEN *Continued*

Abdomen	PTS	Abdomen	PTS	Abdomen	PTS	Abdomen	PTS	Abdomen	PTS	Abdomen	PTS
19 4/8	1.5	24 7/8	6.0	30 2/8	10.4	35 5/8	14.9	41 0/8	19.3	46 3/8	23.8
19 5/8	1.6	25 0/8	6.1	30 3/8	10.5	35 6/8	15.0	41 1/8	19.4	46 4/8	23.9
19 6/8	1.7	25 1/8	6.2	30 4/8	10.6	35 7/8	15.1	41 2/8	19.5	46 5/8	24.0
19 7/8	1.8	25 2/8	6.3	30 5/8	10.7	36 0/8	15.2	41 3/8	19.6	46 6/8	24.1
20 0/8	1.9	25 3/8	6.4	30 6/8	10.8	36 1/8	15.3	41 4/8	19.7	46 7/8	24.2
20 1/8	2.0	25 4/8	6.5	30 7/8	10.9	36 2/8	15.4	41 5/8	19.9	47 0/8	24.3
20 2/8	2.2	25 5/8	6.6	31 0/8	11.1	36 3/8	15.5	41 6/8	20.0	47 1/8	24.4
20 3/8	2.3	25 6/8	6.7	31 1/8	11.2	36 4/8	15.6	41 7/8	20.1	47 2/8	24.5
20 4/8	2.4	25 7/8	6.8	31 2/8	11.3	36 5/8	15.7	42 0/8	20.2	47 3/8	24.6
20 5/8	2.5	26 0/8	6.9	31 3/8	11.4	36 6/8	15.8	42 1/8	20.3	47 4/8	24.7
20 6/8	2.6	26 1/8	7.0	31 4/8	11.5	36 7/8	15.9	42 2/8	20.4	47 5/8	24.8
20 7/8	2.7	26 2/8	7.1	31 5/8	11.6	37 0/8	16.0	42 3/8	20.5	47 6/8	24.9
21 0/8	2.8	26 3/8	7.2	31 6/8	11.7	37 1/8	16.1	42 4/8	20.6	47 7/8	25.0
21 1/8	2.9	26 4/8	7.3	31 7/8	11.8	37 2/8	16.2	42 5/8	20.7	48 0/8	25.1
21 2/8	3.0	26 5/8	7.4	32 0/8	11.9	37 3/8	16.3	42 6/8	20.8	48 1/8	25.2
21 3/8	3.1	26 6/8	7.5	32 1/8	12.0	37 4/8	16.4	42 7/8	20.9	48 2/8	25.3
21 4/8	3.2	26 7/8	7.6	32 2/8	12.1	37 5/8	16.5	43 0/8	21.0	48 3/8	25.4
21 5/8	3.3	27 0/8	7.7	32 3/8	12.2	37 6/8	16.6	43 1/8	21.1	48 4/8	25.5
21 6/8	3.4	27 1/8	7.8	32 4/8	12.3	37 7/8	16.7	43 2/8	21.2	48 5/8	25.6
21 7/8	3.5	27 2/8	7.9	32 5/8	12.4	38 0/8	16.8	43 3/8	21.3	48 6/8	25.7
22 0/8	3.6	27 3/8	8.1	32 6/8	12.5	38 1/8	17.0	43 4/8	21.4	48 7/8	25.8
22 1/8	3.7	27 4/8	8.2	32 7/8	12.6	38 2/8	17.1	43 5/8	21.5	49 0/8	26.0
22 2/8	3.8	27 5/8	8.3	33 0/8	12.7	38 3/8	17.2	43 6/8	21.6	49 1/8	26.1
22 3/8	3.9	27 6/8	8.4	33 1/8	12.8	38 4/8	17.3	43 7/8	21.7		
22 4/8	4.0	27 7/8	8.5	33 2/8	12.9	38 5/8	17.4	44 0/8	21.8		
22 5/8	4.1	28 0/8	8.6	33 3/8	13.0	38 6/8	17.5	44 1/8	21.9		
22 6/8	4.2	28 1/8	8.7	33 4/8	13.1	38 7/8	17.6	44 2/8	22.0		
22 7/8	4.3	28 2/8	8.8	33 5/8	13.2	39 0/8	17.7	44 3/8	22.1		

Thigh	PTS	Thigh	PTS	Thigh	PTS	Thigh	PTS	Thigh	PTS
11 6/8	0.0	16 2/8	7.0	20 6/8	13.7	25 2/8	20.5	29 6/8	27.3
11 7/8	0.2	16 3/8	7.1	20 7/8	13.9	25 3/8	20.7	29 7/8	27.5
12 0/8	0.4	16 4/8	7.3	21 0/8	14.1	25 4/8	20.9	30 0/8	27.7
12 1/8	0.6	16 5/8	7.4	21 1/8	14.3	25 5/8	21.1	30 1/8	27.9
12 2/8	0.8	16 6/8	7.6	21 2/8	14.5	25 6/8	21.3	30 2/8	28.1
12 3/8	1.0	16 7/8	7.8	21 3/8	14.6	25 7/8	21.5	30 3/8	28.3
12 4/8	1.2	17 0/8	8.0	21 4/8	14.8	26 0/8	21.7	30 4/8	28.5
12 5/8	1.4	17 1/8	8.2	21 5/8	15.0	26 1/8	21.8	30 6/8	28.9
12 6/8	1.6	17 2/8	8.4	21 6/8	15.2	26 2/8	22.0	30 7/8	29.0
12 7/8	1.8	17 3/8	8.6	21 7/8	15.4	26 3/8	22.2	31 0/8	29.2
13 0/8	1.9	17 4/8	8.8	22 0/8	15.6	26 4/8	22.4	31 1/8	29.4
13 1/8	2.1	17 5/8	9.0	22 1/8	15.8	26 5/8	22.6	31 2/8	29.6
13 2/8	2.3	17 6/8	9.1	22 2/8	16.0	26 6/8	22.8	31 3/8	29.8
13 3/8	2.5	17 7/8	9.3	22 3/8	16.2	26 7/8	23.0	31 4/8	30.0
13 4/8	2.7	18 0/8	9.5	22 4/8	16.3	27 0/8	23.2	31 5/8	30.2
13 5/8	2.9	18 1/8	9.7	22 5/8	16.5	27 1/8	23.4	31 6/8	30.4
13 6/8	3.1	18 2/8	9.9	22 6/8	16.7	27 2/8	23.6	31 7/8	30.6
13 7/8	3.3	18 3/8	10.1	22 7/8	16.9	27 3/8	23.7	32 0/8	30.8
14 0/8	3.5	18 4/8	10.3	23 0/8	17.1	27 4/8	23.9	32 1/8	30.9
14 1/8	3.6	18 5/8	10.5	23 1/8	17.3	27 5/8	24.1	32 2/8	31.1
14 2/8	3.8	18 6/8	10.7	23 2/8	17.5	27 6/8	24.3	32 3/8	31.3
14 3/8	4.0	18 7/8	10.9	23 3/8	17.7	27 7/8	24.5	32 4/8	31.5
14 4/8	4.2	19 0/8	11.0	23 4/8	17.9	28 0/8	24.7	32 5/8	31.7
14 5/8	4.4	19 1/8	11.2	23 5/8	18.1	28 1/8	24.9	32 6/8	31.9
14 6/8	4.6	19 2/8	11.4	23 6/8	18.2	28 2/8	25.1	32 7/8	32.1
14 7/8	4.8	19 3/8	11.6	23 7/8	18.4	28 3/8	25.3	33 0/8	32.3
15 0/8	5.0	19 4/8	11.8	24 0/8	18.6	28 4/8	25.4	33 1/8	32.5
15 1/8	5.2	19 5/8	12.0	24 1/8	18.8	28 5/8	25.6	33 2/8	32.7
15 2/8	5.4	19 6/8	12.2	24 2/8	19.0	28 6/8	25.8	33 3/8	32.8
15 3/8	5.5	19 7/8	12.4	24 3/8	19.2	28 7/8	26.0	33 4/8	32.9
15 4/8	5.7	20 0/8	12.6	24 4/8	19.4	29 0/8	26.2		
15 5/8	5.9	20 1/8	12.7	24 5/8	19.6	29 1/8	26.4		
15 6/8	6.1	20 2/8	12.9	24 6/8	19.8	29 2/8	26.6		
15 7/8	6.3	20 3/8	13.1	24 7/8	20.0	29 3/8	26.8		
16 0/8	6.5	20 4/8	13.3	25 0/8	20.1	29 4/8	27.0		
16 1/8	6.7	20 5/8	13.5	25 1/8	20.3	29 5/8	27.2		

*Measurements are expressed in inches. PTS, points.

of 1 year a person could lose 104 pounds. Greater weight loss is not recommended because of the potential for injury and increased loss of muscle tissue.

Perhaps the most effective way to reduce calorie intake is to reduce the fat content in the diet. In the current American diet, fat calories represent approximately 42% of all calories consumed. Reducing this value to 30% or less has a significant impact on total calorie consumption and improves other aspects of health such as blood cholesterol level. Thus, a combination of dietary changes and exercise has the best chance of success in weight loss programs.

Bicycling or Using a Stationary Cycle to Lose Weight

Calorie use during cycling increases with the workload. A cycle ergometer shows the workload, and one can determine the rate of calorie expenditure by using Table 40–3. It is important to remember that exercise intensity is dictated by fitness and that it is not always possible to increase the workload to use more calories. The more prudent approach is to increase the duration of the exercise. On a bicycle the rate of calorie expenditure depends on the speed. Bicycling at 10 miles per hour requires approximately 7.0 calories per minute for a 150-pound person.

Walking or Jogging

During walking or jogging, the calories used are directly related to body weight and distance. As the weight of the individual increases, the number of calories expended increases (Table 40–4). The rate of calorie expenditure is less when walking than when jogging. For a person of a given weight the calorie expenditure is calculated by multiplying body weight by 0.52 for walking and 0.81 for running. For example, 0.52×135 pounds = 70 kcal for each mile walked (109 kcal for each mile run).

Table 40–3. RATE OF CALORIE EXPENDITURE WHILE RIDING A CYCLE ERGOMETER

Work		Energy Equivalents		
			Calories	
Kilopoundmeters (Kpm) min	Watts	Oxygen Uptake (liters/min)	kcal/ min	kcal/ hr
150	25	0.6	3.0	180
300	50	0.9	4.5	270
450	75	1.2	6.0	360
600	100	1.5	7.5	450
750	125	1.8	9.0	540
900	150	2.1	10.5	630
1050	175	2.4	12.0	720
1200	200	2.7	14.0	840
1350	225	3.0	15.0	900
1500	250	3.3	17.0	1020
1650	275	3.6	18.0	1080
1800	300	3.9	20.0	1200

Table 40–4. CALORIE REQUIREMENTS FOR WALKING OR JOGGING ONE MILE

Individual Weight (pounds)	Walking (kcal)	Jogging (kcal)
110	58	89
154	81	125
220	115	179

Swimming Programs

To achieve substantial benefits from swimming it is necessary to choose a stroke that can be sustained for at least 20 minutes. For nonexpert swimmers, the breast stroke, side stroke, and back stroke are preferred, as they eliminate the need to coordinate breathing with stroke. Calorie values for swimming are difficult to estimate owing to the wide range of efficiency of swimmers and the fact that body fat decreases the work required to stay afloat. Roughly speaking, as many calories are required to swim 1/4 mile as to run 1 mile.

SUMMARY AND CONCLUSIONS

While all of the data are not in complete agreement, a large body of data published since 1985 suggests that regular aerobic exercise reduces the risk of cancer. Perhaps the data are stronger for colon cancer, but current evidence also supports a decreased risk of breast and reproductive organ cancers as well.

Exercise is also beneficial as a therapeutic and rehabilitative technique. Published reports suggest that regular exercise may help control some of the side effects associated with cancer treatment. In addition, it helps the patient deal with the psychologic problems that accompany this disease. Patients undergoing treatment should be screened before beginning an exercise program and should be supervised during activity. Certain precautions and contraindications should be observed when prescribing exercise for cancer patients.

Finally, by following the information provided here, one can start a regular exercise program safely. It is the exercise itself that is most important; fitness will improve with regular exercise. Exercise should not be viewed as a quick way to change but rather as a way of life.

References

Albanes, D., Blair, A., and Taylor, P. R.: Physical activity and risk of cancer in the NHANES I population. Am. J. Public Health, *79*:744–750, 1989.

Ballard-Barbash, R., Schatzkin, A., Albanes, D., et al.: Physical activity and risk of large bowel cancer in the Framingham study. Cancer Res., *50*:3610–3613, 1990*a*.

Ballard-Barbash, R., Schatzkin, A., Carter, C., et al.: Body fat distribution and breast cancer in the Framingham Study. J Natl Cancer Inst., *82*:286–290, 1990*b*.

Bjorntorp, P.: Classification of obese patients and complication related to the distribution of surplus fat. Am. J. Clin. Nutr., *45*:1120–1125, 1987.

Bjorntorp, P.: The associations between obesity, adipose tissue distribution and disease. Acta Med. Scand., *723*(Suppl.):121–134, 1988.

Blair, S. N., Kohl H. W. III, Paffenbarger, R. S. Jr, et al.: Physical fitness and all-cause mortality: A prospective study of healthy men and women. J.A.M.A. *262*:2395–2401, 1989.

Boissonneault, G. A., Elson, C. E., and Pariza, M. W.: Net energy effects of dietary fat on chemically-induced mammary carcinogenesis in F344 rats. J. Natl. Cancer Inst., *76*:335–338, 1986.

Buettner, L. L., and Gavron, S. J.: Personality changes and physiological effects of a personalized fitness enrichment program for cancer patients. Read at the Third International Symposium on Adapted Physical Activity, New Orleans, LA, Nov. 23–25, 1981.

Cohen, L. A., Choi, K., and Wang, C. X.: Influence of dietary fat, caloric restriction, and voluntary exercise on *N*-nitrosomethylurea–induced mammary tumorigenesis in rats. Cancer Res., *48*:4276–4283, 1988.

Convertino, V., Hung, J., Goldwater, D., et al.: Cardiovascular responses to exercise in middle-aged men after 10 days of bed rest. Circulation, *65*:134–140, 1982.

Despres, J. P., Poulict, M. C., Moorjani, S., et al.: Loss of abdominal fat and metabolic response to exercise training in obese women. Am. J. Physiol., *261*:E159–E167, 1991.

Deuster, P. A., Morrison, S. D., and Ahrens, R. A.: Endurance exercise modifies cachexia of tumor growth in rats. Med. Sci. Sports Exerc., *17*:385–392, 1985.

Eichner, E. R.: Exercise, lymphokines, calories, and cancer. Phys. Sports Med., *15*:109–116, 1987

Elliott, E. A., Matanoski, G. M., Rosenshein, N. B., et al.: Body fat patterning in women with endometrial cancer. Gynecol. Oncol., *39*:253–258, 1990.

Folsom, A. R., Kaye, S. A., Sellers, T. A., et al.: Body fat distribution and 5-year risk of death in older women. J.A.M.A., *269*:483–487, 1993.

Frisch, R. E., Wyshak, G., Albright, N. L., et al.: Lower prevalence of breast cancer and cancers of the reproductive system among former college athletes compared to non-athletes. Br. J. Cancer, *52*:885–891, 1985.

Frisch, R. E., Wyshak, G., Albright, N. L., et al.: Lower lifetime occurrence of breast cancer and cancers of the reproductive system among former college athletes. Am. J. Clin. Nutr., *45*:328–335, 1987.

Frisch, R. E., Wyshak, G., Albright, N. L., et al.: Lower prevalence of nonreproductive cancers among female former college athletes. Med. Sci. Sports Exerc., *21*:250–253, 1989.

Garfinkel, L.: Overweight and cancer. Ann. Intern. Med., *103*:1034–1036, 1985.

Garfinkel, L., and Stellman, S. D.: Mortality by relative weight and exercise. Cancer, *62*(Suppl.):1844–1850, 1988.

Gaskin, T. A., LoBuglio, A., Kelly, P., et al.: Stretch: A rehabilitative program for patients with breast cancer. South. Med. J., *82*:467–469, 1989.

Gauthier, M. M.: Can exercise reduce the risk of cancer? Phys. Sports Med., *14*:171–178, 1986.

Hopkins, G. J., and Carroll, K. K.: Relationship between amount and type of dietary fat in promotion of mammary carcinogenesis induced by 7,12-dimethylbenz-(a)anthracene. J. Natl. Cancer Inst., *62*:1009, 1979.

Howely, E. T., and Franks, B. D.: Health Fitness Instructor's Handbook. 2nd ed. Champaign, IL, Human Kinetics, 1992.

Johnson, J. B., and Wilde-Kelly, A.: A multifaceted rehabilitation program for women with cancer. Oncol. Nurs. Forum, *17*:691–695, 1990.

Klurfeld, D. M., Welch, C. B., Davis, M. J., et al.: Determination of degree of energy restriction necessary to reduce DMBA-induced mammary tumorigenesis in rats during the promotion phase. J. Nutr., *119*:286–291, 1989.

Kohl, H. W., LaPorte, R. E., Blair, S. N.: Physical activity and cancer: An epidemiological perspective. Sports Med., *6*:222–237, 1988.

Kritchevsky, D., and Klurfeld, D. M.: Caloric effects in experimental mammary tumorigenesis. Am. J. Clin. Nutr., *45*:236–242, 1987.

MacVicar, M. G., Winningham, M. L., and Nickel, J. L.: Effects of

aerobic interval training on cancer patient's functional capacity. Nurs. Res., *38*:348–351, 1989.

Moreschi, C.: Beziehungen zwischen Ernahrung und Tumorwachstum. Z. Immunitatsforsch., *2*:651–675, 1909.

Nieman, D. C.: Fitness and Sports Medicine: An Introduction. Palo Alto, CA, Bull Publishing, 1990.

Paffenberger, R. S., Hyde, R. T., Wing, A. L.: Physical activity and incidence of cancer in diverse populations: A preliminary report. Am. J. Clin. Nutr., *45*:312–317, 1987.

Pariza, M. W.: Fat, calories and mammary carcinogenesis: Net energy effects. Am. J. Clin. Nutr., *45*(Suppl.):261, 1987.

Pfalzer, C.: Aerobic exercise for patients with disseminated cancer. Clin. Management Phys. Ther., *8*:28–31, 1988.

Pollock, M. L., Wilmore, J. H., and Fox S. M. III: Exercise in Health and Disease: Evaluation and Prescription for Prevention and Rehabilitation. Philadelphia, W. B. Saunders, 1984.

Rous, P.: The influence of diet on transplanted and spontaneous mouse tumors. J. Exp. Med., *20*:433–451, 1914.

Rous, P.: The influence of dieting upon the course of cancer. Johns Hopkins Hosp. Bull., *26*:146–148, 1915.

Schapira, D. V., Kumar, N. B., and Lyman, G. H.: Abdominal obesity and breast cancer risk. Ann. Intern. Med., *112*:182–186, 1990.

Schapira, D. V., Kumar, N. B., Lyman, G. H., et al.: Upper-body fat distribution and endometrial cancer risk. J.A.M.A., *266*:1808–1811, 1991.

Severson, R. K., Nomura, A. M. Y., Grove, J. S., et al.: A prospective analysis of physical activity and cancer. Am. J. Epidemiol., *130*:522–529, 1989.

Shephard, R. J.: Physical activity and cancer. Int. J. Sports Med., *11*:413–420, 1990.

Siiteri, P. K.: Adipose tissue as a source of hormones. Am. J. Clin. Nutr., *45*:277–282, 1987.

Simopoulos, A. P.: Nutritional cancer risks derived from energy and fat. Med. Oncol. Tumor Pharmacother., *4*:227–239, 1987.

Swanson, C. A., Jones, D. Y., Schatzkin, A., et al.: Breast cancer risk assessed by anthropometry in the NHANES I epidemiological follow-up study. Cancer Res., *48*:5363–5367, 1988.

Tannenbaum, A., and Silverstone, H.: Nutrition in relation to cancer. Adv. Cancer Res., *1*:451, 1953.

Taylor, H. L., Henschel, A., Brozek, J., et al.: Effects of bed rest on cardiovascular function and work performance. J. Appl. Physiol., *2*:233–239, 1949.

Thompson, H. J., Ronan, A. M., Ritacco, K. A., et al.: Effect of exercise on the induction of mammary carcinogenesis. Cancer Res., *48*:2720–2723, 1988.

Tonkelaar, I., Seidell, J. C., Collette, H. J. A., et al.: Obesity and subcutaneous fat patterning in relation to breast cancer in postmenopausal women participating in the diagnostic investigation of mammary cancer project. Cancer, *69*:2663–2667, 1992.

Vena, J. E., Graham, S., Zielezny, M., et al.: Lifetime occupational exercise and colon cancer. Am. J. Epidemiol., *122*:357–365, 1985.

Vena, J. E., Graham, S., Zielezny, M., et al.: Occupational exercise and risk of cancer. Am. J. Clin. Nutr., *45*:318–327, 1987.

Watchie, J.: Expanding the rehab. model to include cancer patients. Paper presented at AACVPR Seventh Annual Meeting, Chicago, IL, October 22–25, 1992.

Willett, W.: The search for the causes of breast and colon cancer. Nature, *338*:389–394, 1989.

Winningham, M. L., MacVicar, M. G., and Burke, C. A.: Exercise for cancer patients: Guidelines and precautions. Phys. Sports Med., *14*:125–134, 1986.

Winningham, M. L., and MacVicar, M. G.: The effect of aerobic exercise on patient reports of nausea. Oncol. Nurs. Forum, *15*:447–451, 1988.

Winningham, M. L., MacVicar, M. G., Bondoc, M., et al.: Effect of aerobic exercise on bodyweight and composition in patients with breast cancer on adjuvant chemotherapy. Oncol. Nurs. Forum, *16*:683–689, 1989.

41

Statistical Methods in Cancer Research

Pippa M. Simpson
John A. Spratt
John S. Spratt

In his review of the penetration of statistical methods into clinical medicine, Cassedy (1984) credits Samuel D. Gross, Frank H. Hamilton, and Jonathan Mason Warren as being the first Americans to report statistical results for surgery in cancer, all in the antebellum period. From that meager beginning, efforts to define in statistical and mathematical terms the story of cancer and its control have continued. As in all true sciences, the development of the appropriate mathematics precedes progress in the science itself, since mathematics is the language of science. The natural mathematical order of the universe and of all its components overrides the relevance of intuitive, subjective, and empirical description in science. The purpose of this chapter, however, is not to review the long and often arduous evolution of mathematics applicable to the understanding and control of human cancer but rather to review some of the methods currently applicable and some of the pitfalls that can occur in their application. As Yancey (1990) points out, many inaccurate conclusions are drawn from studies via statistics, and there are many pitfalls in interpreting results reported in scholarly papers. Baar and Tannock (1989) report on data from a (fictional) study of patients undergoing chemotherapy, where two analyses produce contradictory results.

Another aim is to provide a selected bibliography for further study and a glossary of relevant terms. A vigorous and continual penetration of mathematics into clinical medicine has been foreordained by the rapid evolution of computer technology, with its capacity to manage, consider, and analyze large volumes of data with great speed. This capacity can be brought directly to the physician-patient level, providing immediately available assistance. This technological capacity increasingly infuses mathematics into the "art" of medicine, and, of necessity, future generations of physicians will have to increase their basic knowledge of how mathematics is applicable to clinical medicine and will have to develop increasing levels of computer literacy and competence.

Chapters 15 and 17 contain discussions of mathematics, which will not be duplicated in this chapter. Applications are to be found throughout those sections of text that deal with end results and comparisons. Reviews of statistics evaluating clinical management identify prevalent problems in many published studies (Lavori et al., 1983; and Bailar et al., 1984). The potential invalidity of various studies

resulted from a lack of sufficient detail regarding methods of randomization, inadequate detail about patient sources, failure to use multivariate statistical techniques when applicable, and insufficient use of preliminary statistical models in designing clinical studies. Reported studies often contained insufficient details about patient selection, management protocols, and statistical analysis and interpretation. They often inadequately considered the relevance of covariates to outcome.

Many good articles and books have been published with physicians in mind on clinical studies that focus on clinical trials. *Cancer Clinical Trials* by Buyse et al. (1988) particularly addresses aspects of special interest for readers of this book. Many (e.g., Peto et al., 1976, 1977; Ward et al., 1986; and Bailar et al., 1984, 1992) cover details of careful experimental design and analysis: number of patients required, treatment schedules to be compared, significance levels, reasons for large trials, prior opinions, insignificant differences, treatment allocation ratios, randomized controls, historical controls, exclusions, losses, withdrawals, deviations, ethics, and definition of trial time for each patient. In addition, aspects of analysis are discussed such as the life table, the log rank test, log rank significance levels, prognostic factors, use of prognostic factors, refinement of treatment comparisons, poor methods of analysis, amount of data per patient to be collected, subdivision of the follow-up period, aspects of data collection, assessment of causes of death, endpoints, duration of remissions, and the combining of information from different trials. All the works cited are easy to read and well worth the effort. Breslow and colleagues (1980, 1987) are especially good for a comparison of case-control cancer studies (in their first volume) and cancer cohort studies (in their second).

In this single chapter, only a few statistical high points can be addressed. We refer to the theory available, but emphasize understanding of the basic ideas.

The theory of probability has always played a role in medicine, as in other areas of knowledge. Diagnoses are often made with incomplete certainty and doctors prescribe a particular therapy not with absolute assurance that the patient will recover but because they believe it offers the patient a greater probability of recovery than any other treatment approach. Often, physicians derive from their experience an intuitive idea of the relative chances or probabilities of accurate diagnosis and successful treatment.

Using collected data they may be able to evaluate probabilities more reliably, when such probabilities are derived from equations, using methods of statistics.

PRINCIPLES

Statistical methods, however well-defined or explicit they may be, are of little, if any, value if the data they are designed to analyze are not gathered rigorously. Details of events relevant to the question being examined must be collected accurately. Florence Nightingale recognized these principles and attempted to collect reliable and consistent data (Cook, 1914). She devised forms to collect information on diseases and treatments and persuaded some London hospitals to adopt them. Her hope was that a scheme for collecting hospitals' statistics would be developed so that different treatments might be evaluated accurately. Although much research has been done toward this end, it cannot yet be said, in general, that her hopes have been realized.

Statistical methods involve these interrelated processes:
■ Identification of a problem
■ Formulation of hypotheses to test solutions
■ Experimental planning
■ Collection of the data
■ Analysis of data

This diagram shows the process of statistical research:

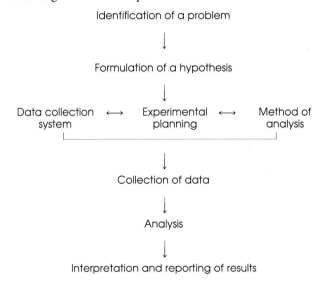

Identification of a Problem

Research activity may be categorized in many ways. It is helpful to define whether a research project has broad goals and is useful, or even necessary, when little is known about a particular area of interest. An investigator must have some knowledge of an area of interest before any refined research can begin or any hypotheses be formulated. In one sense, investigational research can be likened to the survey approach, which is never used to prove anything, but rather to help one become familiar with the area and the associ-

ated problems. Before sophisticated research can be attempted in any area, the investigator must know the territory and may need to do a pilot study to gain some familiarity with it. Once the territory is well known, more refined research can follow. Many retrospective studies of a clinical problem, whether it is of clinical charts or earlier studies, have their main value in exploring the territory.

A clear understanding of terms and their relevance in a study is needed. It may be that survival over a defined period is of interest, but this may be disease-free survival or, even a more complex concept, limited side effect survival. The complexity of verifying benefit of treatment as a response—as opposed to the more objective endpoint of actual survival—can pose a complex statistical problem. Simplifying this problem requires the use of very concise and consistently measurable definitions of response.

One system of proven value is the Karnofsky scale, which defines the performance status of the patient (see Chapter 24). When the Karnofsky index improves significantly, this indicates a measurable benefit. Transient regressions of measurable neoplasms with no improvement in the Karnofsky index are of dubious benefit even if survivorship can be increased. As Oye and Shapiro (1984) report, there is a trend toward treating many common solid tumors by chemotherapy despite the fact that there is little evidence of treatment effectiveness. They reviewed 80 studies, 95% of which used response to chemotherapy as an endpoint. They observed that responders in these studies may have lived longer had they had no treatment and that using response as an endpoint may have biased the conclusions toward overestimating the effectiveness of chemotherapy.

Clear endpoints of the study—both initial and final—should be stated. Criteria for exclusion and inclusion must also be clearly stated. Variations in breast cancer treatment may result in insufficient participation in a study (Deber and Thompson, 1990). This can affect the ''generalizability'' of conclusions and so should be investigated. Because some subjects are *certain* to drop out, a policy to minimize these should be formulated.

Formulation of a Hypothesis

Whether the interest be cost-benefit, quality of life, survival, or response to treatment, a hypothesis, and possibly some subsidiary ones, will be the focus of the study. The formulation of a hypothesis requires understanding which variables are most relevant. A suitable hypothesis is meaningful *and* testable. The formulation of the hypothesis guides the collection of data, so that, ideally, only (but all) data needed to test the hypothesis are collected. The hypothesis, of course, guides the analysis, and this affects decisions on how much information is needed, and in what ways and forms the data are collected. If it is impossible, owing to time or cost constraints, to collect the data needed for specific analysis, the hypotheses may have to be modified. This, in turn, may affect data collection, the design of the experiment, data items and forms.

Types of Errors

Statistics tend to prove results by contradiction. If a study is designed to prove some difference, the aim is to reject the null hypothesis, which is formulated as ''no difference'' or ''no change.'' As with any test, two types of errors can occur. A *Type I* error occurs when something (in the statistical case, the null hypothesis) that is actually true is determined to be false. A *Type II* error occurs when something that is in fact false is determined to be true. Clearly, the optimal situation is to be always right, but in an imperfect world we usually have to settle for balancing the chances of error in some way. The *significance level* is the probability of making a Type I error, and is often denoted as α ($0 \leq \alpha \leq 1$), or a *P* value. Its calculation is based on what test is used. By accepting a 5% chance of error ($P = .05 = \alpha$) the investigator recognizes that there is 1 chance in 20 that by chance alone the study will show a difference. If there truly is a chance, it needs to be quantified exactly before the probability of a Type II error, denoted by β, can be calculated. Often we can specify what would be the minimum difference we would consider clinically significant. Once this is specified, we can calculate a β ($0 \leq \beta \leq 1$). This value will decrease as we take a larger sample or as we increase the probability of a Type I error, since then we will be less likely to accept the null hypothesis. Thus, we can use sample size with a specified significance level to control the *power*, $1 - \beta$, of a test.

Suppose an investigator wishes to see if a newly developed treatment is superior to the standard one. Assume that the 2-year survival rate for the standard treatment is 45%. Preliminary results indicate that the new treatment will result in a 2-year survival rate of 65%. What size samples for the control and experimental groups will the investigator need to test whether the new treatment is, indeed, superior to the standard one? It is further assumed that the investigator will accept the new treatment as superior if the hypothesis is rejected at the 5% level of significance. To compute the required sample size, the investigator must state the *power* of a test, or the ability to detect a true difference of a specified size. A power of 0.5 means the investigator has a 50% chance of accepting the null hypothesis, that there is no difference, when there is really the difference of specified size between the survival rates of the two treatments. Or, in colloquial terms, the investigator has only ''half a chance'' to reject the null hypothesis. Similarly, a power of 0.7 gives the investigator a 30% chance of still accepting that there is no difference when the true difference is of the specified size.

Another way of looking at the power of a test is this: Suppose 100 institutions are simultaneously but independently evaluating the new treatment. Each institution's sample size is sufficient to yield a power of 0.5, assuming each accepts the experimental treatment as better if the difference is significantly different from zero at the 5% level. In this situation, approximately half (0.5) of the institutions will find the new treatment significantly (statistically) better than the standard treatment. Also, half of the institutions will be unable to demonstrate this. Thus, arguments ensue. Indeed, this problem may lie at the heart of many disputes over the value of different treatments. Because many institutions do not have a large enough patient population to be able to compare two treatment methods within a reasonable time frame, there is a tendency toward conducting more cooperative studies. It is generally accepted that a statistical test for any serious research should have a power of at least 0.8. This means that before the experiment is begun, the researchers have at least an 80% chance of statistically rejecting the null hypothesis *if it is false*. Certainly, any investigator who is going to put a great amount of effort into the work will want at least this much of a chance. To be assured of this, he or she will need to select a sample of appropriate size.

Optimal Allocation of Resources

The following increase the power of a study:

■ Use of more sensitive outcome measures
■ Use of important prognostic factors to reduce variability
■ Larger samples

By varying α- and β-levels a planner can get estimates of sample size. Clinical trial design has economic significance. By multiplying a cost per unit (case) by the number of cases, a planner can estimate the project's cost for each possible significance level, power, and sample size. Rosenberg (1983) calculates an optimal allocation ratio, which he defines as the ratio that provides the greatest amount of information (or most statistical power) per dollar. When such cost information is needed for research budgeting, the reader will find Rosenberg's methods a useful approach.

Caveats

Although a study may yield an insignificant result, this may be of interest, especially if the power is reasonable (Angell, 1989). Moreover, statistical significance should always be interpreted in conjunction with clinical significance. A result may not be statistically significant but still be clinically significant, especially if the sample is small. On the other hand, when a sample is large, results may be statistically significant but not clinically so.

Classical hypothesis testing and significance levels have achieved great status in statistical analysis. Nevertheless, it should be borne in mind that they are only part of statistical methodology, including Bayesian theory (Efron, 1985), decision analysis, and exploratory analysis (Morrow, 1991), which may also serve to establish the truth of a hypothesis.

Data Collection

Statistical methods, however well-defined or explicit, are of no value if the data they are designed to analyze are poorly gathered. Statistical methods can be applied properly only when information gathered is sufficiently detailed and accurate. A monitor of the data collection process, especially in multicenter studies, is invaluable for ensuring this.

Before collecting the data for a research project, the purpose of the project should be stated clearly. Data that have been collected without purpose may be useless for hypothesis testing. The method of analysis dictates not only what data should be collected but how they will be recorded and coded. Whether a study is a clinical trial, a survey, or an epidemiologic study, a form is needed to collect the data. Before a final form is designed it is important for the investigator to state specifically (1) the objective of the investigation, (2) the methods of analysis, and (3) the amount of detail necessary for each item to answer questions or hypotheses. Data are not merely analyzed but are analyzed with respect to specific questions, hypotheses, and statistical models. On the assumption that the purpose and method of an investigation are well-defined, in the following section we discuss other important considerations for creating a data collection form.

Investigators are well-advised to consult with someone familiar with computer processing and data management at the outset. Such consultation will clarify aspects of form design and coding, to ensure accurate and easy data entry.

Data Collection System

Form Design

Invalid data or incomplete data are difficult, and often impossible, to correct, even when the defect is noticed early in a study. In designing the form, all efforts should be made to ensure maximum clarity and ease of understanding to avoid such errors. The wording or sequencing of questions can bias the answers, so that the collected data are "tainted." Because simplicity and unambiguity are so important, a form should be subjected to pretesting.

Necessary Information. Each form should contain the patient's or subject's chart number; for consistency, the first entry of the form may be used for this purpose. By using chart numbers, information belonging to a particular patient is always identifiable. Identification by chart numbers also allows certain information to be gained from other forms containing identical questions.

Although it is easier to design questions with open-ended answers, this just "puts off the evil day" since before they can be analyzed, the answers will have to be grouped into a finite number of alternatives, and this exercise can introduce a degree of subjectivity. Moreover, when every response that can be given is predetermined each time the form is filled out, the same alternatives are considered. If any alternatives might need to be explained, such clarification should be provided. Care should be taken to ensure that all possible alternative answers are offered on the form, lest data be incomplete because possible answers are left out. It may be advisable, for example, to perform a preliminary review of hospital charts to help the design of responses.

Information gathering usually involves a tradeoff between cost and utility; however, in some cases it is just as easy to get more precise information as it is to get approximate values. For example, age in years may be just as easy to collect as age by decade of life. For analysis, if only age groups are needed, then answers can be easily and accurately recoded by using software. On the other hand, if in trying to determine a given variable exactly information may be lost because such an answer cannot or will not be given, it may be necessary to ask only for approximate answers (for example, people generally do not like to disclose their exact income).

Because the answer to a question is not always known, the response *unknown* must be an alternative, as must *none* when appropriate.

Sequence of Items. By designing a questionnaire format that follows the sequence in which information appears in a hospital chart or becomes available in the research plan, recording is made simpler and more accurate. It is important to arrange questions to avoid ambiguity of answers. For example, if the patient has not had surgery, there can have been no complications from surgery, and it should be clear that that part of the form need not be filled out.

Clarity. A form should be sufficiently well-written that the investigator will be able to understand it 6 months or 1 year later. It may be necessary to include a special set of definitions or instructions, either on the form or in a glossary.

Avoiding Ambiguity. Each question should be stated as specifically as possible, without ambiguity. This is one of the most difficult problems of questionnaire design. A complex question is best divided into two or more simple ones. Questions should be stated in such a way that they can be answered simply and concisely. Succinct and explicit definitions help.

An answer such as "a combination of the above" usually is not informative and should be avoided. If, say, the investigator desires to collect information on complications, which may be several, each complication should be listed individually with the possible responses: *no*, *yes*, and *don't know*.

Simplicity. Each item should answer only a single question or relate to a single dimension. It is best to have a separate item for gender and for ethnic origin than to combine the two in a single item. It is easier to code each of five symptoms separately than to employ a combination code that could produce 32 different answers. That is confusing and takes time; whereas, if all five variables are listed and the possible answers are *yes*, *no*, and *don't know*, five items are needed, but the same answer will be derived much more quickly. On small items this may not be critical, but it can create great difficulties with larger ones.

Consistency. All coding should be consistent throughout. For example, if on Item 1 the code for *no* is 0 and for *yes* is 1, it should be thus for all *yes-no* items.

Computerization

There are two types of electronic computers, mainframe and personal, (though these days the distinction between them is becoming increasingly blurred). The mainframe computer is run by others, usually at a computer center, not by the investigator, and has the advantage of being more powerful than a personal computer, but the investigator does not have total control.

If there is a very large data set or if extensive statistical analysis is planned, the power of a mainframe may be needed. Moreover, the fact that a mainframe is run by others can be an advantage. A backup of files is usually created automatically, so they are safer. If the computer should be inoperative for a while, it can be expected that in a short time it will be operative again.

Nowadays, with the proliferation of personal computers, many people have easy access to a personal computer of considerable power. Statistical packages as versatile as those on a mainframe are available, and in fact, there are many interactive statistical graphics packages, some three-dimensional (e.g., JMP, Data Desk, and SYSTAT), which enable a researcher to explore the data in an easy, complete, and interesting way. Many good programs are available, including personal computer versions of mainframe packages such as SPSS and SAS. Some care should be taken in choosing a statistical program, since some have not been tested as rigorously as longstanding programs.

Should a computer fail, a compatible computer is usually available, so this creates no problem provided that good housekeeping has been observed with data files and programs. There should be a policy of maintaining regular backup of files. Documentation of all files used should be available. Files on hard disk should be backed up on another medium (for example, floppy disks), which must be kept safe.

Often it is convenient to use a combination of personal and mainframe computers. Data entry can be easier and more accurate using programs available on a personal computer. The data files can then be uploaded to a mainframe. This can be a straightforward procedure, but, again, this is where a data manager may prove invaluable in giving advice so that there is no lengthy delay before data analysis.

Editing

One of the most important errors that can affect an analysis is data entry error. It is important to design the data collection process so that the process of data entry is as straightforward as possible and there are as many checks as possible. There are data collection programs in which a screen can be designed to look like the form on which data are to be recorded and where range and consistency of data can be verified as the data are entered. At the very least, checks should be done after data are entered. Although it may seem simpler to enter data straight into a computer rather than first recording it, great care should then be taken to generate a hard (printed) copy immediately, lest the computer fail and there be no possibility of retrieving the data. Such a misadventure could render a study incomplete and the study's conclusions possibly useless or, at least, less compelling.

Description

A description of the data—such as frequencies and plots—is useful in checking for errors. As Williamson (1989) argues, such tools as the box-plot can be used to explore the underlying structure of data and for checking assumptions that may need to be made for further analysis of the data.

Method of Analysis

Statistical analysis may proceed in many ways, and though in this chapter we offer an overview of statistics, it is important to involve a statistician from the beginning. Possible approaches are not limited to what is available on the more popular statistical packages, and a statistician is likely to know what is feasible and how a program can be generated. Statistical packages or programs are proliferating rapidly and are becoming more sophisticated. The experience with clinical trials has led to ever greater refinement of the methods of design and analysis. The vast improvements in computer technology allow investigators today to make fewer statistical distributional assumptions than their predecessors had to (Efron and Tibshirani, 1991).

Experimental Design

Consideration should be given to how the study is to be done: as a planned, randomized clinical study or an observational epidemiologic study, either retrospective or prospective. In a two-group controlled clinical trial, one of the groups studied is the control group that receives (1) no treatment or (2) the standard treatment. Another group receives the treatment under investigation. By randomizing subjects to the two groups, any effect observed can be attributed to the treatment, rather than to other extraneous variables. If the study is planned and then carried out, it is a *prospective* study, and the definition of variables can be more precise (and, hopefully, missing information can be avoided). If it is *retrospective* (that is, if it uses previously accumulated data), data may have been collected in many ways and standardization may be imperfect. In an observational study, often it may be important to follow comparable groups (cohorts) of subjects over time in what are called *cohort studies.*

Many factors influence the choice of study type—length of time for study, feasibility, ethical aspects, objective, type of study (exploratory, confirmatory or predictive)—to name a few. A properly designed clinical study can be more definitive in demonstrating a cause-and-effect relationship. Mantel (1988) disputes the conclusions of a study associating breast cancer with moderate alcohol consumption. He points out that because the study was not a randomized clinical study, a causal relationship cannot be established but rather only an association, which may be due to other factors. A properly designed epidemiologic study may be the only efficient way to evaluate various factors relating to the outcome of interest. It may be especially useful when combined with a clinical trial.

Clinical trials have a long history. In the 1990s Lawrence (1991) saw the clinical trial as ''a carefully controlled and highly ethical human experiment that is designed to test an hypothesis relative to possible improvements in patient management.'' The goal of any clinical trial is to obtain a result that can be generalized to the population at large.

Bias occurs when consideration is not given in studies to confounding variables, such as the difference between groups. In a study comparing conventional and unconventional treatments for cancer (Cassileth et al., 1991), those people who chose to have the unconventional treatment were initially much sicker. Thus, unless allowances were made for this fact in the analysis, any evaluation of the quality of life would be biased toward the conventional treatment. An estimate of the quality of life for the unconventional treatment might be low not because of the treatment but because of the patient's initial condition.

The potential for biases is constantly present. Hillman and coworkers (1991) point out that bias occurs not only in the conduct of a study but sometimes also in the reporting of economic value of a treatment. Mantel (1988) discusses the problem of bias in two prospective epidemiologic studies of breast cancer. Even in well-designed cohort epidemiologic studies (Gray-Donald and Kramer, 1988), it is often difficult to eliminate bias. Indeed, there may be limits to what can be done.

Measures to Reduce Bias

Collect data in a reliable and accurate way.

Formulate Exclusion Criteria. Confounding variables, size of sample, and generalizability of conclusions should all be considered in formulating precise, applicable exclusion criteria. On the other hand, too stringent exclusion criteria may make it difficult to generate a sample of the required size. In analysis, it may be possible, where necessary, to allow for confounding variables in order to get more generalizable results.

Randomize. Patients who meet the entry requirements for a study should be allocated randomly to groups, as by using random numbers. The scheme should be adhered to strictly. It may be argued that interpretation of the results should be based on "intent to treat." Sommer and Zeger (1991) argue that the *efficacy* of a treatment is different from the *effectiveness* of a treatment, the latter being measured by the "usual" pattern of results obtained when some subjects do not comply with treatment.

If it is known in advance that some attributes are of special interest, groups with these attributes can be sampled. This is called *prestratification*. In a variation of this approach only one member of each treatment group is selected from each attribute group; this is a matched case control study.

Follow Patients for the Duration of the Study. When information is missing for a patient it is possible that the response variable itself is the reason. For example, a patient who is doing particularly well may see no need to visit the physician any longer. Though techniques have been developed to deal with missing values (Little and Rubin, 1987), they cannot replace diligent follow-up.

Blinding. Blinding is a method whereby patient, clinician, or analyst is unaware of what treatment a given patient receives. Usually the word "blinding" describes the fact that the patient does not know which treatment (or the placebo) he or she is getting. "Double blinding" describes the situation when neither the person administering the treatment nor the patient knows. Sometimes blinding may be difficult or impossible, as when treatment involves surgery. Blinding helps to eliminate bias imposed by the *ex-*

pectation (on the part of subject or clinician) of a particular effect.

Chalmers and colleagues (1983) conducted a study related to controlled clinical trials in the management of acute myocardial infarction, but their conclusions could just as well apply to cancer. The report shows that the magnitude of these biases varies with the design of the trial. These investigators analyzed 145 published papers and divided the papers according to the method of case allocation: random selection, blinded (57 papers); random selection, may have been blinded (45 papers); and selection of controls by a nonrandom process (43 papers). At least one prognostic variable was significantly maldistributed in 14% in the first group, in 26.7% in the second group, and in 58.1% in the third group. The authors concluded that their study confirms the importance of blinding.

Ethics

Some physicians may believe that one treatment is superior to another. In that case it would not be ethical for them to do a randomized trial (Passamani, 1991). Taylor and colleagues (1984) discuss one such situation in a study of surgery for breast cancer. There are other possible designs that still minimize bias and that meet ethical requirements. An example is the "play the winner," or adaptive design (Buyse et al., 1988, p. 326), in which a treatment is more likely to be chosen if it appears to be efficacious.

If it is believed that a patient should not be treated by an inferior therapy once a superior one has been identified, it may be preferable to set up a study as a sequential trial where the final sample size depends on the outcome. In such trials results are periodically analyzed, and, depending on some predetermined criteria, the trial is either continued or terminated when the primary objectives have been met. The more often the data are examined, however, the more likely it is that a significant result will be obtained *by chance*. Sequential procedures have to adjust nominal significance levels to a wide variety of stopping rules. Indeed, the data can be examined after each case is treated, and a decision can be made to continue or terminate the experiment. The additional advantage of a sequential trial is that it can reduce the total number of patients required for a study. Such sequential designs are rarely used in cancer studies owing to the length of time between treatment and outcome. The reader is referred to Pasternak's report (1981) for a further discussion and a table of adjusted significance levels when the study is analyzed several times before its completion.

A multistage study may address issues similar to those in a sequential trial. A study can start off with a large sample and with simple goals and in successive stages can become more definitive, with smaller samples.

Quality of Life

The study of Cassileth and coworkers (1991) highlights the concern these days of evaluating treatment outcomes by quality of life as well as by "hard facts."

Costs

The flip side to benefit is cost. More studies in the future will address this concern. This may shift the focus of studies to how findings influence decision theory, which is a wider statistical approach that incorporates hypothesis testing as a particular case, taking into account the cost of different decisions.

Sample Size

Important in the design of any research is determining how many observations are necessary (Ellenberg, 1989). If the number of observations is more than the minimum necessary to test a hypothesis, the extra time and cost involved are wasted. On the other hand, if the number of observations is too few, the investigator may not have enough to test the hypothesis. The goal of this section is to aid the investigator in selecting the proper sample size for the experiment at hand.

Generally, the standard clinical experiment requires a control group and an experimental group. This is called a two-group experiment. Both groups are treated identically, except for the experimental variables being evaluated. Ideally, such studies should be double blinded. The assignment of a patient to a group should be random. Also, if it is known that the experimental treatment is superior to the treatment to be received by the control group, the experiment would be unethical, as the experimental treatment *should* be given to everyone. If it is not known which treatment is truly superior, an experiment is the only scientific way to proceed. For this reason, the investigator will need to use a nondirectional, or two-tailed, test. A one-tailed test can be used validly only if the researcher is unwilling to conclude, regardless of the experimental results, that the new treatment is inferior to the standard treatment.

The tables included in the appendix to this chapter are designed to be used as a ready reference for determining appropriate sample size for a proposed experiment. All values are computed by use of the arc sine transformations of a proportion, as described by Sokal and Rohlf (1969).

ANALYSIS

Chi Square (χ^2) and Comparisons of Proportions

Description

Often in clinical research the investigator wishes to discover whether there is a relationship between two variables, neither of which may be quantifiable. For example, the researcher may wish to test whether there is a relationship between occupation and tumor site. If six tumor sites and four occupations were selected for investigation, a two-way contingency table could be set up, as in Table 41–1. Since neither occupation nor tumor site is a quantifiable variable,

Table 41–1. A TWO-WAY CONTINGENCY TABLE RELATING SITE OF CANCER TO OCCUPATION OF PATIENT

Occupation	Tumor Site					
	Skin	Lung	Mouth	Neck	Breast	Liver
Executive	10	6	0	3	0	1
Laborer	5	0	8	0	7	2
Farmer	1	3	0	9	0	5
Salesman	4	0	9	0	6	0

the order in which the different categories are placed in the figure is unimportant. For example, if the occupational categories were recorded as farmer, executive, laborer, and salesman, rather than the order given in the table, the table would look different but would be just as meaningful. Variables that require no specific sequence are called *nominal* variables. To study the relationship between occupation and tumor site, the frequency of a combination is placed in the appropriate cell. As illustrated in Table 41–1, there are 10 executives with skin tumors, 6 executives with lung tumors, 5 laborers with skin tumors, and 8 laborers with mouth tumors. In a contingency table of this type, each patient should be counted as being in only one cell. This would mean that patients with two different tumor sites could not be used in this study. Or, if it were desired to use a patient with multiple tumors, the patient would be considered for only one site on the basis of some criterion, such as the site of the first tumor to appear. Similarly, if the patient had two occupations, he or she should be classified as belonging to only one occupational category, perhaps the one where more time is spent. If these rules are followed, the sum of all numbers in the contingency table will be equal to the number of patients in the study. When each patient is counted only once in such a contingency table, statistical methods exist for determining whether the two variables (in this example, occupation and tumor site) are related. Similar methods do not exist if a patient is counted as being in more than one cell.

Example

Using this technique, a researcher may be interested in testing whether different methods of classifying breast tumors are related. From data on radical mastectomy cases, a contingency table (Table 41–2) comparing histologic classification and Columbia Clinical stage has been constructed. To determine whether the two variables in the table are related a statistic called chi square (χ^2) must be computed. This is a relatively simple procedure, as follows:

1. Compute the expected value. The expected values are computed under the assumption that the two variables are not related. The expected value (E) for any cell in the table is derived by multiplying the total number in the corresponding row by the total number in the corresponding column and then dividing this result by the total number in the table (N); for this example $N = 445$. For the foregoing

Table 41-2. A TWO-WAY CONTINGENCY TABLE TO DETERMINE THE RELATIONSHIP BETWEEN THE HISTOLOGIC TYPE OF MAMMARY CANCERS AND THEIR CLINICAL STAGE

Columbia Clinical Stage	Histologic Type				Row Totals
	1	*2*	*3*	*4*	
A	5 (3.04)	10 (6.08)	142 (145.08)	12 (14.80)	169
B	0 (2.43)	5 (4.85)	119 (115.89)	11 (11.83)	135
C	3 (1.67)	1 (3.34)	78 (79.84)	11 (8.15)	93
D	0 (0.86)	0 (1.78)	43 (41.22)	5 (4.21)	48
Column totals	8	16	382	39	445

In parentheses are expected values calculated under the assumption that *no* relationship exists between the two variables.

example, the expected value for the cell in the second row and third column is 135 × 382/445 = 115.89

The expected figures for all entries of the table are also shown in Table 41–2 in parentheses, following the observed value.

2. The observed values (O) in the original table are compared with the corresponding expected values, and differences are noted ($O - E$). For example, the first entry in the first row, has O = 5, E = 3.04, O − E = 1.96. The *sign* of the difference (i.e., plus or minus) is disregarded. If the differences are large it is likely that the two variables are related.

3. Square the resulting difference: $(O - E)^2$. Divide by the expected value (E), to get $(O - E)^2/E$. Thus, for the first entry in the first row we have $1.96^2/3.04$.

4. Find the sum of these new values and call this S. For Table 41–2, $S = 13.51$.

5. To determine whether a statistically significant relationship exists between the histologic type of neoplasms and the clinical stage, we need to compute the degrees of freedom (df) associated with this χ^2 as,

$$df = \text{(Number of rows} - 1) \times \text{(Number of columns} - 1).$$ (Equation 1)

For this problem,

$$df = (4 - 1) \times (4 - 1) = 3 \times 3 = 9.$$

6. The level of significance associated with the computed χ^2 value is found in the χ^2 table (Table 41–3). Because, for this problem, there are nine degrees of freedom,

the values on the ninth row are the ones of interest. This row is indicated in the first column, headed *df*. The computed χ^2 value (13.51) falls between the tabled χ^2 values 12.242 and 14.684 in the row with nine degrees of freedom. The levels of significance associated with these two values are $P = .20$ and $P = .10$, respectively. Thus, the probability that the χ^2 value would be this large if there were no relationship between the two variables is between .20 and .10, which may be written as $.10 < P < .20$. As this probability is relatively high, it cannot be inferred that the two variables are related.

Had the χ^2 value been higher so that the $P < .05$ (meaning that the probability was less than one in twenty that the association occurred by chance), it could have been inferred that the two variables were related and it would have been of interest to see in what way they were. To do this, the observed set of values (see Table 41–2) is compared with expected values. To the extent that the observed values differ from the values expected if there is no relationship it may be said that the two variables are related. However, there is no simple, single numerical value by which to express this, so the χ^2 is limited. The type of relation involved, if it is statistically significant, can be understood by comparing the observed values with the expected ones. It will be noted that in the example given all such differences are relatively small; thus, no pattern of relationship is evident.

An investigator may not be fortunate enough to have a large number of observations. It is generally stated in most

Table 41-3. SIGNIFICANCE ASSOCIATED WITH VARIOUS VALUES OF CHI SQUARE

df	p = 0.99	0.98	0.95	0.90	0.80	0.70	0.50	0.30	0.20	0.10	0.05	0.02	0.01
1	0.000157	0.000628	0.00393	0.0158	0.0642	0.148	0.455	1.074	1.642	2.706	3.841	5.412	6.635
2	0.0201	0.0404	0.103	0.211	0.446	0.713	1.386	2.408	3.219	4.605	5.991	7.824	9.210
3	0.115	0.185	0.352	0.584	1.005	1.424	2.366	3.665	4.642	6.251	7.815	9.837	11.345
4	0.297	0.429	0.711	1.064	1.649	2.195	3.357	4.878	5.989	7.779	9.488	11.668	13.277
5	0.554	0.752	1.145	1.610	2.343	3.000	4.351	6.064	7.289	9.236	11.070	13.388	15.086
6	0.872	1.134	1.635	2.204	3.070	3.828	5.348	7.231	8.558	10.645	12.592	15.033	16.812
7	1.239	1.564	2.167	2.833	3.822	4.671	6.346	8.383	9.803	12.017	14.067	16.622	18.475
8	1.646	2.032	2.733	3.490	4.594	5.527	7.344	9.524	11.030	13.362	15.507	18.168	20.090
9	2.088	2.532	3.325	4.168	5.380	6.393	8.343	10.656	12.242	14.684	16.919	19.679	21.666
10	2.558	3.059	3.940	4.865	6.179	7.267	9.342	11.781	13.442	15.987	18.307	21.161	23.209

(Reprinted with permission of Macmillan Publishing Co., Inc., from Fisher, R. A.: Statistical Methods for Research Workers. © 1970, University of Adelaide.)
Abbreviation: df = degrees of freedom.

statistical textbooks that if more than 20% of the expected values are less than 10, the level of significance is poorly estimated by the χ^2 procedure. With small sample sizes, there are alternative tests for relations between variables. For 2-by-2 tables, many statistical packages can calculate the Fisher exact test.

Some statistical packages, for example STATXACT, can calculate exact P values for more general tables. The necessary computations are time consuming if done by hand, and a computer must be used for all but the smallest tables.

The *t* Test and Comparison of Means

Description

During the last half of the 19th century a brewer, William Gosset, devised a statistical method for determining whether two groups are different for a given set of measurements. Fearful lest he hurt his company's reputation, he published the method under the pseudonym Student. Since that time, Student's *t* test has become one of the most used, and perhaps most useful, statistical methods available for everyday use. One use is to test whether the average value for a group of observations is different from the average value for a second group of observations. The *t* test is employed, for example, to test whether the average height of men is different from that of women. The data must conform to the following conditions if the *t* test is to have validity:

Underlying Normal. A set of values is said to be normally distributed if the shape of the histogram of the frequency polygon can be approximated by a certain mathematical equation whose plot is often called the *bell-shaped* or *normal curve*. It is illustrated in Figure 41–1, for the logarithms of survival times for mastectomy patients whose lesion was classified as TNM Stage I. The dashed line represents the smoothed frequency curve that would result if a large number of observations were made. The normal curve is symmetric about the average value and the most frequent interval. The *variability* of the distribution refers to the width of the curve at a given point.

Equal Variability Within Each Group. Equal variability may be interpreted as requiring the shapes of the histograms arising from the two groups being compared to be the same when there are an equal number of observations in each. Often a frequency histogram of data does not

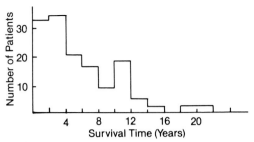

Figure 41–2. Frequency distribution of survival times for TNM clinical Stage I breast cancer patients treated with mastectomy.

produce a bell-shaped curve. This is true, for example, of survival times for breast cancer patients (Fig. 41–2). The curve has a long tail on the right and thus is said to be *skewed positively*. A long tail on the left would demonstrate a *negative skew*. It is obvious that Student's *t* test cannot be used to compare the survival times of two different groups of patients because the distribution curve of survival time is not symmetric and therefore not normal. However, if the survival time for each patient is converted to its logarithm, the log values are approximately normally distributed; the resulting histogram is bell shaped. As these new values (logarithm of survival times) conform to the two rules required for Student's *t* test, they may be compared to test for differences in survival times between two groups of patients. Because every patient in each group must have a value for survival time, all subjects must have died. This is a great drawback if rapid analyses are required for comparing the results of two different treatments, but it has the advantage of being able to detect smaller differences than the life table method.

Example

An illustration of the use of Student's *t* test to compare the survival times of two groups of patients is presented in Table 41–4. The data are from the first eight patients in

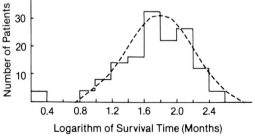

Figure 41–1. The frequency distribution of log-survival times of patients treated with mastectomy for TNM Stage I carcinoma of the breast.

Table 41–4. STUDENTS *t* TEST FOR COMPARING SURVIVAL TIMES OF EIGHT PATIENTS EACH WITH TNM CLINICAL STAGE I AND IV BREAST CARCINOMA

TNM Stage I		TNM Stage IV	
Patient Survival (Mo.)	Logarithm of Survival Time	Patient Survival (Mo.)	Logarithm of Survival Time
300	2.477	6	0.778
42	1.623	14	1.146
269	2.430	3	0.477
32	1.505	21	1.322
93	1.968	26	1.415
93	1.968	51	1.708
76	1.881	20	1.301
69	1.839	24	1.380
$T_1 = 15.691$		$T_2 = 9.527$	
$S_1 = 31.606$		$S_2 = 12.410$	
$N_1 = 8$		$N_2 = 8$	
$A_1 = 1.961$		$A_2 = 1.191$	

each of the TNM clinical Stage I and Stage IV breast tumor groups.

1. The first column under each stage lists survival time, in months, for the patients in each group.

2. The second column under each stage contains the logarithm of the survival time for each patient.

3. T_1 is the sum of the logarithms for patients in the Stage I category and S_1 is the sum of the squares of the logarithms for Stage I patients.

4. A_1 is the average value of the logarithms for the Stage I patients and is defined as follows: $A_1 = T_1/N_1$, where N_1 is the number of patients in the Stage I category.

T_2, S_2, N_2, and A_2 are similarly defined for the patients in the Stage IV category. Once the computations in Table 41–4 have been completed, the value of Student's t is derived from the formula at the bottom of this page.

Interpretation

If there were no difference between the survival rates for the two groups, the probability is less than 1 in 100 that the value of $A_1 - A_2$ would be as great as it is. Therefore it is relatively certain that a real difference exists between the two groups. If the value of t had been 2.33 with 14 degrees of freedom, the same row would have been used in the t table but the level of significance would be between 0.05 and 0.02. In this case, a relatively small sample from each of the two groups being compared was sufficient to demonstrate a difference in survival times. In general, this method of comparing survival rates is more sensitive than the χ^2 method, in that it requires fewer observations to demonstrate a statistically significant difference. The disadvantage is that the survival time for every patient must

be known. As long as any of the patients survive, Student's t cannot be computed. Discarding data from surviving patients would only bias the result and render the analysis meaningless.

Life Tables and Survival Analysis

Description

A graph and life table (actuarial or Kaplan-Meier) are important in the analysis of human survival studies and are particularly useful for comparing end results for different groups of patients. It provides estimates of survival curves even when all patients have not yet died or have withdrawn for other reasons (e.g., because death was due to causes unrelated to breast cancer). Anderson and colleagues (1991) give a description of this method in cancer studies along with a discussion of survival analysis techniques.

A life table is designed to compute the proportion of patients surviving after a given interval, generally 1 year. It is not necessary that 12-month intervals be used, and when the average survival time is relatively short, intervals of 3 or 6 months may be more informative. Intervals need not be of the same length. In Kaplan-Meier survival curves each interval is determined by either a patient's death or withdrawal. If all patients in the group being compared have died, so that survival times are available for all, Student's t test can be used to compare the results, but a life table must be used in making comparisons for groups that still have surviving members.

In general, groups of patients do have survivors, and individuals have usually been followed for different periods. Obviously, survivors who have been followed for only 2 years at the termination of the follow-up period yield no

$$t = \frac{A_1 - A_2}{\sqrt{\frac{(S_1 - A_1 T_1) + (S_2 - A_2 T_2)}{N_1 + N_2 - 2} \times \left(\frac{1}{N_1} + \frac{1}{N_2}\right)}}$$

A numerical illustration of this formula is given for the data from Table 41–4:

$$t = \frac{1.961 - 1.191}{\sqrt{\frac{(31.606 - 1.961 \times 15.691) + (12.410 - 1.191 \times 9.527)}{8 + 8 - 2} \times \left(\frac{1}{8} + \frac{1}{8}\right)}}$$

$$t = \frac{0.770}{\sqrt{\frac{(0.8356) + (1.0636)}{14} \times (0.125 + 0.125)}}$$

$$t = \frac{0.770}{\sqrt{0.033925}}$$

$$t = 4.18$$

To interpret the value of Student's t, we first determine the number of degrees of freedom, $N_1 + N_2 - 2$, and for this example it is $8 + 8 - 2 = 14$. The computed t value (Table 41–5) is greater than any value on the $n = 14$ line, and therefore the level of significance for the computed difference is less than 0.01.

Table 41-5. TABLE OF *t* VALUES

n	p = 0.9	0.8	0.7	0.6	0.5	0.4	0.3	0.2	0.1	0.05	0.02	0.01
1	0.158	0.325	0.510	0.727	1.000	1.376	1.963	3.078	6.314	12.706	31.831	63.657
2	0.142	0.289	0.445	0.617	1.816	1.061	1.386	1.886	2.920	4.303	6.965	9.925
3	0.137	0.277	0.424	0.584	0.765	0.978	1.250	1.638	2.353	3.182	4.541	5.841
4	0.134	0.271	0.414	0.569	0.741	0.941	1.190	1.533	2.132	2.776	3.747	4.604
5	0.132	0.267	0.408	0.559	0.727	0.920	1.156	1.476	2.015	2.571	3.365	4.032
6	0.131	0.265	0.404	0.553	0.718	0.906	1.134	1.440	1.943	2.447	3.143	3.707
7	0.130	0.263	0.402	0.549	0.711	0.896	1.119	1.415	1.895	2.365	2.998	3.499
8	0.130	0.262	0.399	0.546	0.706	0.889	1.108	1.397	1.860	2.306	2.896	3.355
9	0.129	0.261	0.398	0.543	0.703	0.883	1.100	1.383	1.833	2.262	2.821	3.250
10	0.129	0.260	0.397	0.542	0.700	0.879	1.093	1.372	1.812	2.228	2.764	3.169
11	0.129	0.260	0.396	0.540	0.697	0.876	1.088	1.363	1.796	2.201	2.718	3.106
12	0.128	0.259	0.395	0.539	0.695	0.873	1.083	1.356	1.782	2.179	2.681	3.055
13	0.128	0.259	0.394	0.538	0.694	0.870	1.079	1.350	1.771	2.160	2.650	3.012
14	0.128	0.258	0.393	0.537	0.692	0.868	1.076	1.345	1.761	2.145	2.624	2.977
15	0.128	0.258	0.393	0.536	0.691	0.866	1.074	1.341	1.753	2.131	2.602	2.947
16	0.128	0.258	0.392	0.535	0.690	0.865	1.071	1.337	1.746	2.120	2.583	2.921
17	0.128	0.257	0.392	0.534	0.689	0.863	1.069	1.333	1.740	2.110	2.567	2.898
18	0.127	0.257	0.392	0.534	0.688	0.862	1.067	1.330	1.734	2.101	2.552	2.878
19	0.127	0.257	0.391	0.533	0.688	0.861	1.066	1.328	1.729	2.093	2.539	2.861
20	0.127	0.257	0.391	0.533	0.687	0.860	1.064	1.325	1.725	2.086	2.528	2.845
21	0.127	0.257	0.391	0.532	0.686	0.859	1.063	1.323	1.721	2.080	2.518	2.831
22	0.127	0.256	0.390	0.532	0.686	0.858	1.061	1.321	1.717	2.074	2.508	2.819
23	0.127	0.256	0.390	0.532	0.685	0.858	1.060	1.319	1.714	2.069	2.500	2.807
24	0.127	0.256	0.390	0.531	0.685	0.857	1.059	1.318	1.711	2.064	2.492	2.797
25	0.127	0.256	0.390	0.531	0.684	0.856	1.058	1.316	1.708	2.060	2.485	2.787
26	0.127	0.256	0.390	0.531	0.684	0.856	1.058	1.315	1.706	2.056	2.479	2.779
27	0.127	0.256	0.389	0.531	0.684	0.855	1.057	1.314	1.703	2.052	2.473	2.771
28	0.127	0.256	0.389	0.530	0.683	0.855	1.056	1.313	1.701	2.048	2.467	2.763
29	0.127	0.256	0.389	0.530	0.683	0.854	1.055	1.311	1.699	2.045	2.462	2.756
30	0.127	0.256	0.389	0.530	0.683	0.854	1.055	1.310	1.697	2.042	2.457	2.750
χ	0.12566	0.25335	0.38532	0.52440	0.67449	0.84162	1.03643	1.28155	1.64485	1.95996	2.32634	2.57582

(Reprinted with permission of Macmillan Publishing Co., Inc., from Fisher, R. A.: *Statistical Methods for Research Workers*. © 1970, University of Adelaide.)

information for the life table beyond 2 years and are "withdrawn" from the life table at this time.

Example

For ease of computation, an augmented working life table is given in Table 41–6. To facilitate computation, extra columns are used to record intermediate values. The entries for each column in the table are defined as in Table 41–7.

The cumulative survival rate (Column 10) indicates what proportion of persons is expected to survive for a given interval after some starting point (in this case the time of mastectomy). For example, of the 189 patients who had mastectomy, 128 survived 4 years—that is, they were still alive at the beginning of the fifth year. The survival rate through the fourth year is then 128/189 = 0.677, or 67.7%. Some patients underwent operation more recently than 5 years ago, so follow-up is impossible. Such patients are withdrawn alive at the limit of their follow-up period. The method of computing the cumulative survival rate takes this into account. Thus, the 10-year survival rate is 0.459 (45.9%), not (71 − 6)/189 = 0.344 (34.4%).

The standard deviation (σ) of the proportion surviving is given in Column 11. If the number of persons in the group is large, the researcher may be relatively certain (95 times in 100) that the true cumulative survival rate lies between the computed cumulative survival rate and ± 2σ. For example, it is 95% certain that the true 5-year survival rate is 0.608 ± 0.072, or between 0.536 and 0.680. Stated in terms of percentages, it may be said that between 53.6% and 68.0% of the patients are expected to survive 5 years. Similarly, 45.9% ± 2 (3.7%), or between 38.5% and 53.3%, are expected to survive 10 years.

Cumulative Frequency Distribution of Death Rates

Lognormal probability paper is a type of graph paper set up in such a fashion that the user may quickly perceive what proportion of patients have survived for a given interval. The resulting "curve," as in Figure 41–3, approaches a straight line when survival times are distributed lognormally. The data plotted in Figure 41–3 indicate that, of eight patients with clinical Stage IV breast carcinoma who received a mastectomy, 75% lived 6 months or longer, 50% survived at least 20 months, and so on. Of the first 100 patients with Stage I breast tumors who were treated with

Table 41–6. AUGMENTED WORKING LIFE TABLE*

1 Time Interval (y)	2 Number at Beginning of Interval	3 With- drawn Alive	4 Effective Exposed	5 Died in Interval	6 Proportion Dying	7 Proportion Surviving	8†	9†	10 Cumulative Survival Rate	11 σ of Cumulative Rate
0–1	189	0	189	14	0.074	0.926	0.000423	0.000423	0.926	0.019
1–2	175	0	175	15	0.086	0.914	0.000538	0.000961	0.846	0.026
2–3	160	0	160	14	0.088	0.912	0.000603	0.001564	0.772	0.030
3–4	146	0	146	18	0.123	0.877	0.000961	0.002525	0.677	0.035
4–5	128	0	128	13	0.102	0.898	0.000887	0.003412	0.608	0.036
5–6	115	1	114.5	7	0.061	0.939	0.000567	0.003979	0.571	0.036
6–7	107	1	106.5	8	0.075	0.925	0.000691	0.004670	0.528	0.036
7–8	98	12	92	5	0.054	0.946	0.000621	0.005291	0.500	0.036
8–9	81	7	77.5	3	0.039	0.961	0.000523	0.005814	0.480	0.037
9–10	71	6	68	3	0.044	0.956	0.000677	0.006491	0.459	0.037

*EFSCH patients with TNM clinical Stage I carcinoma of the breast. Illustrates computation of cumulative and interval survival of a population with variable duration of follow-up.
†See Table 41–7 for explanation of this column.

mastectomy, 92% lived 12 months or more, 77% 36 months or more, and so on.

From this type of graph, it becomes readily apparent that the survival times for these two groups are different and that Stage I patients survive longer. This is a convenient way of looking at survival data. Other types of transformations achieve similar results for other distributions. If the number of patients in a group is large, the resulting line is often straight, but when the number of patients in a group is small the line is irregular.

The method of testing whether the two survival curves are significantly different when neither group has survivors has been discussed under Student's *t* test. For these data, both axes are unequally spaced. The space between the survival times of the two groups is proportional to the logarithm of the differences between the survival times; that is, it is a logarithmic scale. The spacing between the percentage of survival is arrived at in a somewhat more com-

Table 41–7. EXPLANATION FOR COLUMN NUMBERS IN TABLE 41–6

Column	Explanation
1	Time interval for all entries in the row
2	Number of patients alive at beginning of interval
3	Number of patients withdrawn during interval (includes lost to follow-up*)
4	Column 2 − ½ number in Column 3; effective number of patients exposed during time interval
5	Number of patients who died during interval
6	Column 5 ÷ Column 4; proportion dying during interval
7	1.0 − Column 6; proportion surviving interval
8	Column 6 ÷ (Column 4 − Column 5); intermediate values
9	Sum of all entries in Column 8 to and including this line; intermediate values
10	Product of all entries in Column 7 to and including this line; cumulative survival rate through given interval
11	Column 10 × √Column 9; standard deviation of cumulative survival rate

*Note: Lost patients introduce possible bias and should be held to a minimum.

plex manner. Producing survival curves in this manner allows the researcher to present data in a direct, meaningful manner. An approach toward determining whether a straight line plot on cumulative probability paper is indeed lognormal has been reported previously (Spratt, 1969).

Testing Whether Survival Rates Are Different for Two Different Life Tables

It is possible to determine if the survival rates for two groups of patients computed by the life table method are statistically different. A χ^2 test may be used for this purpose. From each of the two life tables being compared the effective number exposed to risk and the number of patients who die during each interval are determined.

Example

Available data are used to test whether the survival of patients with TNM clinical Stage I carcinoma is different from that of patients with Stage II carcinoma. Table 41–8 illustrates a convenient way to make computations. The definitions of the columns in Table 41–8 are given in Table 41–9.

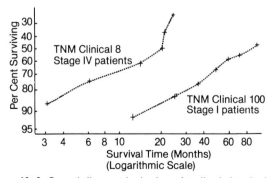

Figure 41–3. Cumulative survival rates of patients treated with radical mastectomy for mammary carcinoma (illustrating the use of logarithms of survival time).

Table 41–8. COMPUTATIONS FOR DETERMINING BY THE χ^2 METHOD WHETHER THE SURVIVAL RATE FROM THE LIFE TABLE OF PATIENTS WITH TNM STAGE I BREAST CARCINOMA IS DIFFERENT FROM THAT OF PATIENTS WITH TNM STAGE II

	Observed										Expected			
	TNM Stage I			TNM Stage II			TNM Combined				TNM Stage I		TNM Stage II	
Interval (Y.)	Effective No. Exposed	No. Dying During Interval	No. Surviving Interval	Effective No. Exposed	No. Dying During Interval	No. Surviving Interval	Effective No. Exposed	No. Dying During Interval	Probability of Dying During Interval	No. Dying During Interval	No. Surviving Interval	No. Dying During Interval	No. Surviving Interval
1	2	3	4	5	6	7	8	9	10	11	12	13	14
1	189	14	175	230	11	219	419	25	.05966	11.28	177.72	13.72	216.28
2	175	15	160	219	24	195	394	39	.09899	17.32	157.68	21.68	197.32
3	160	14	146	195	29	166	355	43	.12113	19.38	140.62	23.62	171.38
4	146	18	128	166	19	147	312	37	.11859	17.31	128.69	19.69	146.31
5	128	13	115	147	9	138	275	22	.08000	10.24	117.76	11.76	135.24
6	114.5	7	107.5	138	19	119	252.5	26	.10297	11.79	102.71	14.21	123.79
7	106.5	8	98.5	116	9	107	222.5	17	.07640	8.14	98.36	8.86	107.14
8	92	5	87	102	7	95	194	12	.06186	5.69	86.31	6.31	95.69
9	77.5	3	74.5	92	5	87	169.5	8	.04720	3.66	73.84	4.34	87.66
10	68	3	65	81.5	2	79.5	149.5	5	.03344	2.27	65.73	2.73	78.77
SUM		100			134					107.08		126.92	

$$\chi_i^2 = (100-107.08)^2/107.08 + (134-126.92)/126.92 = 0.88, P > 0.20$$

The information contained in Columns 1 to 7 of Table 41–8 is derived directly from the life tables of the two groups being compared. Columns 8 and 9 contain the combined information for the two groups. Column 10 is the probability of dying during a given interval for the group as a whole. This is the best estimate of this probability under the assumption that the survival rates are identical for the two groups.

Columns 11 and 13 are the numbers of persons expected to die in each time interval for each group if the rates are identical. Similarly, Columns 12 and 14 are the numbers of

Table 41–9. EXPLANATION FOR COLUMN NUMBERS IN TABLE 41–8

Column	Explanation
1	Time interval from life tables
2	Effective number exposed to risk during time interval for first group, from Column 4 in life table
3	Number of patients dying during time interval for first group, from Column 5 in life table
4	Column 2 − Column 3
5	Effective number exposed to risk during time interval for second group, from Column 4 in life table
6	Number of patients dying during time interval for second group, from Column 5 in life table
7	Column 5 − Column 6
8	Column 2 + Column 5
9	Column 3 + Column 6
10	Column 9 − Column 8
11	Column 2 × Column 10
12	Column 2 − Column 11
13	Column 5 × Column 10
14	Column 5 − Column 13

patients expected to survive. Columns 11 and 14 contain theoretically expected values for the two groups under the assumption that the survival rates are identical.

The χ^2 value is found from the sums for Columns 3, 6, 11, and 13. The χ^2 value corresponds to S and is equal to the sum of $(O - E)^2/E = 0.88$, as given at the bottom of Table 41–8. The degree of freedom (df) is 1. This procedure is known as the *log rank test* (Peto et al., 1976).

The probability that the two survival rates are not different can now be found from the χ^2 table with the proper degrees of freedom. For the example in Table 41–8, there is one degree of freedom. The probability that the χ^2 with one df would be as large as or larger than 0.88 (from Table 41–3) is greater than 0.50. Therefore, no difference between Stage I and Stage II survival rates has been demonstrated. If these two rates truly are different, a larger number of observations is needed to demonstrate this fact.

Discussion

The values computed with Student's *t* or the log rank (χ^2) test, when used to test whether two groups differ, may be interpreted in terms of probability. Suppose two large groups of cancer patients have identical survival times. Suppose further that a small sample is randomly selected from each group and the average survival times for each sample are compared. It is highly unlikely that the two averages would be identical, quite likely that they would be approximately equal, and unlikely that they would be very different. These are the conditions that are intuitively believed by almost everyone, but *unlikely* and *different* are ill-defined and may mean different things to different people.

One object of developing statistical procedures is to define more precisely such nebulous terms. In doing so, some of the terms have been reduced to "standardized" forms. Both Student's t and χ^2 are such standardized terms. If the data from which these statistics are computed have particular characteristics, the relationship between their values and the probability (frequency) of the values occurring may be stated precisely.

Assume that it is possible to obtain from many different hospitals survival times for eight patients who have had mastectomy for TNM clinical Stage I cancer and a similar number for Stage IV disease, and assume further that the survival times for both stages are identical. If a t value is computed for the two stage groups for each hospital, it will be found that most of the ts are small, some are large, and others are intermediate. As a matter of fact, it can be found from the t table that, when there is really no difference between the groups, a t value with 14 degrees of freedom would be greater than 0.128 for 90% of the time, would be 0.692 or greater for 50% of the time, and would be greater than 2.977 for only 1% of the time. Thus, if there were no difference between the survival of patients with Stage I and Stage IV cancers, it is highly unlikely, with a given set of eight patients in each group, that a t ratio between the logarithms of survival times would exceed 2.977. Here, *highly unlikely* means only 1 chance in 100. Since such a large t ratio did occur between the two groups, and it is unlikely to have occurred if there were really no difference, it may be concluded that there is a real difference in the survival times for the two stages.

The χ^2 table is based on similar logic. Supposing that two groups are identical and that a small sample is taken from each group, the researcher may test whether these two samples differ in the proportion of living and dead subjects in each. If this experiment were repeated many times, and there were no actual difference in the 5-year survival rates, the χ^2 values computed would sometimes be small and sometimes large. As this problem has one degree of freedom, it can be found from the χ^2 table that 80% of the time the χ^2 value would be greater than 0.0642, 30% of the time it would be greater than 1.074, and only 1% of the time it would exceed 6.635. The χ^2 table defines the probability that χ^2 would exceed a given value by chance alone, as it is assumed that the groups are identical.

If the computed χ^2 value is much larger than what is expected by chance, it is inferred that it was not caused by chance, and that a real difference exists between the groups. This is the logic behind the method of statistical inference. It is not at all unlike the logic used in medical diagnosis. If a patient is seen who has a certain set of symptoms, certain disease entities are immediately ruled out because they are highly unlikely to be associated with that set of symptoms. The terms "likely" and "unlikely" in this situation are not precisely defined; they are related to the clinician's knowledge and experience. On the other hand, if data are recorded from experience, they can be analyzed to define more precisely the meaning of *likely*. For example, suppose that symptom x is found to be associated with disease y in 84 of 93 cases (prevalence 90.3%), whereas symptom x occurred with disease z in only 15 of 93 cases (16.1%). If such records are kept, the terms "likely" and "unlikely"

are replaced by more objective values, 90.3% and 16.1%, which have the same meaning to different diagnosticians. Interpreting data is of interest in that it enables the user to predict future events. How data are employed to predict or draw inferences about future events depends on what may be assumed about the events involved, such as the known underlying mechanisms relating symptoms and diseases or the characteristics of the patient population. The rules established by these considerations are restated in mathematical terms. This restatement is often called a *mathematical* or *statistical model*. In general, it is difficult, and sometimes impossible, to devise a model that includes all known factors about the phenomenon under study, so the model is only an abstraction. This may seem to be a weakness of mathematical models, but it is a weakness that is shared by human thought as well. The advantages of a mathematical model are that the rules are stated more explicitly and the variation of meanings is reduced. This is a great advantage because many investigators may employ the model to analyze different data and the results may be compared more meaningfully. Just as a person may buy a ready-made suit, researchers can resort to many ready-made statistical models. Also, as some off-the-rack suits fit a given individual better than others, a ready-made statistical model may be selected because the logic on which it is based best conforms to the logic of the problem under study.

The χ^2 and Student's t test are examples of "off-the-rack statistical models." The assumptions on which they are built conform reasonably well to the assumption made about many medical phenomena and they are, therefore, useful in these situations.

Other models that are useful for analyzing survival data are those models that analyze survival for different groups, for example age groups. This is called *stratified survival analysis*, and a traditional approach uses the Mantel-Haentzel statistic (Fleiss, 1986) and variants of it. The calculation of the test statistic is given in many books (Fleiss' is one) and produces a χ^2 value. Table 41–3 can be used to check significance; however, once stratification occurs it is probably better to use other modeling techniques.

Models

In linear regression analysis, a line or plane is fitted to values of a response variable and various other (independent) variables. This idea of some underlying linear relationship between independent variables and the response variable has been generalized to fitting a function of the response variable and resulted in log-linear models, logistic models, and general linear models.

For contingency tables of more dimensions there are log-linear models. This approach, or logistic modeling, can be used where data are ordinal (i.e., have an obvious order) rather than categorical (with no order) (Agresti, 1990). Logistic modeling is especially useful when the response is a survival variable with only two possibilities, since then a byproduct can be an estimate of the odds ratios of various outcomes. A general linear model can be developed to deal with the case where repeated measurements are taken on each patient, but otherwise the situation resembles the χ^2 example, where cross-tabulations summarize the data.

As a generalization of the t test, there is analysis of variance to deal with more than two groups. This approach in turn can be generalized to deal with the case where there are repeated measurements on each patient with nested analysis of variance or multivariate analysis of variance if necessary (Fleiss, 1986).

There has been much interest in survival models, starting with the Cox hazard model (Cox, 1988). In this type of model the assumption is made that, for a patient in the study who is alive after a certain time and with known values for a set of variables, such as type of disease, age, weight etc., the probability of death at that time is represented by the product of (1) the (hazard) function of the studied period and (2) the function (usually linear) of variables.

Many more complex models now exist that deal with the fact that the response may be truncated at either end of the study or dropout may occur. Some can even allow for all kinds of variables, which may themselves be affected by the amount of time on study and more complex hazard functions (Hastie et al., 1992; and Chapman et al., 1992). For example, Aalen (1988) allows for differences among people with regard to susceptibility to a disease. This approach could be used to analyze survival if there are two types of tumors, fast-growing and slow-growing.

The number of possible models has increased with the rapid development of computers. Ravdin and colleagues (1992a, 1992b) used neural networks to predict recurrence of breast cancer. There remains much work to be done in the development of statistical models as well as in translating medical logic to mathematical or statistical statements. Only as medical and statistical professionals continue to collaborate in development of models can more meaningful interpretations of medical data be made.

Adjustments to Level of Significance

Simultaneous Tests of Significance (Analysis of Subgroups)

There are two major types of research: hypothesis testing (when the investigator has devised a hypothesis to be evaluated) and investigation (when the investigator seeks to derive acceptable hypotheses from a set of data). In many cases investigational and confirmatory analysis with hypothesis testing are of interest. Keiding and colleagues (1987) show how a model may be used for both types of analysis in looking at survival times for Danish breast cancer patients.

The implications of tests of statistical significance are different for the two types of research. With a properly defined hypothesis and a properly designed experiment, a statistically significant result (a result that rejects the null hypothesis) may be obtained. A statistically significant result in investigative research, in which the researcher has no prespecified hypotheses but rather selects hypotheses as suggested by the data, can only be suggestive.

Either hypothesis testing or investigation may seek to

test more than one hypothesis. The investigator may test dozens—even hundreds—of hypotheses suggested by the data. In such situations the levels of significance of the tests are not those that would apply had there been only a single hypothesis (Emerson and Fleming, 1990). For example, suppose an investigator has 100 measurements from each of two groups of patients and that there really are no differences between the two groups on these variables. If the investigator computes 100 χ^2 tests on these variables, one could expect five of them to be significant at the 0.05 level by pure chance, with the result that none of the differences may be considered significant. Yet if the investigator does not take this into consideration, and the results are then published, the researcher should not be surprised if other investigators are unable to verify the results. What can be done? First, if the significant hypotheses resulted from investigative research, the investigator may design experiments to be based on totally new data to test each hypothesis that was suggested by the investigative research. Data used to suggest a hypothesis cannot be used to prove it. Second, the experimenter may consider using statistical procedures that allow simultaneous testing of multiple hypotheses. Perhaps the best-known is a Bonferroni correction, where the P value of a test is adjusted by multiplying by the number of related tests done (Fleiss, 1986). This is a very conservative approach, since the result is a highly inflated P value, which in many cases may lead to a conclusion of nonsignificance (Schwager, 1984).

A procedure is readily available for using χ^2 tests of significance (Lindquist, 1956). Consider the example of testing the difference between two groups on 100 independent variables. Compute the 100 χ^2 values as before. Next, add those 100 values and add the 100 associated degrees of freedom, to obtain a total χ^2 value and total degrees of freedom. Find the level of significance of the total χ^2 based on the total degrees of freedom from a χ^2 table. If this is not significant, none of the individual χ^2 values may be considered significant.

Other procedures permit simultaneous testing of multiple hypotheses when variables are distributed normally. These procedures are based upon Hotelling's T^2 test. Another important procedure is Scheffe's S test (Scheffe, 1959). Many packages offer these as options. These procedures are complex and will not be described here. Several references are given in Bancroft (1968). If care is not taken to correct for multiple testing, the use of classic statistical testing procedures will yield erroneous levels of significance when used to test multiple hypotheses simultaneously.

Power Analysis

Computing the Power of a Test

The literature is full of nonsignificant results, and even more are never published. But what does a nonsignificant result mean? Does it mean that no difference exists? Or does it mean the sample size was too small to afford a reasonable chance of a significant result? If an investigator found ''no significant difference'' when using the t test (or another test), should this be taken to mean that there is probably no real difference? Our interpretation of the expression "not significant" has different meanings, depending on the power of the test that was used. The power of a test may always be computed based on the sample size actually employed and a minimum difference that should be discerned.

We present examples to show how the power and significance levels affect sample size, but many power calculations are complex. For example, if the test involves a logistic regression, when survival is examined a power analysis cannot be easily done, and for special cases such as Hsieh (1989) considers, other tables are calculated from simulations. Cohen (1988) has a book and Borenstein and Cohen have a program for a personal computer to do many power calculations. Other programs are also available. This is another instance when a collaborating statistician can give invaluable insight into the process.

For the standard clinical experiment Table 41–10 may be used to determine what size sample is required to test the hypothesis at the 0.05 level of significance with a power of 0.9. For example, if it is assumed that the standard (control) treatment has a 45% ($p_c = 0.45$) 2-year survival rate, and it is believed that the experimental treatment will yield 65% ($p_e = 0.65$) 2-year survival, the required sample size for each group will be 128.2. This is determined by finding in Table 41–10 $p_c = 0.45$ on the row indicated by 0.45 in the left-hand column and the column indicated by 0.65 in the first row. At their intersection is the value 128.2. Thus, 129 patients will be required in each group, for a total of 258 patients. Let p_e be the proportion cured for the experimental group and p_c for the control group. The general hypotheses will be $H_o: p_e = p_c$ and $H_1: p_e \neq p_c$, with values known or estimated for each p_e and p_c. H_o is the null hypothesis and H_1 the alternate hypothesis. Find the value of p_c in the left-hand index and the value of p_e in the top index of Table 41–10. At the intersection is the sample size required for *each* group if the experiment is to have a 90% chance (power = 0.9) of detecting the difference at the 5% level of significance.

As another example, suppose the 2-year survival rates for the control and experimental groups were $p_c = 0.30$ and $p_e = 0.55$. Table 41–10 indicates that 80.2 (i.e., 81) subjects will have to be treated by each method.

Impact of Level of Significance

If the investigator wishes to be more stringent and will accept the hypothesis that the experimental treatment is superior only if it can be demonstrated at the 1% ($\alpha = 0.01$) level of significance, rather than at 5%, Table 41–11 must also be used in conjunction with Table 41–10.

Table 41–11 lists factors by which the number from Table 41–10 is to be multiplied to obtain the required sample size for each of two groups, depending on the power, as indicated on the left-hand index, and the level of significance, as indicated across the top.

For the standard clinical experiment, find the value in Table 41–10 (N_1) that corresponds to the rates of the experimental and control groups, then find the value in Table 41–11 (N_2) that corresponds to the desired level of significance and power. The product of these two values is the sample size (N) required for *each* group. When N is fewer than 20, this value should be increased by 1.

For a two-tailed test, find the place in Table 41–11 where the 0.01 level of significance (α) and the power of 0.9 intersect. Multiply the sample size from Table 41–10 by this value (1.416) to obtain the sample size needed to test the hypothesis at the 0.01 level of significance with a power of 0.9. Thus, for $p_c = 0.30$ and $p_e = 0.55$, the power is 0.9 and the level of significance 0.01. The required sample size for each group for a two-tailed test is

$$N = 80.2 \times 1.416 = 113.6. \qquad \text{(Equation 2)}$$

If the experimenter wants a 99% (power of 0.99) chance of detecting the difference at the 0.01 level of significance and assumes that $p_c = 0.50$ and $p_e = 0.75$, for each group the required sample size would be

$$N = 76.7 \times 2.287 = 175.4 \qquad \text{(Equation 3)}$$

Suppose the two hypothetical cure rates to be compared were $p_1 = 0.25$ and $p_2 = 0.75$; then $N_1 = 20.4$. If the investigator wished, as a preliminary evaluation, to test at the 0.05 level of significance, with a power of 0.7, using a two-tailed test, $N_2 = 0.588$. Then the first estimate of the required sample size would be the following:

$$N = N_1 \times N_2 \qquad \text{(Equation 4)}$$
$$N = 20.4 \times 0.588 \qquad N = 12.0.$$

As this value is less than 20, 1 must be added. The regular sample size for each group is then 13.

One Hypothetical Value

If an investigator wishes to test whether an experimental treatment yields a rate different from a hypothetical rate, only one group (the experimental group) is required. In this case, the desired sample size can be computed according to the previous equations, and this value is then divided by 2 to obtain the final required sample size. The investigator should know that this procedure (single group) has many problems and should be aware of them before planning or executing a single-group experiment.

Pool Power

Suppose two institutions wish to investigate, independently, the value of a new treatment. Assume the standard treatment yields a cure rate of 50% and the new treatment is expected to yield a cure rate of 70%. It is not yet known that the new treatment is better, so the trial is necessary.

Assume that each institution wishes to have a 90% chance of demonstrating that the new treatment is 20 percentage points better than the standard treatment and wishes to demonstrate this at the 1% level of significance. From Tables 41–10 and 41–11 it is found that the required size for each group (control and experimental) is 176 (124.2 × 1.416). Each institution needs a total of 352 patients. Since each institution is performing the experiment independently

Table 41-10. TWO-TAILED SAMPLE SIZE DETERMINATION, α = 0.05, POWER = 0.9

Smallest Proportion	Largest Proportion																	
	0.95	0.90	0.85	0.80	0.75	0.70	0.65	0.60	0.55	0.50	0.45	0.40	0.35	0.30	0.25	0.20	0.15	0.10
0.05	5.4	6.3	7.1	8.0	9.0	10.2	11.5	13.3	15.3	18.0	21.5	24.9	31.5	42.0	59.1	92.6	177.2	567.4
0.10	6.3	7.4	8.5	9.7	11.2	13.0	15.1	17.8	21.1	25.6	30.7	39.9	54.2	79.0	129.0	261.0	910.7	—
0.15	7.1	8.5	9.9	11.7	13.7	16.2	19.3	23.3	27.4	35.0	46.1	63.8	94.8	158.8	331.5	1208.2	—	
0.20	8.0	9.7	11.7	13.9	16.7	20.1	24.7	29.4	38.0	50.8	71.2	107.5	183.1	390.6	1462.0	—		
0.25	9.0	11.2	13.7	16.7	20.4	25.3	30.7	40.0	54.0	76.7	117.2	202.5	438.7	1673.1	—			
0.30	10.2	13.0	16.2	20.1	25.3	31.0	41.0	56.0	80.2	124.2	216.8	475.8	1842.0	—				
0.35	11.5	15.1	19.3	24.7	30.7	41.0	56.6	82.1	128.2	226.4	502.5	1968.4	—					
0.40	13.3	17.8	23.3	29.4	40.0	56.0	82.1	129.6	231.2	518.4	2052.6	—						
0.45	15.3	21.1	27.4	38.0	54.0	80.2	128.2	231.2	523.7	2094.9	—							
0.50	18.0	25.6	35.0	50.8	76.7	124.2	226.4	518.4	2094.9	—								
0.55	21.5	30.7	46.1	71.2	117.2	216.8	502.5	2052.6	—									
0.60	24.9	39.9	63.8	107.5	202.5	475.8	1968.4	—										
0.65	31.7	54.2	94.8	183.1	438.7	1842.0	—											
0.70	42.0	79.0	158.8	390.6	1673.1	—												
0.75	59.1	129.0	331.5	1462.0	—													
0.80	92.6	261.0	1208.2	—														
0.85	177.2	910.7	—															
0.90	567.4	—																

Table 41–11. POWER CONVERSION FACTORS

Power	Level of Significance (Two-Tailed) (α)						
	0.20	*0.10*	*0.050*	*0.02*	*0.01*	*0.002*	*0.001*
0.70	0.311	0.447	0.588	0.773	0.914	1.243	1.385
0.80	0.429	0.588	0.747	0.955	1.112	1.471	1.624
0.90	0.625	0.815	1.000	1.239	1.416	1.819	1.989
0.95	0.815	1.030	1.236	1.500	1.697	2.134	2.320
0.99	1.239	1.501	1.748	2.060	2.287	2.792	3.002

of the other, what results may be expected? Let P be the power or probability that an institution will find the difference significant, and $Q = 1 - P$. Then, because two institutions perform the same experiment independently, the answer is found by expanding the polynomial as follows:

$$(P + Q)^2 = P^2 + 2PQ + Q^2 \qquad \text{(Equation 5)}$$

where $P^2 = .81$ is the probability that both institutions will find the new treatment significantly better; $2PQ = .18$ is the probability that one institution will find the new treatment significantly better, but the other one will not; and $Q^2 = .01$ is the probability that neither will find the new treatment significantly better.

Because two institutions are involved, in total, 704 patients are required. Yet, 18% of the time disagreement will occur, and only 82% of the time will the results from the two institutions agree. Thus, the question would still stand a good chance of not being resolved. In one sense, then, the power of the combined experiments is only .81, rather than .9, as each had thought: the probability of totally missing that the new treatment is better, however, is reduced from .10 to .01. On the other hand, had the two institutions decided to join in the research and pool their observations in a single experiment, with all else being equal, each institution would have to supply only 284 patients. That is, in total only 284 patients would be required for each group to obtain a power of 0.99 to test at the significance level of 0.01. This number may be obtained by multiplying the appropriate values in Tables 41–10 and 41–11:

$$284 = 124.2 \times 2.287. \qquad \text{(Equation 6)}$$

Thus, with 568 patients, the two institutions would be able to demonstrate, jointly, the superiority of the experimental treatment at the 1% level of significance with a power of 0.99. Individually, 704 patients will yield disagreement 18% of the time and a power of 0.81. Of course, there are methods of combining evidence from independent studies that would recover some of the lost power. It is apparent, then, that if many institutions independently perform the experiment, the power of each must necessarily be low, and the chance for disagreement becomes great. Thus, many important questions remain unresolved in this situation. On the other hand, by joining forces definitive answers may be obtained regarding the superiority of new treatments. Not only is the smaller sample size important in itself; the time required to resolve the question is also reduced.

The power of a test is significantly greater when data from several institutions are pooled than when they are analyzed separately, though logistically multicenter studies are more complex. Great care must be taken so that each center conducts the study in a uniform way and so that the results can be legitimately pooled. Even when all precautions are taken, usually there is some center effect, so, in calculating sample size some allowance should be made for this by using a sample at least 10% larger than calculations indicate is appropriate.

Power Needed to Reject a New Treatment

Perhaps too frequently investigators pay little attention to the power of a test. Then, the resulting statistical analyses are often unable to demonstrate differences between competing treatment methods, but it must be kept in mind that the failure to demonstrate a difference does not imply that there is no difference. This is especially true if the statistical procedure has insufficient power because of a relatively small sample size.

Suppose that a standard treatment method yields a 2-year survival rate of 55% and a new procedure is expected to produce a 2-year survival rate of 75%. From Table 41–10 it can be seen that a sample size of 117.2 is required for each of the two treatments to establish a difference at the 0.05 level of significance with a power of 0.9. If the difference is demonstrated in this example by statistical analysis, clinicians may still be hesitant to discard the standard treatment in favor of the new one, as there is a 5% chance that the 0.05 level of significance is the result of chance alone. Thus, the physician may believe that the value of the new treatment has not been proved. On the other hand, if no difference has been demonstrated at the 0.05 level of significance, it is tempting to continue the standard treatment with confidence. But if the specified difference exists, chances are 10% that it will be missed.

In general, if the level of significance is less than 1 minus the power of a test, a bias is given to the standard treatment. This may be correct, but it should not be done without consideration. The bias in favor of the standard treatment is that it is more likely to be accepted. For example, suppose the standard rate and the experimental rate are equally likely to be true and a level of significance, α, is employed. Then, if the standard rate is true, it will be accepted as true $(1 - \alpha)$ of the time. On the other hand, if the experimental rate is true, it will be accepted a proportion of the time equal to the power of the test. Thus, they are equally likely to be accepted if power $= (1 - \alpha)$, or if $\alpha = (1 - \text{power})$. However, if $\alpha < (1 - \text{power})$, then $(1 - \alpha) > \text{power}$, and the standard rate is more likely to be accepted as true. Let α be the probability of making an error when the standard rate is true, and $(1 - \text{power})$ be the probability of making an error when the experimental rate is true. If the cost of each error is the same, the expected cost is minimized when $\alpha = (1 - \text{power})$. As a consequence, if a level of significance of 0.01 is demanded, so that the new treatment will replace the standard treatment with ample confidence and $(1 - \text{power})$ is set equal to the level of significance, the value corresponding to $\alpha = 0.01$ and power $= 0.99$ must be found in Table 41–11. This value is 2.287. The required sample size for each group in this example would be

$$N = 117.2 \times 2.287 = 268.0. \qquad \text{(Equation 7)}$$

If the power is 0.99 and the level of significance 0.01, the resulting analysis will yield a considerably more definitive conclusion than in the previous example. Just as, if the results demonstrate a difference, the difference may be considered real, so also, if no difference is demonstrated, the investigator may be equally confident that any difference between the two survival rates is less than 20% (75% − 55%).

The decision to accept the new treatment, continue with the standard one, or gather more experience, depending on the results of the experiment, is influenced by the proper choices of power and level of significance. This choice in turn is based on the costs involved in making a wrong decision. A wrong decision may be made in two ways: to continue the standard treatment when the experimental treatment is in fact better or to change to the experimental treatment when in fact no difference exists. This is a simplification of the total problem, but it describes its essence. The proper values for power and levels of significance for an experiment depend on what actions will be based on the outcome and the consequence of these actions if the incorrect decision is made.

Decision Analysis

Concern over costs, total treatment time, comparative morbidity, and the preservation of a maximal functional life span require complex algorithms to compare the efficacy of different clinical processes. These must evolve along with quality clinical data and the data management systems essential to clinical decision making (Spratt 1971*a*, 1971*b*, 1975*a*, 1975*b*; and Spratt and Watson, 1973). These algorithms involve the concepts that (1) the clinical process is influenced significantly by the law of diminishing marginal returns, (2) the limits of attainable longevity are known for different cohorts of people, and (3) the actions used in any clinical process may be categorized according to whether the morbidity and costs do or do not accrue to the advantage of the individual. Categories of clinical actions are shown in Tables 41–12 and 41–13. Siminoff and Fetting (1989) looked at how physicians might affect patients' decisions in taking a particular treatment for breast cancer. Decision analysis tries to handle this complexity (Boyd et

Table 41–12. DOWNTIME FACTORS ACCRUING TO THE DISADVANTAGE OF THE PATIENT

A. Time lost in diagnostic effort not leading to beneficial treatment
B. Treatment not restoring or preserving function
C. Treatment not preserving maximum longevity
D. Cost in excess of ultimate value
E. Time consumed in the coordination of interdisciplinary consultation and unbeneficial treatment
F. Time wasted in travel and waiting
G. Time wasted by avoidable morbidity
H. Avoidable mortality from elements of the clinical process
I. Time lost in delaying rehabilitation

(From Spratt, J. S., and Watson, F. R.: The decision-making process in cancer patient care. Cancer, 23:157, 1973. Reprinted with permission.)

al., 1990) in reaching treatment decisions. Recently Hillner and Smith (1991) applied a decision analysis approach in a cohort epidemiologic study of the efficacy and cost-effectiveness of adjuvant chemotherapy for women with ''node-negative'' breast cancer. It can be argued that in all clinical studies a more general concept of outcome should be incorporated into hypothesis testing. This requires putting a ''utility'' value on an outcome. Making precise what is by nature imprecise, seems to be the main barrier to the acceptance of clinical decision analysis (Balla et al., 1989). Simes (1986) suggests an approach that permits a clinician to see the effect of different utilities.

Judgment Analysis

The problem with a general viewpoint of treatment effectiveness is caused mostly by the subjective nature of variables and the subjectivity of weighting outcomes to obtain an overall measure. Sensitivity analysis assesses the effect of different weights. Judgment analysis attempts to derive a model to combine variables in such a way as to be satisfactory to many ''judges.'' Stewart and Joyce (1988) discuss its role in a decision analytic framework. They use statistical models to develop and justify their theory.

Meta-Analysis

Meta-analysis attempts to combine outcomes from different studies. A meta-analysis compares the results of previously

Table 41–13. DOWNTIME FACTORS ACCRUING TO THE ADVANTAGE OF THE PATIENT

A. Diagnostic effort leading to effective treatment of diseases
B. Beneficial treatment to alleviate symptoms, restore function, or preserve longevity at a tolerable cost
C. Beneficial rehabilitation
D. Education and motivation of people to request health services
E. Education and motivation of people to participate effectively in their own health maintenance, health care, and rehabilitation

(From Spratt, J. S., and Watson, F. R.: The decision-making process in cancer patient care. Cancer, 23:156, 1973. Reprinted with permission.)

conducted studies on a given topic. To be credible, it should include both published and unpublished results, otherwise there may be a bias toward positive studies, which are more likely to be published (Angell, 1989; Mann, 1990; and Bangert-Drowns, 1986). Any paper presenting a meta-analysis should make it possible for the reader to make up his or her own mind, since there is more than one way to derive conclusions. For example, some people combine with equal weight randomized trials with nonrandomized ones; this is like comparing apples to oranges. Steinberg and colleagues (1991), in their meta-analysis of the effect of estrogen replacement therapy on the risk of developing breast cancer, only look at published case-control clinical trials, to which they assign quality scores based on three epidemiologist's opinions. They argue against the inclusion of unpublished studies, but their argument does not seem valid. Their conclusions must be taken with reservations despite the otherwise superior quality of their analysis. Jones (1992) discussed meta-analysis of observational epidemiologic studies with reference to breast cancer and highlights its problems.

Meta-analysis may be seen as a way to reconcile conflicting evidence from trials. More importantly, when the proportion of people who respond to a treatment is small, it is difficult to detect a change due to treatment. To embark on a large study is expensive, but meta-analysis may provide support for it.

As discussed in Mann (1990), Peto popularized meta-analysis by using it to investigate the effect of aspirin on heart disease. By synthesizing the literature and reanalyzing the published results in a meta-analysis, he was able to instigate a very large clinical study. When this was done the results coincided with findings of the meta-analysis and were definitive.

The subjectivity involved in deciding which studies are to be included and what weights should be given to the conclusions of each study has not been resolved. The method of analysis is still controversial. If a meta-analysis can reach a conclusion that is not very sensitive to the inclusion or exclusion of various studies and can do so using a simple method such as the Mantel-Haentzel-Peto method based on two-by-two tables, then it is more credible than one that does not have these attributes. Although a meta-analysis ends in conclusions, it should not be seen as the end of an investigation but rather as a supporting argument for further study.

SUMMARY

In this chapter we presented and elaborated on some of the more fundamental statistical methods that can be applied to medical data and that appear most frequently in the literature. Familiarity with these concepts is necessary for critical evaluation of a variety of medical data, but the results of the analysis can be no better than the data themselves.

To evaluate the quality of the data obtained in a clinical trial, the following guidelines (from Simon and Wittes, 1985) are recommended:

1. Authors should discuss briefly the quality control methods used to ensure that the data are complete and accurate. A reliable procedure should be cited for ensuring that data on all patients entered in the study are actually reported. If no such procedures are in place, this fact should be noted. Any procedures employed to ensure that assessment of major endpoints is reliable should be mentioned (e.g., second-party review of responses); otherwise, their absence should be noted.

2. All patients registered on a study should be accounted for. The report should specify for each treatment the number of patients who were not eligible, who died, or who withdrew before treatment began. The distribution of follow-up times should be described for each treatment, and the number of patients lost to follow-up should be given.

3. The study should have the smallest possible "unevaluability" rate for major endpoints. If more than 10% of eligible patients are lost to follow-up or considered unevaluable for response owing to early death, protocol violation, or missing information, we recommend caution in interpreting the results.

4. In randomized studies, the report should include a comparison of survival or other major endpoints for all eligible patients as randomized; that is, with none excluded except those who do not meet eligibility criteria.

5. The sample size should be sufficient to either establish or conclusively rule out effects of clinically meaningful magnitude. For "negative" results in therapeutic comparisons, the adequacy of sample size should be demonstrated by either presenting confidence limits for true treatment differences or calculating statistical power for detecting differences.

6. Authors should state the initial target sample size. They should specify how frequently interim analyses were performed and how decisions to stop accrual and report results were made.

7. All claims of therapeutic efficacy should be based on comparison with a specific control group, except in special circumstances in which each patient is his or her own control. If nonrandomized controls are used, the characteristics of the patients should be presented in detail and compared with those of the experimental group. Potential sources of bias should be discussed.

8. The subjects should be described adequately. Applicability of conclusions to other patients should be addressed. Subset-specific treatment differences must be documented as more than the random results of multiple subset analyses.

9. The methods of statistical analysis should be described in detail sufficient that a knowledgeable reader could reproduce the analysis if the data were available.

GLOSSARY

Type I error: The conclusion that a significant difference exists between two groups when no difference exists—a false positive error. The probability of a Type I error is designated by the Greek letter alpha (α).

Type II error: The conclusion that no significant difference exists between studied groups when a difference does exist—a false negative error. The probability of a Type II error is designated by the Greek letter beta (β).

Statistical power: The probability of detecting a difference in outcome when one exists. The probability of detecting a difference can range from 0 (no chance) to 1 (a perfect study assured of detecting differences that exist). The probability of missing a difference is related to the risk of a Type II error and equals $1 - \beta$.

Phase I trial: The initial assessment in humans of a new drug given by a fixed route and on a prescribed schedule. The three aims are the estimation of human toxicity, selection of dose for a clinical trial to evaluate efficacy, and investigation of clinical pharmacology.

Phase II trial: Assessment of biologic activity of a drug to identify tumor types for which it is promising as treatment. This further evaluates toxicity.

Phase III trial: Assessment of therapeutic efficacy in a well-defined population of patients in comparison with the natural history of the untreated disease or with a standard therapy.

For an expanded glossary of epidemiologic and biostatistical terms the reader is referred to Last's *Dictionary of Epidemiology* (1988), which contains the accepted definitions agreed upon by the International Epidemiological Association stated in concise English with supporting formulae.

References

Aalen, O. O.: Heterogeneity in survival analysis. Statistics Medicine, 7:1121–1137, 1988.

Agresti, A.: Categorical Data Analysis. New York, Wiley, 1990.

Anderson, J. R., Crowley, J. J., and Propert, K. J.: Interpretation of survival data in clinical trials. Oncology, 5:104–110, 1991.

Angell, M.: Negative studies. N. Engl. J. Med., 321:464–466, 1989.

Armitage, P.: Interim analysis in clinical trials. Statistics Medicine, 10:925–937, 1991.

Baar, J., and Tannock, I.: Analyzing the same data in two ways: A demonstration model to illustrate the reporting and misreporting of clinical trials. J. Clin. Oncol., 7:969–978, 1989.

Bailar, J. C. III, and Mosteller, F.: Medical uses of statistics. 2nd Ed. Boston, Massachusetts Medical Society, 1992.

Bailar, J. C. III, Louis, T. A., Lavori, P. W., et al.: Statistics in practice. A classification for biomedical research reports. N. Engl. J. Med., 311:1482, 1984.

Balla, J. L., Elstein, A. S., and Christensen, C.: Obstacles to acceptance of clinical decision analysis. Br. Med. J., 298:579–582, 1989.

Bangert-Drowns, R. L., Review of developments in meta-analytic method. Psychol. Bull., 99:388–399, 1986.

Borenstein, M., and Cohen, J.: POWER: Statistical Power Analysis: A Program. Hillsdale, NJ, L. Erlbaum, 1988.

Boyd, N. F., Sutherland, H. J., Heasman, K. Z., et al.: Whose utilities for decision analysis. Med. Decision Making, 10:58–67, 1990.

Breslow, N. E., and Day, N. E.: Statistical Methods in Cancer Research. Vol. I. Lyon, IARC, 1980.

Breslow, N. E., and Day, N. E.: Statistical methods in cancer research. Vol. II. Lyon, IARC, 1987.

Buyse, M. E., Staquet, M. J., and Sylvester, R. J.: Cancer Clinical Trials, Methods and Practice. Oxford, Oxford University Press, 1988.

Cassedy, J. H.: American Medicine and Statistical Thinking 1800–1860. Cambridge, Harvard University Press, 1984.

Cassileth, B. R., Lusk, E. J., Guerry, D., et al.: Survival and quality of life among patients receiving unproven as compared with conventional cancer therapy. N. Engl. J. Med., 324:1180–1185, 1991.

Chalmers, T. C., Celano, P., Sacks, H. S., et al.: Bias in treatment in controlled clinical trials. N. Engl. J. Med., 309:1358, 1983.

Chapman, J. A., Trudeau, M. E., Pritchard, K. I., et al.: A comparison of all-subset Cox and accelerated failure time models with Cox step-wise regression for node-positive breast cancer. Breast Cancer Res. Treat., 22:263–272, 1992.

Cohen, J.: Statistical power analysis for the behavioral sciences. Hillsdale, NJ, L. Erlbaum, 1988.

Cook, E.: Life of Florence Nightingale. London, MacMillan, 1914.

Cox, D. R., and Oates, D.: Analysis of Survival Data. London, Chapman and Hall, 1988.

Cutler, S. J., and Ederer, F.: Maximum utilization of the life table method in analyzing survival. J. Chron. Dis., 8:699, 1958.

Data Desk, [Computer program]. Ithaca, NY, Data Description Inc., 1992.

Deber, R. B., and Thompson, G. A.: Variations in breast cancer treatment decisions and their impact in mounting trials. Controlled Clinical Trials, 11:353–373, 1990.

De la Place, P. S. (translated by F. W. Truscott and F. L. Emory): A Philosophical Essay on Probabilities. New York, Davis, 1951.

Dixon, D. O.: Prognostic factors and clinical trials. Oncology, 4:116–121, 1990.

Efron, B.: Why isn't everyone a Bayesian [with comments]? Am. Statistician, 40:1–11, 1985.

Efron, B., and Tibshirani, R.: Statistical analysis in the computer age. Science, 253:390–395, 1991.

Ellenberg, S. S.: Determining sample sizes for clinical trials. Oncology, 3:39–46, 1989.

Emerson, S. S., and Fleming, T. S.: Interim Analyses in Clinical Trials, Oncology, 4:126–133, 1990.

Fleiss, J. L.: The Design and Analysis of Clinical Experiments. New York, Wiley, 1986.

Geller, N. L.: Design of phase I and II clinical trials in cancer: A statistician's view. Cancer Invest., 2:483, 1984.

Gray-Donald, K., and Kramer, M. S.: Causality inference in observational vs. experimental studies. Am. J. Epidemiol., 127:885–892, 1988.

Halperin, M., Rogot, E., Gurian, J., et al.: Sample sizes for medical trials with special reference to long-term therapy. J. Chron. Dis., 21:13, 1968.

Hastie, T., Sleeper, I., and Tibshirani, R.: Flexible covariate effects in the proportional hazards model. Breast Cancer Res. Treat., 22:241–250, 1992.

Hillman, A. L., Eisenberg, J. M., Pauly, M. V., et al.: Avoiding bias in the conduct and reporting of cost-effectiveness research sponsored by pharmaceutical companies. N. Engl. J. Med., 324: 1362–1365, 1991.

Hillner, B. E., and Smith, T. J.: Efficacy and cost effectiveness of adjuvant chemotherapy in women with node-negative breast cancer. N. Engl. J. Med., 324:160–168, 1991.

Hsieh, F. Y.: Sample size tables for logistic regression. Statistics Medicine, 8:795–802, 1989.

Hotelling, H.: The generalization of "students" ratio. Ann. Math. Statist., 2:360, 1931.

Jones, D. R.: Meta-analysis of observational epidemiological studies: A review. J. R. Soc. Med., 85:165–168, 1992.

Kaplan, E. L., and Meier, P.: Non-parametric estimation from incomplete observations. J. Am. Statist. Assn., 53:457, 1958.

Keiding, N., Bayeer, T., and Watt-Boolsen, S.: Confirmatory analysis of survival data with left truncation of the life times of primary survivors. Statistics Medicine, 6:939–944, 1987.

Last, J. M.: Dictionary of Epidemiology. 2nd Ed. Oxford, Oxford University Press, 1988.

Lavori, P. W., Louis, T. A., Bailar, J. C. III, et al.: Statistics in practice. Designs for experiments—parallel comparisons of treatment. N. Engl. J. Med., 309:1291, 1983.

Lawrence, W.: Some problems with clinical trials. Arch. Surg., 126:370–378, 1991.

Lindquist, E. F.: Design and Analyses of Experiments. Boston, Houghton Mifflin, 1956, p. 71.

Little, R. J. A., and Rubin, D. B.: Statistical Analysis with Missing Data. New York, Wiley, 1987.

Mann, C.: Meta-analysis in the breech. Science, 249:476–480, 1990.

Mantel, N.: An analysis of two recent epidemiological reports in the New England Journal of Medicine associating breast cancer in women with moderate alcohol consumption. Prevent. Med., 17:672–675, 1988.

Morrow, G. R., Black, P. M., and Dudgeon, D. J.: Advances in data assessment. Cancer, 3:780–787, 1991.

Oye, R. K., and Shapiro, M. F.: Reporting results of chemotherapy trials.

Does response make a difference in patient survival? J. A. M. A., *252*:2722, 1984.

Passamani, E.: Clinical trials—are they ethical? N. Engl. J. Med., *324*:22, 1991.

Pasternak, B. S.: Sample sizes for group sequential cohort and case control study designs. Am. J. Epidemiol., *113*:182, 1981.

Peto, R., Pike, M. C., Armitage, P., et al.: Design and analysis of randomized clinical trials requiring prolonged observation of each patient. I. Introduction and design. Br. J. Cancer, *34*, 585, 1976.

Peto, R., Pike, M. C., Armitage, P., et al.: Design and analysis of randomized clinical trials requiring prolonged observation of each patient. II. Analysis and examples. Br. J. Cancer, *35*:1, 1977.

Ravdin, P. M., and Clark G. M.: A practical application of neural network analysis for predicting outcome of individual breast cancer patients. Breast Cancer Res. Treat., *22*:285–293, 1992b.

Ravdin, P. M., Clark G. M., Hilsenbeck, et al.: A demonstration that breast cancer recurrence can be predicted by neural network analysis. Breast Cancer Res. Treat., *21*:47–53, 1992a.

Rosenberg, M. J.: Cost efficiency in study planning and completion. How many cases? How many controls? Am. J. Med., *75*:833, 1983.

SAS (version 6), [Computer program]. Available SAS Institute: Cary, NC, 1993.

Scheffe, H.: The Analysis of Variance. New York, Wiley, 1959.

Schumacher, M.: Evaluation of non-proportional treatment effects in cancer clinical trials. Cancer Invest. *8*:91–98, 1990.

Schwager, S.: Bonferroni sometimes loses. Am. Statistician, *38*:192–205, 1984.

Simes, R. J.: Application of decision to treatment choices: Implications for the design and analysis of clinical trials. Statistics Medicine, *6*:411–420, 1986.

Siminoff, L. A., and Fetting, J. H.: Effects of outcome framing on treatment decisions in the real world: Impact of framing on adjuvant breast cancer decisions. Med. Decision Making, *9*:262–271, 1989.

Simon, R., and Wittes, R. E.: Methodologic guidelines for reports of clinical trials. Cancer Treat. Rep., *69*:1, 1985.

Sokal, R. R., and Rohlf, F. J.: Biometry: The Principles and Practice of Statistics in Biological Research. San Francisco, W. H. Freeman, 1969, p. 550.

Sommer, A., and Zeger, S. L.: Estimating efficacy from clinical trials. Statistics Medicine, *10*:45–52, 1991.

Spratt, J. S.: The lognormal frequency distribution and human cancer. J. Surg. Res., *9*:151–157, 1969.

Spratt, J. S.: Cost-effectiveness in the post-treatment follow-up of cancer patients. J. Surg. Oncol., *3*:393, 1971a.

Spratt, J. S.: The measurement of the value of the clinical process to the individual by age and income. J. Trauma, *11*:966, 1971b.

Spratt, J. S. Jr.: The relation of ''human capital'' preservation to health costs. Am. J. Econ. Soc., *34*:295, 1975a.

Spratt, J. S.: The physician's role in minimizing the economic morbidity of cancer. Semin. Oncol., *2*:411, 1975b.

Spratt, J. S., and Watson, F. R.: The decision-making process in cancer patient care. Cancer, *23*:155, 1973.

SPSS (version 5), [Computer program]. Available SPSS, Inc.: Chicago, IL, 1993.

StatXact, [Computer program]. Available CYTEL Software Cororation: Cambridge, MA, 1993.

Steinberg, K. K., Thacker, S. B., Smith, S. J., et al.: A meta-analysis of the effect of estrogen replacement therapy on the risk of breast cancer. J. A. M. A., *225*:1985–1990, 1991.

Stewart, T. R., and Joyce, C. R. B.: Increasing the power of clinical trials through judgement analysis. Med. Decision Making, *8*:33–38, 1988.

SYSTAT, [Computer program]. Available SYSTAT, Inc.: Evanston, IL, 1993.

Taylor, K. M., Margolese, R. G., and Soskolne, C. L.: Physicians' reasons for not entering eligible patients in a randomized clinical trial of surgery for breast cancer. N. Engl. J. Med., *310*:1363, 1984.

Wald, A.: Sequential Analysis. New York, Wiley, 1947.

Ward, R. A., O'Connor, T. A., and Simpson, P. M.: Design of Clinical Trials in Handbook of Biomaterials Evaluation. New York, Macmillan, 1986.

Williamson, D. F., Parker, R. A., and Kendrick, J. S.: The box plot: A simple visual method to interpret data. Ann. Intern. Med., *110*:916–921, 1989.

Yancey, J. M.: Ten rules for reading clinical research reports. Am. J. Surgery, *159*:533–539, 1990.

Index

Note: Page numbers in *italics* refer to illustrations; page numbers followed by t refer to tables.